IAL Textbook
of
LEPROSY

Leprosy work is not merely medical relief; it is transforming frustration of life into joy of dedication, personal ambition into selfless service.

— Mahatma Gandhi

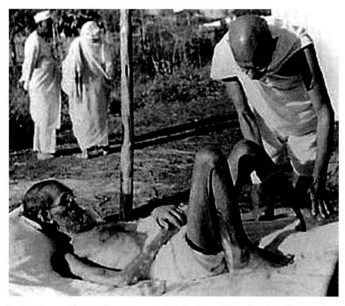

Mahatma Gandhi serving Pandit Parchure Shastri (a renowned scholar of Sanskrit) suffering from leprosy at Sevagram, Wardha in 1939. Shastri was disowned by his family after he contracted the disease. Gandhi kept him at his ashram at Sevagram (against the opposition from inmates), used to nurse his wounds personally and massage his limbs. The same picture was used later in an India postage stamp with words *Leprosy is Curable*. (*Photo courtesy*: Kanu Gandhi)

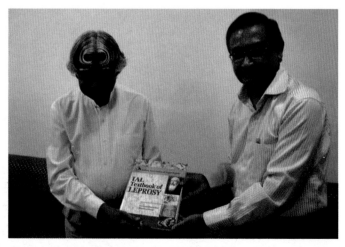

The 1st edition of *IAL Textbook of Leprosy* being presented to Dr APJ Abdul Kalam, Former President of India by Dr Hemanta Kumar Kar, one of the Editors. It is worth mentioning that Honorable Dr Kalam provided a lot of advice to Dr Kar for betterment of the book while it was under preparation. We, all the members of IAL, salute him for his great interest in leprosy and compassion for leprosy affected people.

IAL Textbook
of
LEPROSY

Second Edition

Editors

Bhushan Kumar
MD FRCP (Edin) FRCP (London)
Former Professor and Head
Department of Dermatology, STD and Leprosy
Postgraduate Institute of Medical Education and Research (PGIMER)
Chandigarh, India
kumarbhushan@hotmail.com

Hemanta Kumar Kar
MD MAMS
Professor in Dermatology
North Delhi Municipal Corporation
Medical College, Hindu Rao Hospital
Malka Ganj, New Delhi
Former Director, Medical Superintendent, Dean, Professor and Head
Department of Dermatology, STD and Leprosy
PGIMER and Dr Ram Manohar Lohia Hospital
New Delhi, India
hkkar_2000@yahoo.com

Foreword

SK Noordeen

JAYPEE *The Health Sciences Publisher*

New Delhi | London | Philadelphia | Panama

Jaypee Brothers Medical Publishers (P) Ltd.

Headquarters
Jaypee Brothers Medical Publishers (P) Ltd.
4838/24, Ansari Road, Daryaganj
New Delhi 110 002, India
Phone: +91-11-43574357
Fax: +91-11-43574314
E-mail: jaypee@jaypeebrothers.com

Overseas Offices

J.P. Medical Ltd.
83, Victoria Street, London
SW1H 0HW (UK)
Phone: +44-20 3170 8910
Fax: +44(0)20 3008 6180
E-mail: info@jpmedpub.com

Jaypee-Highlights Medical Publishers Inc.
City of Knowledge, Bld. 237, Clayton
Panama City, Panama
Phone: +1 507-301-0496
Fax: +1 507-301-0499
E-mail: cservice@jphmedical.com

Jaypee Medical Inc.
The Bourse
111, South Independence Mall East
Suite 835, Philadelphia, PA 19106, USA
Phone: +1 267-519-9789
E-mail: jpmed.us@gmail.com

Jaypee Brothers Medical Publishers (P) Ltd.
17/1-B, Babar Road, Block-B, Shaymali
Mohammadpur, Dhaka-1207
Bangladesh
Mobile: +08801912003485
E-mail: jaypeedhaka@gmail.com

Jaypee Brothers Medical Publishers (P) Ltd.
Bhotahity, Kathmandu, Nepal
Phone: +977-9741283608
E-mail: kathmandu@jaypeebrothers.com

Website: www.jaypeebrothers.com
Website: www.jaypeedigital.com

Inquiries for bulk sales may be solicited at: jaypee@jaypeebrothers.com

IAL Textbook of Leprosy

First Edition: 2010
Second Edition: **2016**
ISBN: 978-93-5152-991-0
Printed at: Samrat Offset Pvt. Ltd.

Dedicated to

All those who served the cause of leprosy in whatever capacity and whatever form, to mitigate the sufferings of the unfortunate patients by giving them the most precious gift of time. Looking back, the times were very difficult, experiences harrowing and there was hardly any tool to fight this scourge. They were destined to suffer this in misery and isolation. The only hope in their expectant eyes was the mere thought of arrival of these 'angels' who would touch them, listen to their woes and tried to lift them from despair and fill the void in their hearts.

All those who fearlessly fought the disease and the stigma and have made the world more livable with the eradication of the disease in sight.

May the flock of the devoted grow and so also the compassion for needs of the suffering humanity.

CONTRIBUTORS

Amrita Chauhan MD
Senior Resident
Department of Dermatology
STD and Leprosy
PGIMER and Dr Ram Manohar Lohia Hospital
New Delhi, India

Aparna Palit MD
Professor
Department of Dermatology, STD and Leprosy
Shri BM Patil Medical College
Bijapur, Karnataka, India

Archana Singal MD MNAMS
Professor
Department of Dermatology, STD and Leprosy
University College of Medical Sciences and
Guru Teg Bahadur Hospital
Founder President, Nail Society of India (NSI)
Convener IADVL SIG Genodermatosis
New Delhi, India

Arun C Inamadar MD DVD
Professor and Head
Department of Dermatology, STD and Leprosy
Shri BM Patil Medical College
Bijapur, Karnataka, India

Atul Shah MS (Gen Surgery) MS (Plastic
Surgery) MNAMS (Plastic Surgery)
Ex-Honorary Professor and Head
Department of Plastic Surgery
Grant Medical College and Sir JJ Group of
Hospitals
Mumbai, Maharashtra, India

Balram Sekar MD (Microbiology)
Director
Pasteur Institute of India
Coonoor, Tamil Nadu, India

Bela J Shah MD
Professor and Head
Department of Dermatology, Venereology
and Leprology
BJ Medical College and City Hospital
Ahmedabad, Gujarat, India

Bella Devaleenal
Scientist C
National Institute of Epidemiology
Chennai, Tamil Nadu, India

Ben Naafs MD PhD Dipl TM & H
Dermatovenereologist
Foundation Global Dermatology
Gracht 15 8485 KN Munnekeburen
The Netherlands
Regional Dermatology Training Center
(RDTC) Moshi Tanzania
Instituto Lauro de Souza Lima (ILSL)
Bauru, Brazil

Bhushan Kumar MD FRCP (Edin) FRCP (London)
Former Professor and Head
Department of Dermatology
STD and Leprosy
PGIMER, Chandigarh, India

BK Girdhar MD
Consultant Dermatologist
Shanti Manglick Hospital, Agra
Formerly Head, Clinical Division
National JALMA Institute for Leprosy and
Other Mycobacterial Diseases (ICMR)
Agra, Uttar Pradesh, India

BN Barkakaty
National Consultant (NLEP)
Central Leprosy Division
Directorate General of Health Services
New Delhi, India

CM Agrawal
Deputy Director General (Leprosy)
Central Leprosy Division
Directorate General of Health Services
New Delhi, India

D Kamaraj MSc CDS
WHO Consultant (Rehabilitation)
New Delhi, India

David M Scollard MD PhD
Director, National Hansen's Disease
Programs, USA
Adjunct Professor, Department of Pathology
Louisiana State University, School of Medicine
Baton Rouge, Louisiana, USA

Devinder Mohan Thappa
MD DHA FAMS FIMSA
Professor and Head
Department of Dermatology and STD
JIPMER, Puducherry, India
Former Editor-in-Chief, Indian Journal
of Dermatology, Venereology, and
Leprology (2009-13), Former Vice President,
National Executive of Indian Association
of Dermatologists, Venereologists and
Leprologists (2004-05)
Former President IASSTD (2006-07)

Diana NJ Lockwood MD FRCP
Former Chairperson and Editor
Leprosy Review
Professor of Tropical Medicine
London School of Hygiene and Tropical
Medicine, Keppel St, London, UK

Divya Gupta MD
Senior Resident
Department of Dermatology and STD
JIPMER, Puducherry, India

Dullobho Porichha MD
Medical Coordinator, LEPRA Health in Action
Formerly Consultant Pathologist
Medical Center, Parliament House Annexe
Bhubaneshwar, Odisha, India

Ebenezer Daniel MBBS MS DO MAMS MPH PhD
Former Head, Margaret Brand Chair of the
Ophthalmology Department
SLRTC, Karigiri, Vellore, Tamil Nadu, India
Director of Ophthalmology Reading Center
Ophthalmology Department
University of Pennsylvania
Philadelphia, Pennsylvania, USA

Gigi J Ebenezer MBBS MD
Assistant Professor
Cutaneous Nerve Laboratory
Department of Neurology
Johns Hopkins School of Medicine
Baltimore, Maryland, USA

GN Malaviya MMS MSc DHRM
Scientist G (Retd)
Former Head, Department of Plastic and
Reconstructive Surgery
National JALMA Institute for Leprosy and
Other Mycobacterial Diseases (ICMR)
Agra, Uttar Pradesh, India

Gurmohan Singh MD FAMS FRCP (Edin)
Consultant Dermotologist and
Emeritus Professor
National Academy of Medical Sciences and
Overseas Regional Advisor, Royal College of
Physicians of Edinburgh, UK
The Skin Institute
Varanasi, Uttar Pradesh, India

Hemanta Kumar Kar MD MAMS
Professor in Dermatology
North Delhi Municipal Corporation
Medical College, Hindu Rao Hospital
Malka Ganj, New Delhi
Former Director, Medical Superintendent
Dean, Professor and Head
Department of Dermatology
STD and Leprosy
PGIMER and Dr Ram Manohar Lohia Hospital
New Delhi, India

Indira Nath MD FRCPath DSc (HC Paris 6)
FNA, FASc, FNAS, FAMS, TWAS
Ex-Head and Senior Professor
Department of Biotechnology
All India Institute of Medical Sciences
Formerly Raja Ramanna Fellow and Emeritus
Professor, NIOP
Emeritus Professor
Institute of Pathology (ICMR)
Safdarjung Hospital Campus
New Delhi, India

Joginder Kumar Kataria MD
Consultant
Department of Dermatology, Venereology
and Leprosy
Safdarjung Hospital and Vardhman Mahavir
Medical College, New Delhi, India

Joyce Ponnaiya MBBS MD (Path)
Consultant Pathologist
SLRTC, Karigiri
Ex-Director
Christian Medical College and Hospital
Vellore, Tamil Nadu, India

Kiran Katoch MD
Former Director
National JALMA Institute for Leprosy and
Other Mycobacterial Diseases (ICMR)
Agra, Uttar Pradesh, India

Krishnamurthy Venkatesan MSc PhD
Deputy Director (Sr Grade)/
Scientist F and Head (Biochemistry)
In-charge, Laboratory Division
Department of Biochemistry
National JALMA Institute for Leprosy and
Other Mycobacterial Diseases (ICMR)
Agra, Uttar Pradesh, India

KV Desikan MD FICP
Former Director
National JALMA Institute
for Leprosy and Other Mycobacterial
Diseases (ICMR)
Agra, Uttar Pradesh, India

Linda B Adams DHHS HRSA HSB PhD
Head, Immunology Research Section
US Department of Health and Human
Services
Health Resources and Services
Administration
Healthcare Systems Bureau
National Hansen's Disease Program
Baton Rouge, Louisiana, USA

Luna Azulay-Abulafia MD PhD
Professor
The Universidade do Estado do
Professor
The Instituto de Dermatologia Santa Casa,
Rio de Janeiro, Brazil

Manimozhi Natarajan MBBS DHE Cert.
(Epidemiology) John Hopkins
Medical Coordinator, AIFO India
Bengaluru, Karnataka, India

Marcos Virmond MD PhD
Leprologist, Plastic and Reconstructive
Surgeon
Director, Instituto Lauro de Souza Lima
Bauru, Brazil
President
The International Leprosy Association
Former President
The Brazilian Leprosy Association
Fellow
Brazilian Society of Plastic Surgery
Fellow, Brazilian Leprosy Association

Maria T Pena DHHS HRSA HSB
National Hansen's Disease Programs
Laboratory Research Branch
Baton Rouge, Louisiana, USA

Masanori Matsuoka
Visiting Researcher of Leprosy
Leprosy Research Center
National Institute of Infectious Diseases
Higashimurayama, Tokyo, Japan

Mehervani Chaduvula MD
Blue Peter Research Center (LEPRA)
Cherlapally, Hyderabad, Telangana, India

Mohammad Aleem Arif MD MPH MIPHA
Country Representative for India
Netherlands Leprosy Relief
Amsterdam, The Netherlands

Mohan Natrajan MBBS DD PhD
Deputy Director (SG)
Department of Histopathology
National JALMA Institute for Leprosy and
Other Mycobacterial Diseases (ICMR)
Agra, Uttar Pradesh, India

Namrata Chhabra MD
Senior Resident
Department of Dermatology and STD
University College of Medical Sciences and
Guru Teg Bahadur Hospital
New Delhi, India

Neela Shah MSc DHM
Managing Director
Novartis Comprehensive Leprosy Care
Association
Mumbai, Maharashtra, India

Neena Khanna MD
Professor
Department of Dermatology
STD and Leprosy
All India Institute of Medical Sciences
New Delhi, India

Nirmala Deo MSc PhD
Research Assistant
Department of Biochemistry
National JALMA Institute for Leprosy and
Other Mycobacterial Diseases (ICMR)
Agra, Uttar Pradesh, India

NL Sharma MD
Former Professor and Head
Department of Dermatology
Government Medical College, Shimla
Consultant Dermatologist
National Skin Clinic
Palampur, Himachal Pradesh, India

P Narasimha Rao MD DD PhD
Professor
Department of Dermatology, STD and
Leprosy
Bhaskar Medical College
Hyderabad, Telangana, India

PAM Schreuder MD MSc (London)
Senior Public Health Consultant
Heijedaal 4
6228 GW Maastricht
The Netherlands

Pankaj Sharma MBBS DVD
Ex-Senior Research Officer
Department of Dermatology, STD and
Leprosy
PGIMER and Dr Ram Manohar Lohia Hospital
New Delhi, India

Partha Sarathy Mohanty
Scientist B
National JALMA Institute for Leprosy and
Other Mycobacterial Diseases (ICMR)
Agra, Uttar Pradesh, India

Paul R Saunderson MB BChir MRCP (UK)
DTM & H (London School of Hygiene and Tropical
Medicine), MD (UK)
Medical Director
American Leprosy Missions Greenville
South Carolina, USA

PK Gopal MA PhD
President
International Association for Integration
Dignity and Economic Advancement (IDEA)
India
Erode, Tamil Nadu, India

PL Joshi MD FAMS
Ex-Deputy Director General (Leprosy)
Directorate General of Health Services
Government of India, Ministry of Health and
Family Welfare
New Delhi, India

Pratap Rai Manglani MBBS
Former National Consultant (DPMR)
Central Leprosy Division
Directorate General of Health Services
New Delhi, India

PS Sunder Rao MA, MPH
Consultant Research Director, LEPRA
(India) and Honorary Professor of Research
and Biostatistics, Martin Luther Christian
University
Shillong, Meghalaya, India

PV Ranganadha Rao MBBS DT M & H
(Liverpool, UK)
Technical Officer
WHO Global Leprosy
Programme
WHO SEARO, New Delhi, India

Radhey Shyam Misra MD DD
Senior Consultant Dermato-Cosmetologist
and Leprologist
Skin Care and Cosmetology Center
Sir Ganga Ram Hospital, New Delhi
MCKR Hospital, New Delhi, India

Ragunatha S MD
Assistant Professor
Department of Dermatology, STD and
Leprosy
BLDEA's SBMP Medical College Hospital and
Research Center
Bijapur, Karnataka, India

Rahul Sharma DHHS, HRSA, HSB
National Hansen's Disease Programs
Laboratory Research Branch
Baton Rouge, Louisiana, USA

Rajni Rani PhD
Staff Scientist VI
Molecular Immunogenetics Group
National Institute of Immunology
JNU Campus, New Delhi, India

Ramanuj Lahiri DHHS HRSA HSB
National Hansen's Disease Programs
Laboratory Research Branch
Baton Rouge, Louisiana, USA

Richard W Truman DHHS HRSA HSB
National Hansen's Disease Programs
Laboratory Research Branch
Baton Rouge, Louisiana, USA

RR Rao MBBS DPH
Ex-Assistant Director
Bombay Leprosy Project (BLP)
Vidnyan Bhavan
Mumbai, Maharashtra, India

Ruchi Gupta MD
Senior Resident
Department of Dermatology
STD and Leprosy
PGIMER and Dr Ram Manohar Lohia Hospital
New Delhi, India

S Noto MD MPH (Palermo) MCTM (London)
Dermatologist
Verdellino (BG), Italy

Saba Lambert MBChB (Dundee)
DTMH (Liverpool)
Department of Infectious and Tropical
Diseases
London School of Hygiene and Tropical
Medicine
London, UK

Shubhada S Pandya MBBS PhD
Acworth Leprosy Hospital Society for
Research, Rehabilitation and Education in
Leprosy
Mumbai, Maharashtra, India

Sowmya Kaimal MD
Senior Resident
Department of Dermatology and STD
St John Medical College
Bengaluru, Karnataka, India

Sujai K Suneetha MBBS DCP PhD
Director
Nireekshana ACET, Narayanguda
Hyderabad, Telangana, India

Suman Jain MBBS DCH
Senior Research Consultant, Nireekshana
ACET and Chief Medical Research Officer and
Secretary
Thalassemia and Sickle Cell Society
Hyderabad, Telangana, India

Sumana Barua MD MPH PhD
Team Leader
Global Leprosy Program
WHO-South East Asia Regional Office
New Delhi, India

Sunil Dogra MD DNB FRCP (London)
Additional Professor
Department of Dermatology, STD and
Leprosy
PGIMER, Chandigarh, India

Thomas Abraham BSc MD DVD
Dy-Director and Medical Advisor, GLRA/Swiss
Emmaus India
Chennai, Tamil Nadu, India

U Sengupta PhD FNASc FAMS
Ex-Director, National JALMA Institute for
Leprosy and Other Mycobacterial Diseases
(ICMR), Agra, Uttar Pradesh
Consultant, Stanley Browne Research
Laboratory
The Leprosy Mission
New Delhi, India

UD Gupta MSc PhD
Deputy Director and Scientist E
Laboratory for Animal Experiment
National JALMA Institute for Leprosy and
Other Mycobacterial Diseases (ICMR)
Agra, Uttar Pradesh, India

V Halwai MD (Russia) DDV (CPS)
Senior Medical Officer
Bombay Leprosy Project
Mumbai, Maharashtra, India

V Ramesh MD
Professor and Head
Department of Dermatology
STD and Leprosy
Safdarjung Hospital and Vardhman Mahavir
Medical College, New Delhi, India

Vanaja Prabhakar Shetty PhD
Deputy Director
The Foundation for Medical Research
Mumbai, Maharashtra, India

Vikram Mahajan MD
Professor and Head
Department of Dermatology, STD and
Leprosy
Dr RP Government Medical College
Kangra, Himachal Pradesh, India

Vineet Kaur DNBE Dip GUM (UK) FRCP (Lond)
Consultant Dermatologist and
Vice President, Community Dermatology
Society (India)
Member, Board of Directors
International Skin Care Nursing Group
The Skin Institute
Varanasi, Uttar Pradesh, India

Virendra N Sehgal MD
Ex-Director, Professor and Principal
Lady Hardinge Medical College and Sucheta
Kriplani Hospital, New Delhi
Consultant Dermato-Venereologist
New Delhi, India

VM Katoch MD FNASc FAMS FASc FNA
Ex-Director
National JALMA Institute for Leprosy and
Other Mycobacterial Diseases (ICMR)
Agra, Uttar Pradesh
Former Secretary
Department of Health Research
Ministry of Health and Family Welfare
Former Director General
Indian Council of Medical Research (ICMR)
New Delhi, India

VV Dongre GFAM LMP MBBS DVD DHA DSW
DHE PGD-PR and A PGD-MLS
Senior Consultant, ALERT-India, Mumbai
Honorable Secretary
The Society for the Eradication of Leprosy
Mumbai, Maharashtra, India

VV Pai MBBS DVD FCGP
Director
Bombay Leprosy Project (BLP)
Mumbai, Maharashtra, India

FOREWORD

The publication of the second edition of the *IAL Textbook of Leprosy* is a major landmark achieved by the 65-year-old Indian Association of Leprologists. Thanks to the tremendous efforts put by Dr Bhushan Kumar, Dr HK Kar and all the various contributors to the textbook. It is indeed a great honor for me to write this foreword.

India is not only the home of the largest leprosy problem in the world, but is also the largest center of leprosy work and leprosy research. Generations of Indian leprologists have contributed towards the scientific understanding of the disease, its manifestations, etiology and epidemiology, diagnostic issues, various complications, therapeutic challenges, rehabilitation problems as well as disease control/elimination strategies.

The textbook, through its contributions, very effectively addresses all the challenges currently faced by leprosy work in all its detail, and provides a comprehensive understanding of the disease to the leprologists working exclusively in leprosy, to the dermatologists who are increasingly taking full responsibility for the care of leprosy patients as well to the postgraduate students in various fields who come across leprosy in the course of their work.

Leprosy, in terms of the number of individuals affected may be relatively less now, but nevertheless its complexity is still overwhelming. The textbook addresses the challenges faced by the researchers, clinicians, public health workers, and others very effectively, and it is indeed a step forward in our endeavor to see that the disease is fully understood and effectively dealt with in the laboratory, the clinic, and the field.

SK Noordeen
Former Director
Global Leprosy Elimination Programme
World Health Organization (Geneva)

PREFACE TO THE SECOND EDITION

In the last six years, since the publication of the first edition (2010), leprology has reached a new level of global understanding—both scientific and social. Leprology in the 21st century continues to reflect the major advances in the practice and science of medicine affecting the community in which we live and work.

The main objective of the current edition is to provide clinicians, researchers and everyone associated with leprosy, insights into the latest research and developments on the subject all over the world, and access to an updated and organized database of information. The text has undergone a significant revision to incorporate the advances in the many areas that further our understanding of the disease, particularly in relation to its immunology, genetics and host susceptibility, drug resistance, molecular diagnostics, reactions and biology of *Mycobacterium leprae*, unraveling the immunopathogenic basis of some of the major components of the disease presentation.

For all the reasons of advancement and expanding knowledge, the responsibility of revision attained huge proportions and with this caveat, it looked very difficult to cover everything in the revised edition. Nevertheless, to provide our readers with the most important and up-to-date information in this specialty, significant changes have been made in many of the chapters. To make the picture more complete, additional chapters by international authors of repute in the field of leprosy—Diana Lockwood, Paul Saunderson, Linda Adams and her team, Masanori Matsuoka, David Scollard, Gigi and Daniel Ebenezer, Marcos Virmond, Mohammad Arif, Ben Naafs and his team—have been added to reminisce about the morbidity and the migration the disease caused in the past, significance of animal models in leprosy research, chemotherapy and also the projections for the future; some hopeful prospects and some real and important challenges. Each of the new authors who have contributed to the book, represents the vanguard of our specialty. Readers, we are sure, you will appreciate their expertise in presenting succinctly, the most contemporary information on the subject.

To give a very good visual impression to Asian readers of how the disease will manifest in whites and darker individuals, representative photographs provided by Luna Azulay of Brazil, Ben Naafs from Netherlands and Saba Lambert from Ethiopia have been added. Their valuable contributions are acknowledged.

We are indebted to each and every author for their expert opinions, extensive literature review, lucid writing and communication skills in sharing their experiences. This has resulted in the creation of a comprehensive textbook addressing virtually all the situations, a clinician/surgeon, a scientist or a social worker is likely to encounter while dealing with leprosy patients and the community around as a whole—keeping the narrative in a form which is easily readable and understandable.

We acknowledge our advisers, reviewers and readers whose criticism and views have helped a lot in shaping of this edition to the present form. We are grateful to all of them, Dr VM Katoch does need a special mention. We are fortunate to have a large number of vitally important people who have helped us complete the revised edition. Diana Lockwood comes to our mind immediately; especially her comments on the first edition helped us to reshape our contents in the second edition. Her continued encouragement is highly appreciated.

We especially acknowledge the support of our families who did feel the deficiency, but did not much grudge the lack of deserved attention and time, they were entitled to. They understood our commitment and provided us all the needed support and encouragement to complete the task. Thanks to all of them for their understanding.

We wish to express our appreciation to many associates and colleagues for their help in all areas—academic or nonacademic and at all times: Sunil Dogra, Sendhil Kumaran, Tarun Narang, Amrita Chauhan and Ruchi Gupta, to mention a few.

Special thanks are also due to Shri Jitendar P Vij (Group Chairman), Mr Ankit Vij (Group President), Tarun Duneja (Director–Publishing), KK Raman (Production Manager), Sunil Kumar Dogra (Production-Executive), Neelambar Pant (Production Coordinator), Sarvesh Kumar Singh (Proofreader), Vinod Kumar Sharma (DTP Operator), Pawan Kumar (Graphic Designer) and all concerned team members of M/s Jaypee Brothers Medical Publishers (P) Ltd, New Delhi, India, for their understanding and whole-hearted cooperation.

It is an honor to have been asked to continue to shepherd this important book—thank you members of the IAL for putting your trust in us to deliver.

We bring this edition to you, dear reader, with the hope that you will enjoy reading it and find it a valuable resource. We look forward to the continued impact of leprology in the enhancement of health care for leprosy patients throughout the world.

Bhushan Kumar
Hemanta Kumar Kar

PREFACE TO THE FIRST EDITION

We must justify the addition of another book on leprosy when many good books are already available on the subject. It is not that the Indian leprologists should also publish a book when everyone else has—because knowledge is universal, to be shared and its spread a pious academic act.

However, in the last conference of the Indian Association of Leprologists (IAL) in September 2007 at Kanpur, it was felt that because of various logistic and financial reasons coupled with the dwindling number of leprosy patients all over the globe, revisions of the existing books on the subject were not forthcoming in the post-leprosy elimination era. It was also felt that despite the reduced number of new leprosy patients being detected, changing classification systems, modifications of traditional multidrug therapy schedules, changing the profile of disease presentation, shortage of expertise and shrinking of control program activities, the need was for more up-to-date knowledge and sharper skills to diagnose the patients more confidently and to manage them better to reduce the incidence of complications and deformities; and above all, to understand the patient with leprosy better. More fundamental change is that management of leprosy now has become an integral part of general health care. Therefore, all physicians and new medical graduates/postgraduates are to be equipped as best as is possible with the basic but essential knowledge about the disease than ever before, further justifying the need for a textbook to strengthen still more their basics in the field.

It was in their utmost wisdom that the members of the IAL expressed the need and the desire to have an updated book on leprosy encompassing all aspects of the disease. We would remain eternally grateful to the IAL for choosing us to take on this onerous task in the presence of so many stalwarts who had more experience collected over their lifetime devoted to leprosy.

It was decided to be a multiauthor book because it is impossible for any single author to cover the entire gamut of epidemiology, immunology, immunogenetics, pathology, clinical aspects, management (medical and surgical), and finally the social, legal aspects and rehabilitation, and then give you an insight into the brighter prospects beyond 2010 and future research. Moreover, it was felt that a collection from experts from all over the country will give the book a pleasant hue and the most updated scientific content in their respective areas.

While going through the chapters from renowned leprologists, we did realize that there had been many important and exciting newer advances in the field of diagnostics and therapy. With the rich contributions from the experts, the book is hopefully the most up-to-date collection of the material available in the field which has recently been added to the literature. The number of new drugs, treatment regimens, approaches to management and diagnostics have continued to evolve and are being regularly added giving us more options. We are probably near the top or close to it, if the best has still to come.

We would sincerely believe that the book helps to produce excellent clinicians, educators and researchers not excluding the medical students who should have a better feel of the Indian scenario in relation to other leprosy affected nations. The final decision about the product obviously has to come from the readers—happy reading.

However, we would frankly accept that this textbook is not perfect and in many places may not have the expected details. Because of certain constraints, we could not do better than this—our sincere apologies especially to the luminaries in the field who naturally expected more. We sincerely hope, the next attempt would be more organized and certainly better.

Writing a textbook of this size would be impossible without the very willing cooperation of the contributors and assistance and support of many other people. Although it is not possible to enumerate all—the editors most heartily thank the most experienced and celebrated authors in the field and other colleagues who contributed illustrations and photographs, gave suggestions and most of all, the reviewers who made substantive suggestions to improve the contents and to all those who encouraged us to carry on.

This compilation entailed a tremendous amount of work, but the experience gained and the rewards are priceless.

Hemanta Kumar Kar
Bhushan Kumar

CONTENTS

Section 3: CLINICAL, LABORATORY DIAGNOSIS AND DIFFERENTIAL DIAGNOSIS

Section 9: FUTURE PROSPECTS

SECTION 1

The Disease History and Epidemiology

CHAPTERS

1
CHAPTER

History of Leprosy in India: A Historical Overview from Antiquity to the Introduction of MDT

KV Desikan, Shubhada S Pandya

CHAPTER OUTLINE

- Historic Authentication of Leprosy in India
- The Evolution of Modern Leprology
- Pathology
- The Era of Chaulmoogra/Hydnocarpus Oil Therapy in India
- Leprosy as a Public Health Problem
- ICBELRA in Madras Province
- The Bhore Committee
- Legislation
- The Era of New Drugs
- Developments at Independence
- Indian Social Initiatives and Gandhiji's Support
- The Indian Association of Leprologists
- Surgeons as Trail Blazers

Note: *The use of the term 'leper' in this chapter is solely in its historical context, and not in a derogatory sense.*

INTRODUCTION

In October 1950, at the close of his final sojourn in India, Ernest Muir, the originator of the first antileprosy campaign in India was invited to deliver the Presidential address at the Third All India Leprosy Workers' Conference at Madras. It was a gesture of appreciation—many of the leprosy workers in the audience that day were mentored by him in the 1920s and 1930s. In his address, Muir recalled that it was 30 years to the month that he began leprosy studies at the Calcutta School of Tropical Medicine. While a great deal of knowledge had been acquired about the disease since 1920, said Muir, "[but] *it is questionable if that knowledge has to any extent caused a diminution of leprosy in the country*".[1]

The candid admission implied that independent India had a clean slate on which to inscribe her own antileprosy efforts.

The present chapter recapitulates significant observations and activities of the 19th century in Europe and the British colonial era in India (detailed in the first edition), and presents a wider time frame from antiquity to the introduction of Multi-Drug Therapy in 1981.

HISTORIC AUTHENTICATION OF LEPROSY IN INDIA

Circumstantial evidence of the long presence of leprosy in this country gleaned from Ayurvedic medical descriptions of

Charaka, Susruta and others,[2] and socioreligious practices sanctioned in the *Shastras*, received strong authentication in an archaeological report published in 2009.[3] Skeletal remains of a 40-year old male unearthed at a Vedic burial site dating from 2,000 BC at Balathal, near Udaipur (Rajasthan), bore tell-tale signs of leprosy in the skull (erosion of the margins of the nasal aperture and complete atrophy of the anterior spine) as well as in the postcranial skeleton (Fig. 1.1). The authors of the report proposed that the explanation lay in the customary practice of burial alive of lepers in India in Vedic times (*See* Section on Legislation).

THE EVOLUTION OF MODERN LEPROLOGY

The Norwegian researchers, Daniel Cornelius Danielssen (1815–1894) and Carl-Wilhelm Boeck (1808–1875), who were based in the western seaport of Bergen, must be credited with the first scientific study of leprosy. Their celebrated treatise *Om Spedalskhed* ('On Leprosy', 1847) was published in French translation in 1848.[4] These pioneers proposed a classification of the disease based on the dominant clinical features. They traced the seat of pathology to the nervous system (central and peripheral), and the pathogenesis to an excess of 'albumen' circulating in the blood, which was deposited in the skin and nervous system. It was their pronouncement on the etiology of leprosy that it was hereditary, sometimes supplemented by environmental factors, that was to arouse the greatest controversy in Europe, and echoed in colonial India.

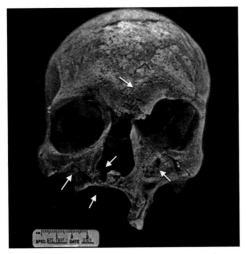

Fig. 1.1: The Skull of the 4,000 year-old leper skeleton found buried in Rajasthan. The skeleton was interred within a large stone enclosure filled with vitrified ash, considered purifying in Vedic tradition.[3]

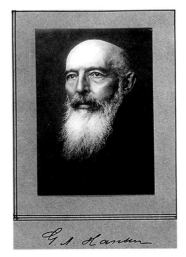

Fig. 1.2: Gerhard Armauer Hansen

Etiological Controversies

In 1895, Armauer Hansen (1841–1912), the discoverer of the *Bacillus* of leprosy, remarked wryly:

"There is hardly anything on earth, or between it and heaven which has not been regarded as the cause of leprosy; and this is but natural, since the less one knows, the more actively does his imagination work".[5]

The disease exhibited apparently contradictory features which directed opinions in different directions, depending on the biases of the observer. For example:

- Although sporadic cases occurred, leprosy was frequently seen in direct as well as collateral descendants of lepers—hence it was due to hereditary transmission of an unspecified structural defect.
- Although a rich man could get leprosy, it most often occurred in poor people living in insanitary environments—hence it was a nonspecific disease of sub-standard environmental and living conditions.
- It was frequent in Asiatic countries such as India, subjugated by European imperialism—hence it was a disease of their low level of 'civilization' and their state of 'degradation'.[6]
- Conjugal leprosy was uncommon, but contrarily the disease appeared to be communicated by contact, direct or mediate, with a leper—hence it was 'contagious', like syphilis, the archetypal contact disease.
- Rudolf Virchow, the father of cellular pathology, was struck by the rarity of leprosy among Norwegian immigrants to the United States, and inclined towards inhospitable 'locality' (climatic and soil conditions) as the explanation. He remained a firm anticontagionist for most of his life, eventually conceding the bacillary origin grudgingly.[7]

- Some observers did not regard the above theories as mutually incompatible, since it seemed conceivable that sub-standard living conditions might weaken a constitution enough to unmask a hereditary predisposition; or that optimum environmental and dietary conditions might protect against the development of leprosy even in 'predisposed' individuals or that *susceptibility* to leprosy (rather than leprosy *per se*) was transmitted through heredity, which in turn facilitated familial spread of the supposed leprous 'contagion'.

Gerhard Armauer Hansen (Fig. 1.2) commenced leprosy work in 1869. After conducting field surveys in leprosy-endemic hamlets in and around Bergen, he noted that sporadic cases had arisen in strangers originally from leprosy-free regions of the country, but resident in Bergen. He became convinced that leprosy was not hereditary but contagious. In 1875, in a critique of the hereditary theory, he postulated that leprosy was a *specific* disease connected with the *Bacillus* discovered by him in 1873.[8]

An important visitor to Hansen's laboratory in 1873–74 was Henry Vandyke Carter (1831–1897) (Fig. 1.3) of the Bombay Medical Service. Carter is unfortunately forgotten by leprologists, although he was the foremost authority on the disease in India in the latter half of the 19th century.

Although until his Norwegian visit Carter leaned towards hereditary etiology, he quickly grasped the profound implications of Hansen's yet-unconfirmed discovery (Fig. 1.4).[9]

Despite the plethora of causation theories, and the efforts of die-hard anticontagionists, and notwithstanding failed attempts to transmit the disease to experimental animals, it became increasingly untenable in late 19th century scientific circles to dismiss the bacterial etiology of leprosy. A ringing endorsement of Hansen's discovery and his long-held opinions on the efficacy of leper segregation as a means of control came in 1897 at the First International Leprosy Congress held at Berlin.[10]

Clinical Features as Basis of Classification

Danielssen and Boeck in 1847 classified leprosy as two main clinical types *Elephantiasis Anaisthetos* and *Elephantiasis Tuberculosa,* with a 'mixed' type, labeled *mixta.* It is interesting that in early 19th Century, East India Company

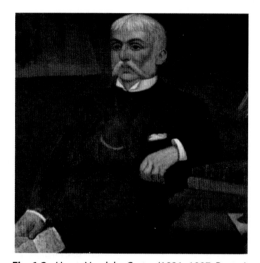

Fig. 1.3: Henry Vandyke Carter (1831–1897, Portrait at Grant Medical College, Mumbai)

physicians were already well aware that leprosy appeared as two such main types.[11,12]

The 'mixed' variety was described and labeled as *Lepra leprosa* by Carter of Mumbai, in his beautiful self-illustrated magnum opus *On Leprosy and Elephantiasis* which was published in 1874. His illustration identifies it as today's 'borderline tuberculoid' (Fig. 1.5).

International Classifications

The advent of influential multinational bodies such as the British Empire Leprosy Relief Association in 1924, the League of Nations Leprosy Commission in 1930 (*See* Section: The Era of Chaulmoogra Oil in India), and the International Leprosy Association in 1931, signaled a progressive 'internationalization' aimed at reconciling medical experience and harmonizing theory and practice across the globe. The most important fora for deliberations on classification were the International Leprosy Congresses, beginning with the Third Congress held at Strassbourg in 1923.

A three-type classification was agreed, based on the consideration that while lepra bacilli were to be found in various other organs of the body, broadly speaking there was,

1. Skin leprosy
2. Nerve leprosy
3. Mixed leprosy.

At the International Congress at Cairo in 1938, the main clinical varieties were delineated. The skin type which was characterized histologically by the 'leproma' populated by lepra cells, became 'lepromatous'—the first example

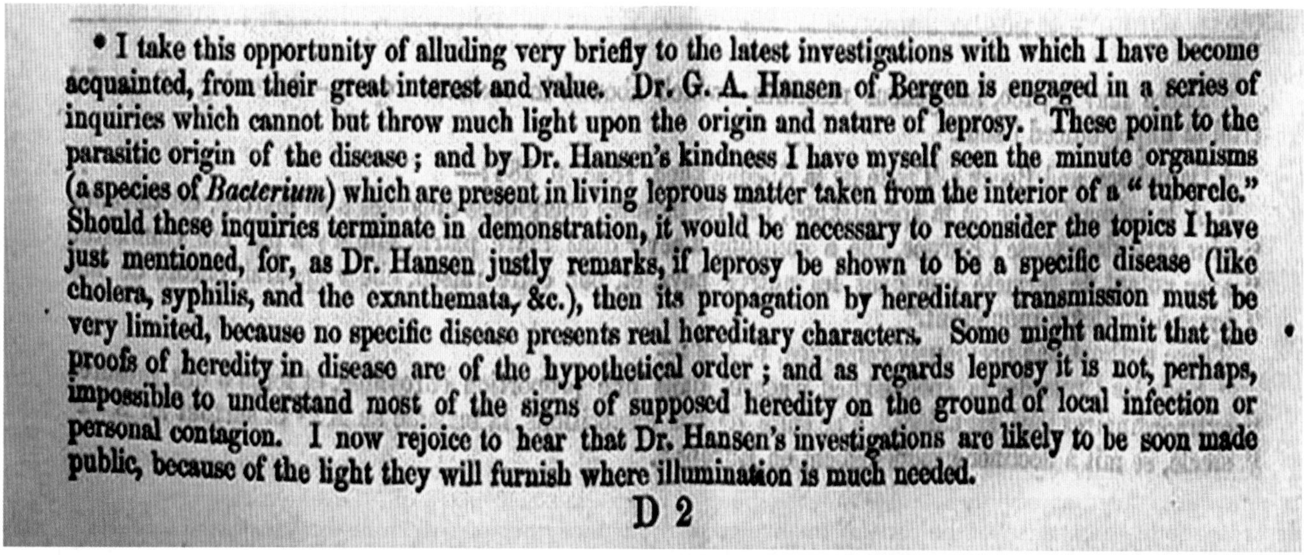

* I take this opportunity of alluding very briefly to the latest investigations with which I have become acquainted, from their great interest and value. Dr. G. A. Hansen of Bergen is engaged in a series of inquiries which cannot but throw much light upon the origin and nature of leprosy. These point to the parasitic origin of the disease ; and by Dr. Hansen's kindness I have myself seen the minute organisms (a species of *Bacterium*) which are present in living leprous matter taken from the interior of a " tubercle." Should these inquiries terminate in demonstration, it would be necessary to reconsider the topics I have just mentioned, for, as Dr. Hansen justly remarks, if leprosy be shown to be a specific disease (like cholera, syphilis, and the exanthemata, &c.), then its propagation by hereditary transmission must be very limited, because no specific disease presents real hereditary characters. Some might admit that the proofs of heredity in disease are of the hypothetical order ; and as regards leprosy it is not, perhaps, impossible to understand most of the signs of supposed heredity on the ground of local infection or personal contagion. I now rejoice to hear that Dr. Hansen's investigations are likely to be soon made public, because of the light they will furnish where illumination is much needed.

D 2

Fig. 1.4: The English-speaking world first learned of Hansen's discovery of the leprosy bacillus in 1873, through HV Carter of the Bombay Medical Service
Source: Carter HV. Report on Leprosy and the Leper Asylums in Norway. London, Her Majesty's Stationery Office; 1874. pp. 27.

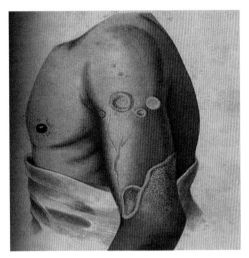

Fig. 1.5: Carter's illustration of Lepra Leprosa
(*See* Reference 16, Plate 11)

of clinicohistological correlation. The two main types, 'lepromatous' and 'neural' were subclassified according to the *degree of advancement* (e.g. L1 for slight lepromatous to L3 for advanced lepromatous; N1 for slight neural to N3 for advanced neural. Combinations and permutations of the subclasses described the mixed forms, e.g. (L3N2). The Congress also suggested "+" and "–" as symbols to indicate bacteriological status.[13]

A significant contribution of the Fifth International Congress at Havana in 1948, was the inclusion of 'indeterminate' leprosy and 'dimorphous' leprosy as categories.[14] The Classification subcommittee at the International Conference at Madrid in 1953, (in which the clinician Robert Cochrane and the pathologist Vasant Khanolkar both working in India, were prominent), recommended that two distinct polar *types* of stable but mutually incompatible leprosy be recognized— 'Lepromatous' and 'Tuberculoid'. Also recommended was that two *groups* be recognized, less distinctive and less stable— 'Indeterminate' and 'Borderline' ('dimorphous'). *Types* and *groups* were further classified into *varieties*. The Lepromatous type and Borderline group were seen to be 'malign'.[15]

The Indian Classification arrived at under the aegis of the Indian Association of Leprologists in 1955 divided leprosy into 6 types, viz. (1) Indeterminate; (2) Maculo-anesthetic; (3) Tuberculoid; (4) Lepromatous; (5) Borderline; and (6) Polyneuritic.[16]

In 1966, Ridley and Jopling devised a Classification for workers with access to investigative facilities.[17] Taking into account the Madrid recommendations, it was a 5-group system which graded leprosy into a clinicohistologic spectrum according to the 'resistance' of the patient. The five groups were designated TT, BT, BB, BL, LL which correlated with decreasing lepromin reactivity and increasing bacteriological index. The Ridley-Jopling Classification has been widely used in research projects.

Leprosy Reactions

So-called 'acute manifestations' in the course of leprosy were also noted by the pioneer leprologists. For example, repeated crops of reddish nodules accompanied by fever were described by Danielssen and Boeck as presenting signs in nodular ('tubercular') leprosy, and were interpreted as pointing to disease dissemination.

A bacteriologic interpretation of the phenomenon was attempted in 1883 by Vandyke Carter in Mumbai, a decade after Hansen's discovery. Carter was struck by the contrast between the often 'scanty' (indolent) constitutional response of the human system to the leprosy *Bacillus* interrupted by 'occasional reproduction of the nodules', with the 'violent' symptoms attending acute infections with 'pathogenetic' (pyogenic) bacteria. He concluded that the 'interruptions' in the course of leprosy were due to 'infection' of the system from reabsorption and 'autoinoculation' of leprous matter from softening nodules.[18]

A foretaste of the modern terminology for the episodic skin eruptions is provided in an early 20th century, German textbook of tropical medicine, in which 'acute inflammatory skin nodules' having their seat in the cutis and subcutis were labeled as a type of 'erythema nodosum' ('rose rash') resulting from bacillary emboli,[19] while the specific term 'erythema nodosum leprosum' (ENL) was first employed by Murata of Japan in 1912. Sir Leonard Rogers of the Bengal cadre of the Indian Medical Service (*See* "The Era of Chaulmoogra/Hydnocarpus Oil Therapy in India"), who was a well-known tropical diseases expert, cited his clinician-collaborator Ernest Muir's description of the clinical picture during acute 'reactionary episodes' (the term 'reaction' was probably employed in the belief that it represented an 'allergic reaction' to the bacterial toxin): "sudden swelling and redness of existing lesions with appearance of new ones with toxemia and fever. This is often followed by spontaneous subsidence".[20]

It was noticed that fever, softening of nodules and fragmentation of intralesional bacilli occurred spontaneously, but more particularly during 'reactions' brought on by putative therapies such as vaccines and salts such as potassium iodide and the salts of chaulmoogra oil. Were spontaneous 'reactionary episodes' evidence of increased immunity to the *Bacillus*? Were episodes occurring in the course of treatment evidence of therapeutic efficacy? Should the severity of a 'reaction' be controlled? All these points were moot. Rogers, an ardent advocate of intravenous treatment with salts of hydnocarpus oil (which he introduced into leprosy therapy in the 1920s) declared that "the intravenous method led to a most important and encouraging advance, for in certain

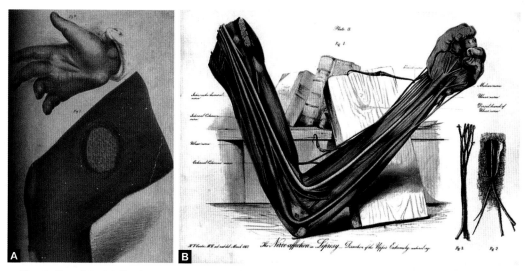

Figs 1.6A and B: (A) Skin lesions and neural involvement; (B) Morbid peripheral neuro-anatomy in leprosy. Note the illustration of intraneural anastomoses (*See* Reference 12, Plates I & IX)

cases, especially marked nodular ones, local inflammatory reactions, sometimes accompanied by fever, took place in the thickened cutaneous lesions, and were followed by rapid absorption of the diseased tissues. Still more striking was the fact that microscopic examination proved that these local reactions were accompanied by active destruction of the innumerable bacilli in the lesions".[21]

Nerve Involvement and Neuropathogenesis

Danielssen and Boeck stated that the nervous system in general was the seat of leprous pathology, as evidenced by diffuse spinal and cranial meningitis as well as peripheral nerve enlargement. But it was Carter working in Mumbai in the early 1860s who cast leprosy as a *sensory* peripheral nerve disease *par excellence.*

The principles which he propounded on neuropathogenesis which were based on close clinical examination and post-mortem dissections (Figs 1.6A and B) carried out at the Jamsetjee Jejeebhoy ("JJ") Hospital at Mumbai are valid even today. Carter stated that leprosy "is probably the only disease known which is confined to the (peripheral) nerves and the sentient skin"; that neither nerve involvement nor enlargement were random, but followed a pattern, e.g. the ulnar at the elbow, the median above the wrist, the cutaneous nerves in their superficial course after they have pierced the deep fascia; that "the nerve centers (the central nervous system) are not necessarily affected".[22]

It is also remarkable that Carter postulated that the progression of the disease within the peripheral nerves was facilitated by intraneural anastomoses an anatomical feature, which was illustrated together with his dissection of the arm nerves.[23]

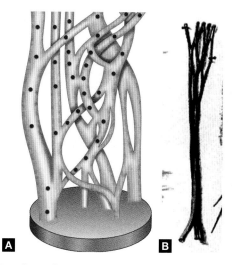

Figs 1.7A and B: Schematic of intraneural anastomoses by a modern neuro-anatomist (*See* Reference 24); (B) Compare with Carter's illustration from Figure 1.6B

Symptoms in the extremities in anesthetic variety of leprosy were in direct relation with the 'neuritis' of the nerves which supplied the benumbed part, wrote Carter. The importance of the intraneural anastomosis in the sequential appearance of sensory and motor signs and symptoms in leprosy originally stated by Carter, were rediscovered and illustrated by a modern neuro-anatomist (Figs 1.7A and B).[24]

Carter also noticed numerous dark 'nuclei' in histologic sections of peripheral nerves and surmised that they were derived from the exudate within the diseased tissue, a fact confirmed by the great pathologist Rudolf Virchow in his own investigations into the 'granulomatous diseases'.[25]

Virchow was of the (mistaken) view that the neural pathology in leprosy was 'trophic' and secondary to the primary pathology in the skin, but he was more percipient when he stated that "compared to the sensory disturbances, the motor change lie in the background". By the first decades of the 20th century leprosy neuropathy was recognized as a specific primary inflammatory and destructive process in the nerve with the *Bacillus* providing the stimulus.

The Estonian researcher Dehio and his pupil Gerlach are associated with arguably the most important late 19th century postulate relating to neuropathogenesis. On the basis of a case observed clinically and minutely examined anatomically, these researchers proposed that in the anesthetic form, the disease commenced in the skin. The local circumscribed anesthesia caused by the spread of the leprous granuloma in the diseased skin, invaded the lymph spaces and lymphatics in the skin and penetrated the tubular tissue spaces in which the most delicate terminal branches of the dermal nerves are distributed. In consequence, the skin nerves within the 'maculae' disintegrated, and the maculae become anesthetic. In the further course of the disease, the granuloma spread upwards by way of the nerve sheaths, creeping gradually to the larger ramifications and finally to the nerve trunks, the muscular atrophy occurring as a consequence (Fig. 1.8). The Dehio-Gerlach hypothesis retains its credibility even today, because it is in harmony with current knowledge of the internal anatomy of limb peripheral nerves.[26]

Nerve Abscess

In 1924, Ernest Muir working in Kolkata documented nerve abscesses in anesthetic leprosy in India and also surgically explored their relation to the funiculi. He pointed out the poor correlation between the degree of nerve enlargement and the severity of fiber damage in such nerves.[27]

PATHOLOGY

In his landmark book *Pathology of Tumours* (published in 1864–65), Virchow described the microscopic picture in a group of nodule-forming ulcerous diseases (syphilis, lupus vulgaris, leprosy), which he labeled the 'granulomas', because they were marked by the growth of 'granulation tissue'.[25] The leprosy granuloma was composed of sheets and masses of small and larger cells, some multinucleated, infiltrating the dermis and extending into the sheath of peripheral nerves in the anesthetic variety. In nodular leprosy, thinning of the epidermis and flattening of the papillae were described, as also the presence of vacuolated ('physaliferous') cells. 'Virchowian leprosy' became a synonym for nodular leprosy, characterized by the so-called 'lepra cell'. Elucidation of the contents of the cell had to await Armauer Hansen's discovery of the *Bacillus* in 1873, almost a decade after Virchow's studies.

Discovery and Properties of the Bacillus

GA Hansen's discovery (in 1873) of the causative organism was a landmark event, ahead of its time (Fig. 1.9). The *Bacillus* was the first to be proposed as the cause of a human disease, but the germ theory in general was yet in its infancy. Using osmic acid to stain cells teased out from a freshly excised leproma obtained from a man with nodular leprosy, Hansen described rod-shaped 'bacteria' within granular cells (Unstained bacilli mounted in distilled water showed vigorous movements, which he mistook for true motility; he also described 'spores').[28]

Despite numerous attempts by Hansen and his contemporaries, no experimental animal proved susceptible to leprosy, and the putative 'leprosy germ' faced skepticism and even outright rejection for several decades. Contrast

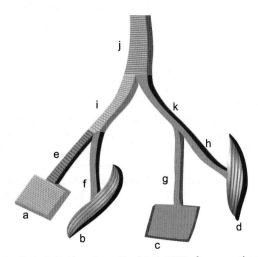

Fig. 1.8: Gerlach-Dehio schematic dated 1897 of neuropathogenesis. Ascent of neuritis from dermal nerve a to mixed nerves (i) and (j), causing muscle paralysis (b) and (d).[26]

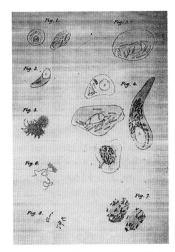

Fig. 1.9: Hansen's depiction of intracellular bacilli.[28]

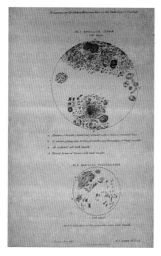

Fig. 1.10: The first display of 'bacillus leprae' and 'bacillus tuberculosis' in India was by Carter in Mumbai in 1883, using the Ehrlich stain.[18]

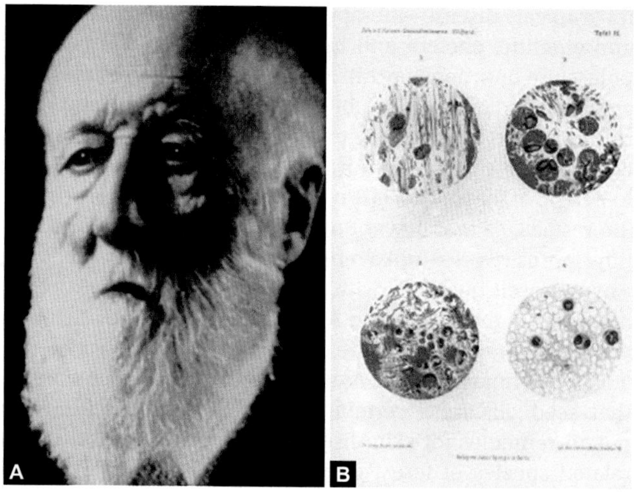

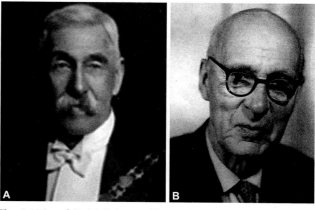

Figs 1.11A and B: (A) Georg Sticker; (B) Stained preparations of nasal smears from inmates of the Homeless Leper Asylum, Mumbai, 1897. (*See* Reference 30)

this with the approbation which greeted Koch's discovery of the tubercle *Bacillus* almost a decade later, fortified by ample experimental authentication and the statement of his 'postulates'. The pathogenicity of *Bacillus leprae* was finally acknowledged on empirical grounds by the international scientific community at the Berlin Congress in 1897.

A notable advance was Paul Ehrlich's introduction of aniline dyes as bacillary stains and acid decolorization, and Ziehl's substitution of carbolic solution for aniline oil, which became standard practice in the demonstration of the so-called 'acid-fast bacilli'.[29] This advance was utilized by Carter in Mumbai in 1883 for the first demonstration in India of the bacilli of tuberculosis and leprosy (Fig. 1.10).[18] Interestingly, all the early investigators noticed that leprosy bacilli were not evenly stained (Fig. 1.10).

In 1897 an important study was conducted at the 'Homeless Leper Asylum' in Mumbai by a German bacteriologist. It confirmed the suspicion that the nose was a nidus for the bacilli. Georg Sticker, a member of the German Commission investigating the plague epidemic then raging in Mumbai, used the opportunity to visit the Asylum to investigate and found bacillary clusters and globi in nasal smears in 128 of 153 inmates (Figs 1.11A and B). He reported these findings at the First International Leprosy Congress held at Berlin in 1897.[30] Incidentally, Robert Koch was also a member of that Commission. Sticker and Koch raised the possibility that nose was the *escape* route of leprosy bacilli.

THE ERA OF CHAULMOOGRA/HYDNOCARPUS OIL THERAPY IN INDIA

With the retirement of Vandyke Carter in 1888, there was a vacuum in scientific leprology in India for almost three

Figs 1.12A and B: (A) Sir Leonard Rogers (1868–1962); (B) Ernest Muir 1880–1974, the guiding spirits in antileprosy work in India in the first half of the 20th century

decades. In 1915, a new center of study arose in Kolkata with the entry of Sir Leonard Rogers (1868-1962) of the Indian Medical Service, and Ernest Muir (1880-1974) a medical missionary (Figs 1.12A and B) into the field. Both men attained worldwide reputations and influence through their prolific writings and the institutions and organizations which they founded or nurtured. Rogers was the spirit behind the establishment of the Calcutta School of Tropical Medicine in 1920 just prior to his retirement from India, by which time he had introduced a new therapy (more accurately an old therapy in a new *avatar*), and he and Muir had outlined a revolutionary approach to leprosy control.

Rogers was one of the most prominent tropical medicine specialists in the Indian Medical Service at the turn of the 20th century, with a reputation grounded in contributions to tropical disease therapeutics, e.g. amebic dysentery and emetine, cholera and hypertonic saline, kala azar and potassium antimony tartrate. It was his ambition to close his career in India in a blaze of glory with another therapeutic triumph—the successful treatment of leprosy. Rogers's collaborator was Ernest Muir, a medical missionary who came to Bengal in the first decade of the 20th century with a primary interest in kala azar. It was Rogers who inducted him into full-time leprosy work. Unlike most missionaries at the time, Muir was very well-qualified, with a postgraduate degree from his *alma mater* the Edinburgh Medical School. The association with Edinburgh was to prove crucial in his leprosy work.

It was a hoary belief in Ayurveda and Indian folk medicine that seed oils from certain indigenous tree species were potent remedies for skin diseases, especially leprosy.[31] Two related species of forest trees, namely *Taraktogenos kurzii* ("chaulmoogra") from the North-East, and *Hydnocarpus wightiana*, ("marotti", "kowti") from the coastal South-West, were the best regarded. The latter ("marotti") was first reported to Western readers in 1687 in a beautifully illustrated tome of the flora of Malabar (Kerala) (Figs 1.13A and B).[32] brought out by the Dutch Governor van Rheede.

The opinions of 19th century physicians employing *Chaulmoogra* and *Marotti* oils were uneven, improvement being variously found to be 'decided', 'impermanent', or none at all. Frequently patients refused to persist with oral treatment because of nausea and gastric irritation. Thus, while the oils continued to be employed, it was by default rather than proven merit and patient satisfaction. Rogers's contribution was to substitute oral administration of the oil with parenteral (injection) administration of a soluble derivative of the oil.

Rogers, who was Professor of Pathology at Calcutta Medical College, utilized technical assistance of Indian organic chemists, settled on the water-soluble sodium salt of the fatty acids of *chaulmoogra*—sodium chaulmoograte. Therapeutic trials were launched in late 1915, and results were published frequently as more patients were added. In some patients given the injection subcutaneously for '6 months and over', Rogers claimed that lost sensation and muscle power had returned. His next 'advance' was intravenous injection of 3% sodium chaulmoograte, which was declared to be not only painless, but better than the subcutaneous route at initiating softening of nodules, clearing bacilli, and overall clinical improvement.[32]

His consolidated report published in India in 1917, contained a tabulated summary of 2 years' experience with sodium chaulmoograte administered subcutaneously and intravenously to 26 patients.[33] Although claiming "2 years' experience", Rogers' Table shows that actually just *2 patients of the 26* had been treated for that length of time! By 1919 sodium chaulmoograte was replaced by sodium hydnocarpate (hydnocarpus oil being more easily available), and by 1920 (Rogers' last year in India), his final patient tally from 5 and 1/2 years ot work with the compounds was 51 cases, of whom 13 had been given the treatment (intravenously and/or subcutaneously) for upwards of a year (Rogers was clearly a master of semantics). He waxed eloquent over the 'unique' ability of this drug of plant origin to induce local 'reactions' and active destruction of leprosy bacilli, but glossed over the serious side effects of intravenous administration—dizziness and fainting, and venous thrombosis.

On retirement in England, Rogers wrote in prestigious journals and lectured before august medical bodies about the 51 patients. In 1924, he invoked the data to launch an ambitious campaign to "STAMP OUT LEPROSY IN THE BRITISH EMPIRE... PROBABLY WITHIN THREE DECADES" (*sic*).[34]

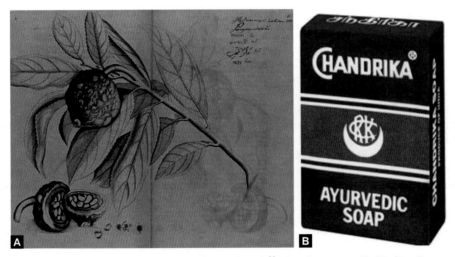

Figs 1.13A and B: (A) Hydnocarpus Wightiana ("marotti") fruit and seeds;[32] (B) Hydnocarpus oil's skin-friendly reputation endures as a constituent of well-known Ayurvedic soap from Kerala

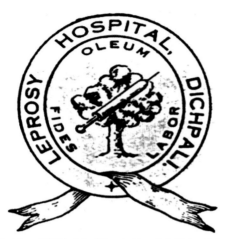

Fig. 1.14: Emblem (1934) of the Victoria Hospital, Dichpali, Nizamabad, incorporating hydnocarpus tree and syringe. The 3-point motto translates as: "Faith, Oil, Work".[36]

It was Britain's imperial duty, Rogers declared, to provide 'our lepers' with the benefits of the latest treatment. The organization which Rogers was responsible for launching was the British Empire Leprosy Relief Association (BELRA). A contemporary, ironically observed that BELRA (today known as LEPRA, a successful nonsectarian international leprosy NGO), was in effect founded on *13 cases treated "for upwards of a year" with the sodium salts!* [35]

The sodium salt treatment had some enthusiastic supporters in India. Muir himself was impressed enough by the initial results he obtained in Mission asylum inmates in Bengal, to agree to Rogers' suggestion to take up full-time leprosy work at the School of Tropical Medicine at Calcutta in 1921, so as to exploit the potential of the therapy. In England, Rogers, as BELRA's Medical Adviser, was particularly gratified by favorable reports on sodium hydnocarpate injection in early leprosy. The Mission Asylum and Hospital at Dichpali, Nizamabad reported that 90% of early cases were discharged 'symptom-free.' Hydnocarpus oil acquired emblematic status in the Hospital (Fig. 1.14).[36]

But Rogers' therapeutic experiments were flawed methodologically even by the standards of his day. Rigorous scientific trials as we know them today were still of the future, but Rogers made no attempt whatever at objectivity. The bluff of *chaulmoogra* enthusiasts such as Rogers was finally called in 1931 when the Leprosy Commission of the League of Nations pointed out that the so-called *remedy* had never been subjected to double-blind controlled clinical trials, and hence "no conclusive evidence exists of the efficacy of *chaulmoogra* as such". [37]

LEPROSY AS A PUBLIC HEALTH PROBLEM

Till the early 20th century, the only method of dealing with leprosy was to isolate the patients in 'leprosy asylums' where they were fed and cared for. *Chaulmoogra* oil therapy gave hope of possible cure. Very early in their collaboration, Rogers and Muir envisioned leprosy eradication through *chaulmoogra* treatment, which they outlined at the Conference of the Mission to Lepers (present "The Leprosy Mission") held at Calcutta in 1920. It was an historic occasion.

Rogers declared

"recent improvements of methods of injections.....have now reached a stage.....when our leper asylums can be converted more into leper colonies and hospitals, to which earlier cases.....will be receiving beneficial treatment with even some hope of ultimate cure"[38]

Muir went a step further stating

"With a view to bring early cases as soon as possible under treatment, every effort must be made through schools and the press to educate the public of the cause, early symptoms and hopefulness of treatment in early cases and inducements should be created to undertake treatment".[38]

Muir joined the newly opened Calcutta School of Tropical Medicine in 1921 as Head of the Leprosy Department, which provided him an unparalleled opportunity to refine his ideas and make improvements in the treatment itself. By 1925, he had demonstrated the feasibility of diagnosis and treatment of early cases at the School's outpatient clinic, which held promise of a wider application of the clinic concept. The concept of the clinic itself was inspired by the pioneering tuberculosis dispensaries set-up by Sir Robert Philip in late 19th century Edinburgh (the city where Muir underwent his medical training).

A unique opportunity came with Rogers' establishment of the British Empire Leprosy Relief Association (BELRA) in 1924 in England, which was followed in the next year by its Indian auxiliary, The Indian Council of BELRA (ICBELRA). Launched through a public appeal by the Viceroy Lord Reading, ICBELRA (the present-day Hind Kusht Nivaran Sangh, HKNS) was generously funded by Indian donations. Muir as Leprosy Expert and Research Worker, authored and supervised a countrywide disease control strategy to optimize the benefits of "the favorable results obtained from the new treatment".

Muir initiated the "Propaganda, Treatment, Survey" (PTS) scheme, as a public health approach to leprosy.[39]

Propaganda was carried out by putting up posters in the clinics and villages. The press was used to spread information about the disease; magic lantern slides were projected before village communities and in schools (Fig. 1.15). *Treatment* was intradermal injection of *chaulmoogra* oil (Fig. 1.16) at clinics in villages. The *Survey* arm of PTS was conducted mainly by Isaac Santra of Sambalpur, Orissa who joined Muir in 1927.

Isaac Santra (1892-1968) (Fig. 1.17) born in Sambalpur, Orissa, obtained his medical degree at Calcutta Medical

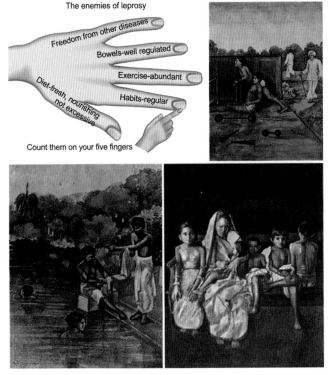

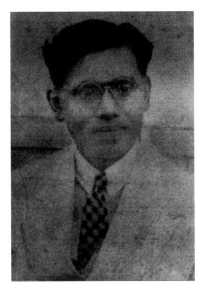

Fig. 1.17: Isaac Santra (1892–1968)

Fig. 1.15: Some Propaganda posters brought out in Kolkata by the Indian Council of the British Empire Leprosy Relief Association, 1930s. (Scans kindly supplied by Ms Irene Allen, LEPRA, UK)

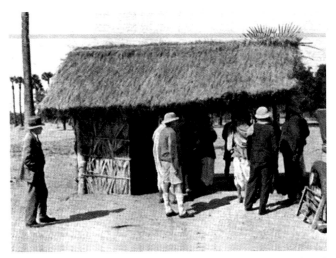

Fig. 1.18: The India Survey Team sets up a leprosy clinic in rural Bengal
Source: Leprosy in India, July 1934

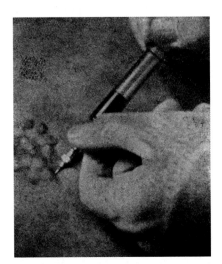

Fig. 1.16: Multiple intralesional injections of hydnocarpus oil were required

College. His entry into leprosy work started in 1920 at the Cuttack Asylum. He joined ICBELRA in 1927 as Propaganda Officer in the "India Survey Team". He visited almost all parts of the country, lecturing on leprosy and exhorting patients to attend the newly-opened leprosy clinics (Fig. 1.18). On

the basis of his sample surveys he warned that leprosy was far more prevalent than indicated in the National Decennial Censuses which were conducted by lay enumerators. Santra was deeply influenced by Muir in the notion of the supposed connection between leprosy and syphilis, as also on the seminal role of industrialization and breaching of traditional social barriers in the spread of leprosy to hitherto disease-free ethnic groups.

In 1950, Santra set-up the "Hathibari Health Home" on 560 acres of timber-rich, irrigated, cultivable land donated by the Government, to serve as a Group isolation and rehabilitation center and hospital. Awarded "Padma Shri" in 1957, he was the first leprosy worker to be honored.[40]

ICBELRA IN MADRAS PROVINCE

Ironically, the most influential critic of *chaulmoogra* oil emerged from BELRA's own ranks. Robert Cochrane (1899–1985), BELRA Medical Secretary, who was initially well-disposed to the therapy, became disillusioned and expressed his opinion forthrightly. He wrote approvingly after an extensive tour of the Indian subcontinent in 1934, that he discerned "an altogether more reasoned outlook" which emphasized leprosy prevention by selective segregation, rather than oil treatment of early cases.[41]

Following on the retirement of Muir from the Tropical School in 1935 and the arrival in the country of Robert Cochrane [(1899–1985) Fig. 1.19A] as Chief Medical Officer of the Lady Willingdon Leprosy Sanatorium, at Chingleput, the center of influence shifted once again, this time from Bengal to Madras Presidency. Cochrane was two decades younger than Muir, and like him, of Scottish descent and medically well-qualified. Cochrane became the chief spokesman for leprosy in India in the immediate preindependence period (1935–1947). He left his imprint on official policy as Director of the Leprosy Campaign for the State, besides training a dedicated band of Indian leprologists. In addition, he catalyzed the entry of specialists from other medical disciplines, e.g. Vasant Khanolkar (pathologist), and Paul Brand (surgeon) into leprosy work.

The Clinic Overshadowed: Resurgence of Segregation

It was under Cochrane's influence in Madras Presidency that leprosy 'prevention' by isolation of the infectious in institutions was pursued most energetically. The leprosy clinic's prime purpose shifted from detection and treatment of the *early* case, to netting persons with *infectious* leprosy for admission into leprosy settlements. The phrase "leprosy can be cured" was studiously avoided in ICBELRA's Madras Provincial Branch campaign, which for practical purposes became Propaganda, Survey, Segregation. Most telling of the change in emphasis was that Muir's landmark "Propaganda, Treatment, Survey" scheme did not merit even a mention in a report to the Government of India, which had Cochrane and the like-minded John Lowe among its authors.[42]

"Revision of Policy... In other words, without effective isolation of all, or at least the great majority of dangerous lepers, there is little hope of controlling and curtailing the disease... more prominence must be given to isolation".

Downgrading the efficacy of the available therapy, Cochrane envisaged prevention by way of leprosy sanatoria, leprosy colonies, domestic isolation, night isolation of infectious lepers outside the village, and leprosy-affected children's sanatoria. He declared that "without adequate (voluntary) institutional accommodation, a complete anti-leprosy system is impossible to organize" (Fig. 1.19B).[43]

In addition to superintending the Lady Willingdon Leprosy Sanatorium at Chingleput, Cochrane successfully lobbied the Provincial health authorities for opening leprosy outpatient departments in public hospitals, and for (noninfectious) leprosy patients suffering from other diseases to be treated in general medical wards. At Christian Medical College, Vellore where he became Principal, leprosy was taught in the undergraduate medical curriculum. He was thus a pioneer in bringing leprosy into the mainstream of medicine.

The preoccupation with isolation originated in Cochrane's skepticism about *chaulmoogra* oil treatment, not treatment *per se*. It is not surprising that the two leprologists, John Lowe and Robert Cochrane, who were to contribute significantly to inaugurating the Dapsone tablet era in India, were products of Indian experience and *chaulmoogra* oil therapy's earliest critics.

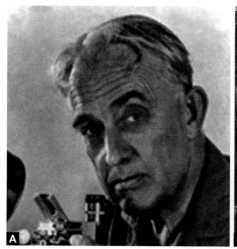 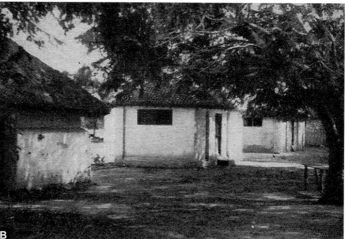

Figs 1.19A and B: (A) Robert Cochrane (1899–1985); (B) Huts for night isolation at Leprosy Asylum, Polambakkam (Tamil Nadu)

Portents of Failure of ICBELRA

Muir in course of time turned skeptical about the efficacy of *chaulmoogra* therapy, and began placing greater emphasis on upkeep of general health and morale to ameliorate leprosy.

By the mid-1930s, patients also appeared increasingly unimpressed by the claimed results of *chaulmoogra* oil-based treatment, added to which was the discomfort and pain associated with intradermal injection. Muir estimated that for every cubic centimeter of the drug injected some 32 punctures were necessary, the dose being 0.5–5 cc (depending on lesion size) once or twice a week (Fig. 1.16).[44]

Their dissatisfaction was expressed in growing absenteeism at leprosy clinics, including that at the Calcutta School itself. Patients were probably disappointed by Muir's advocacy of vigorous exercise, fresh air and nutritious diet which placed the onus of recovery squarely on them.

Lastly, the political scenario in India after 1920 (Montagu-Chelmsford Reforms) was not conducive to the success of ICBELRA's initiative. Provincial governments to whom executive responsibilities for Public Health and Medical Relief were devolved in the reforms had meagre funds, and were not enthusiastic about taking on leprosy among numerous other health and medical responsibilities.

Other ICBELRA Initiatives

Two Muir-guided ICBELRA initiatives are still with us today. The first was the launch in 1929 of the journal *Leprosy in India* (in 1984 re-titled *Indian Journal of Leprosy*); the first such in the country, if not the English-speaking world. *Leprosy Review* (published by BELRA in England) was first published in 1930, while the International Leprosy Association's *International Journal of Leprosy* came out in 1933.

The other innovation was the convening in 1933, of the first leprologists conference in the country, to discuss various problems and suggest guidelines for improvement (Fig. 1.20). Some of the original attendees were instrumental in forming the Indian Association of Leprologists in the post-Independence period (*See* Section "Indian Association of Leprologists").[45]

THE BHORE COMMITTEE

In histories of public health in modern India the favored starting point is the "Health Survey and Development Committee" (known as the Bhore Committee after its Chairman Sir Joseph Bhore), which was constituted in 1943 to prepare for the post-World War scenario. The Committee's Recommendations on Leprosy which are summarized below reflect the long shadow cast by Robert Cochrane:
- Creation of provincial leprosy organizations
- Increase of the existing provision for institutional treatment of outpatients and inpatients
- Development of group isolation colonies

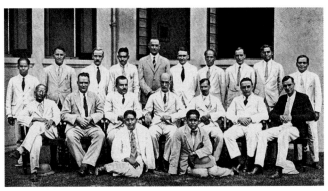

Fig. 1.20: The "First All India Leprosy Conference" held at Calcutta in 1933. The group comprised physicians engaged in leprosy work in India RG Cochrane attended as BELRA Secretary
Seated on floor: BN Ghosh, DN Mukherji
Seated L to R: Sen, J Lowe, CR Avari, E Muir, SN Chatterji, RG. Cochrane, V Rambo
Standing L to R: GR Rao, S Jaikaria, AD Miller, HN Gupta, CS Ryles, HH Gass, PC Verghese, DS Baxter, I Santra, AT Roy

- Substantial financial help to voluntary organizations engaged in antileprosy work
- Establishment of a Central Leprosy Institute for training of doctors, promotion of research, and provision of information on best practices to governments and voluntary organizations.[46] (The Institute was duly set up after Independence at the original Lady Willingdon Leprosy Sanatorium at Chingleput, Tamil Nadu).

Institutions for the Leprosy Afflicted

The leprosy asylum is not an authentic Indian institution. The fact is that sufferers were traditionally lumped with other handicapped or marginalized persons or those considered undesirable, repulsive or otherwise unworthy of normal social intercourse. For such marginalized groups, benevolent rulers and religion-inspired persons established poor-houses known as *dharmashalas,* where the inmates were fed and sheltered and where no restriction was placed on entry and departure. Examples are Jamsetjee Jejeebhoy Dharmashala in 19th Century, Mumbai, and Sant Gadge Maharaj Dharmashala in the 1950s at Pandharpur (Maharashtra).

Leprosy Asylums under British Auspices

The concept of institutions for *special* categories of marginalized groups is a peculiarly European one, and leprosy (and lunatic) asylums were, and are, the tangible symbols of India's colonial encounters. The first institution established under British aegis was at Almora by Sir Henry Ramsay, Chief Commissioner of Kumaon (Uttarakhand) in 1835. While there is no doubt that genuine charitable feeling and pity inspired many such projects, the associated motives were equally important. Firstly, such acts bolstered British colonialism's anxiety to project itself as a caring system amidst 'apathetic' and 'unfeeling' Hindu society. Secondly, by the late 19th century the leprosy asylum became the solution to the fear and loathing caused to well-to-do urban Indian society by crowds of begging lepers infesting the streets of prosperous colonial cities such as Mumbai and Kolkata. Thirdly, by the end of that century leprosy institutions acquired medical justification. Hereditarians saw them as places to ensure sexual segregation of lepers and prevent hereditary transmission; contagionists regarded them as a measure to isolate dangerously contagious person from society; sanitarians thought they were places to reinvigorate and rehabilitate demoralized sufferers in a wholesome environment. For Christian missionaries, who soon dominated the field, leprosy asylums provided scope and space for preaching the gospel.[47]

Moulding the New Man in Mission Asylums

The large-scale involvement of Protestant missionaries with leprosy asylums in India commenced with the founding of "The Mission to Lepers in India and the East" (today known as "The Leprosy Mission") by Wellesley Bailey in 1874.[48] The Mission established its own asylums and also aided other Protestant denominations involved in leprosy work. The asylums at Purulia in West Bengal, Faizabad and Naini in Uttar Pradesh, Vadathorasalur in Tamil Nadu are a few such institutions.

Pioneering agricultural experiments were undertaken by nonmedical missionaries such as George Kerr and his doctor wife Isabel at the Victoria Hospital, Dichpali (Nizamabad), under the guidance of the renowned Sir Albert Howard of the Imperial Agricultural Institute at Pusa (Samastipur), a pioneer of composting and green organic farming.[49]

The approach of another visionary, the Welsh-American missionary Sam Higginbottom, Superintendent of the Naini Leper Asylum, Allahabad (he also founded the Naini Agricultural Institute), was to enhance farm yields by improving and modifying common agricultural equipment. Though an admirer of Gandhiji, Higginbottom differed in envisioning rural revival through improved farming practice and yields rather than encouragement of khadi and village small-scale industries.[50] Asylum inmates thus 'transformed' were expected to become foci of transformed when they were discharged from the asylum and returned to their villages. The aim was to fashion reinvigorated catalysts of Indian revival rather than merely 'cured lepers'.

Homeless Leper Asylum, Mumbai

The Asylum was established in Mumbai in 1890 and was unique in more than one way. Housing over 300 pauper lepers, it was the largest nonsectarian institution in the country.

It was initiated by Harry Acworth ICS, Municipal Commissioner of Mumbai, in order to purge the streets of leper beggars. The seed money was donated entirely by the *shethias* and ordinary citizens of Mumbai and rulers of princely states subservient to the Mumbai Government. Maintenance funds were provided equally by the Provincial Government and the Municipality. As such it was completely nonsectarian. The inmates' religious and caste preferences were respected, and there was no rigid rule on segregation of the sexes. The Asylum was the site of another innovation; it was there that biogas was first used for lighting and sewage farming, adding to the income of the institution.[51] After several name changes over the past 130 years, the institution is today known as the Acworth Municipal Leprosy Hospital (Figs 1.21A and B).

LEGISLATION

Historic Indian Practices with Respect to Leprosy Sufferers

Dharmasastra texts contain an inclusive group of persons debarred from inheriting property, for example, those with mental ailments, blindness, 'black teeth', leprosy, etc. (Fig. 1.22A).[52] It is noteworthy that leprosy sufferers were *never specifically* singled out for disinheritance, they were constituents of a marginalized *group*. Further, in recompense for denial of inheritance the *Sastras* privileged the group by entitling them to maintenance and sustenance by relatives.[53] It has to be admitted that although leprosy sufferers were not thus singled out, generous family spirit was not invariably their lot. Over the centuries, thousands men, women and children must have been expelled from hearth and home to join bands of vagrants, mendicants, the lame, and the halt who congregated near places of worship. In the late 19th and early 20th century, they were conspicuous on the streets of prosperous cities of colonial India.

A notable scripturally sanctioned practice was for pious relatives to aid the suicide of lepers who begged for release from a miserable existence. Common modes of suicide were burning or burial alive in specially prepared pits (Fig. 1.22B), drowning in a river, or plunging off a cliff into the sea (perhaps voluntarily or under duress).[54] *Sant Devidas*, authored by Gujarat's most celebrated literary figure Jhaverchand Meghani (1896–1947), is a fictional account woven around a (forced) leper suicide on the sea-coast off Saurashtra, saved in the nick of time and ministered to by the Sant (1725–1800) in his ashram.[55] Meghani testified that such suicides were not unknown till at least the 1930s.

Secular Legislation in the Colonial Era

The time-line of leprosy history in colonial India shows a sharp politicization of the leprosy problem in the last two decades of the 19th century. The immediate trigger was the death from

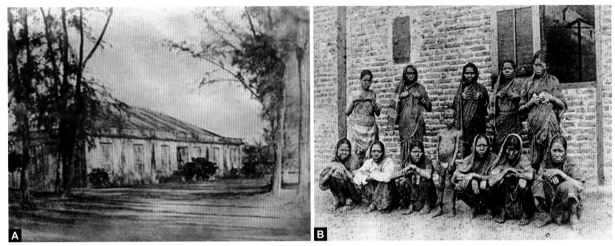

Figs 1.21A and B: (A) Abandoned military barracks were converted into the "Homeless Leper Asylum"
at Mumbai in 1890; (B) The first group of women inmates at the Asylum
Source: From archival collection at Acworth Leprosy Hospital Research Society Mumbai

CHAP. V. On Exclusion from Participation.

Sect. I. On Persons excluded from Inheritance. A vicious son or brother, an outcast, a professed enemy to his father, an eunuch, a leper, a madman, an ideot, an impostor, and a man born blind, deaf, or lame, are excluded, but entitled to maintenance, except the outcast and his offspring. With the same exception, their sons inherit. Eight sorts of leprosy. Obsequies of outcasts and lepers forbidden. Certain diseases are tokens of former sins. Impotence defined. Wives and daughters of excluded persons must be maintained. Exclusion of sons born in the inverse order of classes, or born of any illegal marriage. Hermits are excluded. Divorce of a wife illegally espoused. Exclusion of spurious offspring. Separate claims of sons by different husbands. 298

A

220 CASES IN THE NIZAMUT ADAWLUT.

1810.
Aug. 7th.
SOHAWUN'S
case.

VAKEEL OF GOVERNMENT,
against
SOHAWUN.

Charge—HOMICIDE.

Case of a Hindoo of the Rajpoot tribe, preparing a pit and setting fire to the fuel in it, to enable his father, who was ill with the leprosy. to burn himself. The prisoner held justified under the tenets of the Hindoo law and religion, and also acquitted under the provisions of the Moohummudan law.

THIS trial came on at the Goruckpore sessions the prisoner was arraigned, on the charge of assisting his father Akbar to burn himself alive. From the declaration of the prisoner and the testimony of witnesses, the following appeared to be the circumstances of the case. The father of the prisoner had been afflicted for some time with a leprous disease, from which he suffered so much, that he desired his son (the prisoner) to prepare a pit, and fill it with cow-dung and other fuel, to which he was to set fire, that the deceased might cast himself in and be burnt. The prisoner at first declined; but afterwards, his father becoming still worse, prepared a pit, as he desired, and set fire to the fuel with which he had filled it. He then informed his father (the deceased); who repaired to the spot, and threw himself in; some time after which, the prisoner covered up the mouth of the pit.

The *futwa* of the law officers of the Court of Circuit, declared, that a sentence of *Kissas* was barred, from the circumstance of the deceased having flung himself into the fire, where he was burnt; but that the prisoner was liable to discretionary punishment, for having, in pursuance of his father's directions, prepared the pit, and set fire to the fuel with which he had filled it. The Judge of Circuit did not concur in the above *futwa*; he expressed his sentiments as follows :—" I am assured, that in the case of Hindoos, it (alluding to suicide) is countenanced and enjoined by their religion. It is supposed that the leprosy is a visitation of Providence for some offence or other; and that the souls of the victims are purified by fire from the taint of the disease, and exempted from passing into impure bodies after death. There is also a popular notion, that by this self-devotion, the disease is rooted out of the family." In recommending that the prisoner

B

Figs 1.22A and B: (A)) Civil disabilities on lepers and other groups in the Hindu Law of Inheritance; (B) The Leper and Criminal Law. Case against Sohawun, a son who facilitated the suicide of his grievously suffering leper father by burning alive in a specially prepared pit. The case was heard before the East India Company's Nizamat Adalat (Court of Criminal Justice) at Calcutta in 1810. The accused was acquitted on the Court Kazis and Pundits certifying that the deed was not against the tenets of Mohamedan or Hindu Law leprosy in 1889, of the Belgian priest Father Damien who had lived with the lepers at Molokai in Hawaii for 15 years. The fact that a European had fallen victim to leprosy was seized on by British imperialists, Indian alarmists and contagionists to agitate for segregation of lepers congregating in major Indian cities. However, even in 1889, medical circles in India were not of one mind on the etiology of leprosy. Some contagion-skeptics labeled the mass hysteria as motivated, and warned against police *zoolum* against the hapless leper. In 1890, a 4-member Leprosy Commission was dispatched from London to report on the disease in India and make policy recommendations. The Commissioners concluded that though leprosy was an infective disease, caused by a specific *Bacillus*, and moreover also a contagious disease, there was not sufficient evidence that it was diffused by contagion (contact). The amount of contagion in the surroundings was so small that it could be disregarded. They said, "No legislation is called for on the lines of either segregation or the interdiction of marriages with lepers".[56] The Commission therefore rejected compulsory segregation, but recommended asylums situated near cities to house pauper lepers.

The recommendations of the Commission formed the basis of "The Lepers Act" of 1898, the only leprosy-specific legislation enacted by the British (Fig. 1.23A). Interestingly, the Commission also attempted to culture the *Bacillus*, of course without success.

The well-to-do leper was not compulsorily isolated; the Act initially mandated institutionalization of ulcerous pauper lepers only. Following representations from the Mission to Lepers, its purview was broadened to include *all* pauper lepers. Such persons were arrested and given a 'Certificate' by a competent medical officer before being dispatched to an asylum (Fig. 1.23B). Lepers were also prohibited from plying trades/professions such as butcher, washerman, nurse, etc. Existing institutions were gradually incorporated as statutory leper institutions under the Act. Governments gave grants-in-aid to such asylums, most of which were Mission-run; it was a symbiotic relationship since it was economical for the State, and benefited the missionary enterprise too. However, as a public health measure, the Act was a dead letter.

It was repealed in 1985.

THE ERA OF NEW DRUGS

Sulfones

Diamino diphenyl sulfone (DDS) was synthesized in 1908. In 1937, it was found to be more active than Sulfnilamide against streptococci. Attempts were made to use it in man against streptococcal infection. Used in doses that produced the same blood levels as with sulfonamides it was found to be highly toxic. Efforts were made to produce less toxic derivatives. Feldman and others in 1941 produced Promin which was a derivative of DDS and it was found to have some protective action against tubercle bacilli. It was tried in 1941 for treatment of leprosy at the National Leprosarium, Carville.[57] It was to be given intravenously and the dose was 2.5 g daily. It was soon found that all sulfone derivatives were converted back to DDS in the body indicating that parent DDS itself can be administered. DDS was first used parentarily in 1947 by Cochrane as a 25% suspension in arachis oil.[58] DDS was first used orally by Muir in 1950 as aqueous suspension.[59] It was then generally used as tablets.

Clofazimine

Clofazimine (B663), a dye substance was originally synthesized in Dublin. Its antimicrobial action was shown as early as in 1948 against tubercle bacilli (H37Rv) *in vitro* and also in several experimental animals. The first trial of B663 in human leprosy was carried out by Browne and Hogerzeil in Africa.[60] Subsequently, its anti-inflammatory action was demonstrated by the same authors.[61]

DEVELOPMENTS AT INDEPENDENCE

National Leprosy Control Programme (1955–1981)

In the immediate post-independence period, the most notable effort to address leprosy as a public health problem was that undertaken by Ramchandra V Wardekar at the Gandhi Memorial Leprosy Foundation (GMLF) at Wardha (Fig. 1.24).

The importance of rural leprosy had been recognized as early as 1934 by Muir who set-up the Leprosy Investigation Center at Bankura in Bengal. Here were pioneered 'house to house' surveys and lists were made of all cases detected. Also innovative was Muir's utilization of the services of "trained but unqualified assistants", i.e. paramedical workers.[62]

Wardekar's scheme under GMLF started around Sewagram, later extended to 12 centers in different parts of the country, was also field-based, but extensively deployed well-trained paramedical workers (PMW). The strategy was in principle similar to Muir's PTS, except that the term "Propaganda" (which had an unhealthy connotation with Hitlerian methods) was replaced by 'Education', so it was known as the Survey, Education, Treatment (SET) pattern. House-to-house *Surveys* were carried out as part of the leprosy campaign—every man, woman and child being examined for signs of the disease. *Health Education* was energetically carried out through Information, Education and Communication (IEC). *Treatment* was chemotherapy using oral Dapsone, with regularity of intake by patients being ascertained by PMW (Fig. 1.25).

Wardekar's signal contribution was the systematic incorporation of "PMW" into the National Leprosy Control Programme (NLCP) itself, which had the virtues of flexibility, decentralization, easier access to communities, and cost-effectiveness. NLCP based on the SET pattern was launched

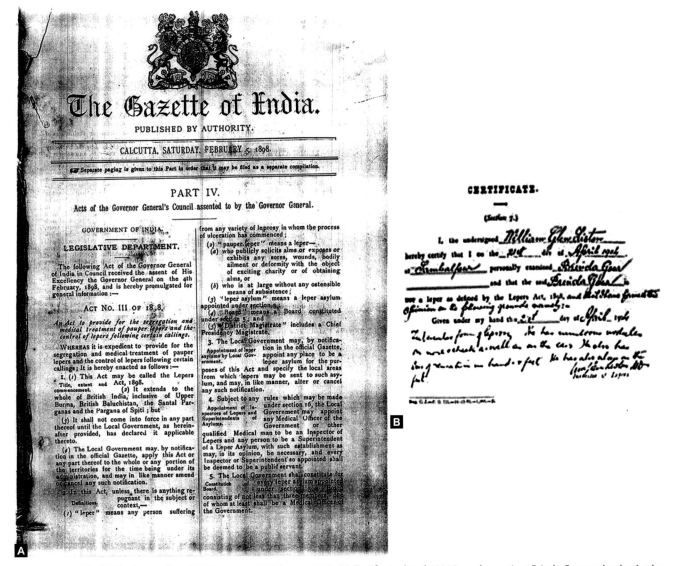

Figs 1.23A and B: (A) The Lepers Act of 1898, gazetted 5 February 1898. (B) Certificate dated 1904 issued to patient Brinda Gaur under the Act by William Glen Liston, Civil Surgeon of Sambalpur, as "Inspector of Lepers"
Photographed with permission in 2006 at the Leprosy Mission Hospital, Chandkuri, Chhattisgarh. Glen Liston (1873-1950) later became Director of the Haffkine Institute, Mumbai, and an authority on plague

in 1955 as a component of the First Five Year Plan. By the Fourth Plan, the entire country was covered by Leprosy Control Units (LCU) and SET centers. An LCU covered a population of one lakh and an SET center covered 15,000.[63]

Ramchandra V Wardekar (1913–1996) (Fig. 1.26) was a student of Grant Medical College, Mumbai, where he obtained MD degree in Pathology. He set-up a laboratory and started private practice in Mumbai and was well off monetarily. However, it did not give him mental satisfaction. He went around to a few places of spiritual atmosphere and finally landed at Wardha, the home town of his wife. He was impressed by a small general hospital at Sewagram, started by Dr Sushila Nayyar and offered his service part-time. While

working there he developed many ideas of rural health. He was taken to Gandhiji. Gandhiji was impressed by his views and enthusiasm and offered him financial support for his projects on condition that he remain at Wardha for at least 25 years. Wardekar agreed. In the meantime, GMLF was established, and Wardekar became its Director. The ensuing years at the Foundation made it possible for him to fulfill his promise to Gandhiji.

At that time leprosy work consisted mainly of admitting patients in asylums and taking care of them. It was Wardekar who conceived the idea of dealing with leprosy as a public health problem and take steps to prevent its spread in the community. This could be achieved by detecting all

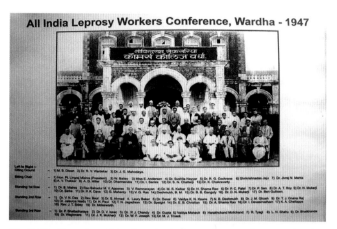

Fig. 1.24: Changing of the Guard at Independence. Influence in leprosy policy shifts from foreign into Indian hands

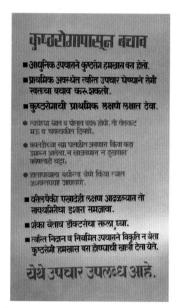

Fig. 1.25: Gandhi Memorial Leprosy Foundation (GMLF) Poster (1950s, in Marathi) on signs and symptoms of leprosy and the availability of treatment at the clinic

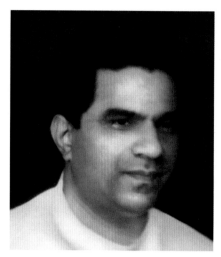

Fig. 1.26: Ramchandra V Wardekar (1913–1996)

Wardekar also leant his weight for repeal of some of the outdated objectionable civil laws against 'lepers' such as the Hindu Marriage Bill, etc. He and the Association fought successfully to prevent the 'sterilization' of the Unfit Bill which was introduced in the parliament in 1964 (Fig. 1.29).

Under his stewardship, GMLF became a leading organization. One important effect was that the government regularly invited GMLF and all NGOs for consultation and participation in national leprosy programs (Fig. 1.27).

INDIAN SOCIAL INITIATIVES AND GANDHIJI'S SUPPORT

Mahatma Gandhi's concern for leprosy sufferers dated from his sojourn in South Africa. The care he provided to the sufferer Parchure Shastri at the Sewagram ashram was immortalized in the photograph easily recognizable by modern Indian leprologists. Gandhiji's example inspired some of his followers to take up leprosy work.

Kushtadham Dattapur, District Wardha (Maharashtra)

It is said that Manohar Diwan (1901-1980) took to leprosy work when he saw a miserable leprosy patient near a well looking for someone to help him with water. Manoharji came to his aid; and thereby changed his life's course (Figs 1.30A and B).

With Gandhiji's encouragement and help Dattapur leprosy home was established in 1936 on a small plot of land near Wardha. A few huts were put up and patients taken in. They were housed, fed and cared for, but no medical work could be undertaken due to the reluctance of local doctors to treat leprosy patients. Diwan himself underwent a training course at the Calcutta School of Tropical Medicine; on his return,

the patients in a defined area and providing them with domiciliary treatment with DDS. This was how the Survey, Education and Treatment (SET) method was started and later taken over by the Government of India as the national policy and implemented all over the country (Fig. 1.27). Subsequently, WHO adopted the method for international work. The SET work needed the service of a large number of PMW. The systematic utilization of PMWs for leprosy control programs was a signal contribution of Wardekar. PMW training program was initiated at Sewagram with necessary syllabus and the Government and the NGOs started many training centers (Fig. 1.28).

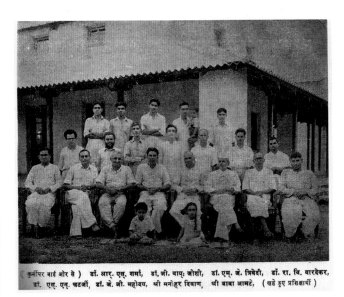

Fig. 1.27: Excerpt of Wardekar's correspondence (1953) with the Planning Commission on the requirements of his leprosy control strategy which "is very much different from the one which has been followed so far". Original document in the archives of GMLF

chaulmoogra oil injection treatment, ulcer dressing and care of limbs were provided. Outpatients were also treated.

It is not surprising that Gandhiji's friend Parchure Shastri spent his last days at Dattapur.

As the work expanded, the Government granted a large area of surrounding land. Public donations and Government

Fig. 1.28: The first paramedical trainees with teachers at Dattapur, 1952. Wardekar is seated at center. Original photograph in Manohar Diwan: Vyakti aur Vichar, Maharogi Seva Samiti, Manohardham, Dattapur, 1981

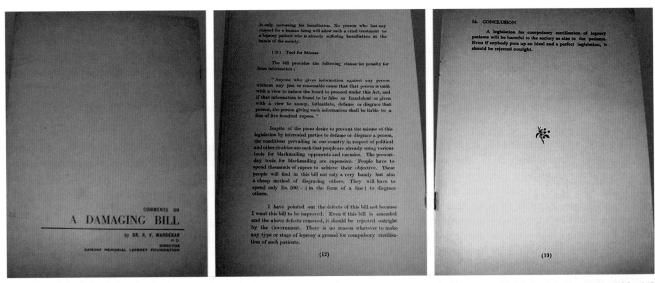

Fig. 1.29: In 1964 The Gandhi Memorial Leprosy Foundation played a leading role in petitioning Parliament and lobbying against Rajya Sabha MP Shakuntala Paranjpye's proposed legislation to sterilize sufferers of leprosy (among other "defective" people) as a public health measure. Original document in the Archives of GMLF

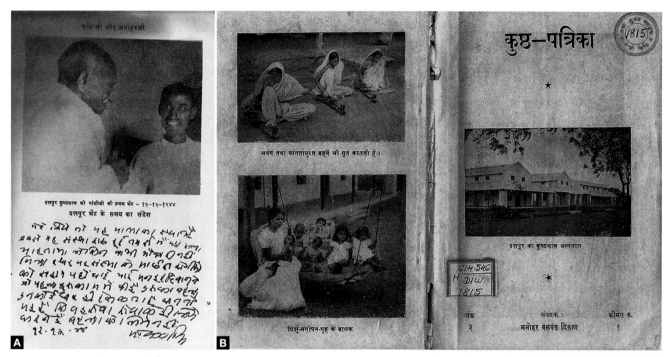

Figs 1.30A and B: (A) Gandhiji with a youthful Diwan; (B) Periodical edited by Diwan and published at Dattapur

grants helped considerably. In the late 1950s, there were more than 800 inmates and an additional settlement was established near village Seldoh, so that far-flung farms would be easily accessible. The activities of the patients at Dattapur centerd on:

Agriculture and Dairy: The inmates worked the fields to produce Jowar and Toor. Bountiful harvests of cotton and oranges, the major commercial crops of the region were obtained. The residue from the cotton-seed oil press was a nutritious cattle feed for the dairy farm.

Village industries on Gandhian lines: Ambar Charkhas (of improved design) were distributed. The yarn spun mostly by women earned them a small income. Handlooms were installed with the help of the Khadi and Village Industries Board.

Education: A hostel was started for girl inmates and daughters of leprosy patients attending high schools were helped with books. The girls were taught handicrafts such as embroidery, knitting, carpet making, etc. The products were sold to visitors and at exhibitions.

A Japanese organization started a hostel for out-station girl students; all their educational needs were provided. They were also taught handicrafts such as knitting, crochet, and making door mats by volunteer teachers.

Medical and Social: The Dattapur institution participated in carrying out the SET based NLCP. An SET center was established in two villages nearby. The work was carried out by an inmate of the colony under the supervision of the Medical Officer.

When the Sewagram Medical College was started, consultants became available to treat leprosy patients suffering from other diseases. Medical students were posted at Dattapur during their internship. Similarly students of local schools were sent to Dattapur to learn about leprosy and participate in the agricultural activities.

Dattapur Kusta Dham was later renamed *Manohar Dham* in honor of Manohar Diwan.

Tapovan—Vidarbha Maharogi Seva Mandal, Amravati (Maharashtra), 1950

Dr Shivajirao Patwardhan (1892–1986) (Fig. 1.31): *Satyagrahi* and homeopath founded the Mandal in 1950. During his frequent periods of imprisonment (1942–1945) he noticed the enforced isolation of a leprosy-affected prisoner. Another moving incident was the sight of the dead body of a leprosy sufferer lying abandoned on the road side, being scavenged by dogs. Yet another incident was when he was informed that a road-side beggar whom he had not seen for many days had committed suicide. These defining experiences and the consent of Gandhiji and Vinoba Bhave encouraged Patwardhan to enter leprosy work in 1946, to rehabilitate the affected at *Tapovan*. As a life-long crusader against injustices to the leprosy affected, Patwardhan sometimes faced influential opposition. In 1950, he started a periodical

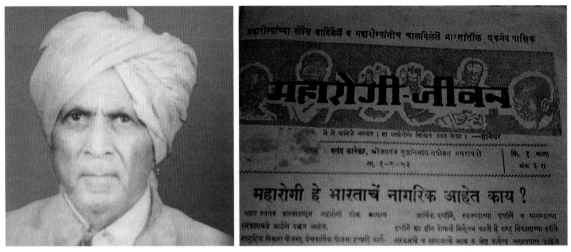

Fig. 1.31: Shivajirao Patwardhan (1892–1986) and the periodical Maharogi Jeevan started by him

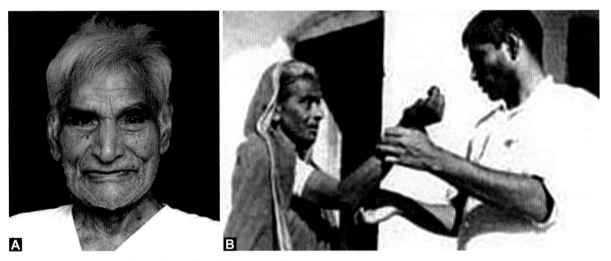

Figs 1.32A and B: (A) Baba Amte; (B) A young Amte examining a leprosy patient

Maharogi Jeevan, as a voice for and by leprosy-affected people.

In 1948, a school was established for leprosy affected children, juvenile delinquents and children of unmarried mothers.

In 1958, *Tapovan* was proposed as a State-approved *"Open Jail"* for leprosy-affected prisoners, where they could be taught skills and occupations in a humane atmosphere, to prepare them for a productive life after their release.

In 1960 with the number of inmates rising to 1,500, the rehabilitation activities were enhanced to include carpentry, spinning, weaving, etc. At meetings in *Tapovan* it was the practice to seat the leprosy-affected together with leprosy workers.

The efforts of the institution enabled leprosy-affected people to obtain concessions from public transport authorities. The first ever marriage between leprosy patients outside an asylum was arranged by Dr Patwardhan.

Anandwan, Warora, District Chandrapur (Maharashtra)

Murlidhar Devidas ("Baba") Amte (1914–2008) (Figs 1.32A and B). The trajectory of *Anandwan* Leprosy Home which was established by Amte in 1949, has some parallels with Dattapur Kushta Dham, as well as unique features. Like Diwan, Amte was a person of strong convictions. He started his career as a criminal lawyer and had a lucrative practice, but he was not happy. He went to Mahatma Gandhi whose work and teaching deeply impressed him. He decided to work for the so-called 'untouchables' who, for centuries were condemned to scavenging and carrying night soil on their heads.

To understand their problems, he undertook scavenging himself for several months. It was during this period that he came upon the badly disfigured body of a leprosy sufferer lying in a lane. The unforgettably pathetic sight decided him on leprosy.

Anandwan was started on land leased from Government near Warora (Maharashtra). With donations from the public and the support of friends, a few small buildings were erected and patients admitted. Several activities were started at Anandwan.

Personality Development: The treatment of leprosy was, in those days, basic. Amte concentrated on personality development and inculcating self-respect in the socially-deprived inmates. It was his hope that thus regenerated patients would return to society with self-reliance, in which endeavor he was fairly successful.

Cultivating the Land: Economic upliftment was most important. Bringing land under cultivation, finding water resources, acquiring the necessary equipment was difficult work, but the fertile fields produced abundantly.

Small-scale Industries: Spinning, weaving, carpet-making were developed. Milk and milk products were produced in the dairy. Sale of the handiwork of the patients was accepted by the society.

Medical: Initially, Amte could not get doctors, leading him to train at the School of Tropical Medicine in Kolkata. Dapsone treatment was initiated.

Education: Baba Amte started a science college in the campus about 55 years ago. Students came from the town, as also sons and daughters of inmates of *Anandwan*. An agricultural college has since been added.

Anandwan has a university, an orphanage, and schools for the blind and the deaf. Currently, the Ashram has over 5,000 residents. The community development project at *Anandwan* is recognized around the world. Besides *Anandwan*, Baba Amte later founded *Somnath* and *Ashokwan* ashrams for leprosy patients. A high standard of medical work is provided in the hospital and operation theater. Surgical correction of deformities became routine.

Crafts Training: In addition to spinning and weaving on handlooms and powerlooms, *dhurri* making was also introduced. Different types of cloths are produced which found a good market.

Dairy: Milk and milk products were produced in the patient-run dairy. The products made by leprosy patients are sold and accepted by society.

A Unique Feature of Anandwan: The most noteworthy characteristic of *Anandwan* is that it houses several thousand persons with various disabilities, but has fully integrated the leprosy-affected on equal terms as the others.

Baba Amte received the highest civilian award from the Government.

Kasturba Kushta Nivaran Nilayam, Malavanthangal District South Arcot (Tamil Nadu)

TN Jagadisan, (1909–1991) (Fig. 1.33) was born into a middle class Brahmin family near Chidambaram, Tamil Nadu. He graduated in English literature in 1930. His first job was at Karachi in a publishing company. In 1941, he manifested the first signs of leprosy, a patch which disappeared temporarily with Ayurvedic treatment. He became a lecturer in a college in Annamalai University and came under the influence of the celebrated orator, freedom activist, the Vice-Chancellor Srinivasa Shastry, whose biography Jagadisan authored in later years. Four years later he decided to work for leprosy-affected people. Through the good offices of Gandhiji's associate Thakkar Bapa, Jagadisan, accompanied by Robert Cochrane, were able to meet Gandhiji at Sewagram, who agreed to provide funds through the Kasturba Smarak Nidhi for a leprosy home at Malavanthangal (District South Arcot), which was named Kasturba Kusta Nivarana Nilayam and administered by Jagadisan, which Cochrane visited frequently.

Jagadisan's leprosy was of the noninfectious type, but left him with deformities. He was cured with dapsone treatment under the care of experts such as Cochrane. Later, surgeon Paul Brand constructed a "Brand new hand" for him.

With independence and the start of NLCP, Jagadisan became Secretary of Hind Kushta Nivaran Sangh. He traveled widely in India. He helped to establish the Polambakkam Leprosy Center run by Belgian workers.

During national and international meetings on social aspects or rehabilitation he promoted social action and reintegration of leprosy patients in the mainstream of society.[64]

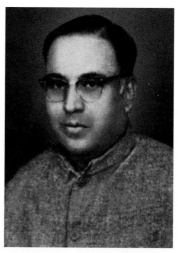

Fig. 1.33: TN Jagadisan (1909–1991)

With the support of sympathizers and help from Kasturba Memorial Trust, the Malavanthangal institution grew, serving the afflicted on Gandhian lines with emphasis on agriculture, spinning and weaving. He titled his autobiography *Fulfilment Through Leprosy.*[65]

THE INDIAN ASSOCIATION OF LEPROLOGISTS

The following is an extract of the first three decades of the Indian Association of Leprologists [IAL (Fig. 1.34)].[66] Notes on some prominent personalities are based on the recollections of one of the authors (KVD).

Genesis

The Association was not the first coming together exclusively of medical men engaged in leprosy work in India (See Section on ICBELRA). At Independence, hopes for Indian initiatives, social as well as medical, were expressed at the first All India Leprosy Workers Conference at Wardha in 1947 (Fig. 1.24). Medical men were hopeful that leprosy control would be put on a firm and formal footing if it were backed by scientifically conducted studies using the newly introduced Dapsone chemotherapy.

The founding of IAL in 1950 marked a parting of ways between nonmedical (though there were many veteran leprosy workers of the Gandhian era), and medical men specializing in leprosy. Referring to the first three (jointly attended) "All India Leprosy Workers' Conferences" held in 1947 (Wardha), 1948 (Kolkata), and 1950 (Chennai), Manohar Diwan of the Maharogi Seva Mandal, Wardha declared that the formation of IAL was a result more of 'enthusiasm' than need. Diwan complained about "the condescension among physicians towards those who work in leprosy (poor leprosy workers) and a sort of inferiority complex among the latter." The bone of contention was the emphasis placed by workers

on isolation and institutionalization: "control by [Dapsone] treatment alone, with isolation abandoned, is an attitude not scientific", claimed Diwan. Matters came to a head when physicians attending the Third All India Leprosy Workers Conference at Chennai in 1950 pushed through a resolution "that [because] social workers are apt to take views and make pronouncements which are unbalanced, this Conference calls upon all social workers to be guarded and constructive, and avoid making statements which conflict with expert medical opinion".

Foundation Members of IAL

Dharmendra, Kolkata	AC Rebello, Mumbai
P Sen, Kolkata	H Shama Rau, Chennai
SN Chatterjee, Kolkata	N Figueredo, Mumbai
BB Ganguly, Lucknow	P Kapoor, Mumbai
KW Waghela, Porbunder	H Paul, Chennai
J Joseph, Chennai	DN Bose, Asansol, West Bengal
DA Lakshman Rao, Bangalore	DN Mukerjee, Raipur
I Santra, Sambalpur, Orissa	NB Pattanayak, Bhubaneshwar
VV Shenoi, Chennai	KR Chatterjee, Kolkata
K Chakravarthy, Kolkata	AT Roy, Purulia, West Bengal

The first Central Council consisted of:
Dharmendra (President), AC Rebello (Vice-President), P Sen (Secretary), H Shama Rau (Honorary Treasurer, replaced by SN Chatterjee in October 1951).

Dharmendra (1900–1991) (Fig. 1.35) was *the* doyen among Indian leprologists, founder member of the Association, its first President, untiring exponent of the Indian viewpoint at international gatherings, and diligent editor of *Leprosy in India (Indian Journal of Leprosy)* till well into his 80s.

"I was born in February 1900; I commenced my medical education at King Edward Medical College at Lahore. During the second year of medical studies I answered Gandhiji's

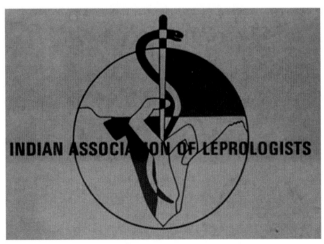

Fig. 1.34: Logo of the Indian Association of Leprologists

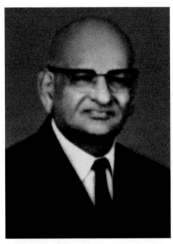

Fig. 1.35: Dharmendra (1900–1991)

call for non-cooperation with the British Raj following the Jallianwala Baug massacre I was initiated into laboratory techniques during employment in Delhi and Simla, but seized an opportunity to join the School of Tropical Medicine at Kolkata".

"After two or three years in laboratory work in various diseases, the Nation's spirit once again came back. I found that in the field of leprosy all the senior workers were foreign (1935), and although I appreciated their dedication, I felt that Indian workers of good calibre could also demonstrate their ability, I joined the leprosy department where I conducted clinical, epidemiological and laboratory studies (including fruitless experiments at culture of the bacillus), before settling into immunology and the Mitsuda reaction".

"While at the School of Tropical Medicine, the Government of India extended his service and in 1955 appointed him Director of the NLCP. Thereafter, he served as the first Director of the Central Leprosy Teaching and Research Institute at Chingleput where he spent about thirteen years. During this period schemes for Dapsone chemoprophylaxis in contacts of lepromatous cases were initiated with Drs Noordeen, Mohamed Ali and Ramanujam".

Some Notable IAL Conferences

Indian association of leprologists' history is epitomized in its Biennial Conferences and other meetings with which it has sponsored or been associated with. In the first twenty-five years of its existence, the biennial meetings and the Leprosy Workers Conferences were held together; administrators and politicians' speeches and messages formed an important part of the inauguration ceremonies. The last joint meeting was held at Baroda in 1976.

First Conference, Puri (Orissa), January 1953
The main subjects for discussion were Classification of Leprosy, the Role of New Drugs in Treatment and Control, Aspects of Pathology, and the Role of BCG Vaccination in Leprosy Control.

Second Conference, Jamshedpur (Bihar), March 1955
The highlights were three technical sessions devoted to Surgical and Physiotherapeutic Measures (PW Brand and his team), Chemotherapy and Leprosy Control (RV Wardekar, SN Chatterjee), BCG Vaccination and Leprosy Control (H Paul, NN Mukerjee), and Classification (Classification Committee of IAL).

A special resolution was adopted, greatly appreciating the reconstructive surgical work of Dr Paul W Brand. IAL became affiliated to the International Leprosy Association.

Sailendra Nath Chatterjee (1899–1989) (Fig. 1.36) learnt leprosy in Muir's Department at the School of Tropical Medicine Kolkata, an institution which he served from 1928 till 1954. As a clinician, his chief interest was in nerve damage in 'maculo-anesthetic' lesions. He was probably

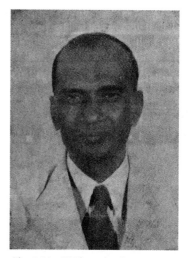

Fig. 1.36: SN Chatterjee (1899–1989)

the first to note thickened cutaneous nerves associated with patches. His papers (some co-authored) may be read with interest even today.[67,68] He emphasized vascular pathology in the development of nerve damage. Chatterjee attended the first conference of Indian leprosy workers held at Kolkata in 1933. He was also a foundation member of IAL; he was elected President at the Second Biennial Conference held at Jamshedpur in 1955.

Third Conference, Gorakhpur, December 1957 (Fig. 1.37)
The focus was on (a) Treatment including reactions, surgery, and the management of eye lesions; (b) Control including the activities of Government agencies, the Gandhi Smarak Nidhi, and the Belgian Mission at Polambakkam; (c) Pathology and Bacteriology including cytochemistry of leprosy and electronmicroscopy of *Mycobacterium leprae*. The Association acquired a new typewriter.

Fifth Biennial Conference, Hyderabad, January 1962
Foreign guests included Drs E Muir, RG Cochrane, TF Davey, SG Browne, JA Doull and K Hamano. The epidemiologist J Doull spoke on "Some Leprosy Questions demanding Field Research".

Dr KV Desikan presented an assessment of field treatment with Dapsone in the experimental projects of the Gandhi Memorial Leprosy Foundation while Drs Dharmendra and KV Ramanujam presented the results of a case-control study of dapsone chemoprophylaxis in intrafamilial and extra-familial child contacts of leprosy patients (lepromatous as well as treated and untreated nonlepromatous).

Conference on the Centenary of Hansen's Discovery 1973
A largely attended conference was organized at Sevagram (Wardha) in October 1973 to mark the "Centennial Celebration of Dr Hansen's Bacillus Discovery". It was sponsored jointly by Hind Kusht Nivaran Sangh, IAL, the National Leprosy

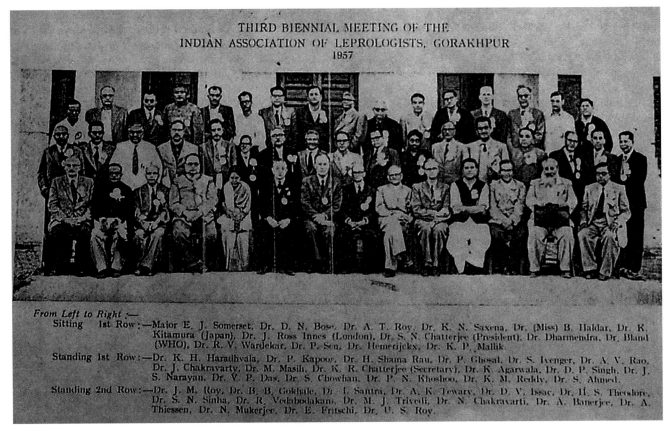

THIRD BIENNIAL MEETING OF THE
INDIAN ASSOCIATION OF LEPROLOGISTS, GORAKHPUR
1957

From Left to Right :—
Sitting 1st Row :—Major E. J. Somerset, Dr. D. N. Bose, Dr. A. T. Roy, Dr. K. N. Saxena, Dr. (Miss) B. Haldar, Dr. K. Kitamura (Japan), Dr. J. Ross Innes (London), Dr. S. N. Chatterjee (President), Dr. Dharmendra, Dr. Bland (WHO), Dr. R. V. Wardekar, Dr. P. Sen, Dr. Hemerijckx, Dr. K. P. Mallik.
Standing 1st Row :—Dr. K. H. Haradhvala, Dr. P. Kapoor, Dr. H. Shama Rau, Dr. P. Ghosal, Dr. S. Ivenger, Dr. A. V. Rao, Dr. J. Chakravarty, Dr. M. Masih, Dr. K. R. Chatterjee (Secretary), Dr. K. Agarwala, Dr. D. P. Singh, Dr. J. S. Narayan, Dr. V. P. Das, Dr. S. Chowhan, Dr. P. N. Khoshoo, Dr. K. M. Reddy, Dr. S. Ahmed.
Standing 2nd Row :—Dr. J. M. Roy, Dr. B. B. Gokhale, Di I. Santra, Dr. A. K. Tewary, Dr. D. V. Issac, Dr. H. S. Theodore, Dr. S. N. Sinha, Dr. R. Vedabolakam, Dr. M. J. Trivedi, Dr. N. Chakravarti, Dr. A. Banerjee, Dr. A. Thiessen, Dr. N. Mukerjee, Dr. E. Fritschi, Dr. U. S. Roy.

Fig. 1.37: Third Biennial Meeting, 1957, held during the Presidentship of SN Chatterjee

Organization and the Leprosy Mission. *It was therefore not a Biennial Conference of IAL.* Noteworthy among the gathering were several immunologists and experimental scientists (T Godal, GP Talwar, I Nath, RG Navalkar, W Kirchheimer). The armadillo, sulfone resistant leprosy, immunological diagnosis of infection, and the high cost of Rifampicin and Clofazimine were some of the subjects discussed.

Tenth Conference, Baroda, April 1976 (Fig. 1.38)
The meeting could have marked the Silver Jubilee of the Association, but strangely no mention was made of the anniversary by any speaker. This Conference was nevertheless a landmark of another kind; it was the last time that IAL and Leprosy Workers held a biennial meeting jointly where KV Ramanujam was elected as President.

KV Ramanujam (1918–2008 (Fig. 1.39) is ranked as an accomplished leprosy clinician, who devoted his life to service of leprosy patients. The events that led to his entering leprosy field (as described by him to KVD) make a striking anecdote. Ramanujam obtained his MBBS degree of Madras University in 1941. At that time, doctors with MBBS degree were very few. His father who was a senior-most police officer in the then Madras Presidency, was naturally very proud and had made all arrangements for his son to start private practice

in Chennai. One day Ramanujam, sitting in a park heard over the radio a talk by Robert Cochrane describing the plight of leprosy patients and the great need of doctors to treat them. This deeply touched the young listener's tender heart and he decided to take up leprosy work. His father was aghast on hearing of it—LEPROSY of all diseases!! His annoyed parents argued, coaxed and tried to persuade him in every possible way to change his mind, but he remained adamant. Ultimately, they gave up—it was Divine will, they concluded. Ramanujam joined Cochrane.

His first posting was at the Silver Jubilee Children's Leprosy Center at Saidapet in Chennai. Soon he was like an elder brother or a father of those children (Fig. 1.40).

Those were the days of *Chaulmoogra* oil intradermal injection therapy. His important contribution was long time follow-up of the children stretching over years, which was presented at the 11th International Leprosy Congress at Mexico in 1978.

When the Government of India established the Central Leprosy Teaching and Research Institute (CLTRI) at Chingleput, Ramanujam was transferred there as the Head of the Clinical Division, which also gave him ample opportunity for research. New drugs on the anvil had to be modified,

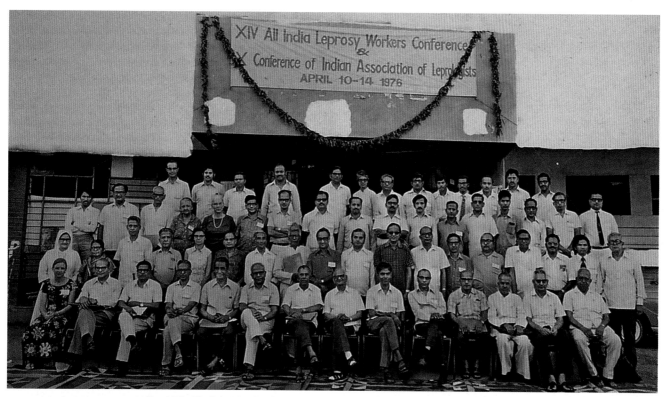

Fig. 1.38: The last Joint Conference of Leprosy Workers and Leprologists, Baroda 1976

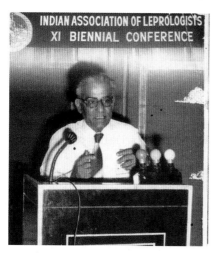

Fig. 1.39: Ramanujam (1918–2008)

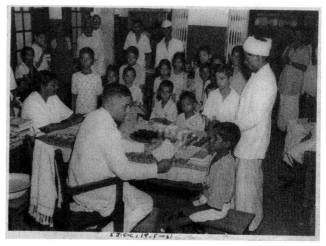

Fig. 1.40: Ramanujam examining at the Children's Leprosy Center at Saidapet

dosages decided. Dapsone (injectable and oral), Sulphetrone, Diasone, Rifampicin, Clofazimine, were closely tried and monitored. Several drugs were also tried for treatment of reaction including some aniline dyes. An important field study was of leprosy in twins.

After retiring from CLTRI, Ramanujam worked in Iran for a couple of years. On returning to India, Scheiffelin Leprosy Research Center at Karigiri requisitioned his services which he could not refuse. He returned to his clinical work for about 3 years.

Vasant Ramji Khanolkar (1895–1978) (Fig. 1.41) was the pre-eminent Indian pathologist and experimentalist from the early 1950s to the mid-1960s, who carved a niche in two main fields: (1) cancer and (2) leprosy. His work was

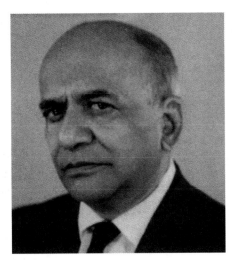

Fig. 1.41: VR Khanolkar (1895–1978)

carried out at the Indian Cancer Research Center, attached to the Tata Memorial Hospital at Mumbai. He was born in Quetta (Balochistan, now part of Pakistan), one of 4 sons of an eminent military Assistant Surgeon in the Indian Medical Department. Khanolkar joined the Grant Medical College, Mumbai, in 1912; he later studied at University College Hospital Medical School, London, securing MD in Pathology in 1923. On return to India, he joined his *alma mater* as Professor of Pathology.

In 1926, he relocated to the newly established Gordhandas Sunderdas Medical College and its affiliated King Edward Memorial Hospital as Chief of Pathology.

From 1941 to 1973, his most productive years, he was Director of Laboratories and Chief of the Indian Cancer Research Center at the Tata Memorial Center, Mumbai.

The credit for recruiting Khanolkar into leprosy pathology must go to the celebrated Robert Cochrane, the self-styled 'catalyst' who also energized Paul Brand (surgeon), Graham Weddell (sensory neurophysiologist), among others. The Cochrane-Khanolkar collaboration dated from as early as 1948, as can be gleaned from Khanolkar's seminal *Studies in the Histology of Early Lesions in Leprosy*, in which he also famously stated: "all leprosy is neural in its inception in as much as the spread of microorganisms is either in or along nerve fibers in the initial stage".[69]

A pertinent observation by Khanolkar was that under certain circumstances, evidence of *M leprae* infection could be discovered in clinically asymptomatic contacts of leprosy-affected individuals—"the silent phase". Another was that in all leprosy types, *M leprae* showed a predilection for the axoplasm of the cutaneous nerves and the inflammatory response tended to be located in richly innervated areas of the dermis (Fig. 1.42).[70] While it required electronmicroscope studies of Weddell to identify parasitization of the Schwann cell in leprosy, Khanolkar's observation of bacillary presence in the axoplasm in lepromatous leprosy was confirmed by Nishiura.

The collaboration with Cochrane was also evident as members in the Classification Committee at the Sixth International Congress of Leprosy at Madrid in 1953, when 'Neuritic' was recognized as an entity within the main types. A joint paper appeared in 1958 on this entity.[71]

Khanolkar's Influence

Association with Khanolkar was responsible for two of his research students to maintain a career-long interest in leprosy: CGS Iyer as Pathologist and Director of the Central Leprosy Teaching and Research Institute, Chingleput (Tamil Nadu); Darab K Dastur as Head of the ICMR Neuropathology Unit at JJ Hospital, Mumbai. It was at the Indian Cancer Research Center, too, that CV Bapat isolated the "ICRC *Bacillus*" from a leprosy nodule. It was shown to have potential as a prophylactic vaccine.

Honors[72]

- Founder-President, Indian Association of Pathologists and Microbiologists.
- Awarded Padma Bhushan in 1955 for contributions to Medicine.
- First President of the National Academy of Medical Sciences; Khanolkar Memorial Oration, of the Academy.
- President, International Union Against Cancer.
- Member, WHO Panels on Cancer and Leprosy.
- Vice-Chancellor of Bombay University 1960–1963.

Charles K Job (1923–2012) (Fig. 1.43): The Christian Medical College (CMC) at Vellore was originally a women's college. When it became coeducational, Job was in the first batch. Since he wanted to work in leprosy, he joined the newly established Schieffelin Leprosy Research Center at Karigiri soon after graduation. He also registered for MD in Pathology at CMC. At SLRC he had to carry out multiple duties since it was difficult to get doctors. He had to attend to clinical as well as laboratory work. When he was appointed Superintendent, he had administrative responsibilities as well. When a leprosy control project was started in Gudiyatham Taluk, he had to be the epidemiologist.

After obtaining MD, Job moved to CMC Hospital as Professor, and later became Head of Pathology. He undertook several research studies mainly in leprosy. He was particularly interested in pathogenesis of nerve damage. In autopsy material, the pattern of nerve involvement at various levels was identified. An important work was the study of nerve lesions under light and electron microscope. Job set up an animal house with mice and was the first in India to conduct mouse foot-pad inoculation work.

In 1981, after retirement from Vellore, Job went to work in the Leprosy Research Center at Carville, USA. Using the armadillo as experimental animal, it was conclusively shown that leprosy bacilli enter their bodies through the

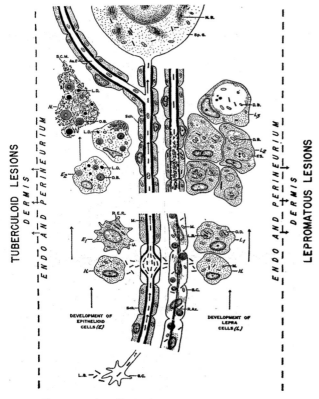

TUBERCULOID LESIONS

LEPROMATOUS LESIONS

DEVELOPMENT OF EPITHELIOID CELLS *(E)*

DEVELOPMENT OF LEPRA CELLS *(L)*

Fig. 1.42: Khanolkar's schematic on axonal centripetal transport of *M. leprae* in dermal nerves[70]

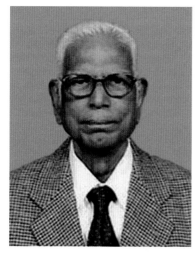

Fig. 1.43: CK Job (1923–2012)

nasal mucosa and abraded skin. With the excellent research facilities available at Carville he conducted several other studies in nerve pathology.

On return to India, Job proceeded to help at St Thomas Hospital in Chettupattu in Tamil Nadu. He built up the

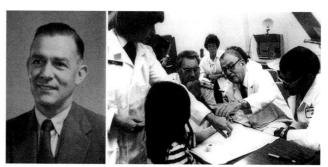

THE RECONSTRUCTION OF THE HAND IN LEPROSY
Hunterian Lecture delivered at the Royal College of Surgeons of England
on
24th October, 1952
by
P. W. Brand, F.R.C.S.
Surgeon, Christian Medical College, Vellore, South India.

LEPROSY IS A disease which affects chiefly two tissues ; skin and peripheral nerves. Through most of his life the patient with leprosy should be a relatively healthy person. His vital organs are not affected, his mind is clear, and his digestion sound. There may be bouts of fever in the acute stages, and distressing complications such as iritis, but these are now readily controllable by the new drugs which the physician has at his disposal.

Fig. 1.44: Paul W Brand FRCS (1914–2003), medical missionary, was introduced by Robert Cochrane to the possibilities of orthopedic correction of limb deformities in leprosy. As Professor at the Christian Medical College, Vellore and Schieffelin Leprosy Center, Karigiri, Brand pioneered/adapted several hand reconstruction techniques, thereby inaugurating a new avenue of service to leprosy sufferers. Equally importantly, Brand pioneered physiotherapy for keeping the joints of paralyzed hands and feet supple, so as to obtain maximum benefit from reconstructive surgery. He brought in several methods of physiotherapy and plantar ulcer care. Equally important was that self-care of hands and feet taught to the patients. Brand trained a large number of doctors; reconstructive surgery, physiotherapy, ulcer care and adapted footwear are an essential part of a treatment program

pathology laboratory and trained technicians. Soon St Thomas Hospital became a well-equipped scientific institution. After working there for about 4 years, he wished to retire but retirement evades any active scientist. He was called to SLRC as a consultant pathologist. He worked ceaselessly and also guided research projects almost till his death.

SURGEONS AS TRAIL BLAZERS

Two surgical specialists stand out in the post-independence period for charting new avenues of service to deformed and disfigured leprosy patients. They were Paul Brand of Vellore (orthopedic surgeon), and Noshir Antia of Pune and Mumbai (plastic surgeon). Each adapted and innovated established operative techniques in this particular field to address the specific neurological and cosmetic sequelae of leprosy. The work of both was recognized by Hunterian lecturerships awarded by the Royal College of Surgeons of England, to Brand in 1952 (Fig. 1.44)[73] and Antia in 1962 (Fig. 1.45).[74,75]

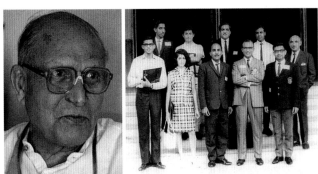

RECONSTRUCTION OF THE FACE IN LEPROSY
Hunterian Lecture delivered at the Royal College of Surgeons of England
on
17th April 1962
by
N. H. Antia, F.R.C.S.
Plastic and Reconstructive Surgery Unit, Sir J. J. Group of Hospitals, Bombay

AT A ROUGH estimate there are ten million people suffering from leprosy in the world to-day. About two million of these are in India. It has also been estimated that over a quarter of these patients require some form of reconstructive surgery. Many of them require multiple operations due to the presence of several deformities. Several of these operations have to be multi-staged. Hence leprosy poses one of the largest, if not the

Fig. 1.45: Noshir Antia (portrait on the left) made the care of leprosy patients in a general hospital acceptable. He built a team (shown on the right) that continues his work. His work on leprosy was recognized by the Royal College of Surgeons of London when they invited him to deliver the prestigious Hunterian Lecture

DEJA VU

The Twelfth IAL Conference held in 1981 at Agra was inaugurated by Dr V Ramalingaswami, Director-General of the Indian Council of Medical Research. In his address, he remarked on the shortcomings in the NLCP, such as inadequate population coverage, inadequate attention to deformities, and high rates of drop-out with Dapsone treatment. Complaints had been voiced, he said, about shortages and irregular supply of the drug, and anxiety expressed about sulfone resistance. He hinted that a sea-change in strategy and administration of the Control Program was the need of the hour.

[**Note**: However, in the personal experience of one of the authors (KVD) who served as a WHO consultant for overseeing NLCP work in two districts, there was full coverage of population in all the Leprosy Control Units which were subjected to repeated house-to-house surveys. Regularity of attendance at clinics and intake of drugs were monitored by paramedical workers. No case of sulfone resistance or shortage of the drug was reported. The NLCP was a field program where mobile teams dispensed treatment in wayside clinics. Attending to deformities, carrying out physiotherapy was left to the NGO's and some Government centers.]

Optimism for a 'Final Solution' to the leprosy problem was generated, each time a new Control Program arrived on virgin territory, or gave way to a 'better' successor—from the *chaulmoogra* oil-based PTS strategy of ICBELRA to the Dapsone monotherapy-based SET pattern of NLCP; from Dapsone-based NLCP to MDT-based NLEP.

Amid the euphoria, one might profitably ponder the sobering argument mooted by LM Bechelli, WHO Leprosy Chief in 1973 that many factors may influence the application of the control measures among these are the socioeconomic, political and hygienic conditions as well as cultural patterns and health infrastructure in leprosy-endemic areas.[76]

ACKNOWLEDGMENTS

The authors thank the staff of the Acworth Leprosy Hospital Society for Research, Rehabilitation and Education in Leprosy (Mumbai) and the Gandhi Memorial Leprosy Foundation (Wardha) for cordial help in locating source material.

REFERENCES

1. Muir E. The past and future of anti-leprosy work in India. Lepr India. 1951;23:8-13.
2. Dharmendra. Leprosy in ancient indian medicine. Int J Lepr. 1947;15:424-30.
3. Robbins G, Tripathy VM, Misra VN, et al. Ancient skeletal evidence for leprosy in India (2000 B.C.). PLoS ONE. 2009; 4(5):e5669.
4. Danielssen DC, Boeck C-W. Traite de la Lepre, Paris, Balliere, 1848.
5. Hansen GA, Looft O. Leprosy in its Clinical and Pathological Aspects, Transl. N. Walker, London: John Wright; 1895. p. 86.
6. British Medical Journal dated 6/12/1862.
7. Pandya SS. Anti-contagionism in leprosy 1844-1897. Int J Lepr. 1998;66:374-84.
8. Hansen GHA. On the aetiology of leprosy. British and Foreign Medico-Chirurgical Review. 1875;55:459-89.
9. Carter HV. Report on Leprosy and the Leper Asylums in Norway. London: Her Majesty's Stationery Office; 1874. p. 27.
10. Pandya SS. The First International Leprosy Conference, Berlin, 1897: The politics of segregation. Indian J Lepr. 2004;76:51-70.
11. Robinson J. On the elephantiasis as it appears in Hindoostan. Medico-Chirurgical Transactions. 1819;10:27-37.
12. Carter HV. On Leprosy and Elephantiasis. London, Eyre and Spottiswoode. 1874. Plate 11.
13. Rogers L, Muir E. Leprosy, Bristol, John Wright and Sons; London; 1940. pp. 172-4.
14. Sehgal VN, Jain MK, Srivastava G. Evolution of the classification of leprosy. Int J Dermatol. 1989;28:161-7.
15. Sixth International Congress of Leprosy. Int J Lepr. 1953; 21:504-10.
16. Classification of Leprosy (Editorial). Lepr India. 1955;27:1-10.
17. Ridley DS, Jopling WH. Classification of leprosy according to immunity. Int J Lepr. 1966;34:255-73.
18. Carter HV. Note on the Pathology of Leprosy. Maharashtra State Archives General Department, Publication No: 14494, Appendix; 1883. p. 7.
19. Scheube B. The Diseases of Warm Countries, Transl. P. Falcke, edited by James Cantlie, 2nd. Rev. Edition, London: John Bale, Sons & Danielsson, Ltd; 1903. pp. 231-89.

20. Rogers L. Leprosy in Tropical Medicine Sir Leonard Rogers and John WD Megaw (Eds) London: J&A Churchill; 1930. pp. 320-44.
21. Rogers L. The Treatment of Leprosy, Indian Medical Gazette. 1920. pp. 125-8.
22. Carter HV. Case of Anaesthetic Leprosy with Post-mortem Examination and Remarks, Transactions of the Medical and Physical Society of Bombay. 1862 ;VII: xxviii-xxix.
23. Carter HV. On the Symptoms and Morbid Anatomy of Leprosy: with Remarks, Transactions of the Medical and Physical Society of Bombay. 1863;VIII: 1-104.
24. Sunderland S. The internal anatomy of the nerve trunks in relation to leprosy. Brain. 1975; 96:865-88.
25. Virchow R. Virchow's Leprosy: From Die Krankhaften Geschwulste (Berlin 1863), Part II; Transl. Fite GL. Int J Lepr. 1954; 22:205-16.
26. Dehio K. On the lepra anaesthetica on the pathogenetical relation of the disease appearances. (Transl. Biswas MG). Lepr India. 1952;24:78-83.
27. Muir E. Nerve Abscess in Leprosy. Indian Medical Gazette. 1924. pp. 87-9.
28. Hansen GA. The Bacillus of Leprosy. Quarterly Journal of Microscopical Sciences. 1880; 20: Plate VIII.
29. Mettler CC. History of Medicine. The Blakiston Company, Philadelphia; 1947. pp. 471-2.
30. Sticker G. Mittheilungen und Verhandlungen der Internationalen Wissenschaftlichen Lepra-Conferenz zu Berlin; 1897. pp. 55-9.
31. Ghosh JC. Indigenous Drugs Of India: Their Scientific Cultivation and Manufacture with Numerous Suggestions Intended for Educationists and Capitalists, Second Edition, Calcutta; 1940. pp. 97-114.
32. van Rheede. Hortus Malabaricus. Amsterdam: 1687, Vol. 1, Plate 36.
33. Sir Leonard Rogers. Preliminary note on the intravenous injection of gynocardates of soda in leprosy. BMJ. 1916;550-2.
34. Sir Leonard Rogers. Two years' experience of sodium gynocardate and chaulmoograte subcutaneously and intravenously in the treatment of leprosy. Indian J Med Res. 1917;5:277-300.
35. British Empire Leprosy Relief Association, Rog/C.13/126-364/Box8. Wellcome Institute of The History of Medicine, London;1924.
36. Tomb JW. Chaulmoogra oil and its derivatives in the treatment of leprosy, Part III. J Trop Med Hyg. 1933;36:201-7.
37. Papers of Isabel Kerr and George McGlashan Kerr. 1911-1956, Centre for the Study of World Christianity, Edinburgh.
38. Report of the Study Tour of the Secretary of the Leprosy Commission in Europe, South America and the Far East, January 1929-June 1930. Geneva, League of Nations No: C.H; 887, 1930. pp. 39-40.
39. Report of a Conference of Leper Asylum Superintendents and Others on the Leper Problem in India, under the Auspices of the Mission to Lepers, Cuttack, Orissa Mission Press; 1920.pp.32-3.
40. Muir E. The Propaganda-Treatment-Survey Centre As a Means of Dealing with Leprosy. Transactions of the Seventh Congress (British India, 1927) of the Far Eastern Association of Tropical Medicine. 1928;2:305-7.
41. Sahu J. One Hundred Years of Leprosy Work in Orissa 1885-1984. Unpublished PhD Thesis, Sambalpur University; 1989.
42. Cochrane RG. Leprosy in India and Ceylon. Lepr Rev. 1934;5:28-32.
43. Report on Leprosy and its Control in India. Central Advisory Board of Health, New Delhi, Government of India; 1942.
44. Cochrane RG. Leprosy control with particular reference to the Madras Presidency. Lepr India. 1945;17:47-57.
45. Muir E. Note on the treatment of leprosy by intradermal Infiltration. Lepr India. 1933;5:20-4.
46. The All India Leprosy Conference. Lepr India. 1933;5:113-6.
47. Report of the Health Survey and Development Committee, Vol. IV: Summary, Government of India Press, New Delhi; 1946. pp.43-5.
48. Kipp RS. The Evangelical Uses of Leprosy. Social Science and Medicine, 1994; xxxix: 165-78.
49. Jackson J Lepers: Thirty-One Years of Work Among Them, Being the History of the Mission to Lepers in India (1874-1905), Marshal Brothers, London; 1905.
50. Howard A. An Agricultural Testament. Oxford University Press; Oxford;1943.
51. Hess GR. Sam Higginbottom of Allahabad: Pioneer of Point Four to India. University Press of Virginia; 1967.
52. Choksy NH. Report on Leprosy and the Homeless Leper Asylum Matunga, Mumbai, 1890-97. British India Printing Works; Mumbai; 1900.
53. Colebrooke HT. Digest of Hindu Law, of Contracts and Successions: with a Commentary by Jagannatha Tercapanchanana. Vol. III. Printed at the Honourable Company's Press, Calcutta; 1801.
54. Glucklich A. Laws for the Sick and Handicapped in the Dharmasastra. South Asia Research. 1984;4:139-52.
55. Macnaghten WH. Reports of Cases Determined in the Court of Nizamat Adalat, Vols. 1 and 2, , Baptist Mission Press, Calcutta; 1828. pp. 220-2.
56. Meghani J. Sant Devidas, Bhavnagar, Prasar; 1938.
57. Leprosy in India: Report of the Leprosy Commission in India 1890-91. Superintendent of Government Printing, Calcutta; 1892.
58. Faget GH, Pogge RC, Johansen FA, et al. Treatment of leprosy with promin: A Progress Report. US Public Health Reports. 1943;58:1729-41.
59. Cochrane RG, Ramanujam K, Paul H, et al. Two and half years experimental work on sulphone group of drugs. Lepr Rev. 1949;20:4-64.
60. Muir E. Preliminary report on DDS treatment of leprosy. Int J Lepr. 1950;18:299-308.
61. Browne SG, Hogerzeil LM. B663 in treatment of leprosy: Preliminary report of a pilot trial. Lepr Rev. 1962;33:6-10.
62. Browne SG. Possible anti-inflammatory action in lepromatous leprosy. Lepr Rev. 1965;36:9-11.
63. Muir E, Chatterji KR. The Bankura Leprosy Investigation Centre. Lepr India. 1934;6:128-32.
64. Desikan KV. Elimination of leprosy and possibility of eradication—Indian scenario, (Editorial). Indian J Med Res. 2012;135:3-5.

65. Srinivasan HV. Obituary—TN Jagadisan. Int J Lepr. 1991;59:656-7.

66. Jagadisan TN. Fulfilment Through Leprosy. Kasturba Kushta Nivaran Nilayam, Malavanthangal P.O. South Arcot District, Tamil Nadu; 1988.

67. Pandya SS. Indian Association of Leprologists: 50 Golden Years (1950-2000). Souvenir distributed at the Golden Jubilee Conference of IAL, Patna; 2001.

68. Muir E, Chatterjee SN. Leprosy nerve lesions of the cutis and sub-cutis. Int J Lepr. 1933;1:129-48.

69. Chatterjee SN. The mechanism of the neural signs and symptoms of leprosy. Lepr India. 1956; 27: 7-20.

70. Khanolkar VR. Studies in the Histology of Early Lesions in Leprosy. Indian Council of Medical Research, Special Report Series No: 19, 1951.

71. Khanolkar VR. Pathology of early lesions in leprosy. In: Cochrane RG and Davey TF (Eds.). Leprosy in Theory and Practice. John Wright and Son: Bristol; 1964.

72. Cochrane RG, Khanolkar VR. Dimorphous polyneuritic leprosy. Indian J Med Sci. 1958; 12:1-9.

73. Pai Sanjay A. VR Khanolkar: Father of Pathology and Medical Research in India. Ann Diag Pathol. 2002;6:334-7.

74. Brand P, Philip Y. Pain: The Gift Nobody Wants. Harper Collins Publishers; 1993.

75. Antia NH. A Life of Change: Autobiography of a Doctor. Delhi: Penguin; 2009.

76. Bechelli LM. Advances in leprosy control in the last 100 years. Int J Lepr. 1973;41:285.

2

CHAPTER

Epidemiology of Leprosy

PL Joshi

INTRODUCTION

Leprosy has been a feared illness since antiquity, due to the havoc it wreaks upon the body. Unlike infections or illnesses that ravage internal organs, such as its closely related counterpart tuberculosis, leprosy preferentially infects cooler parts of the body, particularly the fingers, toes, eyes, nose and testes. The response of the immune system to the infection often leads to an intense inflammation, and in the involved nerve, it causes severe damage, leading to peripheral neuropathy. As a result, the afflicted person progressively loses sensation in these areas, which ultimately leads to tissue breakdown, ulceration and bacterial super infection, followed by the loss of fingers and toes, destruction of the structure of the nose and, in some cases, blindness. Unlike tuberculosis (*M. tuberculosis*), leprosy is not often a direct killer. Instead, due to the predilection of the infective agent for skin and peripheral nerves, the serious but fortunately not very common consequences of leprosy are deformity and disability. This has significant social and economic impact on both the patient and their community. Therefore, early detection and prompt treatment of the disease prevents stigma and discrimination. With treatment, the persons affected with leprosy can lead productive life in the community.

Leprosy remains the most common infection that leads to disability, and its elimination has proven to be difficult, with nearly 250,000 new cases seen worldwide annually, including approximately 100 new cases in the United States each year. The prevalence (total number of cases) has declined dramatically, due to the introduction of dapsone in the 1940s, widespread BCG vaccination for tuberculosis (which also provides protection against *Mycobacterium leprae*), free distribution of multidrug therapy to all newly diagnosed patients worldwide, and improved recognition and diagnostic techniques. However, in recent years, the incidence (the number of new cases) has not changed significantly. Leprosy is a disease of poverty, and 90% of cases occur in the poorest regions of Brazil, Madagascar, Mozambique, Tanzania, India and Nepal. One to two million people are permanently disabled by the disease, many of whom continue to suffer from ostracism and inadequate care.

In the pre-sulfone era, the most prevalent technique to prevent the spread of leprosy was compulsory segregation of those afflicted with the disease. Due to the fear of transmission of the disease to healthy individuals, people infected with leprosy were treated as badly if not worse than criminals: they were housed in the most decrepit settlements, which were often ringed with walls and barbed wires, with no protection from the harsh elements of nature, inadequate food and water, and little if any medical care. Those who sought to leave the leprosaria were hunted down like escaped convicts, and forcibly returned. In some extreme cases, the afflicted were gathered under false pretences, and shot or burned alive *en masse*, particularly, in the 19th and early 20th centuries.

Modern day leprosy dates from 1873 when Armauer Hansen of Norway discovered *M. leprae*. For many years there was no effective remedy for leprosy. The introduction of sulfones in the treatment of leprosy in 1943 marked the beginning of the new era, the era of case finding and domiciliary treatment. Leprosy has since become a curable and controllable disease.

The decades of 1960s and 1970s witnessed great strides in the development of experimental models. In 1960, Shepard discovered that *M. leprae* could multiply to a limited extent when injected into footpads of mice. In 1971, Kirchheimer in USA reported on the successful transmission of leprosy to a South American ant-eater, armadillo. These two discoveries paved way for vast experimental work in leprosy research. Currently, Indian Council of Medical Research (ICMR) "Special Task Force for Research in Leprosy" is supporting Indian scientists in basic, applied and sociobehavioral research in leprosy.

Recognizing leprosy as a national health problem, the Government of India launched the National Leprosy Control Programme (NLCP) in 1954-55 in collaboration with State Goverments to control the spread of the disease and render modern treatment facilities to all leprosy patients, which is currently in operation in the form of National Leprosy Eradication Programme (NLEP).

LEPROSY AND INTERNATIONAL DISEASE CLASSIFICATION

International classification of diseases ICD-10 was endorsed by the Forty-third World Health Assembly in May 1990 and came into use in WHO Member States from 1994. The classification is the latest in a series which has its origins in the 1850s. The first edition, known as the International List of Causes of Death, was adopted by the International Statistical Institute in 1893. WHO took over the responsibility for the ICD at its creation in 1948 when the Sixth Revision was published which included causes of morbidity for the first time. The World Health Assembly adopted in 1967 the WHO Nomenclature Regulations that stipulate use of ICD in its most current revision for mortality and morbidity statistics by all Member States.

The ICD is the international standard diagnostic classification for epidemiological, health management and clinical use. These include the analysis of the general health situation of population groups and monitoring of the incidence and prevalence of diseases and other health problems in relation to other variables such as the characteristics and circumstances of the individuals affected, reimbursement, resource allocation, quality and guidelines. It is used to classify diseases and other health problems recorded on many types of health, and vital records including death certificates and health records. In addition to enabling the storage and retrieval of diagnostic information for clinical, epidemiological and quality purposes, these records also provide the basis for the compilation of national mortality and morbidity statistics by WHO Member States (Box 2.1).

DEFINITION OF LEPROSY

The accepted definition of leprosy as per the 7th WHO Expert Committee on Leprosy (WHO, 1998), is a person having one

Box 2.1: Leprosy in ICD-10 (Version 2007)	
A30	Leprosy (Hansen's disease) *Includes:* Infection due to *Mycobacterium leprae* *Excludes:* Sequelae of leprosy (B92)
A30.0	Indeterminate leprosy (I leprosy)
A30.1	Tuberculoid leprosy (TT leprosy)
A30.2	Borderline tuberculoid leprosy (BT leprosy)
A30.3	Borderline borderline leprosy (BB leprosy)
A30.4	Borderline lepromatous leprosy (BL leprosy)
A30.5	Lepromatous leprosy (LL leprosy)
A30.8	Other forms of leprosy
A30.9	Leprosy, unspecified

or more of the following features, and who is yet to complete the full course of treatment: hypopigmented or reddish skin lesion(s) with definite loss of sensation, nerve thickening with sensory impairment and skin smear positive for acid fast bacilli. The use of such standard definition is important from epidemiological point of view. The definition is partly based on treatment so that any change in the treatment of leprosy will change the epidemiology of the disease. The definition also means that once an individual patient has successfully completed the course of treatment that individual is no longer considered as a case.

GEOGRAPHICAL DISTRIBUTION AND PREVALENCE

During the middle ages, leprosy was widespread in almost all countries` in the world. Thereafter, it declined slowly in many European countries, partly due to strict isolation and partly due to improvement in the standards of living and quality of life of the people. In the present era, the fall in prevalence rate is mainly due to an improvement in the management of cases, very low rate of relapse, high cure rate, absence of drug resistance and shorter duration of treatment with multidrug treatment (MDT). Happily, the overall target for the global elimination of leprosy has been attained.

Global

The distribution of new cases detected in 2013 across WHO Regions was similar to the findings in previous years. The South East Asia Region accounted for 71% of new cases detected worldwide, with 16% from Americas, 9% from African region and 2% from Eastern Mediterranean and Western Pacific regions. Table 2.1 presents by region the number of new cases detected annually from 2005–2013 in different WHO regions. Compared to the previous years, in 2013 a decline was observed in the number of new cases reported mainly in the South East Asia region. Marginal increases of new cases were also noted in the African and Western Pacific regions. Altogether 17,203 less new cases were detected in 2013 than in 2012.

If innovative case finding methods are introduced to access areas and population groups which are difficult to reach, together with improved data management, an increase in detection of new cases can be expected.

Globally, 14,409 new grade 2 deformity (G2D) cases were reported during the year 2012 as compared to 13,289 cases in year 2013. The G2D rate per 100,000 population ranged from 0.05 in Western Pacific region to 0.43 in South East Asia region (Table 2.2 and Fig. 2.1). The global G2D rate was recorded at 0.25 per 100,000 population in the year 2012 as compared to 0.23 in year 2013. The number of new cases reported is important as it indicates presence of infection in the community.

South East Asia Region

The report reveals that out of 18 countries reporting more than 1000 cases globally, six are from the SEA region (Bangladesh: 3,141; India: 126,913; Indonesia: 16,856; Myanmar: 2,950; Nepal: 3,225; and Sri Lanka: 1,990). India contributed over 80% of new cases detected in the year 2012. In South East Asia, DPR Korea reported zero incidence in year 2013. Situation of leprosy in other countries of the region is shown in the Table 2.3.

India

Leprosy prevalence has always been uneven geographically, even within a country or within a State or tehshil. In India, during the 1980s prior to the introduction of MDT, the

Table 2.1: Trends in detection of new cases of leprosy by WHO regions

WHO region	2005	2006	2007	2008	2009	2010	2011	2012	2013
Africa	45,179	34,480	34,468	29,814	28,935	23,345	20,213	20,599	20,911
Americas	41,952	47,612	42,135	41,891	40,474	37,740	35,852	36,178	33,084
Eastern Mediterranean	3,133	3,261	4,091	3,938	4,029	4,080	4,357	4,235	1,680
South East Asia	201,635	174,118	171,576	167,505	166,115	156,254	160,132	166,445	155,385
Western Pacific	7,137	6,190	5,863	5,859	5,243	5,055	5,092	5,400	4,596
Total	**299,036**	**265,661**	**258,133**	**249,007**	**244,796**	**228,474**	**226,626**	**232,857**	**215,656**

Table 2.2: Number of cases of leprosy (rate/100 000 populations) with grade-2 disabilities among new cases reported, by WHO region, 2007–2013

WHO region[a]	Year[b]						
	2007	2008	2009	2010	2011	2012	2013
African	3,570 (0.51)	3,458 (0.51)	3,146 (0.41)	2,685 (0.40)	2,300 (0.26)	2,709 (0.40)	2,552 (0.43)
Americas	3,431 (0.42)	2,512 (0.29)	2,645 (0.30)	2,423 (0.27)	2,382 (0.27)	2,420 (0.28)	2,168 (0.25)
Eastern Mediterranean	466 (0.10)	687 (0.14)	608 (0.11)	729 (0.12)	753 (0.12)	700 (0.12)	191 (0.05)
South-East Asia	6,332 (0.37)	6,891 (0.39)	7,286 (0.41)	6,912 (0.39)	7,095 (0.39)	8,012 (0.43)	7,964 (0.43)
Western Pacific	604 (0.03)	592 (0.03)	635 (0.04)	526 (0.03)	549 (0.03)	568 (0.03)	386 (0.02)
Total	**14,403 (0.26)**	**14,140 (0.25)**	**14,320 (0.25)**	**13,275 (0.23)**	**13,079 (0.22)**	**14,409 (0.25)**	**13,289 (0.23)**

[a] Reports from the European Region are notincluded.
[b] Values are numbers (rate/100 000 population).

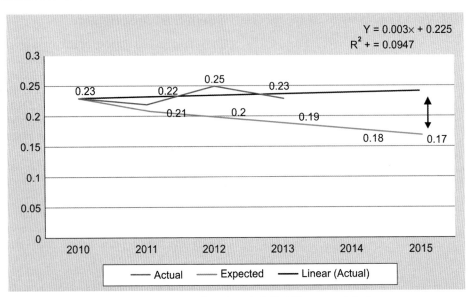

Fig. 2.1: Linear regression of grade 2 disability cases globally

Table 2.3: Trends in the detection of number of new leprosy cases in 14 countries reporting ≥ 1000 new cases annually from 2006 to 2013, globally

Country	2006	2007	2008	2009	2010	2011	2012	2013
Bangladesh	6,280	5,357	5,249	5,239	3,848	3,970	3,688	3,141
Brazil	44,436	39,125	38,914	37,610	34,894	33,955	33,303	31,044
Cote d'Ivoire	976	1,204	998	884	NR	770	1,030	1,169
Democratic Republic of Congo	8,257	8,820	6,114	5,062	5,049	3,949	3,607	3,744
Ethiopia	4,092	4,187	4,170	4,417	4,430	NR	3,776	4,374
India	139,252	137,685	134,184	133,717	126,800	127,295	134,752	126,913
Indonesia	17,682	17,723	17,441	17,260	17,012	20,023	18,994	16,856
Madagascar	1,536	1,644	1,763	1,572	1,520	1,577	1,474	1,569
Myanmar	3,721	3,637	3,365	3,147	2,936	3,082	3,013	2,950
Nepal	4,235	4,436	4,708	4,394	3,118	3,184	3,492	3,225
Nigeria	3,544	4,665	4,899	4,219	3,913	3,623	3,805	3,385
Philippines	2,517	2,514	2,373	1,795	2,041	1,818	2,150	1,729
Sri Lanka	1,993	2,024	1,979	1,875	2,027	2,178	2,191	1,990
United Republic of Tanzania	3,450	3,105	3,276	2,654	2,349	2,288	2,528	2,005
Total (%)	243,477	237,652	231,047	225,442	211,261	210,655	220,810	206,107
	(92)	(92)	(93)	(92)	(92)	(93)	(95)	(96)
Global Total	**265,661**	**258,133**	**249,007**	**244,796**	**228,474**	**226,626**	**232,857**	**215,656**

southern states of Tamil Nadu and Andhra Pradesh had the highest prevalence. Today, hyperendemic areas of India are in the north and east. Currently, seven States in India, namely, Bihar, Uttar Pradesh, Chhattisgarh, Jharkhand, Maharashtra, Odisha and west Bengal contribute almost 3/4th of the total leprosy burden (74.9% new leprosy cases detected). Several reasons could be cited for south Indian states to have reached elimination faster: earlier implementation of MDT and better coverage, and timely release from treatment (RFT) are the major service delivery factors. Better nutrition, greater awareness and early reporting for treatment, as well as improved hygiene could also be responsible. Now the focus of the program has shifted from endemic States to high priority districts and blocks. India achieved elimination target in December 2005. Total number of new cases recorded in year 2013 was 126,913 with 3.4% of cases having grade 2 disability.

AGENT

The causative agent of leprosy, *Mycobacterium leprae*, was identified by Armauer Hansen in 1873. It is an obligate intracellular pathogen that mainly infects macrophages and Schwann cells, though it also multiplies in muscles and vascular endothelium, and can infect other tissues such as the eye and testis. Unlike tuberculosis, which also results from infection with a *Mycobacterium (M. tuberculosis)*, leprosy is not often a direct killer. Instead, due to the infective agent's predilection for skin and peripheral nerves, the common severe consequences of leprosy are deformity and disability which, have significant social and economic impact. *Mycobacterium leprae* is an acid-fast, straight/ slightly curved rod shaped gram-positive bacillus which can be seen in clumps or bundles on microscopic examination. They are slow growing bacilli and one bacillus divides into two every 12–14 days. They do not produce toxins and occur both extracellularly as well as intracellularly with affinity for Schwann cells and cells of reticuloendothelial system. They can remain dormant in various body sites and tissues causing relapse.

The organism is killed by boiling and autoclaving. Its susceptibility to air, cold, water, drying and disinfectants is uncertain. *M. leprae* can survive outside the human body for up to 45 days depending upon the environmental conditions.

M. leprae grows best in cooler tissues like the skin, peripheral nerves, upper respiratory tract and testes, sparing warmer areas. They are found in large quantities in skin of earlobes, face and buttocks. Bacillary load is the highest in lepromatous cases. Number of antigens have been detected in *M. leprae*, the most significant of which is the phenolic glycolipid (PGL-1) detected by serological tests. Successful transmission of *M. leprae* has been observed in experimental animals like 9-banded armadillo and nude mouse. *M. leprae* can be grown experimentally by injecting them into the foot pad of mice. However, it has not yet been shown to grow in artificial medium. The natural life span of the bacillus in human body is not exactly known, but persisters have been isolated from patients even after 10 years of release from therapy.

HOST FACTORS

Age

Leprosy can occur at any age, but is more commonly seen in the age group between 20 and 30 years. In endemic areas, the infection generally takes place during childhood. In low endemic areas, the infection may occur in adulthood or later part of life. Increased proportion of child leprosy cases in the population has epidemiological significance as it indicates presence of active transmission of the disease in the community. As transmission of the disease declines, it is seen more often in the older age group. Age distribution of lepromatous cases generally shows that the disease has a later onset as compared with nonlepromatous cases.

Gender

Leprosy occurs in both the sexes. However, males are affected more as compared to females, generally in the proportion of 2:1. Sex difference is least among children below 15 years and is more marked among adults. More number of male cases could be attributed to their greater mobility and increased opportunity for contact. Males are also more willing in reporting to the health facility for seeking treatment.

Migration

Due to migration of population from rural to urban areas, leprosy cases have increased in urban areas in recent years. The urban slums have a distinct geographic and population characteristic, common to all urban areas. The population density in the slums is very high (10,000–15,000 per sq. km), most of the inhabitants are migrants from distant villages, the hygienic and living conditions are poor, breathing space is greatly compromised (8–10 or even more people sharing the same room) and other utilities. The conditions are nearly the same, both at home and place of work, in many situations both premises are the same.

Two types of leprosy carriage can be noted: (1) the two way traffic, to and from the villages and slums, and (2) one way from slums to middle class localities where the population density and living conditions are different from those in slums. Most of the household helps and maids working in middle class urban localities are originating from slums inhabited by migrant population from the villages.

Household and Other Contacts

The most consistent and most studied risk factor for development of leprosy is contact status. Intensity and physical distance from an index lepromatous leprosy case were directly associated with increased risk of developing leprosy.

Ethnicity

The association between the epidemiology of leprosy and ethnicity has been a topic of interest but there are no groups immune to leprosy although the rate of disease differs. Types/forms of the disease vary between ethnic groups: in Micronesia the frequency of disability is very low whereas in China it is very high. Involvement of the lower branches of the facial nerve occurs more often in China but it is very rare elsewhere, and some reactional states such as Lucio phenomenon occur mainly in Americas. These observations suggest that there may be genetically determined differences in the immune response to *M. leprae* infection.

Immunity

Occurrence of the disease depends on susceptibility/ immunological status of an individual. Large proportion of early lesions in leprosy heal spontaneously. Such self healing lesions suggest acquired immunity. Cell mediated immunity is responsible for resistance to infection with *M. leprae*. Only a few persons (about 1%) exposed to infection develop disease. Subclinical infections also contribute to development of immunity. A certain degree of immunity also appears likely through infections with other related mycobacteria. There is no evidence to suggest that leprosy patients are more susceptible to tuberculosis and vice versa. However, there is good evidence that BCG vaccine can provide some protection against leprosy. Trials have shown that BCG offers significant but varying levels of protection.

Leprosy is like tuberculosis in that in the majority of cases, infection does not lead to clinical disease and when the disease does develop, much of the damage is not caused by the infecting organism, but rather by the immune responses of the host to the infecting organism.

In leprosy, the significance of the host response to infection is illustrated by the broad clinical spectrum observed amongst those that develop the disease. At one pole is tuberculoid leprosy, characterized by strong cell-mediated immunity, a Th1 CD4+ cytokine profile (IL2, IFN-γ), very few bacteria and localized lesions. At the other pole is lepromatous leprosy, characterized by a lack of cell-mediated immunity, Th2 CD4+ response (IL4 and IL5), a strong humoral response, disseminated progressive disease and large numbers of bacilli. Thus, tuberculoid patients can be thought of as those exhibiting the most resistance whereas lepromatous patients are exhibiting the least. This is not to say that the pathogenesis associated with the more resistant pole is necessarily milder; strong Th1 responses in tuberculoid pole can result in rapid and severe nerve damage.

Genetic Factors and Susceptibility

Leprosy is a disease of very low infectivity and high morbidity. Only few people exposed to infection develop clinical signs of the disease. For this, the role of genetic factors in leprosy has been under consideration for a long time and investigated thoroughly. General genes are involved in the response of the host to the mycobacteiral antigens. While some play an adaptive role in innate immunity, others play a role in adaptive immune response. Since several molelcules are involved, they probably play an integral role in determining the immune response of the host to the infectious agent. Studies suggest that, among monozygotic (identical) twins if one has leprosy, the other almost always had leprosy, while this was not the case with dizygotic twins. Monozygous (MZ) twins share all the genes while dizygous (DZ) twins share half the genes. The often quoted study of leprosy occurrence among twins, from Chakravarty and Vogel in 1973, was conducted in endemic areas of Andhra Pradesh and West Bengal. The study included a total of 102 twins affected by leprosy. As shown in Table 2.4, in 59.7% of the monozygotic twins affected by leprosy, both the twin children developed leprosy, and among dizygotic twins, in only 20% cases, both the twins developed leprosy. The concordance was not limited to the disease *per se;* it was reflected also in the type of the disease developed. Further, among the twins concordant for leprosy, 86.5% twins were concordant for leprosy type. These studies suggest genetic susceptibility to the disease. This is supported by another observation that the rate of conjugal leprosy is very low.

The goal of identification of host genetic factors responsible for susceptibility to leprosy can be approached in at least two ways: firstly, candidate gene studies can be carried out on genes of known function that have a possible biological role in the control of infection or disease. A second approach utilizes a non-targeted genome-wide linkage analysis, in which increased sharing of chromosomal regions by affected individuals leads to identification of positional candidates. How *M. leprae* targets Schwann cells, exactly how it brings about nerve damage and how it is killed in macrophages have not been fully elucidated. It is possible that host genes which influence these processes may influence the outcome of infection. It is clear, however, that

Table 2.4: Study of concordance in 102 twin pairs for leprosy concordance, and for leprosy type

Concordance for leprosy			Concordance for leprosy type			
Gender	MZ (62)	DZ (40)	Only the twins concordant for leprosy			
Male	24 (60.0%)	5 (22.7%)	Zygosity	Concordant for type	Discordant for type	Total
Female	13 (59.1%)	1 (16.7%)	MZ	32 (86.5%)	5 (13.5%)	37
M+F	—	2 (16.7%)	DZ	6 (75%)	2 (25.0%)	8
Total	**37 (59.7%)**	**8 (20.0%)**	**Total**	**38**	**7**	**45**

Abbreviations: MZ, monozygotic; DZ, dizygotic.

the development of appropriate cell-mediated immunity is important in the control of mycobacterial disease.

Familial Clustering

The occurrence of leprosy has been found more in certain clusters of communities and especially in family clusters. The community clusters can be explained in terms of environmental factors of exposure, e.g. local mycobacterial flora, and other environmental conditions to which all community people are exposed. But for the family clusters it becomes difficult to explain whether it is due to similar environmental conditions or due to the close familial (genetic) relatedness, close contact with an affected family member or a combination of all. Also it has been shown that the probability of finding familial occurrence of leprosy is higher in families that include a lepromatous patient, than in those where it does not.

Nutrition

Although intensive control programs reduced the prevalence of leprosy worldwide, new cases of this infectious disease are still detected in several of the poorest areas of the world. Therefore, the disease is also known as a disease of poverty. To be able to control the disease, it is important to know which aspects of poverty play a role in transmission and acquiring clinical signs of disease. A study conducted in Bangladesh showed that a recent period of food shortage was the only socioeconomic factor that was found related to leprosy disease and not poverty as such. Malnutrition is known to lower immunity and make people more vulnerable to infectious diseases. It was concluded that malnutrition as an aspect of poverty played an important role in the development of the clinical signs of leprosy.

ENVIRONMENTAL FACTORS

Humidity favors survival of the mycobacterium in the environment. The bacilli remain viable for about 9 days in dried nasal secretions and for almost 46 days in moist soil at room temperature. Thus, risk of transmission increases with humid conditions.

Socioeconomic Factors

Leprosy is a social disease and is generally associated with poverty related factors such as overcrowding, lack of education, lack of personal hygiene, lack of ventilation, etc. which favor transmission of the disease. However, it may affect persons from any socioeconomic group. Fear of leprosy, guilt, stigma and discrimination associated with the disease in the community and unfounded prejudices regarding leprosy force a person to hide the disease and contribute to delay in seeking treatment, leading to development of deformities

and also promote transmission of the disease. Even today, in spite of availability of enormous scientific information about leprosy, the legend is deeply rooted in the minds of people at all level of society that it is highly contagious and incurable. People still associate leprosy with gross deformities affecting hands and feet which could have been otherwise prevented by early diagnosis and treatment with MDT or could have been corrected with reconstructive surgery and regular physiotherapy.

Risk Factors

A number of studies have attempted to identify the determinants of leprosy by assessing the risk factors in either case control or cohort studies. A case control study in Brazil (Kerr-Pontes, 2006) found a range of risk factors associated with leprosy; these included low education, poor hygiene, and food shortages. BCG scar was found to be protective. A cohort study in Indonesia, identified household crowding as a risk factor as well as household contact status. Leprosy has been regarded as a disease associated with poverty and these analytical studies provide documentary evidence for this.

DISABILITY

The epidemiology of disability associated with leprosy has become a topic in its own right. This is important as it focuses attention on the disability and not just the infection. The most frequently used method of assessing disability is using the WHO disability grading. This grading is not based on treatment and can be used at diagnosis, at completion of treatment and to monitor response to treatment. Disability is more common in MB leprosy than PB leprosy and any existing nerve impairment is a predictor of further disability. Grade 2 disability rate control is the new global target for leprosy.

TRANSMISSION

Source of Infection

Man is the only natural reservoir of *M. leprae* and the only source of infection is an untreated case of leprosy. Multibacillary cases are more important source of infection compared to paucibacillary cases. However, all active leprosy cases should be considered as potential sources of infection. It is now well known that, wild animals like armadillos, mangabey monkeys and chimpanzees show infections with *M. leprae*. However, it is least likely that leprosy in wild animals could be a serious threat to human beings.

Portal of Exit

The bacilli are shed from nose, upper respiratory tract and the skin. Respiratory tract, especially nose is the major portal of exit of *M. leprae* from the body of an infectious person.

Millions of bacilli are discharged from the nasal mucosa of a bacteriologically positive case during sneezing. Considerable number of bacilli are shed from the nose especially when there are nasal ulcers. Patients harbor most bacilli in their skin, but are seldom shed from intact skin. Large number of lepra bacilli are found in sweat glands, sweat ducts, sebaceous glands and hair follicles. However, bacilli can be shed from broken skin and ulcers of lepromatous cases. Only a small percentage (less than 3%) of these escaping bacilli are viable even in untreated patients.

Portal of Entry

Respiratory route is the major portal of entry for the lepra bacilli. The possibility of infection by entry through skin, particularly broken skin cannot be ruled out.

Mode of Transmission

Various modes of transmission of the leprosy are described, but the exact contribution of each mode is still not established with certainty. The main likely modes of transmission are:

- *Inhalation (droplet infection)*: The transmission of leprosy bacilli from person to person is mainly due to nasal droplet infection.
- *Contact*: To a smaller extent, the disease may also be transmitted by skin to skin contact. As leprosy bacilli can survive in favorable environmental conditions for quite a long duration, the hypothesis that it can be transmitted by indirect contact also cannot be entirely ruled out.
- *In utero transmission*: There have been reports of detection of leprosy in infants of very young age. Brubaker et al. reported a series of about 50 patients with leprosy below 1 year age, most of them with indeterminate and BT disease. The youngest age of a reported leprosy case from Martinique was 3 weeks. Another young child with histopathologically proven tuberculoid leprosy was reported by Noordeen. In the series by Brubaker et al., only 50% cases had their mother with clinical leprosy or history of leprosy, suggesting that about half the mothers had subclinical infection. In all such cases, the possibility could be that the disease presented after a very short incubation period, if the infection occurred after birth; or the infection occurred *in utero*. High levels of IgG, IgM antibodies to *M. leprae* have been demonstrated in a higher percentage of 3-24 months old infants born to lepromatous mothers. Occasional *M. leprae* have been demonstrated in placenta and cord blood in humans and armadillos. Despite all this body of evidence supporting uterine transfer of infection, one does very rarely come across infected babies of mothers with untreated lepromatous leprosy.
- *Transmission through ingestion (breast milk)*: The possibility has always been expressed in the past that leprosy could be transmitted through ingestion of infected milk. The presence of *M. leprae* in the breast milk of mothers with lepromatous leprosy also raised this possibility. The impressive investigative work by Pedley showed leprosy bacilli in the epithelial linings of lactating mammary glands which are excreted in milk. They also estimated that through a feed of 4 oz; the baby would ingest about 2 million leprosy bacilli. Despite all these observations, the fact remains that as of date, there is no definite evidence that (i) breast milk with viable leprosy bacilli acts as a source of infection and also (ii) that such an infected breast milk induces any protective immune response in the child.
- *Inoculation following trauma*: A number of cases have been reported where development of leprosy was linked to the trauma of various kinds. Appearance of leprosy lesions has been observed after thorn prick, tattooing, vaccination, roadside injury, after dressing of a wound in a leprosy hospital, dog bite, and following injury sustained by a surgeon during operating a lepromatous leprosy patient. Although it may be difficult to demonstrate the presence of *M. leprae* over the objects or instruments involved in producing trauma in the instances mentioned, but this itself is sufficient to know that the development of leprosy lesions were related to the site of trauma and the trauma sites served as the entry points for leprosy bacilli.

INCUBATION PERIOD

Incubation period or latent period for leprosy is variable and unusually long. It may vary from few weeks to even 20 years. However, average incubation period for the disease is considered to be 5-7 years. A patient with paucibacillary leprosy may have shorter incubation period.

DIAGNOSIS

Diagnosis of leprosy is most commonly based on the clinical signs and symptoms. These are easy to observe and elicit by any health worker after a short period of training. In practice, persons with such complaints report on their own to the health center. Only in rare instances, there is a need to use laboratory and other investigations to confirm a diagnosis of leprosy. In an endemic country or area, an individual should be regarded as having leprosy if he or she shows *One* of the following cardinal signs:

- Skin lesion consistent with leprosy and with definite sensory loss, with or without thickened nerves
- Nerve thickening with sensory loss
- Positive skin slit smears—for AFB.

The skin lesions can be single or multiple, usually less pigmented than the surrounding normal skin. Sometimes, the lesion is reddish or copper-colored. A variety of skin lesions may be seen but macules (flat), papules (raised), or nodules are common. Sensory loss is a typical feature of leprosy.

The skin lesion may show loss of sensation to pin prick and/or light touch. Thickened nerves, mainly peripheral nerve trunks constitute another feature of leprosy. A thickened nerve is often accompanied by other signs as a result of damage to the nerve. There may be loss of sensation in the skin and weakness of muscles supplied by the affected nerve. In the absence of these signs, nerve thickening by itself, without sensory loss and/or muscle weakness is often not a reliable sign of leprosy. Positive skin smears: though seen in a small proportion of cases, are diagnostic of the disease.

A person presenting with skin lesions or with symptoms suggestive of nerve damage, in whom the cardinal signs are absent or doubtful should be called a 'suspect case' in the absence of any immediately obvious alternate diagnosis. Such individuals should be told the basic facts of leprosy and advised to return to the center if signs persist for more than 6 months or if at any time worsening is noticed. Suspect cases may be also sent to referral clinics with more facilities for diagnosis.

CLASSIFICATION OF LEPROSY

The classification of leprosy is also used in describing the epidemiology of leprosy. Various classifications have been used in the past and they have often differed between countries. Currently the most commonly used classification is the PB (paucibacillary leprosy) and MB (multibacillary leprosy). This is used universally as it is also used in the treatment regimen required for each form of the disease, 6 months of rifampicin and dapsone for PB and 12 months of rifampicin, clofazimine and dapsone for MB disease (WHO 2006). The other classification is the Ridley and Jopling classification, which is used for research purposes to classify the full spectrum of leprosy from polar tuberculoid to polar lepromatous leprosy. This classification requires an accurate clinical description and information on microbiology, immunology and histology. It is rarely used in routine leprosy programs.

EPIDEMIOLOGICAL INDICATORS FOR MONITORING

The main objective of the leprosy eradication/control program is to cure people with leprosy, to stop the transmission of the disease and to prevent disabilities. Health indicators are measures (mostly quantitative) aimed at summarizing the health situation and the performance of the health system, measuring and monitoring progress towards achievement of the objectives and facilitating the evaluation of policies and initiatives undertaken by the leprosy eradication/control program. Indicators should be easy and should directly show how far a result or objective is being achieved. There are several epidemiological and operational indicators for monitoring leprosy control activities. The most important indicators are prevalence, incidence, proportion of new cases

presenting with Grade 2 disability, and treatment outcome. New cases with Grade 2 disability point to delay in diagnosis; treatment oucome tells how many patients have successfully completed treatment among those diagnosed. To interpret these indicators, the following must be specified: the criteria used for diagnosis; inclusion of indeterminate leprosy or postponing diagnosis until one of the cardinal signs is positive; the definition of **case**, **cure**, **defaulter**, the population, and the time. A **case** of the leprosy is a person presenting clinical signs of leprosy who has yet to complete a full course of treatment. A patient is defined as **cured** when he has successfully completed his course of treatment. **Defaulters** are defined as those who were not able to complete the course of treatment within given time.

Prevalence

Prevalence is the total number of leprosy cases in a defined population at a specified time. It gives the total quantum of case load in an area and is a useful indicator in planning healthcare activities in the specified area. However, if one needs to take an idea about the comparative account of leprosy prevalence in different areas, then this indicator does not convey the clear picture. For that purpose, another indicator (called as rate) is used which expresses the number of leprosy cases in a unit population, e.g. cases per one thousand, or ten thousand or one lakh or one million population. When the leprosy prevalence was very high in the pre-MDT era, the rates used to be expressed in terms of per 1000; e.g. in Kanpur Dehat district, the prevalence of leprosy was 18 per one thousand during 1980. Later on following reduction of number of cases after the success of MDT, the reference is made to leprosy elimination criteria of less than 1 per ten thousand population, which itself is derived from the nonstatus of the disease as a public health problem of less than 100 cases per one million population.

Prevalence is not a very reliable epidemiological indicator of leprosy, as it is subject to a number of confounding factors. It reflects only the leprosy cases registered for chemotherapy, and no account is given of the patients who are undetected or those who abandoned their treatment some time ago. Registered prevalence is also subject to change abruptly if the treatment duration is changed suddenly, e.g. when the treatment duration of WHO recommended MDT for MB leprosy was changed in 1997 from 2 years to 1 year. At best it serves as an indicator of treatment load of the health service at a given time.

Criteria of Leprosy Elimination

WHO defines the "elimination of leprosy" as the achievement of prevalence rate below 1 case per 10,000 population (Fig. 2.2). Although adopted in most of the leprosy control programs globally, this definition has some problems, which are discussed here.

Leprosy (a public health problem)	
Population	1 million
No. of cases	100
Prevalence	1 per ten thousand

Fig. 2.2: The criteria of leprosy elimination as a public health problem defined by WHO, usually expressed as less than 1 case per 10,000 population

- The rate of 1 case per ten thousand is completely arbitrary.
- The rate intended (when the elimination strategy was launched) was based on the actual prevalence and not the prevalence of registered cases.
- The strategy of elimination was based on the assumption that transmission would be reduced, once the prevalence reached below a certain threshold. There is no scientific basis for such a hypothesis when the fall in prevalence is the result of shortening of the duration of treatment; rather than of a declining incidence of the disease. Hence, the prevalence rate is often irrelevant.

Incidence

This indicates the number of newly detected cases in a defined population over a defined period of time (usually one year). For comparison in different areas, like prevalence, incidence is expressed in terms of number of cases per unit population in one year. Incidence is the most effective indicator of the transmission of disease. It gives an account of the population at risk of getting the disease. If any disease control program aims at prevention, the goal must be to reduce the incidence. Thus, incidence is a far better indicator than prevalence to judge the success of a disease control program.

In case of leprosy, the true incidence is difficult to obtain because it depends on the thoroughness of case finding/reporting; and can also be confounded by over-diagnosis. Usually, the newly registered cases are considered as substitutes for incidence. Since the incidence is also influenced by age, reporting of case detection should be expressed in two age groups above and below 15 years age. They can also be grouped separately as paucibacillary and multibacillary, or by presence or absence of deformities.

Annual New Case Detection Rate

The annual new case detection rate (ANCDR) is the indicator used in leprosy control program and indicates the new cases recorded in an area per one lakh population over a period of one year. Since actual incidence is difficult to estimate due to operational reasons, the case detection is considered as a proxy indicator of incidence. Case detection rate should also form the basis for evaluation of requirement for MDT supply.

Age and Sex Specific Prevalence and Incidence Rates

These indicators are used to remove the age and gender related bias in reporting the data of leprosy cases. It is well known, that leprosy is comparatively less common in children and women. The male predominance is observed in adults but in children the gender distribution is nearly equal. Also leprosy is less common among children, more truely for lepromatous type, most common disease form among children is borderline tuberculoid.

MB Proportion

It is the percentage of multibacillary cases among the total number of new leprosy cases detected during the reporting year. People with MB leprosy are considered to be more infectious, and thus more likely to be responsible for leprosy transmission. The proportion of MB cases among newly detected cases is usually high at the beginning of the leprosy control program, due to the fact that MB cases would have accumulated over the years, and the PB cases would have undergone self-healing in many cases. The definition of MB case itself has undergone considerable changes over the years. In 1981, the MB-MDT was recommended for any case that fell in LL, BL and BB type of Ridley Jopling classification; or any case that had bacteriological index of 2+ or more at any site. In 1988, all cases with BI smear positivity were to be considered as MB. From 1995 onwards, the definition of MB is any case with more than 5 patches with anesthesia, in addition to any one BI smear positivity (if facility is available). As a result of these changes in definition, the proportion of MB cases is increasing over the years. Moreover, MB leprosy is less frequent among females and children; the MB proportion is likely to be influenced by age and sex composition of the population under consideration. MB proportion is also a good indicator for estimation of drug requirements.

Lepromatous Rate

The proportion of cases with lepromatous leprosy, among the total number of cases was the indicator in use in pre-MDT era when the definition of MB case was different than from that of today. Wide geographical differences were seen in the proportion of MB cases across the world, ranging from 5–70%. There did not seem to be any correlation between the total prevalence in the population area and the proportion of lepromatous cases. Since the redefinition of MB case in last decade, the lepromatous rates of pre-MDT era is no longer relevant.

Child Proportion

This is the percentage of children among all new cases detected during the reporting year.

As children leprosy patients will have very less time since getting infection, a high child proportion would indicate an active and recent transmission of the disease. Since most of the child leprosy cases fall in paucibacillary type, the case detection through self-reporting is bound to be low, as the patches are hardly noticeable in majority of the cases. If active case finding is pursued, this proportion would be higher.

Deformity Rate

This is expressed in terms of percentage of patients with deformities among newly detected cases in a period of one year. This is expressed separately for different grades of deformities, as per the WHO grading (0,1,2). This indicates the delay in time between a case getting infected and getting diagnosed and treated. This rate is usually high at the beginning of the leprosy control activities due to accumulation of backlog cases, and it stabilizes subsequently. Decreasing this rate is one of the major objectives of the control program.

Basic Reproduction Rate

This is an indicator of disease transmission, though not used very often. It is a measure of new cases arising from the index cases. For a disease to be considered as an epidemic, the basic reproduction rate (BRR) must be more than one. It may be used to monitor disease control.

Treatment Completion Rate

This is the proportion of cases who complete the treatment in the stipulated time, i.e. 6 pulses of PB-MDT in 9 months; and 12 pulses of MB-MDT in 18 months period. This is a very sensitive indicator since the effectiveness of MDT totally depends on this single factor, that the treatment is taken regularly and in time. Irregular treatments and defaults make the person prone to getting the disease complications. For a leprosy control program, it is extremely necessary to keep this rate as high as possible. If this rate is below 85% in any control program, the strategy calls for a review.

RELAPSES

Relapses indicate treatment failure, which could generally be caused by inadequate dosage and/or duration of treatment, and irregular intake of drugs. Reinfection is also a possible cause of relapse, though it is difficult to confirm with the technology available in the national programs. In addition, the threat of drug resistance, although reported sporadically in the recent past, cannot be ignored. Globally more relapses are being reported and more countries have been reporting relapse cases. A total of 3,427 relapses were reported from 105 countries in 2012. It would be useful to continuously monitor relapse cases in relation to treatment completion and drug resistance in all national programs of various countries.

SUMMARY

WHO has twice updated the global leprosy control strategy since 2006, to further reduce the disease burden due to leprosy in collaboration with national health programs of member countries, partner organizations and other donor agencies. Detection of all cases in a community and completion of treatment using MDT are the basic tenets of the enhanced global strategy.

Communities in leprosy endemic areas have benefited greatly from the implementation of MDT, which has enabled the disease to be cured and has reduced the number of cases, with (G2D). Consequently stigma associated with leprosy and resultant discrimination against those affected have been reduced. There have also been economic benefits, with reduction of health system costs incurred for disability care, reconstructive surgery, and rehabilitation. Nevertheless, surveillance of drug resistance, research to develop shorter regimens and efficient and affordable prophylaxis, need to be continued or initiated in order to sustain the gains achieved and further reduce the disease burden due to leprosy.

FURTHER READING

1. Achilles EK, Hagel M, Dietrich M. Leprosy accidentally transmitted from a patient to a surgeon in a non-endemic area. Ann Int Med. 2004;141:51.
2. Bechelli LM, Martinez DV. Further information on the leprosy problem in the world. Bull World Health Org. 1972;46:523-36.
3. Brandsma JW, Yoder L, Macdonald M. Leprosy acquired by inoculation from a knee injury. Lepr Rev. 2005;76:175-9.
4. Brubaker ML, Meyers WM, Bourland J. Leprosy in children under one year of age. Int J Lepr Other Mycobact Dis. 1985;53: 516-23.
5. Chakravarti MR, Vogel FA. Twin study on leprosy. In: Becker PE (Ed), Topics in Human Genetics Vol.1, Publisher: Georg Thieme Verlag, Stuttgrat, 1973:pp.1-123.
6. Chatterjee BR. The importance of urban slums in leprosy. In: Chatterjee BR (Ed). Leprosy, Etiobiology of Manifestations, Treatment and Control. Leprosy Field Research unit, Jhalda, West Bengal (Pub.) 1994: pp. 5.
7. Dharmendra. Contact with intact skin as a common mode of transmission of leprosy. Lepr India. 1980;52:472-74.
8. Enhanced global strategy for further reducing the disease burden due to leprosy (Plan period 2011–2015), New Delhi, WHO, regional Office for South East Asia, 2009.
9. Gelber RH. Leprosy (Hansen's disease). In: Harrison's Principles of Internal Medicine, 15th edition, Volume 1. Braunwald E, Hauser SL, Fauci AS, et al (Eds). McGraw Hill (Pub), New Delhi, 2003:pp.1035-40.
10. Ghorpade A. Inoculation indeterminate leprosy localized to a smallpox vaccination scar. Lepr Rev. 2007;78:398-400.
11. Girdhar BK. Skin to skin transmission of leprosy. Indian J Dermatol Venereol Leprol. 2005;71:223-5.
12. Gupta CM, Tutakne MA, Tiwari VD. Inoculation leprosy subsequent to dog bite. Indian J Lepr. 1984;56:919-21.
13. ILEP. The interpretation of epidemiological indicators in leprosy. Technical Bulletin 2001; ILEP, London: pp.3.

14. Job CK, et al. Leprosy: Diagnosis and Management. Hind Kusht Nivaran Sangh. 1975.

15. Job CK, Sanchez RM, Hastings RC. Lepromatous placentitis and intrauterine fetal infection in lepromatous 9-banded armadillo. Lab Invest. 1986;56:44-8.

16. Job CK. Transmission of Leprosy. Indian J Lepr. 1987;59:1-8.

17. Kapoor P. Epidemiologic survey of leprosy in Maharashtra State (India). Lepr India. 1963;35:83-9.

18. Kerr-Pontes LRS, Barreto ML, Evangelista CMN, et al. Socioeconomic, environmental, and behavioural risk factors for leprosy in North-east Brazil: results of a case-control study. Int J Epidemiol. 2006;35:994-1000.

19. Melsom R, Harboe M, Duncan ME. IgA, IgG and IgM anti-*M. leprae* antibodies in babies of leprosy mothers during first 2 years of life. Clin Exp Immunol. 1982;49:532-42.

20. Mittal RR, Handa F, Sharma SC. Inoculation leprosy subsequent to roadside injury. Indian J Dermatol Venereol Leprol. 1976;42:175-7.

21. Montestruc E, Berdonneau R. Two new cases of leprosy in infants in Martinique (in French). Bull Soc Pathol Exot Filiales. 1954;47:781-3.

22. Noordeen SK. In: Thangaraj RH (Ed). A Manual of Leprosy, 2nd edition. The Leprosy Mission, New Delhi,1980.

23. Noordeen SK. The epidemiology of leprosy. In: Hastings RC (Ed). Leprosy, 2nd edition. Churchill Livingstone (Pub.), London. 1994: pp.31.

24. Park JE. Leprosy. In: Park K (Ed), Textbook of Preventive & Social Medicine, 16th edition. Banarsidas Bhanot (Pub.), Jabalpur (India), 2000: pp.242.

25. Pedley JC. Presence of *M. leprae* in the nipple secretion and lumina of hypertrophied mammary glands. Lepr Rev. 1968; 39:67-73.

26. Sehgal VN, Rege VL, Vediraj SN. Inoculation leprosy subsequent to smallpox vaccination. Dermatologica. 1970;141:393-6.

27. Thangaraj RH. A Manual of Leprosy, 3rd edition. South Asia, The leprosy Mission (Pub.), New Delhi, 1983:pp.3-9.

28. Valla MC. Lepre et grossesse. Thesis, University of Lyon, France, 1976.

29. Van Brakel WH, de Soldenhoff, Mc Dougall AC. The allocation of leprosy patients into paucibacillary and multibacillary groups for multidrug therapy, taking into account the number of body areas affected by skin, or skin and nerve lesions. Lepr Rev. 1992;63:231-45.

30. Wagener DK, Schauf V, Nelson KE, et al. Segregation analysis of leprosy in families of northern Thailand. Genet Epidemiol. 1988;5:95-105.

31. Waters MFR, Rees RJ, Mc Dougall AC, et al. Ten years of dapsone in lepromatous leprosy: clinical, bacteriological and histological assessment and the finding of viable leprosy bacilli. Lepr Rev. 1974;45:288-98.

32. Weekly Epidemiological Record (WER), WHO, 30th August 2013, Vol. 88, 35, pp. 365-80.

33. WHO Weekly Epidemiological Record No 20, 2001.

34. WHO Weekly Epidemiological Record No 28, 2000.

35. WHO. International classification of diseases (ICD) Version 2007. Available at http://apps.who.int/classifications/apps/icd/icd10 online/.

36. WHO. International classification of diseases (ICD). Available at http://www.who.int/classifications/icd/en/.

37. WHO. Natural history of leprosy. In: Technical Report Series No.716, WHO, Geneva, 1985: pp.21.

Global Leprosy Situation: Historical Perspective, Achievements, Challenges and Future Steps

Sumana Barua

Every person has a role to play in reducing the leprosy disease burden and removing the age old scourge from the globe. We need to enhance awareness about the early signs of the disease, make MDT available and encourage acceptance of the affected at home, school or at the workplace—

**Dr Poonam Khetrapal Singh,
Regional Director, WHO South East Asia Region**

LEPROSY: A BRIEF OVERVIEW

Leprosy is a chronic infectious disease caused by *Mycobacterium leprae*. Though human being is the main source of infection, nine banded Armadillo is incriminated as a reservoir of infection, at least in some parts of the world. Incubation period is long, ranging generally from 5–7 years. Some element of uncertainty lingers with regard to mode of transmission, though most investigators believe that transmission occurs from person to person through nasal droplet infection. The disease is rarely seen in children below the age of 5 years. Among communicable diseases, it is one of the leading causes of permanent physical disabilities.

Leprosy control is based on breaking the chain of transmission by treating the patient, a potential source of infection, which is rather a secondary preventive strategy that warrants detection and treatment of all cases in the community. Elementary to this is an effective surveillance measuring the prevalence of the disease and occurrence of new cases, the two sensitive indicators to understand the

natural history of the disease and epidemiology of leprosy in different parts of the world.

World Health Organization acquires data on annual basis from national leprosy programs of member states, with the help of Regional advisors from the WHO Regional Offices worldwide, and International Federation of Anti Leprosy Associations (ILEP). The global leprosy situation after due analysis, is published through WHO weekly epidemiological record (WER), which is the official reference publication on leprosy situation worldwide, for leprosy program managers, civil societies working in leprosy, academicians and researchers.

Detection of leprosy patients in time before nerve impairment sets in, is the crucial factor that signifies the effectiveness of leprosy control, and is measured by number or rate of new leprosy cases with visible deformities or grade 2 disabilities (G2D cases). Early reporting for consultation, diagnosis or treatment essentially depends on the awareness level in the community and responsive nature to illness by an individual. This needs to be constantly monitored and enhanced in order to reduce disease burden measured in terms of visible deformities (G2D Cases) among new cases. It is important to note that uninterrupted availability of multidrug therapy (MDT), is the mainstay of leprosy control. WHO made it available for national programs through the support of The Nippon foundation (TNF) (from 1995 to 1999) and presently from Novartis Foundation for Sustainable Development from the year 2000 onwards.

Yohei Sasakawa, WHO Goodwill Ambassador for elimination of leprosy spearheads reduction of stigma initiatives. Mr Sasakawa advocates for meaningful and greater participation of persons affected by leprosy in all services to the affected and to facilitate constitution and operationalization of forums or fora, the leprosy programs, besides funding number of leprosy projects including that of WHO.

Key challenges are continuous occurrence of new cases, potential risk of drug resistance and complacency among health staff in addressing leprosy program. Though BCG vaccination demonstrated protection to some extent against leprosy, preventive chemotherapy or vaccine development may hasten the process of reduction of occurrence of new cases. Research to discover biological, serological and clinical markers, which define susceptibility to leprosy among healthy and predict nerve function impairment is the need of the hour. Though, not discounting the robustness of MDT and its efficacy, it is prudent at this point in time to continue a scientific quest for new drugs which can kill *Mycobacterium leprae* quickly and completely.

HISTORY OF THE DISEASE

Leprosy is a disease of great antiquity and was well-recognized in the oldest civilizations of Egypt, China and India. The first known written reference to leprosy appeared in an Egyptian papyrus document written around 1550 BCE.[i]

Throughout history, leprosy has been feared and misunderstood, and has resulted in significant stigma and isolation of those who are afflicted. It was thought to be a hereditary disease, a curse, or a punishment from God. During the Middle Ages, those with leprosy were forced to wear special clothing and ring bells to warn others of their entry or even their presence around.

Origin and Early Spread

The origin and early spread of leprosy is however, largely a matter of surmise. "It is not possible to declare with certainty in what country leprosy started.[1] It can be considered that leprosy was prevalent centuries ago in India, China, Egypt and other parts of Africa, it was also found in Europe and the New World and Pacific islands.

Leprosy was described in ancient literatures to varying extent. In the ancient Indian medical literature, in 600 BCE with details of clinical features like loss of sensation, numbness, tingling, using diverse terminologies. "Kushtha" an expression of dermatological manifestation and leprosy is still commonly referred to in many parts of India. Egyptian literature also shows reference to leprosy as 'Uchedu' in Ebers Papyrus written about 1555 BCE. Some researchers have also discussed mention of the name 'Ghon's swelling'[2] and the association of 'Ghon's swelling' (Gas gangrene or weeping eczema) though it was debated later.[3] Ping is probably closer to leprosy as presented in Chinese literature. Chao's Pathology published in 7th Century CE.[ii] Biblical literature describes leprosy as 'Zaraath' (a Hebrew word) in The Old Testament and as 'leprosy' (a Greek word) in The New Testament. The Arabic literature used the word 'Juzam' or 'lepra arabum' while referring to leprosy.[4]

The spread of leprosy was mentioned in "thousand Golden Remedies" compiled by Physicians of Ming Dynasty (1368–1643 CE), which mentioned that contact with leprosy patients is the route for spread for infection. It further explained that unhygienic housing, use of utensils and bed of patients are the circumstances, which lead to spread of the infection. Since then the evidence of practice of ostracism or isolation is available, through many anecdotes, and even from religious books from different parts of the world including Europe and Mediterranean countries. This continued for centuries, the leprosy care getting mired in sheer denial of the illness, ignorance about its treatment and prefixed wrong notions about the disease. It would be difficult to weigh the benefit of isolation practiced over centuries, in the light of the tragedy a patient experiences. In the name of isolation, people were taken away from home, couples were separated and children removed from their parents.

Mercantile routes cannot be discounted either. Though there is no clear cut mention of disease spread, some of the papers from medical historians have provided an evidence that leprosy was at its peak in Europe in 12th century CE. It can be concluded that spread of leprosy can be attributed to movement of population groups belonging to Military, Mercantile and Missionaries.

HISTORY OF TREATMENT OF LEPROSY

Chaulmoogra oil has been the mainstay of leprosy treatment according to, 'Sushruta Samhita' of 600 BCE, which was also mentioned in western medicine late in 19th century CE. 'Tuvarka', the Indian plant was identical with Hydnocarpus Wightiana, from which *Chaulmoogra* oil was extracted. The oil was used to be taken orally, rubbed on the skin lesions and later was used as an injection also.

---

[i]BCE is Before Common/Current/Christian Era, equal to the BC (Before Christ).
[ii]CE is Common Era (also Current Era or Christian Era), is an alternative naming of the traditional calendar era or Anno Domini (abbreviated AD).

In 1941, Guy Faget, the medical officer in charge of National Leprasorium in Carville, Lousiana, started administering 'Promin', a sulfone drug. Though this treatment also involved painful injections, but demonstrated effective treatment if not complete cure for leprosy. Though sulfones were synthesized in early 1900s, enough evidence was not available for their induction in the treatment of leprosy, it was not possible to culture *M. leprae* in the laboratory and research evidence was not available. Another derivative of sulfone, 4,4-diaminodiphenyl sulfone (DDS, otherwise known as Dapsone) was considered in 1947 and in early 1950s. Introduction of dapsone kindled a ray of hope for cure of leprosy. Administration of Dapsone was considered suitable for treating large number of patients. It was an oral medication, given once a week (due to its suspected toxicity) and had a long shelf-life. The problems of dapsone toxicity were managed by altering dosages.

Gradually in two decades of starting dapsone mono-therapy, challenges in treating leprosy started surfacing. Many patients with high bacteriological load remained positive. And in 1964, the first confirmed case of dapsone resistance was reported from Malaysia. In 1977, primary drug resistance was documented.

In 1921, the US Public Health Service established the nation's first leprosarium, located in what is now known as Carville, Louisiana. The leprosarium served as an institution for people with leprosy and a hospital for experiments with treatments for leprosy as well as a laboratory to study the organism. The center, which became known simply as "Carville", became a refuge for leprosy patients and one of the premier centers of scientific research and testing in attempts to find a cure for the disease.

Similar centers isolating persons affected were also recorded in the history in many countries, including India and Hawaii.

The **Culion Leper Colony**[iii] was a former leprosarium located on Culion, an island in the Palawan province of the Philippines. It was established by the US government in order to get rid leprosy from the Philippine islands through the only method known at the time, i.e. isolating all existing cases and gradually phasing out the disease from the population. In addition to segregating the disease from the rest of the population, the island was later established in order to offer a better opportunity for people afflicted by leprosy to receive adequate care and modern treatments. By 1830, approximately four hundred lepers were patients in Leper Colonies established by Catholic priests at Manila, Cebu and Nueva Caceras. By Act 1711 of the Philippine Commission passed September 12 1907, Victor G Heiser was given full responsibility of the segregation program. Heiser was given the responsibility of locating segregating and moving any known person afflicted with Leprosy in the Philippines to Culion. Religious organizations on the island influenced the role of marriage and consequently parenthood in patients' lives.

Under the appointment-ship of Governor General Leonard Wood, Culion continued to expand its staff and facilities and continued using *Chaulmoogra* oil for treatment into the 1920s and 1930s. Culion's decline began with staff layoffs during the financial crisis of 1933. After 1935 only leprosy patients who preferred life at Culion as opposed to life at leprosarium closer to their region were shipped to Culion. Due to advanced treatment methods and the influence of regional clinics.

Source: http://en.wikipedia.org/wiki/Culion_leper_colony

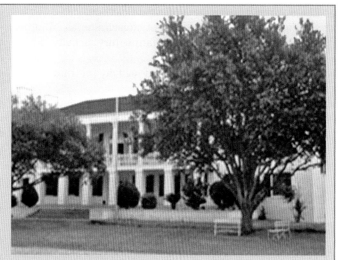

Leprosarium, Carville, Louisiana

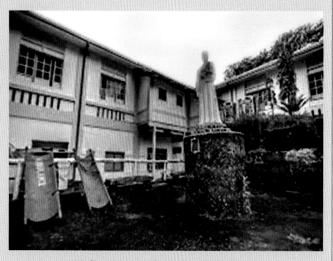

Culion Leper Colony, The Philippines

[iii] Culion leper colony in Palawan, The Philippines was established by US Govt. in 1906.

WHO expert committee through its reports from third and fourth meetings advised more research and data about drug resistance in all parts of the world and simultaneously reviewed information about new drugs becoming available. B663 or Clofazimine, a riminophenazine drug was reported as being therapeutically active against *M. leprae* and also having lowered the incidence of *erythema nodosum leprosum (ENL)* reactions. Rifampicin was reported to be therapeutically active (1970) in all patients irrespective of dapsone resistance.[4]

The key milestones reached between 1960 and 1970, which made significant changes in the chemotherapy of leprosy are mentioned below:[5]

- In 1964, the first case of dapsone-resistant leprosy was demonstrated by the mouse footpad method.
- During the 1960s, the efficacy of clofazimine as an anti-leprosy drug and its anti-inflammatory activity were reported.
- In 1970, the rapid bactericidal activity of rifampicin against *M. leprae* was demonstrated.
- Although it had been known since the earliest days of the chemotherapy of leprosy that multibacillary patients can relapse if they stop treatment, it was only in 1974 that the existence of persisting viable *M. leprae* was detected for the first time in lepromatous patients treated for 10–12 years with Dapsone monothreapy. Thus, the concept of 'persisters' was established.

GLOBAL LEPROSY SITUATION

Annual statistics on leprosy for the year 2013 with information on new cases detected, number of new cases with visible deformities (G2D cases), number of children, women and treatment completion rates of patients with multibacillary (MB) leprosy were reported by 102 countries from five WHO regions. Mid-year population estimates for the year 2014 were drawn from data published by the World population prospects, (accessed in July 2014)* was used as denominator for calculating prevalence rate and rates for new case detection and grade 2 disabilities due to leprosy in different countries and WHO regions.

Table 3.1 presents leprosy prevalence at the end of March 2014 and new case detection at global level during the year 2013 in different regions. A decreasing trend in both prevalence and new case detection, globally, is observed when compared to the previous year. The prevalence of leprosy at the end of March 2013 was 189,017 (0.34) when compared to 180,618 (0.32) at the end of March 2014.

Table 3.2 presents number of new cases detected in different WHO Regions annually from 2006 to 2013. When compared to the previous years, in 2013, a decrease was observed in number of new cases reported mainly in Eastern Mediterranean and South-East Asian regions. Decrease in number of new cases was also noted in American and Western Pacific regions, though marginally. Altogether, there was a decrease by 17,201 new cases in 2013 than in the previous year.

Innovative case finding methods introduced to reach out to hard to reach areas and difficult to reach population groups, improving data management would have probably led to increase in detection of new cases.

Table 3.3 presents new case detection trends from 14 countries, which reported more than 1,000 cases during 2006 to 2013. These 14 countries, contributed to 96% of total new cases reported worldwide in 2013. However, the three major endemic countries (Brazil, India and Indonesia) reported a

Table 3.1: Registered prevalence of leprosy and number of new cases detected in 102 countries or territories, by WHO Region, 2013		
WHO region[a]	**Number of cases registered (prevalence/10,000 population), first quarter of 2014[b]**	**Number of new cases detected (new-case detection rate/100,000 population), 2013[c]**
African	22,722 (0.38)	20,911 (3.50)
Americas	31,753 (0.36)	33,084 (3.78)
Eastern Mediterranean	2,604 (0.05)	1,680 (0.35)
South-East Asia	116,396 (0.63)	155,385 (8.38)
Western Pacific	7,143 (0.04)	4,596 (0.25)
Total	**180,618 (0.32)**	**215,656 (3.81)**

[a]No reports received from the European region.
[b]The prevalence rate is the number of cases on treatment/10,000 population at the beginning of 2014.
[c]The new case detection rate is the number of new cases/100,000 population during the year 2013.

*World Population Prospects: The 2010 revision (vol. I, comprehensive tables, pp224-233....) New York, United Nations Secretariat, Population Division, Department of Economic and Social Affairs, 2011.(http://esa.un.org/wpp/Documentation/pdf/WPP2010_volume-II_Demogaphic-Profiles.pdf, accessed in July 2013.

Table 3.2: Trends in the detection of new cases of leprosy, by WHO Region, 2006–2013

WHO region	2006	2007	2008	2009	2010	2011*	2012	2013
African	34,480	34,468	29,814	28,935	25,345	20,213	20,599	20,911
Americas	47,612	42,135	41,891	40,474	37,740	36,832	36,178	33,084
Eastern Mediterranean	3,261	4,091	3,938	4,029	4,080	4,357	4,235	1,680
South-East Asia	17,418	171,576	167,505	166,115	156,254	160,132	166,445	155,385
Western Pacific	6,190	5,863	5,859	5,243	5,055	5,092	5,400	4,596
Total	**265,661**	**258,133**	**249,007**	**244,796**	**228,474**	**226,626**	**232,857**	**215,656**

Table 3.3: Trends in the detection of leprosy in 14 countries reporting more than or equal to 1,000 new cases from 2006–2013, globally

Country	2006	2007	2008	2009	2010	2011*	2012	2013
Bangladesh	6,280	5,357	5,249	5,239	3,848	3,970	3,688	3,141
Brazil	44,436	39,125	38,914	37,610	34,894	33,955	33,303	31,044
Cote d'Ivoire	976	1,204	998	884	NR	770	1,030	1,169
Democratic Republic of Congo	8,257	8,820	6,114	5,062	5,049	3,949	3,607	3,744
Ethiopia	4,092	4,187	4,170	4,417	4,430	NR	3,776	4,374
India	139,252	137,685	134,184	133,717	126,800	127,295	134,752	126,913
Indonesia	17,682	17,723	17,441	17,260	17,012	20,023	18,994	16,856
Madagascar	1,536	1,644	1,763	1,572	1,520	1,577	1,474	1,569
Myanmar	3,721	3,637	3,365	3,147	2,936	3,082	3,013	2,950
Nepal	4,235	4,436	4,708	4,394	3,118	3,184	3,492	3,225
Nigeria	3,544	4,665	4,899	4,219	3,913	3,623	3,805	3,385
Philippines	2,517	2,514	2,373	1,795	2,041	1,818	2,150	1,729
Sri Lanka	1,993	2,024	1,979	1,875	2,027	2,178	2,191	1,990
United Republic of Tanzania	3,450	3,105	3,276	2,654	2,349	2,288	2,528	2,005
Total (%)	243,477	237,652	23,1047	225,442	211,261	210,655	220,810	206,107
	(92)	(92)	(93)	(92)	(92)	(93)	(95)	(96)
Global Total	**265,661**	**258,133**	**249,007**	**244,796**	**228,474**	**226,626**	**232,857**	**215,656**

Updated data for 2011.

total of 12,236 less number of new cases in 2013 than that of 2012. Eight of the 14 countries reported reduced number of new cases between 2012 and 2013 and these are Bangladesh, Ethiopia, Myanmar, Nepal, Nigeria, the Philippines, Sri Lanka and United Republic of Tanzania. The remaining three counties reported increased number of new cases between 2012 and 2013 and these are Cote d'Ivoire, Democratic Republic of Congo and Madagascar.

The histogram (Fig. 3.1) conspicuously marks the localization of the disease prevalence in 14 countries reporting more than 1,000 cases amounting to 96% of global leprosy burden when compared to the rest 99 countries reporting the rest 4% of cases.

Epidemiology

During the year 2013, globally, 215,656 new leprosy cases were detected. Early case detection still remains the only tool available to reach the target set by the current Enhanced Global Strategy: a significant reduction in new case detection is noticed in Eastern Mediterranean and Western Pacific regions.

Enhanced global strategy for further reducing disease burden due to leprosy (2011-2015) set a target of reducing G2D rate to one third of that of 2010. The G2D rate was 0.23 per 100 000 people in 2010 and it should reach 0.17 as per the estimate based on interpolation using linear trend per

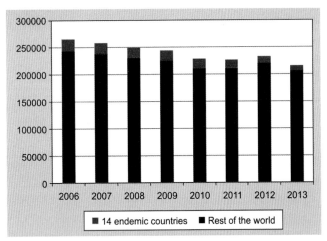

Fig. 3.1: Histogram showing new case detection in 14 endemic countries compared to the rest of the world from 2006-2013

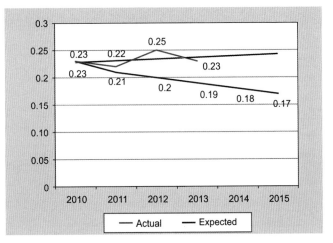

Fig. 3.2: Trends of grade 2 disability cases 2010-2013

Table 3.4: Number of cases of leprosy (rate/100,000 populations) with grade-2 disabilities among new cases reported, by WHO region, 2007–2013[a]

WHO Region[a]	Year[b]						
	2007	*2008*	*2009*	*2010*	*2011*	*2012*	*2013*
African	3,570 (0.51)	3,458 (0.51)	3,146 (0.41)	2,685 (0.40)	2,300 (0.26)	2,709 (0.40)	2,552 (0.43)
Americas	3,431 (0.42)	2,512 (0.29)	2,645 (0.30)	2,423 (0.27)	2,382 (0.27)	2,420 (0.28)	2,168 (0.25)
Eastern Mediterranean	466 (0.10)	687 (0.14)	608 (0.11)	729 (0.12)	753 (0.12)	700 (0.12)	191 (0.05)
South-East Asia	6,332 (0.37)	6,891 (0.39)	7,286 (0.41)	6,912 (0.39)	7,095 (0.39)	8,012 (0.43)	7,964 (0.43)
Western Pacific	604 (0.03)	592 (0.03)	635 (0.04)	526 (0.03)	549 (0.03)	568 (0.03)	386 (0.02)
Total	**14,403 (0.26)**	**14,140 (0.25)**	**14,320 (0.25)**	**13,275 (0.23)**	**13,079 (0.22)**	**14,409 (0.25)**	**13,289 (0.23)**

[a]Reports from the European Region are notincluded.
[b]Values are numbers (rate/100,000 population).

100,000 population by end of 2015. With 13,289 new cases with G2 D cases detected in 2013, the G2 D case rate actually shows an increase to 0.23 per 100,000 persons. The trends of grade 2 disability cases is presented in Figure 3.2 and Table 3.4.

EVOLUTION OF GLOBAL LEPROSY STRATEGIES: TO ENSURE RELEVANT TECHNICAL ASSISTANCE FROM WHO

Breaking the chain of the transmission remains the basic principle of leprosy control. Hence, detection of all cases in the community and treatment of cases with MDT, before infection is spread to the healthy is the most crucial factor for success of leprosy control. Key responsibility of WHO is to provide technical assistance and since 1950s WHO has spearheaded consultations, discussions and research in defining leprosy control strategies at global level and facilitated development of strategies for different national programs. The evolution of global leprosy strategies demonstrates adaptation of relevant technical advancements in accordance with the epidemiology of the disease. Leprosy control was based on containment of infection through isolation of patients for ages till the introduction of Dapsone in early 1950s. For over 30 years, the disease control progressed on Dapsone monotherapy showing hope to many patients requiring treatment. Recognition of resistance to Dapsone led to the introduction of MDT in the early 1980s. MDT besides being robust, has reduced the duration of treatment considerably and thereby resulting in a vast reduction of prevalence. Recognizing the achievement of leprosy programs worldwide, the 44th World Health Assembly (WHA), adopted in May 1991, a resolution to eliminate leprosy as a public health problem by the year 2000. Elimination of leprosy as a public health problem has been defined as prevalence rate of the disease to less than 1 case per 10,000 people. Most of the countries have achieved the goal of elimination, and India reached the set goal in December 2005.[6]

WHO, in continuum to previous global leprosy strategies, brought out two global strategies since 2006, essentially focusing on further reducing the disease burden due to leprosy, in consultation with national programs of member states, partner organizations and donors. Detection of all cases in a community and completion of prescribed MDT were rather the basic tenets of the 'Enhanced Global Strategy' for further reducing disease burden due to leprosy—2011-2015, which is currently guiding the national leprosy programs globally. The 'Enhanced Global Strategy' was developed in 2009, in consultation with national program managers, partners in leprosy program like International Federation of Anti-leprosy Associations (ILEP) and representatives of the people affected by leprosy. Sustaining expertise and further improving number of skilled leprosy staff was another facet of the strategy. Besides reduction of disease burden, the strategy also emphasized on improving participation of persons affected, in leprosy services and reduction of stigma against the disease.

MEASURE FOR DISEASE BURDEN DUE TO LEPROSY

Many indicators and changes in situations related to leprosy can be used for measuring the disease burden. The Enhanced Global Strategy for further reducing disease burden (2011-2015) has many indicators, such as those for monitoring progress; case detection and patient management as a target. Targets should have epidemiological and operational considerations. Targets provide accountability and enable program planning. They are important for political commitment and securing resources. However, there is a potential for misuse as data may be manipulated. Thus, a target should be robust, and should have means in place to check the validity of the target. A key feature of the target is that it must have been obtained by consensus, and be owned by the community and populations concerned. In addition, a target should be evidence based, realistic, attainable, reasonable, measurable and valid, and linked to implementation. Targets are tools for influencing policy. Among the various options, choosing for leprosy, the target of reducing new cases with grade 2 disabilities (G2D) per 100,000 population is challenging. The rationale for choosing the target is as follows:

- It promotes early case detection. This reduces delay in diagnosis, and thus has an impact on disability and transmission.

- It addresses concern about under detection.
- It reduces stigma and discrimination.
- It reduces service costs of disability care and rehabilitation.
- It promotes prevention of disability (POD) activities.
- It promotes collaboration.
- It is a robust measure.
- It is acceptable to partners and to those affected by leprosy.

Thus, it has been proposed to have not just a target but also a time scale (2011-2015), which will coincide with the timeframe of the UN Millennium Development Goals (MDGs). Programs can make adjustments and pay more attention to early case detection and POD activities. The enhanced global strategy set a target of reducing new cases with visible deformity or grade 2 disabilities (G2D) per 100,000 people by 35% by 2015 compared to the G2D rate of 2010. WHO expert committee on leprosy, a body of internationally recognized experts, in its eighth report, recommended a target of incidence of new cases with grade 2 disabilities or visible deformities among new cases to less than one case per million population by the year 2020.

For Leprosy, the vision, goal, target and indicators could be synopsized as follows:

Vision: A world without leprosy.

Goal: Dramatically reduce the global burden of leprosy by 2015 in line with **Millennium Development Goals** (MDGs).

Target: Linked to the MDGs and endorsed by National Program Managers, WHO, International Federation of Anti-leprosy Association (ILEP), The Nippon Foundation, Novartis Foundation for sustainable development, International Association for Integration, Dignity and Economic Advancement (IDEA)
To reduce rate of new cases with Grade-2 disabilities by at least 35% by 2015.

Indicators:

- New case detection: Number of new cases, proportion of cases with G2D, proportion of children, proportion of multibacillary (MB) disease and proportion of women.
- Quality of patient management: Treatment completion, proportion of correct diagnosis, proportion of treatment defaulters, number of relapses, proportion of new disability.

REMAINING CHALLENGES IN FURTHER REDUCING THE DISEASE BURDEN

Although considerable progress has been made in controlling and reducing the disease burden in medical terms, much needs to be done to reduce the disease burden due to physical, mental and socioeconomic consequences of leprosy on the affected individuals and communities. The major challenges being currently faced are:

- Removing sense of complacency that seems to have set in control programs after initial success.
- In most endemic countries referral systems are weak.

- Developing effective tools/tests to detect cases early, including tools/tests for early recognition and management of leprosy reactions.
- Much needs to be done in the field of prevention of disabilities and rehabilitation.
- Improving information, education and communication (IEC) components of the program to be locally relevant, cost-effective and sustainable.
- Accessibility in the three major endemic countries- vast areas.
- Developing alternative treatment regimens to combat the threat of drug-resistance.
- Developing effective vaccines for the prevention of leprosy.

INTERNATIONAL LEPROSY SUMMIT

An international leprosy summit from 24 to 26 July 2013 was organized jointly by WHO Global Leprosy Programme (GLP) and The Nippon Foundation to get political commitment reaffirmed by countries, those that reported more than 1,000 new cases annually.

The snapshot on leprosy situation at the end of 2012 form annual statistics from 115 countries indicates marginal increase in new case detection with 232,857 new leprosy cases worldwide and 14,409 with visible deformities among them. Comparison with previous years does not show significant deviation statistically barring detection of 6,231 more new cases. Nevertheless, the trend of new cases detection for the past 5 years shows that 15 to 20 countries report more than 1,000 cases and 95% of leprosy is limited to these countries. It is prudent to note that India in South East Asia contributes to 58% of global new case load. The 5-year trend also indicates a very small decline in new cases detection from 249,007[1] in 2008 to 232,857 in 2012.*

Observing the situation, an 'International Leprosy Summit' was conceptualized (24–26 July, 2013) by Dr Samlee Plianbangchang, Regional Director, WHO-South East Asia Region and Mr Yohei Sasakawa, WHO Goodwill Ambassador for Leprosy Elimination inviting participation of Honorable Ministers of Health from 17 endemic countries who reported more than 1,000 case annually, to make a statement and discuss, sign in and announce declaration at Bangkok in July 2013. The declaration and the statements vindicated the need for improved political commitment, allocation of more resources, and involvement of partners from different backgrounds and inclusion of persons affected by leprosy (Figs 3.3 and 3.4). The Bangkok Declaration is presented at the end of the chapter (Annexure 1).

The summit also discussed the situation of leprosy as on today in terms of figures and brainstormed on defining further strategies. Diverse factors, limitation of disease distribution to small number of countries, need for further

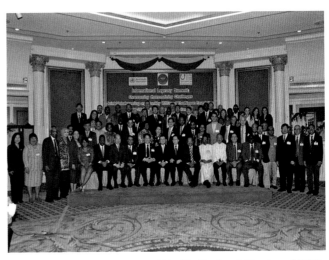

Fig. 3.3: Honorable Ministers of Health, Regional Director of WHO-South East Asia Region, WHO Goodwill Ambassador, members of Partner organizations in International Leprosy Summit–released Bangkok Declaration

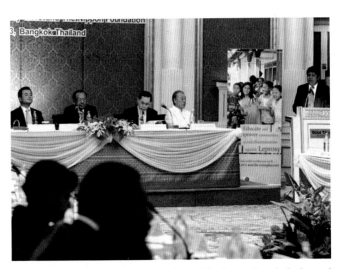

Fig. 3.4: Honorable Ministers of Health from Bangladesh and Thailand, Regional Director of WHO-South East Asia Region, Goodwill Ambassador and the Team Leader, WHO-Global Leprosy Programme are seen during the Bangkok Declaration.

improving preventive measures and continued need to support research were flagged up for further discussions to define global leprosy strategy towards leprosy free world.

The final conclusion of the Bangkok summit are presented below for ease of reference.

Conclusion and Recommendations: International Leprosy Summit

The Summit noted challenges facing countries in reducing the burden of leprosy. Such challenges include: reducing

*Leprosy update 2011; WHO Weekly epidemiological record 2nd September 2011, No 36 2011, 8, 389-400

grade 2 disabilities in new cases through early case detection; access to equitable and quality health care, including rehabilitation and referral systems; the need to strengthen human resources; raising awareness about leprosy; promoting leprosy, wherever appropriate, as an integral part of neglected tropical diseases; and reliable information systems.

- With a view to overcoming the remaining challenges, countries renewed their commitment to reducing the burden of leprosy.
- The commitment and contribution of national and international partners in overcoming the burden of leprosy was acknowledged, and the importance of further strengthening partnerships was emphasized.
- The Summit emphasized the importance of involvement and participation of communities and people affected by leprosy, including efforts to reduce stigma and discrimination.
- The Summit emphasized the need for adequate resources for supporting program implementation.
- The Summit recognized the continuing need for supporting research in leprosy.

Recommendations

The Summit recommends full implementation of the Bangkok Declaration—Towards a leprosy-free world—in all countries. While agreeing that reaffirming improved political commitment and mobilizing increased resources are essential for improving the program implementation, however, adopting local problem specific strategies at sub-national levels (provinces, districts, municipalities) to address diverse factors influencing leprosy situation in the 16 high burden countries is crucial at this juncture for further reducing the disease burden due to leprosy in accordance with Enhanced Global Strategy and recommendations of WHO Expert Committee on leprosy.[6]

NEED TO CHANGE THE IMAGE OF LEPROSY IN THE COMMUNITY

It is crucial to change the negative perception of leprosy and encourage patients to come forward for treatment as soon as they note a suspicious skin patch. The objective of information campaigns could be to raise the suspicion index in the community and to initiate an informed decision to seek treatment on appearance of such a suspicious skin lesion. The need is to bring in a paradigm shift in thinking about leprosy based on the scientific facts like curability of the disease and the misconception of linking disability with infectivity of the disease. These two achievements will gradually improve acceptance of leprosy as a curable disease and the disability management as an acceptable home-based care strategy.

It is time to improve the knowledge of the decision makers and responsible members in the community to change their impression about leprosy. It is particularly important for policy makers, judiciary and health professionals.

WHO developed Guidelines for strengthening participation of persons affected by leprosy in leprosy services is to promote greater involvement of the affected person and reduce stigma in the community. Meaningful involvement of persons affected by leprosy in programs will help in all constituents of leprosy program from detecting cases early enough to reducing stigma against the disease and to promote social integration. The participation of the persons affected will also help in operationalization of enhanced global strategy and policy formulation.

Inclusion of persons affected by leprosy and promoting community based initiatives are very promising practices which would give an opportunity to improve the leprosy control program and facilitate mainstreaming of persons affected by leprosy in the community. These two strategies in addition to continuing the MDT program will help all the countries to sustain the gains achieved and cross the last mile "Towards A Leprosy-Free World".

POLICY GUIDANCE BY WHO FOR MEMBER STATES NATIONAL LEPROSY PROGRAMS

WHO guides the member states in formulating technical policies to address key health issues and to facilitate implementation of national programs. The technical policy is laid down in the recommendation of WHO Technical Expert Committee on Leprosy, which meets periodically. The members are appointed by Director General of WHO to serve on the committee for recommending technical policies after debating on the prevailing situation of leprosy, globally and in different countries in the light of technical advancements stemming from research and development to make the leprosy program more effective so as to reach the set targets and goal of leprosy program. WHO Expert committee meetings on Leprosy are called by Director General, WHO depending on the need basis.

The recommendations of the WHO technical Expert Committee are published as WHO technical report series on leprosy and remain as key references for implementation of the program. The first WHO Technical Expert Committee Meeting was held in 1952 and the report was brought out in 1953. The meeting recommended abolition of compulsory isolation of leprosy patients and that leprosy control should be based on early case detection and ambulatory regular treatment of patients.

In further meetings, e.g. in 1965 WHO Expert committee advised that countries with limited resources should concentrate their efforts on treatment and follow-up on infectious cases and surveillance on their contacts.

Integration of leprosy services into general health services was introduced and it emphasized on regular availability of MDT at all health facilities.

The latest WHO Expert Committee Meeting on leprosy was organized in Geneva in 2010, which brought out its eighth report as 'WHO Technical Report Series 968'. The major conclusions and recommendations of the committee are summarized (see box) according to the four specific purposes of the Expert Committee Meeting.[7]

KEY MESSAGES ON LEPROSY

Raising awareness to focus on initiating response to early symptoms of leprosy and covering persons and population groups at risk of developing leprosy is the need of the hour in leprosy control. Materials to disseminate key messages about leprosy were available in different formats. WHO Global Leprosy Programme, carried out a study to define "Key messages" about leprosy. The document is the product of a systematic participatory field study to design the material

---

WHO Technical Expert Committee on Leprosy (2010), Eighth report (Technical Report Series No. 968)
Conclusions and recommendations

The global leprosy situation
1. The global leprosy situation is now best described by the patterns and trends in new case detection; however, caution is needed in interpreting these data and efforts are needed to continuously improve their quality.
2. Globally, and in most countries, there has been a steady decline in new case detection; the rate of decline varies between countries.
3. The age and sex, classification and disability of new cases vary considerably between countries for reasons that include epidemiological and operational factors.

Current status with regard to developments
4. The current strategy for leprosy control is based on early case detection and MDT treatment.
5. The uneven distribution of leprosy within countries represents an opportunity to focus on areas of higher endemicity as well as on underserved communities.
6. Surveillance of contacts through examination and education, with or without chemoprophylaxis, is increasingly important as the numbers of new cases decline.
7. Integration of leprosy activities into general health services, supported by referral systems including supervision is vital to further reduction in the burden of leprosy.
8. Standard MDT regimens remain the mainstay of leprosy chemotherapy, although there are second-line and promising new anti-leprosy drugs.
9. The relapse rates after MDT completion remain very low, but some Rifampicin-resistant strains of *M. leprae* have been identified; a surveillance program for drug resistance is therefore required.
10. Trials of treatment regimens using new drugs are recommended.
11. It is essential that WHO–funded drug trials in leprosy be reported in timely fashion in peer-reviewed journals.
12. To further reduce the burden of leprosy, research based in new molecular tools, improved diagnostic tests, improved MDT, studies of subclinical infection, and trials of prevention and treatment of reactions and nerve function impairment are recommended.
13. Support for operational, social and implementation research should continue because of its potential to improve the quality of leprosy services, particularly in community-based rehabilitation.
14. The focus on issues of equity, social justice, human rights, sigma and gender, together with the increasing contribution from people affected by leprosy is recommended.

Latest evidence and existing indicators
15. The main indicators to be used for monitoring progress relate to case detection, disability assessment and treatment completion, and these indicators are to be interpreted together.
16. The new indicator of grade 2 disability in new cases detected per million population is recommended as it focuses attention on early case detection, treatment and disability prevention; however, more operational experience is required in the use of this indicator.
17. The current treatment completion indicator based on MDT provision needs to be revised to reflect adherence to treatment through an end-of-treatment review.

Further reducing disease burden of leprosy
18. Maintaining high levels of BCG immunization in newborns is important in the prevention of leprosy.
19. Adoption by individual countries of the target to reduce grade 2 disability in new cases per million population by 35% between 2011–2015 will help to maintain commitment to further reducing the burden of leprosy.
20. A global goal of reducing the disease burden of leprosy to 1 new G2D cases per million population by 2020 is recommended to maintain long-term commitment through partnerships with governments, NGOs, communities, WHO, academia, industry and people affected by leprosy. This is to be a global, rather than a national goal.

and test it for acceptance in the general public. The theme lies in informing people at large that leprosy is curable, MDT is available at all health facilities and the early signs of leprosy, which should be prompting medical consultation.

The key messages document is enclosed as Annexure 2.

FURTHER STEPS IN DEFINING GLOBAL LEPROSY STRATEGY 2016–2020

The Enhanced Global Strategy for further reducing the disease burden due to leprosy (2011–2015) concludes in 2015. At this point in time WHO Global Leprosy Programme is planning wider and deeper consultations with all stake holders in leprosy program to define a new strategy covering the period, 2016 to 2020.

A mid-term review is planned during the year 2013-14 and consultation programs are being organized using a set of Terms of References to define the goal, and target for the plan period of 2016 to 2020. Feedback from consultations will be discussed in WHO Technical Advisory Group on leprosy initially, and then discussed with national program managers in different regions.

The information acquired will also be discussed in the light of recent technological advances in leprosy, operational challenges and with the current political climate. WHO actively promotes meaningful participation of people affected in leprosy services. In the area of stigma reduction and developing community-based initiatives, inputs on stigma reduction and enhancing participation of people affected will be sought from the organizations with necessary expertise, so that, it would be appropriately included in the next global strategy covering the period from 2016 to 2020.[8]

LIST OF PUBLICATIONS ON LEPROSY BY WHO GLOBAL LEPROSY PROGRAMME

Strategy and Operational Guidelines:
- Monitoring Enhanced Global Leprosy Strategy, 2012
- Enhanced Global Strategy for Further Reducing the Disease Burden due to Leprosy (Plan Period: 2011–2015)
- Enhanced Global Strategy for Further Reducing the Disease Burden due to Leprosy (2011–2015) Operational Guidelines
- Enhanced Global Strategy for Further Reducing the Disease Burden due to Leprosy: Questions and Answers
- Guidelines for Strengthening Participation of Persons Affected by Leprosy in Leprosy Services, 2011
- Monitoring Grade-2 Disability Rate and Applicability of Chemoprophylaxis in Leprosy Control, 2009
- Guidelines for Global Surveillance of Drug Resistance in Leprosy, 2009
- Leprosy Elimination Monitoring: Guidelines for Monitors, 2000

- Prevention of Disabilities in Patients with Leprosy: A Practical Guide, 1993.

TECHNICAL REPORT SERIES: WHO EXPERT COMMITTEE ON LEPROSY

- WHO study group introducing Multidrug Therapy (MDT).
- Question and Answers; Enhanced global strategy for further reducing the disease burden due to leprosy, WHO SEARO publication; SEA-GLP.2012.01.
- WHO Technical Report Series 968; Eighth report; October 2010.

WHO TECHNICAL ADVISORY GROUP ON LEPROSY CONTROL: MEETING REPORTS

- Report of the Eleventh Meeting, New Delhi, India, September 2011.
- Report of the Tenth Meeting, New Delhi, India, April 2009.
- Report of the Ninth Meeting, Cairo, Egypt, March 2008.

GLOBAL PROGRAM MANAGERS' MEETING REPORTS

- Meeting of Global Leprosy Program Managers, New Delhi, India, September 2011.
- Report of the Global Program Managers' Meeting on Leprosy Control Strategy, New Delhi, India, April 2009.

SENTINEL SURVEILLANCE FOR DRUG RESISTANCE IN LEPROSY: MEETING REPORTS

- Sentinel Surveillance for Drug Resistance in Leprosy: Report of the WHO Global Leprosy Programme Meeting, Cotonou, Benin, November 2012.
- Report of Meeting on Sentinel Surveillance for Drug Resistance in Leprosy, Hyderabad, India, August 2011.
- Meeting on Sentinel Surveillance for Drug Resistance in Leprosy: A Report, Tokyo, Japan, November 2010.
- Sentinel Surveillance for Drug Resistance in Leprosy: Report of the Workshop, Paris, France, October 2009.
- Report of the Workshop on Sentinel Surveillance for Drug Resistance in Leprosy, Hanoi, Viet Nam, October 2008.

TRAINING MANUALS

- Workshop for Health Service Managers in charge of Leprosy Control Programmes, 2008
  - Facilitator Guide
  - Participant Guide.
- I can do it myself! Tips for people affected by leprosy who want to prevent disability, 2007.

ANNEXURE 1

BANGKOK DECLARATION TOWARDS A LEPROSY-FREE WORLD
International Leprosy Summit–Overcoming the Remaining Challenges,
Bangkok, Thailand, 24–26 July 2013

We, the Ministers of Health from the 17 high-burden leprosy countries in all WHO regions, with relevant stakeholders, and the World Health Organization;

Appreciating the enormous strides made in the reduction of the global burden of leprosy over the past 25 years, including the attainment of the global goal of elimination of leprosy as a public health problem as defined in the World Health Assembly resolution WHA 44.9 (in 1991), to reduce the prevalence of leprosy to less than 1 case per 10,000 population;

Acknowledging the huge reduction of disease burden through the widespread implementation of multidrug therapy (MDT) among other prevention and control and care approaches;

Further acknowledging the contribution of all partners involved in leprosy work;

Believing that the long experience of the leprosy control program in achieving the goal of elimination of leprosy as a public health problem globally will be used to improve the interventions against other neglected tropical diseases;

Concerned, however, with the continuing occurrence of new leprosy cases annually in significant numbers in various countries and also with the continued existence of hyperendemic areas within countries that have led to the consequent stagnation of the leprosy situation over recent years;

Noting with concern the rising complacency consequent to perceiving the leprosy problem as relatively small, and that such complacency results in reduced political commitment, relegated priority, and decreased resources towards dealing effectively with this public health problem;

Recognizing the set target in the current enhanced global strategy for further reducing the disease burden due to leprosy (2011–2015), following the recommendations of the WHO Expert Committee on Leprosy in its eighth report, and considering the World Health Assembly resolution WHA 66.12 (2013), on Neglected Tropical Diseases, which includes leprosy, and that urges Member States to implement the WHO roadmap for accelerating the work to overcome the global impact of such diseases;

We, the Ministers of Health from the 17 high-burden leprosy countries in all WHO regions, with relevant stakeholders, and the World Health Organization;

1. *Declare* that it is time for the leprosy-endemic countries, as well as their international and national partners, to reaffirm their commitments and reinforce their participation towards addressing leprosy in order to ensure a leprosy-free world at the earliest;

2. *Urge* governments and all interested parties to accord higher priority for activities towards a leprosy-free world, and allocate increased resources in the coming years, in a sustainable manner, and in doing so:
   a. Aim to reduce the burden of leprosy and ultimately move towards a leprosy-free world;
   b. Apply special focus on high-endemic geographic areas within countries through vigorous and innovative approaches towards timely case detection and treatment completion aiming to achieve leprosy elimination as a public health problem at subnational levels;
   c. Achieve the global target of reducing the occurrence of new cases with visible deformity (grade 2 disability) to less than one case per million population by the year 2020;
   d. Prevent occurrence of disability through early detection as well as limiting disabilities among already disabled persons;
   e. Involve communities and the forums of persons affected by leprosy in the process of strategy formulation and implementation of leprosy care, including physical, social and economic rehabilitation and social integration, as per WHO guidelines[1];
   f. Promote empowerment of persons affected by leprosy and ensure effective implementation of United Nations resolutions A/RES/65/215, Elimination of Discrimination Against Persons Affected by Leprosy and their Family Members, and A/HRC/15/30 Principles and Guidelines for the Elimination of Discrimination against Persons Affected by Leprosy and their Family Members.
   g. Monitor the progress towards attainment of targets through a mechanism at the national level with technical support from WHO and other relevant partners;

3. Reaffirm our political commitment and guidance towards a world free of leprosy.

Bangkok, 24 July 2013

WEEKLY EPIDEMIOLOGICAL RECORD (WER)

- Annual leprosy statistics:
  - WER, 88, No. 35, 30 August 2013: Global leprosy: update on the 2012 situation.
  - WER, 87, No.34, 24 August 2012: Global leprosy situation, 2012.
  - WER, 86, No.36, 2 September 2011: Leprosy update, 2011.
  - WER, 85, No.35, 27 August 2010: Global leprosy situation, 2010.
  - WER, 85, No.6, 5 February 2010: Leprosy fact sheet (revised February 2010).
  - WER, 84, No.33, 14 August 2009: Global leprosy situation, 2009.
  - WER, 83, No.33, 15 August 2008: Global leprosy situation, 2008.

ANNEXURE 2

WHO GLOBAL LEPROSY PROGRAMME

Leprosy is curable

Free treatment is available at health centres

Leprosy is caused by a germ.
It is not a curse.
It is not hereditary.

Casual touch, like shaking hands or playing together or working in the same office, will not transmit or spread leprosy.

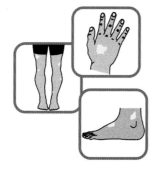

Leprosy usually starts as a patch without sensation
- **no feeling of touch and pain**
- **can be anywhere on the body.**

It is important to see a health worker or a doctor as soon as you notice any of these skin changes.

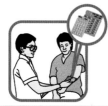

Leprosy can be cured with medicines within 6–12 months.
Multidrug therapy (MDT) taken regularly:
- **ensures complete cure**
- **prevents deformities**
- **stops transmission to other individuals.**

World Health Organization
Regional Office for South-East Asia

People affected by leprosy can lead a normal and dignified life like any other person.

- WER, 82, No.25, 22 June 2007: Global leprosy situation, 2007.
- Sentinel surveillance for drug resistance
  - WER, 86, No.23, 3 June 2011: Surveillance of drug resistance in leprosy, 2010.
  - WER, 85, No.29, 16 July 2010: Surveillance of drug resistance in leprosy, 2009.

- WER, 84, No.26, 26 June 2009: Drug resistance in leprosy: reports from selected endemic countries.

REFERENCES

1. Scott HH. The influence of slave trade in the spread of tropical diseases. Trans Roy Soc Med Hyg. 1943;37:169.

2. Dharmendra. Leprosy in ancient Indian Hindu medicine. Lepr India. 1940;12:19.
3. Ebbel B. The Papyrus Ebers. 1937, Copenhagen.
4. Anderson JG. Studies in the Mediavel Diagnosis of Leprosy, A thesis for the Doctorate in Medicine. Published as supplement to Danish Medical Bulletin 1969; Vol.16.
5. Lechat MF. The saga of Dapsone. Multidrug Therapy against leprosy, Development and implementation over the past 25 years. WHO/CDS/CPE/2004.05.
6. Sansarricq H, Pattyn SR. Improved Knowledge and new hopes; Multi Drug Therapy against leprosy, Development and implementation over the past 25 years. WHO/CDS/CPE/2004.05.
7. WHO Technical Report Series 968. WHO Expert Committee on Leprosy, Eighth report. October 2010. pp.53.
8. Guidelines for strengthening participation of persons affected by leprosy in leprosy services, WHO Regional Office for South-East Asia (SEA-GLP-2011.2).

Changing National Scenario, National Leprosy Control Programme, National Leprosy Eradication Programme, and New Paradigms of Leprosy Control

CM Agrawal, BN Barkakaty

PREFACE

Although leprosy has been known to be prevalent in India from antiquity, the disease received due attention when Government of India (GOI) started the Control Programme in 1955. Subsequently, with availability of multiple drug therapy (MDT) as a cure for leprosy, National Leprosy Eradication Programme (NLEP) was started in the year 1983-84. Since then, through different plan periods, the NLEP as a centrally sponsored scheme went through various stages of planning and implementation of different strategies. The program achieved an appreciable milestone in December 2005, when the prevalence of leprosy reached below 1 case per 10,000 population at the national level. Modified Leprosy Elimination Campaigns (MLECs) conducted between 1998 and 2004 helped in quickening the process of elimination.

After elimination at national level, the program continued with services provided in an integrated set-up through the primary healthcare system. Elimination at state and district level was aimed. New paradigms in leprosy control were brought in during 2007-08. The nongovernmental organizations (NGOs) played key role in the fight against leprosy. Partners like the World Health Organization (WHO), the World Bank, International Federation of Antileprosy Associations (ILEP), Novartis, Sasakawa India Health Foundation, Danida-Assisted National Leprosy Eradication Program (DANLEP), etc. also provided crucial support to the Indian program.

VISION

"Leprosy-free India" is the vision of the NLEP.

MISSION

The NLEP's mission is to provide quality leprosy services free of cost to all sections of the population, with easy accessibility through the integrated healthcare system, including care for disability after cure of the disease.

PROGRESS THROUGH DIFFERENT STAGES

National Leprosy Control Programme

The foundations were laid for the beginning of organized leprosy work in India with the establishment of the Indian Council of the British Empire Leprosy Relief Association in 1925 (renamed as Hind Kusht Nivaran Sangh in 1947). A committee appointed by the GOI in 1941 reviewed the extent of the leprosy problem in the country and made specific recommendations for antileprosy work. This was followed by another Expert Committee in 1954 that gave rise to concrete plans for the control of leprosy in India, including legislation. Prior to the launching of the National Leprosy Control Programme (NLCP) in 1955, though antileprosy activities were available in the country, they were primarily concerned with the treatment of patients, and were organized by charitable missions and nongovernmental agencies. The physical facilities available were far from satisfactory. It was estimated that, on an average, there was one clinic per 3 lac population, which again varied greatly from state-to-state. This, however, was undertaken by several independent agencies such as voluntary organization, religious institutions and charitable trusts without any plan and coordination to provide services on a rational basis. Lack of any organized efforts triggered off the governmental action to control the disease through the establishment of the NLCP in 1955, based on the recommendations of an Expert Committee.

National Leprosy Eradication Programme

The late Prime Minister of India, Smt Indira Gandhi, in her address to the World Health Assembly in May, 1981, made an appeal to all the developed countries, to help in leprosy eradication. While addressing a joint meeting of the Cabinet Committee on Science and Technology and Science Advisory Committee to the Cabinet in May, 1981, she again asked the Indian scientists to develop a leprosy eradication strategy. In pursuance of this determination, the Ministry of Health and Family Welfare constituted a Working Group to devise a new strategy and action plan for the control and ultimate eradication of leprosy. Dr MS Swaminathan, the then Member, Planning Commission, was the Chairman, and eminent scientists, leprologists and social scientists were the members of this committee.

Following the recommendations of the Working Group, it was considered that a stage had arrived for undertaking an eradication program for leprosy in the next 20 years, to achieve the goal of leprosy eradication by the turn of the century, taking advantage of the twin developments of great advances in chemotherapy of leprosy and extended reach of mass media. Consequently, the program was redesignated from one of controlling leprosy to that of its eradication.

The National Leprosy Eradication Programme was launched in 1983. The program passed through different stages with changes in strategy and focus as below:

Elimination Strategy

At the 44th World Health Assembly held in 1991, WHO and its member states committed themselves to eliminate leprosy as a public health problem by the year 2000, elimination being defined as prevalence below one case per 10,000 population. The GOI was also a signatory to this commitment. To enhance the process of elimination, the first World Bank supported project on NLEP was started in the year 1993-94, where the project supported the vertical program structure formulated by GOI for the high endemic districts, while in the moderate and low endemic districts, Mobile Leprosy Treatment Units (MLTUs) were established. The project was completed on March 31, 2000 with further 6 months' extension to complete the preparation of proposal for 2nd phase project. During this phase, against a target of 2 million cases, 3.8 million leprosy cases were newly detected and on the whole 4.4 million leprosy cases were cured with MDT.

The global target of leprosy elimination by end of the year 2000 was attained although prevalence rate in India in March 2001 remained at 3.7/10,000 population. The Second World Bank supported National Leprosy Elimination Project was started for a period of 3 years from 2001-02.

This phase was implemented with the objectives towards:
- Decentralization of NLEP responsibilities to states/union territories (UTs) through State/District Leprosy Societies
- Accomplish integration of leprosy services with general healthcare system (GHS), and
- Achieve elimination of leprosy at national level by the end of the project.

This project envisaged following strategy towards leprosy elimination in India:
- Decentralization of NLEP to states and districts
- Integration of leprosy services with GHS
- Leprosy training of GHS functionaries
- Surveillance for early diagnosis and prompt MDT, through routine and special efforts
- Intensified information, education and communication (IEC) activities using local and mass media approaches
- Prevention of disability (POD) and care
- Monitoring and evaluation on regular (monthly/quarterly/annually) basis as well as with special efforts such as independent evaluation, leprosy elimination monitoring, annual survey(s) and validation of progress towards leprosy elimination, etc.

Well-planned activities were efficiently implemented in close association of various NLEP partners, viz. State and UTs Governments, World Bank, WHO, ILEP, DANLEP, NGOs and Community, private medical practitioners and various concerned Government ministries/departments such as Information and Broadcasting, Social Justice and Empowerment, Education, Railways, Defence/Paramilitary, Labor and Industries, etc.

The 2nd National Leprosy Elimination Project successfully ended on December 31, 2004. Major initiatives taken during 2nd phase NLEP were:
- State leprosy societies (SLS) were formed in all the states/UTs except in eight small states/UTs where the HQ district leprosy society functions as SLS for that state/UT. In the country, all the districts were covered through 576 district leprosy societies (DLS).
- Release of NLEP fund as grant-in-aid to all the SLS and adequate quantity of antileprosy drugs (MDT) supply to states/UTs were maintained. Funds were also provided to the State Governments as cash assistance for maintenance of cost of vertical units created during the particular plan period and also through DLS for meeting the cost of other treatment activities.
- A nationwide IEC through mass media (TV, AIR, newspapers) was undertaken through M/s LINTAS (SOMAC) at cost of ₹ 11.32 crores. In addition, state/district leprosy societies were made responsible to plan, implement, monitor and supervise rural/local IEC up to periphery on continuous basis, while actively involving the *Panchayats*, village level functionaries, schools, women and other community-based organizations. Various community educational as well as advocacy activities were

in full swing throughout the country. A comprehensive IEC strategy had been developed for ensuring multilayered focused campaign in prioritized areas and issued to the states.

- Integration of leprosy services with GHS had been operationalized with daily availability of diagnosis and MDT of leprosy patients up to primary health centers (PHCs)/subcenters. Process of merging the existing vertical NLEP staff with GHS initiated.
- The general healthcare system (medical and paramedical) functionaries had been trained on leprosy (technical + IEC) in all the districts and urban areas in the country.
- Guidelines on Simplified Information System under NLEP were issued to all the states/UTs for their implementation by September 2002.
- The pattern of assistance for voluntary leprosy survey, education and treatment (SET) scheme had been modified (2004).
- All the states/UTs through their respective leprosy societies were equipped and empowered with all requisite guidelines, manpower and their capacity building, equipment and various procurements, etc. for achieving the national objectives of leprosy elimination by the year 2005.
- Strategy for implementation of NLEP activities in urban areas were developed and sent to the states for implementation.

At the end of the second project as on March 31, 2005, the prevalence rate was 1.34/10,000.

Modified Leprosy Elimination Campaign

Modified Leprosy Elimination Campaign approach was first started in India during 1997-98 with the objective to generate mass awareness about leprosy in the general population, to give training to the General Healthcare Service staff who were not involved for leprosy service delivery so far and to detect the hidden leprosy cases in all the states/UTs and to put them under MDT. The campaign was a roaring success and helped in detection of as high as 4.5 lac new leprosy cases who received treatment with MDT immediately.

Subsequently, four other MLECs were carried out in the country. New cases detected during the five MLECs were put under treatment with MDT. Details of the detected cases are given in Table 4.1.

These MLECs not only helped in bringing out 9.9 lac new leprosy cases for treatment and cure in a short period of time, but also in increasing leprosy awareness among the masses to a high level, which contributed in bringing out hidden cases of leprosy under treatment and reducing stigma to the disease. Further, these campaigns helped in capacity building of the general healthcare staff for their skill development in case detection which contributed to better performance

Table 4.1: New cases detected during the five modified leprosy elimination campaigns

MLEC	Year	No. of new cases detected
I	1997–98 (Jan-Mar '98) 1998–99 (April-Sept '98)	88,510 } 450,798 362,288
II	1999–2000 (Jan-Mar '00)	213,732
III	2001–2002 (Oct '01-Feb '02)	164,970
IV	2002–2003 (Aug '02-Mar '03)	104,184
V	2003–2004 (Feb '04-Mar '04) 2004–2005 (April-May '04)	46,806 } 57,702 10,896
	Total	**991,386**

under the integrated leprosy services provided by the primary healthcare facilities.

The changes in prevalence rate (PR) and annual new case detection rate (ANCDR) since 1993-94 in relation to the five MLECs conducted till the elimination was achieved in December 2005 are shown in Figure 4.1.

Final Push Strategy

The World Health Organization developed the Strategic Plan for the Final Push towards Elimination of Leprosy (2000–2005). The components under the strategic plan were:

- Reducing the reservoir of infection by improving access to MDT services.
- Curing patients and preventing suffering and disabilities.
- Essential technical support.
- Phasing out.

In order to make a "final push" to detect and cure all the remaining leprosy cases in the World and thereby eliminate leprosy from every country by the year 2005, a Global Alliance for the Elimination of Leprosy (GAEL) was created in November 1999 with initiative of WHO. The first meeting of GAEL was held in New Delhi, India on January 30-31, 2001, under the chairmanship of the Union Minister of Health, India. The meeting recommended that the members of the GAEL collaborate in the true spirit of partnership in order to eliminate leprosy as a public health problem from every country by the year 2005.

The Government of India sets the goal of elimination of leprosy, i.e. to reduce the number of cases to less than 1/10,000 population by the year 2005, in the National Health Policy 2002.

Strategic plan of action (2004-05): During the year 2004-05, the program focus was shifted from states to high and medium endemic districts and blocks. A strategic plan of action was drawn up with the following focus:

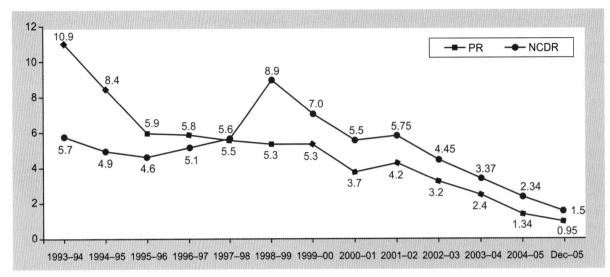

Fig. 4.1: Changes in prevalence rate and annual new case detection rate (1993-94 to Dec 2005)

- Intensified focused action with strong supervisory support in 72 high priority districts with PR greater than 5/10,000 and 16 moderately endemic districts but with more than 2,000 leprosy cases detected during 2003-04.
- Increased efforts put on IEC, Training and Integrated Service Delivery in identified high endemic localities of 86 medium priority districts.
- In 836 blocks in the country with PR greater than 5/10,000 as on March 31, 2004, a 2-week long Block Leprosy Awareness Campaign was conducted through intensified IEC and through leprosy counseling centers at subcenter level during the period October-December 2004 to ensure follow-up of existing leprosy patients and self-reporting of new cases.

The outcomes of the strategic plan of action (2004-05) were very encouraging as indicated below:

Indicators	March 2004	March 2005
States achieved elimination	17	24
Districts with PR >5/10,000	72	7
Blocks with PR >5/10,000	836	150

As a result of the hard work and meticulously planned and executed activities, the country achieved the goal of elimination of leprosy as a public health problem, defined as less than 1 case per 10,000 population, at the national level in the month of December, 2005. As on December 31, 2005, PR recorded in the country was 0.95/10,000 population.

New Paradigms in Leprosy Control

Post-elimination, NLEP needed to expand the scope of leprosy services provided to the patients, their families and community at large. The aims and objectives under the 11th Plan (2007–2012) call for further reducing the leprosy burden in the country, provide quality leprosy services, enhance disability prevention and medical rehabilitation (DPMR), increase advocacy towards reduction of stigma and stop discrimination and strengthen monitoring and supervision. These objectives are also in conformity with the global strategy issued by WHO (2006–2010).

In view of the need to sustain leprosy services for many years to come, there has to be a shift from a campaign like elimination approach, towards the long-term process of sustaining integrated high-quality leprosy services, which in addition to case detection and treatment with multidrug therapy, also include POD and rehabilitation. There was an opportunity for this process to build on the gains made by the elimination campaigns, such as increased awareness of leprosy, political commitment and involvement of general health services.

To get the program move in the desired direction, the new paradigms in NLEP were started in the year 2007, which have the following components:
- Burden of leprosy
  - Incidence of disease (case detection rate)
  - Registered prevalence of disease
  - Persons with leprosy-related disability.
- Improving quality of services
  - Accessible to all who need them
  - Patient-centered and protect rights of the patient
  - Address each aspect of case management
  - Follow the principles of equity and social justice.
- Integration of leprosy services with PHC system for sustainability
  - General healthcare system takes full responsibility
  - Creating community awareness about the disease, its curability and availability of MDT services in the integrated set-up.

- Referral services and long-term care
  - Good linkage of peripheral level staff with referral units
  - Good linkage of referral level staff with specialist clinics
  - More emphasis on long-term care.
- Improving community awareness and involvement
  - Information, education and communication should encourage self-reporting of new cases and reduce stigma and discrimination
  - Active involvement of community through involvement of *Panchayati Raj* institutions and village health and sanitation committees.
- Prevention and management of impairment and disabilities
  - Reassessment of persons living with leprosy-related disabilities needed
  - These persons should have access to services through programs dealing with other disabling diseases
  - Use of locally produced and esthetically acceptable footwear.
- Support of National Rural Health Mission (NRHM).

Under the NRHM, institutional mechanisms have been created at each level to support national health programs and improve delivery of healthcare services. At village level, there are multistakeholders—village health and sanitation committee to decide the health priorities in the village and their appropriate solution. There is also an accredited social health activist (ASHA) for every village. She is a female volunteer belonging to the same village, selected by the community. ASHA could be utilized for early detection of suspected cases of leprosy, referral of such cases to nearest health center for confirmation and completion of treatment. *Rogi Kalyan Samities* at PHC, community health center and district hospitals are autonomous registered bodies constituted at each level to facilitate in management of hospitals and delivery of quality care to patients. *Rogi Kalyan Samiti* is authorized to procure drugs at local level in emergency, out of the funds available with *Samiti*. Lepra reaction in persons affected with leprosy is an emergency condition which can occur during the treatment or post-treatment period or at any other time, and requires immediate treatment with a complete course of prednisolone as well as other supportive drugs. Any delay in treatment of reaction may lead to further damage to affected nerves resulting in deformity/disability. Similarly, medical rehabilitation of persons affected with leprosy may be supported by the *Rogi Kalayan Samities*. District Health Mission which is chaired by the president of *Zila Parishad* may be helpful for advocacy of the program.

- Rehabilitation
  - Community-based rehabilitation
  - Ensuring inclusion of leprosy-disabled persons in Government scheme for disabled persons
  - Leprosy-disabled persons and persons with other disabilities to have access to general rehabilitation services and physical medicine and rehabilitation departments which are being established
  - Nongovernmental organizations providing service to leprosy-disabled persons should provide services to persons with other disabilities.
- Indicators for monitoring and evaluation
  - New case detection rate (NCDR) indicate effectiveness of disease controlling activities and estimate MDT requirement. Quarterly assessment of NCDR needed
  - *Treatment completion/cure rate*: Indicate how well leprosy patients are being served. Needs to be calculated separately for paucibacillary (PB) and multibacillary (MB) cases by cohort analysis
  - *Registered prevalence*: Temporary indicator—only for target of elimination.
- Additional indicators for case detection:
  - Proportion of new cases presenting with grade II deformities/impairments at the time of diagnosis
  - Proportion of child cases among new cases
  - Proportion of MB cases among new cases
  - Proportion of female cases among new cases.
- Indicators for patient management and follow-up:
  - Proportion of new cases verified as correctly diagnosed
  - Proportion of treatment defaulters
  - Number of relapses
  - Proportion of patients who develop new/additional deformity during MDT.

Eleventh Five Year Plan (2007-2012)

At the beginning of the 11th Plan, the country had ANCDR of 12.07/100,000 population. Prevalence rate in March 2007 was 0.72/10,000 population. Out of 35 states/UTs, only 26 achieved the level of elimination. Till then 487 (79.7%) of total 611 districts had also achieved elimination.

The status of elimination in states/UTs till 2007 is indicated in the maps given in Figure 4.2.

The NLEP program strategy under 11th Plan was modified in comparison to the previous plans, keeping in view the WHO Global Strategy, 2006-2010. The strategy under 11th Plan constituted of: (1) provision of high quality leprosy services for all persons affected by leprosy (PAL), through GHS including referral services for correction of complications and chronic care; (2) involvement of ASHA under NRHM for leprosy work; (3) enhanced DPMR services for deformity in leprosy affected persons; (4) enhanced advocacy in order to reduce stigma and stop discrimination against leprosy affected persons and their families; (5) capacity building among health service personnel in integrated setting both for rural and urban areas; and (6) strengthen the monitoring and supervision component of the surveillance system.

At the end of the 11th Plan, the country achieved ANCDR of 10.35/100,000 population. Prevalence rate in March 2012 was 0.68/10,000 population. Out of 35 states/UTs, 33

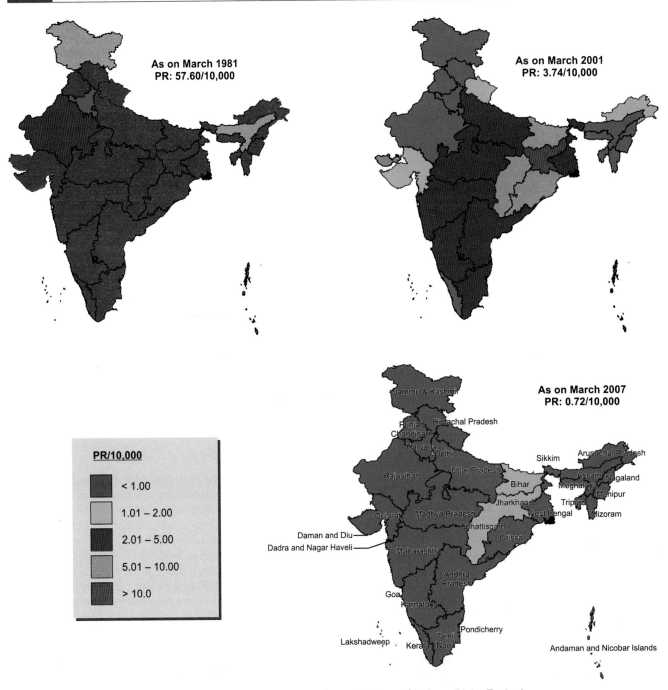

Fig. 4.2: Status of leprosy elimination achieved in 29 out of 35 States/Union Territories

states/UTs achieved the level of elimination. Till then, 543 (84.6%) of a total 642 districts had also achieved elimination. The map in Figure 4.3 indicates the prevalence rates as on March 2012.

Impact of the program activities during the 11th Plan may be summarized as: (1) seven states/UTs achieved leprosy elimination status; (2) ANCDR decreased from 14.27/100,000 in 2005-06 to 10.35/100,000 in 2011-12; (3) prevalence rate decreased from 1.34/10,000 in 2004-05 to 0.68/10,000; (4) treatment completion rate improved from 90.34 in 2006-07 to 92.93 in 2010-11; (5) reconstructive surgery (RCS) conducted on 14,373 persons affected by disability due to leprosy; (6) high endemic districts (ANCDR >10/100,000 population) reduced from 275 districts in 2005-06 to 209 districts.

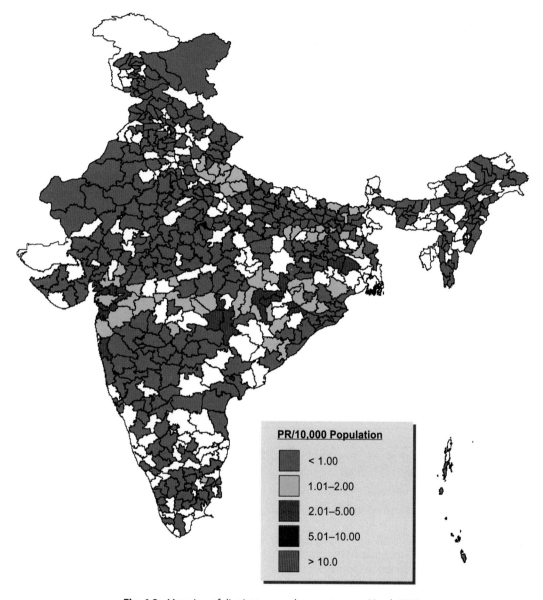

Fig. 4.3: Mapping of district to prevalence rate as on March 2012

Trends in new case detection and other parameters are depicted in Table 4.2 and Figure 4.4.

Trends in ANCDR and prevalence rate may be seen in Figure 4.4.

Current scenario (as on March 2013): After elimination, number of new cases has come down, but the disease is still prevalent with moderate endemicity in about 19% of the districts.

Thirty three states/UTs have achieved leprosy elimination status. Only one state (Chhattisgarh) and one UT (Dadra and Nagar Haveli) are yet to achieve elimination. Three states namely Bihar, Maharashtra, and West Bengal which had achieved elimination earlier have shown slight increase in prevalence rate as on March 2013 because of Special Activity Plan (SAP) 2012. Further, out of 649 districts, 528 (81.4%) have also achieved elimination level. In 2012-13, total 134,752 new leprosy cases were detected and put under treatment as compared to 127,295 leprosy cases detected during corresponding period of previous year giving ANCDR of 10.78 per 100,000 population. Among the new cases detected in 2012-13, the proportions were: MB cases (49.9%), female (37.7%), children (9.9%) and grade 2 disability (3.4%). For correction of disability due to leprosy, 94 institutions (Government 52 and NGO 42) have been recognized for RCS

Table 4.2: Trends in annual new case detection rate, grade 2 deformity and disability						
Year	New cases	ANCDR per 100,000	Cases on record	PR per 10,000	No. of Grade II deformity	Disability %
2005-06	161,457	14.3	95,150	0.84	3,015	1.87
2006-07	139,252	12.1	82,801	0.72	3,130	2.25
2007-08	137,685	11.7	87,228	0.74	3,477	2.53
2008-09	134,184	11.2	86,331	0.72	3,763	2.80
2009-10	133,717	10.9	87,190	0.71	4,117	3.08
2010-11	126,800	10.5	83,041	0.69	3,927	3.10
2011-12	127,295	10.4	83,687	0.68	3,865	3.04
2012-13	134,752	10.8	91,743	0.73	4,650	3.45

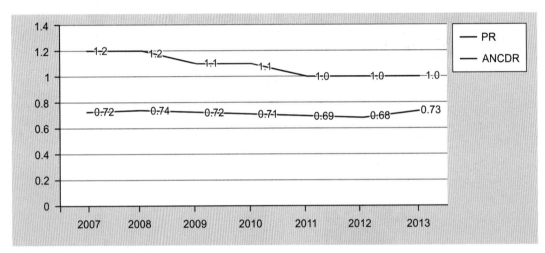

Fig. 4.4: Trends in annual new case detection rate and prevalence rates (2007–2013)

in the country. During 2012-13, 2,413 reconstructive surgeries were performed for correction of disability in leprosy affected persons. A total of 443 (68.3%) districts out of total 649, have ANCDR less than 10 per 100,000 population and 87 districts have ANCDR greater than 20/100,000. Only 14 districts with ANCDR greater than 50/100,000 population are in Chhattisgarh (2), Gujarat (4), Maharashtra (3), West Bengal (1), Dadra and Nagar Haveli (1), Orissa (2), and Delhi (1).

Challenges: The program faces a number of challenges to achieve the desired objectives; these can be clubbed as under:

- Technical
  - Slow decline in disease burden (new cases)
  - Increase in number of new leprosy cases in Bihar, Maharashtra, Chhattisgarh, West Bengal, and Dadra and Nagar Haveli
  - Reduction in grade 2 disability rate per million population in a few states only
  - Varied incidence of disease as well as the deformities associated with leprosy in different states/UTs, calling for State-specific attention.
- Operational
  - Decreasing priority at subnational level
  - Sustaining leprosy expertise at periphery
  - Poor quality through integrated service delivery
  - Early detection (voluntary reporting) in remote, tribal, hard-to-reach and insurgent affected areas
  - Treatment completion in urban area
  - Referral services at secondary level
  - Availability of dedicated staff at district level
  - Slow clearance of backlog for reconstructive surgeries
  - Delay in release of funds from State NRHM to districts resulting in nonexecution of planned activities.
- Social/economic/cultural
  - Stigma still exists even in educated and well-to-do families resulting in delayed detection

- Participation of persons affected (disabled) in disability services
- Closure of leprosy homes and colonies which keeps the discrimination to continue.

Twelfth Five Year Plan (2012–2017)

Keeping the above status and challenges in view, the 12th plan was prepared with thrust in achieving elimination of leprosy in all the districts of the country and reduction in grade 2 disability through POD and RCS.

Objectives of the 12th Plan are: (1) Elimination of leprosy, i.e. prevalence of less than 1 case per 10,000 population in all districts of the country; (2) strengthen disability prevention and medical rehabilitation of PAL; and (3) reduction in the level of stigma associated with leprosy.

Strategies of the 12th Plan:
- Decentralized integrated leprosy services through GHS.
- Early detection and complete treatment of new leprosy cases.
- Carrying out household contact survey in detection of MB and child cases.
- Involvement of ASHA in the detection and complete treatment of leprosy cases under NRHM for leprosy work.
- Strengthening of DPMR services.
- Information, education and communication activities in the community to improve self-reporting to PHC and reduction of stigma.

Strategic changes in the program: The disease also has a long incubation period and therefore, needs a longer period of surveillance. Since the program aims for eradication, i.e. zero endemicity of leprosy as the ultimate goal, sustained control measures need to be continued for some more time.

Certain strategic changes have been made in the NLEP during the 12th Plan period. These are:
- During 11th Plan, elimination of leprosy in all the State/UTs was the main objective. Elimination of leprosy in all the districts has now been planned.
- Case detection and treatment for further reducing leprosy burden was aimed till the 11th Plan. Focused attention in high endemic districts for ensuring elimination is planned during the 12th Plan. Active house-to-house search in identified localities in a planned manner is also a part of the SAP.
- Expansion of DPMR services was started during the 11th Plan period. Reduction in disability in new cases by early detection and complete treatment on time will be the focus along with increased correction of disabilities now.
- Strengthening of monitoring and supervision component within the GHS was practiced in previous plans. Strengthening of monitoring and supervision component in the high endemic districts with additional manpower support at Block PHC/urban area level is planned now.
- Enhanced advocacy to reduce stigma and stop discrimination was practiced during the 11th Plan. Focus will now be on reduction in stigma and discrimination through awareness campaigns and involvement of PAL as well as the community.

Result-based planning: The NRHM issued guidelines to the states/UTs regarding decentralized planning through district health plans. To make the NLEP plan more compliant to the NRHM guidelines, the states/UTs were advised that annual plans should be prepared as a result-based plan. The results to be achieved at the end of the 12th Plan are:
- Improved early case detection.
- Improved case management.
- Reduced stigma.
- Development of leprosy expertise sustained.
- Research supported evidence-based program practices.
- Improved monitoring, supervision and evaluation system
- Increased participation of PAL in society.
- Program management ensured.

Government support:
- The plan budget has been substantially increased from ₹ 219.00 crores in 11th Plan to ₹ 500.00 crore in the 12th plan.
- The states/UTs have been given power to ascertain their requirement and prepare their annual plan accordingly.
- Additional human resources for NLEP implementation in the state/district/block/urban areas have been provided under the 12th plan.
- The NGO schemes in NLEP have been introduced w.e.f. April 1, 2014 replacing the existing modified SET scheme (2004).

Partner support:
- International Federation of Antileprosy Associations provides support to the NLEP in implementation of the plans with aim to achieve the results. The Memorandum of Understanding (MOU) between the ILEP and GOI extending support till March 2017 has been signed on August 16, 2013.
- The World Health Organization also provides support by supplying MDT requirement for free distribution to all PAL and organizing annual conference for state leprosy officers.
- Novartis India also provides support in the field of DPMR, mainly through RCS, training of surgeons, free supply of grip aids for hand deformity and self-care kits.
- Other NGOs like the Association for Leprosy Education, Rehabilitation and Treatment (ALERT), India and the National Forum of Persons Affected also support the program through field activities.

CONCLUSION

The Government is aware about the fact that there may be more cases hidden than the cases reported voluntarily. During the 12th Five Year Plan, provision for two rounds of house-to-house search has been kept particularly in blocks identified by the states/UTs, in consultation with the partners in NLEP. The task is huge and the time is running short. Active support from all stakeholders is required to assist the states/districts in their planning and implementation, so that the desired results can be achieved in time. This will help the cause for reducing the disease burden in the country.

FURTHER READING

1. National Leprosy Eradication Programme (NLEP) in India, Status Report, 1985-86.
2. NLEP in India: Guideline for multidrug treatment in endemic districts, 1993.
3. NLEP in India: Guideline for multidrug treatment in non-endemic districts, 1994.
4. Report on the 1st Modified Leprosy Elimination Campaign under NLEP, DGHS, Leprosy Division, New Delhi, 1999.
5. Report on the 2nd Modified Leprosy Elimination Campaign under NLEP, DGHS, Leprosy Division, New Delhi, 2000.
6. Report on the 3rd Modified Leprosy Elimination Campaign under NLEP, DGHS, Leprosy Division, New Delhi, 2002.
7. Report on the 4th Modified Leprosy Elimination Campaign under NLEP, DGHS, Leprosy Division, New Delhi, 2003.
8. Report on the 5th Modified Leprosy Elimination Campaign under NLEP, DGHS, Leprosy Division, New Delhi, 2005.
9. Experience in Implementation of Modified Leprosy Elimination Campaign in India. Leprosy Review, 2000.
10. The Push towards Elimination of Leprosy, WHO Strategic plan, 2000-2005.
11. NLEP, Revised project implementation plan for phase II of World Bank support, 2000.
12. NLEP, Programme Implementation Plan (PIP) for continuation of NLEP from 1st April 2005 to 31st March 2007.
13. NLEP, Programme Implementation Plan (PIP) for 11th Five Year plan (2007-2012).
14. New paradigms in NLEP, Guidelines to States/UTs.
15. NLEP, Progress Report for the year 2012-13.
16. WHO, Weekly epidemiological record No. 35, 88; 2013. pp. 365-80.
17. NLEP, Programme Implementation Plan (PIP) for 12th Five Year plan (2012-2017).

EDITORS' VIEWS

Leprosy: Postamalgamation/Integration.

Leprosy services were integrated into the GHS more than a decade ago. Subsequently, there have been studies that have evaluated the impact of this amalgamation on leprosy services and control in India.[1-5] Most studies consider that integration enhances treatment coverage, while others felt that integration can affect performance negatively. Integrating the control strategies is believed to have the potential of minimizing costs, improving access, expanding coverage, ensuring equity and sustainability. Stigmatization has been a big hindrance to the control processes and integration of leprosy services into the existing healthcare system. Reverse integration or integrating other healthcare services into existing leprosy services could be a solution. By doing this, leprosy patients can have access to important services they need, such as eye care, counseling and rehabilitative physiotherapy from one point instead of going to general healthcare facilities where they feel stigmatized. There are opportunities for partnership and integration at many levels including surveillance, monitoring, drug distribution, treatment delivery, training, health information, health promotion, program evaluation and research. Greater synergy between leprosy and other tropical/communicable diseases by governments, NGOs, and international funding agencies can achieve greater efficiencies in the use of scarce resources. This also offers new opportunities for leprosy control to be more integrated with the control of other infections that experience similar challenges.

Integration of leprosy control activities with GHS has its own set of problems. The vast diversity in health and socioeconomic situations across states in India influences its implementation. Results from a follow-up operational research studies from India undertaken in 2006-2007 to assess the level of integration, on predetermined indicators related to referral services, training of health functionaries, availability of diagnostics, treatment, MDT dispersal and counseling guidelines in health facilities, recording and reporting by GHS staff, MDT stock management and involvement of health subcenters in different Indian provinces, show low training levels of medical officers and lower training levels of multipurpose workers leading to missed cases, problems of shortage of medicines, nonavailability of MDT in the nearest subcenter, lack of staff, no counseling guidelines in many centers and involvement of subcenters, in case referral, recording and dispensing MDT was nil to poor in some states.[1] Other studies showed a significant increase in the mean age of registration, percent multibacillary (clinical criteria) and grade 2 disabilities in postintegration period.[2] Patients were concerned about limited clinic hours, long waits and delayed treatment.[3] Disabled patients indicated how they were troubled by stigmatization of their condition. Program managers mentioned limited support for needed research and some emphasized the potential threat of emerging drug resistance.[4] Another issue was attainment of the needs of the program versus needs of the patient which some feel are not fulfilled as some cases are missed by medical officers in GHS, and if the missed case is of MB, it may be a cause of more problems in the future.[6]

However, in majority of the areas, the proportion of bacteriological positive cases did not change, which is a positive sign of effective coverage in the postintegration scenario in this population.[5] However, increase in proportion of cases with grade 2 deformities observed in tertiary care centers is a matter of concern and suggests continued need for referral hospitals for their management and also population-based overall assessment. Some experts have also blamed oversimplification of the management which has compromised the clinical services and led to pooling of these cases.[3] In the context of a declining disease burden, capacity development becomes important due to declining clinical expertise in leprosy. Adequate training of staff, an effective referral network, and supportive supervision are essential for timely and effective diagnosis and treatment of the disease and its complications. In the postintegration phase, leprosy is taking a back seat due to passing on the baton of managing the disease to general physicians, who have other "important" diseases to cater to.

Comments

With decreasing prevalence worldwide, adequate capacity and competence building in leprosy now is essential for the future of leprosy control. The objective has now shifted from prevalence of registered cases to reduction in new case detection and more recently to reducing disability in new cases. However, sustainability would be a challenge, as the problem appears to get smaller. With a shift from a well-supported, high-priority specialized program to one integrated with GHS, leprosy elimination too is facing problems of sustainability. The responsibility now lies with all aspects of the general healthcare system; however, active support and assistance is required from all stakeholders in planning and implementation, so that the desired results can be achieved in time. While integration of leprosy control with GHS has resulted in attainment of the needs of the program, certain aspects like hidden cases in the urban and remote rural areas need attention. During the 12th Five Year Plan, therefore provision for two rounds of house-to-house search has been kept particularly in blocks identified by the states/ UTs, in consultation with the partners in NLEP. The focus should be more on early detection of leprosy cases and curing them rather than on achieving the present elimination target. There is need for clear instructions, closer monitoring and supportive supervision at each level, district downwards, more so for PHC and subcenter, for successful integration. Focused research on interventions to reduce transmission and disability is the need of the hour. Pilot studies are underway to explore the ethical and logistic aspects of implementing chemo/immune-prophylaxis as an integral part of national programs and on the development of diagnostic tests and new vaccines. The most important step in eradication of any communicable disease is to knock out the last case. This can be achieved essentially by community participation for which vigorous IEC activities are required. It is only the enlightened public that can provide the solution to any social or public health problem.

However, unlike other infections, the impact of control programs for leprosy is limited due to many factors. Owing to its long incubation period, individuals incubating the disease may already harbor many bacilli, and these individuals might have transmitted *Mycobacterium leprae* to others (especially household contacts) long before their disease becomes clinically detectable. So, we have to be vigilant, otherwise we may face a situation like tuberculosis making a comeback with AIDS.

All stakeholders should strive for building capacity and competence. The roles of different levels of healthcare workers in leprosy control must be clearly defined and addressed accordingly. The following strategies would be helpful:[7,8]

- Development of national conceptual framework for leprosy control.
- Community mobilization in hyperendemic areas.
- Awareness program for primary health care.
- Linking leprosy control with basic dermatology.
- Needs-based, task-oriented training.
- Reliable expertise at national/regional resource centers.
- Continued political commitment.

In addition to all this, we should continue to conduct situation analysis and training needs assessment, review national guidelines for leprosy control, network with capacity building in basic dermatology and strengthen National Resource Centers for Leprosy.

REFERENCES

1. Pandey A, Rathod H. Integration of leprosy into GHS in India: a follow-up study (2006-2007). Lepr Rev. 2010;81:306-17.
2. Ganapati R, Pai VV, Tripathi A. Can primary health centres offer care to the leprosy-disabled after integration with general health services?—a study in rural India. Lepr Rev. 2008;79:340-1.
3. Pandey A, Rathod H. Integration of leprosy in general health system vis-à-vis leprosy endemicity, health situation and socioeconomic development: observations from Chhattisgarh and Kerala. Lepr Rev. 2010;81:121-8.
4. Jaeggi T, Manickam P, Weiss MG, et al. Stakeholders perspectives on perceived needs and priorities for leprosy control and care, Tamil Nadu, India. Indian J Lepr. 2012;84:177-84.
5. Daniel S, Arunthathi S, Rao PS. Impact of integration on the profile of newly diagnosed leprosy patients attending a referral hospital in South India. Indian J Lepr. 2009;81:69-74.
6. Singal A, Sonthalia S. Leprosy in post-elimination era in India: difficult journey ahead. Indian J Dermatol. 2013;58:443-6.
7. Oliveira MLW, Fernandes NC. Best practices: from a broad approach to field application on leprosy patient care. Paper presented at 18th International Leprosy Congress: Hidden Challenges. 16-19 September (L-001-pp. 41). Brussels.
8. Schmotzer C. Building capacity and competence for leprosy within integrated programmes. Paper presented at 18th International Leprosy Congress: Hidden Challenges. 16-19 September (L-002-pp. 41). Brussels.

SECTION 2

Basic Scientific Considerations and Pathology

CHAPTERS

5

CHAPTER

Immunogenetics of Leprosy

Rajni Rani

INTRODUCTION

Leprosy, caused by *Mycobacterium leprae (M. leprae)*, presents in the form of a spectrum of different manifestations. On one pole of the leprosy spectrum are patients with paucibacillary tuberculoid leprosy (TT) and on the other pole, we see patients with multibacillary lepromatous leprosy (LL). In between the two polar forms of leprosy, there are cases showing variable features of tuberculoid and lepromatous lesions, which could clinically be classified into borderline tuberculoid (BT), borderline borderline (BB) and borderline lepromatous (BL) forms of the disease. While clinically different manifestations can be easily recognized, there are demonstrable differences in the immune response against *M. leprae* antigens in the patients. Most healthy people exposed to *M. leprae* are resistant to the infection and with an effective immune response do not develop the disease.[1] On the other hand, while all leprosy patients show variable humoral immune response, predominant cell-mediated immune response (CMI), is observed in the tuberculoid end, i.e. TT and BT.[2]

Nerve damage is seen throughout the spectrum. One wonders, when the infectious agent is the same, why different people get different forms of the disease. Obviously, there are host factors which are involved in differential immune responses to the infectious agent, giving rise to differential manifestations of leprosy. Several recent reviews discuss the host genetic factors in leprosy and leprosy reactions.[3-8] There are several proteins/molecules, which are involved in the immune responses; these proteins are coded for by different genes which are polymorphic in nature.

Many patients with leprosy may undergo sudden activation of immune responses, affecting mainly the skin and peripheral nerves. These are known as the 'reactional states', which may occur before diagnosis, during treatment, or after MDT.[9] These reactions can be classified into type 1 reaction (T1R) or reversal reaction and type 2 reaction (T2R) or erythema nodosum leprosum (ENL). In T1R, there may be an acute inflammation of pre-existing skin lesions or appearance of new lesions and/or neuritis. T1R has been observed predominantly among BT, BB, BL forms of leprosy. ENL or T2R, however, is observed in multibacillary patients with predominantly Th2 immune responses, toward the lepromatous pole (BL and LL) of the disease.

The most common genes involved in immune responses, which have been shown to be polymorphic are major histocompatibility complex (*MHC*) genes, MHC class-I chain related genes A (*MICA*), transporters associated with peptide loading 1 and 2 (*TAP1* and *TAP2*), low molecular weight proteases 2 and 7 (*LMP2* and *LMP7*), cytokine genes, protein tyrosine phosphatase nonreceptor type 22 (*PTPN22*) and toll-like receptors (*TLRs*) to name a few.

When an infection takes place, the infectious agent is endocytosed by the macrophages/dendritic cells or the antigen presenting cells (APCs), and its proteins are processed and presented on the surface of the APCs in the context of MHC molecules. The peptides of the antigen (which have been processed after endocytosis) are presented by the MHC molecules in their peptide binding grooves to the T-cell receptor on T helper (Th) cells, which in turn secrete cytokines and activate B lymphocytes to become plasma cells or precursor cytotoxic T-cells, to become effector cytotoxic T-cells, and the immune response is generated, which may differ in type and strength depending on several genes involved in generating the immune responses.

GENES AND PROTEINS OF THE MAJOR HISTOCOMPATIBILITY COMPLEX

The human MHC, human leukocyte antigen (HLA) system is the most polymorphic system of the human genome with more than 9,500 alleles. It codes for glycoprotein molecules, which are expressed on all nucleated cells and are responsible for the recognition of nonself from self. The function of MHC molecules is to present exogenous and endogenous antigens in the form of peptides to the T-cells for subsequent immune response to take place. There are several genes for the HLA, which are tightly linked to each other in such a way that they are inherited en-bloc most of the time. A set of genes on a chromosome that are inherited together en-bloc is termed as a haplotype. *HLA* genes are located on chromosome 6p21.3 (Fig. 5.1). The gene map of the *MHC* region of man was published in 2006.[10] This is the most gene-dense region of the human genome and spans about four megabases (3,838,986 bp to be precise). At least 224 known genes are identified in this region with 128 known to be expressed; 40% of these expressed genes have immune related functions.[10]

There are two types of MHC molecules: MHC class-I and class-II, which differ from each other in their constituents as well as their functions. The MHC is the most polymorphic region of the human genome and this polymorphism is required for the survival of the species since MHC has a significant role in generation of adaptive immune responses against infectious agents and tumors.

Major Histocompatibility Complex: Class-I Genes and Proteins

Major histocompatibility complex class-I genes are expressed on all nucleated cells in the form of cell surface glycoproteins. The classical class-I genes in humans are *HLA-A*, *HLA-B* and *HLA-C*. Besides, there are nonclassical class-I genes *HLA-E*, *-F* and *-G*. Classical and nonclassical class-I genes are organized in the telomeric region of the chromosomal segment 6p21.3 (telomere → centromere *HLA-F*, *-G*, *-A*, *-E*, *-C* and *-B*) (Fig. 5.2A). The alleles of *HLA* loci are codominant. The classical class-I genes are very polymorphic with 2,365 alleles for *HLA-A* locus, 3,005 alleles for *HLA-B* locus and 1,848 alleles for *HLA-C* locus and these numbers are increasing with the discovery of new alleles everyday (Fig. 5.2B). On the other hand, nonclassical class-I genes are less polymorphic with only 13, 22 and 50 alleles for *HLA-E*, *-F* and *-G*, respectively.[11,12]

The MHC class-I molecule is a heterodimer of a heavy alpha chain (about 40–45 KDa) and the light chain beta-2-microglobulin (β_2m) of 12 KDa.[13] While the genes for the heavy chain of the MHC class-I molecule are encoded on chromosome 6, the gene for β_2m is encoded on human chromosome 15. The MHC class-I molecule can be divided into (i) membrane distal domains, (ii) membrane proximal domains, (iii) transmembrane domain and (iv) the cytoplasmic tail (Fig. 5.3), which are encoded by different exons of the gene. The membrane distal domains are two polymorphic domains, alpha 1 (α1) and alpha 2 (α2) domains, which are encoded by second and the third exons of the alpha chain gene; α3 domain, on the other hand, is membrane proximal domain and is encoded by exon 4 of the alpha chain gene. Exon 5 codes for the transmembrane domain, exon 6 for cytoplasmic tail, and exons 7 and 8 for the 3′ untranslated region (UTR). The α1 and the α2 domains form the peptide binding groove of the molecule. The peptides that are presented by the MHC molecules have allele specific motifs, which mean that certain peptides can be presented by certain MHC molecules. This is determined by anchors present on the peptide binding grooves where the peptides go and bind through hydrogen bonds. Specific motifs on the peptides determine which peptides would bind to which MHC molecule.[14,15]

For the antigen to be presented, it needs to be processed and loaded on to the peptide binding groove of the MHC molecule. Cytosolic or viral proteins are degraded in the cytoplasm by a complex of proteosomes called LMP2 and LMP7. LMP2 and LMP7 are involved in proteolytic degradation of the antigen into small peptides.[16-18] Simultaneously, the MHC class-I molecules are being synthesized in the endoplasmic reticulum (ER). The short peptides are loaded on to the newly formed MHC class-I molecules in the ER with the help of TAP1 and TAP2.[19] Now, the fully loaded MHC molecule is transported to the cell surface through golgi. An MHC class-I molecule without a peptide is unstable and degrades.[17,18] The fully loaded MHC class-I molecule presents antigen to the cytotoxic T-cells (CD8+ T-cells). As stated earlier, the peptides bound to different MHC molecules have allele specific motifs, this suggests that an immune response to a particular antigen depends on the types of MHC molecules present in an individual, which are involved in antigen presentation.

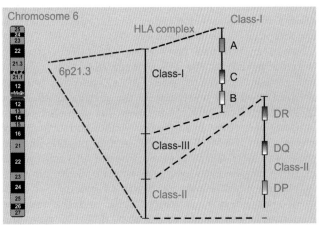

Fig. 5.1: Chromosomal localization of human leukocyte antigens (HLA) class I and II

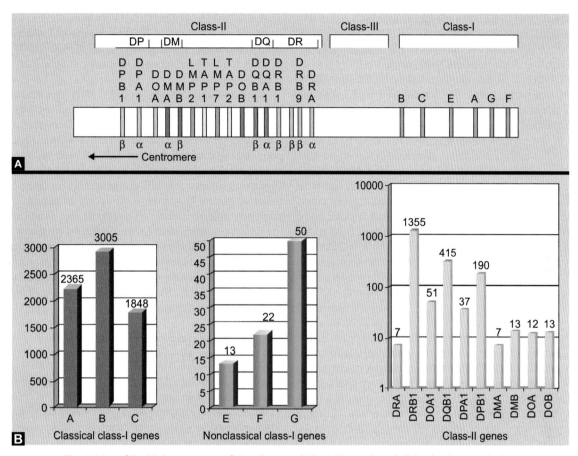

Figs 5.2A and B: (A) Organization of HLA class I and II loci; (B) Number of alleles for class I and II loci

Hence, some people mount a good immune response to the infectious agent, clear the infection and become immune to further infection, while others may develop the disease or develop chronic infection depending on many other factors besides the peptides of the infectious agent being presented by MHC molecules.

Major Histocompatibility Complex: Class-II Genes and Proteins

Major histocompatibility complex class-II genes in humans are *HLA-DR, -DP* and *-DQ*, which code for the HLA class-II glycoproteins. The MHC class-II molecule is a heterodimer of two polypeptide chains: an alpha (25–33 KDa) and a beta chain (24–29 KDa).[20,21] Unlike MHC class-I, both alpha and beta chains of the class-II molecule are encoded on chromosome 6 (Fig. 5.2A). *DRB1* gene encodes DR beta chain while *DRA1* encodes DR alpha chain with 1,355 *DRB1* alleles and 7 *DRA1* alleles. Similarly, *DQB1* and *DPB1* encode beta chains of DQ and DP molecules with 416 and 190 alleles, respectively, and *DPA* and *DQA* encode the alpha chains of

DP and DQ molecules with 37 and 51 alleles, respectively (Fig. 5.2B).[11] Interestingly, the MHC class-II region has several pseudogenes, which are *HLA-DP, DQ* and *DR* beta and alpha chains related genes. Besides, there are *HLA-DMA, DMB* and *DOA* and *DOB* genes located in the HLA-DR region with 7, 13, 12 and 13 alleles, respectively.[12] The HLA DR region on the chromosome is more complicated with 9 *DRB* genes starting for functional *DRB–DRB9*, some of which are functional and others are pseudogenes.

While HLA class-I molecules are expressed on all nucleated cells, HLA class-II molecules are expressed on APCs, like macrophages, dendritic cells, B cells, thymic epithelium and activated T cells.[22] The function of MHC class-II molecules is to present antigen to the Th cells. This is the initiation of an adaptive immune response. When a nonself antigen is presented to CD4+ Th cells, they get activated and secrete certain cytokines, like interferon gamma (IFN-γ) and TNF-alpha in case of Th1 cells, and IL-4, IL-5 and/or IL-6 in case of Th2 cells. While the cytokines secreted by Th1 cells in turn activate the cytotoxic T-cells, which have already seen the antigen in the context of HLA class-I, Th2 cytokines activate the B-cells to become plasma cells which make the antibodies against antigen they have seen. Thus, an immune response takes place, which varies in strength depending on the host factors and the peptides being presented.

The DR molecule is also synthesized in the ER. The alpha chain and the beta chains are synthesized and invariant chain (*Ii*) is attached to the peptide binding groove of the newly synthesized molecule so that no other peptide from the ER binds to the peptide binding groove of the MHC class-II molecule.[23] The alpha1 and beta1 domains of the alpha and beta chain constitute the peptide binding cleft of the MHC class-II molecule (Fig. 5.3). An antigen/infectious agent is phagocytized and a phagosome-lysosome fusion takes place where lysosomal cysteine proteases cathepsin S and L play an important role in degradation of the antigen into small peptides and result in epitope generation. The MHC class-II molecule gets synthesized in the ER and is transported through the golgi to the endosomal-lysosomal compartment where the *Ii* is degraded by cathepsin S and a small peptide of the invariant chain[23,24] called CLIP (class-II associated invariant chain peptide) is still bound to the peptide binding groove of the MHC class-II molecule. The CLIP is replaced by the antigenic peptide with the help of another MHC molecule called HLA-DM.[25] *HLA-DM* is also encoded on the MHC class-II region on chromosome 6 and has a very specialized function of editing the peptide repertoire to be presented by MHC class-II molecules. HLA-DO, which was thought to be negative regulator of HLA-DM, actually collaborates

with HLA-DM to optimize the epitope selection and thus it is a detrimental factor in final repertoire of the peptides that would be presented by the MHC class-II molecule.[26-31] Finally, the fully loaded MHC class-II molecule goes and expresses on the cells' surface.

There are about 50,000–100,000 MHC molecules on each cell. Most MHC molecules are occupied by self peptides and the T-cells are tolerized against them during thymic education. However, during infection a number of foreign peptides are presented by the MHC molecules and immune response takes place against them. Sometimes, the infectious agent may mimic the self-antigens and, in such cases, the infection is able to survive without any antagonistic immune response against them, resulting in the establishment of the infection. Sometimes, even with an immune response against the infectious agent, the infectious agent may thrive as the infection becomes more dominant as compared to the immune response and that depends on a lot of factors other than the MHC, like the cytokine genes and other genes involved in the immune responses.

NOMENCLATURE OF THE HUMAN LEUKOCYTE ANTIGEN

There are more than 9,500 alleles for different *MHC* loci. So, a system has been developed to identify the *MHC* alleles. Initially the HLA antigens were typed using serological assays when antibodies were derived from multiparous women who

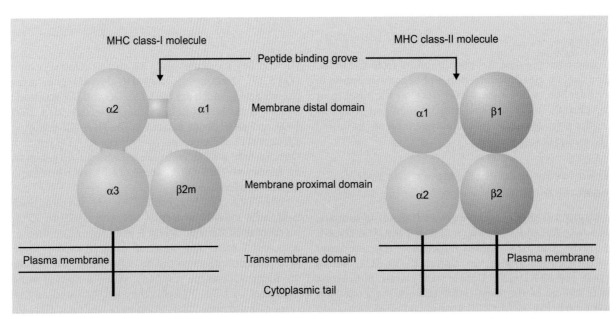

Fig. 5.3: Structural arrangement of MHC class I and II molecules, showing the alpha chain of class-I molecule with three domains α1, α2 and α3, domains which are noncovalently associated with β2m. MHC class-II structure has an alpha chain and a beta chain with two domains each: α1, α2 and β1, β2. α1 and α2 domains of the MHC class-I molecule make the peptide binding groove, which is the most polymorphic region of the whole molecule. For class-II, α1 and β1 domains form the peptide binding groove and α1 domain of alpha chain and β1 domain of beta chain are the most polymorphic regions of the class-II molecule

developed anti-HLA antibodies against their husbands' HLA antigens (since the fetus is haploidentical to the mother). At that time, the HLA antigens were given numbers like HLA-A1, A2, A3, A9, A10, A11, A19, and so on for A locus and HLA-B4, B5, B6, B7, B8, B12, B13, B14, B15, B16, B17, B18, B21, B22, etc. You will notice that the numbers after the A locus and B locus are not in continuation. This is because initially when HLA was discovered, the numbers were given to the antigens which were discovered in continuation. However, later it was discovered that these antigens belonged to two different loci, which were called HLA-A and B loci. The numbers remained the same but their locus was added before the numbers to clarify the locus.

Now, with the advent of molecular techniques, we know the sequences of these antigens and it was realized that each of these serologically defined antigens are actually a cluster of several alleles which differ from each other in certain nucleotide sequences. Most of the variability is seen in the second exons of the genes of *MHC class-II* loci and exons 2 and 3 for the genes of *class-I* loci, since these exons code for the peptide binding groove of the MHC molecules. So, based on the nucleotide sequences, the alleles are named after their serological counterparts. For example, if there are 10 alleles for serologically defined HLA-A1, based on their nucleotide sequences, the alleles would be called *HLA-A*01:01, A*01:02, A*01:03, A*01:04*, and so on. However, the nomenclature is slightly different for MHC class-II alleles. Both the alpha chain and the beta chain of the class-II alleles are polymorphic, so the nomenclature shows whether one is referring to the alpha chain or beta chain allele. For instance, alleles of antigen DR1 can be written as *DRB1*01:01, DRB1*01:02, DRB1*01:03* and so on. Here *DR* is the locus, *B1* stands for the beta chain gene 1 (since there are nine *DRB* loci, one needs to clarify the locus) and the number is separated by a star (*).

The first two numerals after the * show the serological specificity. The next set of digits is used to list the subtypes, numbers being assigned in the order in which DNA sequences have been determined. Alleles, whose numbers differ in the two sets of digits, must differ in one or more nucleotide substitutions that change the amino acid sequence of the encoded protein. Alleles that differ only by synonymous nucleotide substitutions (also called silent or noncoding substitutions) within the coding sequence are distinguished by the use of the third set of digits. Alleles that only differ by sequence polymorphisms in the introns or in the 5' or 3' UTRs that flank the exons and introns are distinguished by the use of the fourth set of digits. If there is an N at the end, it shows a null allele. Table 5.1 depicts how to decipher the HLA alleles. However, for all practical purposes we will be discussing about the alleles up to four digits only in this chapter.

HUMAN LEUKOCYTE ANTIGEN AND LEPROSY

With the above introduction, it will become easy to understand the association of HLA alleles present in leprosy

Table 5.1: Nomenclature for the HLA system: how are the alleles named[42]

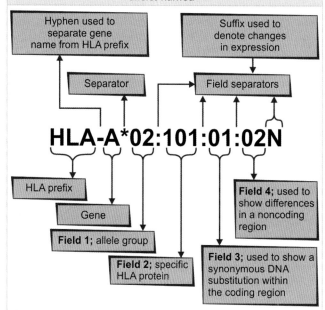

Nomenclature	Indicates
HLA	The HLA region and prefix for an HLA gene
HLA-DRB1	A particular HLA locus, i.e. *DRB1*
HLA-DRB1*13	A group of alleles which encode the DR13 antigen or sequence homology to other *DRB1*13 alleles*
HLA-DRB1*13:01	A specific HLA allele
HLA-DRB1*13:01:02	An allele that differs by a synonymous mutation from *DRB1*13:01:01*
HLA-DRB1*13:01:01:02	An allele which contains a mutation outside the coding region from *DRB1*13:01:01:01*
HLA-A*24:09N	A 'null' allele, an allele which is not expressed
HLA-A*30:14L	An allele encoding a protein with significantly reduced or 'low' cell surface expression
HLA-A*24:02:01:02L	An allele encoding a protein with significantly reduced or 'low' cell surface expression, where the mutation is found outside the coding region
HLA-B*44:02:01:02S	An allele encoding a protein which is expressed as a 'secreted' molecule only
HLA-A*32:11Q	An allele which has a mutation that has previously been shown to have a significant effect on cell surface expression, but where this has not been confirmed and its expression remains 'questionable'

patients. Several studies on leprosy have been done either on families with index cases of leprosy or case control studies. The initial studies on association of HLA with leprosy were done on class-I antigens. Most studies done earlier used conventional serological techniques and the results have been inconsistent.[32-39] However, A11 and B40 seem to be significantly increased consistently in a few of these studies in Indians.[39] In southern Brazilian population, an association has been reported with *HLA-A*11, HLA-B*38, HLA-C*12* and *HLA-C*16* with leprosy *per se*. Also, *HLA-B*35, HLA-C*04,* and *HLA-C*07* frequencies were different between LL and tuberculoid TT patients. However, the p values for these associations did not remain significant after adjusting for multiple comparisons.[40] In another Brazilian study, *MHC class-II* allele *HLA-DRB1*16* was marginally significantly increased ($p = 0.05$) and *HLA-DRB1*11* allele was reduced in the leprosy group, though not significantly.[41] However, this association also would not stand after the *p* value is corrected for multiple corrections. The major drawback in these studies was small numbers of samples.

Association of MHC class-II alleles has been shown to be consistent in almost all the studies. HLA-DR3 has been shown to be associated with TT patients in Surinam, Venezuela and Mexico.[43-45] Most studies show an association of HLA-DR2 with leprosy, *per se*. However, earlier studies showed association of HLA-DR2 with TT[46-48] while later studies showed an association of DR2 with LL as well.[32,38,49-57] Most of these studies were done using serological techniques. With the advent of molecular typing of HLA, one can study different alleles of DR2. HLA-DR2 has several alleles which are subdivided into two broad categories: *DRB1*15* and *DRB1*16*, which could be further subdivided into *DRB1*15:01, DRB1*15:02, DRB1*15:03*, etc., and *DRB1*16:01, DRB1*16:02*, etc. We studied the multibacillary leprosy patients consisting of lepromatous, BL and paucibacillary TT patients. The results show that while one of the alleles of DR2, *DRB1*15:01* was significantly increased in LL patients,[54,56] *DRB1*15:02* was significantly increased in tuberculoid patients[54,58] as compared to healthy controls. However, *DRB1*07:01* was significantly reduced in multibacillary patients as compared to controls and the tuberculoid patients who have similar frequency of *DRB1*07:01*, as in healthy controls.[54] A study in Argentinean leprosy patients, however, showed *DRB1*14:01* and *DRB1*14:06* to be significantly increased in leprosy patients.[59] Recently, *HLA-DRB1*04:05* has been shown to be associated with resistance to multibacillary leprosy in Taiwanese population.[60]

HLA-DRB1 genes are in linkage disequilibrium with or in simpler terms closely linked to *HLA-DQA1* and *DQB1* genes, which code for DQ alpha and beta chains, respectively. *DRB1*15:01* and *DRB1*15:02* are in linkage disequilibrium with *HLA-DQB1*06:01*, and *DQA1*01:02* and *DQA*01:03*. The product of *DQB1*06:01* gene forms the heterodimer with the products of *DQA*01:02* or *DQA*01:03*. We observed

DQA1*01:03 to be significantly increased in LL patients while *DQA1*01:02* was significantly increased in BL patients, suggesting that the products of alleles *DQB1*06:01-DQA1*01:03* and *DQB1*06:01-DQA1*01:02* present different peptides of *M. leprae* leading to differential immune responses and thus resulting in differential manifestations of the disease, i.e. LL and BL, respectively.[54]

As previously mentioned tuberculoid patients have milder form of the disease as they resemble the healthy control MHC profile at some places, whereas they also resemble the MHC profile of the LL patients. Interestingly, *DQB1*05:03* was significantly reduced in TT patients as compared to controls. This suggests that while the TT patients have predisposing MHC alleles, there are differences as well as similarities in their HLA profiles with that of healthy controls, which renders them to have good immune response against the infectious agent resulting in milder form of the disease. These data suggest certain fine differences involving *DQA1* and *DQB1* alleles which seem to separate the three subtypes of LL, BL and TT types of leprosy.[54]

OTHER GENES INVOLVED IN SUSCEPTIBILITY TO LEPROSY

MHC Class-I Chain Related Genes A

Major histocompatibility complex class-I region has another set of genes which are involved in innate immunity. These are *MICA and MHC class-I chain related genes B (MICB)*, which are encoded 46.4 kb and 110 kb centromeric to *HLA-B* locus, respectively. They are conserved in many mammals but are not found in rodents. MIC molecules are highly glycosylated, stress induced proteins with structure similar to MHC class-I molecules with three extracellular domains $\alpha1$, $\alpha2$ and $\alpha3$, one transmembrane and cytoplasmic domain. However, unlike MHC class-I molecules, they do not need β_2m to stabilize the molecule. $\gamma\delta$ T cells, NK cells and CD8+ $\alpha\beta$ T cells which express NKG2D receptor respond to MICA and MICB, and these may also contribute to innate immune response against mycobacteria. *MICA* and *MICB* are highly polymorphic with 93 and 40 alleles, respectively. A small study done in south Chinese patients suggested that an HLA-linked disease-resistant gene to LL is in strong linkage disequilibrium with the *HLA-B46/MICA-A5* haplotype.[61] Tosh et al.[62] have shown that *MICA*5A5.1* allele is associated with leprosy susceptibility in south Indians. This allele encodes a protein that lacks the cytoplasmic tail providing a possible mechanism for defective immune surveillance against mycobacteria.[62] A recent case-control study by do Sacramento et al.[63] assessed whether the MICA alleles influence susceptibility for leprosy or affect the subtype of the disease in a population of southern Brazil. They reported that *MICA*027* allele is associated with a protective effect for leprosy per se, while the *MICA*010* and *MICA*027* alleles are associated with protection against multibacillary leprosy.

Transporters Associated with Peptide Loading

The genes for the TAP are localized in the HLA class-II region. TAP1 and TAP2 have a very important function of translocating the peptide from the cytosol onto the newly synthesized MHC class-I molecule in the ER. *TAP2* has been shown to have three polymorphic sites at codons 379, 565 and 665, which result in eight *TAP2* alleles which are called *A, B, C, D, E, F, G* and *H*. *TAP-2B* has been reported to be associated with TT form of leprosy in north india.[64]

Cytokine Genes

Cytokines are the mediators of the immune responses that interact in integrated networks.[65] Single nucleotide polymorphisms (SNPs) at certain defined regions in different cytokine genes have been associated with differential expression of the genes.[66-70] A recent review by Jarduli et al.[71] discusses the literature available on association of SNPs in different cytokine genes in leprosy, which is briefly discussed as follows:

Tumor Necrosis Factor-alpha Gene

Tumor necrosis factor-α (TNF-α) is proinflammatory, pleiotropic cytokine produced by macrophages with its gene being localized on the MHC chromosome in between the class-I and class-II region, the class-III region. Certain *SNPs* in the promoter of the *TNF-α* gene have been shown to be associated with the amount of cytokine that would be produced, for example, at position *–308*, there could be either a *G* nucleotide or an *A* nucleotide. *–308A* allele has been associated with higher production of TNF-α while *–308G* allele has been associated with lower production of TNF-α.[67,72-74] However, several other studies did not find this SNP to have functional implications.[75-78] Kroeger et al.[72] showed that the elevated levels of TNF-α were produced by the *–308A* allele, when certain types of cells were stimulated with certain stimuli, and that was probably the reason for controversial results obtained by different investigators. In terms of association of the *–308* SNPs with leprosy too, there are controversial results. While in Indians from West Bengal and north India, *–308A* has been reported to be predisposing[79,80] for LL, in Brazil, Nepal and some other populations the same allele has been associated with protection from LL and leprosy *per se*.[81-86] However, these associations could not be reproduced in Karonga district of Malawi, Mexican mestizos and French Polynesian families.[5,87-89] TNF-α is an important cytokine involved in activation of macrophages, which in turn are involved in killing of the mycobacteria and also in granuloma formation, which helps in containment of the mycobacteria. However, these different results from different populations could be a result of differences in the genetic background of the patients and also different strains of mycobacteria infecting the patients. Hence, more studies need to be done to unequivocally show the role of this *SNP* in manifestation of leprosy.

Interleukin-10

Interleukin 10 (IL-10) is a regulatory cytokine involved in the regulation of inflammatory immunological reactions. Several *SNPs* have been reported in *IL-10* gene, which include $A^{-1082}G$, $T^{-819}C$, $C^{-592}A$.[90] There are contradictory reports again with respect to association of these *SNPs* with leprosy. While in Mexican patients there was no significant association,[89] *IL-10 -819T* allele and *TT* genotype have been associated with leprosy in Brazilian populations.[82,91] However, *IL-10-819 CC* and *CT* and *–592 CC* and *CA* were associated with leprosy in Colombian patients.[92] Besides these well-known SNPs, some other SNPs have also been studied in the promoter region of *IL-10*, which include $T^{-3575}A$, $A^{-2849}G$ *and* $C^{-2763}A$ in leprosy patients by Moraes et al.[93] and they observed that the haplotype *–3575A/–2849G/–2763C* was associated with protection from leprosy and from more severe forms of the disease. On the other hand, the *IL-10* haplotype *–3575T/–2849A/–2763C* was found to be associated with susceptibility to leprosy *per se*. The extended haplotype *IL10 –3575T/–2849G/–2763C/–1082A/–819C/–592C* conferred resistance to leprosy *per se* in Indian leprosy patients and *IL-10* haplotype *–3575T/–2849G/–2763C/–1082A/–819T/ –592A* was associated with development of severe form of leprosy. The role of *IL-10* promoter *SNPs* in Brazilian and Indian population strongly suggests the involvement of *IL-10* locus in the outcome of leprosy.[84,94]

Interleukin-12, Interferon-γ, Interleukin-4 and Interleukin-6 Genes

Interleukin-12 and IFN-γ are proinflammatory cytokines involved in CMIs; however, IL-4 is a Th2 cytokine which has a role in humoral immunity. IL-12 is a heterodimeric cytokine composed of p35 and p40 subunits and is required for induction of Th1 responses.[95] Polymorphisms in the genes coding for these cytokines have been studied for susceptibility to leprosy with variable results. While *IL-12 p40 3'UTR 1188 A/C* polymorphism has been shown to be associated with greater susceptibility to LL in patients from western Mexico,[96] no association was observed in Mexican patients from Sinaloa[97] and Korea patients.[98]

IFN-γ $A^{+874}T$ (*rs2430561*) has been associated with expression of IFN-γ with *T* allele, showing higher production as compared to *A* allele. *IFN-γ +874T* has been associated with protection from leprosy in patients from São Paulo and Rio de Janeiro, in two independent studies conducted by Cardoso et al.[99] On the other hand, no association of *+874 T/A* allele was observed in Chinese patients.[100] Wang et al. studied the *CA-repeat* alleles in *IFN-γ* and they observed that the alleles CA_{10} was significantly increased in leprosy patients with CA_{13} and CA_{15} being in significantly higher frequencies in multibacillary patients compared to the control group.[100]

Three polymorphisms in *IL4* have been reported which include $T^{-590}C$ in the promoter region, polymorphism $C^{+33}T$ in *exon 1*, and *variable number of tandem repeats (VNTR)* polymorphism in *intron 3*. *IL4–590TC* and *CC* genotypes and the *–590C* allele were reported to be protective from leprosy in a Chinese study.[101]

Since the expression of IL-6 was enhanced in both T1R and T2R,[9] three tag SNPs (rs2069832, rs2069840, rs2069845) were studied in leprosy patients from central Brazil and all three SNPs were associated with T2R, while no association of IL-6 SNPs was observed with T1R. SNP rs2069832 is closely linked to a functional SNP rs1800795 localized at the negative regulatory domain in the promoter region of IL-6, which was also associated with T2R. The C allele at both the loci were associated with T2R.[9]

Toll-like Receptor 1 and 2

Toll-like receptors (TLRs) are important cell surface molecules that are involved in innate immune response and recognize the pathogens through specific patterns, which results in facilitating transcription of certain genes that regulate adaptive immune responses. Since they provide the first line of defense against microbes, they have been studied in leprosy. Of the ten TLRs, TLR2 has been shown to control the production of cytokines, cell signaling and resistance to *M. leprae*. Kang et al.[102] have reported the detection of a *C* to *T* mutation in *TLR2*, resulting in arginine (Arg) to tryptophan (Trp) at highly conserved amino acid 677 in LL. Further, Kang et al.[103] reported that the innate immune response of monocytes against *M. leprae* is mediated by TLR2 and suggested that the mutation in the intracellular domain of *TLR2* gene is associated with IL-12 production in LL. Bochud et al.[104] subsequently investigated the role of TLRs in recognition of *M. leprae* and studied the significance of *TLR2 Arg(677) Trp SNP*. They reported an impaired function of the variant *TLR2Arg(677)Trp* which provides a molecular mechanism for the poor cellular immune response associated with LL and may have important implications for understanding the pathogenesis of other mycobacterial infections. Kang et al.[105] further studied the cytokine responses against *M. leprae* in peripheral blood mononuclear cells (PBMCs) with the *TLR2* mutation *Arg677Trp*. In leprosy patients with the *TLR2* mutation, production of IL-2, IL-12, IFN-γ, and TNF-α by *M. leprae*-stimulated PBMC were significantly decreased and IL-10 was significantly increased, compared with that in groups with wild-type *TLR2*. This observation suggests that the *TLR2* signal pathway plays a critical role in the alteration of cytokine profiles in PBMC from leprosy patients and the *TLR2* mutation *Arg677Trp* provides a mechanism for the poor cellular immune response associated with LL.

Interestingly, a follow-up study was done by Malhotra et al.[106] to study the role of *Arg677Trp* polymorphism in Indian leprosy patients. Genotyping results after direct polymerase chain reaction (PCR) sequencing showed that the *TLR2 Arg677Trp* polymorphism associated with LL in the Korean population was not a true polymorphism of the *TLR2* gene. They concluded that the so-called functional mutation has resulted from the duplication of *TLR2 exon 3* present approximately 23 kb upstream of *TLR2* and shares 93% homology with *exon 3* of *TLR2*. These results suggest that *TLR2* polymorphism needs to be studied with caution in future, because of the presence of variations in the duplicated (pseudogene) region representing *exon 3* of the *TLR2* gene. The absence of any variant in the conserved promoter and intracellular signaling regions of the *TLR2* gene in their study indicates a need to investigate other regulatory mechanisms which could control TLR2 function.[106]

Recently, Wong et al. conducted a gene-centric microarray study, where they genotyped SNPs in over 2,000 genes and identified TLR1 and HLA-DRB1/DQA1 as major leprosy susceptibility genes.[107] Krutzik et al.[108] investigated the expression and activation of TLRs in leprosy and observed that TLR2-TLR1 heterodimers mediated cell activation by killed *M. leprae* where, IFN-γ and granulocyte-macrophage colony-stimulating factor (GM-CSF) enhanced TLR1 expression in monocytes and dendritic cells, respectively. On the other hand, IL-4 downregulated TLR2 expression. Both TLR2 and TLR1 had stronger expression in the paucibacillary lesions as compared with the disseminated multibacillary form of the disease. These data show that regulated expression and activation of TLRs at the site of disease contributes to the host defense against microbial pathogens.[108]

Misch et al. reported a common human polymorphism in *TLR1* (*T1805G, I602S*) that regulates cytokine production when stimulated with lipopeptide and it also influences the cellular innate immune response to mycobacteria. They showed that the *1805G* variant does not mediate an inflammatory response to *M. leprae in vitro* and that this polymorphism is associated with protection from reversal reaction.[109] *1805G* allele has been shown to be protective against leprosy *per se* in two additional studies from India and Turkey.[107,110] An additional *SNP in TLR1* gene at amino acid position 248 (rs4833095) which causes a substitution of asparagine to serine (N248S) has been studied. In this study from Bangladesh, homozygous genotype SS was more frequent and the heterozygous SN genotype was less frequent in patients with leprosy than in control subjects.[111]

An association of reversal reaction (T1R) with a *SNP in TLR2* at position +597 C/T (*rs3804099*) and a microsatellite located between 162–100 bp upstream of the start codon have been reported in three ethnic groups from Ethiopia. While *+597T* allele has been shown to be protective, homozygosity for the 280 bp allelic length of the microsatellite strongly increased the risk of T1R or reversal reaction in all three ethnic groups.[112] Misch et al. studied a common polymorphism in *TLR1* ($T^{1805}G$) and reported that *1805G* variant (rs5743618) is associated with protection from reversal reaction.[109] Additionally, TLR1, N248S (*rs4833095*) has been shown to be associated with reversal reactions and/or ENL reactions, with serine coding allele to be protective in Bangladeshi population, although the sample size for T2R cases in this study was too small.[111]

Vitamin D Receptor

Vitamin D receptor (VDR) is a ligand dependent transcription factor that belongs to the super family of the nuclear hormone receptors.[113] The ligand for VDR is vitamin D_3, i.e. 1,25-$(OH)_2D_3$, which mediates its biological actions through VDR. Binding of 1,25-$(OH)_2D_3$ induces conformational changes in VDR, which promotes its heter-dimerization with retinoid X receptor (RXR), followed by translocation of this complex into the nucleus. The RXR-VDR heterodimer binds to the vitamin D_3 responsive elements (VDRE) in promoter regions of 1,25-$(OH)_2D_3$ responsive genes,[114] which in turn results in the regulatory function of 1,25-$(OH)_2D_3$. In the absence of classical responsive elements, 1,25-$(OH)_2D_3$ may control the expression of some genes, like cytokine genes, by targeting inducible transcription factors like *NFAT* in IL-2 in a sequence specific manner.[115] 1,25-$(OH)_2D_3$ has been shown to have an important immunomodulatory role since it represses transcription of *IL-2*,[116,117] *IFN-γ*,[118] *GM-CSF*[119] and *IL-12*[120] and up regulates the production of Th2 cytokines IL-4 and TGF-β1,[121] thereby inhibiting the overall Th1 responses. It has been shown to enhance the development of Th2 cells via a direct effect on naive CD4 cells.[114] Besides, 1,25-$(OH)_2D_3$ has also been shown to modulate the expression of *HLA class-II* alleles on monocytes and human bone cells[122-124] *VDR* gene is localized on chromosome 12q 13–14 with several *SNPs*, which include the T > C *SNP* in *exon 2* initiation codon detected with *FokI* restriction enzyme,[125] the A > G *SNP* detected with *Bsm*[126] and G > T *SNP* detected with *Apa*[127] located in *intro 8*, and a silent C > T *SNP*[128] detected with *TaqI*, located in *exon 9*. The alleles of the SNPs are named based on the presence or absence of the restriction site. For example, presence of restriction site for *Fok1* is denoted by *"f"* while absence of restriction is denoted by *"F"*, similarly presence of the restriction site for *Taq1* is denoted by *"t"* while its absence is denoted as *"T"*. Roy et al.[129] have reported an association of genotype *"tt"* with tuberculoid and *"TT"* with LL. Fitness et al.[87] reported that in Karonga the *"tat"* genotype was associated with susceptibility to leprosy *per se*. In Mali and Nepal, no association was found for the *VDR* genotype with either LL or TT or leprosy *per se*.[86] Goulart et al. observed an association between *"t"* allele and negative lepromin test and positive bacterial indices.[130] *FokI* and *TaqI* genotypes have been reported to be independent determinants of *VDR* mRNA and protein levels.[131] More functional studies are required to be done to establish the role of *VDR* gene in manifestations of leprosy.

Natural Resistance Associates Macrophage Protein 1 or Solute Carrier Family 11 Member 1

Natural resistance associates macrophage protein 1 encoded by *NRAMP1* gene maps to chromosome 2q35 and influences the antimicrobial activity of macrophages. Abel et al.[132] reported segregation of *NRAMP1* haplotypes into affected siblings was significantly nonrandom in 16 Vietnamese families, however, not so in four Chinese families. Similarly, in case-control studies from India[129] and Mali[133] no association of *NRAMP1* was observed in leprosy patients. However, in Mali study, a deletion of *4 bp* in the *3' UTR* was associated with leprosy type,[133] heterozygotes were more frequent among multibacillary than paucibacillary leprosy cases. Thus, variation in or near the *NRAMP1* gene may exert an influence on the clinical presentation of leprosy, possibly by influencing cellular immune response type.

A recent study on Brazilian population reported that *274 C/T* polymorphism of the *NRAMP1* gene may aid in determining the susceptibility to type 2 reactions among leprosy patients, since *274T* was associated with T2R and the presence of *274C* allele was associated with T1R.[134]

GENOME WIDE ASSOCIATION STUDIES

Numerous studies have been done on candidate genes based on their functions, however, many genes which may have a role to play in manifestations of different diseases may have been ignored, due to either unknown functions or not suspected to be associated with the disease. Genome wide association studies (GWAS) provide a high throughput genotyping technology that can screen thousands of polymorphic *SNPs* and microsatellites throughout the genome. The advantage of using this technology is that one does not need a prior knowledge of the genes to be associated with the disease. Strong associations with the chromosomal regions may be used to determine the probable genes localized in the region of interest (i.e. the regions showing strong associations) using the draft human genome sequence. Very few studies on genome wide associations have been done on different diseases, primarily due to the costs involved in such studies. Zhang et al.[135] conducted the first GWAS in 2009 and reported significant associations of *SNPs* in the genes *CCDC122* (the gene encoding coiled-coil domain containing 122), *C13 or f31* (the gene encoding chromosome 13 open reading frame 31), *NOD2* (nucleotide-binding oligomerization domain containing 2), *TNFSF15* [the gene encoding TNF (ligand) superfamily member 15], *HLA-DR*, *RIPK2* (the gene encoding receptor-interacting serine-threonine kinase 2) and *LRRK2* (the gene encoding leucine-rich repeat kinase 2) with leprosy. Also, the associations of *SNPs* in *C13 or f31*, *LRRK2*, *NOD2*, and *RIPK2* were stronger with multibacillary leprosy than with paucibacillary leprosy, and they concluded that genes in the *NOD2*-mediated signaling pathway (which regulates the innate immune response) are associated with susceptibility to infection with *M. leprae*.[135] A subsequent study was carried out by Wong et al.[136] on Indian and West African leprosy patients, where they genotyped the *SNPs* that were implicated by Zhang et al.[135] While they confirmed the associations between leprosy and *SNPs* at C13 or f31 and CCDC122, they did not observe association of leprosy with the other four non-major histocompatibility complex genes related to the NOD2 pathway (NOD2, RIPK2, TNFSF15 and LRRK2). Their results suggest that there is heterogeneity among populations.

Zhang et al.[137] further performed another genome-wide association study with increased number of controls and replicated the top 24 SNPs in three independent replication samples from China. Two loci that were not previously associated with leprosy in the earlier GWAS, *IL23R* and *RAB32* were identified in this study. They further identified evidence of interaction between the *NOD2* and *RIPK2* loci, the protein complex encoded by these genes (*NOD2-RIPK2* complex) is involved in activating the *NF-kappa B* pathway as a part of the host defense response to infection.[137]

Liu et al.[138] conducted a large three-stage candidate gene-based association study of 4,363 *SNPs* in 30 TLR and *caspase recruitment domain* (CARD) genes in leprosy samples of Chinese Han population. During the first stage of 4,363 *SNPs* investigation, eight *SNPs* showed suggestive association ($p < 0.01$) in their previously published GWAS data sets.[135] During stage-two on independent series of patients and controls, only two of the eight *SNPs*, *rs2735591* and *rs4889841* showed significant association ($p < 0.001$). However, only *rs2735591* (next to BCL10) showed significant association in the third stage on an independent series of patients and controls, which showed significant association in the combined validation samples, which was significant even after correction. In addition, they also demonstrated the lower expression of BCL10 in leprosy lesions than normal skins and a significant gene connection between BCL10 and the eight previously identified leprosy loci that are associated with *NFκB*, a major regulator of downstream inflammatory responses. Thus, a novel susceptibility locus on 1p22 was reported, which implicates BCL10 as a new susceptibility gene for leprosy, highlighting the important role of both innate and adaptive immune responses in leprosy.[138,139]

PARK2/PACRG Genes

Genome wide association study on 86 multiplex leprosy families from south Vietnam with multibacillary and paucibacillary patients showed strong evidence for linkage in chromosomal region 6q25–27. This was confirmed by family-based association analysis in an independent panel of 208 Vietnamese leprosy simplex families. Of seven microsatellite markers underlying the linkage peak, alleles of two markers (*D6S1035* and *D6S305*) showed strong evidence

for association with leprosy ($p = 6.7 \times 10^{-4}$ and $p = 5.9 \times 10^{-5}$, respectively).[140]

In a follow-up study, Mira et al.[141] investigated this region further by using a systematic association scan of the chromosomal interval most likely to harbor this leprosy susceptibility locus. In 197 Vietnamese families, they found a significant association between leprosy and 17 markers located in a block of approximately 80 kb overlapping the 5'-regulatory region shared by the Parkinson's disease gene *PARK2* (also known as *parkin*) and the coregulated gene *PACRG*. Presence of two *SNPs* (*rs1040079*) and *PARK2-e1* (–2599), of the 17 risk alleles was highly predictive of leprosy. This was confirmed in Brazilian leprosy patients in whom the same alleles were strongly associated with leprosy. Variants in the regulatory region shared by *PARK2* and *PACRG*, therefore, act as common risk factors for leprosy.[141] This was followed by an Indian study, where Malhotra et al.[142] showed that *T* allele of *SNPs PARK2_e01 (–2599)* and 28 kb target_2_1 was significantly associated with susceptibility to leprosy *per se* ($p = 0.03$ and 0.03, respectively). Haplotype analysis for the two alleles studied by previous investigators showed a lack of significant association of any haplotype with cases or controls. The noninvolvement of major risk *SNPs* in the regulatory region of *PARK2* and *PACRG* locus with leprosy susceptibility in Indian and Chinese population highlights the differential effect of these SNPs in regulating genetic susceptibility to leprosy in different populations.[142,143]

Chromosomal Regions 10p13 and 20p12

Siddiqui et al.[144] reported a genetic linkage scan of the genomes of 224 families from South India, containing 245 independent affected sib pairs with paucibacillary leprosy. Using 396 microsatellite markers, they found significant linkage [maximum lod score (MLS) = 4.09, $p < 2 \times 10^{-5}$] on chromosome 10p13 for a series of neighboring microsatellite markers, providing evidence for a major locus for this prevalent infectious disease. Mira et al.[140] confirmed these results in paucibacillary patients from Vietnam. Eichbaum et al.[145] showed by *in situ* hybridization and PCR based somatic cell hybrid mapping, that human macrophage mannose receptor gene (MRC1) is localized on this chromosome 10p13 region. The macrophage mannose receptor is a transmembrane protein that is expressed on the surface of mature macrophages[146] that mediates endocytosis of glycoproteins from pathogens with terminal mannose and fucose structures present on their cell surface.[147] *MRC* has been shown to be responsible for uptake of mycobacterial lipoglycan lipoarabinomannan for the presentation by CD1b molecules to LAM-reactive T-cells.[148] This pathway links recognition of microbial antigens by a receptor of the innate immune system to the induction of adaptive T-cell responses.[149] This suggests that *MRC1* may have a role in immune response to *M. leprae*.

Table 5.2: Different genetic markers found associated with different types of leprosy

S. No.	Gene-allele, Chromosomal localization	Type of leprosy	Function of the gene	Reference
1.	HLA-DR2 Ch6p21	Tuberculoid	To present peptides for immune response	46–48
2.	HLA-DR2 Ch6p21	Lepromatous	Same as above	32, 38, 49–56
3.	HLA-DR3 Ch6p21	Tuberculoid	Same as above	43–45
4.	HLA-DRB1*1501 (allele of DR2) Ch6p21	Multibacillary	Same as above	54, 56
5.	HLA-DRB1*1502 (allele of DR2) Ch6p21	Tuberculoid	Same as above	54,58
6.	HLA-DQB1*0601 Ch6p21	LL, BL, TT	Same as above	54
7.	HLA-DQA1*0103 Ch6p21	LL	Same as above	54
8.	HLA-DQA1*0102 Ch6p21	BL	Same as above	54
9.	HLA-DRB1*0701 Ch6p21	Reduced in lepromatous leprosy	Same as above	54
10.	HLA-DRB1*1401, HLA-DRB1*1406 Ch6p21	Leprosy *per se*	Same as above	59
11.	MICA-A5 Ch6p21	Resistant to LL	Role in innate immunity	61
12.	MICA-5A5.1 Ch6p21	Tuberculoid	Role in innate immunity	62
13.	MICA*010, *027 Ch6p21	Protection from multibacillary leprosy	Role in innate immunity	63
14.	TNF-α-308A Ch6p21	LL	Associated with high secretion of TNF-α	79, 80
15.	TNF-α-308A Ch6p21	Protective from LL, TT and leprosy *per se*	Associated with high secretion of TNF-α	81, 82, 86
16.	TNF-α-308A Ch6p21	No association	Same as above	5, 87–89
17.	IL-10-819T, TT Ch1q31–q32	Leprosy *per se*	Regulation of immune response	82, 91
18.	IL-10-819CC −592CC and CA Ch1q31–q32	Leprosy *per se*	Regulation of immune response	92
19.	IL-10 −3575T/−2849A/−2763C Ch1q31–q32	Protection from leprosy	Regulation of Immune response	93, 94
20.	IL-12 p40 3′UTR 1188A/C Ch5q31.1–33.1	Lepromatous leprosy	Immune response	96

Contd...

Contd...

S. No.	Gene-allele, Chromosomal localization	Type of leprosy	Function of the gene	Reference
21.	*IL-12 p40* *3ÚTR 1188A/C* Ch5q31.1–33.	No association with leprosy	Immune response	97, 98
22.	*IFN-γ +874T* Ch12q14	Protection from leprosy	Immune response	99
23.	*IFN-γ +874T* Ch12q14	No association with leprosy	Immune response	100
24.	*IFN-γ CA repeats* Ch12q14	Multibacillary leprosy	Immune response	100
25.	*IL-4-590TC and CC* Ch5q31.1	Protective from leprosy	Immune response	101
26.	*TLR2-1 strong expression* Ch4q32–Ch 4p14	Paucibacillary versus multibacillary	Innate immune response	108
27.	*TLR1 1805G* Ch4p14	Protection from reversal reaction	Innate immune response	109
28.	*TLR2 Arg677Trp* Ch4q32	Lepromatous	Innate immune response	102–104
29.	Vitamin D receptor *Taq 1* site Ch12q 13–14	Gene *tat* in tuberculoid and TT in lepromatous	Binds to $1,25\text{-}(OH)_2D_3$ to induce its regulatory functions	87,129
30.	*NRAMP1(SLC11A1)* Ch2q35 4 bp deletion in 3′ UTR	Heterozygous more frequent in multibacillary than paucibacillary	Influences the antimicrobial activity of macrophages	133
31.	*PARK2/PACRG* SNPs (*rs1040079*) and *PARK2-e1 (–2599)* Ch6q25-27	Leprosy *per se*	Ubiquitin E3 ligase involved in delivery of ubiquitinated proteins to the proteosomal complex	141, 142
32.	*MRC1*, microsatellite markers Ch10p13	Paucibacillary	Mediates endocytosis of glycoproteins from pathogens with terminal mannose and fucose structures present on their cell surface	144, 145
33.	*MRC1 G396S* Ch10p13	Leprosy *per se* and multibacillary type	Same as above	150
34.	Chromosomal region 20p12 D20S835	Protection from leprosy	Function not known	151
35.	Chromosomal region 20p12 D20115	Leprosy *per se*	Function not known	151
36.	*PTPN22 C1858T* SNP Ch1p13	Multibacillary and paucibacillary	A gain-of-function mutant with more potent negative regulation of T cell signaling	158

Further, Alter et al. studied a nonsynonymous *SNP* in *exon 7* of the *MRC1* gene *G396S* in unrelated Vietnamese subjects, and in simplex and multiplex leprosy families. They observed significant under-transmission of the serine allele of the *G396S* polymorphism with leprosy *per se* (p=0.036) and multibacillary leprosy (p=0.034). In Brazilian leprosy cases, they observed significant association of the glycine allele of the *G396S* polymorphism with leprosy *per se* (p = 0.016) and multibacillary leprosy (p = 0.023).[150]

Tosh et al.[151] reported a second region of linkage on chromosome 20p12 at marker *D20S115* with a significant maximum logarithm of odds score of 3.48 (p = 0.00003). The transmission linkage disequilibrium test (TDT) showed that another marker *D20S835* was associated with protection from leprosy.

PTPN22

PTPN22 encodes for an 807 amino acid residue protein called lymphoid tyrosine phosphatase (LYP) which has been shown to negatively regulate T cell signaling.[152] A SNP in the *PTPN22* gene at nucleotide position 1858 C > T (codon 620) resulting in an arginine to tryptophan (*CGG to TGG*) transition has been shown to be a gain-of-function mutant with more potent negative regulation of T-cell signaling through reduced Lck-mediated phosphorylation of the T-cell receptor zeta chain (*TCRξ*), reduced tyrosine phosphorylation of LAT and reduced activation of Erk2.[153] The mutant, LYP-Trp 620 has been associated with several autoimmune diseases.[154-156] However, Chapman et al.[157] have shown its involvement in invasive pneumococcal disease and gram-positive bacterial disease. Due to its involvement in down-regulation of T-cell functions and in invasive bacterial diseases, one could hypothesize that LYP-Trp620 may have a role in manifestation of mycobacterial diseases as well.

Hence, to study the role of *PTPN22 C1858T SNP*, 153 leprosy patients consisting of 103 LL (including BL) patients and 50 tuberculoid (including BT) patients from north India were compared with 365 ethnically matched healthy controls.[158] The frequency of *1858T* allele was significantly increased in both lepromatous ($p < 0.00006$) and tuberculoid ($p < 0.001$) leprosy patients as compared to normal healthy controls. We also studied the role of predisposing *HLA* alleles in combination with the *PTPN22* alleles, *DRB1*15:01* along with both *PTPN22 1858CC* and *CT* was significantly increased in lepromatous patients. There was no significant difference between tuberculoid patients and controls with respect to simultaneous presence of *DRB1*15:01* and *PTPN22 1858* genotypes. However, a significantly higher number of the tuberculoid patients had predisposing *DRB1*15:01* ($p < 0.04$) and *PTPN22 1858CT* ($p < 0.001$) independent of each other. Interestingly, the protective *DRB1*07:01* along with *PTPN22 1858CC* was significantly reduced in lepromatous patients as compared to controls ($p < 1 \times 10^{-6}$) and tuberculoid patients ($p < 0.0001$). In spite of a significant increase of *PTPN22 1858CT* in tuberculoid patients as compared to controls, a significant increase of *HLA DRB1*07:01* along with *PTPN22 1858CC* (both protective) as compared to lepromatous patients who have increased frequencies of both *PTPN22 1858CC* and *PTPN22 1858CT* along with *DRB1*15:01*, suggests that these genes play an integrated role in manifestation of different forms of leprosy through their functional roles in antigen presentation and inhibition of T cell responses.[158]

Thus, while predisposing, *MHC* alleles may be involved in inefficient antigen presentation, *LYP-Trp620* allele may have a pathogenic role in hyporesponsiveness of T-cells due to anomalies in early T-cell signaling, resulting in clinical manifestations of leprosy *per se*. Contrary to our expectations, significantly higher number of the tuberculoid patients had *PTPN22 1858CT* suggesting that there may be early T-cell defects in these patients resulting in a compromised immune response to the infectious agent, which manifests in the milder form of the disease, since most healthy people exposed to *M. leprae* are resistant to the infection and with an effective immune response do not develop the disease.[1]

CONCLUSION

It is clear from the above discussion that several genes are involved in host's response to the mycobacterial antigens. While some may have a role in adaptive immune responses (like *HLA, TAP2, VDR, PTPN22*), others may have a role in innate immunity (*NRAMP1, TLR2, MICA, TNF-alpha, MRC1*). Since several molecules are involved, they seem to play integrated roles in determining the immune response to the infectious agent. Depending on the alleles of different genes (Table 5.2) that an individual possesses, one may get a milder or severe form of the disease or may be able to resist the infection totally. However, some of the studies listed above have been done in either a few populations or on a few numbers of subjects in some populations, hence, large scale studies are required to confirm the associations before the actual pathways could be formulated as to how these genes interact in integrated networks to fight against the infection.

REFERENCES

1. Bongiorno MR, Pistone G, Noto S, et al. Tuberculoid leprosy and type 1 lepra reaction. Travel Med Infect Dis. 2008;6(5):311-4.
2. Ridley DS, Jopling WH. Classification of leprosy according to immunity. A five-group system. Int J Lepr Other Mycobact Dis. 1966;34(3):255-73.
3. Schurr E, Alcais A, de Leseleuc L, et al. Genetic predisposition to leprosy: a major gene reveals novel pathways of immunity to *Mycobacterium leprae*. Semin Immunol. 2006;18(6):404-10.
4. Mira MT. Genetic host resistance and susceptibility to leprosy. Microbes Infect. 2006;8(4):1124-31.
5. Fitness J, Tosh K, Hill AV. Genetics of susceptibility to leprosy. Genes Immun. 2002;3(8):441-53.
6. Moraes MO, Cardoso CC, Vanderborght PR, et al. Genetics of host response in leprosy. Lepr Rev. 2006;77(3):189-202.
7. Misch EA, Berrington WR, Vary JC, et al. Leprosy and the human genome. Microbiol Mol Biol Rev. 2010;74(4):589-620.
8. Fava V, Orlova M, Cobat A, et al. Genetics of leprosy reactions: an overview. Mem Inst Oswaldo Cruz. 2012;107 (Suppl 1):132-42.
9. Sousa AL, Fava VM, Sampaio LH, et al. Genetic and immunological evidence implicates interleukin 6 as a susceptibility gene for leprosy type 2 reaction. J Infect Dis. 2012;205(9):1417-24.
10. Horton R, Wilming L, Rand V, et al. Gene map of the extended human MHC. Nat Rev Genet. 2004;5(12):889-99.
11. Robinson J, Waller MJ, Fail SC, et al. The IMGT/HLA database. Nucleic Acids Res. 2009;37:D1013-7.
12. Robinson J, Halliwell JA, McWilliam H, et al. The IMGT/HLA database. Nucleic Acids Res. 2013;41:D1222-7.
13. Bjorkman PJ, Saper MA, Samraoui B, et al. Structure of the human class-I histocompatibility antigen, HLA-A2. Nature. 1987;329(6139):506-12.

14. Falk K, Rotzschke O, Stevanovic S, et al. Allele-specific motifs revealed by sequencing of self-peptides eluted from MHC molecules. Nature. 1991;351:290-6.

15. Garrett TP, Saper MA, Bjorkman PJ, et al. Specificity pockets for the side chains of peptide antigens in HLA-Aw68. Nature. 1989;342(6250):692-6.

16. Spies T, Bresnahan M, Bahram S, et al. A gene in the human major histocompatibility complex class II region controlling the class I antigen presentation pathway. Nature. 1990;348:744-7.

17. Van Kaer L. Pillars article: antigen presentation: discovery of the peptide TAP. J Immunol. 2008;180(5):2723-4.

18. Cresswell P, Ackerman AL, Giodini A, et al. Mechanisms of MHC class-I restricted antigen processing and cross-presentation. Immunol Rev. 2005;207:145-57.

19. Groothuis TA, Griekspoor AC, Neijssen JJ, et al. MHC class-I alleles and their exploration of the antigen-processing machinery. Immunol Rev. 2005;207:60-76.

20. de Vries RR, van Rood JJ. Immunobiology of HLA class-I and class-II molecules. Introduction. Prog Allergy. 1985;36:1-9.

21. Brown JH, Jardetzky TS, Gorga JC, et al. Three-dimensional structure of the human class-II histocompatibility antigen HLA-DR1. Nature. 1993;364:33-9.

22. Holling TM, Schooten E, van Den Elsen PJ. Function and regulation of MHC class-II molecules in T-lymphocytes: of mice and men. Hum Immunol. 2004;65(4):282-90.

23. Cresswell P. Antigen processing and presentation. Immunol Rev. 2005;207:5-7.

24. Costantino CM, Ploegh HL, Hafler DA. Cathepsin S regulates class-II MHC processing in human CD4+ HLA-DR+ T cells. J Immunol. 2009;183(2):945-52.

25. Denzin LK, Cresswell P. HLA-DM induces CLIP dissociation from MHC class II alpha beta dimers and facilitates peptide loading. Cell. 1995;82(1):155-65.

26. van Ham SM, Tjin EP, Lillemeier BF, et al. HLA-DO is a negative modulator of HLA-DM-mediated MHC class II peptide loading. Curr Biol. 1997;7(12):950-7.

27. Ullrich HJ, Doring K, Gruneberg U, et al. Interaction between HLA-DM and HLA-DR involves regions that undergo conformational changes at lysosomal pH. Proc Natl Acad Sci U S A. 1997;94:13163-8.

28. Gruneberg U, Van Ham SM, Malcherek G, et al. The structure and function of the novel MHC class II molecule, HLA-DM. Biochem Soc Trans. 1997;25:208S.

29. Poluektov YO, Kim A, Sadegh-Nasseri S. HLA-DO and its role in MHC class II antigen presentation. Front Immunol. 2013;4:260.

30. Poluektov YO, Kim A, Hartman IZ, et al. HLA-DO as the optimizer of epitope selection for MHC class II antigen presentation. PLoS One. 2013;8:e71228.

31. Kim A, Ishizuka I, Hartman I, et al. Studying MHC class II peptide loading and editing in vitro. Methods Mol Biol. 2013;960:447-59.

32. Kim SJ, Choi IH, Dahlberg S, et al. HLA and leprosy in Koreans. Tissue Antigens. 1987;29(3):146-53.

33. Mohagheghpour N, Tabatabai H, Mohammad K, et al. Histocompatibility antigens in patients with leprosy from Azarbaijan, Iran. Int J Lepr Other Mycobact Dis. 1979;47(4):597-600.

34. Chiewsilp P, Athkambhira S, Chirachariyavej T, et al. The HLA antigens and leprosy in Thailand. Tissue Antigens. 1979;13(3):186-8.

35. Fine PE, Wolf E, Pritchard J, et al. HLA-linked genes and leprosy: a family study in Karigiri, South India. J Infect Dis. 1979;140(2):152-61.

36. Wolf E, Fine PE, Pritchard J, et al. HLA-A, B and C antigens in South Indian families with leprosy. Tissue Antigens. 1980;15(5):436-46.

37. Agrewala JN, Ghei SK, Sudhakar KS, et al. HLA antigens and erythema nodosum leprosum (ENL). Tissue Antigens. 1989;33(4):486-7.

38. Rani R, Zaheer SA, Mukherjee R. Do human leukocyte antigens have a role to play in differential manifestation of multibacillary leprosy: a study on multibacillary leprosy patients from north India. Tissue Antigens. 1992;40(3):124-7.

39. Shankarkumar U, Ghosh K, Badakere S, et al. Novel HLA class-I alleles associated with Indian leprosy patients. J Biomed Biotechnol. 2003;2003(3):208-11.

40. Franceschi DS, Tsuneto LT, Mazini PS, et al. Class-I human leukocyte alleles in leprosy patients from Southern Brazil. Rev Soc Bras Med Trop. 2011;44(5):616-20.

41. Correa Rda G, de Aquino DM, Caldas Ade J, et al. Association analysis of human leukocyte antigen class II (DRB1) alleles with leprosy in individuals from São Luis, state of Maranhão, Brazil. Mem Inst Oswaldo Cruz. 2012;107 Suppl 1:150-5.

42. Marsh SG. Nomenclature for factors of the HLA system, update June 2010'. Int J Immunogenet. 2011;38(1):77-81.

43. van Eden W, de Vries RR, D'Amaro J, et al. HLA-DR-associated genetic control of the type of leprosy in a population from surinam. Hum Immunol. 1982;4(4):343-50.

44. van Eden W, Gonzalez NM, de Vries RR, et al. HLA-linked control of predisposition to lepromatous leprosy. J Infect Dis. 1985;151(1):9-14.

45. Gorodezky C, Flores J, Arevalo N, et al. Tuberculoid leprosy in Mexicans is associated with HLA-DR3. Lepr Rev. 1988;58(4):401-6.

46. van Eden W, de Vries RR, Mehra NK, et al. HLA segregation of tuberculoid leprosy: confirmation of the DR2 marker. J Infect Dis. 1980;141(6):693-701.

47. de Vries RR, Mehra NK, Vaidya MC, et al. HLA-linked control of susceptibility to tuberculoid leprosy and association with HLA-DR types. Tissue Antigens. 1980;16(4):294-304.

48. Miyanaga K, Juji T, Maeda H, et al. Tuberculoid leprosy and HLA in Japanese. Tissue Antigens. 1981;18(5):331-4.

49. Visentainer JE, Tsuneto LT, Serra MF, et al. Association of leprosy with HLA-DR2 in a Southern Brazilian population. Braz J Med Biol Res. 1997;30(1):51-9.

50. Schauf V, Ryan S, Scollard D, et al. Leprosy associated with HLA-DR2 and DQw1 in the population of northern Thailand. Tissue Antigens. 1985;26(4):243-7.

51. Serjeantson SW. HLA and susceptibility to leprosy. Immunol Rev. 1983;70:89-112.

52. Cem Mat M, Yazici H, Ozbakir F, et al. The HLA association of lepromatous leprosy and borderline lepromatous leprosy in Turkey. A preliminary study. Int J Dermatol. 1988; 27(4):246-7.

53. Todd JR, West BC, McDonald JC. Human leukocyte antigen and leprosy: study in northern Louisiana and review. Rev Infect Dis. 1990;12(1):63-74.

54. Rani R, Fernandez-Vina MA, Zaheer SA, et al. Study of HLA class II alleles by PCR oligotyping in leprosy patients from north India. Tissue Antigens. 1993;42(3):133-7.

55. Izumi S, Sugiyama K, Matsumoto Y et al. Analysis of the immunogenetic background of Japanese leprosy patients by the HLA system. Vox Sang. 1982; 42:243-7

56. Joko S, Numaga J, Kawashima H, Namisato M, Maeda H. Human leukocyte antigens in forms of leprosy among Japanese patients. Int J Lepr Other Myobac Dis. 2000;68:49-56.

57. Zhang F, Liu H, Chen S, et al. Evidence for an association of HLA-DRB1*15 and DRB1*09 with leprosy and the impact of DRB1*09 on disease onset in a Chinese Han population. BMC Med Genet. 2009;10:133.

58. Mehra NK, Rajalingam R, Mitra DK, et al. Variants of HLA-DR2/DR51 group haplotypes and susceptibility to tuberculoid leprosy and pulmonary tuberculosis in Asian Indians. Int J Lepr Other Mycobact Dis. 1995;63(2):241-8.

59. Borrás SG, Cotorruelo C, Racca L, et al. Association of leprosy with HLA-DRB1 in an Argentinean population. Ann Clin Biochem. 2008;45(Pt 1):96-8.

60. Hsieh NK, Chu CC, Lee NS, et al. Association of HLA-DRB1*0405 with resistance to multibacillary leprosy in Taiwanese. Hum Immunol. 2010;71(7):712-6.

61. Wang LM, Kimura A, Satoh M, et al. HLA linked with leprosy in southern China: HLA-linked resistance alleles to leprosy. Int J Lepr Other Mycobact Dis. 1999;67(4):403-8.

62. Tosh K, Ravikumar M, Bell JT, et al. Variation in MICA and MICB genes and enhanced susceptibility to paucibacillary leprosy in South India. Hum Mol Genet. 2006;15(19):2880-7.

63. do Sacramento WS, Mazini PS, Franceschi DA, et al. Frequencies of MICA alleles in patients from southern Brazil with multibacillary and paucibacillary leprosy. Int J Immunogenet. 2012;39(3):210-5.

64. Rajalingam R, Singal DP, Mehra NK. Transporter associated with antigen-processing (TAP) genes and susceptibility to tuberculoid leprosy and pulmonary tuberculosis. Tissue Antigens. 1997;49(2):168-72.

65. Bidwell J, Keen L, Gallagher G, et al. Cytokine gene polymorphism in human disease: on-line databases. Genes Immun. 1999;1(1):3-19.

66. Asderakis A, Sankaran D, Dyer P, et al. Association of polymorphisms in the human interferon-gamma and interleukin-10 gene with acute and chronic kidney transplant outcome: the cytokine effect on transplantation. Transplantation. 2001;71(5):674-7.

67. Louis E, Franchimont D, Piron A, et al. Tumour necrosis factor (TNF) gene polymorphism influences TNF-alpha production in lipopolysaccharide (LPS)-stimulated whole blood cell culture in healthy humans. Clin Exp Immunol. 1998;113(3):401-6.

68. Pociot F, Briant L, Jongeneel CV, et al. Association of tumor necrosis factor (TNF) and class II major histocompatibility complex alleles with the secretion of TNF-alpha and TNF-beta by human mononuclear cells: a possible link to insulin-dependent diabetes mellitus. Eur J Immunol. 1993;23(1):224-31.

69. Fishman D, Faulds G, Jeffery R, et al. The effect of novel polymorphisms in the interleukin-6 (IL-6) gene on IL-6 transcription and plasma IL-6 levels, and an association with systemic-onset juvenile chronic arthritis. J Clin Invest. 1998;102(7):1369-76.

70. Burzotta F, Iacoviello L, Di Castelnuovo A, et al. Relation of the -174 G/C polymorphism of interleukin-6 to interleukin-6 plasma levels and to length of hospitalization after surgical coronary revascularization. Am J Cardiol. 2001;88(10):1125-8.

71. Jarduli LR, Sell AM, Reis PG, et al. Role of HLA, KIR, MICA, and cytokines genes in leprosy. Biomed Res Int. 2013;2013:989837.

72. Kroeger KM, Carville KS, Abraham LJ. The –308 tumor necrosis factor-alpha promoter polymorphism effects transcription. Mol Immunol. 1997;34(5):391-9.

73. Wilson AG, Symons JA, McDowell TL, et al. Effects of a polymorphism in the human tumor necrosis factor alpha promoter on transcriptional activation. Proc Natl Acad Sci USA. 1997;94(7):3195-9.

74. Knight JC, Udalova I, Hill AV, et al. A polymorphism that affects OCT-1 binding to the TNF promoter region is associated with severe malaria. Nat Genet. 1999;22(2):145-50.

75. Stuber F, Udalova IA, Book M, et al. -308 tumor necrosis factor (TNF) polymorphism is not associated with survival in severe sepsis and is unrelated to lipopolysaccharide inducibility of the human TNF promoter. J Inflamm. 1995-1996;46(1):42-50.

76. Brinkman BM, Zuijdeest D, Kaijzel EL, et al. Relevance of the tumor necrosis factor alpha (TNF alpha) –308 promoter polymorphism in TNF alpha gene regulation. J Inflamm. 1995-1996;46(1):32-41.

77. Somoskovi A, Zissel G, Seitzer U, et al. Polymorphisms at position -308 in the promoter region of the TNF-alpha and in the first intron of the TNF-beta genes and spontaneous and lipopolysaccharide-induced TNF-alpha release in sarcoidosis. Cytokine. 1999;11(11):882-7.

78. Kaijzel EL, Bayley JP, van Krugten MV, et al. Allele-specific quantification of tumor necrosis factor alpha (TNF) transcription and the role of promoter polymorphisms in rheumatoid arthritis patients and healthy individuals. Genes Immun. 2001;2(3):135-44.

79. Roy S, McGuire W, Mascie-Taylor CG, et al. Tumor necrosis factor promoter polymorphism and susceptibility to lepromatous leprosy. J Infect Dis. 1997;176(2):530-2.

80. Ali S, Chopra R, Aggarwal S, et al. Association of variants in BAT1-LTA-TNF-BTNL2 genes within 6p21.3 region show graded risk to leprosy in unrelated cohorts of Indian population. Hum Genet. 2012;131(5):703-16.

81. Santos AR, Almeida AS, Suffys PN, et al. Tumor necrosis factor promoter polymorphism (TNF2) seems to protect against development of severe forms of leprosy in a pilot study in Brazilian patients. Int J Lepr Other Mycobact Dis. 2000;68(3):325-7.

82. Santos AR, Suffys PN, Vanderborght PR, et al. Role of tumor necrosis factor-alpha and interleukin-10 promoter gene polymorphisms in leprosy. J Infect Dis. 2002;186(11):1687-91.

83. Moraes MO, Duppre NC, Suffys PN, et al. Tumor necrosis factor-alpha promoter polymorphism TNF2 is associated with a stronger delayed-type hypersensitivity reaction in the skin of borderline tuberculoid leprosy patients. Immunogenetics. 2001;53(1):45-7.

84. Franceschi DS, Mazini PS, Rudnick CC, et al. Influence of TNF and IL10 gene polymorphisms in the immunopathogenesis of leprosy in the south of Brazil. Int J Infect Dis. 2009;13(4):493-8.

85. Cardoso CC, Pereira AC, Brito-de-Souza VN, et al. TNF -308G>A single nucleotide polymorphism is associated with leprosy among Brazilians: a genetic epidemiology assessment, meta-analysis, and functional study. J Infect Dis. 2011;204(8):1256-63.

86. Sapkota BR, Macdonald M, Berrington WR, et al. Association of TNF, MBL, and VDR polymorphisms with leprosy phenotypes. Hum Immunol. 2010;71(10):992-8.

87. Fitness J, Floyd S, Warndorff DK, et al. Large-scale candidate gene study of leprosy susceptibility in the Karonga district of northern Malawi. Am J Trop Med Hyg. 2004;71(3):330-40.

88. Levee G, Schurr E, Pandey JP. Tumor necrosis factor-alpha, interleukin-1-beta and immunoglobulin (GM and KM) polymorphisms in leprosy. A linkage study. Exp Clin Immunogenet. 1997;14(2):160-5.

89. Velarde Felix JS, Cazarez-Salazar S, Rios-Tostado JJ, et al. Lack of effects of the TNF-alpha and IL-10 gene polymorphisms in Mexican patients with lepromatous leprosy. Lepr Rev. 2012;83(1):34-9.

90. Turner DM, Williams DM, Sankaran D, et al. An investigation of polymorphism in the interleukin-10 gene promoter. Eur J Immunogenet. 1997;24(1):1-8.

91. Pereira AC, Brito-de-Souza VN, Cardoso CC, et al. Genetic, epidemiological and biological analysis of interleukin-10 promoter single-nucleotide polymorphisms suggests a definitive role for –819C/T in leprosy susceptibility. Genes Immun. 2009;10(2):174-80.

92. Cardona-Castro N, Sanchez-Jimenez M, Rojas W, et al. IL-10 gene promoter polymorphisms and leprosy in a Colombian population sample. Biomedica. 2012;32(1):71-6.

93. Moraes MO, Pacheco AG, Schonkeren JJ, et al. Interleukin-10 promoter single-nucleotide polymorphisms as markers for disease susceptibility and disease severity in leprosy. Genes Immun. 2004;5(7):592-5.

94. Malhotra D, Darvishi K, Sood S, et al. IL-10 promoter single nucleotide polymorphisms are significantly associated with resistance to leprosy. Hum Genet. 2005;118(2):295-300.

95. Tone Y, Thompson SA, Babik JM, et al. Structure and chromosomal location of the mouse interleukin-12 p35 and p40 subunit genes. Eur J Immunol. 1996;26(6):1222-7.

96. Alvarado-Navarro A, Montoya-Buelna M, Munoz-Valle JF, et al. The 3′ UTR 1188 A/C polymorphism in the interleukin-12p40 gene (IL-12B) is associated with lepromatous leprosy in the west of Mexico. Immunol Lett. 2008;118(2):148-51.

97. Jesus Salvador VF, Jose Guadalupe RM, Luis Antonio OR, et al. Lack of association between 3′ UTR 1188 A/C polymorphism in the IL-12p40 gene and lepromatous leprosy in Sinaloa, Mexico. Int J Dermatol. 2012;51(7):875-6.

98. Lee SB, Kim BC, Jin SH, et al. Missense mutations of the interleukin-12 receptor beta 1(IL12RB1) and interferon-gamma receptor 1 (IFNGR1) genes are not associated with susceptibility to lepromatous leprosy in Korea. Immunogenetics. 2003;55(3):177-81.

99. Cardoso CC, Pereira AC, Brito-de-Souza VN, et al. IFNG +874 T>A single nucleotide polymorphism is associated with leprosy among Brazilians. Hum Genet. 2010;128(5):481-90.

100. Wang D, Feng JQ, Li YY, et al. Genetic variants of the MRC1 gene and the IFNG gene are associated with leprosy in Han Chinese from Southwest China. Hum Genet. 2012;131(7):1251-60.

101. Yang D, Song H, Xu W, et al. Interleukin 4-590T/C polymorphism and susceptibility to leprosy. Genet Test Mol Biomarkers. 2011;15(12):877-81.

102. Kang TJ, Chae GT. Detection of Toll-like receptor 2 (TLR2) mutation in the lepromatous leprosy patients. FEMS Immunol Med Microbiol. 2001;31(1):53-8.

103. Kang TJ, Lee SB, Chae GT. A polymorphism in the toll-like receptor 2 is associated with IL-12 production from monocyte in lepromatous leprosy. Cytokine. 2002;20(2):56-62.

104. Bochud PY, Hawn TR, Aderem A. Cutting edge: a toll-like receptor 2 polymorphism that is associated with lepromatous leprosy is unable to mediate mycobacterial signaling. J Immunol. 2003;170(7):3451-4.

105. Kang TJ, Yeum CE, Kim BC, et al. Differential production of interleukin-10 and interleukin-12 in mononuclear cells from leprosy patients with a toll-like receptor 2 mutation. Immunology. 2004;112(4):674-80.

106. Malhotra D, Relhan V, Reddy BS, et al. TLR2 Arg677Trp polymorphism in leprosy: revisited. Hum Genet. 2005;116(5):413-5.

107. Wong SH, Gochhait S, Malhotra D, et al. Leprosy and the adaptation of human toll-like receptor 1. PLoS Pathog. 2010;6:e1000979.

108. Krutzik SR, Ochoa MT, Sieling PA, et al. Activation and regulation of Toll-like receptors 2 and 1 in human leprosy. Nat Med. 2003;9(5):525-32.

109. Misch EA, Macdonald M, Ranjit C, et al. Human TLR1 deficiency is associated with impaired mycobacterial signaling and protection from leprosy reversal reaction. PLoS Negl Trop Dis. 2008;2(5):e231.

110. Johnson CM, Lyle EA, Omueti KO, et al. Cutting edge: A common polymorphism impairs cell surface trafficking and functional responses of TLR1 but protects against leprosy. J Immunol. 2007;178(12):7520-4.

111. Schuring RP, Hamann L, Faber WR, et al. Polymorphism N248S in the human Toll-like receptor 1 gene is related to leprosy and leprosy reactions. J Infect Dis. 2009;199(12):1816-9.

112. Bochud PY, Hawn TR, Siddiqui MR, et al. Toll-like receptor 2 (TLR2) polymorphisms are associated with reversal reaction in leprosy. J Infect Dis. 2008;197(2):253-61.

113. Evans RM. The steroid and thyroid hormone receptor superfamily. Science. 1988;240(4854):889-95.

114. Boonstra A, Barrat FJ, Crain C, et al. 1alpha,25-dihydroxy vitamin D3 has a direct effect on naive CD4(+) T cells to enhance the development of Th2 cells. J Immunol. 2001;167(9):4974-80.

115. Takeuchi A, Reddy GS, Kobayashi T, et al. Nuclear factor of activated T cells (NFAT) as a molecular target for 1alpha,25-dihydroxyvitamin D3-mediated effects. J Immunol. 1998;160(1):209-18.

116. Bhalla AK, Amento EP, Serog B, et al. 1,25-Dihydroxyvitamin D3 inhibits antigen-induced T cell activation. J Immunol. 1984;133(4):1748-54.

117. Alroy I, Towers TL, Freedman LP. Transcriptional repression of the interleukin-2 gene by vitamin D3: direct inhibition of NFATp/AP-1 complex formation by a nuclear hormone receptor. Mol Cell Biol. 1995;15(10):5789-99.

118. Cippitelli M, Santoni A. Vitamin D3: a transcriptional modulator of the interferon-gamma gene. Eur J Immunol. 1998;28(10):3017-30.

119. Lemire JM. Immunomodulatory role of 1,25-dihydroxyvitamin D3. J Cell Biochem. 1992;49(1):26-31.

120. D'Ambrosio D, Cippitelli M, Cocciolo MG, et al. Inhibition of IL-12 production by 1,25-dihydroxyvitamin D3. Involvement of NF-kappaB downregulation in transcriptional repression of the p40 gene. J Clin Invest. 1998;101(1):252-62.

121. Cantorna MT, Woodward WD, Hayes CE, et al. 1,25-dihydroxyvitamin D3 is a positive regulator for the two anti-encephalitogenic cytokines TGF-beta 1 and IL-4. J Immunol 1998;160(11):5314-9.

122. Rigby WF, Waugh M, Graziano RF. Regulation of human monocyte HLA-DR and CD4 antigen expression, and antigen presentation by 1,25-dihydroxyvitamin D3. Blood 1990;76(1):189-97.

123. Skjodt H, Hughes DE, Dobson PR, et al. Constitutive and inducible expression of HLA class II determinants by human osteoblast-like cells in vitro. J Clin Invest. 1990;85(5):1421-6.

124. Israni N, Goswami R, Kumar A, et al. Interaction of vitamin D receptor with HLA DRB1 0301 in type 1 diabetes patients from North India. PLoS One. 2009;4(12):e8023.

125. Gross C, Eccleshall TR, Malloy PJ, et al. The presence of a polymorphism at the translation initiation site of the vitamin D receptor gene is associated with low bone mineral density in postmenopausal Mexican-American women. J Bone Miner Res. 1996;11(12):1850-5.

126. Morrison NA, Yeoman R, Kelly PJ, et al. Contribution of trans-acting factor alleles to normal physiological variability: vitamin D receptor gene polymorphism and circulating osteocalcin. Proc Natl Acad Sci U S A. 1992;89(15):6665-9.

127. Faraco JH, Morrison NA, Baker A, et al. ApaI dimorphism at the human vitamin D receptor gene locus. Nucleic Acids Res. 1989;17(5):2150.

128. Durrin LK, Haile RW, Ingles SA, et al. Vitamin D receptor 3'-untranslated region polymorphisms: lack of effect on mRNA stability. Biochim Biophys Acta. 1999;1453(3):311-20.

129. Roy S, Frodsham A, Saha B, et al. Association of vitamin D receptor genotype with leprosy type. J Infect Dis. 1999;179(1):187-91.

130. Goulart LR, Ferreira FR, Goulart IM. Interaction of TaqI polymorphism at exon 9 of the vitamin D receptor gene with the negative lepromin response may favor the occurrence of leprosy. FEMS Immunol Med Microbiol. 2006;48(1):91-8.

131. Ogunkolade BW, Boucher BJ, Prahl JM, et al. Vitamin D receptor (VDR) mRNA and VDR protein levels in relation to vitamin D status, insulin secretory capacity, and VDR genotype in Bangladeshi Asians. Diabetes. 2002;51(7):2294-300.

132. Abel L, Sanchez FO, Oberti J, et al. Susceptibility to leprosy is linked to the human NRAMP1 gene. J Infect Dis. 1998;177(1):133-45.

133. Meisner SJ, Mucklow S, Warner G, et al. Association of NRAMP1 polymorphism with leprosy type but not susceptibility to leprosy per se in west Africans. Am J Trop Med Hyg. 2001;65(6):733-5.

134. Teixeira MA, Silva NL, Ramos Ade L, et al. NRAMP1 gene polymorphisms in individuals with leprosy reactions attended at two reference centers in Recife, northeastern Brazil. Rev Soc Bras Med Trop. 2010;43(3):281-6.

135. Zhang FR, Huang W, Chen SM, et al. Genomewide association study of leprosy. N Engl J Med. 2009;361(27):2609-18.

136. Wong SH, Hill AV, Vannberg FO. Genomewide association study of leprosy. N Engl J Med. 2010;362(15):1446-7.

137. Zhang F, Liu H, Chen S, et al. Identification of two new loci at IL23R and RAB32 that influence susceptibility to leprosy. Nat Genet. 2011;43(12):1247-51.

138. Liu H, Bao F, Irwanto A, et al. An association study of TOLL and CARD with leprosy susceptibility in Chinese population. Hum Mol Genet. 2013;22(21):4430-7.

139. Liu H, Irwanto A, Tian H, et al. Identification of IL18RAP/ IL18R1 and IL12B as leprosy risk genes demonstrates shared pathogenesis between inflammation and infectious diseases. Am J Hum Genet. 2012;91(5):935-41.

140. Mira MT, Alcais A, Van Thuc N, et al. Chromosome 6q25 is linked to susceptibility to leprosy in a Vietnamese population. Nat Genet. 2003;33(3):412-5.

141. Mira MT, Alcais A, Nguyen VT, et al. Susceptibility to leprosy is associated with PARK2 and PACRG. Nature. 2004;427(6975):636-40.

142. Malhotra D, Darvishi K, Lohra M, et al. Association study of major risk single nucleotide polymorphisms in the common regulatory region of PARK2 and PACRG genes with leprosy in an Indian population. Eur J Hum Genet. 2006;14(4):438-42.

143. Li J, Liu H, Liu J, et al. Association study of the single nucleotide polymorphisms of PARK2 and PACRG with leprosy susceptibility in Chinese population. Eur J Hum Genet. 2012;20(5):488-9.

144. Siddiqui MR, Meisner S, Tosh K, et al. A major susceptibility locus for leprosy in India maps to chromosome 10p13. Nat Genet. 2001;27(4):439-41.

145. Eichbaum Q, Clerc P, Bruns G, et al. Assignment of the human macrophage mannose receptor gene (MRC1) to 10p13 by in situ hybridization and PCR-based somatic cell hybrid mapping. Genomics. 1994;22(3):656-8.

146. Harris N, Peters LL, Eicher EM, et al. The exon-intron structure and chromosomal localization of the mouse macrophage mannose receptor gene Mrc1: identification of a Ricin-like domain at the N-terminus of the receptor. Biochem Biophys Res Commun. 1994;198(2):682-92.

147. Taylor ME, Drickamer K. Structural requirements for high affinity binding of complex ligands by the macrophage mannose receptor. J Biol Chem. 1993;268(1):399-404.

148. Nejentsev S, Godfrey L, Snook H, et al. Comparative high-resolution analysis of linkage disequilibrium and tag single nucleotide polymorphisms between populations in the vitamin D receptor gene. Hum Mol Genet. 2004;13(15):1633-9.

149. Prigozy TI, Sieling PA, Clemens D, et al. The mannose receptor delivers lipoglycan antigens to endosomes for presentation to T cells by CD1b molecules. Immunity. 1997;6(2):187-97.

150. Alter A, de Leseleuc L, Van Thuc N, et al. Genetic and functional analysis of common MRC1 exon 7 polymorphisms in leprosy susceptibility. Hum Genet. 2010;127(3):337-48.

151. Tosh K, Meisner S, Siddiqui MR, et al. A region of chromosome 20 is linked to leprosy susceptibility in a South Indian population. J Infect Dis. 2002;186(8):1190-3.

152. Hasegawa K, Martin F, Huang G, et al. PEST domain-enriched tyrosine phosphatase (PEP) regulation of effector/memory T cells. Science. 2004;303(5658):685-9.

153. Vang T, Congia M, Macis MD, et al. Autoimmune-associated lymphoid tyrosine phosphatase is a gain-of-function variant. Nat Genet. 2005;37(12):1317-9.

154. Bottini N, Musumeci L, Alonso A, et al. A functional variant of lymphoid tyrosine phosphatase is associated with type I diabetes. Nat Genet. 2004;36(4):337-8.

155. Begovich AB, Carlton VE, Honigberg LA, et al. A missense single-nucleotide polymorphism in a gene encoding a protein tyrosine phosphatase (PTPN22) is associated with rheumatoid arthritis. Am J Hum Genet. 2004;75(2):330-7.

156. Kyogoku C, Langefeld CD, Ortmann WA, et al. Genetic association of the R620W polymorphism of protein tyrosine phosphatase PTPN22 with human SLE. Am J Hum Genet. 2004;75(3):504-7.

157. Chapman SJ, Khor CC, Vannberg FO, et al. PTPN22 and invasive bacterial disease. Nat Genet. 2006;38:499-500.

158. Rani R, Singh A, Israni N, et al. The role of polymorphic protein tyrosine phosphatase non-receptor type 22 in leprosy. J Invest Dermatol. 2009;129(11):2726-8.

Bacteriology of Leprosy

B Sekar

INTRODUCTION

Leprosy is an ancient, clinically well-recognized disease. Though leprosy was known to the mankind as a contagious disease since olden times, nothing was known about its causative agent till mid-nineteenth century. The coincidental development of microscopy and the emergence of "germ theory" favored the young Norwegian physician GHA Hansen to demonstrate, in 1873 by microscopy, the presence of rod-shaped bodies in unstained preparation of nodular lesions from leprosy patients.[1] Though Danielssen, in 1847, came across globi, solid and beaded rods, coccoid forms, etc., both within and outside of the cells in leprosy lesions, but because of his strong faith in the hereditary nature of the disease, he failed to associate his findings with cause of the disease.[2] Although it was one of the first organisms demonstrated by microscopy, it has not yet been possible to cultivate it *in vitro*, in an artificial media, till today.

In 1960, Charles C Shepard demonstrated a limited growth of *Mycobacterium leprae* in the footpad of mouse.[3] This landmark discovery proved to be a major contribution as it made possible the screening of drugs, assessment of their efficacy and detection of drug-resistant strains. Mouse footpad experiments paved a way for understanding many biological properties of *M. leprae*. Further, RJW Rees showed enhanced growth of *M. leprae* in the footpad of thymectomized-irradiated (nude) mice in the year 1966.[4]

In 1971, Kirchheimer and Storrs demonstrated unlimited multiplication of *M. leprae* in nine-banded armadillo (a Southern American rodent).[5] Subsequently, in 1976, Draper developed a procedure for the purification of *M. leprae* from armadillo tissues.[6] This made available a large number of *M. leprae* for the immunological and molecular biological studies carried out in the present era. Many attempts have been made to cultivate *M. leprae in vitro* but all of them turned futile and, as such, no artificial medium is available as yet for the *in vitro* cultivation of *M. leprae*.

Following the genome sequencing of *M. tuberculosis*, the genome sequencing of *M. leprae* was completed in 2000, by Cole, which enabled us to understand its biology in more detail. *M. leprae* has undergone a reductive evolutionary process through adaptation to its intracellular parasitic lifestyle. Comparative analysis of the genome sequences with *M. tuberculosis* established that gene deletion and decay in *M. leprae* have resulted in the formation of 1,116 nonfunctional pseudogenes, resulting in an elimination of many key metabolic activities of *M. leprae*.[7] Thus, *M. leprae* barely maintains its existence with a minimal gene set.[8]

MYCOBACTERIA

These are a group of bacteria, initially thought to be a fungus (*myco* = fungus), well known for their unique character of acid-fastness. These bacteria do not stain readily, but once stained, resist the decolorization with acid/alcohol. Hence, they are called as acid-fast bacteria (AFB). The acid-fastness is due to the presence of a chemical in the cell wall called "mycolic acid". Amongst different species of mycobacteria some are pathogenic, e.g. *M. tuberculosis*, *M. leprae*, *M. marinum*, *M. scrofulaceum*, etc.; and some are saprophytic (nonpathogens), e.g. *M. fortuitum*, *Mycobacterium w* (now renamed after complete genomic sequencing as *M. indicus pranii*), etc. Some of the mycobacteria are fast growers *in vitro* and some are slow growers. *M. leprae* is physiogenetically placed somewhere in between *M. tuberculosis* and *M. avium-intracellular-scrofulaceum (MAIS) complex.*

Mycobacterium leprae

It is a rod-shaped bacterium, measuring 1–8 microns in length and 0.3 microns in diameter, with parallel sides and rounded ends. It is strongly acid-fast when stained by Ziehl-Neelsen method. In skin smears towards the (immunocompromized) lepromatous (LL) end of the disease spectrum, *M. leprae* are predominantly found in clumps or globi within the macrophages (lepra cells). Inside these cells *M. leprae* multiply unrestricted, which may contain hundreds of bacilli arranged in parallel arrays, placed side by side by the presence of surface lipids (glial substances) suggesting "bundle of cigars". Globi are characteristically seen in the smears of borderline lepromatous (BL) and LL patients. These are spherical conglomeration of rods, presenting in unusually symmetrical circumference, the wet mount reveals a membrane confining the rods, giving a spherical shape to the cluster. Though it is thought to be the characteristic of leprosy, such phenomenon is reported to be occurring in *M. avium* infected specimens from severely immune compromised acquired immunodeficiency syndrome (AIDS) patients. This would imply that the globus phenomenon manifests in situations where the environment is favorable for a rapid multiplication, free of immunobactericidal/bacteriostatic mechanisms—such an environment, with deficient or immune compromised cellular immunity as exists in LL leprosy and AIDS patients.[2]

Cellular Morphology

M. leprae is a nonmotile, nonspore forming, microaerophilic, acid-fast staining bacterium that usually forms slightly curved or straight rods. Electron microscopy (EM) revealed the details of the ultrastructure of *M. leprae*, which is found to have the following structures:

Cell wall: This outer coat protects bacteria from environment and gives definite shape to the bacterial cell. It has an inner electron-dense and an outer electron-transparent layer. The cell wall is a covalently linked peptidoglycan-arabinogalacton-mycolic acid complex; similar in composition to all mycobacterial cell walls.[8-10]

The cell wall in the core contains peptidoglycan, composed of chains of alternating N-acetylglucosamine and N-glycolylmuramate linked by peptide cross-bridges, which are linked to the galactan layer by arabinogalactan. Three branched chains of arabinan are in turn linked to the galactan, forming along with the peptidoglycan layer, an electron-dense zone around *M. leprae*. Mycolic acids

are linked to the terminals of arabinan chains to form the inner leaflet of a pseudolipid bilayer. The outer leaflet is composed of an array of intercalating mycolic acids of trehalose monomycolates (TMM) and mycoserosoic acids of phthiocerol dimycocerosates (PDIMs), as well as phenolic glycolipids (PGLs), forming the electron-transparent zone. Phosphatidylinsitol mannosides and phospholipids are released from the cell wall after synthesis, forming a capsule-like region. The dominant lipid in the cell wall, which gives *M. leprae* immunological specificity, is PGL-1.[11] Recent studies suggest that PGL-1 is involved in the interaction of *M. leprae* with laminin of Schwann cells, suggesting a role for PGL-1 in peripheral nerve-bacillus interactions.[12]

Annotations of *M. leprae* genome and comparative genomic studies with other mycobacterial genomes have produced insight into the putative genes needed to direct the synthesis of this complex cell wall biopolymer. Most of the genes necessary to build the peptidoglycan-arabinogalactan-mycolate polymer appear to be present in the *M. leprae* genome and fit a reasonable strategy for its construction (Fig. 6.1).[13]

The plasma membrane is covered by a cell wall core made of peptidoglycan covalently linked to the galactan by a linker unit of arabinogalactan. Three branched chains of arabinan are in turn linked to the galactan. Mycolic acids are linked to the termini of the arabinan chains to form the inner leaflet of a pseudolipid bilayer. An outer leaflet is formed by the mycolic acids of TMM and mycocerosic acids of PDIMs and PGLs-as shown. A capsule, presumably composed largely of PGLs and other molecules, such as PDIMs, phosphatidylinositol mannosides and phospholipids, surrounds the bacterium. Lipoglycans, such as phosphatidylinositol mannosides, lipomannan (LM) and lipoarabinomannan (LAM), known to be anchored in the plasma membrane, are also found in the capsular layer, as shown in Figure 6.1.

Cell membrane: This structure seems to contain proteins which control the active and passive transport of substances across, between inside and outside of the cell. Enzymes synthesizing the cell wall and capsular lipids are also present. There is evidence for the presence of phospholipids, characteristic of membrane of cultivable mycobacteria, including members of phosphatidylinositol mannosides (PIM).[14,15] Biochemical fractionation studies identified two major polypeptides—major membrane protein-I (MMP-I) and major membrane protein-II (MMP-II)—associated with the cell membrane of *M. leprae*.[16] MMP-I is a 35 kDa protein independently identified as a serologically active component recognized by murine monoclonal antibodies specific to *M. leprae*.[17] A study by Triccas et al. with r35 kDa antigen indicated proliferative response predominantly from paucibacillary (PB) leprosy patients and healthy contacts of leprosy.[18] The gene encoding for *M. leprae* 35 kDa has been identified, isolated and characterized.[19] It was further shown that 35 kDa protein has no homologue within

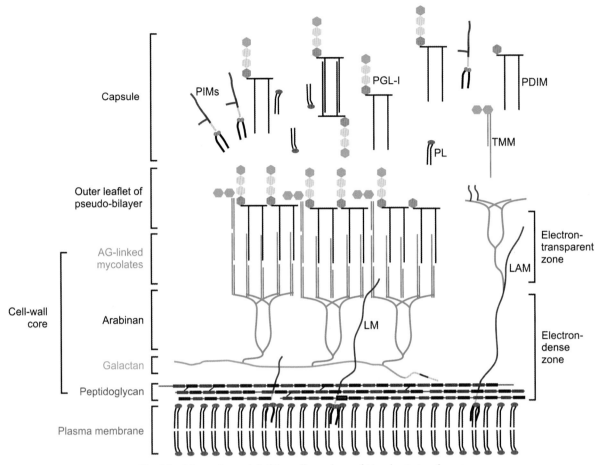

Fig. 6.1: Schematic model of the cell envelope of *Mycobacterium leprae*

Abbreviations: PIMs, phosphatidylinositol mannosides; PGL-1, phenolic glycolipid-1; PDIMs, phthiocerol dimycocerosates; PL, phospholipids; TMM, trehalose mono-mucolates; LAM, lipoarabinomannan; LM, lipomannan

Source: Scollard DM, Adams LB, Gillis TP, et al. The continuing challenges of leprosy. Clin Microbiol Rev. 2006;19(2):338-81.

the *M. tuberculosis* complex, but it has a homologue in *M. avium.* MMP-II was originally identified from *M. leprae* as a major native protein and was recognized to be identical to mycobacterial bacterioferritin. MMP-II protein has a large molecular mass of 380 kDa, which has a feroxidase-center residue and was conserved among *M. leprae, M. tuberculosis* and *M. avium.* The homology at the amino acid level is about 86% among them.

Cytoplasm: Earlier studies of fractionation by *sodium dodecyl sulphate* (SDS)-polyacrylamide gel electrophoresis revealed the presence of three major proteins in cytoplasmic extracts of *M. leprae.*[16] They were found to be a doublet at 28 kDa, a second one with a molecular weight of 17 kDa and the third corresponded to GroES heat shock protein found also in cell wall fractions. Studies on the protein composition of *M. leprae* based on serological techniques resulted in identification of another component; with 65 kDa antigen appearing particularly prominent.[20] A 65 kDa protein (identified as the *M. leprae* homologue of the GroEL heat shock protein)[21]

is generally found in an extensively degraded form in *M. leprae* preparations. Proteins with a molecular mass of 10–12 kDa from *M. leprae* and *M. tuberculosis* were originally found to carry separate species-specific epitopes identified with monoclonal antibodies. An analysis of their sequence showed 90% identity between *M. leprae* and *M. tuberculosis* and 44% homology with the GroES heat shock protein of *Escherichia coli.*[22] The protein induced a strong delayed-type hypersensitivity and threonine 1 (Th1) cytokine production. Monoclonal antibody studies have also identified an 18 kDa protein which is structurally related to a loosely conserved family of low molecular weight heat shock proteins.[23]

Capsule: Electron microscopy confirmed the observation of capsule around *M. leprae* in tissues by light microscopy. It contains bacterial lipid found to be in large amounts in infected tissues. The two main bacterial lipids present are (1) Phthiocerol dimycocerosate, a highly apolar substance, which seems to have a purely passive protective function, (2) Phenolic glycolipid 1, a specific glycolipid for *M. leprae*

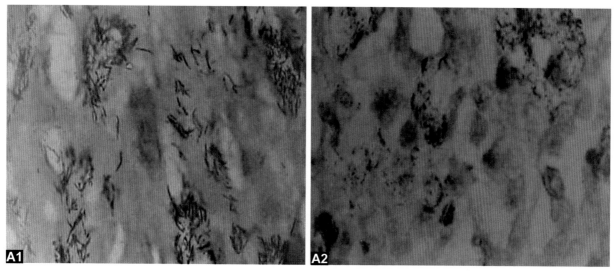

Figs 6.2A1 and A2: *Mycobacterium leprae* in skin smear demonstrated by Ziehl-Neelsen staining; (A1) Solid bacilli and (A2) nonsolid (fragmented/granular) bacillli

found to be active serologically.[24] The PGL-1 is found in abundance in infected tissue (armadillo liver and skin of LL patient). *M. leprae* secretes this glycolipid locally and may constitute the characteristic foamy appearance seen within the macrophages of LL patients. PGL-1 is highly immunogenic, generating immunoglobulin M (IgM) class of Ig, demonstrable in 60% of tuberculoid (TT) and 90% of LL patients. Enzyme linked immunosorbent assay (ELISA) test to detect the specific antibody (anti-PGL) has been used as a serological test for leprosy.

Solid Bacteria

M. leprae is a strong acid-fast bacterium which appears bright pink on Ziehl-Neelsen staining. In practice, in a stained smear, *M. leprae* shows highly polymorphic morphology. Few are brightly and uniformly stained with parallel sides, rounded ends, length being five times the breadth, such bacteria are called "solid bacteria". Mostly *M. leprae* in smear appears irregularly stained and fragmented or granular. Mouse foot pad experiments have shown that the solid bacteria are viable bacteria, whereas the morphologically imperfect (fragmented and granular) forms are usually considered to be dead. This was even cited by Hansen "As the bacilli at first multiply in the cells, and the breaking down appears most definitely and freely when the cells are crammed full of bacilli. It is equally possible that it is the result of diminished nutrition, and as they break down more rapidly in the internal organs, it is also possible, indeed probable, that the higher temperature in these organs favors disintegration. The transformation into granules is considered as degeneration and that the bacilli are altered dead".[25] Electron microscopic study further confirmed that in case of irregularly stained bacteria the contents of the cytoplasm disappeared, were severely distorted and the plasma membrane incomplete.

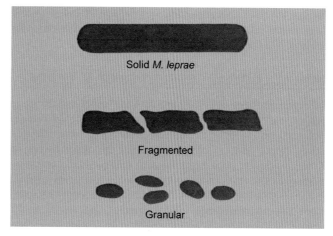

Fig. 6.2B: Schematic model of solid and nonsolid lepra bacilli

These findings are the basis for the morphological index (MI), which gives an idea of solid, fragmented and granular forms in a smear (Figs 6.2A1, A2 and B).

PYRIDINE EXTRACTION

M. leprae smears on treating with pyridine, lose the ability to stain subsequently with carbol fuchsin and thereby appear nonacid fast. This property of pyridine extraction is considered unique for *M. leprae.*[26]

$$M.\ leprae \xrightarrow{\text{ZN staining}} \text{Acid-fast}$$

$$\underset{\text{Pyridine}}{+} \xrightarrow{\text{ZN staining}} \text{Nonacid-fast}$$

However, some nonleprosy mycobacteria have been reported to lose their acid fastness after pyridine treatment and, also, not all the bacilli of leprosy smears may lose the red stain.[27] *Nocardia* recovered from LL showed such characteristics. So this test may be regarded as an optional confirmatory test, provided the culture growth is 'pure'; without any coexisting cultivable mycobacteria.

CLINICAL SPECTRUM OF LEPROSY

Leprosy exhibits a diverse manifestation from a highly resistant TT type to poorly resistant LL type. Ridley and Jopling, in 1962, described five overlapping groups of leprosy based on the immunological status of the patients. It extends from tuberculoid type (TT) through, borderline tuberculoid (BT), midborderline (BB), borderline lepromatous (BL), to the lepromatous type (LL).

The LL and TT are relatively stable and the BL, BB and BT types are unstable. Of these, the BB type is more inconsistent form and encountered less often.[28,29]

The indeterminate leprosy patients do not fall in the Ridley-Jopling spectrum because of the unpredictable behavior and lack of specific clinicohistological features necessary for inclusion in the spectrum.

IMMUNOLOGICAL PROPERTIES OF *M. LEPRAE*

M. leprae induces both humoral and cell-mediated immune responses. The immunogenic components of *M. leprae* include polysaccharides and proteins. Polysaccharide components induce mainly humoral immune response. Proteins induce both humoral and cell-mediated immune response. The immunogens in *M. leprae* form two distinct groups; cytoplasmic antigens and antigens actively secreted from the mycobacterial cell. A species specific phenolic glycolipid PGL-1 has been identified in *M. leprae,* which has immunogenic properties.

The variety of *M. leprae* antigens identified using monoclonal antibodies include 18 kDa, 28 kDa, 7 kDa, 14 kDa, 36 kDa, 65 kDa and 70 kDa antigens which could possibly express immune response. The 65 kDa antigen was the first *M. leprae* antigen to be cloned and characterized.[30]

PATHOGENESIS OF *M. LEPRAE*

M. leprae is an obligate intracellular parasite. It grows very slowly *in vivo* and *in vitro* in macrophage cultures.

In immunocompetent individuals, the growth of *M. leprae* is arrested due to effective cellular immunity. After uptake of *M. leprae* in the macrophages follows the intracellular multiplication, some antigens of *M. leprae* are processed and presented as peptides in the groove of human leukocyte antigen (HLA) class-II molecules on the macrophage surface to induce T-cell activation. The accumulation of an increased number of T-lymphocytes and simultaneous release of interleukins from activated T-cells results in macrophage activation. Thus, the macrophages limit the further multiplication or kill the intracellular *M. leprae*.

In some individuals, *M. leprae* infection leads to LL leprosy due to inefficient cell-mediated immunity (CMI) response. This immunodeficiency is due to predisposing genetic factors and extent of exposure to *M. leprae*; and is highly specific. This specific immunodeficiency persists even after prolonged chemotherapy and it is, therefore, considered to be responsible for the increased risk of relapse or reinfection in these patients.

METABOLISM OF *M. LEPRAE*

The microbiological interest of understanding the metabolism of *M. leprae* has been to formulate a special medium that could support *in vitro* growth of the bacilli; to learn more about the intrinsic metabolic pathways and to utilize them for developing newer antileprosy drugs. Earlier works of Rees and Young have portrayed some information on the anabolic and catabolic pathways needed for the survival of the bacterium.[31] However, with the complete sequencing and annotation of *M. leprae* genome, an improved understanding of metabolic capabilities of *M. leprae* now exists (Box 6.1).[32-34]

Inspection of the 3.27 MB genome sequence of *M. leprae* (of an armadillo-derived Indian isolate of the leprosy bacillus) identified 1,605 genes encoding for proteins; and 50 genes for stable ribonucleic acid (RNA) species. Comparison with the genome sequence of *M. tuberculosis* revealed an extreme case of reductive evolution, since less than half of the *M. leprae* genome contains functional genes while inactivated or pseudogenes are highly abundant. The level of gene

Box 6.1: Salient features of metabolism of *Mycobacterium leprae* as deduced from its genome[34]
Uniquely for a host-dependent pathogen the biosynthetic pathways for purine and pyrimidine nucleotide are complete.
Biosynthetic pathways for lipids and amino acids are also complete with the exception that *M. leprae* is a methionine auxotroph.
Only central pathways of carbon and energy metabolism are complete but alternative pathways are degenerate.
The coenzymes central to the most universal metabolic pathways-NADH cannot be recycled to NAD by the usual oxidative respiratory route.
Redundancy seen in *M. tuberculosis* is often lost in *M. leprae*, as most paralogues seen in *M. tuberculosis* are pseudogenes (nonfunctional) in *M. leprae*.
Defense against toxic radicals is severely degenerate, as neither katG nor the narGHJI cluster is functional.
None of the few (142) additional genes found only in *M. leprae*, appears to conquer additional metabolic pathways.

duplication was approximately 34% and on classification of the proteins into families, the largest functional groups were found to be involved in the metabolism and modification of fatty acids and polyketides, transport of metabolites, cell envelope synthesis and gene regulation.[33]

Annotation of the genome identified genes showed that *M. leprae* has the capacity to generate energy by oxidizing glucose to pyruvate through the Embden-Meyerhof-Parnas (EMP) pathway. Acetyl-coenzyme A from glycolysis enters the Krebs cycle producing energy in the form of ATP. In addition to using glycolysis for energy production, these organisms rely heavily upon lipid degradation and the glyoxylate shunt for energy production. In this regard, *M. leprae* contains a full complement of genes for beta oxidation but compared to *M. tuberculosis*, very few genes capable of lipolysis. Acetate has been lost to *M. leprae* as a carbon source, since only pseudogenes are present for acetate kinase, phosphate acetyltransferase and acetyl-coenzyme A synthase.[34]

Overall, *M. leprae* has much fewer enzymes involved in degradative pathways for carbon and nitrogenous compounds than *M. tuberculosis*. This is reflected in the paucity of oxidoreductases, oxygenases, and short-chain alcohol dehydrogenases and their probable regulatory genes. In addition, other major problems associated with metabolism of *M. leprae* are that the bacilli have lost anaerobic and microaerophilic electron transfer systems; and that the aerobic respiratory chain is severely curtailed, making it impossible for *M. leprae* to generate adenosine triphosphate (ATP) from the oxidation of nicotinamide adenine dinucleotide phosphate (NADH). In contrast to the reduction in catabolic pathways, the anabolic capabilities of *M. leprae* appear relatively unharmed. For example, complete pathways are predicted for synthesis of purines, pyrimidines, most amino acids, nucleosides, nucleotides, and most vitamins and cofactors. The maintenance of these anabolic systems suggests that the intracellular niche that *M. leprae* has found for itself may not contain these compounds or transport systems.[11]

BIOLOGICAL PROPERTIES OF *M. LEPRAE*

The understandings about the biological properties of *M. leprae* have come from the mouse footpad experiments.

Bacterial Growth and Cell Division

Growth

Despite repeated failures in achieving *in vitro* cultivation of *M. leprae* by various scientists over the last 125 years[35] many investigators have continued their attempts in growing *M. leprae in vitro*.[36] Many of such attempts have been reported from India. Some of them have reported the isolation of coccoids and L-phase like forms[36] and repeated isolation of *Nocardia* like organisms from leprosy lesions.[37] Interestingly, in many of these *in vitro* attempts, organisms belonging to *MAIS* complex have also been isolated. It was suggested that it could be due to the fact that skin of leprosy patients is colonized by the members of this complex.[38] However, *M. leprae* has never been grown on artificial media but maintained in axenic cultures in what appears to be a stable metabolic state for a few weeks.[39]

As a result, propagation of *M. leprae* has been restricted to animal models, including the armadillo[40] and normal, athymic and gene knockout mice.[41] These systems have provided the basic resources for genetic, metabolic and antigenic studies of the bacillus. Growth of *M. leprae* in mouse foot pads also provides a tool for assessing the viability of a preparation of bacteria and testing the drug susceptibility of clinical isolates.[39,42]

Generation Time

It is the time taken by a bacterium to divide into two cells. In case of *M. leprae* the generation time during the logarithmic multiplication is calculated to be 11–13 days. Thus, *M. leprae* has a slow rate of multiplication, in contrast to *M. tuberculosis*, and other slow growing cultivable mycobacteria which have a generation time of 20 hours. This may be the reason for the long incubation period of leprosy. Reductive evolution, gene decay and genome downsizing all may explain the unusually long generation time and account for our inability to culture the leprosy bacillus.[33]

Temperature for Optimum Growth

M. leprae has a preference for temperature less than 37°C for its optimal growth. Many studies showed the optimum growth of *M. leprae* in footpad at 27°–30°C.[43] Clinical evidence also shows that leprosy predominantly involves skin, nasal mucosa, peripheral nerves, where the temperature is lesser than core body temperature.

M. leprae causes a natural, systemic infection in nine-banded armadillos (*Dasypus novemcinctus*), whose core body temperature is 33°–34°C. This obligate pathogen has been shown to maintain its metabolic activity in axenic medium, cultured murine and human macrophages and primary rat Schwann cells for several weeks at 33°C, but rapidly loses this activity at 37°C. A possible explanation for the inability of *M. leprae* to survive at elevated temperatures is that it is unable to mount a protective heat stress response.[44]

Minimum Infective Dose

Mouse foot pad experiments show that the minimum infective dose ranges from 1–10 solidly staining (viable) bacteria.[45]

Viability and Stability

M. leprae retains its viability at 4°C in biopsies or tissue suspensions for 7–10 days. In dried nasal discharges viability is maintained for 7 days at 20.6°C and 43.7% humidity.[46]

They can remain dormant in the host tissues. *M. leprae* in skin of dead armadillo was observed to live up to 3 weeks and in soils of their dwellings up to 5 weeks.[47] *M. leprae* remains viable for up to 5 months, particularly under humid atmospheric conditions; even 3 hours a day exposure to sunlight for 7 days could not kill the bacteria and at 26.7°C and 77.6% humidity, they could survive for 14 days.[48] So, it is clear that large numbers of viable bacteria are being continuously discharged from active LL patients and with the stability in the outside environment, act as a potential source of infection. *M. leprae* can be preserved in laboratories by cryopreservation in liquid nitrogen (at –190°C) for indefinite period of time.

Even on passage from one mouse foot pad to another over a period of many years, the pathogenicity of *M. leprae* is unaltered. Also *M. leprae,* isolated from disseminated infection of armadillo or immunodeficient mice; and inoculated into the immunocompetent adult mouse, have shown the usual characteristics of limited growth in footpad.

Strain Variations in *M. leprae*

Advances in molecular typing will make it feasible not only to study the global and geographical distribution of distinct clones of *M. leprae*, but also to explore correlation between the *M. leprae* and the type of disease manifested, and provide insight into historical and phylogenetic evolution of the bacillus.[49]

Whole genome sequencing of *M. leprae* revealed tandem repeats scattered through the genome either in intragenic, intergenic regions within pseudogenes that could be potential markers for genotyping *M. leprae*. Short tandem repeats (STR) are patterns of two or more nucleotides, which are repeated in the genome and are placed adjacent to each other. STR based polymorphisms have been used as a powerful typing tool for differentiating several organisms.[50-52] These STR vary in copy number creating polymorphism of variable length.

Variable numbers of tandem repeats (VNTR) are tandem repeats sequence repeated multiple times, which vary in copy number in different strains creating variable length polymorphisms. Primers flanking the variable region can be designed for amplification and sequencing.

A single nucleotide polymorphism (SNP) is a change or variation in a single nucleotide (A, T, G, C) of the deoxyribonucleic acid (DNA). This change occurs during DNA replication and is used as evolutionary marker. SNPs, which have revealed a global pattern of distinct types of *M. leprae* strains (SNP types 1–4), have been identified. Monot et al.,[49] in their study observed the SNP frequency of *M. leprae* to be as 1 per 28 kb indicating the well conserved and highly clonal

nature of the bacteria. SNP typing may assist in understanding important factors, such as disease susceptibility, location of real loci in the bacteria and the epidemiology of the disease.

To determine suitability of VNTRs for differentiating *M. leprae*, Truman et al.[53] examined PCR systems to amplify five distinct VNTR loci and elucidated their applicability for molecular typing using 12 *M. leprae* strains derived from patients, as well as from armadillos and mangabey monkey. They found reproducible diversity at four VNTR loci. Namely, alleles for the GAA VNTR varied in copy number from 10–16, those for AT varied in copy number from 10–16, those for GTA varied in copy number from 9–12 and those for TA varied from copy number 13–20. In contrast, no variation was observed for CG VNTR.

Recently, the method that can be used to type *M. leprae* isolates by the use of 16 VNTR loci, and as few as 10 cells as the starting material, has been developed and validated, which largely meets the need for an inexpensive typing method.[54] There are several reasons why VNTR typing is superior to SNP typing for investigating the epidemiology of *M. leprae*. First, VNTR loci evolve much faster than SNPs, with the consequence being that VNTR typing reveals considerably more genetic heterogeneity than examination of an equivalent number of SNPs. For instance, in their survey of 400 *M. leprae* strains using 84 informative SNP sites, Monot et al.,[55] identified only 16 unique SNP types, whereas Hall[56] identified 465 strains, which included 417 unique VNTR types. The availability of complete *M. leprae* genome sequences has permitted the identification of over 50 potentially useful VNTR loci, from which a panel of 16 was characterized in great detail.[54]

To date, those 16 VNTR loci have been used in six independent survey studies in Brazil, China, Colombia, India, the Philippines and Thailand.[57-62] However, because the data were reported independently, there has been no analysis of the results taken as a whole. To take it forward, Barry et al.[56] attempted to provide a comprehensive analysis of the relationships among the strains in order to investigate the patterns of transmission and migration of *M. leprae*. Since phylogenetic analysis found to be inadequate, Barry et al.[56] have developed an alternative method, i.e., structure-neighbor clustering, which assigns isolates with the most similar genotypes to the same groups and, subsequently, subgroups, without inferring how the strains descended from a common ancestor, by using simulated data and detecting expected epidemiological relationships from experimental data.

Their results suggest that most *M. leprae* strains from a given country cluster together and that the occasional isolates assigned to different clusters are a consequence of migration. Further, they reported three genetically distinguishable populations among isolates from the Philippines, as well as evidence for the significant influx of strains to that nation from India. It is suggested that the reference strain TN originated from the Philippines and not from India, as was previously believed. Further evidences are required to qualify their findings.

Recent studies on strain typing of *M. leprae* based on VNTR and SNP typing from different countries reported distinct genotypes. In China, a study conducted in Guangdong province of China, by Li et al.,[63] on *M. leprae* isolates collected from both local cases and emigrant cases, showed that most isolates from local patients belong to SNP type 1, and SNP type 3 isolates were found in a small part of local isolates. However, all the emigrants belong to SNP type 3—whether it was SNP type 1 or SNP type 3 from Guangdong local isolates, their VNTR profiles are close and the main differences are in the alleles at ML-1, (TA)10 and (GGT)5. They hypothesized that the transmission of strain with SNP type 1 is associated with Silk Road on the Sea and required to confirm whether the transmission of patients with SNP type 3 in Guangdong are from the second transmission of the emigrant patients.

In a similar study carried out in China by Weng et al.,[64] it was observed that VNTR linked strains are of type 1 in Guangdong, Fujian and Guangxi in Southern China. Second, a subset of VNTR distinguishable strains of type 3 coexists in these provinces. Although majority of the Guangdong strains are of SNP type 1 or a version of SNP type 3 seen in neighboring Jiangxi and Guangxi, six out of 22 strains diverged. Third, type 3 strains with *rpoT* VNTR allele of four, detected in Japan and Korea were discovered in Jiangsu and Anhui in the East and in Western Sichuan bordering Tibet. Fourth, considering the overall genetic diversity, strains of endemic countries of Qiubei, Yunnan; Xing Yi, Guizhou and across Sichuan in Southwest were related. However, closer inspection showed distinct local strains and clusters. The authors concluded that altogether, these insights, primarily derived from VNTR typing reveal multiple and rather overlooked paths for spread of leprosy into, within and out of China, and invoke attention to historic maritime routes in the South and East China Sea.

In India, Turankar et al.[65] conducted SNP based molecular typing of *M. leprae* from multicase families and their surroundings to understand transmission of leprosy, using slit-smear and soil samples, collected from a high endemic area in Purulia, West Bengal, India. SNP typing of *M. leprae* from all *rlep* PCR positive subjects showed SNP type 1 genotype, from the studied slit-smear and soil samples. Subtyping of the samples showed subtype D. This study put forward that either the contacts were infected by the patients or both patients and contacts had the same source of infection. It also revealed that the *M. leprae* type in the soil in the inhabitant areas where patients resided were of the same type as found in the patients.

In West Africa, Busso et al.,[66] performed SNP genotyping in samples as part of the sentinel surveillance for drug resistance network, carried out in Mali and Benin. All the strains studied were classified as SNP type 4, the most common in West Africa, 33 of these type 4 strains were subtyped N (78%), five (12%) were O and four (10%) belong to the P subtype.

In Nepal, Thapa et al.,[67] have done molecular epidemiology investigation on 220 patients diagnosed at Anandaban Leprosy Hospital, Nepal. A total of 22 VNTR loci including loci with short (TA) arrays were added along with few novel minisatellites. A recently developed non-DNA sequence based, real-time PCR high resolution melt analysis technique was used for rapid SNP typing (as 1, 2, 3 or 4). In Nepal, the major SNP types were 1 and 2. VNTR strain types with novel allele combinations, not seen elsewhere, were identified. The VNTR strain types were highly resolved, although three major subgroups could be detected. Several loci, in particular (GGT) 5 and 21-3, had characteristic alleles associated with the SNP type 1 or 2. There was no apparent association between the proportion of SNP type 1 or 2 with caste or location or gender or clinical type.

EXPERIMENTAL ANIMAL MODELS FOR *M. LEPRAE*

(*For detail see Chapter 13 on Experimental Leprosy: Contributions of Animal Models to Leprosy Research*)

With the nonavailability of an artificial media for *in vitro* growth of *M . leprae*, cultivation of *M. leprae* in mouse foot-pad and the inoculation of armadillos with *M. leprae* still plays an important role in understanding the biological properties of *M. leprae*.[5,68] Extensive utilization of these two animal models has made possible many of the remarkable advances in recent years in leprosy research.

Mouse

Immunocompetent Rodents

In 1960, Arthur C Shepard demonstrated that *M. leprae* multiply to a limited extent in the hind foot pads of immunologically intact mice. The observation on the manner of multiplication of *M. leprae* in mouse foot pads shows a characteristic pattern, as elaborated below:
- *Lag phase*: Lasting for 3-6 months after inoculation, showing no multiplication of *M. leprae*.
- *Logarithmic phase*: Usually starts 6 months after inoculation, showing active multiplication of *M. leprae* up to 10^5 per footpad.
- *Stationary phase*: Usually after 12 months, showing no further multiplication.

Experiments concluded that in an adult immunocompetent mouse, an inoculum size of less than 10^4 can be inoculated, and once the multiplication reaches more than 10^6, it starts acting as an immunogen in the mouse, preventing further multiplication of lepra bacilli.

Immunodeficient Mouse

In artificially immunosuppressed or naturally immunodeficient mice, after the inoculation of the size of more than 10^5, the multiplication of *M. leprae* reaches beyond 10^6 and they also show prolonged survival and grossly evident clinical lesion at the site of inoculation.[69]

Many immunosuppressed/immunodeficient animal models have been studied. They are:
- Adult thymectomized-irradiated mice
- Nude mice
- Other rodents studied
  - Neonatally thymectomized rat
  - Congenitally athymic rat.

OTHER EXPERIMENTAL ANIMALS

Armadillo

Nine-banded armadillo (*Dasypus novemcinctus* Linn.) found in Southern United States was shown to develop LL leprosy when experimentally infected by Kirchheimer and Storrs in 1971.[5] On inoculation of 10^8 *M. leprae* intravenously into armadillo, it develops generalized progressive disease with up to 10^{10} lepra bacilli/g of tissue in liver, spleen and lymph nodes.

Nonhuman Primates

Experimental inoculation was shown to result in disseminated leprosy in chimpanzees,[70] white handed gibbons,[71] and rhesus monkeys.[72] Sooty mangabey monkeys developed extensive infiltration with clawing of toes during the course of disease;[73] and African green monkeys developed lesions of multibacillary (MB) leprosy and polyneuritic leprosy within 4–6 months.[72,74]

DRUG RESISTANCE

Bacteriological proof of the emergence of drug resistance strain of *M. leprae* as a cause of relapse in treated patients was dependent on the application of mouse foot pad techniques. This involves identifying multiplication of bacteria in treated mice receiving diets containing doses of the drug in excess of the minimum effective dose (MED) for the respective drug. The first bacteriological proof of drug resistance to diamino diphenyl sulphone (DDS) was demonstrated when *M. leprae* from three relapsed LL patients receiving DDS were not inhibited from multiplying in DDS treated mice at a dose 1,000-fold above the MED for DDS.[75] The emergence of drug resistance per se during treatment (referred to as secondary drug resistance) is confined to MB leprosy. This is due to the fact that the frequency of drug-resistant mutants in a bacterial population is never greater than one per million bacteria; and the bacterial population of this size is only present in patients with MB leprosy. Primary DDS resistance refers to the patients who have never received DDS but present with a DDS-resistant strain of *M. leprae*. The first case of primary DDS resistance was reported from Ethiopia[76] and has, since,

been reported from many countries around the world, where secondary DDS resistance is common.

Rifampicin, although a highly bactericidal drug and being used in leprosy since 1970, two Rifampicin-resistant mutants had been reported by 1976.[77] Later, Rifampicin resistance was reported among 39 cases of relapse by Grosset et al. in 1989.[78] Rifampicin-resistant *M. leprae* appear to be single-step mutants. All these earlier patients had received monotherapy with Rifampicin. Although DDS resistance, along with Rifampicin resistance; has been reported elsewhere, Rifampicin resistance among patients receiving multidrug therapy (MDT) has been recently reported from India.[79] However, a report from Southern India demonstrated 19% of 265 *M. leprae* isolates from biopsied samples of leprosy patients resistant to Dapsone, Rifampicin, or Clofazimine. All the resistant strains reported in this study had low rifampicin resistance (against 0.003% of rifampicin in diet).[80]

Resistance against clofazimine has been reported in few studies.[81-84] Resistance against Ofloxacin has also been reported in 1996.[85]

Molecular Mechanism of Drug Resistance

(*See Chapter 40 on Drug Resistance in Leprosy*)

Dapsone is a synthetic sulfone, structurally and functionally related to Sulfonamide drugs and targets dihydropteroate synthase, a key enzyme in the folate biosynthesis pathway in bacteria, by acting as a competitive inhibitor of p-aminobenzoic acid.[86,87] Dapsone has also been shown to target the folate biosynthetic pathway of *M. leprae*.[88]

Specific mutations within the highly conserved p-aminobenzoic acid binding sites of *Escherichia coli* dihydropteroate synthase, encoded by *folP* gene, result in the development of dapsone resistance.[89] The new evidence from the *M. leprae* genome sequencing project has indicated that *M. leprae* possesses two *folP* homologues (*folP1* and *folP2*). Through surrogate genetic studies with *M. smegmatis*, the relationship between dapsone resistance and the dihydropteroate synthase of *M. leprae* has been established.[90] Mis-sense mutations within codons 53 and 55 of the sulfone resistance determining region of *folP*1, result in the development of high-level dapsone resistance in *M. leprae*. Similar observation has also been reported from India.[91]

Rifampicin is the key bactericidal component of all recommended antileprosy chemotherapeutic regimens. The target for Rifampicin in mycobacteria and *E. coli* is the β-subunit of the RNA polymerase, encoded by rpoB.[92-94] Comparison of the deduced primary structure of β-subunit proteins from several mycobacteria to that of *M. leprae* demonstrated that *M. leprae* shares six highly conserved functional regions common to this enzyme in mycobacteria.

Mycobacterial resistance to Rifampicin correlates with the changes in the structure of the β-subunit of the DNA-dependent RNA polymerase, primarily due to mis-sense mutations within codons of a highly conserved region of the *rpoB* gene, referred to as the Rifampicin resistance-determining region.[93-95] Rifampicin resistance in *M. leprae* also correlates with mis-sense mutations within this region of *rpoB*.[92,96] Substitutions within codon Ser425 have been shown to be the most frequent mutations associated with the development of the rifampicin-resistant phenotype in *M. leprae*.

Clofazimine is a substituted iminophenazine with antimycobacterial activity for which the mechanism has not been fully elucidated.[85] Clofazimine attains high intracellular levels in mononuclear phagocytic cells, its metabolic elimination is slow, it has an anti-inflammatory effect and the incidence of resistance to it in *M. leprae* is low. It is highly lipophilic and appears to bind preferentially to mycobacterial DNA. Binding of the drug to DNA appears to occur principally at the base sequences containing guanine, thus explaining the preference of Clofazimine for the G+C-rich genomes of mycobacteria over human DNA. Lysophospholipids appear to mediate the activity of Clofazimine in some Gram-positive bacteria.[97] However, it is unclear whether this mechanism of action is operational in *M. leprae*. Since Clofazimine may act through several different mechanisms, it is not difficult to understand why only a few cases of Clofazimine-resistant leprosy have been reported over the years.[82-84]

LABORATORY DIAGNOSIS OF LEPROSY

Since majority of the cases of leprosy are PB in nature and also *M. leprae* is not cultivable, the laboratory diagnosis of leprosy and determination of the viability of *M. leprae* have always been a challenge. Over the years, with the developments in technology, many attempts have been made to improvise one laboratory technique over the other. These include microscopic staining methods, metabolic assays, radiolabeled techniques, molecular methods, etc.

Slit–Skin Smear

Laboratory investigations of leprosy patients for diagnosis, classification and monitoring of chemotherapy have traditionally been depending on slit-skin smear examinations.

Skin smear examinations is carried out by slit-scrape technique. The chosen skin site is cleaned with cotton soaked in spirit and allowed to dry. Next, the skin is pinched up into a fold between the index finger and thumb, exerting enough pressure to stop or minimize bleeding. A clean cut, about 5 mm long and deep enough (3 mm), to get into the infiltrated layer of the dermis, is made with a sterile scalpel. Then the blade of the scalpel is turned through 90° and using the blunt edge of the blade the side of the cut is scraped two or three times sufficiently, to obtain tissue pulp from below the epidermis. This material is then transferred from the tip of the scalpel blade to a glass microscopic slide, where it is spread in a circular motion by the flat of the blade to produce a uniform and moderately thick smear over an area of 5–7 mm

in diameter. Two to four smears may be placed on a single slide and carefully labeled. Then the smear is stained by acid-fast staining, preferably undertaken at room temperature. The smears are microscopically examined to measure the bacterial load in the form of bacteriological index (BI). This method helps in the estimation of total number of *M. leprae*, both viable and dead, present in the sampled tissue. MI is a method done for the estimation of the proportion of viable *M. leprae* amongst the bacterial population in a patient.[98] This investigation is less sensitive as it requires a minimum 1×10^4 to 3×10^4 AFB/mL.

Fluorescein Diacetate–Ethidium Bromide Staining

Live cells can split fluorescein diacetate (FDA) to fluoresce green, while dead cells take the red ethidium bromide (EB) stain. The proportion of stained green cells by this staining method has been observed to correlate with viable populations in several eukaryotic and prokaryotic cells. These techniques have been standardized for mycobacteria, including *M. leprae*, for use in direct clinical specimens, as well as for assessing the growth/viability in macrophages. Their application to LL leprosy patients shows that this parameter is good for monitoring the trends of chemotherapy responses. This technique can, therefore, be used to confirm relapse, provided sequential samples are studied and statistical limits defined. The persistence of green staining signals for some time after death, and lack of its applicability to patients with PB leprosy are the main limitations of this method.[99]

Determination of Bacillary Adenosine Triphosphate Biomass

Estimation of ATP content has been established as an important parameter for determination of viable biomass of different mammalian, other eukaryotic and bacterial species. Techniques for ATP assays for mycobacteria, including *M. leprae*, have been developed. By optimizing the techniques for extraction and assay conditions, ATP assay has been observed to detect even as low as 100 viable mycobacterial cells. This technique has been successfully applied to monitor the trends of responses to chemotherapy, as well as to demonstrate persisters.[99]

Assays Using Radiolabeled Substrate

Several *in vitro* methods based on incorporation/utilization of various substrates in cell free media conditions have been published. These assays are based on uptake of labeled dopamine (DOPA), thymidine or incorporation of ^{14}C palmitic acid into phenolic glycolipid of *M. leprae*. The measurement of oxidation of ^{14}C-palmitic acid to $^{14}CO_2$ by *M. leprae* is done using Buddemeyer type counting system or BACTEC 400 system. These assays have been reported to be useful for drug sensitivity screening using bacilli harvested from patients and experimental animals.[99]

Molecular Identification by Polymerase Chain Reaction

Rapid molecular assays for detection of *M. leprae* directly from patient specimen using available *M. leprae* genetic data have been developed. These assays have been based on the amplification of *M. leprae* specific DNA fragment. Many *M. leprae* genes and sequences like *hsp18, ag36, groEL, 16S ribonucleic RNA (rRNA), RLEP*, etc., have been targeted in the development of polymerase chain reaction (PCR). These techniques have been applied not only in skin biopsy samples but also to several different specimen, like skin smear, nasal smear, paraffin-embedded skin biopsy samples, blood, nerve lesions, ocular lesions, etc. RNA analysis using 16S rRNA and reverse transcription PCR has the added benefit of measuring viability of *M. leprae* also. These PCR-based and reverse transcription PCR-based techniques have shown a specificity of 100% and a sensitivity ranging from 34–80% in PB form of leprosy and greater than 90% in MB form of leprosy.[11]

Newer Methods for Testing Viability

Recently, using the commercial kit LIVE/DEAD® Bact Light™ combined with flow cytometry, Guerrero et al.,[100] in Colombia have attempted to assess the viability of *M. leprae* in samples from MB patients treated with MDT to obtain the cut-point to distinguish nonviable versus viable populations. The viable bacterial population was observed to be different between those treated with 12 doses and 24 doses, favoring treatment of 24 months. Further, 56.7% patients after 24 months of treatment with WHO-MDT had viable bacilli.

Based on the principle that real-time PCR (RT-PCR) has the potential to detect RNA, which indirectly indicates the viability status of the organism, Turankar et al.,[101] attempted to detect viable bacilli from environmental samples in the inhabitants area of active leprosy cases, in endemic pockets of Purulia, West Bengal, India. RT-PCR for 16S rRNA gene was performed to detect viable *M. leprae*, from samples positive for *rlep* region of *M. leprae* DNA. 48.6% of soil samples and 46.5% water positive for *M. leprae* DNA showed presence of viable bacilli. Moist environment had higher presence of viable bacilli, in comparison to dry environment, indicating that *M. leprae* survive better in moist places. Further, samples collected from the control area, where no active leprosy case resided, showed no viable bacilli. Authors conclude that leprosy patients discharge or shed viable *M. leprae* into their surrounding environment (soil and water), which may act as potential reservoir for *M. leprae* that may play a role in the focal transmission of the disease.

Mycobacterium lepromatosis

In 2008, Han et al.,[102] reported isolation of a new mycobacterium species from two Mexican patients, who died in Phoenix, Arizona, the United States of America (USA) with diffuse lepromatous leprosy (DLL) and extensive necrotizing skin lesions. Biopsies from both lesions showed vasculitis with acid fast bacilli in macrophages. The diagnosis in both cases was compatible with Lucio reactions. Han et al. proposed the name *M. lepromatosis* for the disease-causing agent because of the close genetic relationship to *M. leprae* and the apparent association with DLL. The AFB (strain FJ924) from case 1 was identified by the amplification of 16S rRNA gene by PCR, cloned and sequenced. Three other genes were amplified and sequenced directly without cloning: housekeeping genes *hsp65* (65 kDa heat shock protein), *rpoB* (for RNA polymerase β-subunit) for further phylogenetic analysis and the *rpoT* gene (for RNA polymerase σ factor) for analysis of tandem repeats. In case 2, the paraffin-embedded tissue blocks, were sent to laboratories for genetic analysis.

Each species has a signatory 16S rRNA gene and that an approximately 3% sequence divergence between closest species forms the main criterion for species definition. BLAST analysis of the 1,504-bp 16S rRNA gene of strain FJ924 showed that the organism was most closely related to, but distinct from, *M leprae* [matching 1,475 of 1,506 bp (97.9%)]. A phylogenetic tree showed that it descended along with *M. leprae* from a common ancestor that had branched from other mycobacteria. Based on their comparative genetic analysis, the authors concluded that the genetic differences were significant enough to propose a novel species. Further analysis of other genes among *M. leprae* strains, *rpoT* has been shown to contain three or four tandem repeats of the sequence GACATC. The *rpoT* from FJ924, while matching 88% (449/510) overall with *M. leprae*, also contained four such repeats. In addition, FJ924 *rpoT* also contained three repeats of the sequence CGAGCCACCAATACAGCATCT, which appears unique and absent in the *M. leprae* genome.

Han et al.[103] further analyzed the sequences of 20 genes and pseudogenes (22,814). Overall, the level of matching of these sequences with *M. leprae* sequences was 90.9%, which substantiated the species-level difference; the levels of matching for the 16S rRNA genes and 14 protein-encoding genes were 98% and 93.1%, respectively, but the level of matching for five pseudogenes was only 79.1%. Robust phylogenetic trees constructed using concatenated alignment of five conserved protein-encoding genes placed *M. lepromatosis* and *M. leprae* in a tight cluster with long terminal branches, implying that the divergence occurred long ago. These results thus indicate that *M. lepromatosis* and *M. leprae* diverged 10 million years ago.

Further, Cabrera et al.[104] reported that during the drug resistance surveillance study of archived leprosy biopsy specimens from Monterrey, Mexico, it was observed that the specimen (Mx1-22A) from the case of DLL gave negative test results for PCR targeting the *M. leprae folP1* and *gyrA* loci and also for *M. leprae* specific RLEP repetitive sequence, confirming the absence of *M. leprae* DNA, although the sample yielded a product when *rpoB* primers were used. Upon analysis of the sequences of the *rpoB* gene there were multiple mismatches with the *M. leprae* sequence but there was 100% identity with the corresponding sequences of *M. lepromatosis* FJ924.

Further, genetic analysis using the primers described by Han et al., together with additional sets of primers that could amplify the *sigA* sequences from both the *M. leprae* and *M. lepromatosis* species FJ924, led to the unambiguous identification of sample Mx1-22 as *M. lepromatosis*. Like *M. leprae*, *M. lepromatosis* cannot be cultured on artificial media; it also shares other features, such as an unusually low GC content for a *Mycobacterium* (57.8%), the presence of pseudogenes, unique AT-rich insertions in the 16S rRNA gene, and identical six-base tandem repeats in *sigA*. Cases of *M. lepromatosis* infection have exhibited much higher morbidity and even mortality rates than cases of *M. leprae* infection. However, with the exception of direct DNA sequencing of the *Rifampin* resistance determining region (RRDR), none of the current PCR tests for *M. leprae* can detect *M. lepromatosis*, which means that cases of infection by this newly described leprosy bacillus may go undetected, thus jeopardizing patient recovery.[104]

CONCLUSION AND FUTURE PROSPECTS

M. leprae, even though being one of the oldest micro-organisms identified, has been bundled with many unanswered puzzles. Now, the bacteriology of leprosy is becoming clearer after the sequencing of the genome of *M. leprae* was completed. Molecular microbiology has begun to explain some intrinsic factors like the fastidious nature of *M. leprae* and its predilection for an intracellular life. Still there are many gray areas in the comprehension of biology of *M. leprae* to be unraveled. The challenges in the laboratory diagnosis can be addressed with the development of highly sensitive and specific molecular tools. The inherent problems of time consuming and laborious nature of the conventional Mouse foot pad technique in determining the viability and screening of the drug susceptibility may be overcome by further refinement of the PCR-based molecular assays in near future. However, the inability to grow *M. leprae in vitro* would still continue to be an enigma for the bacteriologists. It is hoped that after the successful genome mapping of *M. leprae*, the knowledge gained in *M. leprae* genomics, proteomics and bioinformatics may be integrated for better understanding of the puzzles around *M. leprae*.

REFERENCES

1. Pallamary P. Translation of 'Spedalskhedens Arsager' (cause of leprosy) by G Armauer Hansen, from Norsk magazine for Laegervidenskaben 1874;4:76-79. Int J Lepr Other Mycobact Dis. 1955;23:307-9.
2. Chatterjee BR. *Mycobacterium* leprae and the bacteriology of Leprosy. In: Chatterjee BR. Leprosy: Etiobiology of Manifestations, Treatment and Control. Calcutta: Statesman Commercial Press; 1993. pp. 42-80.
3. Shepard CC. The experimental disease that follows the injection of human leprosy bacillus into foot pads of mice. J Exp Med. 1960;112:445-54.
4. Rees RJW. Enhanced susceptibility of thymectomized and irradiated mice to infection with *Mycobacterium leprae*. Nature (London). 1966;211:657-8.
5. Kirchheimer WF, Storrs EE. Attempts to establish the armadillo (*Dasypus novemcintus* Linn.) as a model for the study of leprosy. Report of lepromatoid leprosy in an experimentally infected armadillo. Int J Lepr Other Mycobact Dis. 1971;39:693-702.
6. Draper P. Cell walls of *Mycobacterium leprae*. Int J Lepr Other Mycobact Dis. 1976;44:95-8.
7. Cole ST, Eiglmeier K, Parkhill J, et al. Massive gene decay in the leprosy bacillus. Nature. 2001;409:1007-11.
8. Vissa V, Brennan PJ. The genome of *Mycobacterium leprae*: a minimal mycobacterial gene set. Genome Biology. 2001;2:1-7.
9. Daffe M, McNeil M, Brennan PJ. Major structural features of the cell wall arabinogalactans of *Mycobacterium*, *Rhodococcus*, and *Nocardia* spp. Carbohydr Res. 1993;249:383-98.
10. Draper P, Kandler O, Darbre A. Peptidoglycan and arabinogalactan of *Mycobacterium leprae*. J Gen Microbiol. 1987;133:1187-94.
11. Scollard DM, Adams LB, Gillis TP, et al. The continuing challenges of leprosy. Clin Microbiol Rev. 2006;19:338-81.
12. Ng V, Zanazzi G, Timpl RJ, et al. Role of the cell wall phenolic glycolipid-1 in the peripheral nerve predilection of *Mycobacterium leprae*. Cell. 2000;103:511-29.
13. Brennan PJ and Vissa V. Genomic evidences for the retention of the essential mycobacterial cell wall in the otherwise defective *Mycobacterium leprae*. Lepr Rev. 2001;72:415-28.
14. Young DB. Detection of mycobacterial lipids in skin biopsies from leprosy patients. Int J Lepr Other Mycobact Dis. 1981;49:198-204.
15. Minnikin DE, Dobson G, Draper P. The free lipids of *Mycobacterium leprae* harvested from experimentally infected nine-banded armadillos. J Gen Microbiol. 1985;131:2007-11.
16. Hunter SW, Rivoire B, Mehra V, et al. The major native proteins of the leprosy baillus. J Biol Chem. 1990;265:14065-8.
17. Ivanyi J, Sinha S, Aston R, et al. Definition of species-specific and cross reactive antigenic determinants of *Mycobacterium leprae* using monoclonal antibodies. Clin Exp Immunol. 1983;52:528-36.
18. Triccas JA, Roche PA, Winter N, et al. A 35 kDa protein is a major target of the human immune response to *Mycobacterium leprae*. Infect Immun. 1996;64:5171-7.
19. Winter N, Triccas JA, Rivoire B, et al. Characterization of the gene encoding the immunodominant 35 kDa protein of *Mycobacterium leprae*. Mol Microbiol. 1995;16:865-76.

20. Engers HD, Abe M, Bloom BR, et al. Results of a World Health Organization sponsored workshop on monoclonal antibodies to *Mycobacterium leprae*. Infect Immun. 1985,48:603-5.

21. Young DB, Lathigra R, Hendrix R, et al. Stress proteins are immune targets in leprosy and tuberculosis. Proc Natl Acad Sci USA. 1988;85:4265-70.

22. Rivore B, Pessolani MC, Bozie CM, et al. Chemical definition, cloning and expression of the major protein of the leprosy bacillus. Infect Immun. 1994;62:2417-25.

23. Nerland AH, Mustafa AS, Sweetser D, et al. A protein antigen of *Mycobacterium leprae* is related to a family of small heat shock proteins. J Bacteriol. 1988;170:5919-21.

24. Hunter SW, Fujiwara T, Brennan PJ. Structure and antigenicity of the major specific glycolipid antigen of *Mycobacterium leprae*. J Biol Chem. 1982;257:15072-8.

25. Hansen GHA, Looft C. Leprosy: in its clinical and pathological aspects (translated by Norman Walker). Bristol: Wright; 1895.

26. Fisher CA, Barksdale L. Elimination of acid fastness but not the gram positive of leprosy bacilli after extraction with pyridine. J Bacteriol. 1971;106:707-8.

27. Slosarek M, Sula L, Theophilus S, et al. Use of pyridine for differentiating *Mycobacterium leprae* from other mycobacterium in direct microscopy. Int J Lepr Other Mycobact Dis. 1978;46:154-9.

28. Ridley DS, Waters MF. Significance of variations within lepromatous leprosy group. Lepr Rev. 1969;40:77-81.

29. Ridley DS. The pathogenesis and classification of polar tuberculoid leprosy. Lepr Rev. 1982;53:19-26.

30. Young RA, Mehra V, Sweetser D, et al. Genes for the major protein antigens of leprosy parasite *Mycobacterium leprae*. Nature. 1985;316:450-2.

31. Rees RJW, Young DB. The microbiology of leprosy. In: Hastings RC (Ed). Leprosy, 2nd edition. Churchill Livingstone Publication; 1994. pp. 49-83.

32. Brosch R, Gordon SV, Eiglmeier K et al. Comparative genomics of the leprosy and tubercle bacilli. Res Microbiol. 2000; 151:135-42.

33. Eiglmeier K, Simon S, Garnier T, et al. The integrated genome map of *Mycobacterium leprae*. Lepr Rev. 2001;72:462-9.

34. Wheeler PR. The microbial physiologist's guide to the leprosy genome. Lepr Rev. 2001;72:399-407.

35. Yoshie Y. Advances in the microbiology of *Mycobacterium leprae* in the past century. Int J Lepr Other Mycobact Dis. 1973;51:361-7.

36. Chatterjee BR. *Mycobacterium leprae* and the bacteriology of Leprosy. In: Chaterjee BR (Ed). Leprosy-Etiobiology of Manifestations, Treatment and Control. Calcutta: Statesman Commercial Press; 1993. pp. 42-80.

37. Chakraborty AN, Dastidar SG. Leprosy-derived chemo-autotrophic nocardioform (CAN) bacteria closely resemble or are identical with *Mycobacterium leprae* on mycolate and other lipid profile. Indian J Lepr. 1992;64:529-36.

38. Sharma RK, Katoch K, Sharma VD, et al. Isolation and characterization of cultivable mycobacteria from leprosy skin. Indian J Lepr. 1995;67:321-5.

39. Truman RW, Krahenbuhl JL. Viable *M. leprae* as a research reagent. Int J Lepr Other Mycobact Dis. 2001;69:1-12.

40. Truman R. Leprosy in wild armadillos. Lepr Rev. 2005;76:198-208.

41. Krahenbuhl JL, Adams LB. Exploitation of gene knockout mice models to study the pathogenesis of leprosy. Lepr Rev. 2000;71:S170-5.

42. Shepard CC, Chang YT. Effect of several anti-leprosy drugs on multiplication of human leprosy bacilli in footpads of mice. Proc Soc Exp Biol Med. 1962;109:636-8.

43. Shepard CC. Temperature optimum of *M. leprae* in mice. J Bacteriol. 1965;90:1271-5.

44. Williams DL, Pittman TL, Deshotel M, et al. Molecular basis of the defective heat stress response in *Mycobacterium leprae*. J Bacteriol. 2007;189(24):8818-27.

45. McRae DH, Shepard CC. Relationship between the staining quality of *M. leprae* and infectivity for mice. Infect Immun. 1971;3:116-20.

46. Davey RF, Rees RJ. The nasal discharges in leprosy, clinical and bacteriological aspect. Lepr Rev. 1974;45:121-34.

47. Harris EB, Landry M, et al. Viability of *M. leprae* in soil and dead armadillo tissue and it's significance. Presented at: 13th International Leprosy Congress. The Hague; 1988. pp. 100.

48. Desikan KV, Sreevatsa S. Effect of adverse environmental conditions of *Mycobacterium leprae*. Indian J Clin Biochem. 1997;12(Suppl):89-92.

49. Monot M, Honora N, Garnier T, et al. On the origin of leprosy. Science. 2005;308:1040-2.

50. Klevytska AM, Price LB, Schupp JM, et al. Identification and characterization of variable tandem repeats in the Yersinia pestis genome. J Clin Microbiol. 2001;39:3179-85.

51. Supply P, Warren RM, Banuls AL, et al. Linkage disequilibrium between minisatellite loci supports clonal evolution of *Mycobacterium tuberculosis* in a high tuberculosis incidence area. Mol Microbial. 2003;47:529-38.

52. Keim P, Price LB, Klevytska AM, et al. Multiple- locus variable-number tandem repeats analysis reveals genetic relationships with *Bacillus anthracis*. J Bacteriol. 2000;182:2928-36.

53. Truman R, Fontes AB, de Miranda AB, et al. Genotypic variation and stability of four variable-number tandem repeats and their suitability for discriminating strains of *Mycobacterium leprae*. J Clin Microbiol. 2004;42:2558-65

54. Gillis T, Vissa V, Matsuoka M, et al. Characterisation of short tandem repeats for genotyping *Mycobacterium leprae*. Lepr Rev. 2009:80:250-60.

55. Monot M, Honore N, Garnier T, et al. Comparative genomic and phylogeographic analysis of *Mycobacterium leprae*. Nat Genet. 2009;41:1282-9.

56. Hall BG, Saliphante SJ. Molecular epidemiology of *Mycobacterium leprae* as determined by structure-neighbor clustering. J Clin Microbiol. 2010;81:96-8.

57. Cardona-Castro N, Beltran-Alzate JC, Romero-Montoya IM, et al. Identification and comparison of *Mycobacterium leprae* genotypes in two geographical regions of Colombia. Lepr Rev. 2009;80:316-21.

58. Fontes AN, Sakamuri RM, Baptista IM, et al. Genetic diversity of *Mycobacterium leprae* isolates from Brazilian leprosy patients. Lepr Rev. 2009;80:302-15.

59. Sakamuri RM, Harrison J, Gelber R, et al. A continuation: study and characterisation of *Mycobacterium leprae* short tandem repeat genotypes and transmission of leprosy in Cebu, Philippines. Lepr Rev. 2009;80:272-9.

60. Shinde V, Newton H, Sakamuri RM, et al. VNTR typing of *Mycobacterium leprae* in South Indian leprosy patients. Lepr Rev. 2009;80:290-301.

61. Srisungnam S, Rudeeaneksin J, Lukebua A, et al. Molecular epidemiology of leprosy based on VNTR typing in Thailand. Lepr Rev. 2009;80:280-9.

62. Xing Y, Liu J, Sakamuri RM, et al. VNTR typing studies of *Mycobacterium leprae* in China: assessment of methods and stability of markers during treatment. Lepr Rev. 2009;80:261-71.

63. Li M, Wang X, Su T, et al. Study on genotyping of *Mycobacterium leprae* in Guangdong Province in China, Presented at: International Leprosy Congress; 2013 Sept 16 – Sept 19; Brussels, Belgium. Abstract. No: P-033.

64. Weng X, Xing Y, Liu J, et al. Molecular, ethno-spatial epidemiology of leprosy in China: Novel insights for tracing leprosy in endemic and non endemic provinces. Presented at: International Leprosy Congress; 2013 Sept 16 – Sept 19; Brussels, Belgium. Abstract. No: O-117.

65. Turankar RP, Lavania M, Chaitanya VS, et al. Single nucleotide polymorphism based molecular typing of *M. leprae* from multi-case families of leprosy patients and their surroundings to understand the transmission of leprosy. Presented at: International Leprosy Congress; 2013 Sept 16 – Sept 19; Brussels, Belgium. Abstract. No: P-032.

66. Busso P, Singh P, Kodio M, et al. Drug resistance study and genotyping in *M. leprae* strains from Mali and Benin, West Africa. Presented at: International Leprosy Congress; 2013 Sept 16 – Sept 19; Brussels, Belgium. Abstract. No: P-035.

67. Thapa P, Khadge S, Li W, et al. *Mycobacterium leprae* strain types in Nepal. Presented at: International Leprosy Congress; 2013 Sept 16 – Sept 19; Brussels, Belgium. Abstract. No: P-499.

68. Storrs EE, Walsh GP, Burchfield HP. Development of leprosy in the armadillo: new model for bio medical research. Science. 1974;183:851-2.

69. Prabakaran K, Harris EB, Kirchheimer WF. Hair less mice, human leprosy and thymus-derived lymphocytes. Experientia. 1975;31:784-5.

70. Gunders AE. Progressive experimental infection with *Mycobacterium leprae* in chimpanzee: a preliminary report. J Trop Med Hyg. 1958;61:228-30.

71. Waters MF, Bakri IB, Isa HJ, et al. Experimental leprosy in a white handed gibbon (Hylobates lar): successful inoculation with leprosy bacilli of human origin. Br J Exp Pathol. 1978;59:551-7.

72. Wolf RH, Gormus BJ, Martin LN, et al. Experimental leprosy in three species of monkeys. Science. 1985;227(4686):529-31.

73. Meyers WM, Binford CH, Brown HL. Leprosy in wild armadillos. In: Comparative pathology of zoo animals. Symposium on comparative pathology of zoo animals; 1978 Oct; Washington DC: Smithsonian Institution; 1980. pp. 247-51.

74. Baskin GB, Gormus BJ, Martin LN, et al. Experimental leprosy in a rhesus monkey: necropsy findings. Int J Lepr Other Mycobact Dis. 1987;55:109-15.

75. Pettit JH, Rees RJ. Sulphone resistance in leprosy. An experimental and clinical study. Lancet. 1964;2:673-4.

76. Pearson JM, Haile GS, Rees RJ. Primary dapsone-resistant leprosy. Lepr Rev. 1977;48:129-32.

77. Jacobson RR, Hastings RC. Rifampicin-resistant leprosy. Lancet. 1976;2:1304-5.

78. Grosset JH, Guelpa-Lauras CC, Bobin P, et al. Study of 39 documented relapses of multibacillary leprosy after treatment with rifampin. Int J Lepr Other Mycobact Dis. 1989;57:607-14.

79. Hasanoor Reja AH, Biswas N, Biswas S, et al. Report of rpoB mutation in clinically suspected cases of drug resistant leprosy: a study from Eastern India. Indian J Dermatol Venereol Leprol. 2015;81:155-61.

80. Ebenezer GJ, Norman G, Joseph GA, et al. Drug resistant *Mycobacterium leprae*—results of mouse footpad studies from a laboratory in South India. Indian J Lepr. 2002;74:301-12.

81. Kar HK, Bhatia VN, Harikrishnan S. Combined clofazimine and dapsone-resistant leprosy: a case report. Int J Lepr Other Mycobact Dis. 1986;54:389-91.

82. Shetty VP, Uplekar MW, Antia NH. Primary resistance to single and multiple drugs in leprosy: a mouse footpad study. Lepr Rev. 1996;67:280-6.

83. Mehta VR. Leprosy resistant to multi-drug-therapy (MDT) successfully treated with ampicillin-sulbactam combination—a case report. Indian J Med Sci. 1996;50:305-7.

84. de Carsalade GY, Wallach E, Spindler J, et al. Daily multidrug therapy for leprosy: results of a fourteen year experience. Int J Lepr Other Mycobact Dis. 1997;65:37-44.

85. Ji B, Perani EG, Petinom C, et al. Clinical trial of ofloxacin alone and in combination with dapsone plus clofazimine, for treatment of lepromatous leprosy. Antimicrob Agents Chemother. 1994;38:662-7.

86. Richey DP, Brown GM. The biosynthesis of folic acid. IX. Purification and properties of the enzymes required for the formation of dihydropteroic acid. J Biol Chem. 1969;244:1582-92.

87. Seydel JK, Richter M, Wempe E. Mechanism of action of the folate blocker diamino-diphenyl-sulfone (dapsone, DDS) studied in *E. coli* cell-free enzyme extracts in comparison to sulfonamides (SA). Int J Lepr Other Mycobact Dis. 1980;48:18-29.

88. Kulkarni VM, Seydel JK. Inhibitory activity and mode of action of diamino-diphenyl-sulfone in cell-free folate-synthesizing systems prepared from *Mycobacterium lufu* and *Mycobacterium leprae*: A comparison. Chemotherapy. 1983;29:58-67.

89. Dallas WS, Gowen JE, Ray PH, et al. Cloning, sequencing, and enhanced expression of the dihydropteroate synthase gene of *Escherichia coli* MC4100. J Bacteriol. 1992;174:5961-70.

90. Williams DL, Spring L, Harris EB, et al. Dihydropteroate synthase of *Mycobacterium leprae* and dapsone resistance. Antimicrob Agents Chemother. 2000;44:1530-7.

91. Sekar B, Arunagiri K, Nirmal Kumar B, et al. Detection of mutations in the rpoB and *folp 1* gene of *M. leprae* using molecular methods. Presented at: 17th International Leprosy Congress; 2008 Jan 30 - Feb 4; Hyderabad, India. Abstract No.: O-99.

92. Honore N, Cole ST. Molecular basis of rifampin resistance in *Mycobacterium leprae*. Antimicrob Agents Chemother. 1993;37:414-8.

93. Telenti A, Imboden P, Marchesi F, et al. Detection of rifampicin-resistance mutations in *Mycobacterium tuberculosis*. Lancet 1993; 341:647-50.

94. Williams DL, Waguespack C, Eisenach K, et al. Characterization of rifampin resistance in pathogenic mycobacteria. Antimicrob Agents Chemother. 1994;38:2380-6.

95. Musser JM. Antimicrobial agent resistance in mycobacteria: molecular genetic insights. Clin Microbiol Rev. 1995;8:496-514.

96. Cambau E, Bonnafous P, Perani E, et al. Molecular detection of rifampin and ofloxacin resistance for patients who experience relapse of multibacillary leprosy. Clin Infect Dis. 2002;34:39-45.

97. De Bruyn EE, Steel HC, Van Rensburg EJ, et al. The riminophenazines, clofazimine and B669, inhibit potassium transport in gram positive bacteria by a lysophospholipid-dependent mechanism. J Antimicrob Chemother. 1996; 38:349-62.

98. World Health Organization-Leprosy Unit. The Smear. In: Laboratory Techniques for leprosy. Geneva: WH/CDS/LEP/86.4.1987.pp. 21-5.

99. *In vitro* methods for rapid monitoring of drug therapy and drug resistance in Leprosy. ICMR Bull. 2001;31:73-84.

100. Guerrero MI, Colorado CL, Muvdi S, et al. Novel methodology for assessing the viability of *Mycobacterium leprae* in samples from multi-bacillary patients treated with MDT-WHO in the Federico Lleras Acosta Dermatology Centre in Bogota Colombia. Presented at: International Leprosy Congress; 2013, Sept 16 - Sept 19; Brussels, Belgium. Abstract No: O-078.

101. Turankar RP, Lavania M, Chaitanya VS, et al. Reverse transcription-PCR based detection of viable *M. leprae* from environmental samples in the inhabitant areas of active leprosy cases: A cross sectional study from endemic pockets of Purulia, West Bengal. –Presented at: International Leprosy Congress; 2013 Sept 16 - Sept 19; Brussels, Belgium. Abstract No: O-179.

102. Han XY, Seo YH, Sizer KC, et al. A new *Mycobacterium* species causing diffuse lepromatous leprosy. Am J Clin Pathol. 2008;130:856-64.

103. Han XY, Sizer KC, Thompson EJ, et al. Comparative sequence analysis of *Mycobacterium leprae* and the new leprosy-causing *Mycobacterium lepromatosis*. J Bacteriol. 2009;191:6067-74.

104. Cabrera LV, Escalante-Fuentes WG, Gomez-Flores M, et al. Case of diffuse lepromatous leprosy associated with *Mycobacterium lepromatosis*. J Clin Microbiol. 2011;49(12):4366-8.

7

CHAPTER

Immunological Aspects

Indira Nath, Mehervani Chaduvula

INTRODUCTION

Leprosy is an infectious disease whose clinical manifestation is highly influenced by the immune response of the subject and is a model disease in clinical medicine for understanding human host defenses against intracellular pathogens. The leprosy spectrum is one of the clearest examples of the same pathogen leading to varied clinicopathological presentations in man. The host response to leprosy bacillus determines the subsequent clinical features was pointed out in 1954 when Mitsuda first showed that intradermal injection of killed *M. leprae* led to a skin reaction 3–4 weeks later with erythema and swelling at the site. Such reaction was observed only in the patients with tuberculoid and not those with lepromatous leprosy (LL), indicating that the inflammatory response of the subject to the bacillus was dependent on the host immune response. Later, Dharmendra showed that a lipid free soluble factor from the leprosy bacilli also produced such a reaction in the shorter time period of 48–72 hours. Whereas, the Mitsuda test measures the ability of the host to mount a granulomatous response, the time kinetics of the Dharmendra test matches the delayed type hypersensitivity (DTH) reaction and explains the time difference between the two tests. Neither of the tests are strictly leprosy specific as individuals who have not been exposed to leprosy may show positive skin reaction. Nevertheless, these tests may have been the earliest markers for delayed hypersensitivity in the leprosy spectrum similar to the purified protein derivative (PPD) antigen used for the Mantoux test in tuberculosis.

Further evidence for the varied immune response emerged through histopathological examination of dermal lesions. Though the histopathology of the skin patch from leprosy patients was described in great detail by Indian and Latin American pathologists, Ridley and Jopling drew attention to the finer details reflecting immunological features based on lymphocyte and macrophage populations in the skin lesions.[1] Since these cells were being discovered at that time to be the major players in an immune response, Ridley-Jopling classification which divided the leprosy spectrum into five groups became popular among immunologists and laboratory-based researchers. However, it may be pointed out that subsequent studies in immune responses do not uphold the immunologists' enthusiasm of the Ridley-Jopling classification as differences are not observed in many of the *in vitro* investigations between borderline and polar counterparts. It is also considered too complicated to be used in the field. Nevertheless, this classification continues to be used in laboratory based research. As the Section 3 on Clinical and Laboratory Diagnosis points out that the most significant feature of the classification is the stability of clinical features in polar forms of tuberculoid (TT) and lepromatous (LL) leprosy whereas, the borderline forms; borderline tuberculoid (BT), borderline borderline (BB) and borderline lapromatous (BL) are unstable and show a greater propensity to develop leprosy reactions.

GENERAL IMMUNE RESPONSES

The defense against pathogens/external agents is first initiated by the innate immune response and subsequently after a lag period by the acquired immune response. Both function through cells as well as soluble factors which are usually glycoproteins. The innate response requires macrophages and their lineage as well as natural killer cells. Though the cells recognize many pathogens via general molecular pattern recognition, complement receptors and toll-like receptors

(TLR) are of relevance in leprosy. The innate system also includes complement and some cytokines as soluble factors. The acquired immune response in contrast involves highly specific interaction through ligand receptor interaction. The major players are lymphocytes, dendritic cells, macrophages and their lineage. The soluble factors released subsequently can be exquisitely specific as in antibodies, or lead to general nonspecific functions as with cytokines. Though the cell recognition is specific, the cytokines released may affect other pathogens and also cause immunopathological derangements in the tissues through bystander effects. Moreover, the acquired immune system retains a memory of its first encounter with the pathogen through memory cells and subsequent encounter with the same pathogen produces a more rapid and enhanced response. It is being increasingly recognized that these two systems are not totally compartmentalized and that there is overlap in some critical areas.

Lymphocytes are known to be of two major types on the basis of cell surface markers and functions. The B-cells bearing immunoglobulin (Ig) surface marker, produce antibodies and lead to humoral immunity that can capture circulating free microbes. Antibodies cannot cross living cell membrane and thus are unable to attack microbes that live within cells (intracellular pathogens). T-cells have the surface CD3 marker and are responsible for cellular immunity [cell-mediated immunity (CMI)/DTH required for limiting and killing intracellular pathogens such as those causing leprosy, tuberculosis, typhoid and leishmaniasis. The subsets of T-cells achieve this mainly by differentiating to effector cells that function directly in killing (CD8, cytotoxic T-cells) through granules present in them or through production of cytokines or biological modulators which are varied and have multiple functions. The CD4+, T helper cells help B-cells to produce antibodies against protein antigens and have an immunoregulatory role. Macrophages, the very cells that carry pathogens within them are required to present antigens to T-cells, which are unable to recognize and respond to pathogens or pathogen products unless they were presented by macrophages along with self-antigens such as histocompatibility antigens [human leukocyte antigen (HLA)]. Thus, it is evident that lesions of tuberculoid leprosy had more lymphocytes and macrophages which had been transformed into epithelioid cells, manifest cellular immunity and explain why they do not show leprosy bacilli in the lesions. The lymphopenic lesions of LL on the other hand show bacilli filled macrophages which lack the ability to kill bacilli efficiently.

Taken together with skin tests; the implications for leprosy are, that the tuberculoid leprosy patients have T-cell immunity/DTH to the pathogen, whereas lepromatous subjects have antibodies but little or no T-cell functions. Thus, began the saga of immunology of leprosy.

This chapter would focus mainly on T-cell-mediated immune responses as they are more important from immunopathological viewpoint. The antibody (humoral) responses are discussed in Chapter 20 on Serological and Molecular Diagnoses. Experimental models of leprosy have included thymectomized and nude mice,[2] as well as the armadillo, which is currently proving to be a useful model to study nerve damage, genetics, transmission of disease and limited information on immune responses.

IMMUNOLOGICAL FEATURES OF LEPROSY
Innate Immunity

Diseases are rarely caused by the direct attack of a pathogen; they result usually by complex interaction of the pathogen and the host. The initial or immediate host response to a pathogen is called the innate immune response, which has been difficult to study in man as leprosy has a long incubation period. However, some clues have emerged both from experimental models and from the associations observed with genetic studies. The entry of pathogens into macrophages or their lineage is not necessarily antigen specific and is mediated by the common phagocytosis. Attachment of the pathogen to the cell membrane and the type of phagocytosis may vary for different pathogens.[3]

Entry is the first step for intracellular lifestyle of pathogens such as *M. leprae*. In leprosy, receptors to complement fragments of CR1, CR3 and CR4 help in phagocytosis. Phenolic glycolipid-1 (PGL-1) an *M. leprae* specific cell wall lipid is recognized by complement 3.[4] It would appear that susceptibility to leprosy may be linked to genes that are involved in macrophage functions in the mouse, such as iron transporter natural resistance-associated macrophage protein 1 (NRAMP 1), which assists in viability/multiplication of pathogen within the macrophage and in iron transport into the phagosome. The human homologue of the gene encoding the protein has been identified to chromosome 2q35 (Table 7.1).[5] The gene associated with early onset Parkinson's disease *PARK2/PACRG* responsible for the synthesis of a ligase in the proteosome pathway has been recently identified as susceptibility gene in the Vietnamese and Brazilian population, suggesting its role in innate immune based defect.[6]

Toll-like receptors are a highly conserved family of proteins present on macrophages and dendritic cells which seem to play a role both in innate and acquired immune responses. They are crucial for recognition of microbial pathogens. Since they are transmembrane molecules, they may also play a role in signaling following their engagement. The cytoplasmic tail is linked to transcription factors such as nuclear factor kappa-light-chain-enhancer of activated B-cells (NFkB), which induces many cytokines. *TLR2* and *TLR4* recognize mycobacteria and release IL-12, a cytokine that induces proinflammatory cytokines such as interferon

Table 7.1: Gene polymorphisms involved in innate and acquired immune responses in leprosy patients from various populations

S. No.	Gene/function of product	Position/country	Reference no.	Conclusion
1.	TNF-α	−308 (G→A) and −238 promoter region/Brazil	28	TNFα allele frequencies significantly lower in leprosy than control subjects
2.	IL-10	−819 (C→T) promoter region/Brazil	28	Homozygous genotype significantly higher in tuberculoid leprosy
3.	IL-10	−3575T/−2849G/−2763C/−1082A/−592 (C→A) and −819 (C→T)/ India	80	Resistance to leprosy
		Minor haplotype in promoter region −3575A/−2849G/−2763C/−/ Brazil	28	Resistance to leprosy
4.	PARK2/PACRG	6q25-q26 susceptibility locus, 5′ region of PACRG, PARK2 / Vietnam, Brazil	6, 68	Major risk factors for leprosy susceptibility is detrimental to M. leprae survival. Role in the pathogenesis of nerve damage
5.	NRAMP1 + Mitsuda test	Polymorphism (GT)(n) in the promoter region of the NRAMP1 gene/Brazil	69	The NRAMP1 promoter genotype 22 and 23 combined with negative Mitsuda test showed greater chance of developing leprosy
6.	TAP1,2	Polymorphism,SNP India	75	TAP1 637G susceptibility to leprosy
7.	TLR1 (Toll receptors)	N248 S SNP, S248 and I620S/ Bangladesh	70	N248 SNP variant diminished the response of TLR1 Homozygous S248 increases and SN decreased susceptibility to leprosy. S248 allele and I620 S association more frequent with reversal reactions
	TLR1	Isoleucine –serine mutation, TLR1àT1805G/Nepal	81	1805G allele was associated with protection from RR. 1805 genotypes GG or TG had a reduced risk of RR in comparison to genotype TT
8.	TLR2	a. TLR2 597C→T b. 1350T→C, c. 280 bp microsatellite marker/ Ethiopia	82	597C→T susceptibility to reversal reaction 597T allele-protective effect Homozygosity for the 280 bp homozygous-risk of reversal reaction
	TLR2	Arg677Trp mutation in TLR2 gene/ Korea	83	IL-12 decrease in LL
	TLR2	Arg677Trp mutation in TLR2 gene/ Korea	71	Cytokines-decrease in IL-2, IL-12, IFN-γ, and TNF-α by M. leprae-stimulated PBMC: increase in IL-10
9.	TLR4	TLR4 896G>A [D299G] and 1196C>T [T399I])/Ethiopia	72	TLR4 SNPs - protection against leprosy
10.	IFN γ	CA repeat microsatellite/Brazil	84	The alleles contribute a role in leprosy
11.	IL12R (IL12-p40)	3′UTR 1188 A/C/Mexico	78	Susceptibility to LL independent of IL-12
12.	IL12Rβ2	Multiple SNPs detected within the 5′ flanking region of IL12RB2/Japan	79	Implicated in leprosy spectrum
13.	IL17F	SNP 7488T>C India	85	Susceptibility to leprosy

Abbreviations: TNF, tumor necrosis factor; IL, interleukin; NRAMP, natural resistance-associated macrophage protein; TLR, toll-like receptor; SNP, single nucleotide protein; IFN, interferon.

gamma (IFNγ) (Table 7.2). The latter along with granulocyte-macrophage colony-stimulating factor (GM-CSF) enhance *TLR1* expression which leads to an inflammatory response through the production of tumor necrosis factor alpha (TNFα). Th2 cytokines seem to inhibit activation of the TLRs. Activation of monocytes and dendritic cell *TLR2* has been observed with 19 kDa and 33 kDa lipopeptides of *M. leprae*. PGL-1 the specific glycolipids of the leprosy bacillus leads to low release of TNFα, IL-1β and IL-10 and increase in negative regulatory molecules such as monocyte chemoattractant protein-1 (MCP-1) and IL1Ra. The overlap of innate and acquired responses occurs when IL-4 and IL-10 down regulate TLR2 expression. It is of interest that *TLR1* and *TLR2* expression is high in skin lesions of tuberculoid leprosy.

C-type lectin receptors present on mature macrophages (such as the mannose receptor) bind carbohydrate moieties, mannose-capped lipoarabinomannan on *Mycobacterium tuberculosis* and *M. leprae* and influence macrophage functions such as phagocytosis, prostaglandin E2 (PGE2), nitric oxide (NO) and TNFα production.[7] Dendritic cell-specific intercellular adhesion molecule-3-grabbing nonintegrin (DC-SIGN),[8] langerin granules of Langerhans cells have also been implicated in the uptake of nonpeptide mycobacterial antigens.[9] Vitamin D has antimicrobial properties and contributes to innate immunity. Cytokine IL-10 induces phagocytosis whereas IL-15 reduces phagocytosis but promotes vitamin D-mediated antimicrobial pathway.

Schwann cells (SCs) are another group of cells of the macrophage lineage which reside in peripheral nerves. *M. leprae* is the only bacterium that infects them. Schwann cell dystroglycans interact with PGL-1 of the bacillus for interiorization.

Acquired Immunity

In addition to the *in vivo* studies as indicated by the skin tests described above, it has been shown (Table 7.2) that T-cell numbers were reduced in LL and failed to respond to *M. leprae* antigens. Indian subjects also showed a general depression of T-cell functions in addition to the antigen specific ones as reflected by low lymphocyte transformation to T-cell mitogens such as concanavalin A and phytohemaglutinin (PHA). Whereas the specific unresponsiveness was long lasting and persistent for many years after bacillary clearance by drugs, the general unresponsiveness and T-cell numbers returned to normal.[10] Lepromatous patients had unique and exquisitely antigen specific unresponsiveness is indicated by the fact that the T-cell response to other antigens and related antigens of the tuberculosis pathogen is unimpaired. The mechanisms underlying this continue to be a source of intense

Table 7.2: Immunological features of leprosy and leprosy reactions, in circulation and in supernatants of antigen-induced peripheral blood mononuclear cell cultures

Features	Tuberculoid leprosy	Lepromatous leprosy	RR	ENL
Total T-cells no.	Normal	Decreased	Normal	Normal
B-cells no.	Normal	Increased	Normal	Normal
Lymphoproliferation to: Mitogen *M. leprae*-specific PPD	Normal High Normal	Low Low/nil Normal	High High Normal	High High Normal
M. leprae-specific cytokines IL-1 IL-2 IL-12 IL-10 IL17A/F IL-21, IL-22 IFNγ TGFβ IL-2 receptor IP-10	 Normal/high High High Low High High High Low/nil ND Low/nil	 Low Low/nil Low High Low Low Low/nil High ND Low/nil	 Normal High High Low High High High Low High High	 Normal High High Low High High High Low High Low
Th phenotype	Th1+Th0 Th17+	Th2+Th0 FOXp3+ Treg+	Th1	Th1

Abbreviations: RR, reversal/Type 1 reaction; ENL, erythema nodosum leprosum/Type 2 reaction; PPD, purified protein derivative; IL, interleukin; IFN, interferon; TGF, tumor growth factor; ND, not done.

research. In contrast to T-cell functions, it would appear that antibody responses of both general and antigen specific type are enhanced in lepromatous and reduced in tuberculoid leprosy patients. In the former, there is a polyclonal B-cell response as even autoantibodies are observed in circulation. However, it must be pointed that the latter are not associated with manifestations of autoimmune disease in leprosy. Thus, it is evident that leprosy shows an inverted relationship between humoral and T-cell-mediated immunity. Moreover, the presence of antibodies is associated with presence of bacilli in LL indicating thereby that protection to this disease is not mediated by antibodies. This is in conformity with the finding that antibodies do not penetrate living cell membrane and thus have no effect on intracellular pathogens such as *M. leprae.* However, they may play a role in capturing bacilli or their products when they are released in tissues or circulation. They may also lead to immune complexes as observed in lepromatous patients when the abundant bacillary antigens associate with the circulating antibodies under appropriate conditions. Antibodies being biological markers of infection can be exploited for diagnosis of the disease or clinical complications (*See* Chapter 20 on Serological and Molecular Diagnosis).

Cell surface CD3 molecule distinguishes all T-cells. In addition, the presence of CD4 and CD8 respectively indicate subsets of helper and cytotoxic/suppressor T-cells. Such cells have been shown to be in normal numbers in tuberculoid leprosy. Both conventional *ab* and nonconventional *gd* T-cell receptor (TCR) may be present in these cells. Whereas, CD4 cells recognize antigen in conjunction with MHC class II, CD8 cells use major histocompatibility complex (MHC) class I. All nucleated cells have MHC class I whereas MHC class II is restricted to antigen presenting cells such as macrophages, dendritic cells and Langerhans cells in the skin. Functional subpopulations also exist based on the type of cytokines that T-cells produce. Cytokines are glycoproteins which are also designated after international consensus as interleukins (ILs) followed by a number, i.e. IL-1, IL-2, etc. Some may have the name defined by their major function, e.g. interferons. Cytokines IL-2 and IFNγ were produced by peripheral blood mononuclear cell (PBMC) on stimulation with *M. leprae-*specific antigens in tuberculoid but not in lepromatous patients.[11,12] In contrast, the latter showed release of IL-10 by both CD8 T-cells[13] and macrophages.[14] Cytokine release was influenced by dendritic cells as compared to monocytes from the same patients.[15] Moreover, IL-2 was shown to be inhibited by soluble factors released by monocytes or macrophage populations.[15] That cytokines played an important role in protection against leprosy was indicated by rapid bacillary clearance by IFNγ and IL-2 injections in dermal and subcutaneous sites of lesions in lepromatous patients as well as by mounting a delayed type reaction with PPD injections.[16,17]

Immunological Unresponsiveness

The basis for T-cell based-immunological unresponsiveness in LL continues to evade consensus even though it has been intensely studied using the state of art concepts and methodologies of a given time. Genetic basis of leprosy has been extensively investigated in leprosy (*See* Chapter 5: Immunogenetics of Leprosy). It is of interest that the HLA class II genes have been implicated in susceptibility to leprosy initially using serological[18] and subsequently molecular tools.[19] This class of HLA is important for presentation of antigens to T-cells. Nevertheless, it is generally accepted that this unresponsiveness is not due to central tolerance or deletion of *M. leprae*-specific T-cells.

Though T-cells of lepromatous subjects do not respond to antigens of whole bacilli, nevertheless many of them respond to synthetic peptides based on the predicted amino acid sequence of the *M. leprae* genome. In a certain situation, such as erythema nodosum leprosum (ENL), T-cells can be shown to emerge in the periphery both in peripheral blood and in dermal lesions in the unresponsive LL indicating that residual T-cell functions may be present. It is thought that the lack of T-cell responsiveness is due to peripheral factors. It was initially suspected that antibody-mediated suppression may be a feature, but that theory lost ground subsequently. In the 1980s, the concept of suppressor T-cells gained popularity as evidence for their role in experimental tolerance was shown.

The presence of CD8 T-cells was thought to indicate suppressor T-cells by some groups both in circulation and in lesions.[20] Immune suppression was detected *in vitro* by different methodologies by various workers.[21] Studies on Indian patients showed that in lepromatous patients macrophages[22,23] or macrophage factors[24] suppressed T-cell lymphoproliferation and IL-2 production. Such factors were nonspecific and consisted of PGE2, thromboxane, leukotrienes and IL-10. This evidence was further supported by the *in vitro* reversal of suppression in lepromatous lymphocytes with the use of human leukocyte antigen (HLA) matched tuberculoid macrophages and antagonists to the soluble factors. PGL the specific antigen of the leprosy bacillus was also thought to be responsible for T-cell suppression.[20] However, Indian studies showed PGL to be generally suppressive in lymphoproliferative assays but could not explain the unique antigen specificity noted in LL.[25] The concept of suppressor T-cells lost credibility in basic immunology in the 1990s as no phenotype or gene could be associated with this function. Currently, the concept of negative regulation is making reappearance in the form of FOXP3 regulatory T-cells which would be discussed later.

The peripheral unresponsiveness in leprosy can be overcome both *in vitro* and *in vivo* as shown above with HLA matched cell cultures wherein tuberculoid monocytes were able to reconstitute lymphoproliferation of lepromatous subjects.[23] Moreover, during leprosy reactions, lepromatous subjects develop T-cell activation and entry of T-cells into lesions as described further in this Chapter.

The discovery of Th phenotypes by the cloning of murine T-cell subsets, which showed mutually exclusive cytokine patterns responsible for cellular or humoral immunity was an attractive concept in diseases such as leprosy which has an inverted relationship between the two types of immune responses. Th1 and Th2 subsets of CD4 cells produce mutually exclusive, IFNγ, a marker of DTH and IL-4 which promotes antibodies respectively and are thus considered responsible for delayed type hypersentivity or humoral immunity (Fig. 7.1). Such clear polarization of subsets is seen mainly in the mouse and under only special situations in man, e.g. helminthic infections and allergies. When both cytokines are produced the phenotype is considered to be Th0. In initial studies, tuberculoid leprosy patients were shown to have Th1 subset, whereas Th2 seemed to be the predominant subset in LL.[26] However, our[27] as well other studies from Latin America and Mexico showed that there was a mixture of Th phenotypes in leprosy patients using both enzyme-linked

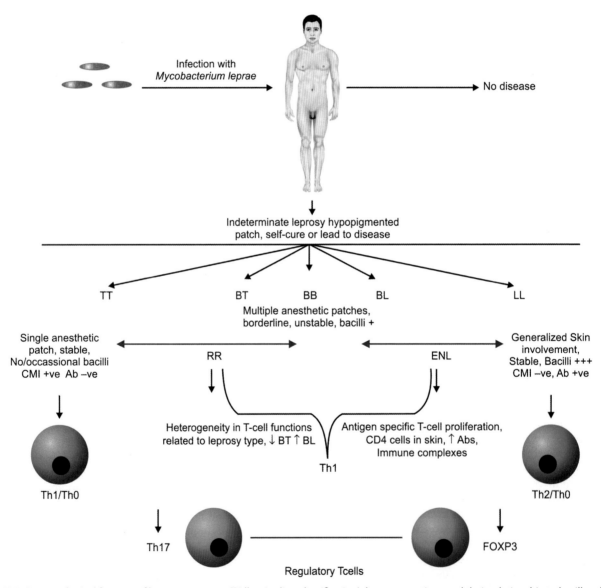

Fig. 7.1: Immunological features of leprosy spectrum (Ridley-Jopling classification), leprosy reactions and their relationship to bacillary load

Abbreviations: TT, polar tuberculoid; BT, borderline tuberculoid; BB, borderline borderline; BL, borderline lepromatous; LL, polar lepromatous leprosy; RR, type1/reversal; ENL, type 2/erythema nodosum leprosum reactions; Th1, T helper 1; Th2, T helper 2; Th0, T helper 0; Th17, T helper 17; FOXP3, fork head box P3.

immunosorbent assay (ELISA) and reverse transcription polymerase chain reaction (RT-PCR) for expression of cytokine genes. Though 50% of tuberculoid patients had Th1 others had Th0 phenotype. Similarly Th0 was again noted in 40% of LL patients with the remainder having Th2 phenotype.[27] There were no clinically detectable differences between patients having polarized Th phenotypes from those having the mixed Th0 functional phenotype.[27] Our group also showed that monocyte derived IL-10 and PGE2 played a role in Th2 phenotype in LL.[12] Thus, it would appear that there is a trend toward Th1 and Th 2 respectively in tuberculoid and LL. However, this may not be absolute or a paradigm.

The roles of costimulatory molecules such as B7, CD40/CD40L and CD28 have also been investigated as an explanation for the Th phenotype paradigm but definitive evidence for their direct effect is still awaited.[28] In conclusion, it is evident that the mechanisms underlying the antigen-specific unresponsiveness may be many and differ in various populations studied in the various laboratories. Consensus is lacking as to which the principle mechanism is underlying unresponsiveness.

Recently, other phenotypes such as Th17 or Th9 are being described, which produce respectively IL-17 that promotes inflammation and IL-9, which is involved in autoimmunity. CD4+ Th17+ cells have been shown to be increased more in tuberculoid as compared to LL both in the lesions and in the peripheral blood using gene expression studies and histochemistry. IL-17 isoforms and associated cytokines such as IL-21 and IL-22 which help in differentiation of Th17 cells also showed increase in culture supernatants of antigen stimulated peripheral blood mononuclear cells. This was further confirmed by the Th17 associated transcription factor retinoid receptor related orphan receptor. Of interest is the finding that Th17+ cells form a third subset of Th cells as they were seen in patients with non-Th1 and non-Th2 profiles.[29] Thus, this population may constitute the initial immune response to the leprosy bacillus before Th polarization has taken place; alternatively it may represent a constant nonpolarized state in some leprosy patients. That the Th17 cells may play a role in protective immunity is indicated by their greater presence in tuberculoid leprosy.

Another CD4+ CD25+ cell having the *FOXP3* transcription factor in the nucleus has been shown to have a regulatory role (Treg) and is involved in the downregulation of immune response in autoimmune diseases (Fig. 7.2). Recent reports from our laboratory and others have shown an increase in *FOXP3+* Treg cells in LL as compared to tuberculoid leprosy in both antigen stimulated peripheral blood and skin lesions using gene expression and flow cytometry studies.[30-32] More importantly, they secrete tumor growth factor beta (TGFβ)[30-32] or IL-10[31] which may be responsible for their suppressor role. The earlier studies that implicated monocytes derived factors as agents of suppression can be reconciled with the presence of Treg cells as it has been reported that prostaglandins,

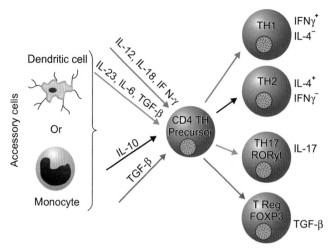

Fig. 7.2: The development of Th phenotypes, regulatory T-cells and related cytokines from a CD4 precursor cell induced by antigen and cytokines released by accessory cells

Abbreviations: IFN, interferon; IL, interleukin; TGF, tumor growth factor.

leukotrienes and thromboxanes play a role in the induction of *FOXP3* gene expression and induced Treg function in human CD4+ T-cells.[33] In summary, it is evident that T-cell biology involves a complex interaction between effector and regulatory cells and is a double-edged sword which may lead to protection through elimination of the pathogen and/or immunopathology as a result of tissue damage caused by DTH.

LEPROSY REACTIONS

Leprosy reactions are acute inflammatory episodes which occur in 10–20% of Indian patients and are seen more frequently (40–50%) in Latin America and Mexico where the severity of tissue injury is also greater. Since severe inflammation is a hall mark of reactions, injury to the neighboring nerves may occur which requires immediate medical attention to prevent nerve damage and deformity. Leprosy reactions can occur spontaneously but are mainly observed during or after institution of multidrug therapy (MDT). They are of two major clinical types: (1) Type 1 or reversal reactions (RR) which are localized to the dermal patch and neighboring nerve and occur mostly in patients with borderline leprosy, i.e. BT, BB and BL, (2) Type 2 reactions or ENL occurring predominantly in patients in the lepromatous end of the spectrum, i.e. BL and LL. Patients develop crops of tender erythematous nodules over the body and have accompanying systemic symptoms of fever, joint pain and neuropathy. In some patients, ENL episodes occur multiple times in spite of antireaction treatment with steroids or thalidomide.

In Type 1 reactions, T-cell-mediated responses toward *M. leprae* are activated resulting in an inflammatory response in the areas of the skin and nerves affected by the disease. From the point of clearing bacteria, such increased cellular immune responses may be beneficial, because they promote bacterial killing mechanisms. However, the accompanying inflammation in and around the infected nerve tissue can result in severe and irreversible damage within a matter of days. It is not clear what initiates this spontaneous and natural T-cell activation. During reactions, the PBMC of patients show increased lymphoproliferation to the *M. leprae* antigens as well as increased expression and release of proinflammatory cytokines such as IL-1, IL-2, IL-12, IFNγ and TNFα. These features are also noticed in the dermal lesions and nerves where increased infiltration by CD4 cells has also been observed. Recent evidence has indicated that IP-10 a chemokine induced by IFNγ seems to be a biomarker for Type 1 reactions as it is consistently observed to increase in the serum during or just prior to RR.[34-36] Some cytokines such as TNFα, IL-6, IL-10, IL-12 and soluble receptors of IL-2 have been demonstrable in circulation. Recent studies from our laboratory indicate that Th17 cells are increased and FOXP3+ Treg cells are decreased in Type 1 reactions. ENL or Type 2 reactions were initially thought to be due to immune complex deposition in the vessels and it was suggested that ENL was due to Arthus reaction.[37] Such deposition is not consistently demonstrable and conventional immune complex disease is not a clinical feature in ENL. Vasculitis is observed in ENL with Ig and complement in the vessel walls in the skin and nerves. Our and other studies have drawn attention to antigen specific T-cell activation, and release and expression of IFNγ and IL-12.[26,38,39] As mentioned above, lesions also show entry of T-cells,[40] lymphoproliferation and cytokine release after stimulation *in vitro* with *M. leprae* antigens. In addition, some studies have shown increase in IL-4, IL-6, IL-8 which are chemotactic for neutrophils and consistent with histological evidence of neutrophil infiltration in ENL lesions. However, such emergence of T-cells/functions in circulation or lesions does not reverse the negative skin test seen in LL patients and points to the gap between cellular immunity and the ability to develop delayed hypersensitivity in the skin. The latter involves other factors that lead to inflammation and the infected skin may lack such factors which would result in clinical hallmarks of DTH, viz. erythema and induration.

The trigger for the spontaneous development of antigen-specific immune responses in leprosy reactions has been a puzzle. Molecular recognition may vary during the natural course of diseases. With a view to investigate whether there were cryptic/hidden sites in the bacillus in the natural state which become exposed at such times, synthetic peptides covering the entire region of an immunologically active recombinant protein designated Lsr2[41] and A15[42] were designed. The Lsr2 first described by us has now been observed in many mycobacteria and other organisms. Intense research over the decade has shown it to be a transcription regulator with roles in biofilm formation, drug resistance and other functions. Screening leprosy sera with Lsr2 synthetic peptides in ELISA demonstrated that specific amino acid sequences were recognized during and prior to ENL.[43] Whereas, antibodies to sequence NAA (asparagine, alanine, alanine, respectively) were seen only in active ENL patients, antibodies to RGD (arginine, glycine, aspartic acid, respectively) were recognized before and during the reaction. Motif GVTY (glycine, valine, threonine, tyrosine, respectively) was also recognized in ENL, but its recognition was masked by flanking glutamic acid.[44] T-cell responses to peptides of Lsr2 have also been demonstrated in healthy contacts and stable leprosy patients. About 40% lepromatous patients who showed no responses to antigens of whole leprosy bacillus nevertheless recognized specific peptides of Lsr2 indicating that immune responses to part of the bacillus may be intact.[45] Of interest was the change in peptide/T-cell epitope recognition when ENL was observed in these anergic patients.[46] Moreover, the *in vitro* recognition of Lsr2 peptides continued to be seen well after the subsidence of the clinical signs of ENL following antireaction therapy, indicating that subclinical immune perturbations continue and may explain recurrence of reaction states in some patients.

Another model for the understanding of the reactions may be via the therapeutic approach. As indicated above, mounting delayed type response with PPD or intralesional injection of IFNγ reduces bacillary load in the skin within 3–6 weeks and also precipitates ENL as observed in Brazilian patients. Thalidomide, another effective drug for steroid resistant ENL patients has been shown to inhibit TNFα, IgM response, but increased IL-2 and apoptosis of neutrophils. Cyclosporine seems to also clinically improve ENL by inhibition of IL-2 and other cytokines.

In summary, it would appear that there is emergence of T-cell responses in reactional states. Antibodies and T-cells that recognize molecular motifs in the pathogen are also seen concurrently. Exploiting the cryptic motifs of the pathogen recognized by T-cells of lepromatous subjects may provide tools for vaccine design or boosting the immune response in the hitherto anergic patients. Taken together with earlier data of increased levels of polyclonal antibodies at the LL end of the spectrum, it is possible that T-cell activation leading to cytokine mediated killing of bacilli may release pathogen related antigens which then bind with existing antibodies to create immune complexes. T-cell recognition of motifs within the leprosy bacillus may indicate strategies to be used for diagnosis as well as vaccine targets.

IMMUNOPATHOLOGY OF DERMAL LESIONS

The leprosy lesion in the skin has also been studied for understanding immunopathology.[47,48] As mentioned above, the descriptions of earlier pathologists had given clues that the granuloma seen in tuberculoid leprosy has an immunological basis. In tuberculoid leprosy the granuloma shows the presence of lymphocytic cuff around the epithelioid cell center and lacks leprosy bacilli. The converse features are observed in the LL where lymphopenia is a hallmark and the macrophages lacking evidence of activation are filled with bacilli. Using cell surface markers defining the cell types, it was established that the lymphocytes were mainly of the CD4+ T-cells known commonly as helper T-cells as they are required to provide help to B-cells to produce antibodies against protein antigens. Such cells were both in the periphery of the granuloma as well as scattered among the epithelioid cells. CD8+ T-cells were fewer but formed a distinct ring around the epithelioid cells. CD8+ cells were known to be cytotoxic particularly in the transplant graft site and in malignancies and also considered by some to have suppressive functions in leprosy. In recent times in the animal model particularly, CD8+ cells were thought to have a containing role in mycobacterial infections such as tuberculosis. Surprisingly, B-cells are in low numbers even in LL.

About 90% of peripheral lymphocytes are T lymphocytes which exist as different subpopulations and have the αβ receptor (TCR), which recognizes protein antigens in association with major histocompatibilty (MHC/HLA) class II molecules. A small subset (< 1%) have an unconventional γδ TCR which has antigen specificity and plays an additional role. It detects bacterial lipid antigens in association with nonclassical MHC class Ib and CD1 molecules. The γδ T-cells are increased in mucosal epithelia which may be the entry point for most pathogens. They appear to recognize mycobacterial glycolipids in particular, and have been identified in leprosy lesions during reactions. They seem to have a regulatory role and appear before the conventional T-cells suggestive of their role in innate immunity. Conventional α/β TCR bearing T-cells are commonly seen in lesions and PBMC. γδ T-cells which constitute less than 1% of peripheral lymphocytes appear to be concentrated in leprosy granulomas.[49] CD1 molecules bind hydrocarbon chain of lipids and present them to CD1 restricted T-cells. Such T-cells have been shown to be increased in TT and Type 1 reaction skin lesions.[50]

In addition, Langerhans cells, another class of antigen presenting cells, present in the epidermis appear to migrate into the tuberculoid leprosy granulomas as CD6+ cells and are seen to be scattered among the lymphocytes.[40] Such migration may reflect a mode for transport of antigens from the skin to the lymph nodes for presentation to the appropriate T-cells to initiate cell-mediated immunity. The lymphocytes in the skin reaction to lepromin, also show the predominance of CD4 T-cells. This is not surprising as soluble antigens do not use the MHC class I pathway and therefore would not engage CD8 T-cells. In reactional states, the dermal lesions show an increase in CD4 T-cells and enhanced MHC class II on Langerhans cells. It is of interest that the earlier lymphopenic

LL lesions also showed entry of CD4 T-cell.[40] Local antibody release of IgG and IgM have also been demonstrated in leprosy lesions and from lesional cell cultures.[51] *TLR1* and *TLR2* are expressed more in tuberculoid lesions.[52]

Cytokine expression, as evidenced by mRNA detection has also been observed in dermal lesions. The tuberculoid leprosy granulomas show expression of interferon gamma (IFNγ) suggestive of a Th1 bias whereas lepromatous lesions had evidence of Th2 cytokines. Interestingly, during both reversal (Type 1) and erythema nodosum (ENL, Type 2) reactions, there is a distinct polarization to Th1 type as seen, both in our as well as other studies. The lesions in both type 1 and 2 reactions showed not only an increase in CD4 T-cells as mentioned above but also the expression of Th1 cytokine IFNγ and IL-12 p40, indicating a shift in Th type in ENL. That cytokines such as IFNγ are relevant for killing/clearance of leprosy bacilli is further endorsed by studies where genetically engineered IFNγ injected into dermal lesions showed a faster clearance of bacilli as compared to a control group that received only MDT. The lesional cells were shown to have enhanced arginine dependent NO synthetase in the injected sites which is a well-recognized radical responsible for killing organisms and damaging tissues.[53] Immunocytochemical demonstration of inducible nitric oxide synthase (iNOS) was also shown independently in leprosy lesions.[54] More importantly, such injected sites showed a clearance of bacilli and the entry of CD4 T-cells.[55] These changes were observed as early as 3 weeks after IFNγ injections indicating the effectiveness of cytokines as compared to combination of multiple antileprosy drugs which produce one log reduction of bacilli in the skin only after 1 year of therapy. Increase in Th17+ cells in tuberculoid leprosy and FOXP3+ cells in LL lesions have been shown.[29-31]

NERVE DAMAGE IN LEPROSY: THE IMMUNE MECHANISMS

Involvement of peripheral nerves is a hallmark of leprosy. *M. leprae* is the only bacterium that infects the nerves. Though occasionally bacilli in the mouse brain have been reported, it is the peripheral nervous system that is the target of immunologically mediated tissue destruction. Though the clinical and pathological features of leprosy neuropathy were well-known to the mechanism of interaction between *M. leprae* and peripheral nerves, in particular the SC, were described only in the last decade.

Entry of leprosy bacillus into SC is through multiple mechanisms. Mannose-capped lipoarabinomannan has been shown to bind to α-dystroglycans of SC. MLpLBP21 a cell wall fraction binds to α-laminin on the surface of SC. PGL-1 has also been shown to bind in a laminin 2 dependent manner to the SC of a SC line as do many other mycobacterial species without causing infection in human nerves. Following ingestion, as expected interiorization occurs and prevents the bacilli from being killed by antibodies. In patients, the infected nerves may be damaged by concurrent immunological and inflammatory events. Intraneural macrophages are capable of secreting a wide array of cytokines and chemokines, some of which may be deleterious to the nerve. TNF-α and TNF-α messenger ribonucleic acid (mRNA) have been observed in leprosy nerve lesions both in stable and reactional states. In some cases they may act synergistically with other cytokines to initiate apoptosis of SC. In addition, pro-inflammatory cytokines such as TNF-α also contribute to demyelination. Oliveira et al.[56] demonstrated the presence of *TLR2* on the human SC line ST88-14 and on SCs in the leprosy skin. Activation of SCs *in vitro* with a synthetic lipopeptide of the putative *M. leprae* 19 kDa lipoprotein lpqH, ML1966, triggered apoptosis which is in conformity with SC apoptosis seen in leprosy lesions. These observations indicate that activation of TLR-2 on SCs may contribute to nerve damage in leprosy and draw attention to the overlap of innate and adaptive immunity during the development of nerve damage.

In type 1 reactions, DTH reactions were induced against *M. leprae* antigenic determinants released from SCs, leading subsequently to damage of the nerve. Chronic ENL often leads to nerve damage, probably induced by local immune complex deposition with granulocyte attraction leading to tissue damage, and complement activation. *M. leprae* infected SCs play a role in the pathogenesis of nerve damage. In long-term cultures, human SCs were shown to express MHC class I and II, intercellular adhesion molecule 1 (ICAM-1), and CD80 surface molecules which are known to be involved in antigen presentation. Sperings et al.[57] showed that human SCs processed and presented native *M. leprae* bacilli as well as recombinant *M. leprae* proteins and peptides to MHC class II-restricted CD4+ T-cells. Such activated T-cells subsequently lysed the infected SCs. *M. leprae* infected SCs predominantly produced IL-4 and IL-10 (Th2 type) and failed to produce the proinflammatory cytokines (Th1).

That inflammation is the main component for nerve damage in reactional states particularly in Type 1 reactions has also been shown elegantly in patients using imaging techniques such as high resolution ultrasonography (Fig. 7.3). Intraneural blood flow signals indicative of increased blood flow as well as intraneural edema caused during inflammation has been observed in peripheral nerves during reactions.[58]

Nonimmune Mechanism of Nerve Damage

Mycobacterium leprae colonizes SC by attaching to the G domain of laminin-α2 chain (LN-α2), a protein constituent of the extracellular basal lamina, and its receptor α-dystroglycan, a component of the dystroglycan (DG) complex in the SC plasma membrane.[59] Other receptors may also be involved in the *M. leprae*-SC interaction, since blocking of the DG complex with purified α-DG in competition assays did not

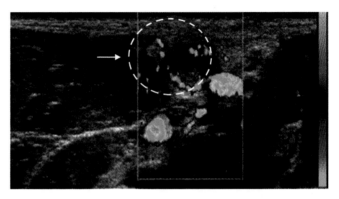

Fig. 7.3: High-resolution sonography and color Doppler image of right popliteal nerve showing intraneural blood flow signals (arrow and circle) indicative of inflammation in a patient with Type 1/reversal reaction

completely inhibit adhesion of *M. leprae*. The bacterial ligand that binds to the laminin-DG complex is thought to be PGL-1 glycolipid found only in *M. leprae*. Thus, PGL-1 is important for the bacillary invasion of SCs via the basal lamina in a laminin-2 dependent pathway. It is thought to act as a second receptor on *M. leprae* in which the combined action of *LBP21* and PGL-1 appears to provide sufficient energy of binding and thereby ensure safe entry of *M. leprae* into the SC. DG complexes link the basal lamina to the actin cytoskeleton of SC through membrane-associated linker proteins called dystrophins. They are believed to lend mechanical stability to SC and the nerve axons and may also transduce signals from the exterior to the interior of the cell.[60]

Contact-dependent demyelination induced by *M. leprae* in nerve tissue culture in the absence of immune cells has been described by Rambukkana et al.[61] suggesting a role for nonimmune mechanisms during the initial stage of nerve infection. Using a rat SC/axon coculture system, they reported rapid demyelination following adherence of *M. leprae* to SCs in the absence of immune cells. It can be easily interpreted to be a contact-dependent mechanism dependent on PGL-1,[62] a component of the *M. leprae* cell wall. It has been suggested in cultures that myelin-associated SC seem to be relatively free from *M. leprae* infection, whereas nonmyelinating SC were heavily colonized. Whether only nonmyelinated SCs permit infection by *M. leprae* is currently controversial though other studies have shown no such distinction.[63] Moreover, earlier ultrastructure studies on nerves from leprosy patients had demonstrated clearly the presence of the bacilli inside the SCs of myelinated axons.[64]

The major toxic effector molecule known to kill *M. leprae* is NO, and NO has been demonstrated in the inflammatory infiltrates of nerves in leprosy lesions.[65] Nitrotyrosine, an end product of the metabolism of NO, has also been observed in nerves in BL lesions, and this molecule has been associated with lipid peroxidation of myelin leading to demyelination of nerves in other diseases.[66] In association with the active inflammation of leprosy neuritis, reduced immunostaining for neurofilaments, nerve growth factor receptor, and other neural components has been described.

IMMUNOGENETICS OF LEPROSY

That genetic predisposition rather than environmental factors may predispose to leprosy has been considered for decades, but consensus for the type of genetic susceptibility was not available. It is well-known that household contacts are at a higher risk for developing leprosy. Moreover, only 0.1–1% of the exposed population gets the disease; patients with a particular leprosy type rarely change to another indicating that the immune response to the disease is set early in the host. Bacillus Calmette-Guérin (BCG) vaccination protects at different levels in diverse populations. One of the first evidence for the role of genetics was provided by Chakravarthy and Vogel[67] who showed that monozygotic as compared to dizygotic twins had a greater propensity to develop the same leprosy type.

Modern genetic methods have made possible human genome studies to identify susceptibility regions. Many markers, some relevant to the immune response and other unrelated ones became available. Their weakness lies in the fact that no single genetic factor has been shown to be common and universal to all ethnic groups. Nevertheless, they point toward a multifactorial genetic control (Table 7.1) that may affect multiple pathways of the defense mechanisms against infections. It is clear that polymorphism in genes affecting both innate and acquired immunity is identifiable in various populations indicating that leprosy may be a polygenic disease. But consensus is lacking on the details of how the immune system initiates, maintains and regulates the antigen specificity which is unique to leprosy and the leprosy spectrum.

Innate Immunity

With the deciphering of the human genome, whole gene scans and single nucleotide polymorphisms (SNPs) have been used to test high risk or susceptibility to diseases. Genome wide scans have identified a susceptibility to tuberculoid leprosy in chromosomal region 10p13.[6,68] More recently, genes associated with Parkinson's disease, *PARK2*, an ubiquitin E3 ligase which is involved in the delivery of polyubiquitinated proteins to the proteosomal complex and poxvirus anaphase promoting complex regulator (PACR) also regulating proteosome have been shown to be risk factors for leprosy in Vietnamese and Brazilian populations. The susceptibility locus was mapped to chromosome 6 region q25-q26. 17 SNP markers were found in the 5′ regulatory region of both genes and two of any of the 17 risk alleles was highly predictive of

leprosy. However, a similar study conducted in India failed to show association indicating population differences. The role of the genes in the pathogenesis of leprosy is not fully deciphered (Table 7.1).

Natural resistance-associated macrophage protein 1, which is present on macrophages is important for antigen presentation. The promoter genotypes 22 and 23 were found to be unfavorable when combined with a negative Mitsuda test in leprosy patients.[69]

Toll-like receptors are transmembrane molecules, which engage the lipid antigens of mycobacteria/pathogens and signal cytokine induction via NF-kB. *TLR1*, *TLR2* and *TLR4*, have been studied in leprosy.[52] N248 SNP variant of *TLR1* diminishes but does not totally abolish the response to bacterial agonists whereas *S248* variant enables normal functioning. The homozygous *S248* genotype increases the susceptibility to leprosy whereas the heterozygous SN genotype decreases and NN genotype shows none. *S248* allele and *I620S* are also more frequent in patients with RR. In humans, the 1805G variant does not mediate an inflammatory response to the leprosy bacillus *in vitro* and is associated with protection from reversal reaction. These data suggest that a common variant of *TLR1* is associated with altered adaptive immune responses to *M. leprae* as well as to the clinical outcome.[70]

That innate and adaptive responses can overlap is indicated by the mutation in *TLR2*. A mutation substituting arginine with tryptophan at residue 677 in one of the conserved regions of *TLR2* was shown to have a role in susceptibility to lepromatous, but not tuberculoid leprosy. Later, this mutation was shown to abolish intracellular signaling and activation of NF-kB after exposure of different cell types to *M. leprae* and *M. tuberculosis* leading to decreased production of IL-2, IL-12, IFNγ, and TNFα by *M. leprae* stimulated PBMC as compared with groups with wild-type *TLR2*. Moreover, the cells from patients with the *TLR2* mutation showed increased production of IL-10, which is known to suppress inflammation and Th1 type response. There was no significant difference in IL-4 production between the mutant and wild-type during stimulation. Thus, these results suggest that the *TLR2* signal pathway plays a critical role in the alteration of cytokine profiles in leprosy patients and that the *TLR2* mutation *Arg677Trp* provides a mechanism for the poor cellular immune response associated with LL.[71] In contrast, TLR4 SNPs are associated with protection against leprosy.[72] Toll-like receptors, have also been implicated in nerve damage.[56]

Other immune related genes include variants of vitamin D receptor (VDR),[73] transporter associated with antigen processing 1 (TAP1) and TAP2[74,75] important for antigen processing within the cell as well as cytotoxic T-lymphocyte antigen 4 (CTLA4) known to be a coreceptor in T-cells, macrophage associated NRAMP1[76] and COL3A.[77]

Acquired Immunity

Interleukin-12 polymorphism is associated with greater susceptibility to LL in patients from western Mexico, independently of IL-12 p40 and p70 expression levels.[78] SNPs within the 5' flanking region of *IL12RB2* affect the degree of expression of this gene and may be implicated in individual differences in CMI responsiveness to mycobacterial antigens, leading to lepromatous or tuberculoid leprosy. *IL12RB2*[79] TNFα2 allele frequency was significantly higher among control subjects than among all patients with leprosy or in the LL group. IFNγ mutated alleles contribute a role in leprosy postinfection and polymorphism of its receptor has been reported.

TNFα produced by macrophages appears to be important for resistance to leprosy[73] and as indicated above plays a role in the pathology associated with leprosy reactions. IL17F polymorphism where single nucleotide change from T to C has been shown at position 7448 to be associated with susceptibility to leprosy.[36] MHC class I molecules are delivered from cytosol to endoplasmic reticulum for further antigen binding which requires a heterodimeric protein called TAP. Recently, *TAP1* gene variant *637G* has been shown to be a susceptibility factor in leprosy.[75] Interestingly most studies on polymorphism indicate susceptibility to the leprosy disease and do not distinguish between the clinical types of the leprosy. It is possible that epigenetic differences may exist or alternatively, the critical polymorphisms are yet to be discovered.

CONCLUSION

Understanding the mechanisms that underlie the immunology of leprosy continue to be a challenge. In conclusion, it is possible that many of the differences reported in immunology of leprosy by different laboratories may be due to genetic differences in populations studied and the environmental stimuli that determine the innate immune response and the subsequent acquired immunity to the leprosy bacilli. Such findings draw attention to the need for local and multicenter research to define the profile of patients, and thereby design immunodiagnostics, vaccines and appropriate therapy for a given population.

REFERENCES

1. Ridley DS, Jopling WH. Classification of leprosy according to immunity -a five-group system. Int J Lepr Other Mycobact Dis. 1966;34:255-73.
2. Scollard DM, Adams LB, Gillis TP, et al. The continuing challenges of leprosy. Clin Microbiol Rev. 2006;19:338-81.
3. Nath I. Immune mechanisms of intracellular pathogens. Encyclopedia of Life Sciences. John Wiley & Sons Ltd; 2008.
4. Schlesinger LS, Horwits MA. Phenolic glycolipid-1 of *Mycobacterium leprae* binds complement C3 in serum and mediates phagocytosis by human monocytes. J Exp Med. 1991;174:1031-8.
5. Skamene E, Gros P, Forget A, et al. Genetic regulation of resistance to intracellular pathogens. Nature. 1982;297:506-9.
6. Mira MT, Alcaïs A, Van Thuc N, et al. Chromosome 6q25 is linked to susceptibility to leprosy in a Vietnamese population. Nat Genet. 2003;33:412-5.
7. Chatterjee D, Roberts AD, Lowell K, et al. Structural basis for the capacity of lipoarabinomannan to induce secretion of tumor necrosis factor. Infect Immun. 1992;60:1249-53.
8. Maeda YM, Gidoh M. Ishii N, et al. Assessment of cell mediated immunogenicity of *Mycobacterium leprae*-derived antigens. Cell Immunol. 2003;222:69-77.
9. Hunger RE, Sieling PA, Ochoa MT, et al. Langerhans cells utilize CD1a and langerin to efficiently present nonpeptide antigens to T-cells. J Clin Invest. 2004;113:701-8.
10. Nath I, Curtis J, Sharma AK, et al. Circulating T-cell numbers and their mitogenic potential in leprosy-Correlation with mycobacterial load. Clin Exp Immunol. 1977;29:393-400.
11. Haregewin A, Godal T, Mustafa AS, et al. T-cell conditioned media reverse T-cell unresponsiveness in lepromatous leprosy. Nature. 1983;303(5915):342-4.
12. Misra N, Selvakumar M, Singh S, et al. Monocyte derived IL 10 and PGE2 are associated with Th 2 cells and *in vitro* T-cell supression in lepromatous leprosy. Immunol Lett. 1995;48:123-8.
13. Salgame PR, Mahadevan PR, Antia NH. Mechanism of immunosuppression in leprosy: presence of suppressor factor(s) from macrophages of lepromatous patients. Infect Immun. 1983;40:1119-26.
14. Nath I, Vemuri N, Reddi AL, et al. The effect of antigen presenting cells on the cytokine profiles of stable and reactional lepromatous leprosy patients. Immunol Lett. 2000;75:69-76.
15. Nath I, Jayaraman T, Sathish M, et al. Inhibition of Interleukin-2 production by adherent cell factors from lepromatous leprosy patients. Clin Exp Immunol. 1984;58:531-8.
16. Sampaio EP, Moreira AL, Sarno EN, et al. Prolonged treatment with recombinant interferon gamma induces erythema nodosum leprosum in lepromatous leprosy patients. J Exp Med. 1992;175:1729-37.
17. Kaplan G, Laal S, Sheftel G, et al. The nature and kinetics of a delayed immune response to PPD in the skin of lepromatous leprosy patients. J Exp Med. 1988;168:1811-24.
18. De Vries RRP, Van Rood JJ, Lai Afat RFM, et al. Is susceptibility to tuberculoid leprosy due to a recessive HLA linked gene? Immune Mechanisms and Diseases. New York and London: Academic Press; 1979. p. 283.
19. Rani R, Zaheer SA, Mukherjee R. Do human leukocyte antigens have a role to play in differential manifestation of multibacillary leprosy patients from north India. Tissue Antigens. 1992;40:124-7.
20. Mehra V, Brennan PJ, Rada E, et al. Lymphocyte suppression in leprosy induced by unique M. leprae glycolipid. Nature. 1984;308(5955):194-6.
21. Ottenhoff TH, de Vries RR. HLA class II immune response and suppression genes in leprosy. Int J Lepr Other Mycobact Dis. 1987;55:521-34.
22. Salgame PR, Birdi TJ, Mahadevan PR, et al. Role of macrophages in defective cell mediated immunity in lepromatous leprosy. I. Factor(s) from macrophages affecting protein synthesis and

lymphocyte transformation. Int J Lepr Other Mycobact Dis. 1980;48:172-7.

23. Nath I, Van Rood JJ, Mehra NK, et al. Natural suppressor cells in human leprosy: The role of HLA-D identical peripheral lymphocytes and macrophages in the *in vitro* modulation of lymphoproliferative responses. Clin Exp lmmunol. 1980;42:203-10.

24. Sathish M, Bhutani LK, Sharma AK, et al. Monocyte derived soluble suppressor factor(s) in patients with lepromatous leprosy. Infect lmmun. 1983;42:890-9.

25. Prasad HK, Misra RS, Nath I. Phenolic glycolipid-1 of *Mycobacterium leprae* induces general suppression of Con A responses unrelated to leprosy type. J Exp Med. 1987;165:239-44.

26. Yamamura M, Wang XH, Ohmen JD, et al. Cytokine patterns of immunologically mediated tissue damage. J Immunol. 1992;149:1470-5.

27. Misra N, Murtaza A, Walker B, et al. Cytokine profile of circulating T-cells of leprosy patients reflect both indiscriminate and polarised Th subsets: Th phenotype is stable and uninfluenced by related antigens of *Mycobacterium leprae*. Immunology. 1995;86:97-103.

28. Santos AR, Suffys PN, Vanderborght PR, et al. Role of tumor necrosis factor-alpha and interleukin-10 promoter gene polymorphisms in leprosy. J Infect Dis. 2002;186(11):1687-91.

29. Saini C, Ramesh V, Nath I. CD4+ Th17+ cells discriminate clinical types and constitute a third subset of non Th1, non Th2 T-cells in human leprosy. PLoS Negl Trop Dis. 2013;9(7)e2338.

30. Saini C, Ramesh V, Nath I. Increase in TGF-β secreting CD4+CD25+FOXP3+T regulatory cells in anergic lepromatous leprosy patients. PLoS Negl Trop Dis. 2014;8(1):e2639.

31. Palermo ML, Pagliari C, Trindade MA, et al. Increased expression of regulatory T-cells and down regulatory molecules in lepromatous leprosy. Am J Trop Med Hyg. 2012;86:878-83.

32. Kumar S, Naqvi RA, Rani R, et al. CD4+ CD25+ Tregs with acetylated Foxp3 are associated with immune suppression in human leprosy. Mol Immunol. 2013;56:513-20.

33. Baratelli F, Lin Y, Yang SC, et al. Prostaglandin E2 induces FOXP3 gene expression and T regulatory cell function in human CD4+ T-cells. J Immunol. 2005;175:1483-90.

34. Stefani MM, Guerra JG, Sousa AL, et al. Potential plasma markers type 1 and type 2 leprosy reactions: a preliminary report. BMC Infect Dis. 2009;9:75.

35. Scollard DM, Chaduvula M, Martinez A, et al. Increased CXCL10 levels and gene expression in type 1 leprosy reactions. Clin Vacc Immunol. 2011;18:947-53.

36. Chaitanya VS, Jadhav RS, Lavania M, et al. Interleukin 17F single nucleotide polymorphism (7488T>C) and its association with susceptibility to leprosy. Int J Immunogenet. 2014;41(2):131-7.

37. Wemambu SN, Turk JL, Waters MF, et al. Erythema nodosum leprosum: a clinical manifestation of the arthus phenomenon. Lancet. 1969;2(7627)933-5.

38. Laal S, Bhtnani LK, Nath I. Natural emergence of antigen reactive T-cells in lepromatous leprosy patients during erythema nodusurn leprosum. Infect Immun. 1985;50:887-92.

39. Sreenivasan P, Misra RS, Wilfred D, et al. Lepromatous leprosy patients show T helper 1-like cytokine profile with differential expression of interleukin-10 during type 1 and 2 reactions. Immunology. 1998;95:529-36.

40. Narayanan RS, Bhutani LK, Sharma AK, et al. Normal numbers of T6 positive epidermal Langerhans cells across the leprosy spectrum. Lepr Rev. 1984;55:301-8.

41. Laal S, Sharma YD, Prasad HK, et al. Recombinant protein identified by lepromatous sera mimics native *M. leprae* in T-cell responses across the leprosy spectrum. Proc Natl Acad Sci U S A. 1991;88:1054-8.

42. Sela S, Thole JER, Clark-Curtiss JE, et al. Identification of *Mycobaterium leprae* antigens from a cosmid library: characterization of a 15-kilodalton antigen that is recognized by the humoral and cellular immune system in leprosy patients. Infect Immun. 1991;59:4117-24.

43. Singh S, Narayanan NP, Jenner PJ, et al. Sera of leprosy patients with type 2 reactions recognise selective sequences in *Mycobacterium leprae* recombinant LSR protein. Infect Immun. 1994;62:86-90.

44. Singh S, Jenner PJ, Narayanan NP, et al. Critical residues of *Mycobacterium leprae* LSR recombinant protein discriminate clinical activity in Erythema Nodosum Leprosum Reactions. Infect Immun. 1994;62:5702-5.

45. Chaduvula M, Murtaza A, Misra N, et al. Peptides of Lsr2 of *Mycobacterioum leprare* show hierarchial resposes in lymphoproliferative assays with selective recognition by anergic lepromatous leprosy patients. Infect Immun. 2011;80:742-52.

46. Saini C, Prasad HK, Rani R, et al. Lsr2 of mycobacterium leprae and its synthetic peptides elicit restitution of T-cell responses in Erythema Nodosum Leprosum and Reversal Reactions in patients with lepromatous leprosy. Clin Vacc Immunol. 2013;20:673-82.

47. Narayanan RB, Bhutani LK, Sharma AK, et al. T-cell subsets in leprosy lesions: in situ characterisation using monoclonal antibodies. Clin Exp Immunol. 1983;51:421-9.

48. Modlin RL, Hofman FM, Taylor CR, et al. T lymphocyte subsets in the skin lesions of patients with leprosy. J Am Acad Dermatol. 1983;8:182-9.

49. Uyemura K, Ho CT, Ohmen JD, et al. Selective expansion of V delta 1 + T-cells from leprosy skin lesions. J Invest Dermatol. 1992; 99:848-52.

50. Rosat JP, Grant EP, Beckman EM, et al. CD1-restricted microbial lipid antigen-specific recognition found in the CD8+ alpha beta T-cell pool. J Immunol. 1999;162:366-71.

51. Beuria MK, Mohanty KK, Katoch K, et al. Determination of circulating IgG subclasses against lipoarabinomannan in the leprosy spectrum and reactions. Int J Lepr Other Mycobact Dis. 1999;67:422-8.

52. Krutzik SR, Ochoa MT, Sieling PA, et al. Activation and regulation of Toll-like receptors 2 and 1 in human leprosy. Nature Med. 2003;9:525-32.

53. SivaSai KS, Prasad HK, Misra RS, et al. Effect of Interferon gamma administration on lesional monocytes/macrophages in lepromatous leprosy patients. Int J Lepr. 1993;61:259-69.

54. Khanolkar-Young S, Snowdon D, et al. Immunocytochemical localization of inducible nitric oxide synthase and transforming growth factor-beta (TGF-beta) in leprosy lesions. Clin Exp Immunol. 1998;113:438-42.

55. Kaplan G, Mathur NK, Job CK, et al. Effects of multiple interferon γ injections on the disposal of *Mycobactrium leprae*. Proc Natl Acad Sci U S A. 1989;86:8073-7.

56. Oliveira RB, Ochoa MT, Sieling PA, et al. Expression of Toll-like receptor 2 on human Schwann cells: a mechanism of nerve damage in leprosy. Infect Immun. 2003;71:1427-33.

57. Spierings E, De Boer TT, Zulianello L, et al. Novel mechanisms in the immunopathogenesis of leprosy nerve damage: the role

of Schwann cells, T-cells and *Mycobacterium leprae*. Immunol Cell Biol. 2000;78:349-55.

58. Jain S, Visser LH, Praveen TL, et al. High resolution sonography: a new technique to detect nerve damage in leprosy. PLoS Negl Trop Dis. 2009;3:498.
59. Rambukkana A, Salzer JL, Yurchenco PD, et al. Neural targeting of *Mycobacterium leprae* mediated by the G domain of the laminin alpha 2 chain. Cell. 1997;88(6):811-21.
60. Rambukkana A, Zanazzi G, Tapinos N, et al. Contact-dependent demyelination by *Mycobacterium leprae* in the absence of immune cells. Science. 2002;296:927-31.
61. Rambukkana A. *Mycobacterium leprae*-induced demyelination: a model for early nerve degeneration. Curr Opin Immunol. 2004;16:511-8.
62. Ng V, Zanazzi G, Timpl R, et al. Role of the cell wall phenolic glycolipid-1 in the peripheral nerve predilection of *Mycobacterium leprae*. Cell. 2000;103:511-29.
63. Hagge D, Robinson SO, Scollard D, et al. A new model for studying the effects of *Mycobacterium leprae* on Schwann cell and neuron interactions. J Infect Dis. 2002;186:1283-96.
64. Job CK. Pathology of peripheral nerve lesions in lepromatous leprosy–A light and electron microscopic study. Int J Lepr Other Mycobact Dis. 1971;39:251-68.
65. Khanolkar-Young S, Rayment N, Brickell PM, et al. Tumour necrosis factor-alpha (TNF-alpha) synthesis is associated with the skin and peripheral nerve pathology of leprosy reversal reactions. Clin Exp Immunol. 1995;99:196-202.
66. Schon T, Hernández-Pando R, Negesse Y, et al. Expression of inducible nitric oxide synthase and nitrotyrosine in borderline leprosy lesions. Br J Dermatol. 2001;145:809-15.
67. Chakravarti MR, Vogel FA. Twin study on leprosy. In: Becker PE (Ed). Topics in Human Genetics. Stuttgrat: Georg Thieme Verlag; 1973: pp. 1-123.
68. Mira MT, Alcaïs A, Nguyen VT, et al. Susceptibility to leprosy is associated with PARK2 and PACRG. Nature. 2004;427:63-40.
69. Ferreira FR, Goulart LZ, Silva HD, et al. Susceptibility to leprosy may be conditioned by an interaction between NRAMP1 promoter poly-morphisms and the lepromin response. Int J Lepr Other Mycobact Dis. 2004;72:457-67.
70. Schuring RP, Hamann L, Faber WR, et al. Polymorphism N248S in the human Toll-like receptor 1 gene is related to leprosy and leprosy reactions. J Infect Dis. 2009;199:1816-9.
71. Kang TJ, Yeum CE, Kim BC, et al. Differential production of interleukin-10 and interleukin-12 in mononuclear cells from leprosy patients with a Toll-like receptor 2 mutation. Immunology. 2004;112:674-80.
72. Bochud PY, Sinsimer D, Aderem A, et al. Polymorphisms in Toll-like receptor 4 (TLR4) are associated with

protection against leprosy. Eur J Clin Microbiol Infect Dis. 2009;28(9):1055-65.
73. Roy S, Frodsham A, Saha B, et al. Association of vitamin D receptor genotype with leprosy type. J Infect Dis. 1999;179:187-91.
74. Rajalingam R, Singal DP, Mehra NK. Transporter associated with antigen-processing (TAP) genes and susceptibility to tuberculoid leprosy and pulmonary tuberculosis. Tissue Antigens. 1997;49:168-72.
75. Shinde V, Marcinek P, Rani DS, et al. Genetic evidence of I TAP1 gene variant as a susceptibility factor in Indian leprosy patients. Hum Immunol. 2013;74:803-7.
76. Gruenheid S, Gros P. Genetic susceptibility to intracellular infections: Nramp1, macrophage function and divalent cations transport. Curr Opin Microbiol. 2000;3:43-8.
77. Kaur G, Sachdeva G, Bhutani LK, et al. Association of polymorphism at COL3A and CTLA4 loci on chromosome 2q31-33 with the clinical phenotype and in-vitro CMI status in healthy and leprosy subjects: a preliminary study. Hum Genet. 1997;100:43-50.
78. Alvarado-Navarro A, Montoya-Buelna M, Muñoz-Valle JF, et al. The 3'UTR 1188 A/C polymorphism in the interleukin-12p40 gene (IL-12B) is associated with lepromatous leprosy in the west of Mexico. Immunol Lett. 2008;118:148-51.
79. Ohyama H, Ogata K, Takeuchi K, et al. Polymorphism of the 5' flanking region of the IL-12 receptor beta2 gene partially determines the clinical types of leprosy through impaired transcriptional activity. J Clin Pathol. 2005;58:740-3.
80. Malhotra D, Darvishi K, Sood S, et al. IL-10 promoter single nucleotide polymorphisms are significantly associated with resistance to leprosy. Hum Genet. 2005;118:295-300.
81. Misch EA, Macdonald M, Ranjit C, et al. human TLR1 deficiency is associated with impaired mycobacterial signaling and protection from leprosy reversal reaction. PLoS Negl Trop Dis. 2008;7;2(5):e231.
82. Bochud PY, Hawn TR, Siddiqui MR, et al. Toll-like receptor 2 (TLR2) polymorphisms are associated with reversal reaction in leprosy. J Infect Dis. 2008;197:253-61.
83. Kang TJ, Lee SB, Chae GT. A polymorphism in the toll-like receptor 2 is associated with IL-12 production from monocyte in lepromatous leprosy. Cytokine. 2002;21:20(2):56-62.
84. Reynard MP, Turner D, Junqueira-Kipnis AP, et al. Allele frequencies for an interferon-gamma microsatellite in a population of Brazilian leprosy patients. Eur J Immunogenet. 2003;30:149-51.
85. Chaitanya VS, Lavania M, Nigam A, et al. Cortisol and proinflammatory cytokine profiles in type 1 (reversal) reactions of leprosy. Immunol Lett. 2013;156:150-67.

Biochemical Aspects of Leprosy

Krishnamurthy Venkatesan, Nirmala Deo

INTRODUCTION

Leprosy, also called Hansen's disease, is a chronic granulomatous infection principally affecting the skin and peripheral nerves caused by the obligate intracellular organism *Mycobacterium leprae*. The clinical manifestations of the disease are primarily due to: (1) bacterial progression in the host, and (2) immunologic and biochemical responses of the host to a chronic infection. It is primarily an infection of the peripheral nerves with secondary skin manifestations. One may, therefore, wonder how biochemical studies can be relevant in leprosy. However, biochemical investigations show that the situation is not so simple, but far more complex. Changes noted in biochemical, hematological and serological profiles, consequent to either the infection by leprosy bacilli including the occurrence of reactions; as well as following treatment, are important in understanding the consequences of the disease.

It is interesting to note that biochemical studies in leprosy were initiated over 60 years ago, two decades before the effective treatment with dapsone was introduced in leprosy. The limitation in leprosy research due to the inability to grow *M. leprae in vitro* was overcome by the availability of armadillo derived *M. leprae* in the pregenomics era. However, the scenario of understanding biochemistry of the leprosy bacillus and hence the disease, has become much better after the annotation of the genome of the causative organism *M. leprae*. The global leprosy scenario has witnessed significant change toward optimism with the advocating of WHO recommended multidrug therapy (MDT) in 1982. This chapter gives a bird's eye view of the morphology, cell wall chemistry, genomics, etc. of the causative organism *M. leprae*,

host-parasite interactions, changes in the hematological, serological and biochemical profiles as a result of this infection.

MYCOBACTERIUM LEPRAE

Cellular Morphology

Mycobacterium leprae, the etiological agent of leprosy, is a nonmotile, nonspore-forming, microaerophilic, acid-fast-staining bacterium that usually appears as slightly curved or straight rods. In size and shape, it closely resembles the tubercle bacillus. They occur in large numbers in the lesions of lepromatous leprosy (LL), chiefly in masses within the lepra cells, often grouped together like "bundles of cigars" or arranged in a palisade. Most striking are the intracellular and extracellular masses, known as globi, which consist of clumps of bacilli in a capsular material. Under the electron microscope the bacillus appears to have a great variety of forms. The most common is a slightly curved filament 3-10 μm in length containing irregular arrangements of dense material; sometimes in the shape of rods. Short rod-shaped structures can also be seen (identical with the rod-shaped inclusions within the filaments) along with dense spherical forms. Some of the groups of bacilli can be seen to have a limiting membrane.[1]

It is believed that only leprosy bacilli which stain uniformly with carbol-fuchsin as solid acid-fast rods are viable, and the bacilli which stain irregularly are probably dead and degenerating. These differences are valuable pointers in biopsy specimens to observe the effects of treatment. In patients receiving standard multidrug therapy (MDT), a very high proportion of bacilli are killed within days, which suggests that many of the manifestations of leprosy, including reactions which follow the initial treatment, must be due in part to antigens released from the dead organisms rather than from the living ones. Therefore, there is a need for drugs which will help the body to quickly dispose of dead leprosy bacilli. Two indices which depend on observation of *M. leprae* in smears from skin or nasal mucosa are useful in assessing the quantum of infection, the viability of the organisms and the progress of the patient under treatment. They are the bacteriological index (BI) indicating the density of bacilli in a smear and the morphological index (MI) giving the ratio of live to dead bacilli.[1]

Chemical Composition of Cell Wall of *M. leprae*

The cell wall of the organism is a covalently linked peptidoglycan-arabinogalactan-mycolic acid complex similar in composition to all mycobacterial cell walls.[2,3] Draper analyzed the chemical composition of cell walls of *M. leprae* and found a rare combination of glycine and diaminopimelic acid (DAP) which has not so far been shown to occur in other mycobacteria, and is considered to be an important characteristic of the organism.[4] *M. leprae* cell wall core contains peptidoglycan, composed of chains of alternating N-acetylglucosamine and N-glycolylmuramate linked by peptide cross-bridges, which is then linked to the galactan layer by arabinogalactan. Three branched chains of arabinan are in turn linked to the galactan, forming along with the peptidoglycan layer, an electron-dense zone around *M. leprae*. Mycolic acids are linked to the termini of arabinan chains to form the inner leaflet of a pseudolipid bilayer. The outer leaflet is composed of a rich array of intercalating mycolic acids of trehalose monomycolates and mycoserosoic acids of phthiocerol dimycocerosates as well as phenolic glycolipids (PGLs), forming the electron-transparent zone.[5,6]

The chemical composition of this immunologically active phenolic glycolipid resembles mycoside-A produced by *Mycobacterium kansasii*. However, the terminal trisaccharides in the phenolic glycolipids (PGLs) of *M. leprae* are different. They are 3.6-di-*O*-methyl-ß-D-glucopyranosyl (1→4)-2,3-di-*O*-methyl-α-*L*-rhamnopyranosyl-(1→2)-3-*O*-methyl-α-*L*-rhamnopyranose in phenolic glycolipid, and 3,6-di-*O*-methyl-ß-D-glucopyranosyl-(1→4)-3-*O*-methyl-α-*L*-rhamnopyranosyl-(1→2)-3-*O*-methyl-α-*L*-rhamnopyranosyl in phenolic glycolipid III. Since these are highly specific for *M. leprae*, these are found useful in the serodiagnosis of leprosy. A capsule presumably composed of largely PGLs and other molecules such as phthiocerol dimycocerosates (PDIMs), phosphatidylinositol mannosides, and phospholipids surrounds the bacterium. Lipoglycans such as phosphatidylinositol mannosides, lipomannan (LM), and lipoarabinomannan (LAM), known to be anchored in the plasma membrane, are also found in the capsular layer.[7]

Growth and Metabolism

As of date, it has not been possible to grow *M. leprae* on artificial media. However, they can be maintained in axenic cultures perhaps in a stable metabolic state for a few weeks.[8] Consequently, propagation of *M. leprae* has been restricted to only animal models, including the armadillo and normal, athymic, and gene knockout mice.[9,10] Genetic, metabolic and antigenic studies of the bacillus have all been conducted using the organisms provided by these systems. Growth of *M. leprae* in mouse footpads has also been providing a tool for assessing the viability of a bacterial preparation and testing the drug susceptibility of clinical isolates.[11] Metabolic studies have been/are being conducted on *M. leprae* to explore the possibility of formulating a special media that could support *in vitro* growth of the bacilli and the knowledge on its metabolic pathways could help in developing new antileprosy drugs. Consequent to completed sequencing and annotation of *M. leprae* genome, a better knowledge of the metabolic capabilities of *M. leprae* is now available.[12-14]

Mycobacterium leprae has the capacity to generate energy by oxidizing glucose to pyruvate through the Embden-Meyerhof-Parnas (EMP) pathway. Acetyl-coenzyme A from glycolysis enters the Krebs cycle, producing energy in the form of adenosine triphosphate (ATP). The genome analysis as well as biochemical studies in *M. leprae* and *M. tuberculosis* suggest that these organisms, in addition to glycolysis, rely heavily upon lipid degradation and the glyoxylate shunt for energy production. *M. leprae* contains a full complement of genes for beta oxidation, but, compared to *M. tuberculosis*, has very few genes capable of lipolysis. Since only pseudogenes are present for acetate kinase, phosphate acetyltransferase, and acetyl-coenzyme A synthase, *M. leprae* fails to use acetate as a carbon source. *M. leprae* overall has fewer enzymes involved in degradative pathways for carbon and nitrogenous compounds than *M. tuberculosis*. The paucity of oxidoreductases, oxygenases, and short-chain alcohol dehydrogenases and their probable regulatory genes in *M. leprae* reflects this fact. In addition, other major problems associated with the metabolism of *M. leprae* are loss of anaerobic and microaerophilic electron transfer systems and severe limiting of the aerobic respiratory chain in *M. leprae*. Consequently, it is impossible for *M. leprae* to generate adenosine triphosphate (ATP) from the oxidation of NADH. In contrast to the reduction in catabolic pathways, the anabolic capabilities of *M. leprae* appear relatively unharmed. To cite few examples, complete pathways are predicted for synthesis of purines, pyrimidines, most amino acids, nucleosides, nucleotides, and most vitamins and cofactors.[15,16]

Genome of *M. leprae* vis-à-vis that of *M. tuberculosis*

The source of DNA for sequencing *M. leprae* genome was of the *M. leprae* originally purified from the skin lesions of a multibacillary (MB) leprosy patient from Tamil Nadu, India (TN strain), and subsequently extracted from the liver of a nine-banded armadillo. Comparison of the genome of *M. leprae* with that of its close relative *M. tuberculosis* suggests that *M. leprae* has undergone an extreme degree of reductive evolution.[15,17] This is firmly reflected by its smaller genome (3.3 Mb for *M. leprae* versus 4.4 Mb for *M. tuberculosis*) and a major reduction in G+C content (58% for *M. leprae* versus 66% for *M. tuberculosis*). The annotated genome of *M. leprae* contains only 1,614 open reading frames potentially encoding functional proteins, compared to 3,993 open reading frames predicted in *M. tuberculosis*. *M. leprae* genome possesses 1,133 inactivated genes (genes lost through mutation, or pseudogenes), compared to six pseudogenes in *M. tuberculosis*[18] and a large number of genes apparently have been entirely deleted from the genome of *M. leprae*. The result of massive gene loss has left *M. leprae* with less than 50% of its genome encoding functional genes whereas in *M. tuberculosis* 90% of the genome encodes functional genes. Also 34% of *M. leprae* proteins identified in silico appear to be the products of gene duplication events or share common domains.[19] Downsizing of the genome has its own consequence of the elimination of several metabolic pathways, making the pathogen need very specific growth requirements. The largest functional groups of genes in *M. leprae* are those involved in gene regulation, metabolism and modification of fatty acids and polyketides, cell envelope synthesis, and transport of metabolites.[13,15,17]

The ability of any microorganism to acquire iron from environment is essential for its pathogenic lifestyle. But it appears that *M. leprae* has a major deficiency in this aspect as entire *mbt* operon appears to have been deleted. So *M. leprae* is unable to make iron-scavenging siderophores mycobactin/exochelin.[15] Although genes known to be involved in iron acquisition are not obvious in its genome, *M. leprae* utilizes iron as shown by the presence of genes for cytochrome *c* (*ccsAB*), a ferredoxin (*fdxCD*), biosynthesis of the heme group (*hem* genes), a hemogloblin-like oxygen carrier (*glbO*), the iron storage bacterioferritin *bfrA*, and *ideR*, the iron regulation protein dependent on intracellular iron.[14] Intact polymorphic G+C-rich sequence- or major polymorphic tandem repeat-related repetitive sequences are not found in the genome of *M. leprae* and only a limited number of proline-proline-glutamic acid and proline-glutamic acid proteins are present.[18]

Molecular Identification of *M. leprae*

Rapid molecular-type assays have been developed for detection of *M. leprae* directly from patient specimens using available genetic data.[19-21] These assays have been based primarily on the amplification of *M. leprae*-specific sequences using polymerase chain reaction (PCR) and identification of the *M. leprae* DNA fragment. Many different *M. leprae* genes have been utilized in the development of PCR assays

for detection of *M. leprae* in clinical specimens. RNA analysis using 16S rRNA and reverse transcription-PCR has the added benefit of measuring post-treatment viability.[22,23] PCR has been found very useful in the detection and identification of *M. leprae* and when coupled with mutation detection analyses, it has the ability to provide rapid drug susceptibility results from clinical specimens. (More details in Chapter 20: Serological and Molecular Diagnosis of Leprosy).

Genotypic Variations in *M. leprae*

Genetic markers are increasingly found useful in establishing species- and strain-specific markers for assessing exposure to *M. leprae* and tracing transmission patterns. These genetic tools can also help in improving our understanding of the epidemiology of leprosy. A wide range of molecular markers have been applied to understand genotypic variations in *M. leprae*. Restricted fragment length polymorphism analysis of *M. leprae* isolates using different combinations of restriction enzymes and probes as well as sequencing of the internal transcribed spacer region of the 16S-23S rRNA operon yielded no polymorphic DNA sequences.[24,25] Based on the analysis of chromosomal DNAs encoding all or part of the 12 kDa, 18 kDa, 28 kDa, 65 kDa and 70 kDa proteins of *M. leprae* as well as *M. leprae* specific sequence using DNA probes, Williams et al. concluded that their isolates contained no polymorphism.[26] Polymorphism in another locus *polA* and variation in the number of TTC repeats have been described.[27,28] Variation in the number of copies of the 6 bp tandem repeat in the *rpoT* gene have been reported in 100 strains from north Indian patients. The variation in a GACATC repeat in the *rpoT* gene have also been described, but the value of these elements for differentiating possible *M. leprae* strains appears to be limited at present.[29,30] Based on the frequency of TTC repeats located downstream of a putative sugar transporter pseudogene, Shin et al. reported evidence for diversity among *M. leprae* isolates obtained from several patient biopsy samples in the Philippines.[31]

Pregenomic Study of a Few Enzymes of *M. leprae*

Consequent to the continued failure in attempts to culture *M. leprae*, the complete understanding of this fascinating mycobacterium has been eluding the scientists till annotation of *M. leprae* genome was completed in 2000. Today, however, some very useful basic information has been made available by their persistent efforts. While carrying out certain investigations on the metabolic properties of the leprosy bacilli isolated from leprous nodules and examining the activities of oxidative enzymes and enzyme related to amino acid metabolism in *M. leprae* suspension, Prabhakaran and Braganca were able to show for the first time, the presence of oxidative enzymes such as succinic oxidase, lactic dehydrogenase, peroxidase, etc. in *M. leprae* and that the bacillus is capable of getting its energy requirement with their help.[32,33] Prabhakaran made a very important finding that *M. leprae* possesses dihydroxyphenylalanine (DOPA) oxidase, an enzyme, which oxidises DOPA and this enzyme is highly specific to *M. leprae,* as he could not detect this enzyme activity in eight other mycobacteria studied.[34] However, there is still a debate over the validity of Prabhakaran's claim of the presence of DOPA oxidase in *M. leprae.*

Apart from DOPA oxidase activity attempts to identify other enzymes have also been made. Shetty et al. reported the presence of gamma glutamyl transpeptidase (enzyme catalysing the transfer of glutamyl groups) in suspensions prepared from biopsy materials obtained from leprosy patients.[35] Dhople carried out some taxonomic studies with a view to compare the biochemical properties of *M. leprae* with those of certain slow as well as rapid growing mycobacteria. The enzymes assayed were catalase, at room temperature and at 68°C and pH 7.0, arylsuphatase (3 and 14 days) and urease. Catalase was found to be present in *M. leprae,* arylsuphatase could be demonstrated on the 14th day and urease was not found.[36]

HOST–*M. LEPRAE* INTERACTIONS

The clinical and immunological manifestations and the associated hematological, serological and biochemical changes in leprosy patients can be well understood only with an insight into the finer aspects of the interactions of the causative organism, *M. leprae* with the host. In the past 10–15 years, lot of studies have been conducted on the interactions of *M. lepare* with the Schwann cells (SCs), macrophages, dendritic cells (DCs) and endothelial cells which could explain the pathogenesis and progress/spread of the *M. leprae* infection.

Interactions with the Schwann Cell and Mechanisms of Nerve Injury

Mycobacterium leprae has a unique host cell tropism in that, it preferentially infects and grows within Schwann cell (SC) surrounding the axons of the nerve cells. It is therefore, postulated that nerve damage in leprosy; and the resultant deformities and disabilities related to the disease, result from *M. leprae* invasion of human SC.[37-39] In patients with advanced leprosy, both myelinated and nonmyelinated Schwann cells are infected by *M. leprae* although some reports have suggested some preference for nonmyelinated SC. Several potential mechanisms of binding of *M. leprae* to the SC have been elucidated. Antibodies directed against the polysaccharide and lipid components of *M. leprae* inhibited adhesion to SCs, while those directed against both surface and cytoplasmic protein epitopes did not show any such effect, indicating that the association of *M. leprae* with SCs may be mediated by more than one of its cell surface molecules.[40]

A host molecule laminin-2 is the initial target for *M. leprae* seeking the Schwann cell niche. Laminin molecule comprises of α2, β1 and γ1 chains and is anchored to SC via the laminin receptor, alpha dystroglycan (α-DG). The globular (G) domain of the laminin α2 chain is the specific subunit with which *M. leprae* interact.[41] It is relevant that the natural sites of *M. leprae* infection in the human is the Schwann cells, striated muscle and the placenta where laminin α2 is distributed.[42] The specific receptor for *M. leprae* on Schwann cells is α–DG receptor.[43] Phenolic glycolipid (PGL-1), a molecule unique to *M. leprae* cell wall, has been shown to specifically bind to the laminin via its terminal trisaccharide *in vitro.*[15,44] Another specific putative bacterial adhesion, H1p/LBP21, potentiates interaction of *M. leprae* with the SC.[42]

After *M. leprae* adhere to the SC surface, they are slowly ingested as evidenced by the studies using denervated rat SC cultures and SC-neuron co-cultures,[45] and several protein kinases (except cAMP-dependent kinases) have been demonstrated to be essential for the ingestion.[46] The findings of these studies have shown that acidification of vesicles containing lethally irradiated (killed) *M. leprae* proceeded normally; while acidification was minimal when live *M. leprae* were used, suggest that viable *M. leprae* can interfere with normal endocytic maturation of the SCs. Infection of SC with whole viable *M. leprae* appears to favor survival of SC rather than apoptosis.[47] But binding of a *M. leprae*-derived lipoprotein to toll-like receptor 2 (TLR2) expressed by human SC is set to result in apoptosis.[48]

It has been reported that following adherence/binding of *M. leprae* to SCs in the absence of immune cells, a rapid demyelination occurs perhaps through a contact-dependent mechanism dependent on cell wall PGL-1.[47,49] The immune responses on *M. leprae* infected SCs have been described in detail by Scollard.[40] Based on the studies reported in this review, it appears that human Schwann cells express major histocompatibility complex (MHC) class II molecules after infection with *M. leprae* and the infected SCs appear to be able to process and present *M. leprae* antigens to CD4+ T cells. In addition to MHC class II molecules, human SCs can also express MHC class I, intercellular adhesion molecule 1 (ICAM-I), and CD80 surface molecules involved in antigen presentation. The nerve infected with *M. leprae* can also be affected by concurrent immunological/inflammatory events, through cytokines and chemokines. Molecules like tumor necrosis factor alpha (TNF-α), other proinflammatory cytokines and nitric oxide have also been reported to be involved in apoptosis and demyelination of SCs.[40]

Interactions of Macrophages with *M. leprae*

As an obligate intracellular pathogen, the principal host cells for *M. leprae* are the mononuclear phagocytes or macrophages where they can survive and replicate. The mechanism by which it resists destruction by phagocytes is not fully understood. The possibilities in the context of oxidative killing are:

- An ability to combat phagocytic microbicidal activity by inhibiting the respiratory burst
- An inability to stimulate the production of reactive oxygen metabolism
- Prevention of the interaction of the oxygen metabolites with the bacillus following phagocytosis; or
- Resistance to the oxygen metabolites. A disarrangement of nonoxidative antimicrobial systems cannot be ruled out.[7]

The basic biology of macrophage interactions with *M. leprae* has been reviewed excellently by Krahenbuhl and Adams.[50] The macrophage is a primitive cell type being found in both early and advanced life forms, and possesses a variety of functions, such as phagocytosis of invaded bacteria, production of cytokines, antigen presentation and tumor killing. In human leprosy a reduced chemotactic activity has been reported, although an enhanced migration of leukocytes from LL patients to antigens of *M. leprae* has been observed in mice. Phagocytosis has been reported to be normal in human leprosy.[51] Macrophages in specific tissue and infection sites can play an important role in pathogenesis of leprosy by releasing cytokines, including TNF-α consequent to their stimulation by whole *M. leprae* and/or its cell wall components[52] and by bridging, as antigen-presenting cells, the innate and acquired immunity of the host by evoking T-cell and B-cell responses.[42] It has also been shown that PGL-1, when added to human mononuclear cells exposed to *M. leprae,* stimulates them to produce TNF-α.[53]

Macrophages from LL patients exposed to *M. leprae,* showed reduced protein synthesis, unlike those from tuberculoid leprosy patients or normal individuals.[54] Both cured and active LL patients have defective macrophages, unable to respond to live *M. leprae* to produce superoxide anion, in contrast to the situation with the cells from normal healthy individuals.[55] Macrophages cultured from the peripheral blood of normal individuals, tuberculoid leprosy patients and long-term-treated, bacteriologically negative LL patients are able to release hydrogen peroxide on stimulation with *M. leprae.* But macrophages from bacteriologically positive LL patients produce considerably lower levels of hydrogen peroxide even with demonstrable stimulation of these cells with *M. leprae.* This differential stimulation of macrophages appears to be largely specific to *M. leprae.* It is possible that while other factors aid survival of *M. leprae* in the macrophages, hydrogen peroxide may not be highly effective in the killing of bacteria in infected patients.[56]

Interaction with Dendritic Cells

Though *M. leprae* is known to reside in SCs and macrophages, many other cell types such as DCs and endothelial cells also appear to harbor the organism. Infection of the monocyte-derived DCs *in vitro* with foot-pad derived *M. leprae* are

able to effectively phagocytose *M. leprae* and the DCs are able to present *M. leprae* specific antigens, including PGL-1.[57] Langerhans cells, a subset of DCs that initiate the immune responses in the skin, are more efficient at *M. leprae* antigen presentation than monocyte-derived DCs.[58] Major membrane protein II (MMP-II), an isolated and purified *M. leprae* protein, has been found to be highly immunogenic.[59] This protein stimulated the DCs directly and is suggested to result in high levels of T-cell activation when used to pulse the monocyte-derived DCs.[59,60]

Mycobacterium leprae and Endothelial Cells

Mycobacterium leprae has been reported to be present in the endothelium of the skin, nervous tissue and nasal mucosa, indicating that endothelial cell may be a site for *M. leprae* persistence and replication.[61,62] Based on a seminal study using armadillo model of *M. leprae* to determine the extent to which the bacilli could be found in endothelial cells, Scollard et al. have suggested that the endothelial cells in the epineurial and perineurial blood vessels could be a reservoir for actively replicating *M. leprae* that would subsequently infect SCs in the adjacent tissue. Their findings implicate that some mechanism of *M. leprae* attachment to the endothelial cells could be required for the establishment of infection and that *M. leprae* can reach the peripheral nerve tissue through the blood stream.[63]

HEMATOLOGICAL, SEROLOGICAL AND BIOCHEMICAL CHANGES IN PATIENTS WITH LEPROSY

The clinical manifestations of leprosy are primarily due to: (1) bacterial progression in the host, (2) immunologic responses of the host, and (3) the peripheral nerve damage due to either or both bacterial progression and immunologic responses of the host. Although typically, leprosy causes manifestations in the skin and peripheral nerves; leading to disability and deformity, it also affects multiple organs. Extensive work has been done on the evaluation of changes in hematolgical, serological and blood biochemical profile. Many of such reported studies are of sequential nature. The studies have been conducted across the leprosy clinical spectrum highlighting the profound changes in LL and reactional episodes, particularly erythema nodosum leprosum (ENL).

Hematological Profile in Leprosy

Hematological profile has been studied in adult leprosy patients with different clinical spectrum of leprosy, in various stages of the disease and treatment. Hemoglobin, packed cell volume, and serum iron are significantly lower among LL patients as compared with nonlepromatous patients.

The serum B_{12} levels were significantly higher among the lepromatous group. No significant changes were observed in serum iron levels in relation to disease and treatment status. With rising bacterial load, there was a trend toward lower hemoglobin concentration, higher vitamin B_{12} level and lowered serum folate levels.[64,65] Hematological changes like anemia, leukocytopenia and thrombocytopenia have been reported in a case of florid LL with bone marrow suppression due to the disease and these abnormalities were reversed by MDT for leprosy.[66]

Methemoglobinemia and hemolytic anemia were the principle side effects observed with dapsone long-term treatment. The hematological alterations occur in leprosy patients taking dapsone either as a single drug (DDS group) or as part of a MDT in combination with Rifampicin and Clofazimine. Decrease of hemoglobin in patients taking MDT for leprosy is very frequent. Deps et al. have reported that Dapsone used in the MDT regimen for leprosy patients decreases the hematocrit and hemoglobin levels due to a low-grade hemolysis, which can result in significant anemia. In their study, hemolytic anemia was observed in 24.7% of patients on MDT and occurred within the first 3 months in 51% of these.[67] In another study, reticulocytes were found to be elevated in 90% of the patients. Severe eosinophilia was also found. Heinz bodies have also been detected in 6.6% of the patients. The osmotic fragility test showed a reduction in cell resistance. The hematological side effects of Dapsone are significant even at doses currently used to treat leprosy (100 mg/day). Rifampicin and Clofazimine, however, do not increase the incidence of these effects during long-term treatment.[68]

Serological Profile in Leprosy

Sera of patients with LL have been studied for the presence of a variety of antibodies and immune complexes (ICs).[69] Significantly higher frequencies of heterophile, Hanganutziu-Deicher and Forssman antibodies were found in the sera of LL patients. The frequency of antibodies to cardiolipin was the highest and the frequency of rheumatoid factor was marginally high. Circulating ICs were demonstrated in 54% and 43% of the patients' sera by Raji-cell test and anti-antibody inhibition test, respectively. Analyses of immunoglobulin classes of IC showed that IgG was predominant in IC of patients with leprosy reaction (LR) and IgM in patients without LR. IC bind to various cells of the immune system that bear Fc receptors and they may be quickly cleared from the circulation, especially if they are larger in size. IC may be formed in tissues other than blood, where from they were not detected.[70]

In a study on leprosy patients from Papua New Guinea, serum antibodies to human collagen [anti-cardiolipin antibodies (ACA)] were detected by hemagglutination assay,

with variation in the prevalence of elevated titers of 1:4 or more, according to clinical spectrum of leprosy.[71] The gradient was significant from high prevalence in the immunodeficient polar lepromatous patients (53%); to a low prevalence at the tuberculoid end of the clinical spectrum (9%). It is not clear whether these antibodies are implicated either in the pathogenesis of leprosy, or in the prolongation and intensification of inflammatory reactions involving collagen at sites such as the skin, nerves, and glomerular basement membrane, and if so; to what extent.

A study on the prevalence of autoantibodies in patients by enzyme-linked immunosorbent assay (ELISA) has shown that SS-B (anti-La) antibodies, antibodies to mitochondria, and cardiolipin were most prevalent in the sera.[72] The study further observed that antimitochondrial antibodies, distinct from those seen in biliary cirrhosis, and antiphospholipid antibodies with variable ligand activity to B2GIP were frequent in the sera of leprosy patients. Autoantibodies reacting with testicular germinal cells of spermatozoa have been reported in both tuberculoid and lepromatous patients.[73,74] While these studies have reported postitivity of antispermatozoal antibodies in the sera in 39–77% in LL patients and 33–40% of tuberculoid patients. Kumar and Majumdar have shown a low degree of positivity (23.3%) in BL/LL patients using a sensitive ELISA. So, it is possible that in addition to prolonged disease, there must be other unidentified causes responsible for the reported testicular dysfunction and histopathological abnormalities.[75]

It has been reported that antibodies to (MMP-II) derived from *M. leprae* could be used to diagnose leprosy. MMP-II positivity has been reported in the sera of 82–98% of MB leprosy patients and 39–48% of PB leprosy patients from Japan and Indonesia .[76,77]

A study by Singh et al. has shown specific levels of anti-host keratin antibodies (AkAbs) in leprosy patients across the spectrum and explored its correlation with clinical manifestation of the disease. AkAbs level was significantly high in all the groups of leprosy patients except TT/BL in comparision to healty contacts. A study on TT, BL, LL, T1R and ENL patients have provided the evidence for the existence of molecular mimicry between cytokeratin-10 of keratin (host protein) and 65 kDa heat shock protein (HSP) (groEL2) of *M. leprae*. A positive correlation of antihost keratin antibodies level with the number of lesions of leprosy patients have been shown.[78]

Patients with MB leprosy had significantly higher anti-ceramide antibody serum levels compared to paucibacillary leprosy patients and healthy controls. Since multibacillary leprosy is associated with nerve damage, which contribute to myelin alteration and ceramide is a constituent of myelin sheath, the role of anticeramide antibody as a marker for nerve damage should be explored.[79]

Biochemical Changes in the Host

Hepatic Involvement

Of the various organs studied in leprosy, liver happens to be the most intensively investigated. The involvement of liver by way of formation of granuloma is a well-known feature in lepromatous leprosy and liver involvment has also been reported in cases of TT leprosy. The earlier studies were based on single parameters for liver function.[80-82] Increase in thymol turbidity and cephalin-cholesterol flocculation and reversal of albumin:globulin (A/G) ratio have been reported in the sera of lepromatous leprosy (LL) patients, with minimal changes in the TT spectrum. Serum transaminase levels in LL have been found to be elevated. In a study of hepatic involvement and hepatitis B surface antigenemia in leprosy, HbsAg was detected in 7.54% of lepromatous leprosy patients.[83] There was also a decrease in albumin and increase in globulin levels with significant decrease in A:G ratio. Serum glutamic pyruvate transaminase (SGPT) levels were significantly raised in lepromatous leprosy patients. Histopathological changes were present in 57.1% of lepromatous leprosy and 23.8% of tuberculoid leprosy patients.[83]

Serum Protein Profile

A variety of methods including electrophoresis have been employed to study the serum protein profile. It is difficult to list all the published reports. Briefly, total serum proteins are significantly raised in lepromatous group and in reactional forms of leprosy. This hyperproteinemia is mainly due to hyperglobulinemia which is present in all forms of leprosy with progressive rise from TT to LL and the highest values are noted in ENL. Highest values for plasma fibrinogen was observed in ENL patients while rest of the groups of leprosy showed progressive rise in the parameter from TT to LL.[84-87]

Gupta et al. have studied serum proteome of leprosy patients undergoing ENL reactions and compared it with that of healthy noncontact controls. Differentially expressed proteins were identified by matrix-assisted laser desorption ionization time-of-flight MALDI-TOF and MALDI-TOF-MS (Mass Spectrometry). Significant increase in one of the isoforms of alpha 2 chain of haptoglobin was observed in ENL. Hp 0-0 phenotype was detected in 21.4% of the ENL patients undergoing treatment.[88] A comparative analysis of the serum proteome by two-dimensional gel electrophoresis (2DGE) followed by mass spectrometry has shown the differential expression of acute-phase protein, α_1 acid glycoprotein (AGP; also known as orosomucoid) in the sera of leprosy patients. The AGP levels in untreated leprosy patients and ENL cases were significantly higher than in lepromatous leprosy (LL), reversal reaction (RR) and healthy controls. The acidic glycoforms of AGP were differentially expressed in untreated ENL cases. The levels of AGP decreased to normal levels after treatment with MDT and thalidomide. A stage-dependent increase in AGP in a LL patient who progressed into ENL stage, has validated AGP as an ENL-specific biomarker and treatment indicator.[89]

Lipid Profile

The ability to synthesize different lipid moieties and their distribution through plasma to all the body tissues seems to be altered in leprosy.[90] Misra et al. found a general lowering in total serum lipids, cholesterol and phospholipids but increase in serum triglyceride in LL.[91] On the contrary, a lowering in the levels of serum triglyceride in MB patients has also been reported.[92] Sritharan et al. opined that the decrease could be explained by the decreased adrenocortical functions in LL patients which may result in decreased activity of lipogenic and glycolytic enzymes.[93] Low incidence of atherosclerosis and coronary heart disease in patients of leprosy has been related to elevation of high-density lipoprotein (HDL) cholesterol and reduction of total cholesterol in patients with high bacterial indices. Ahaley et al. documented lowered serum cholesterol levels in patients of leprosy.[90] On the other hand, Gokhale and Godbole observed higher levels in their study.[94] Bansal et al. found significant increase in the values of HDL cholesterol in multibacillary patients patients in their series.[92] Sritharan et al. also observed an increase in HDL-cholesterol and a decrease in the level of LDL cholesterol in active LL patients.[95] Gupta et al. have documented decreased values of low-density lipoprotein (LDL) cholesterol in leprosy, more so in the LL group.[96] M. leprae, is thought to be the mycobacterium most dependent on host metabolic pathways, including host-derived lipids. In lepromatous leprosy lesions, there was preferential expression of host lipid metabolism genes, including a group of phospholipases, and that these genes were virtually absent from the mycobacterial genome. Host-derived oxidized phospholipids were detected in macrophages within lepromatous lesions and these oxidized phospholipids and HDL regulate innate immunity in leprosy.[97]

Renal Involvement and Kidney Function

Leprosy is well-known for its multi-visceral involvement though M. leprae ordinarily does not invade the renal parenchyma, yet considerable functional impairment in leprosy has been reported. Presence of edema, proteinuria, and biochemical abnormalities more so in the reactional phase have been reported.[98] Renal involvement in leprosy was first described by Mitsuda and Ogawa in 1937.[99] They described nephritis of all kinds in leprosy and also observed that renal failure was a frequent cause of death in their patients. Though renal involvement occurs throughout the spectrum of leprosy, it is more often seen in patients with lepromatous leprosy, especially those with history of frequent attacks of type 2 reactions, in which deposition of immune complexes occurs in kidneys. In a study of renal profile of leprosy patients, proteinuria was seen in 20% of patients while glomerular filtration rate (GFR) was low in 27% patients.[100] Renal biopsy specimens showed various types of nephritis: mesangioproliferative glomerulonephritis, membranoproliferative, and chronic interstitial nephritis. Mesangioproliferative glomerulonephritis was the predominant lesion, no acid fast bacillus, amyloid deposit, or granulomas were seen. Proliferative glomerulonephritis reported in patients with ENL could be a part of IC deposition in glomerular capillary walls. Immunofluoroscent staining for immune deposits were seen in the vessel walls and renal tubules apart from the glomeruli. In the glomeruli granular deposits were found to be localised in the mesangium to a larger extent and/or along the capillary walls. This pattern of staining is typical of an immune complexes glomerulonephritis. Renal involvement in experimental animals infected with *M. leprae* is almost comparable to human leprosy.[101]

Connective Tissue Catabolism

Estimation of hydroxyproline and hexosamine levels of skin tissue from patients with different types of leprosy and in different phases revealed a significant increase in the two constituents in LL during reactive phase.[102] Urinary levels of hydroxyproline were also found to be significantly elevated. Cherian et al. carried out longitudinal study of hydroxyproline excretion by leprosy patients and made similar observations. These findings are suggestive of a possible breakdown of connective tissues during reactive phases of LL.[103] Naik et al. have confirmed the increased urinary excretion of hydroxyproline levels in leprosy reactions.[104]

Endocrine Function

The endocrine manifestations caused by leprosy have long been recognized but underestimated, even by specialists. The endocrine dysfunction in leprosy has been extensively reviewed recently.[105] The testes are the most commonly affected endocrine organs. Leprosy may lead to azospermia, sterility and gynecomastia. A significant increase in gonadotrophins has been reported with significantly low level of testosterone in leprosy patients.[106] Increase in levels of luteinizing hormone (LH), follicle-stimulating hormone (FSH) and testosterone has been reported by Rea.[107] A study on the ovarian function in female patients with MB leprosy has reported increased mean levels of LH and FSH vis-à-vis controls.[108] Koshy and Karat reported normal basal pituitary-adrenal functions in LL patients.[109] However, response to the administration of metapyrone and synacten indicated a poor adrenal reserve in patients with chronic leprosy reactions. Balakrishnan et al. observed a significant lowering in 17-ketosteroids as well as 17-hydroxycorticosteroids in LL patients during reactive phase and a subnormal response

to ACTH administration, suggestive of a certain degree of adrenocortical insufficiency in leprosy reactions.[110] Using insulin hypoglycemia and ACTH stimulation tests Dash et al. failed to demonstrate any evidence of adrenal cortical insufficiency in any of the types of leprosy and in acute leprosy reactions.[111] Thus, most of the investigators who have studied hormone function in patients with gynecomastia, have got evidence for adrenocortical dysfunction. However, mention should be made of a report by Dass et al. who investigated the androgenic status of leprosy patients with gynecomastia. They noticed that plasma testosterone levels were significantly diminished along with inflammatory degenerative fibrotic changes in testes.[112]

Structural abnormalities of the thyroid, amyloid deposits, have been reported in leprosy, but the data on functional abnormalities of thyroid gland are controversial. Rolston et al.[113] and Yumnam et al.[114] reported normal serum levels of triiodothyronine (T3) and thyroxine (T4), and thyroid-stimulating hormone (TSH) in leprosy, while Garg et al.[115] and Kheir et al.[116] observed lower mean T3 and T4 levels and higher mean TSH levels in leprosy patients compared to the controls. Sehgal noticed a normal uptake of radioactive iodine by thyroid tissues from leprosy patients.[117]

A study on the functional status of pituitary–gonadal hormones and their relationship to the pattern of inflammatory cytokines in the lepromatous (LL/BL) and tuberculoid (TT/BT) poles of leprosy reported significantly higher levels of gonadotropins (LH and FSH), interleukin (IL)-1β, IL-6, TNF-α and C-reactive protein (CRP) concentrations and erythrocyte sedimentation rate (ESR) in LL/BL leprosy patients than in controls.[118] LH and FSH were positively correlated with IL-1β, IL-6 and TNF-α, and CRP concentrations and ESR. Plasma testosterone levels were significantly decreased in LL/BL patients. The significant correlations between gonadotropins and testosterone and cytokines in leprosy patients suggest that cytokines may have a direct influence at testicular level and may be of pathogenetic significance in leprosy and in other inflammatory states involving reproductive dysfunction. Hypercalcemia and abnormal 1,25 (OH) dihydroxy vitamin D, parathyroid hormone (PTH), and parathyroid hormone-related protein (PTHrP) concentrations have been reported in only a few patients with borderline and LL leprosy.[119-121]

The most common metabolic bone disease, osteoporosis, is of special importance in leprosy because of the risk of bone fracture in patients who already have neural lesions and both specific and nonspecific bone changes that result in deformities and disabilities.[122] Radiological osteoporosis changes have been detected in almost 40% of leprosy patients and with the measurement of bone mineral density (BMD), the incidence of osteoporosis might be higher.[123] Bone mass loss has recently been reported to be an early event in leprosy patients.[124]

Minerals and Trace Elements

Apart from the study on functional aspects of the different organs, isolated observations on certain blood constituents like minerals in leprosy patients have also been made. Some of them do have clinical implications. Significant decrease of serum calcium in LL seems to be related with the extent of leprosy lesions and duration. Serum calcium and magnesium were significantly decreased in all types of leprosy cases and LL patients showed highly significant decrease in serum magnesium level.[125-128] In chronic infections as well as conditions associated with an excess circulating oestrogens, increase in serum copper and decrease in serum zinc are generally observed. Similar observations on serum copper and zinc have been made by other investigators.[129-132] Foster et al. have reported significantly higher serum levels of titanium, silicon, potassium and platinum, lower levels of phosphorus in red blood cells and decreased whole blood levels of phosphorous, selenium, antimony and silver in leprosy patients.[126] Significantly low serum iron and total iron binding capacity have been reported in LL patients.[133-134]

Glucose Tolerance

Glucose tolerance test (GTT) has been carried out in patients in patients with tuberculoid, borderline, LL and those with leprosy reactions. A normal curve was common in tuberculoid leprosy while a flat glucose tolerance curve was observed in borderline and LL. However, diabetic curve was common in leprosy reactions. Fasting blood sugar was low in LL and it tended to be marginally high in leprosy reactions. Also flat GTT curves are observed in those with duration of disease between 7 months and 12 months while diabetic curve was more common in those with disease duration of more than 2 years.[135,136]

SERUM ENZYMES

Apart from transaminases, which have been referred to under liver function tests, a number of other enzymes in serum have also been investigated in leprosy patients. Normal to decreased levels of serum alkaline phosphatase, lipase and amylase have been reported to be generally in the normal range.[137] Saito noticed an elevation of LDH_4–LDH_5 isozyme fractions in serum of patients with progressive LL, probably as a result of injury to tissues like liver, skeletal muscle and skin which are rich in these enzymes.[138]

A significant lowering in serum cholinesterase activity has also been noticed in leprosy patients.[139] The mean values of butyryl cholinesterase (BuChE) in sera of all forms of leprosy are lower than in normal sera, when each group was compared with the normal mean, the value was not significantly different for any group except pure neuritic leprosy, thus the specific relationship of BuChE to nerve damage needs further investigation.[140] Balakrishnan in a study of serum enzymes

in the reactive phase of LL noticed a consistent increase in aldolase, creatine phosphokinase, LDH and serum glutamic oxaloacetic transaminase.[141] All these observations are suggestive of a generalized breakdown of tissue constituents in active LL and in particular, the reactive phase of LL.

There are reports on the blood and tissue levels of lysosomal enzymes, viz. lysozyme, beta-glucuronidase and N-acetyl beta-glucosaminidase correlating the levels with activity of the disease in adult and pediatric leprosy. Increase in the level of circulatory hydrolytic enzymes could be a tissue damaging factor and may be responsible for many of the lesions seen in leprosy.[142-146]

Oxidative and Antioxidant Status

A constellation of reactive oxygen species (ROS) capable of damaging cellular constituents is generated in excess during the chronic, inflammatory, neurodegenerative disease process of leprosy. The consequences of this lead to enhanced oxidative stress and lower antioxidant status. The serum lipid peroxidation products (LPO), serum LDH and important free radical scavenging enzymes, i.e. superoxide dismutase (SOD), catalase and antioxidant glutathione levels; and total antioxidant status have been studied in different types of leprosy patients. The levels of lipid peroxidation product, malondialdehyde (MDA), and LDH increased significantly in MB patients, and both gradually decreased with clinical improvement following MDT. The serum levels of SOD, catalase and glutathione, and the total antioxidant status decreased significantly in MB patients, in comparison with normal human volunteers (NHVs).[147] High free radical activity and low antioxidant levels observed in MB leprosy patients indicate that there is an oxidative stress in MB cases, irrespective of the treatment status and there is a suggestion of a suitable antioxidant therapy to the MB leprosy patients to prevent possible tissue injury.[148,149] Coadministration of vitamin E along with MDT decreases oxidative stress and activate the antioxidant status in leprosy patients.[150] Significant rise in serum MDA in both PB and MB leprosy has been seen when compared with controls. While vitamin E level was significantly low in both MB and PB leprosy patients, vitamin C level was found to be significanyly decreased in MB leprosy patients only compared to controls. It has been suggested that MDA levels can be used to monitor prognosis, treatment and control of leprosy.[151] The levels of LPO and MDA have been reported to be significantly increased in leprosy patients with chronic hepatitis in comparison with other patients, indicating the presence of high free radical activity in these patients. Concentrations of antiproteases-α-antitrypsin (α1AT), α1-acid glycoprotein (α1-GP), α2-macroglobulin (α2-MG), and haptoglobin (HP) were also significantly elevated in these patients. The degree of hepatitis activity was found to be related with increase in antiproteases, LPO and MDA.[152]

Nitric Oxide Metabolites

Nitric oxide (NO) known to contribute to pathogenesis of severe neurological diseases has been detected in tissues and urine of leprosy patients. Nitric oxide metabolites (stable end products of NO—nitrites and nitrates, estimated by a simple cadmium reduction method) have been found to be increased in the sera of MB leprosy patients and in patients with type 1 reaction as compared to healthy controls. These levels reduced significantly after treatment.[153]

The changes in biochemical profile including hematological and serological alterations in leprosy affected persons have been studied extensively during the last seven decades and these have been presented precisely in the chapter.

REFERENCES

1. World Health Organization. (2009). Microbiology of *M. leprae*. [online] Available from *www.who.int/lep/microbiology/en/index.html*. [Accessed May, 2014].
2. Draper P, Kandler O, Darbre A. Peptidoglycan and arabinogalactan of *Mycobacterium leprae*. J Gen Microbiol. 1987;133(5):1187-94.
3. Vissa VD, Brennan PJ. The genome of *Mycobacterium leprae*: a minimal mycobacterial gene set. Genome Biol. 2001;2:1023-30.
4. Draper P. Cell walls of *Mycobacterium leprae*. Int J Lepr Other Mycobact Dis. 1976;44(1-2):95-8.
5. Hunter SW, Brennen PJ. A novel phenolic glycolipid from *Mycobacterium leprae* possibly involved in immunogenicity and pathogenicity. J Bacteriol. 1981;147(3):728-35.
6. Draper P, Payne SN, Rees RJ. Isolation of a characteristic phthiocerol dimycocerosate from *Mycobacterium leprae*. J Gen Microbiol. 1983;129(3):859-63.
7. Brennan PJ. Mycobacterium leprae—the outer lipoidal surface. J Biosci. 1984;6:685-9.
8. Truman RW, Krahenbuhl JL. Viable *M. leprae* as a research reagent. Int J Lepr Other Mycobact Dis. 2001;69(1):1-12.
9. Truman R. Leprosy in wild armadillos. Lepr Rev. 2005;76(3):198-208.
10. Krahenbuhl J, Adams LB. Exploitation of gene knockout mice models to study the pathogenesis of leprosy. Lepr Rev. 2000;71:S170-5.
11. Shepard CC, Chang YT. Effect of several anti-leprosy drugs on multiplication of human leprosy bacilli in footpads of mice. Proc Soc Exp Biol Med. 1962;109:636-8.
12. Brosch R, Gordon SV, Eiglmeier K, et al. Comparative genomics of the leprosy and tubercle bacilli. Res Microbiol. 2000;151(2):135-42.
13. Eiglmeier K, Simon S, Garnier T, et al. The integrated genome map of *Mycobacterium leprae*. Lepr Rev. 2001;72(4):462-9.
14. Wheeler PR. The microbial physiologist's guide to the leprosy genome. Lepr Rev. 2001;72(4):399-407.
15. Cole ST, Eiglmeier K, Parkhill J, et al. Massive gene decay in the leprosy bacillus. Nature. 2001;409(6823):1007-11.
16. Scollard DM, Adfams LB, Gillis TP, et al. The continuing challenges of leprosy. Clin Microbiol Rev. 2006;19(2):338-81.
17. Eiglmeier K, Parkhill J, Honore N, et al. The decaying genome of *Mycobacterium leprae*. Lepr Rev. 2001;72(4):387-98.
18. Cole ST. Comparative mycobacterial genomics. Curr Opin Microbiol. 1998;1(5):567-71.
19. Gillis TP, Williams DL. Polymerase chain reaction and leprosy. Int J Lepr. 1991;59(2):311-6.
20. Katoch VM. Molecular techniques for leprosy: present applications and future perspectives. Indian J Lepr. 1999;71(1):45-59.
21. Scollard DM, Gillis TP, Williams DL. Polymerase chain reaction assay for the detection and identification of *Mycobacterium leprae* in patients in the United States. Am J Clin Pathol. 1998;109(5):642-6.
22. Haile Y, Ryon JJ. Colorimetric microtitre plate hybridization assay for the detection of *Mycobacterium leprae* 16S rRNA in clinical specimens. Lepr Rev. 2004;75:40-9.
23. Kurabachew M, Wondimu A, Ryon JJ. Reverse transcription-PCR detection of Mycobacterium leprae in clinical specimens. J Clin Microbiol. 1998;36:1352-6.
24. Clark-Curtiss JE, Walsh GP. Conservation of genomic sequences among isolates of *Mycobacterium leprae*. J Bacteriol. 1989;171:4844-51.
25. de Wit MY, Klatser PR. *Mycobacterium leprae* isolates from different sources have identical sequences of the spacer region between the 16S and 23S ribosomal RNA genes. Microbiol. 1994;140:1983-7.
26. Williams DL, Gillis TP, Portaels F. Geographically distinct isolates of *Mycobacterium leprae* exhibit no genotypic diversity by restriction fragment-length polymorphism analysis. Mol Microbiol. 1990;4:1653-9.
27. Fishi H, Cole ST. The *Mycobacterium leprae* genome: systematic sequence analysis identifies key metabolic enzymes, ATP dependent transporter system and a novel pol(A) locus associated with genomic variability. Mol Microbiol. 1995;16:909-19.
28. Lavania M, Katoch VM, Singh HB, et al. Genetic polymorphism among *Mycobacterium leprae* strains from Northern India using TTC repeats. Indian J Lepr. 2005;77:60-5.
29. Lavania M, Katoch K, Singh, HB, et al. Predominance of three copies of random repeats in *rpo*T gene of *Mycobacterium leprae* from Northern India. Infect Genetics Evolution. 2007;7:627-31.
30. Matsuoka M, Maeda S, Kai M, et al. *Mycobacterium leprae* typing by genomic diversity and global distribution of genotypes. Int J Lepr. 2000;68:121-8.
31. Shin YC, Lee H, Walsh GP, et al. Variable numbers of TTC repeats in *Mycobacterium leprae* DNA from leprosy patients and use in strain differentiation. J Clin Microbiol. 2000;38:4535-8.
32. Prabhakaran K. Metabolism of *M. leprae* separated from human nodules. Int J Lepr. 1967;35:34-41.
33. Prabhakaran K, Braganca MB. Glutamic acid decarboxylase activity of *M. leprae* and occurrence of gamma-aminobutyric acid in skin lesions of leprosy. Nature. 1962;196:589-90.
34. Prabhakaran K. Specificity of O-Diphenol oxidase in *M. leprae*. An identification test. Lepr India. 1976;48:19-23.
35. Shetty KT, Antia NH, Krishnaswamy PJR. Occurrence of glutamyl transpeptidase activity in several mycobateria including *Mycobacterium leprae*. Int J Lepr. 1981;49:49-56.
36. Dhople AM. Taxonomic studies on *M. leprae*. Lepr India. 1983;55:39-44.
37. Skinsnes OK. *Mycobacterium leprae* and its affinity for nerves. Int J Lepr. 1971;39:762-5.

38. Stoner GL. Importance of the neural predilection of *Mycobacterium leprae* in leprosy. Lancet. 1979;10:994-6.

39. Job CK. Nerve damage in leprosy. Int J Lepr. 1989;57:532-9.

40. Scollard D. The biology of nerve injury in leprosy (Review). Lepr Rev. 2008;79:242-53.

41. Rambukkana A, Salzer JL, Yurchenco PD, et al. Neural targeting of *Mycobacterium leprae* mediated by the G domain of the laminin α2 chain. Cell. 1977;88:811-21.

42. Barker LP. *Mycobacterium leprae* interactions with the host cell: recent advances (Review). Indian J Med Res. 2006;123:748-59.

43. Rambukkana A, Yamada H, Zanassi G, et al. Role of α-dystroglycan as a Schwann cell receptor for *Mycobacterium leprae*. Science. 1998;282:2076-9.

44. Ng V, Zanazzi G, Timpl R, et al. Role of the cell wall phenolic glycolipid-1 in the peripheral nerve predilection of *Mycobacterium leprae*. Cell. 2000;103:511-29.

45. Hagge DA, Oby Robinson S, Scollard D, et al. A new model for studying the effects of *Mycobacterium leprae* on Schwann cell and neuron interactions. J Infect Dis. 2002;186:1283-96.

46. Alves L, de Mendonca Lima L, da Silva Maeda E, et al. *Mycobacterium leprae* infection of human Schwann cells depends on selective host kinases and pathogen–modulated endocytic pathways. FEMS Microbiol Lett. 2004;238:429-37.

47. Rambukkana A, Zanassi G, Tapinos M, et al. Contact-dependent demyelination by *Mycobacterium leprae* in the absence of immune cells. Science. 2002;296:927-31.

48. Oliviera RB, Ochoa MT, Sieling PA, et al. Expression of Toll-like receptor 2 on human Schwann cells: a mechanism of nerve damage in leprosy. Infect Immun. 2003;71:1427-33.

49. Rambukkana A. *Mycobacterium leprae* induced demyelination: a model for early nerve degeneration. Curr Opin Immunol. 2004;16:511-8.

50. Krahenbuhl JL, Adfams LB. The role of the macrophage in resistance to the leprosy bacillus. Immunol Ser. 1994;60:281-302.

51. Kumar B, Vaishnavi C, Ganguly NK, et al. Macrophage chemotaxis in *Mycobacterium leprae* infected mice. Indian J Med Res. 1987;85:125-9.

52. Susuki K, Fukutomi Y, Matsuoka M, et al. Differential production of interleukin 1 (IL-1), IL-6, tumor necrosis factor, and IL-1 receptor antagonist by human monocytes stimulated with *Mycobacterium leprae* and M. bovis BCG. Int J Lepr. 1993;61:609-18.

53. Charlab R, Sarno EN, Chatterjee D, et al. Effect of unique *Mycobacterium leprae* phenolic glycolipid (PGL-1) on tumor necrosis factor production by human mononuclear cells. Lepr Rev. 2001;72:63-9.

54. Mahadevan PR, Antia NH. Biochemical alteration in cells following phagocytosis of *M. leprae*—the consequence—a basic concept. Int J Lepr. 1980;48:167-71.

55. Marolia J, Mahadevan PR. Superoxide production from macrophages of leprosy patients after stimulation with *Mycobacterium leprae*. J Biosci. 1987;12:273-9.

56. Marolia J, Mahadevan PR. *Mycobacterium leprae* mediated stimulation of macrophages from leprosy patients and hydrogen peroxide production. J Biosci. 1988;13:295-303.

57. Hasimoto K, Maeda Y, Kimura H, et al. *Mycobacterium leprae* infection in monocyte-derived dendritic cells and its influence on antigen-preenting function. Infect Immun. 2002;70:5167-76.

58. Hunger RE, Sieling POA, Ocoa MT, et al. Langerhans cells utilize CD1a and langerin to efficiently present nonpeptide antigens to T-cells. J Clin Invest. 2004;113:701-8.

59. Makino M, Maeda Y, Ishii N. Immunostimulatory activity of major membrane protein–II from *Mycobacterium leprae*. Cell Immunol. 2005;233:53-60.

60. Maeda Y, Mukai T, Spencer J, et al. Identification of immunomodulating agent from *Mycobacteium leprae*. Infect Immun. 2005;73:2744-50.

61. Mcdougall AC, Rees RJ, Weddell AG, et al. The histopathology of lepromatous leprosy in the nose. J Pathol. 1975; 115:215-26.

62. Coruh G, McDougall AC. Untreated lepromatous leprosy: histopathological findings in cutaneous blood vessels. Int J Lepr. 1979;47:500-11.

63. Scollard DM, McCormick G, Allen JL. Localization of *Mycobacterium leprae* to endothelial cells of epineurial and perineurial blood vessels and lymphatics. Am J Pathol. 1999;154:1611-20.

64. Karat AB, Rao PS. Hematological profile in leprosy. Part I general findings. Lepr India. 1977;49:187-96.

65. Karat AB, Rao PS. Hematological profile in leprosy. Part II-Relationship to severity of disease and treatment status. Lepr India. 1978;50:18-25.

66. Binitha MP, Saritha S, Riyaz N, et al. Pancytopenia due to lepromatous involvement of the bone marrow:Successful treatment with multidrug therapy. Lepr Rev. 2013;84:145-50.

67. Deps P, Guerra P, Nasser S, et al. Hemolytic anemia in patients receiving daily dapsone for the treatment of leprosy. Lepr Rev. 2012;83:305-7.

68. Queiroz RHC, Melchior Jr E, De Souza AM, et al. Hematological and biochemical alterations in leprosy patients already treated with dapsone and MDT. Pharmaceutica Acta Helvetiae. 1997;72:209-13.

69. Kano K, Aranzazu A, Nishimaki T, et al. Serological and immunohistological studies on lepromatous leprosy. Int Archs Allergy Appl Immun. 1981;64:19-24.

70. Vaishnavi C, Kaur S, Kumar B, et al. Circulating immune complexes in normal and immunosuppressed mice infected with *Mycobacterium leprae*. Indian J Lepr. 1982;58:5229.

71. McAdam KJ, Fudenberg HH, Michaeli D. Antibodies to collagen in patients with leprosy. Clin Immunol Immunopathol 1978; 9:16-21.

72. Guedes-Barbosa LS, Gilbrut B, Shoenfeld Y, et al. Autoantibodies in leprosy sera. Clin Rheumatol. 1996;15:268.

73. Saha KD Gupta I. Immunologic aspects of leprosy with special reference to the circulating antispermatozoal antibodies. Int J Lepr. 1975;45:28-37.

74. Wall JR, Wright DM. Antibodies against testicular germinal cells in lepromatous leprosy. Clin Exp Immunol. 1974;17:519.

75. Kumar B, Majumdar S. Circulating anti-spermatozoal antibodies in leprosy (correspondence). Int J Lepr. 1991; 59:3346.

76. Maeda Y, Mukai T, Kai M, et al. Evaluation of major membrane protein-II as a tool for serodiagnosis of leprosy. FEMS Micrbiol Lett. 2007;272:2025.

77. Hatta M, Makino M, Ratnawati, et al. Detection of serum antibodies to *M. leprae* major membrane protein-II in leprosy patients from Indonesia. Lepr Rev. 2009;80:4029.

78. Singh I, Yadav AR, Mohanty KK, et al. Molecular mimcry between HSP65 of *Mycobacterium leprae* and cytokeratin 10 of the host keratin; Role in pathogenesis of leprosy. Cellular Immunol. 2012;278:63-75.

79. Singh K, Singh B, Ray PC. Anti-ceramide antibodies in leprosy: marker for nerve damage? J Infect Dev Ctries. 2010;4:378-81.

80. Naik S, Kumar B, Kaur S, et al. Cold reactive lymphocytotoxic antibodies in patients with tuberculoid and lepromatous leprosy. Int J Lepr. 1987;55:273-6.

81. Verghese A, Job CK. Correlation of liver function with pathology of liver in leprosy. Int J Lepr. 1965;33:342-8.

82. Dhople AM, Balakrishnan S. Liver function tests in leprosy. Indian J Med Res. 1968;36:1552-8.

83. Nigam PK, Gupta GB, Khare A. Hepatic involvement and hepatitis B surface antigen (HbsAg) in leprosy. Indian J Dermatol Venereol Leprol. 2003;69:32-4.

84. Parvez M, Sharda DP, Jain AK, et al. A study of serum proteins in leprosy. Lepr India. 1980;52:374-82.

85. Kurade N, Dhamanaskar PK, Jadhav VH, et al. Protein profile in leprosy. Indian J Med Sci. 2001;55:319-25.

86. Baji PS, Kher JR, Ganeriwal SK, et al. Electrophoretic patterns of proteins in lepromatous leprosy. Lepr India. 1982;54:82-94.

87. Ramu G, Balakrishnan S. Plasma fibrinogen and fibrinolytic activity in lepromatous leprosy. J Assoc Physicians India. 1977;25:133-8.

88. Gupta N, Shankernarayan NP, Dharmalingam K. Serum proteome of leprosy patients undergoing erythema nodosum leprosum reaction: regulation of expresson of the isoforms of haptoglobin. J Proteome Res. 2007;6:3669-79.

89. Gupta N, Shankeranarayanan NP, Dharmalingam K. α₁-Acid glycoprotein as a putative biomarker for monitoring the development of the Type II reactional stage of leprosy. J Med Microbiol. 2010;59:400-7.

90. Ahaley SK, Sardeshmukh AS, Suryakar AN, et al. Correlation of serum lipids and lipoproteins in leprosy. Int J Lepr. 1992;64:91-7.

91. Misra UK, Venkitsubramanian TA. Serum lipids in leprosy by silicic acid column choromatography. Int J Lepr. 1964;32:248-59.

92. Bansal SN, Jain VK, Dayal S, et al. Serum lipid profile in leprosy. Indian J Dermatol Venereol Leprol. 1997;63:78-81.

93. Sritharan V, Venkatesan K, Bharadwaj VP, et al. Serum lipid profile in leprosy. Lepr India. 1979;51:515-20.

94. Gokhale SK, Godbole SH. Serum lipolytic enzyme activity and serum lipid partition in leprosy and tuberculosis. Indian J Med Res. 1975;45:327-36.

95. Sritharan V, Bharadwaj VP, Venkatesan K, et al. High density lipoprotein cholesterol (HDL-C) analysis in leprosy patients. Lepr Rev. 1984;55:167-71.

96. Gupta A, Koranne RV, Kaul N. Study of serum lipids in leprosy. Indian J Dermatol Venereol Leprol. 2002;68:262-6.

97. Cruz D, Watson AD, Christopher S, et al. Host-derived oxidized phospholipids and HDL regulate innate immunity in human leprosy. J Clin Invest. 2008;118:2917-28.

98. Thomas G, Karat AA, Rao PS, et al. Changes in renal functions during reactive phase of lepromatous leprosy. Int J lepr. 1970;38:45-6.

99. Mitsuda K, Ogawa M. A study of one hundred and fifty autopsies on cases of leprosy. Int J Lepr. 1937;5:53-60.

100. Aggarwal HK, Sharma P, Jaswal TS, et al. Evaluation of renal profile in patients of leprosy. J Indian Acad Clin Med. 2004;5:316-21.

101. Vaishnavi C, Ganguly NK, Kumar B, et al. Renal involvement in *Mycobacterium leprae* infected mice. Histopathological, bacteriological and immunofluorescence studies. Indian J Lepr. 1987;59:416-25.

102. Balakrishnan S. Some aspects of collagen metabolism in leprosy. Indian J Med Res. 1970;58:1044-9.

103. Cherian MG, Karat ABA, Radhakrishna, AN. Urinary excretion of hydroxyproline in leprosy. Clin Chem Acta. 1969;25:395-401.

104. Naik SS, Tanksiile KG, Ganapati R. Study of urinary nitrogenous constituents in reactions in leprosy. Indian J Med Res. 1971;65:193-200.

105. Leal AM, Foss NT. Endocrine dysfunction in leprosy (Review). Eur J Clin Microbiol Infect Dis. 2009;28:1-7.

106. Kannan V, Vijaya G. Endocrine testicular functions in leprosy. Horm Metab Res. 1984;16:146-50.

107. Rea TH. A comparative study of testicular involvememnt in lepromatous and borderline lepromatous leprosy. Int J Lepr. 1988;56:383-8.

108. Khanna N, Ammini AC, Singh MK, et al. Ovarian function in female patients with multibacillary leprosy. Int J Lepr. 2003;71:101-5.

109. Koshy TS, Karat ABA. Assessment of pituitary adrenal functions in lepromatous leprosy. Lepr India. 1973;45:12-7.

110. Balakrishnan S, Ramanujam K, Ramu G. Adrenocotical function tests in lepra reaction Indian J Med Res. 1974;62:1166-70.

111. Dash RJ, Sriprakash ML, Kumar B, et al. Adrenal cortical reserve in leprosy. Indian J Med Res. 1985;82:388-92.

112. Dass J, Murugesan K, Laumas KR, et al. Androgenic status of lepromatous patients with gynaecomastia. Int J Lepr. 1976;44:469-74.

113. Rolston R, Mathews M, Taylor PM, et al. Hormone profile in lepromatous leprosy. A preliminary study. Int J Lepr. 1981;49:31-6.

114. Yumnam IS, Kaur S, Kumar B. Evaluation of thyroid functions in leprosy.I. Thyroid function tests. Lepr India. 1977;49:485-91.

115. Garg R, Agarwal JK, Singh G, et al. Thyroid function in leprosy. Indian J Lepr. 1990;62:215-8.

116. Kheir MM, Ahmed AM, Elsarrag AA. Thyroid functional status in leprosy patients in Sudan. East Mediterr Health J. 2001;7:79-83.

117. Sehgal VN, Basu AK. Thyroid function in leprosy as determined by uptake of radio active iodine. Int J Lepr. 1967;35:58-64.

118. Leal AM, Magalhães PR, Souza CS, et al. Pituitary-gonadal hormones and interleukin patterns in leprosy. Trop Med Int Health. 2006;11:1416-21.

119. Couri CB, Foss NT, Dos Santos CS, et al. Hypercalcemia secondary to leprosy. Am J Med Sci. 2004;328:357-9.

120. Hoffman VN, Korzeniowski OM. Leprosy, hypercalcemia, and elevated serum calcitriol levels. Ann Intern Med. 1986;105:890-1.

121. Vidal MC, Botasso OA, Lehrer A, et al. Altered calcium-binding ability of plasma proteins as the cause of hypocalcemia in lepromatous leprosy. Int J lepr. 1993;61:586-9.

122. Thappa DM, Sharma VK, Kaur S, et al. Radiological changes in hands and feet in disabled leprosy patients: a clinico-radiological correlation. Indian J Lepr. 1992;62:58-6.

123. Chouduri H, Thappa DM, Kumar RH, et al. Bone changes in leprosy patients with disabilities/deformities (a clinico-radiological correlation). Indian J Lepr. 1999;71:203-15.

124. Ribiero FB, Pereira F de A, Muller E, et al. Evaluation of bone and mineral metabolism in patients recently diagnosed with leprosy. Am J Med Sci. 2007;334:322-6.

125. Nigam P, Mukhija RD, Agrawal A, et al. Serum cations (calcium and magnesium) in leprosy. Indian J Lepr. 1985;57:529-33.

126. Rao KN, Gupta JD, Sehgal VN, et al. Trace elements in the sera of leprosy patients. Indian J Lepr. 1985;57:556-61.

127. Saxena N, Sharma RP, Singh VP. Study of serum calcium and magnesium in leprosy. Indian J Dermatol. 1989;34:48-51.

128. Foster R, Sanchez A, Foulkes J, et al. Profile of blood elements in leprosy patients. Indian J Lepr. 1991;63:12-33.

129. Venkatesan K, Kannan KB, Bharadwaj VP, et al. Serum copper and zinc in leprosy and effect of oral zinc therapy. Indian J Med Res. 1983;78:37-41.

130. Narang APS, Kumar B, Kaur I, et al. Serum copper and ceruloplasmin levels in leprosy. Trends Elem Med. 1988;5:70-1.

131. George J, Bhatia VN, Balakrishnan S, et al. Serum zinc/copper ratio in subtypes of leprosy and effect of oral zinc therapy on reactional states. Int J Lepr. 1991;59:20-4.

132. Mennen U, Howells C, Wiese AJ. Serum zinc, sodium, calcium, magnesium and potassium levels and standard diet in leprosy oatients. Indian J Lepr. 1993;65:415-21.

133. Bharadwaj VP, Venkatesan K, Ramu G, et al. Serum iron and total iron binding capacity in leprosy patients. Lepr India. 1978;50:11-7.

134. Saxena N, Sharma RP, Singh VS. Serum iron and total iron binding capacity in leprosy patients. Indian J Lepr. 1990;62:219-22.

135. Garg R, Agrawal JK, Bajpai HS, et al. Glucose tolerance test in leprosy. Indian J Lepr. 1990;62:50-4.

136. Bharadwaj VP, Venkatesan K, Ramu G, et al. Glucose tolerance and serum free fatty acid levels in leprosy. Indian J Med Res. 1979;69:567-70.

137. Balakrishnan S. Biochemical aspects of leprosy. Erwin Stindl Memorial Oration-organised by Greater Calcutta Leprosy Treatment & Health Education Scheme (GRECALTES) in collaboration with OXFAM (India) Trust: Grecaltes: Calcutta; 1986: pp. 6-40.

138. Saito N. Lactic dehydrogenase isozymes in leprosy patients. (1) Serum lactic dehydrogenase. Lepr India. 1972;44:82-9.

139. Gokhale BB, Desai BL. Cholinesterase activity in leprosy. Lepr India. 1960;32:22-4.

140. Suneetha LM, Karunakar V, Karuna S, et al. Serum Butyrylcholine esterase activity in leprosy. Int J Lepr. 2004;72:324-6.

141. Balakrishnan S. Biochemical aspects of reactional states in leprosy. Lepr India. 1976;48:406-12.

142. Venkatesan K, Bharadwaj VP, Ramu G, et al. Serum beta-glucuronidase in leprosy—a preliminary report. Indian J Med Res. 1979;69:553-6.

143. Naik SS, Gurnani S. Serum lysozyme in leprosy. Indian J Lepr. 1980;52:501-7.

144. George J, Rajendran M, Bhatia VN. Serum beta-glucuronidase in subtypes of leprosy. Indian J Med Res, 1990;91:106-10.

145. Vaishnavi C, Dhawan V, Ganguly NK, et al. Hydrolytic enzymes in leprosy sera. J Hyg Epidemiol Microbiol Immunol. 1992;36: 401-4.

146. Nandan D, Venkatesan K, Katoch K, et al. Serum beta-glucuronidase levels in children with leprosy. Lepr Rev. 2007;78: 243-7.

147. Prabhakar MC, Santhikrupa D, Manasa N, et al. Status of free radicals and antioxidants in leprosy patients. Indian J Lepr. 2013;85:5-9.

148. Reddy YN, Murthy SV, Krishna DR, et al. Oxidative stress and anti-oxidant status in leprosy patients. Indian J Lepr. 2003; 75:307-16.

149. Jyothi P, Riyaz N, Nandakumar G, et al. A study of oxidative stress in paucibacillary and multibacillary leposy. Indian J Dermatol Venereol Leprol; 2008.pp.74:80.

150. Vijayaraghavan R, Suribabu CS, Sekar B, et al. Protective role of vitamin E on the oxidative stress in Hansen's disease (Leprosy) patients. Eur J Clin Nutr. 2005;59:112-8.

151. Trimbake SB, Sontakke AN, Dhat VV. Oxidative stress and antioxidants vitamins in leprosy. Int J Res Med Sci. 2013; 1:226-9.

152. Naumov V, Mesniankina Q, Aprishkina M. Metabolic disorders in subsided cases of multibacillary types of leprosy. 18th International Leprosy Congress-Hidden Challenges. 16-19 September, 2013, Brussels (Belgium), Abstract No.O-005: p. 40.

153. Boga P, Shetty V, Khan Y. Nitric Oxide metabolites in sera of leprosy patients across the spectrum of leprosy. Indian J Lepr. 2010;8:123-9.

Pathological Aspects of Leprosy

Dullobho Porichha, Mohan Natrajan

INTRODUCTION

Leprosy a chronic disease of low infectivity is caused by *Mycobacterium leprae,* an acid fast bacillus (AFB). Clinically it manifests as a wide range of skin and nerve lesions the later sometimes causing more suffering due to permanent damage. In the fully evolved stage, the main tissue manifestation of leprosy is the formation of distinct granulomas as a result of acute to chronic inflammation. As space occupying lesions, these granulomas cause considerable host tissue damage, mostly affecting the skin and nerves. Hence, leprosy is also known as a granulomatous disease. *M. leprae* has a unique affinity for the peripheral nerves, in which it initially colonizes.[1-3] The pathogenic process mostly starts in the peripheral nerves and many workers view leprosy, primarily as a neural disease with Schwann cell as the main target.[4,5] Khanolkar was of the view that leprosy is neural in inception. In the words of Fite there is no non-neural leprosy.[6] *M. leprae* is not known to possess any toxin, and the histopathology changes are mostly due to the host immune response or lack of it, to the bacillus and its antigens. It is an intracellular bacillus and lymphocytes and mononuclear phagocytes mostly participate in the defense through the cell-mediated immune (CMI) responses. Bulk of the host tissue damage is due to delayed hypersensitivity and hence leprosy is also regarded as an immunologic disease,[3] and its pathology is now immunopathology. The process of immune-pathogenesis is briefly referred to at the appropriate places. The development of leprosy is graphically seen as four overlapping layers namely genetic, biochemical, cellular and clinical. Histopathology and the participating cells have been known for long but the knowledge about their foundation or basis is now greatly strengthened. There is an extensive scientific exploration in the field of molecular mechanisms or dynamics related to

cell identities, intercellular communications and genetics of an array of related molecules. A passing reference of these developments seems inevitable.

NEED FOR HISTOPATHOLOGY

Histopathology essentially captures the disease in question at the time of biopsy and provides insights into the disease process. Conventionally, it involves the examination of formalin fixed paraffin embedded sections processed and stained with hematoxylin and eosin. Additional special stains, immunohistochemistry and immunoelectron microscopy are now available as added tools. Besides this, application of several procedures related to molecular biology on tissue sections is becoming a routine in many laboratories. These developments make histology more informative and increasingly useful. These tests have contributed greatly to the understanding of leprosy and continue as one of the main pillars in the growth of immunopathology. Some of these tests form the "gold standard" for diagnosis, particularly in the face of ambiguities. The present day applications of histopathology are several and include:

- Confirmation of diagnosis in a clinically ambiguous or suspect case, including special stains and immunohistochemistry.
- Diagnosis of a reaction state, differentiation of type 1 from type 2 reactions and relapse.
- Accurate classification by defining the spectral position of a given case for the purpose of therapy and research.
- Assessment of disease activity, response to therapy including cure.
- Application of the technique related to immunology and molecular biology.

Role of Immunohistochemistry

In most of its applications, conventional histopathology adequately fulfills its role. However, there are certain situations where other supportive procedures or techniques are required for more accurate decision. It may be recalled that there are two distinct aspects of the histological diagnosis of leprosy: (1) ascertaining the morphology and (2) detection of the pathogen. When the disease has evolved into a granuloma and acid fast bacilli are seen, confirmation of diagnosis is seldom difficult. In the pregranulomatous and postgranulomatous stages cardinal signs are ambiguous and negative for AFB. In such situations diagnosis becomes difficult. Literature reveals the confirmation rates through biopsy in several studies to be 29–58% in early and clinically suspect leprosy[7] while, if the sections are of good size and all stages of the disease included, the ambiguity of diagnosis could be narrowed to around 15%.[8] Accuracy of histopathologic diagnosis greatly depends on quality skin sections and Fite-Faraco stain. There cannot be any compromise on these two.

Methods enhancing sensitivity for both the morphology and pathogen through histopathology are now increasingly available. Techniques targeting the morphological aspect include the usage of additional stains like stain for nerves, quantitative morphometry and the use of semi-thin sections. There are also now available more sensitive and specific methods of detecting pathogens or their components on routinely processed tissue specimens. The technique of immunohistochemistry can be used to detect different antigens, applying either monoclonal or polyclonal antibodies (Fig. 9.1). Available multistep procedures make these studies highly sensitive. Several of such procedures using immunohistochemical methods have demonstrated mycobacterial antigens in AFB negative tissue sections from leprosy lesions.[9-12] Technological advances have made it possible to use the techniques of molecular biology on routinely processed tissue specimens.[13] The *in situ* hybridization procedure can be used to detect pathogen specific nucleic acid sequences within tissue sections. Several studies have employed the procedure to detect the presence of pathogens and many have used nonradioactive systems on paraffin sections. Some of the procedures have been employed in the diagnosis of early and clinically suspect leprosy (Fig. 9.2) with satisfactory results.[14] The procedures of immunohistochemistry and *in situ* hybridization can be performed in any histopathology set-up, if the reagent costs are met with.

Polymerase chain reaction (PCR) has been used in conjunction with hybridization to detect *M. leprae* specific nucleic acid sequences with good results.[13,15,16] This also achieves amplification in tissue specimens and is even more sensitive than the *in situ* hybridization procedure. While routine histopathology confirmed only 32% and 20% respectively in early and suspect leprosy cases, with direct *in*

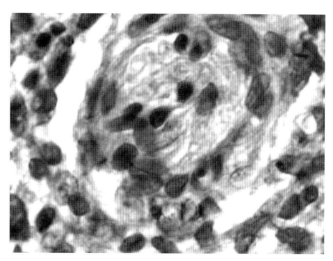

Fig. 9.1: Mycobacterial antigen in a dermal nerve (histochemical stain ×1000)

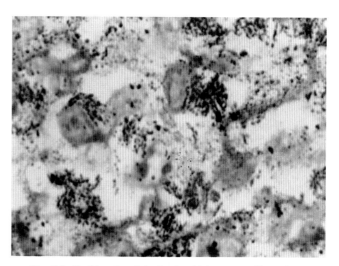

Fig. 9.2: Positive signals indicating *M. leprae* specific antigen (hybridization ×1000)

situ PCR the corresponding positivity rates could be enhanced to 70.6% and 60%. The result confirms the superiority of the procedure over routine histopathology.[17]

HISTOLOGY OF VARIOUS TYPES OF LEPROSY (TABLE 9.1)

The white blood cells (WBCs) mainly take part in defense against the microorganisms. Depending on the invading organism a particular group of WBCs better suited for the situation, become more active and counter the offender by their own strategies. It will be worthwhile to briefly introduce the WBCs which play a major role against *M. leprae* and how they protect or destroy the host tissue resulting in leprosy.

Table 9.1: Histopathological characteristics of various types of leprosy

Types Parameter	Indeterminate	Tuberculoid	Borderline tuberculoid	Borderline borderline	Borderline lepromatous	Lepromatous
Granuloma	Absent	Epithelioid cells	Epithelioid cells	Mixed cellular	Macrophages	Macrophages
T-lymphocytes	++++	++++	+++	++	++	+
Epithelioid-cells	Absent	++++	+++	++	+	Absent
Giant cells	Absent	+++	++++	Absent	Absent	Absent
Macrophage	Absent	Absent	+	++	+++	++++
Bacterial index	Negative	Negative	1+	2–3+	3–4+	5–6+
Nerves	Only lymphocytes	Destroyed	Damaged	Identifiable	Preserved for long	Late destruction
T helper cells	?	Th1 pattern	Th1 pattern	Mixed Th1/Th2	Th2 pattern	Th2 pattern
B-cells/Plasma cells	Absent	Absent	Absent	? Present	Present	Present
Cytokines		IL 2, 6, 12, 18, 10, INF γ, TNF-α	Same as in tuberculoid leprosy	Mixed	IL 4, 5, 8, 10	Same as in borderline lepromatous
Reactions	Absent	Reversal reaction	Reversal reaction	Reversal reaction	Reversal reaction/ENL	ENL

Cells Participating of Leprosy Lesions

Both in defeat and victory granuloma formation is the hallmark in leprosy. A granuloma is defined as a compact aggregate of macrophages or cells derived from them.[3] Monocytes of bloodstream migrate to the tissues as per the need, and transform to macrophages which are tissue based phagocytes. In response to the presence of *M. leprae* a granuloma develops by interaction of the macrophages and lymphocytes when there is immunity, otherwise it is formed by only macrophages. Macrophages belong to an extensive system of cells and tissues called the reticuloendothelial system, presently renamed as mononuclear phagocytic system (MPS). These cells contribute to both the innate (natural) and adaptive (acquired) immunity.[18] As long as in the bloodstream, monocytes are less aggressive round cells appearing as if peace time travelers in the blood. When they migrate to the tissue to deal with organisms or any unwanted element, they are like fighters on the front. They increase in size, develop pseudopodia and start phagocytozing anything that comes on their way. Macrophage literally means a "big eater" and the cells are worthy of the name. There are also cells of macrophage lineage as permanent resident, mostly in the organs facing frequent traffic by microbes. Reticulum cells of connective tissues, follicular cells of the lymph glands, Langerhans cells of the epidermis and Kupffer cells of liver are some examples.

Lymphocytes are of various subsets. After birth in the bone marrow, some lymphocytes from the bone marrow mature in thymus gland and are known as "thymus derived" or T lymphocytes. They are further divided into helper and regulator T lymphocytes, renamed as CD4+ and CD8+ cells respectively on the basis of cluster defined molecules on their surface. If the immunity is effective, macrophages being activated by CD4+ cells eliminate the bacilli or foreign material and transform into epithelioid cells. As an inherent tendency several epithelioid cells also fuse to form giant cells. This process of eliminating the organisms is executed by only immune cells and hence it is called cell-mediated immunity (CMI). Depending on the predominant cell type, a granuloma is called either macrophage or epithelioid cell type (to be described later).

Another subset of lymphocytes matures in the bone marrow in the mammals, and populates different tissues as B lymphocytes. The letter, "B" denotes "bursa derived" as these cells were first discovered in the bursa found in the cloacae of birds. Bone marrow itself is bursa equivalent in the humans. Some of them mature to plasma cells and produce antibodies which take part in humoral immune response, which is sometimes destructive. Though leprosy specific B-cells have been demonstrated in the active skin lesions, their role is not clear.[19] Presence of lymphocytes as such does not help much in diagnosis except in indeterminate leprosy. Schwann cells are important as main target cells of *M. leprae* and contributors to CMI in limited situations. A recent study estimated density of mast cells in Fite-Faraco stain, which stains the cells purple. Other studies reviewed in this connection showed inconsistent correlation with individual types of leprosy across the spectrum though the borderline group showed slightly higher number.[20] Mast cells secrete strong mediators of inflammation and their role may be relevant in reaction-prone borderline cases and deserve in depth study. Though some authors restrict the word granuloma to aggregates of only epithelioid cells, in leprosy the word includes that of macrophages also. Granuloma fraction (GF) is the percentage of dermis-width occupied by the lesion. It is estimated by focusing granuloma in its highest width under low power and expressed as multiple of 10. It can more accurately be measured by help of a planimeter. Sometimes, it is used in assessing the size as response to therapy.[21]

Granuloma formation is often nonspecific and its exact pathogenesis is not understood. In conditions, such as sarcoidosis and Crohn's disease, the etiology is unknown though evidence is building in favor of *Mycobacterium paratuberculosis* as the agent for the later. In diseases as leprosy and TB, it is an immune response to specific bacilli. Evolution of epithelioid cell is an indication of good cellular immune response. In leprosy, the formation of granuloma is preceded by a stage of only lymphocytic infiltration called indeterminate leprosy.

Indeterminate Leprosy

Evolution wise indeterminate leprosy is a pregranulomatous stage.[22] This is an early lesion not as per duration of the disease but disease evolution. Ridley suggested early and late stages of indeterminate leprosy.[23] The former shows occasional AFB either in normal nerve, arrector pilorum muscle, hair follicles, subepidermal zone (SEZ) and/or perivascular infiltrate. The features of late stage indeterminate leprosy are neural inflammation evidenced by lymphocyte infiltration (Fig. 9.3) or Schwann cell proliferation. In the former, varying number of lymphocytes is seen in the perineural sheath but the nerve parenchyma are well appreciated in the longitudinal section.

Sometimes the nerve fiber in a neurovascular bundle is hardly detectable as it is almost replaced by the lymphocytes (Fig. 9.4). The entire nerve may at times appear as a band of lymphocytes.

Schwann cells have the tendency to proliferate as they react to any injury or presence of bacilli. In normal nerves these cells show baton shaped nuclei oriented longitudinally. Once they proliferate, the nuclear orientation is lost and the nerve loses the wavy pattern. In the cases belonging to second stage, occasional AFB may be found on thorough search. Lymphocyte infiltration of other appendages is a feature for suspicion. These are not diagnostic and warrant examination of more sections.

Histological change of indeterminate cases is known to precede the clinical manifestations by 3–6 months.[24] Clinical manifestations are not evident until as high as 30% nerve fibers are damaged in a nerve[25] and these can be viewed as an advantage of histology over clinical signs. From the days of Havana International Congress, this type of leprosy remains a much discussed subject so far as the nomenclature, evolution and clinicopathologic disparity are concerned. These aspects are referred in an elaborate review.[26] Since *M. leprae* is the only bacterium to parasitize a peripheral nerve, the above neural changes are diagnostic of indeterminate leprosy.[27] These indicate good immunity while presence of few *M. leprae* in perivascular monocytes or macrophages indicates lack of CMI. About 70% of the indeterminate leprosy are known to heal spontaneously[28] and the rest develop into granuloma either epithelioid cell or macrophage type. As it is difficult to predict which cases would self-heal or evolve into a granuloma, all cases with confirmed diagnosis need treatement.

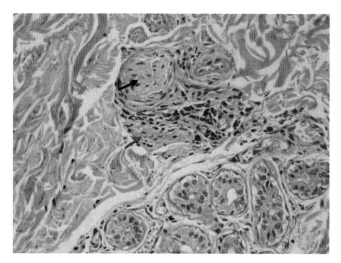

Fig. 9.3: Indeterminate leprosy. Nerve twigs are indicated by black and perineural lymphocytes by red arrow (H & E × 400)

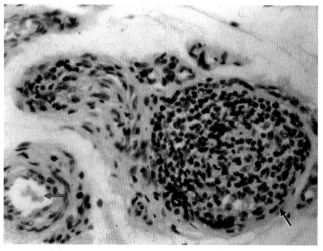

Fig. 9.4: Indeterminate leprosy. The nerve in a neurovascular unit is replaced by lymphocytes. The black and red arrows respectively show a stretched perineurium and blood vessel (H & E × 400)

Splitting of the Spectrum and Classification

As stated early, *M. leprae* is not known to possess any toxin to directly damage the host tissue.[29] The tissue response to the bacilli and their antigens depends on host immunity which is not an all-or-none phenomenon. Higher the number of the CD4[+] cells higher is activation of macrophages and elimination of the bacilli. After the job accomplished, these macrophages differentiate to epithelioid cells or else they continue as macrophages rearing *M. leprae*. Hence, at the time of detection a granuloma consists of either epithelioid cells or macrophages or a mixture of both cell types representing respectively two polar and one borderline types of disease. The histology is completely different though stable in two polar forms. In a particular population their numbers are limited and naturally each occupies a narrow segment in the spectrum. In between the two, lies a wide stretch of borderline leprosy always unstable due to continuing attempts of immunocytes to contain the bacilli. The result is moment to moment change, so dynamic that there may be coexistence of different histology in a single biopsy and/or in different skin lesions from the same patient.[30] If the cellular response is too intense leading to acute inflammation, it is called Type 1 reaction (T1R). In totality, the picture is an ever-changing borderline segment seen between two completely different pictures at the poles. It is rightly said, "leprosy is a spectrum as well as a syndrome with its dynamic immune response or lack of it".[31] Added to this, low mortality, longer disease span and widely spread clinical, histological and immunological, features make leprosy a suitable model for studying spectral manifestations. Cochrane as early as 1961 correlated the histological and clinical features at arbitrary points on the spectrum.[32] Spectral concept is also sometimes referred in diseases like tuberculosis, dermal leishmaniasis, some systemic mycosis such as South American blastomycosis and rarely in onchocerciasis,[22] though there is no evidence of their wider use as in leprosy.

The spectrum of leprosy has been metaphorically compared to *salami*[33]: a spicy meat dish served in slices. It can be sliced into any numbers. Ridley-Jopling classification according to immunity includes tuberculoid leprosy (TT), borderline tuberculoid (BT), borderline borderline (BB), borderline lepromatous (BL) and lepromatous leprosy (LL) types[34] representing five slices. A seven-type grouping was also subsequently proposed by addition of sub-polar TTs and LLs.[35] The WHO classification[36] into multibacillary (MB) and paucibacillary (PB) are like two thick slices and seems to be a rediscovery of the simplicity followed in early days.[37] Historically classification of leprosy has been a matter of active debate in almost all forums. Leprologists from India proposed their own system under the leadership of Dharmendra, who has reviewed the issue in a full article.[38] Discussion in this chapter is confined to only five types of leprosy as given in Ridley-Jopling classification.

Tuberculoid Leprosy (TT)

Histology of TT is characterized by a granuloma consisting of epithelioid cells, giant cells and lymphocytes each varying in number and distribution. It seems to be a replica of CMI. Macrophage has a dual function. In the first phase, it captures and kills the bacilli, processes the antigens and presents with a molecule of major histocompatibility complex II (MHC II) to CD4[+] cells. It acts as antigen presenting cell (APC).[18] The naïve CD4[+] cells receive antigen-MHC and differentiate to T helper 1 (Th1) cells[39] promoted by interleukins 12 and 18 secreted by the macrophages. This helps in production of INFγ and TNF-α along with interleukins 2 and 15 which are T-cell growth factors.[40,41] Some Th1 cells produce different lymphokines which recruit fresh macrophages, activate and retain them until the bacilli are destroyed and the disease gets arrested. This is further supported by CD8[+] cytotoxic cells which destroy the host cells sheltering the bacilli. Their job completed the macrophages along with those, probably arriving in excess to what is required transform to epithelioid cells (Fig. 9.5). These are less phagocytic but rich in hydrolytic enzymes leading to autolysis.[42] Epithelioid cells have the tendency to fuse to form giant cells. In an elaborate article Wiersema and Binford[43] have dealt with various points which identify leprosy amongst epithelioid cell granulomas. Jadassohn seems to be the first to have described the tissue changes with tubercle formation and used the term 'tuberculoid' for such lesions.[44] Wade latter delineated the tuberculoid pole in the spectrum on the basis of histopathology.[45]

Regarding morphology, the granuloma of TT always erodes a chunk of epidermis by obliterating the subepidermal clear zone (Fig. 9.6). Lymphocyte number is high and often they make a dense mantle around a core of epithelioid cells forming a compact organized granuloma. Differentiating epithelioid cells from macrophages requires experience especially when the latter cells are young. Sometimes associated giant cells can be a helpful clue to differentiate. Epithelioid cells are elongated, have bean-shaped vesicular nuclei and densely stained eosinophilic cytoplasm. The cell borders interdigitate and hence appear indistinct. Giant cells are scanty and predominantly of Langhans type. Granuloma is often extensive occupying the entire width of the dermis with more or less round margin indicating arrest of the spread. Conspicuous absence of the nerve in the granuloma, due to complete effacement is the usual finding though occasionally remnants of neural elements may be seen especially by staining with S-100 antigen. If a nerve is clearly identifiable, it is generally a large one situated in the deeper dermis with parenchyma completely replaced by the epithelioid cells and central caseation (Fig. 9.7). It is interesting to find that caseation is mostly confined to nerve lesions.[43] The damage is so rapid that lamination of the perineurium, an attempt to repair is difficult to find. One frequent finding is coexistence of a normal and completely damaged nerve or an abscess overlying normal fascicles.

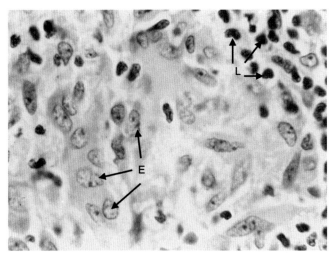

Fig. 9.5: Early epithelioid cell (E) differentiation with supporting lymphocyte (L) (H & E × 1000)

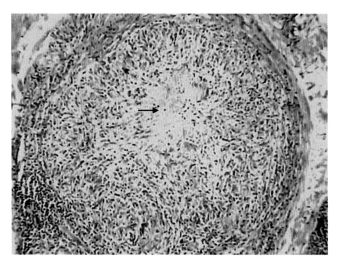

Fig. 9.7: TT leprosy. Shows caseation necrosis at the center of a nerve (H & E × 100)

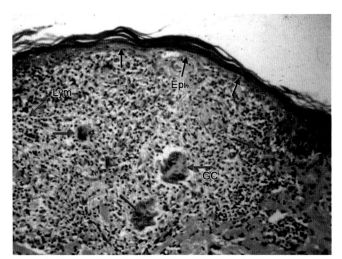

Fig. 9.6: TT leprosy. Epithelioid cell granuloma erodes SEZ (black arrows) and shows dense lymphocytes (red arrows), some Langhans GCs (H & E × 100)

In the lesion, the lymphocytes exhibit two types of distribution. Those in the core are identified as the CD4+ while, those in the outer mantle are CD8+. Strong cellular hypersensitivity is confirmed by a positive LTT.[22,46] Caseation is also an evidence of heightened hypersensitivity. Section is negative for AFB.

Borderline Tuberculoid Leprosy (BT)

The most important transitional stage in the evolution of leprosy is when an indeterminate case transforms to borderline generally the duration of which depends on CMI. A large number of cases are BT when detected and subsequently the number decreases due to both reversal

reactions and downgrading. A manifestation of delayed type hypersensitivity (DTH), epithelioid cell differentiation starts with mild acute inflammation in many cases (Fig. 9.5). This type of disease is a potential risk for tissue damage due to high propensity for DTH and a high tendency to downgrade, though carry the virtue to upgrade with treatment. Some of these facets are dealt in detail in a "point of view" article.[47]

Borderline tuberculoid lesion shows an epithelioid cell granuloma with some admixture of macrophages and lymphocytes. The focalization is lacking and the epithelioid cells are loosely distributed. Some show satellite lesions. In early cases, the granuloma is often branching with projecting spurs along the neurovascular bundles (Fig. 9.8). Lymphocyte number is moderate with fairly good number of giant cells scattered amongst them (Fig. 9.9). The giant cells are often of foreign body type. Nerves are replaced by granuloma but sometimes they are enlarged with stretched out or fragmented perineurium. Clear SEZ is a rule though a spur of the granuloma abuts the epidermis at some point. AFB stain sometimes shows few fragmented bacilli with bacterial index of granuloma (BIG) of around 1+ to 2+.

Borderline Borderline Leprosy (BB)

Granuloma of mid-borderline case shows a mixture of epithelioid cells and macrophages with predominance of the former. Lymphocytes are scattered and lesser in number compared to the other two cell populations. SEZ is always clear. Nerves are not completely destroyed with surviving Schwann cells visible within the granuloma. Transverse section of few nerves may show cut-onion appearance (Fig. 9.10). As the process of damage is slow the perineural cells attempt to repair by proliferation resulting in a multilayer structure the genesis of which is described in an illustrative article.[48]

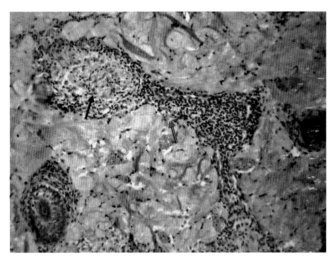

Fig. 9.8: BT leprosy. Shows a band of lymphocytes along a nerve (red) and foci of early epithelioid cell differentiation (black arrow) (H & E × 100)

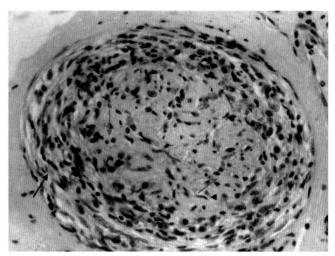

Fig. 9.10: BB leprosy. A nerve shows lamination due to multi-layering of perineurium (black arrows). The nerve parenchyma is replaced by lymphocytes (red arrows) and epithelioid cells and macrophages (blue arrow). H & E × 400

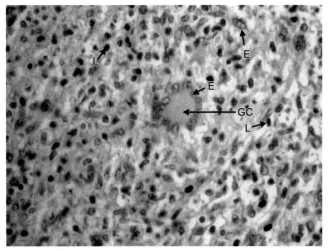

Fig. 9.9: A granuloma of typical BT leprosy. Shows scattered epithelioid cells (E) and lymphocytes (L) . A giant cell (GC) is evolving to Langhans type. Granuloma lacks focalization (H & E × 400)

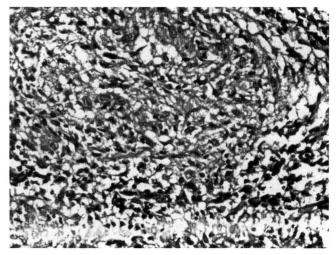

Fig. 9.11: BB leprosy showing a granuloma with epithelioid cells, macrophages and lymphocytes. There is also an element of T1R (H & E × 400)

Nerve parenchyma is intact with much of the cellular activities seen in prominently laminated perineurium. Giant cells are absent and this finding often helps in differentiating it from BT. BB leprosy being at the middle is mostly seen with some element of T1R (Fig. 9.11). Tissue change is highly unstable and transient. Accordingly proportion of cases recorded is low. Epidermis is usually normal with a clear SEZ. AFB is always present with higher density in nerves with a BIG about 3+.

Borderline Lepromatous Leprosy

The granuloma consists predominantly of macrophages with isolated clumps of epithelioid cells. The macrophages are young with uniform size, brightly stained eosinophilic cytoplasm and prominent nucleolus. Initially granuloma is perivascular and then expands around the neurovascular units (Figs 9.12A and B). It is sometimes difficult to differentiate between nascent macrophages and epithelioid cells though the latter are in compact clumps and devoid of bacilli in sections with AFB stain. Lymphocytes are sparse and scattered over most part of the granuloma. Occasionally few aggregates of lymphocytes are seen at some foci as if a group of surviving war prisoners awaiting trial. Nerves are conspicuous by concentric perineural cell proliferation presenting a cut-onion appearance. Occasional segment of nerve may be intact even though surrounded by the granuloma (Fig. 9.13). SEZ is free. Bacilli are always plenty

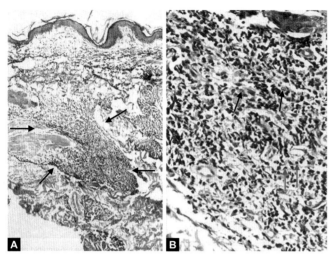

Figs 9.12A and B: BL leprosy. (A) A branching granuloma and clear SEZ (H & E × 40); (B) A higher power view of macrophages (H & E × 100)

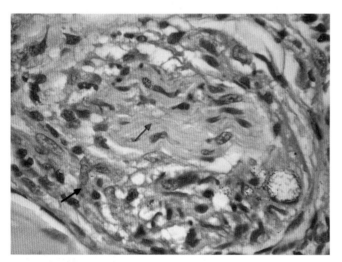

Fig. 9.13: BL leprosy showing surviving neural element (red arrow) in a macrophage granuloma (black arrow) (Fite-Faraco stain × 1000)

including small globi with BIG of about 4⁺. Early foamy change of macrophages gradually starts with aging of the disease.

Lepromatous Leprosy (LL)

Macrophage granuloma is a distinct feature of lepromatous leprosy (LL). As per the present view, *M. leprae* is transmitted through aerosol and deposited in the nose or any breach on the skin. When in the tissues, it is phagocytozed mostly by macrophages. If the CMI is ineffective, the bacilli are not destroyed due to failure of mounting the adaptive immunity. Being protected and nurtured by these cells, they multiply unchecked. With increase in the number of organisms the macrophages ultimately die, releasing hundreds of

M. leprae to be engulfed by fresh macrophages. So long there is multiplication of the organisms, the influx of the cells continues. In an advanced case, the entire dermis may contain a layer of macrophages loaded with bacilli. The piling of macrophages and other inflammatory cells even lift up the overlying skin producing areas of diffusely infiltrated skin, plaques and nodules. Such accumulation of macrophages is a granuloma by definition. The organisms also multiply in other phagocytes of MPS and facultative phagocytes such as endothelial cells and Schwann cells. Granuloma of active LL is mostly packed with macrophages. The cells are monotonously uniform with brightly stained eosiophilic cytoplasm (Fig. 9.14). The granuloma is expansive with high GF and due to the pressure from accumulating cells the epidermis often becomes flattened. A compressed strip of subepidermal clear zone always demarcates the granuloma and epidermis.

Few CD4⁺ or CD8⁺ lymphocytes are seen scattered in the sea of macrophages. Macrophages of aged granuloma vary in size and shape showing foamy cytoplasm. In Fite-Faraco stain, the cells show plenty of bacilli many of them bloated with globi of solid and fragmented AFBs (Fig. 9.15). Most of the cases also show AFB in the cells of the hair follicles. In rare LL cases, AFB even as globi is seen in cells of epidermis (Fig. 9.16).[49,50] In such cases, dissemination of *M. leprae* through normal shedding of epidermal cells cannot be ruled out. Bacilli are innumerable with BIG of 5⁺–6⁺.

Available molecular techniques have demonstrated few and scattered mRNA for interleukins 4, 5 and 10 in the granuloma indicating Th2 pattern CD4⁺ response.[40] Factors leading to lack of immune response are immune deviation from Th1 to Th2 pattern, T-cell unresponsiveness and suppression by macrophages and their factors. There is indication that down regulation could be through another set

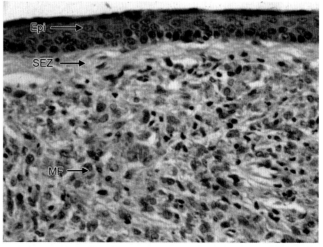

Fig. 9.14: LL leprosy showing nascent macrophages, clear SEZ, flat epidermis and scarce lymphocytes (Fite-Faraco stain × 400)

of CD4[+] cells having forkhead box protein 3 (Fox3p) transcript in the nucleus.[51] The cause of unresponsiveness remains unresolved, though there is general consensus that the defect is not central and not reversible.

Histoid Leprosy

Histoid leprosy is considered as a variant of LL. Described in 1963 by Wade.[52] It presents clinically as localized crops of shiny nodules of different sizes. The nodules are sometimes large and pedunculate. In sections they show hypercellular granuloma composed predominantly of spindle-shaped cells. These cells give an impression of expanding centrifugal growth

compressing the fibrous tissue into a clear "pseudocapsule". The young cells are uniformly arranged in compact bundles and whorls mimicking a histiocytoma (Fig. 9.17), from which the name histoid is derived.[52] The cells are highly bacillated with predominantly solid organisms (Fig. 9.18), arranged in parallel stacks, familiarly known as "histoid habitus" (arrows Fig. 9.18).

Some of the cases show areas with predominately polygonal cells which resemble conventional macrophages. Surprisingly some lesions show nests of epithelioid cells with almost no organisms in them.[52,53] Some call such islands of cells as "epithelioid contaminants". These features initially described by Wade were described latter by other workers.[53-55]

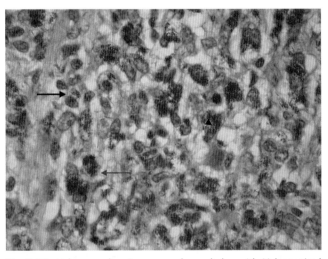

Fig. 9.15: LL leprosy showing macrophages laden with *M. leprae* (red arrow) and scarce lymphocytes (black arrow). (Fite-Faraco stain × 1000)

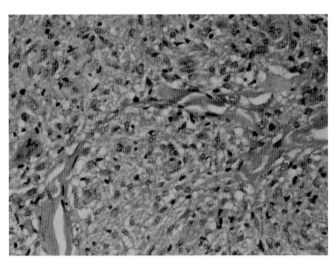

Fig. 9.17: Histoid leprosy showing hypercellular granuloma packed with spindle-shaped macrophages (H & E × 400)

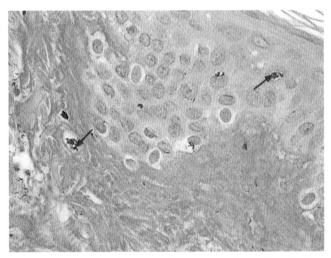

Fig. 9.16: LL leprosy showing *M. leprae* within the epidermal cells (Fite-Faraco stain × 1000)

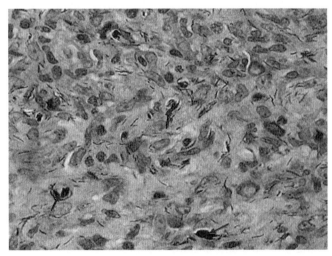

Fig. 9.18: Histoid leprosy showing predominantly solid bacilli in histoid habitus (Fite-Faraco stain × 1000)

The histoid lesions are speculated to have evolved in course of downgrading, from a tuberculoid stage or due to the influence of immunity, operating locally. Electron microscopic studies have confirmed the origin of the spindle-shaped cells from macrophages.[56] During the days of dapsone-monotherapy with emerging resistance,[57] many cases presented nodular type of LL with cellular features, suggestive of histoid lesions.

Experience with the Classifications

Out of several proposed in the evolutionary process, Ridley-Jopling classification at institutions and WHO MB-PB grouping in the field are used at this point of time. Both systems are complimentary for the program. The experience on use of these two classifications has been reviewed in an editorial by Lockwood et al.[58] There are references of both over and under treatments through using these two systems. Ridley-Jopling classification is followed mostly in the institutions, in spite of some over treatment judged as per WHO schedule, as it is probably on the safer side. This was expected while comparing the use of systems meant for different situations: field and institution, the latter also catering to referral. More importantly repeated changes in the criteria of MB PB grouping and case definition in initial years made lot of difference in addition to making outcome analysis of MDT difficult.

As per some recent publications on clinico-pathologic correlation, the concordance ranged from 57%[59] to 94%.[60] Another study reviewing the clinical criterion indicated that the sensitivity of MB group (WHO) can be improved by addition of two more clinical criteria: (1) number of body area affected (NBAA) and (2) size of largest skin lesion (SLSL).[61] Clinicopathological agreement generally depends on use of standard criteria and proficiency of both clinician and the pathologist. Ridley-Jopling classification along with its criteria has been well endorsed, about half century back by several studies undertaken globally after publication of the two articles. The criteria described seem to be of standard, considering the bizarre spectral manifestation of leprosy. In any study, if there is wide disparity the clinician and the histologist may discuss together to identify the reasons if any. The experience so far is: more the criteria more the confusions. Clinical and histopathology which takes care of bacterial aspects also, seem adequate for the field and referral needs until other tools are widely available.

REGRESSING LESIONS

The process of regression is well-appreciated in macrophage granuloma. The cytoplasm becomes foamy giving a soap-bubble appearance due to accumulation of fat (Fig. 9.19), thought to be released from the disintegrating bacilli as well as host cells.[62] Finally, there is accumulation of large "Lepra cells" of Virchow, containing mostly granular bacilli

some within vacuoles (Fig. 9.20). This phenomenon is like disposables moving from smaller to larger bins for final disposal or isolating them from the host tissue through vacuolated giant cells—what a noble way of waste disposal![63] Death of bacilli results in decrease of macrophages due to the arrest of both multiplication and influx of cells. Once the cells constituting the granuloma disappear the space is filled by adipose tissue with small aggregates of lymphocytes. Few bundles of nerves showing fibrosis, atrophic hair follicles and glandular structures are seen embedded in the adipose tissue. Some nerves show hyaline change depending on the age of the granuloma. The epidermis remains flat and thinned out.

Morphology of the epithelioid cells does not change with their age. The number decreases due to death. The size of the

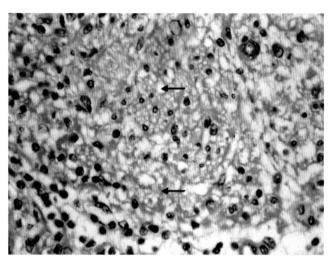

Fig. 9.19: Regressing LL. Shows granuloma with foamy cells and soap bubble appearance (H & E × 400)

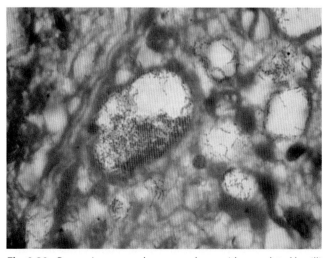

Fig. 9.20: Regressing macrophage granuloma with granulated bacilli in a giant vacuoles: (Fite-Faraco stain × 1000)

cell aggregates also shrinks. The lifespan of cells constituting a granuloma from shortest to longest is: giant cell, epithelioid cell, macrophage in active lesion and macrophage in regressing lesion.[3] Hence, in a regressing granuloma, the giant cells are the first to disappear leaving behind epithelioid cells and lymphocytes. The aggregate of epithelioid cells gradually shrinks due to loss of epithelioid cells and finally only clumps of lymphocytes are left. Any of these stages without edema and evidence of cellular activity indicates a regressing lesion (Fig. 9.21). Regressing TT granuloma with such features indicates vanishing DTH. Hence, substantial number of such lesions is self-healing.[64] It is a beauty that, even after the granuloma is dismantled, aggregates of lymphocyte survive for long as sincere sentinels.

Shrinkage of granuloma has been claimed as an important outcome in therapeutic trials with *Mycobacterium w (now called M. indicus pranii)* vaccine and some such trials reviewed.[65] In addition to rapid clinical improvement, vaccine supplement was found to hasten reduction rate of GF in BT, BB and BL cases and also increased epithelioid cells conversion in BB and BL cases.[65]

REACTIONS IN LEPROSY

Reactions are periodic episodes of acute inflammation caused by immune responses to *M. leprae* or its antigens. These episodes superimpose on the chronic course of leprosy. Depending on the immunological mechanism, these reactions have been classified into two types: (1) Reversal reaction (RR) and (2) Erythema nodosum leprosum (ENL). Jopling renamed them as type 1 and type 2 reactions respectively.[66] RR occurs in the borderline cases, and ENL occurs in BL and LL cases, both reflecting immunological instability. Whatever tissue responses observed during such episodes are mostly a reflection of host tissue damages and hence they are hypersensitivity responses by definition. Type IV dealed type hypersensitivity (DTH) and type III immune-complex mediated of Coombs and Gell classification[67] are respectively known as type 1 and type 2 reactions in leprosy.

Type 1 Reaction

Type 1 reaction (T1R) is associated with sudden alteration of CMI, associated with possible shift in the position of the patient in the leprosy spectrum. T1R is usually observed in the borderline spectrum of the disease and rarely occurs in LL (sub-polar). If there is an increase in the immunity (*de novo* or after therapy) the shift is from BL to the tuberculoid pole, and it is called upgrading or RR. Sudden reduction in immunity and resultant shift toward lepromatous pole is called downgrading reaction. In clinical practice, the distinction may not be clearly evident, and the laboratory tests including histopathology may not be helpful in differentiating the two components of type 1 reactions. As a result downgrading component is less frequently discussed.

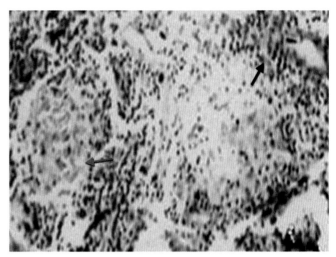

Fig. 9.21: Regressing tuberculoid leprosy showing collar of densely packed lymphocytes (black arrow) around a nest of epithelioid cells (red arrow) H & E × 100

Reversal reaction (RR) being acute in nature, the lesions show all the cardinal signs of acute inflammation, such as redness, swelling, local warmth and tenderness, over the skin lesions. Reaction in skin is often associated with neuritis with resultant pain, tenderness and swelling which are well-appreciated in the nerve trunk.

Clinical features of reaction, viz. redness and swelling also reflect in histology, due to superimposition of acute inflammation on a granuloma. Redness on skin patch is seen in the tissue section as increased hyperemia with dilated blood vessels and lymphatics while swelling is due to flooding of tissues with edema and fresh infiltration of lymphocytes, macrophages and neutrophils. Edema is both intracellular and extracellular. In spite of the new cell influx, the edema fluid disorganizes the collagen bundles and makes the granuloma appear sparsely cellular (Fig. 9.22). More and more macrophages differentiate into epithelioid cells and giant cells. The latter are generally of foreign body type with bizarre shapes and sizes (Fig. 9.23). The cell population of the granuloma becomes so disorganized that the overall impression is described as a "tissue panic" (Figs 9.22 and 9.23). In severe cases there is focal erosion of the epidermis and focal fibrinoid necrosis in the dermis. Sometimes the necrosis is so extensive that a part or whole of the skin lesion sloughs out. This process also occurs in the nerve trunks giving rise to caseation and nerve abscess. The reaction in the nerves is more severe, and is thought to be due to high lipid content in the neural tissue. The non-yielding perineurium increases the pressure of the inflammatory exudates and hastens the destruction of nerve components. During reaction, the bacilli and cells sheltering them are destroyed along with the damage of host tissue as its price. This is the upgrading (reversal) component.

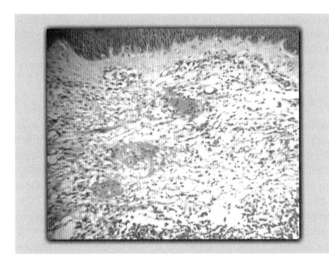

Fig. 9.22: BT leprosy in T1R showing epithelioid cells and foreign body GCs with massive edema (H & E × 100)

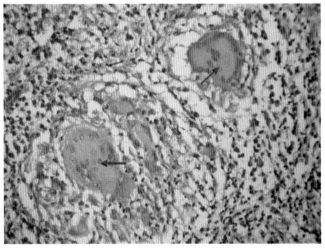

Fig. 9.23: BT in T1R showing large bizarre looking FB type giant cells with epithelioid cells disorganized as if in 'panic' in massive edema (H & E × 400)

According to the prevalent criteria, in a study only 48% of the clinically diagnosed cases of T1R showed the histological features suggestive of T1R. This emphasizes the need for standardization of the histopathological criteria to help support the clinical diagnoses of T1R.[68,69]

If T1R is a fight of immune cells against the bacilli, RR is a win for the host CMI. There is also risk of defeat in spite of fight in which CMI fails to contain the invaders. The bacillary multiplication overpowers the immune mechanism. Result is downgrading during or after TIR[66] ending up in LL.

Regarding the cytokine profile and their function, what has been described in TT is true for T1R with increase in proinflammatory cytokines as IL1, 2, 12, 18, TNF-α and INFγ.[70]

IP-10, and INFγ chemokine are known as the biomarkers for T1R. The details of cellular and cytokine dynamics have been described by Britton and Lockwood in a seminar paper.[71] In another article staining pattern of several antigens of *M. leprae* involved in T1R in both skin and nerve has been described along with their significance.[72] While demonstrating that the staining pattern is similar in these two tissues, they found the intracellular staining to be more intense in macrophages compared to that of Schwann cells. Of the antigens described, two are of particular interest: the 28 kd antigen seems to be strongly associated with T1R as it is absent in new and treated cases with no reaction. The other, lipoarabinomannan (LAM) persists in the lesions for long time and seems to explain the late reactions occurring years after completion of treatment.[72] In the TT patients there is high CMI but no LAM while in LL cases there is plenty of LAM but no CMI. It is only in the borderline cases both the elements are present to trigger and make RR more explosive.

Ridley and Radia in a study on the course of reaction in borderline leprosy have described four stages. The stages are early, acute, late and resolving.[73] When considered with another article, "Leprosy as a model of subacute and chronic immunologic diseases" by Turk,[22] the tuberculoid and borderline segment of leprosy makes a spectrum of inflammation acute to chronic with an intervening subacute stage. The tissue morphology of DTH constitutes a spectrum of inflammation within a larger spectrum of immunity. The tissue response to this is an epithelioid cell granuloma reflecting a sensitized state against *M. leprae*. It is almost similar to the sequential tissue response described in lepromin test.[74]

Lepromin Test (Reaction)

It is a skin test elicited by injection of killed *M. leprae* prepared from highly bacillated nodules from patients, and presently from tissues of armadillo, due to the paucity of the human tissues. A positive reaction generates an erythema with induration at the site to be read between 48 and 72 hours. This is called early or Fernandez reaction. A late reaction peaking at the fourth week is the formation of a nodule known as late reaction or Mitsuda reaction[75] named after the scientist who first described the reaction in 1919. On histology, the lesion starts as acute inflammation with edema, increased vascularity and infiltration of neutrophils, which are replaced by lymphocytes by 48 hours. By the third week there is development of epithelioid cells which organize into a compact granuloma by the end of fourth week,[76] similar to that found in TT.

Decades after the description of Mitsuda reaction, Dharmendra fractionated *M. leprae* from human leproma to prepare purified antigen which would produce skin reaction akin to that of tuberculin. The soluble protein fraction known as Dharmendra lepromin generated similar reaction within 48–72 hours and was more specific than earlier antigen.[77]

The process of testing includes intradermal injection of 0.1 mL of crude suspension of the bacilli and reading the test after 72 hours for erythema and induration (Fernandez reaction), and at fourth week (Mitsuda reaction) for development of a nodule, or ulceration as it occurs in a very strongly positive response. The result is graded as under:

No nodule	Negative
1–2 mm across	Doubtful +/−
3–5 mm	+
Over 5 mm	++
Ulceration	+++

In an immune competent person, the early lepromin reaction indicates a state of sensitization against *M. leprae,* and was often regarded as evidence of prior infection. The late reaction is thought to be an indication of CMI in patients and normal persons. Incidence of LL is higher in subclinically infected Mitsuda negative persons. The test is positive in TT and BT with increased intensity in T1R and negative in other types of leprosy and it further provides an immunologic support in the classification of disease. The antigen could enjoy only limited field trials and is becoming oblivious due to some of its limitations, while tuberculin positivity is still regarded as new infection of TB. The main limitations are low specificity, paucity of human leproma and the reduced availability of test subjects. Attempts are being made now to develop second generation test based on *M. leprae* soluble antigen lipoarabinomannan (MLSA-LAM) and ML cw antigen to test T-cell proliferation and CMI.[78]

Immune Reconstitution Inflammatory Syndrome and Leprosy HIV Coinfection

Through an editorial Lockwood and Lambert briefly dealt with the coinfection of HIV and leprosy, histopathology and immune reconstitution inflammatory syndrome (IRIS).[79] The coinfection was viewed as a threat of increasing incidence of lepromatous type of leprosy, while on the virtue side there was a hope that the incidence of RR would decrease in borderline cases. As per the information available so far, neither of the presumptions came true. There is also no evidence of leprosy incidence increasing as an opportunistic infection similar to TB. Regarding the change in the morphology and constituent cells in the coinfected persons, there were epithelioid cell and macrophage granulomas, respectively in tuberculoid and lepromatous cases, typical of respective leprosy types,[80,81] except borderline cases on highly active antiretroviral therapy (HAART). IRIS is a new dimension to T1R developing in cases coinfected with leprosy and HIV under treatment with HAART. It is a paradoxical deterioration of the disease due to reactivation of lost or dormant CMI response or a dormant disease. Lockwood and Lambert had recently reviewed 23 cases of IRIS recorded since 2003, mostly from Brazil and India. The commonly affected type is borderline leprosy which has already experienced a bout of T1R. The authors also proposed a definition for leprosy associated IRIS, the criteria being: onset of leprosy or reaction, within 6 months of starting antiretroviral therapy (ART); advanced HIV infection; low CD4+ count before treatment and its increase with treatment.

Erythema Nodosum Leprosum

Erythema Nodosum Leprosum occurs in cases of high bacillary load and hence LL and BL cases only suffer from these episodes. It is an immune complex mediated disease implicating B-cells and clinically manifesting as Arthus phenomenon.[82] There is also evidence for the role of T helper cells because there is an increase in the ratio of CD4+ and CD8+ cells in the lesions. In addition, there is activation of antigen specific T-cells, release and expression of INFγ and IL-12 in the lesions.[70] Fresh infiltration of T-cells also corroborates these findings.[83] The possibility is that building up of antigen load by T-cell mediated killing may be contributing to immune complex formation. ENL often involves capillary rich organs, such as nerves, testes, joints, eyes, kidneys and lymph nodes and these organs share ENL overlapping macrophage granuloma. The prominent clinical features are appearances of highly inflamed skin nodules in crops which in severe cases become pustules and may even ulcerate. This is accompanied by pain and tenderness of all the aforesaid organs and fever with other constitutional symptoms.

The histology is that of acute inflammation superimposed on the granuloma. The granuloma is populated by plasma cells which produce antibodies which instead of protection cause tissue damage through formation of immune complexes. Tissue injury is due to deposition of these complexes, in the wall of arterioles and venules resulting in vasculitis (Fig. 9.24).[84] Sometimes there is massive accumulation of these cells enough to form microabscesses and ulcers. Vasculitis causes local ischemia and in severe cases completely blocks blood supply leading to necrosis.

By immunohistochemistry, large amount of antigens have been demonstrated in the extravascular compartment and foamy macrophages,[85] and such findings in sections negative for AFB indicate the role of residual antigens. These episodes are accompanied by high levels of circulating TNF-α often causing systemic toxicity.[86] In recent years, several proinflammatory cytokines along with their transcripts, playing critical role have been demonstrated in the tissues. The prominent among them are interleukin 6, 10 and 17[40] beside the well-established interleukin 1 and TNF-α.

Lucio Leprosy

Lucio leprosy was first described by Rafael Lucio in 1851. It was rediscovered and extensively studied by Latapi and colleagues in Mexico almost a century later.[87] This condition is manifested by ulcerative type of skin lesions occurring in diffusely infiltrated type of LL. The features are similar to ENL

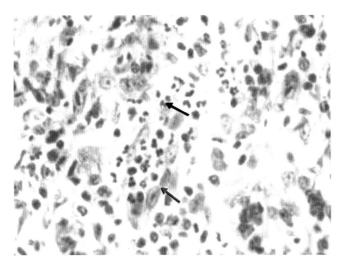

Fig. 9.24: LL with ENL showing macrophage granuloma indicating vasculitis (red arrow) and neutrophils (black arrow)

with histology of vasculitis, thrombosis and other features of acute inflammation. Thrombosis chokes the vessels leading to local ischemia and sloughing ulcers—familiarly known as Lucio phenomenon. This type of reaction is more common in Mexico compared to other parts of the world. It can be considered as a special variety of ENL, thought to be a result of endothelial cell damage caused by *M. leprae* within[88] and the release of antigens from the endothelial cells.[29]

In 2008, two patients of Mexican origin died while under treatment in the intensive care unit in Phoenix, Arizona, USA. The clinical features, histological and bacteriological findings published in the American Journal of Clinical Pathology were compatible with Lucio phenomenon.[89] A subsequent paper published the comparative sequence analysis of *M. leprae* and the new leprosy causing *Mycobacterium*.[90] The authors viewed the genetic difference to be significant enough to propose this isolated strain as a novel species naming *M. lepromatosis*. Through an editorial Gillis et al.[91] reviewed the findings of all parameters published in these papers, and concluded that the experiments and data needed to confirm that these are new species, causing leprosy are not complete.

RELAPSE IN LEPROSY

Relapse is the recurrence of the disease after cure. As stated by Desikan, definition of cure according to the perception of the patients and treating physician is a state of relief from symptoms and disappearance of the signs.[92] It is difficult to apply these criteria in leprosy due to fixed duration therapy and delayed resolution of lesions in several cases.[93] A state of cure need to be defined after which return of the disease would amount to relapse. In leprosy, the histological criteria of cure or proxy cure would be disappearance or

inactivity of the granuloma, and reappearance of an active epithelioid cell granuloma is relapse, in tuberculoid cases. In lepromatous cases formation of an active granuloma need to be accompanied by bacterial features such as: negative case becoming positive, increase of bacterial index (BI) by log 2+ or increase of solid staining bacilli in the lesion. Bacterial parameters are not in practice in the field making data building fairly difficult. Other histological clues are: features of histoid leprosy; branching, satellite and nascent granulomas on a regressed background; and hypercellular granuloma.[94] The terms reactivation, reinfection, relapse and even new reaction in a quiescent PB leprosy could mean return of disease. The histology, constituent of component cells and the shade of inflammation of relapse do not differ much from an active disease. Reappearance on a regressed background is that matters. To systematically address the problem of relapse, the surveillance mechanism in the program needs to be strengthened. As reported by Shetty et al.,[95] out of 62 cases studied for relapse in their research center, 58% of cases were referred by NGOs; 25% by private practitioners and only about 16% by government institutions. As per their observations all types of cases stand the risk of relapse. Initiative needs strengthening in the program.

INVOLVEMENT OF OTHER ORGANS

Depending on the immunity of a person, leprosy manifests either as a localized or generalized disease. Its targets are Schwann cells and cells of the MPS by virtue of their innate property to phagocytose *M. leprae*. Peripheral neural tissue and macrophages are distributed in the entire skin and mucous membrane, whose low temperature favors the multiplication of the bacillus. Rich capillary network, idiosyncrasies of both *M. leprae*, host defense cells make the following organs affected with varying frequency and severity in addition to what has been discribed.[96,97]

Nerve Involvement in Leprosy

Histological changes of nerve have been mentioned along with the types of leprosy. Some special attributes are only mentioned here. *M. leprae* has a special affinity to colonize the Schwann cells and subsequently nerves are destroyed through more than one mechanism.

The histopathology of nerves is identical to what is found in the skin lesion of a particular type of leprosy in the spectrum.[96] Distribution of several crucial antigens and cytokines in both skin and nerve lesions is also mostly similar.[27,72] In spite of this similarity, the pathology in nerves differs from that of skin as mentioned below:
- Lack of lymphatics and tough basal lamina with nerve sheaths prevent attack by immune cells on the bacilli in the Schwann cells for a long time.[25]

- Once detected by immune cells, the reaction becomes more severe and the nerve fibers are damaged as bystander in the DTH induced inflammatory exudates. Lipid content of the myelin acts as an adjuvant to make the reaction more explosive within a nonexpansive perineurial sheath. Result is strangulation with rapid damage of the nerve.
- The Schwann cells also in some situations dedifferentiate and thought to contribute as APC and get destroyed by macrophages activated through CD4+ cells.
- Intense DTH results in frequent caseation in nerves with cold abscess in some cases.
- Inactive does not mean inactive nerve pathology. In other words inactive histology in skin lesions does not mean caseation of inflammation in the nerve.[63]
- Nerve damage through silent neuropathy—an insidious functional impairment is not uncommon.
- Nerves sometimes show more bacilli compared to skin, especially when *M. leprae* are scarred by CMI. Schwann cell is a sanctuary for them though the safety is short lived.

Pure neural leprosy is commonly found in India, though the extent of the disease reported is variable. According to report by Noordeen about 6% of cases in South India belong to this category but in endemic areas it could be as high as one-sixth of the total cases.[98] Clinically where this type of leprosy is to be placed in the spectrum is not well ascertained. These cases commonly belong to TT, BT group as it was placed as a sub-group of non-lepromatous leprosy in Indian classification. Histology that can be assigned to all types except pure LL has been reported. Both macrophage and epithelioid cell granulomas in the mucous membrane of nose were reported in 20 (51%) of 39 cases of primary neuritic leprosy (PNL) by Suneetha et al. from Schieffelin Institute of Health Research and Training Centre, Karigiri.[99] It indicates wider pathological changes sometimes accompanying PNL. Out of 36 cases claiming to have suffered from PNL, diagnosis was established only in 21 cases by electromyography (EMG), PCR, phenolic glycolipid-1 (PGL1) and clinical findings as histology was negative in them. Carpel tunnel syndrome and diabetes mellitus were the main differential diagnosis.[100] It has been reported that around 15% of the patients with PNL may develop one or two skin lesions, as TT or BT at any stage of PNL, generally after the beginning of treatment.[101] All leprosy being neural, skin lesions may be a temporary phenomenon superimposed on a longer neural pathology.

Nose and Larynx

Nasal mucosa is an important receptive as well as disseminative site for *M. leprae*. Though the interior of the nose is commonly affected in LL, occasional epithelioid cell granuloma has been reported.[102] The detailed morphology of granuloma and the BI are similar to that found in the skin.

In late stages, nasal bones and cartilages get destroyed and replaced by fibrosis. The result is the typical collapse of the bridge of the nose, a deformity typical of LL. Nasal secretions are known to contain an enormous amount of bacilli.

Hoarseness of voice which is rare these days is a typical clinical feature of advanced LL. This was due to the submucosal granuloma manifesting as diffuse infiltration, plaques and nodules extending up to vocal cords. ENL in such cases was sometimes life-threatening if there is no facility for tracheostomy.

Oral Cavity

The oral cavity is frequently involved in LL. The clinical lesions consist of diffuse infiltration, plaques and nodules depending on the severity of leprosy. These lesions are seen in the hard and soft palate, uvula inner aspect of lips and gums. Most frequently affected regions are cheek and hard palate sometimes with perforation of the latter in advanced stage.[103] Alveolar bone loss is frequent. Dental caries and periodontal diseases are very common. Oral ulcers are frequent and loss of incisor teeth is premature. Alveolar bone is affected by macrophage granuloma loaded with bacilli. Overall oral hygiene is poor resulting in dental caries and periodontal diseases.[104] Histology is similar to what is found in the lesions of nasal cavity.

Lymph Nodes

Macrophages and cells of their lineage namely, Kupffer cells in liver, littoral cells in spleen and reticulum cells in bone marrow phagocytose lepra bacilli and they keep on multiplying in these organs if CMI is ineffective. Histology of lymph nodes draining the skin lesion of leprosy is infiltrated by the cells of the corresponding type of leprosy granulomas. LL shows numerous miliary lepromas and in advanced cases enlarged glands are studded with multiple lesions. In initial stages, macrophages replace the paracortical areas, and the marginal medullary sinuses occupying the bulk of the gland if the disease is advanced. Macrophages show plenty of AFB. In tuberculoid cases only, the nodes draining leprosy lesions are commonly affected and show epithelioid cell granuloma negative for AFB. Caseation necrosis is rare—a feature which helps differentiating it from tuberculosis. Many atypical mycobacteria, fungi and parasites produce epithelioid cell granuloma and staining for the organisms and molecular techniques help in differentiation.[96,105,106] Differentiation from sarcoidosis, a condition more frequent now is often difficult. Thickening of the lymph node capsule is a constant feature in any type of leprosy. During ENL, the lymph glands swell up with acute inflammatory exudates and cells. These cells sometimes form microabscess, rarely a large one draining outside through a sinus.

Spleen

As an organ of the reticuloendothelial system (RES), spleen is often involved in lepromatous segment of leprosy. Though, both the red and white pulps are replaced by miniature macrophage granulomas, the latter are more prominent in the periarteriolar region. The replacement of lymphocyte of the thymus dependent areas by macrophages, led some to point at the role of spleen in generalized depression of CMI in LL.

Liver

Involvement of liver is next only to lymph nodes, with similar granulomatous change. The discrete initial infiltrates are predominantly seen around the portal triads and central veins. The Kupffer cell hyperplasia is generally a prominent feature. Cirrhotic changes have been reported in early studies.[96] There is a report that the liver function tests become abnormal though the test results do not correlate with the BI of the patient.[107] Cases reported with leprous hepatitis show conventional epithelioid cell granuloma without any caseation.[108]

Testes

Low temperature is favorable for the multiplication of *M. leprae* with initial perivascular accumulation of lymphocytes and macrophages. The inflammatory process gradually spreads to the interstitial tissue leading to edema and accumulation of acute inflammatory cells. When chronic, the basement membrane is thickened and the seminiferous tubules are destroyed. There is focal destruction of germinal layer and cessation of spermatogenesis. The supporting sertoli cells survive longer. Sometimes the entire tubule is atrophied, destroyed and replaced by fibrosis and hyalinization.[96,109] The damage to the tissue is hastened during ENL. For reasons not known the interstitial Leydig cells survive longer with some degree of hyperplasia. In the tissue sections any of the stages described above can be observed depending on the extent of the disease. The macrophages would be laden with *M. leprae*. Evidence involving ovary or other organs of female genital tract is lacking.

Eyes

Eyes are damaged in leprosy primarily due to *M. leprae* and macrophage infiltration in LL and also secondary to nerve damage in borderline leprosy. In LL and BL, microgranulomas are found in cornea, conjuctiva, iris and ciliary body. Iris is rich in small muscles, unmyelinated nerves and a cooler temperature—all providing a congenial milieu for multiplication of *M. leprae* and formation of microgranulomas. These are called "iris pearls" as they appear on slit lamp examination. Iris pearls are well appreciated along the rim of the pupil.[110,111] Beading of the corneal nerves is one of the earlier lesions. The histology of these iris pearls and beads shows aggregates of macrophages containing AFB, lymphocytes and plasma cells. With advanced disease, these spread to all parts of the eye including retina. The smooth muscle and endothelial cells also show bacilli and with added macrophages, they form perivascular nodules. During ENL, the miniature granulomas particularly of anterior segment show edema and infiltration of neutrophils. This if repeated ends up in anterior and posterior synechiae and corneal opacity through epidermalization. Fibrin plugged, an irreversibly constricted pupil results in blindness. Often silent, a state of chronic iridocyclitis harboring *M. leprae,* lasts longer than the skin smear negativity, and AFB could be demonstrated after completion of MDT. Smooth muscle disruption and myotic pupil are better demonstrated on histology.[112]

In borderline leprosy particularly during reaction, ophthalmic branch of trigeminal nerve, and zygomatic branch of facial nerves are destroyed resulting in anesthesia of cornea and lagophthalmos respectively. Loss of this dual protection subjects the cornea to dryness and repeated injuries. Gradually there follow corneal ulceration, perforation, panophthalmitis and blindness.

Kidneys

Due to paucity of biopsy specimens, kidney involvement in leprosy is mostly inferred from functional deficits.[107] Deposition of immune complexes, complements and immunoglobulins is detected by special stains mostly during ENL. Such episodes are accompanied by function deficit as evidenced by proteinuria, hematuria, passage of abnormal casts and increased serum urea and creatinine.[113] On the basis of biopsy findings glomerulonephritis has been reported in all types of leprosy except tuberculoid, indeterminate and pure neuritic cases.[114] Histochemical stains on tissue sections from cases of glomerulonephritis have proved the cause to be mostly immune complex deposition. Other common abnormalities reported are glomerulosclerosis and amylodosis in LL and BL cases.[115]

Bones and Joints

Bones are mostly affected in LL. The common sites are subarticular region of all small bones of feet and hands, bones and cartilages of nose, maxila and mandible. Periosteum of several bones and joints are affected especially during type 2 reaction (T2R), immobility increasing with the chronic disease.[96] Anesthesia adds to the loss or resorption of phalanges and the occurrence of repeated ulcers. Feet and hands are common sites of chronic ulcers leading to osteomyelitis and nonhealing ulcers. Infection and osteoporosis compounded by stresses lead to pathological fractures leading to distortion of normal structure and function. Histopathology shows miniature macrophage granulomas replacing the trabeculae of spongy bones. In children, there is lepromatous periostitis leading to multilayering of the periosteum infiltrated by macrophages and osteoclasts, often showing AFB.[116] Being rich in reticuloendothelial tissue, bone marrow is a fertile soil for macrophages, resident bacilli and predominant plasma cells. More disturbingly, the bacteria persist long even after the battle is won in the skin and other tissues.[117] In reality, leprosy as a disease licks the skin but bites the nerves and bones leaving a deformed face and crippled skeleton as its permanent imprint.

Adrenal Gland

Adrenal glands are associated with leprosy through the corticosteroid axis. In autopsy studies many small macrophage granulomas have been found both in cortex and medulla[96] without any record of functional deficit or loss of adrenal reserve. There is evidence of reversible type of hormonal insufficiency during reactions.[118] During T2R, features of shock have been reported resulting in occasional death.

Amyloidosis

Secondary amyloidosis is a condition in which amyloid is deposited in certain organs due to a chronic disease. It is common particularly in LL. Though the reported incidence is low in India, leprosy is one of the common causes.[96] Liver, spleen, kidney and adrenal glands are most commonly affected organs. Amyloid deposition is attributed to repeated ENL and plantar ulcers. The nature of amyloid in leprosy is composed of the polymerized serum amyloid A (AA) protein but not immunoglobulins.[119] Amyloid in tissue sections is stained by metachromatic stains as methyl violet and toluidine blue. It has also affinity for Congo red which gives green birefringence in polarized light.

ACKNOWLEDGMENTS

The authors are thankful to Dr J Subbanna, Chief Executive, LEPRA Society, Dr KV Desikan for their encouragement. We are grateful to Dr Vanaja P Shetty, Director, The Foundation of Medical Research, Dr Minakshi Bhardwaj, Consultant Pathology, PGIMER for sharing some of the microphotographs.

REFERENCES

1. Nayar A, Narayanan JS, Job CK. Histopathological study of early skin lesion in leprosy. Arch Pathol. 1972;94(3):199-204.
2. Binford CH. The histologic recocgnition of early lesions in leprosy. Int J Lepr Other Mycobact Dis. 1971;39(2):225-30.
3. Ridley DS. Skin Biopsy in Leprosy, 1st edition. Basle: Documenta Geigy, Ciba Geigy Limited; 1977:p.18.
4. Khanolkar VR. Studies in the histology of early lesions in leprosy. Indian Council of Medical Research, Special Report Series, New Delhi; 1951: pp. 1-18.
5. Antia NH. Leprosy—a disease of Schwann cells. Lepr India. 1982;54(4):599-604.
6. Fite GL. Leprosy from the histopathologic point of view. Arch Pathol Lab Med. 1943;35:611-44.
7. Fine PE, Job CK, Lucas SB, et al. Extent, origin and implications of observer variation in the histopathological diagnosis of suspected leprosy. Int J Lepr Other Mycobact Dis. 1993;61(2):270-82.
8. Porichha D, Mishra AK, Dhariwal AC. Ambiguities in leprosy histopathology. Int J Lepr Other Mycobact Dis. 1993;61(3):428-32.
9. Ramu G, Karthikeyan S, Balakrishnan S et al. Histological and immunological correlates of suspected leprosy lesions. Indian J Lepr. 1996;68(2):155-9.
10. Barbosa Ade A, Silva TC, Patel BN et al. Demonstration of mycobacterial antigens in skin biopsies from suspected leprosy cases in the absence of bacilli. Pathol Res Pract. 1994;190(8):782-5.
11. Huerre M, Desforeges S, Bobin P, et al. Demonstration of PGL 1 antigens in skin biopsies in indeterminate leprosy patients, comparison with serological anti PGL 1 levels. Acta Leprol. 1989;7(Suppl 1):125-7.
12. Natrajan M, Katoch K, Katoch VM et al. Enhancement in the histological diagnosis of indeterminate leprosy by the demonstration of mycobacterial antigens. Acta Leprol. 1995;9(4):201-7.
13. Katoch VM. Molecular techniques for leprosy: present application and future perspectives. Indian J Lepr. 1999;71(1):45-59.
14. Natrajan M, Katoch K, Katoch VM, et al. In situ hybridization in the histological diagnosis of early and clinically suspicious leprosy. Int J Lepr Other Mycobact Dis. 2004;72(3):296-305.
15. de Wit NYL, Faber WR, Krieg SR, et al. Application of a polymerase chain reaction for the detection of *Mycobacterium leprae* in skin tissues. J Clin Microbiol. 1991;29(5):906-10.
16. Natrajan M, Katoch K, Katoch VM, et al. Histopathological diagnosis of early and suspicious leprosy by in situ PCR. Indian J Lepr. 2012; 84(3):185-94.
17. Reja AHH, Biswas N, Biswas S, et al. Fite-Faraco staining in combination with multiplex polymerase chain reaction: a new approach to leprosy diagnosis. Indian J Dermatol Venereol Leprol. 2013;79(5):693-700.
18. Abbas AK, Lichtman AH. Innate immunity: Basic Immunology, 2nd edition. New Delhi: Saunders-Elsevier; 2005.p.30.
19. Iyer AM, Mohanty KK, van Egmond D, et al. Leprosy specific B cells within cellular infiltrate in active leprosy lesions. Hum Pathol. 2007;38(7):1065-73.
20. Chatura KR, Sangeetha S. Utility of Fite-Faraco stain for both mast cell count and bacillary index in skin biopsies of leprosy patients. Indian J Lepr. 2012;84(3):209-15.
21. Cree IA, McDougall AC, Coghill G, et al. Quantitation of the granuloma fraction in leprosy skin biopsies by planimetry. Int J Lepr Other Mycobact Dis. 1985;53(4):582-6.
22. Turk JL. Leprosy as a model of subacute and chronic immunologic diseases. J Invest Dermatol. 1976;67(3):457-63.

23. Azulay RD. Histopathology of skin lesions in leprosy. Int J Lepr Other Mycobact Dis. 1971;39 (2):244-50.

24. Ridley DS. Classification of leprosy. In: BR Chatterjee (Ed). Window in Leprosy, 1st edition. Wardha: Gandhi Memorial Leprosy Foundation; 1978:pp.105-19.

25. Pearson JMH, Ross WF. Nerve involvement in leprosy: pathology, differential diagnosis and principles of management. Lepr Rev. 1975;46(3):199-212.

26. Sehgal VN, Srivastava G. Indeterminate leprosy: A passing phase in the evolution of leprosy. Lepr Rev. 1987;58(3):291-9.

27. Shetty VP, Mistry NF, Antia NH. Current understanding of leprosy as a peripheral nerve disorder: significance of involvement of peripheral nerve in leprosy. Indian J Lepr. 2000; 72 (3):339-50.

28. Lara CB, Nolasco JO. Self healing, abortive and residual forms of childhood leprosy and their probable significance. Int J Lepr. 1956;24 (3):245-63.

29. Harboe M. The immunology of leprosy. In: Hastings RC (Ed). Leprosy, 1st edition. London: Churchill Livingstone; 1984.p.53.

30. Ganapati R, Desikan KV. Simultaneous occurrence of different types of leprosy in a patient—a case report. Lepr India. 1974; 46:148-51.

31. Chatterjee BR. Immunopathogenesis of leprosy—facts and artifacts. In: Chatterjee BR (Ed). Leprosy-Etiobiology of Manifestations, Treatment and Control.Jhalda, West Bengal: Leprosy Field Research Unit; 1993; pp. 128-51.

32. Cochrane RG. The correlation of the histopathological picture with the clinical signs. Ciba Symp. 1961;9:238-47.

33. Rea TH, Levan NE. Current concept in the immunology of leprosy. Arch Dermatol. 1977;113 (3):345-52.

34. Ridley DS, Jopling WH. Classification of leprosy according to immunity. A five-group system. Int J Lepr Other Mycobact Dis. 1966;34 (3):255-73.

35. Ridley DS, Waters MFR. Significance of variation within the lepromatous group. Lepr Rev. 1969;40 (3):143-52.

36. Chemotherapy of Leprosy for Control Programmes: Report of a WHO Study. Group (WHO Technical Report Series, No. 675). Geneva, 1982.

37. Hansen GA, Looft C. Leprosy: in its clinical and pathological aspects. Bristol: John Wright and Sons; 1895.p.67.

38. Dharmendra. Classification of leprosy. In: Hastings RC (Ed). Leprosy, 1st edition. London: Churchill Livingstone; 1985. p.837.

39. Nath I, Murtuja A, Singh S. The role of cytokines in leprosy. In T cell subsets and cytokine interplay in infectious diseases. Basle: Karger; 1996: pp.189-200.

40. Yamamura M, Wang XH, Ohmen JD et al. Cytokine patterns of immunological mediated tissue damage. J Immunol. 1992;149 (4):1470-75.

41. Jullien D, Sieling PA, Uyemura K et al. IL-15, an immunomodulator of T cell responses in intracellular infection. J Immunol. 1997;158(2):800-806.

42. Pappadimetriu JM, Spector WG. The origin, properties and fate of epithelioid cells. J Pathol. 1971;105 (3):187-203.

43. Wiersema JP, Binford CH. The identification of leprosy among epithelioid cell granulomas of skin.Int J Lepr Other Mycobact Dis. 1972;40(1):10-32.

44. Jadassohn J. Uebertuberculoide Verranderrungen in der Haut beinichttuberoser Lepra. Proc. VI German Congress of Dermatology, 1898.Reprinted in English translation by L Meyer, Int J Lepr. 1960;28:444-52.

45. Wade HW. Tuberculoid changes in leprosy. Int J Lepr. 1934;2:7-38.

46. Bjune G, Barnetson RStC, Ridley DS, et al. Lymphocyte transformation test in leprosy; correlation of the response with inflammation of lesions. Clin Exp Immunol. 1976;25(1):85-94.

47. Porichha D. Tuberculoid leprosy—one phenomenon with many perceptions. Indian J Lepr. 1997;69(2):183-8.

48. Pearson JMH, Weddel AG. Perineurial changes in untreated leprosy. Lepr Rev. 1975;46(1):51-67.

49. Harada K. Biopsy of skin lesions in leprosy. Tokyo: NEC Documentex Ltd; 1995. p.24.

50. Ghorpade AK. Transepidermal elimination of *Mycobacterium leprae* in histoid leprosy: a case report suggesting possible participation of skin in leprosy transmission. Indian J Dermatol Venereol Leprol. 2011;77(1):59-61.

51. Nath I. Immunological aspects. In: Kar HK, Kumar B (Eds). IAL Text Book of Leprosy, 1st edition. New Delhi: Jaypee Brothers Medical Publishers (P) Ltd; 2010:pp.60-73.

52. Wade HW. The histoid variety of lepromatous leprosy. Int J Lepr. 1963;31:129-42.

53. Bhutani LK, Bedi TR, Malhotra YK, et al. Histoid leprosy in North India. Int J Lepr Other Mycobact Dis. 1974; 42 (2):174-81.

54. Desikan KV, Iyer CGS. Histoid variety of lepromatous leprosy. A histopathologic study. Int J Lepr Other Mycobact Dis. 1972;40(2):149-156.

55. Porichha D, Bhatia VN. Epithelioid and polygonal cells in histoid leprosy. Indian J Lepr. 1987;59(2):191-3.

56. Job CK, Chacko CJG, Taylor PM. Electronmicroscopic study of histoid leprosy with special reference to its histogenesis. Lepr India. 1977;49(4):467-71.

57. Pettit JHS, Rees RJW, Ridley DS. Studies on sulphone resistance in leprosy-:.Detection of cases. Int J Lepr Other Mycobact Dis. 1966;34(4):375-90.

58. Lockwood DN, Sarno E, Smith WC. Classifying leprosy patients. Searching for the perfect solution? Lepr Rev. 2007;78(4):317-20.

59. Bijjaragi S, Kulkarni V, Suresh KK, et al. Correlation of clinical and histopathological classification of leprosy in post elimination era. Indian J Lepr. 2012;84(4):271-5.

60. Giridhar M, Arora G, Lajpal K, et al. Clinicopathological concordance in leprosy-a clinical, histopathological and bacteriological study of 100 cases. Indian J Lepr. 2012;84 (3):217-25.

61. Gupta R, Kar HK, Bharadwaj M. Revalidation of various clinical criteria for the classification of leprosy-a clinical pathological study. Lepr Rev. 2012;83(4):354-62.

62. Job CK, Chandi SM. Differential diagnosis of leprosy: a guide book for histopathologists. Karigiri Leprosy Education Programme. SLRTC, Karigiri. 2001.

63. Porichha D, Mukherjee A, Ramu G. Neural pathology in leprosy during treatment and surveillance. Lepr Rev. 2004;75(3):233-41.

64. Noordeen SK. Evolution of tuberculoid leprosy in a community. Indian J Lepr. 1975;47(1):85-93.

65. Kamal R, Natrajan M, Katoch K, et al. Clinical and histopathological evaluation of the effect of addition of immunotherapy with Mw vaccine to standard chemotherapy in borderline leprosy. Indian J Lepr. 2012;84(4):287-306.

66. Jopling WH. Leprosy reactions (reactional states). Handbook of Leprosy. London: William Heinemann Medical Books; 1971. p.42.

67. Roitt IM. Hypersensitivity reactions. In. Essential Immunology, Blackwell Science Ltd; 1988.p.193-214.

68. Patnaik N, Agarwal S, Sharma S, Pandhi D. Evaluation of key histological variables in skin biopsies of patients of borderline leprosy with type 1 lepra reaction. Indian J Dermatol Venereol Leprol. 2014;80:402-8.

69. Thomas M, Ponnaiya J, Emmanuel M, et al. Type 1 reaction in leprosy—a histopathological analysis. Indian J Lepr. 2013;85(1):1-4.

70. Sreenivasan P, Mishra RS, Wilfred D, et al. Lepromatous leprosy patients show T helper 1-like cytokine profile with differential expression of interleukin 10 during type 1 and type 2 reactions. Immunology. 1998;95(4):529-36.

71. Britton WJ, Lockwood DNJ. Leprosy. Lancet. 2004;363:1209-19.

72. Lockwood DNJ, Colston MJ, Khanolkar Young SR. The detection of Mycobacterium leprae protein and carbohydrate antigens in skin and nerve from leprosy patients with Type 1 (reversal) reactions. Am J Trop Med Hyg. 2002;66(4):409-15.

73. Ridley DS, Radia KB. The histological course of reactions in borderline leprosy and their outcome. Int J Lepr Other Mycobact Dis. 1981;49(4):383-92.

74. Desikan KV, Mukherjee A, Ramu G. et al. Sequential histological study of lepromin reaction. Int J Lepr Other Mycobact Dis.1983;51(4)473-80.

75. Mitsuda K. On the value of skin reaction to a suspension of leprous nodules. Int J Lepr. 1953;21:347-58.

76. Thomas J, Joseph M, Ramanujam K, et al. The histology of the Mitsuda reaction and its significance. Lepr Rev. 1980;51(4):329-39.

77. Dharmendra. The immunological skin tests in leprosy. Part I. The isolation of a protein antigen of Mycobacterium leprae. 1942. Indian J Med Res. 2012;136(3):7p following 502.

78. Brennan PJ. Skin test development in leprosy: progress with first generation skin test antigens and an approach to the second generation. Lepr Rev. 2000;71 (Suppl):S50-4.

79. Lockwood DNJ, Lambert SM. Leprosy and HIV, where are we at? Lepr Rev. 2010;81(3):169-75.

80. Pereira GA, Stefani MM, Araujo Filho JA, et al. Human immunodeficiency virus 1 and Myccobacterium leprae co infection: HIV-1 subtypes and clinical immunologic and histopathologic profile in a Brazilian cohort. Am J Trop Med Hyg. 2004;71(5):679-84.

81. Sampaio EP, Caneshi JR, Nery JA, et al. Cellular immuneresponse to Mycobacterium leprare infection in human immunodeficiency virus infected individuals. Infect Immun. 1995;63(5):1848-54.

82. Wemambu SNC, Turk JL, Waters MFR, et al. Erythema nodosum leprosum. A clinical manifestation of Arthus phenomenon. Lancet. 1969;2(7627):933-5.

83. Laal S, Bhutani LK, Nath I. Natural emergence of antigen reactive T-cells in lepromatous leprosy patients during erythema nodosum leprosum. Infect Immun. 1985;50(3):887-92.

84. Job CK, Gude S, Macaden VP. Erythema nodosum leprosum. A Clinico-Pathologic Study. Int J Lepr. 1964;32:177-84.

85. Ridley MJ, Ridley DS. The immunopathology of erythema nodosum leprosum. The role of extravascular complexes. Lepr Rev. 1983;54(2):95-107.

86. Sarno E, Grau GE, Vieira LM, et al. Serum levels of tumor necrosis factor-alpha and interleukin-1 beta during leprosy reactional states. Clin ExpImmunol. 1991;84(1):103-8.

87. Latapi F, Zamora AC. The spotted leprosy of Lucio.An introduction to the clinical and histological study. Int J Lepr. 1948;16:421-9.

88. Vargas-Ocampo F. Diffuse leprosy of Lucio and Latapi: a histologic study. Lepr Rev. 2007;78(3):248-60.

89. Han XY, Seo YH, Sizer KC et al. A new Mycobacterium species causing diffuse lepromatous leprosy. Am J Clin Pathol. 2008;130 (6):856-64.

90. Han XY, Sizer KC, Thompson EJ, et al. Comparative sequence analysis of Mycobacterium leprae and the new leprosy-causing Mycobaterium lepromatosis. J Bacteriol. 2009;191(19):6067-74.

91. Gillis TP, Scollard DM, Lockwood DNJ. What is the evidence that the putative Mycobacterium lepromatosis species causes diffuse lepromatous leprosy? Lepr Rev. 2011;82(3):205-9.

92. Desikan KV. The risk of relapse after multi drug therapy in leprosy. Lepr Rev. 1997;68(2):114-6.

93. Job CK, Jayakumar J, Asccoff M. Delayed resolution versus treatment failure in paucibacillary leprosy patients under six months fixed duration multidrug therapy. Indian J Lepr. 1997;69(2):131-42.

94. Porichha D, Brahmne HG, Mahapatra DC, et al. Cellularity of macrophage granuloma and morphological Index. Indian J Lepr. 1996;68(3):217-22.

95. Shetty VP, Wakade AV, Ghate SD, et al. Clinical, bacteriological and histopathological study of 62 referred relapse cases between January 2004 and December 2009 at the Foundation for Medical Research, Mumbai. Lepr Rev. 2011;84:235-43.

96. Desikan KV, Job CK. A review of postmortem findings in 37 cases of leprosy. Int J Lepr Other Mycobact Dis. 1968;36(1):32-44.

97. Job CK, Karat AB, Karat S. The histopathological appearance of leprous rhinitis and pathogenesis of septal perforation in leprosy. J Laryngol Otol. 1966;80(7):718-32.

98. Noordeen SK. Epidemiology of polyneuritic type of leprosy. Lepr India. 1972;44:90-6.

99. Suneetha S, Arunthathi S, Job A, et al. Histological studies in primary neuritic leprosy: changes in the nasal mucosa. Lepr Rev. 1998;69(4):358-66.

100. Rodriguez G, Pinto R, Gomez Y, et al. Pure neuritic leprosy in patients from a high endemic region of Colombia. Lepr Rev. 2013;84(1):41-50.

101. Kumar B, Kaur I, Dogra S, et al. Pure neuritic leprosy in India: an appraisal. Int J Lepr Other Mycobact Dis. 2004;72(3):284-90.

102. Chacko CJG, Bhanu T, Victor V, et al. The significance in changes in nasal mucosa in indeterminate, tuberculoid and borderline leprosy. Lepr India. 1979;51(1):8-22.

103. Kumar B, Yande R, Kaur I, et al. Involvement of palate and cheek in leprosy. Indian J Lepr. 1988;60(2):280-4.

104. Rawlani SM, Rawlani S, Degwekar S, et al. Oral health status and alveolar bone loss in treated leprosy patients of central India. Indian J Lepr. 2011;83(4):215-24.

105. Turk JL, Waters MFR. Immunological significance of changes in lymphnodes across the leprosy spectrum. Clin Exp Immunol. 1971;8(3)363-76.

106. Kar HK, Mohanty HC, Mohanty GN, et al. Clinico-pathological studies of lymph node involvement in leprosy. Lepr India. 1983;55(4):725-38.

107. Gharpuray SM, Gharpuray MB, Kelkar SS. Liver function in leprosy. Lepr India. 1977;49(2):216-20.

108. Singh P, Koranne RV. Systemic involvement in tuberculoid leprosy—pathogenesis of leprosy. Lepr India. 1979;51(4):451-8.

109. Liu TC, Qiu JS. Pathological findings on peripheral nerves, lymph nodes and visceral organs of leprosy. Int J Lepr Other Mycobact Dis. 1984;52(3):377-83.

110. Ridley DS, Job CK. The pathology of leprosy. In: Hastings RC (Ed). Leprosy. London: Churchil Livingstone; 1984.p.128.

111. Brand EM, Ffitche TJ. Eye complications of leprosy. In: Hastings RC (Ed). Leprosy. London: Churchil Livingstone; 1984.p.228.

112. Daniel E, Ebenezer G J, Job CK. Pathology of iris in leprosy. Br J Ophthalmol. 1997;81(6):490-2.

113. Kaur S. Renal manifestations of leprosy. Indian J Lepr. 1990;62(3):273-80.

114. Date A. The immunological basis of glomerural disease in leprosy—a brief review. Int J Lepr Other Mycobact Dis. 1982;50(3):351-4.

115. Nakayama EE, Ura S, Fleury RN, et al. Renal lesions in leprosy: a retrospective study of 199 autopsies. Am J Kidney Dis. 2001;38(1):26-30.

116. Job CK. Pathology of leprous osteomyelitis. Int J Lepr. 1963;31:26-33.

117. Sen R, Sehgal PK, Singh U, et el. Bacillaemia and bone marrow involvement in leprosy. Indian J Lepr. 1989;61(4):445-52.

118. Dash RJ, Sriprakash ML, Kumar B, et al. Adrenal cortical reserve in leprosy. Indian J Med Res. 1985;82:388-92.

119. Bryceson A, Pflaltzgraff RE. Clinical Pathology, 3rd edition. London: Churchill Livingstone; 1990.p.20.

Structure, Electrophysiological and Ultrasonographic Studies of Peripheral Nerve

Sujai K Suneetha, P Narasimha Rao, Suman Jain

INTRODUCTION

Leprosy is essentially a disease of the nerves. Most of the disabilities associated with the disease are due to involvement and damage to peripheral nerves. In this context, an understanding of the structure and function of the nerve is in order.

STRUCTURE AND FUNCTION OF PERIPHERAL NERVE

A peripheral nerve is composed of two cellular elements, the neuron and the Schwann cell, both of which are derived from embryonic ectoderm.[1] Neuron is the functional unit of the nervous system and is involved in transmitting nerve messages to all parts of the body. Neurons are basically made up of a cell body, dendrites and an axon. The cell body contains organelles that maintain its life. Dendrites are short processes from the cell body, and are responsible for receiving information and passing it on to the cell body. Dendritic processes almost always undergo branching. The axon passes information away from the cell body. Axons remain unbranched for a long length and only undergo branching towards the end of their process (Fig. 10.1). A nerve fascicle is formed when multiple axons are grouped together and many such fascicles constitute a peripheral nerve.

Structure of the Axon

The axon is a long tubular extension of the neuron. The axon is covered by the neurolemmal membrane and contains fluid axoplasm. The axon carries information from the cell body to the periphery. Each neuron has only one axon. Sensory neurons have long dendrites and a short axon, motor neurons have the opposite.

The cell body of the axons in a peripheral nerve is located in the dorsal root ganglion for sensory nerves; in the ventral horn of the spinal cord or brain stem for motor nerves and in the autonomic ganglion for autonomic nerves.

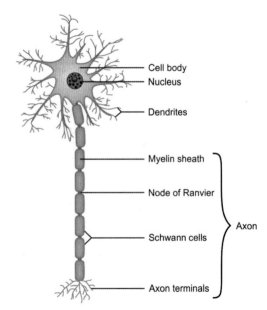

Fig. 10.1: Neuron

Schwann Cells and Myelination of Nerves

Myelin is a sheath of lipid that covers an axon. The myelin sheath protects the axon as well as speeds up the impulse along the length of the axon. Myelin is produced by the Schwann cell that encircles the axon. Schwann cell is vital for the life and the function of an axon. Schwann cells have an electron dense basal lamina which closely encircles the axon on its surface. Successive Schwann cells cover an axon right from its origin in the spinal nerve root almost to its periphery. Mature Schwann cells produce myelin in response to a stimulus from the axon. Schwann cells are also capable of utilizing degraded products of myelin breakdown to resynthesize fresh myelin. The Schwann cell membrane encircles the axon in a spiral fashion to produce multiple layers of the membrane like an onion peel. Thus, the myelin sheath is formed from the lipid and protein of the cell membrane of the Schwann cell. The outermost layer of the myelin sheath is the Schwann cell with its nucleus, cytoplasm and its outer cell membrane called neurolemma.

Along the length of a nerve multiple Schwann cells surround the axon. The neurolemma of two adjoining Schwann cells dips down to the axon to produce short gaps where the axon is not enclosed by myelin. These are called nodes of Ranvier. These points are the places where the myelin sheath of one Schwann cell ends and the next begins. This is also the point at which any collateral branches of the axon leave the main axon.

The axons covered by a myelin sheath and individual Schwann cells are called myelinated nerves. There are unmyelinated nerves where multiple axons are subserved by one Schwann cell with the multiple axons embedded in invaginations of the Schwann cell. These axons are not enclosed beyond the initial stage of enfolding and, therefore, are enclosed by only a single or a few layers of Schwann cell plasma membranes without the formation of a thick lipoprotein sheath constituting myelin.[2] Since multiple layers of myelin are not present around each axon, they are less protected and more importantly they conduct electrical impulse along the axon much slower than myelinated axons. Although the Schwann cells of myelinated and unmyelinated nerves are similar in many aspects, the Schwann cells of unmyelinated axon lack lysosomes and could be the reason why *Mycobacterium leprae* survive and are present in large number in unmyelinated nerves.[3] Myelination of a nerve is an important event for both protection of axon as well as for the quick conduction of nerve impulses. Myelin predominantly contains glycolipids, galactocerebrosides and sulphatides. Gangliosides and myelin protein *P* zero (P_0) are specific for peripheral nerves. Neurobiological studies on the Schwann cell discuss the importance of adhesion molecules like neurofascins, gliomedin, contactins, and neuronal cell adhesion molecule (NrCAM) in maintaining Schwann cell/axon integrity.[4]

STRUCTURE OF NERVE (FIG. 10.2)

A peripheral nerve is formed when multiple axons—both myelinated and unmyelinated—are grouped together into a nerve fascicle. Greater the number of axons in a fascicle and greater the number of fascicles in a nerve, greater is the diameter of the peripheral nerve. On light microcopy, the axon can be visualized only by silver impregnation staining. Electron microscopically, the cytoplasm of the axons contain neurofilaments, mitochondria, longitudinally-oriented endoplasmic reticulum, neurotubules, and small vesicles and granules containing neurotransmitters and neuropeptides.[5]

The axons are long processes and since their terminal ends are distant from the cell body, they are insulated from other axons by endoneurial connective tissue consisting of type I and type II collagen fibrils, fibroblasts, a few mast cells, macrophages and endoneural fluid.

A number of axons are grouped together to form a fascicle and each such fascicle is surrounded by dense connective tissue called perineurium. The perineurium is made up of multiple layers of perineural cells, type I and type II collagen fibrils and elastic fibers, in circumferential, oblique and longitudinal orientation. Each layer of perineural cells has a basal lamina containing laminin and fibronectin. The innermost layer of perineural cells have tight intercellular bridges that maintain the blood nerve barrier and preserve the endoneurial environment. The blood nerve barrier, when broken, provides a point of entry for inflammatory cells and other soluble factors, including cytokines, chemokines and immunoglobulins.[6] Many nerve fascicles are enclosed together in a connective tissue covering called epineurium. The epifascicular epineurium encircles the entire nerve and the interfascicular epineurium separates the different fascicles. The epineurium consists of type I and type III collagen fibrils, fibroblasts, elastic fibers and mast cells.

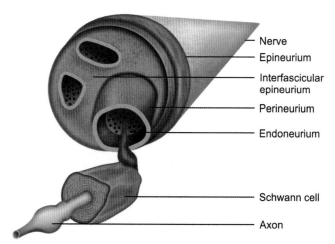

Fig. 10.2: Structure of a nerve

Even if the sensitive living axons are damaged in the nerves, the conduit made up of epineurium and perineurium will often survive and provide a pathway for their regrowth.

Axons often remain within the same fascicle throughout their course. Sometimes they leave one fascicle and enter another fascicle, and continue their course in the adjacent fascicle. The interchange of axons between fascicles may help to minimize the functional deficits caused by partial destruction of a few fascicles.

The axon may give off branches along its course and at its termination. It either forms a synaptic junction with dendritic process of adjoining neurons or with the effectors cells of muscles and glands. In the skin, the axon terminates as sensory nerve endings. A nerve contains bundles of nerve fibers, either axons or dendrites, surrounded by connective tissue. The fascicles of a nerve trunk divide and reunite repeatedly to produce nerve plexuses along the length of a nerve. This results in mixing of constituent fibers of different groups at successive levels producing eventually sensory, motor and mixed nerves.[7] Sensory nerves contain afferent fibers [towards the central nervous system (CNS)], long dendrites of sensory neurons. Motor nerves have efferent fibers (from the CNS), long axons of motor neurons. Mixed nerves contain both types of fibers.

A nerve also has blood vessels enclosed in its connective tissue wrappings. The blood supply to a nerve is from arteries that enter the epifascicular epineurium and then traverse into the interfascicular epineurium. A few of these divide into arterioles, which penetrate the perineurium obliquely and enter the endoneurium. In the endoneurium they divide into smaller capillaries that are longitudinally oriented. These capillaries have tightly interlocked endothelial cells that maintain the blood nerve barrier. Venules drain the blood and return it to the heart. There are no lymphatics in the endoneurium and perineurium. Lymphatics are present only in the epineurium.

TYPES OF NERVES

Nerves that supply the skin and other structural tissues, such as muscle and bone, are called "somatic nerves". Nerves that supply visceral organs, such as the lungs, heart, liver and kidney, are "visceral nerves". These nerves are largely autonomic in function. Axons that carry information from the periphery to the CNS are called "afferent nerves" or "afferent fibers" or "sensory nerves". Axons that carry information from the CNS to produce effects in the periphery, such as contraction of a muscle, are called efferent nerves or motor nerves.

Nerves (axons) are also classified according to their conduction velocities. The conduction velocities are directly related to the size of the fibers, i.e. the larger fibers transmitting the impulse faster than the smaller fibers. The conduction velocity is also dependent on the myelination of the axons—with myelinated fibers transmitting faster than unmyelinated fibers (Table 10.1).

When a peripheral nerve is stimulated electrically and the electrical activity recorded, a wave is generated (Fig. 10.3). The size of the wave generated reflects the number of axons in the nerve and the shape of the wave reflects the type of axons present. The wave form produced by a mixed peripheral nerve, that has all type of fibers, reveals three principal peaks—A, B and C.[8] The A wave is the quickest to appear after stimulation and is produced by the rapidly conducting axons which conduct the impulse in the range of 12–120 m/s. These are called "A" fibers. The A wave is actually made up of four smaller peaks Aα, Aβ, Aγ and Aδ waves, each of which represents a smaller subgroup of rapidly conducting axons.

The B wave is produced by slightly slower conducting axons classified as "B" fibers, which have a conduction velocity in the range of 4–70 m/s. This is followed by the "C" wave, which is produced by slowly conducting axons or "C" fibers, with conduction velocities in the range of 0.5–2 m/s.

Table 10.1: Classification of nerve fibers

S. No.	Name	Type of fiber	Diameter (µm)	Conduction velocity (m/s)	Functions involving	Touch	Pressure	Pain	Temp
1.	A-alpha	Myelinated	13–22	70–120	Alpha-motoneurons, muscle spindle primary endings, golgi tendon organs	+	–	–	–
2.	A-beta	Myelinated	8–13	40–70	Kinesthesia, muscle spindle, secondary endings, vibration sense	+	+	–	–
3.	A-gamma	Myelinated	4–8	15–40	Gamma-motoneurons	+	+	–	–
4.	A-delta	Myelinated	1–4	5–15	Crude touch	+	+	+	+
5.	B	Myelinated, autonomic impulses	1–3	3–14	Preganglionic autonomic	–	–	–	–
6.	C	Nonmyelinated	0.1–1	0.5–2	Postganglionic autonomic	+	+	+	+

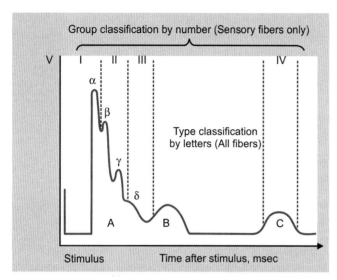

Fig. 10.3: Neurogram of peripheral nerve showing various components of the compound action potential

A and B fibers are myelinated axons of different diameter and differing conducting velocities. Larger myelinated axons carry impulses faster than smaller myelinated axons. "C" fibers are unmyelinated, of small diameter and with slow conduction velocities.

Functionally, Aα, Aβ fibers represent motor fibers to voluntary muscles and few sensory fibers that transmit position sensation from skeletal muscle. Aβ fibers mediate touch, vibration and pressure sensation from the skin. Aδ fibers are sensory fibers that carry pressure, pain and temperature sensation from skin.

C fibers are unmyelinated sensory fibers that arise in all tissues of the body and carry pain, temperature and pressure sensations. Because Aβ fibers have large diameters, they are sometimes called large diameter afferent fibers, and Aδ and C fibers are called small diameter afferent fibers.

Another way of classifying nerves relates specifically to sensory fibers. In this system sensory fibers are grouped into group I, II, III and IV, depending on their conduction velocities. The group I-IV fibers have conduction velocities corresponding to Aα, Aβ, Aδ and C fibers, respectively. Group III and IV fibers mediate pain and temperature sensations, while group II fibers mediate pressure and touch.

NERVE SUPPLY TO THE SKIN

The skin is innervated by cutaneous branches of musculocutaneous nerves that arise segmentally from the spinal nerves. In skin of the face, branches of the trigeminal nerves are responsible for cutaneous innervation. The main nerve trunks enter the subcutaneous tissues, divide, and form a branching network at the dermal-subcutaneous junction. This deep nerve plexus enters the dermis from the subcutaneous tissue and travels along with the blood vessels in the neurovascular bundles. As they traverse the dermis, they become thinner and give off fine branches to the skin adnexal structures, like sweat glands, hair follicles, smooth muscle, sebaceous glands and sensory receptors. Most of these fibers are unmyelinated nerves. Subsequently, the nerve fibers reorganize into small nerve bundles, which ascend along with the blood vessels and lymphatic vessels to form a network of interlacing nerves beneath the epidermis, the superficial nerve plexus of the papillary dermis.[9]

The cutaneous nerves contain sensory or autonomic nerve fibers. The sensory nerves carry afferent impulses from the periphery to their cell body in the dorsal root ganglia, or for the face, to the trigeminal ganglion. Cutaneous sensory neurons are unipolar; one branch of a single axon extends from the cell body toward the periphery, and the second one extends towards the CNS. As many as a thousand afferent nerve fibers may innervate 1 cm^2 of the skin. The sensory supply follows well-defined dermatomes; however, an overlapping innervation may occur. Autonomic nerve fibers are distributed along with the sensory nerves until they branch out into the terminal autonomic plexus, which supplies skin glands, blood vessels and arrectorpili muscles.

In routine histology sections the nerves appear as wavy structures with slender Schwann cell nuclei. Axons and myelin require special stains, like silver impregnation and solochrome cyanine stain, for morphological study.

NERVE ENDINGS

Nerve endings can be differentiated into three types: (1) Free unexpanded endings, (2) Expanded tips, e.g. Merkel's discs, and (3) Encapsulated tips, such as Pacinian and Meissner corpuscles. All autonomic and many sensory nerve fibers terminate as free endings, which consist of axons surrounded by Schwann cell processes. The basal laminas of a few of these Schwann cells are in contact with the outer layer of the epidermis. Only in case of certain pathological conditions and trauma, these nerve endings have been seen to penetrate the epidermis.

There are differences in the arrangement of nerves in hairy and nonhairy skin. In hairy skin, most nerves terminate either as free endings in the epidermis or as endings associated with hair follicles, which may be free or encapsulated.[10] In nonhairy skin, free nerve endings as well as sensory end-organs, such as the Meissner corpuscles, are present. They are touch receptors present in the dermal papillae, especially at the tips of fingers, which consist of layers of flattened Schwann cells. Pacinian corpuscles are pressure-sensitive organs present in subcutis. Mucocutaneous junction contains similar mucocutaneous sensory organs. All these sensory end-organs are innervated by myelinated nerves.

Millions of sensory receptors detect changes which occur inside and outside the body. The receptors on the skin monitor sensations such as light touch, pain and temperature (hot and cold). Deep receptors monitor vibration, joint position and deep pain. In the internal environment, receptors detect variations in pressure, pH, carbon dioxide concentration and levels of important metabolites. All of this gathered information is the sensory input or sensory function. Sensory input is converted into electrical signals called nerve impulses that are transmitted to the brain. There the signals are brought together to create sensations, to produce thoughts, or to add to memory. Decisions are made based on the sensory input.

Based on the sensory input and integration, the nervous system responds by sending signals to muscles, causing them to contract, or to glands, causing them to produce secretions. Muscles and glands are called effectors because they cause an effect in response to directions from the nervous system. This is the output or motor function.

DAMAGE TO PERIPHERAL NERVES

Damage to neural tissue due to trauma, or during neuropathy, elicits certain responses, which in the peripheral nerve largely affect Schwann cells function. There are mainly three pathological responses: (1) Segmental demyelination, (2) Wallerian degeneration, and (3) Axonal degeneration.

1. *Segmental demyelination*: This affects only the myelin that is present between two nodes of Ranvier, while the denuded axons remain unaffected. Demyelination produces delay in nerve conduction and directly affects the integrity and function of the axons they subserve.

2. *Wallerian degeneration*: This involves degeneration of the whole nerve fibers distal to the site of injury or inflammation. Proliferation of Schwann cells in the form of long columns, known as bands of Bungner, leads to the repair of neural tissue. These columns guide the regenerating axon to grow distally from the site of lesion. Within 4 weeks, the newly formed axon gets encapsulated completely by myelin. However, in case of severe damage to axon and myelin, they fail to regenerate and the gap instead gets filled with connective tissue. The first sign that characterizes Wallerian degeneration is that the sheath cell nuclei and the Schmidt-Lanternann clefts in the myelin become more prominent.

   In addition to the longitudinal orientation of the proliferating Schwann cells, another type of development, found especially in chronic neuropathies, is noticed. It involves a concentric arrangement of the Schwann cell processes and connective tissues around a central myelinated fiber. This arrangement is known as an "onion bulb". These are formed by a combination of proliferation and rearrangement of Schwann cells along with degeneration of axons associated with the proliferation of fibroblasts and fibrosis.

3. *Axonal degeneration*: Axonal damage and degradation of myelin as a result of trauma produces myelin debris that needs to be eliminated. This is accomplished by phagocytosis by Schwann cells.

Compartmentation: Regeneration of neural tissue leads to an altered configuration of the fascicles where the larger fascicles get replaced by smaller ones by a process known as compartmentation. In this, Schwann cells and endoneurial fibroblasts elongate and resemble perineural cells.

MYCOBACTERIUM LEPRAE AND NEURAL PREDILECTION

M. leprae survives and proliferates in the cooler parts of the body—in macrophages of skin and in Schwann cells of peripheral nerves where they traverse superficially. A diagnosis of leprosy is made based on the presence of *M. leprae* in the skin and demonstrable nerve involvement and damage.

There are different ways in which *M. leprae* may reach peripheral nerves. *M. leprae* may enter the respiratory tract as a droplet infection and inhabit the nasal mucosa. They may be carried by macrophages into the vascular sinuses in the nose and from there spread to the nerves at the sites of predilection via the bloodstream.

M. leprae may enter the skin at points of microulcerations and enter naked nerve endings and traverse centripetally up the nerve; Khanolkar referred to this as "like fish swimming against the stream".[11] When the organism reaches the peripheral nerve it may enter the endoneurial blood flow and then ultimately parasitizes the Schwann cells. Alternatively, they may be engulfed by the peripheral cells and then pass inwards into the endoneurium and Schwann cells.[12]

Among bacteria, *M. leprae* has the unique ability to infect Schwann cells and axons. The nerve, in general, is an immune protected site. The lack of lymphatics and the presence of blood nerve barrier within the nerve provide high degree of protection from immune surveillance.[13] A near-perfect host parasite relationship is observed between the *M. leprae*, which are nontoxic bacilli with a long generation time and the ability to achieve dormancy, and the Schwann cells which are ideal host for their survival and multiplication. Schwann cells are not functionally akin to macrophages and have low ability to process and present antigen to T lymphocytes which enhance killing of the engulfed *M. leprae*. However, it should be noted that although the phagocytic potential of Schwann cells is relatively low, they are able to ingest mycobacteria and destroy them more rapidly than polymorphonuclear cells. They tend to retain the organism and antigen for long time and only in the presence of a local inflammatory response, there is a bacterial killing and accompanying damage to nerves.[14-17] A C-type lectin, CD209, which is expressed on macrophages and Schwann cells, could also be a common mechanism by which macrophages and Schwann cells bind and internalize *M. leprae*.[18]

Recent studies have revealed that *M. leprae* gains entry to peripheral nerves via the terminal sensory "C" fiber, Schwann cells and a further vertical spread occurs along the Schwann cell column. *M. leprae* binds to the G domain of the laminin α2-chain (LN-α2), which is expressed on the surface of the Schwann cell-axon unit.[19] Dystroglycan and its associated molecules on the Schwann cells play a role in demyelination and other early events of nerve damage.[20]

One of the main causes of nerve damage among several other pathogenic mechanisms is the mechanical damage due to the large influx of cells and fluid, and/or immunological damage. A likely immunopathogenic mechanism of Schwann cell and nerve damage in leprosy is that infected Schwann cells process and present antigens of *M. leprae* to antigen-specific, inflammatory type 1 T-cells and that these T-cells subsequently damage and lyse infected Schwann cells.[21] Diminishing levels of neuropeptides and changes in the cytokine profile affect the cortisol-sensitivity of infiltrating T-cells, and modulate the cortisol-cortisone shuttle so that the inflammatory site becomes resistant to physiological levels of anti-inflammatory adrenocortical steroids.[22] It would be useful to understand the mechanisms involved in inflammatory responses to *M. leprae*, particularly in the context of nerve damage, and also the relationship between infection, inflammation and the nature of damage to nerve fibers to help identify drugs specifically directed at these mechanisms.

Studies of early untreated leprosy have shown that *M. leprae* are primarily seen in the Schwann cells of nonmyelinated fibers. The reason for such preferential lodgment is not known, but could be related to lack of lysosomes in these Schwann cells. Once enclosed, a vertical spread along abundant overlapping of cell processes occurs. Studies have shown that segmental type of demyelination, independent of bacterial load, predominates in both tuberculoid and lepromatous leprosy, which is the main cause for the functional deficit.[23] Demyelination in leprosy is usually not conspicuous, being better detected by the examination of teased fiber. Teased fiber studies have affirmed the two distinct types of demyelination, a primary segmental demyelination occurring in localized areas due to action exerted by inflammatory cells; a secondary demyelination occurring as a sequel to atrophic changes in axonal compartment.[24] This secondary demyelination is considered by some as the cause for silent nerve damage observed in leprosy.

The ocular manifestations of leprosy are attributed to the presence of the bacilli and/or their antigens within the eye or secondary to neuritis of zygomatic branch of the facial nerve or the ophthalmic branch of the trigeminal nerve. Quantitative assessment of the visibility of unmyelinated corneal nerves in a large cohort of leprosy patients have revealed a significant reduction in the visibility of these nerves as the spectrum of the disease moved from the tuberculoid to the lepromatous pole.[25] Corneal nerves exhibiting morphological changes, such as beading and thickening, have been observed in lepromatous leprosy patients.[26]

Fibrosis in leprosy nerves was reported by many authors and was reported in as high as 73% of nerve biopsies in pure neural leprosy patients.[27] It was observed to involve all the three compartments of nerve, the epineurium, perineuriun and endoneurium, in varying degrees. While some studies detected increased type 1 collagen replacing type III collagen normally seen with lamellatedperiaxonal fibrosis surrounding both myelianted and unmyelinated fibres,[28]others associated fibrosis of leprosy nerves with *M leprae* induced alterations of fibroblasts.[29] All these changes lead to nerve fiber loss in leprosy. Thus, the reasons for ensuing nerve fiber loss in leprosy could be explained either as a consequence of the inflammatory process in the nerve resulting in fibrosis and/or of demyelination due to functionally impaired and *M. leprae* infected Schwann cell. An increase in tryptase-rich mast cells was observed in the epineurium, which is rich in type I collagen. This leads to collegenisation through the increased mast cell tryptase activity.[30]

It is generally observed that the nerves of lower extremity are more frequently and severely affected than in the upper extremity in both PB and MB patients of leprosy.

ELECTROPHYSIOLOGICAL STUDIES ON PERIPHERAL NERVES IN LEPROSY

The study of the electrophysiological activity of resting and contracting skeletal muscle with the help of electromyography (EMG) and the conduction of the nerve impulse along the peripheral nerve, also called *Nerve Conduction Study* have become most useful diagnostic tools in the assessment of nerve function in leprosy, as well as in other peripheral nerve disorders. These studies were responsible for a complete reappraisal of neuromuscular diseases as these provide vital information to confirm or alter a clinical diagnosis and prevent a serious diagnostic error. It is only possible to learn these techniques by practical experience; however, it is worthwhile to understand the theory behind them. Hitherto EMG and nerve conduction studies required large and sophisticated instrumentation that necessitated high levels of expertise. More recently, these have become commonly performed bedside/outpatient procedures in many neurological centers. Nonetheless, these instruments are still not in routine use in regular leprosy clinics.

ELECTROPHYSIOLOGICAL STUDY BY EMG

EMG helps in detection and recording of the electrical activity from a portion of a muscle by recording of motor unit potentials. Needle EMG is the usual method followed in the study of leprosy patients. It is carried out by insertion of a twin core needle electrode into the muscle. The electrical potentials in the muscle are observed on an oscilloscope at three points; during the insertion of needle, with the muscle at rest and during full muscle contraction. The muscle to be sampled is selected depending on the clinical diagnosis. The muscles usually examined in leprosy are, abductor pollicis brevis for testing the function of the median nerve, abductor digiti minimi for testing the ulnar nerve and extensor digitorum brevis for testing the lateral popliteal nerve. EMG is to be performed separately for each muscle to be tested. [31]

In the normal EMG, complete electric silence is observed at rest. With minimal voluntary contraction, individual motor unit potentials are seen, which represents the summation of membrane action potentials of many muscle fibers. With increasing active contraction of the muscle, firing rate increases indicating increased motor fiber recruitment, referred to as a complete interference pattern.

If the nerve supply to a muscle is damaged by disease of either ventral horn cell, nerve root or peripheral nerve, the muscle is denervated to a variable extent and the resulting EMG findings are known as 'chronic partial denervation' pattern. As each ventral horn cell and its axons supply a group of muscle fibers, called motor unit, when such group of axons are damaged, as happens in leprosy neuritis, a discrete and limited group of muscle fibers cease to function. It has been shown that surviving neurons are capable of branching and taking over adjacent denervated muscle fibers over a period of time, at least partially. The denervated muscle fibers are observed to be very irritable and show spontaneous electrical activity. On needle insertion in such muscles, in the EMG the normal brief injury potentials are greatly prolonged (increased insertional activity) and occasionally continue in a burst of decreasing frequency and amplitude (pseudomyotonic run). When the needle is held still in the resting muscle, fibrillation potentials occur in the partially denervated muscle which are usually monophasic and of longer duration. Occasionally, contractions of entire muscle producing fasciculation potentials are observed. When such a muscle contracts, gaps appear in the normal interference pattern of the EMG readings. Sometimes large and polyphasic potential are observed during active contraction of partially denervated muscle. In summary, in an abnormal EMG indicating neuropathy, findings include fibrillation, fasciculation, giant motor unit potentials and incomplete interference or reduced recruitment pattern. It should be stated that in cases of myopathy (in contrast to neuropathy) the EMG demonstrates motor unit potentials that are lower in amplitude and shorter in duration than normal, and there is a reduced interference pattern.

Principle of Nerve Conduction Studies[32,33]

The basic requirements for motor nerve conduction studies are that a suitable muscle be available and that its nerve supply can be stimulated at two points along its course.

The time taken for the stimulus to travel to the nearest muscle is known as distal latency and includes not only the time taken for the impulse to travel down the nerve but also the delay at the end-plate and initiation of contraction. If the nerve is then stimulated higher up, a second latency can be obtained, the difference in the time taken being an accurate measurement of the time taken for the impulse to traverse a measured length of nerve. From this conduction velocity (m/s) is obtained. Most commonly nerve conduction studies are performed in ulnar, median, peroneal and tibial nerves. In general, nerve action potentials in upper limb are more easily elicited than in lower limbs. The interpretation of electrophysiological functions of nerve trunks is usually based on the analysis of three basic parameters—velocity, latency and amplitude of the evoked response. Amplitude represents a summation of activity of the axons within a nerve trunk.

Percutaneous stimulation for nerve conduction study is performed with surface electrodes placed at appropriate anatomic locations along the course of nerve segment being studied. The general principle of nerve conduction study is that the recording or active electrode is placed over muscle or nerve segment to be studied. While the reference electrode for motor response is positioned off and distal to the muscle being tested on a nearby bone or tendon, whereas the reference electrode for sensory response is placed distal to and on the nerve segment being studied. The ground electrode which is usually a metal plate that provides a large surface area of contact with patient serves as a reference zero potential and helps to reduce stimulus artifacts. The ground electrode is usually placed on the body prominence between the stimulating and recording electrodes.

Stimulating electrodes are usually two metal electrodes or felt pad electrodes placed 1.5–3.0 cm apart. However, in conventional nerve conduction studies, monopolar needle electrodes can be used, which has certain advantages like: 1. Smaller stimulus intensity is required, 2. Nerve can be stimulated more selectively, and 3. Nerves that lie deep anatomically, can also be stimulated.

Motor Nerve Conduction Study

Peripheral nerve may be stimulated by passing electrical current through the skin, resulting in a synchronized muscle contraction. When recorded by surface electrodes, this is called the compound muscle action potential (CMAP). Motor responses are recorded over muscle being studied. The active (recording electrode—E1)) should be placed over motor point of the muscle so that clear negative defection is recorded when electrostimulation is applied to the nerve supplying that muscle. For example, E1 is to be placed on skin surface of abductor pollicis brevis for testing median nerve motor nerve action potential. The reference electrode (E2) should be placed off the muscle on nearby tendon or bone. Standard recording and reference electrodes are about

1.0 cm in diameter. For standardization or comparisons, E1 and E2 used in CAMP recording should be of the same size.

Sensory Nerve Conduction Study

A compound nerve action potential produced by electrical stimulation of afferent nerve may be recorded over peripheral sensory nerves in a number of areas. Sensory nerve action potentials can be measured in two ways—orthodromically and antidromically. Here the main requirement is a nerve near enough to the surface so that potentials can be picked up by a surface electrode and anatomically constant in position, allowing needle electrodes to be inserted adjacent to it. The reference electrode usually is the same type as recording electrode, and in antidromic studies it is placed distal to the recording electrode. For orthodromic recording the reference electrode is placed proximal to the recording electrode. Recording and reference electrode used for sensory responses, usually, are surface electrodes with spring ring, disc or bar. These different types of electrodes may be used inter-changeably for recording and stimulating purposes.

In recent years, due to improvements in the apparatus, very small action potentials in almost any cutaneous nerve can now be detected above background activity, using antidromic or orthodromic excitation, and standardized variations for size of potential and latency. Moreover, multi channel EMG machines, which are available widely, can perform recordings for both sensory nerve conduction velocities (SNCV) and motor nerve conduction velocities (MNCV).

APPLICATION OF ELECTROPHYSIOLOGICAL STUDIES IN LEPROSY

Peripheral nerve trunk involvement in leprosy is very common and manifests as sensory, motor or autonomic deficit. However, by the time it becomes clinically manifest, the damage to the nerve fascicles present within the nerve is quite advanced. If the preclinical nerve damage can be detected early, the deformities and disabilities can be prevented to a large extent. A stage of functional blockade of conduction of nerve impulse almost always precedes visible pathological changes in the nerve.[34]

The role of electrophysiological evaluation of nerve function in the diagnosis and assessment of different neuropathies is well established. There are number of studies of motor and sensory nerve conduction which have shown that marked slowing of conduction may occur in leprosy affected nerves.[35-38] In addition, a significant slowing of motor nerve conduction velocities has also been reported in clinically normal nerves in leprosy.[39] Such patients can appear normal in routine clinical examination and may progress to clinical nerve damage when a certain quantum of nerve fibers are damaged. Along with reduction in nerve conduction velocity, changes in latency and amplitude were also observed. Changes in sensory nerve conduction were more pronounced. Sensory latencies and amplitude changes were more severe than motor latencies and amplitudes in cases with manifest muscle paralysis.[40]

When sensory conduction velocity (SCV) was studied in leprosy patients and normal subjects, slowing of conduction velocity was shown in all nerves of leprosy patients with no difference between tuberculoid and lepromatous patients. This study concluded that the SCV in radial cutaneous nerve is reliable as an early diagnostic test for leprosy.[41] A pathological study combined with electrophysiology revealed that the slowing of nerve conduction is a reflection of demyelination rather than axonal damage.[42] It is the fast conducting fibers that are taken into account while measuring nerve conduction velocities; therefore if slow conducting fibers are predominantly damaged the findings may be altered.[43]

In a multi center study on 115 leprosy patients who had nerve damage or a reaction of recent onset at diagnosis, sensory and motor amplitudes and Warm Detection Thermal tests (WDT) were most frequently abnormal. Among the nerves tested, the sural and posterior tibial were the most frequently involved. WDT were much more frequently affected than Cold Detection Thermal tests (CDT) in all nerves tested. The thresholds of all test parameters differed significantly between controls and patients, while only some differed between patients with and without reaction. Concordance between Voluntary Muscle Testing (VMT) and motor conduction velocities was good for the ulnar nerve, but was low in a proportion of median and peroneal nerves. However, a proportion of nerves with abnormal Semmes Weinstein (SW) monofilament sensory test results tested normal on sensory nerve conduction tests.[44] This study concluded that nerve conduction studies and WDT appear to be most promising for the early detection of leprous neuropathy as warm sensation was more frequently affected than cold sensation, indicating that unmyelinated C fibers are more frequently affected than small myelinated A-delta fibers. In another multicenter study involving 188 multibacillary (MB) patients, sensory nerve conduction and WDT were found to be promising tests for improving early detection of neuropathy in leprosy patients, as they often became abnormal, 12 weeks or more, before an abnormal monofilament test. This study also concluded that the changes in monofilament test and VMT score mirrored changes in neurophysiology, confirming their validity as screening tests.[45]

In a follow-up study of 17 MB and 15 paucibacillary (PB) leprosy patients on regular MDT therapy over a period of 1 year,[46] it was observed that, overall, 13% of MB and 20% of PB cases showed signs of deterioration clinically and/or electrophysiologically. In further follow-up of these patients no significant improvement in the sensory conduction in both the MB and PB groups of nerves was observed, while motor conduction showed a significant improvement at the first 6-monthly follow-up in the nerves of MB patients. In the early stages of leprosy, sensory fibers undergo damage earlier than motor fibers resulting in a greater reduction of sensory conduction velocity when compared to motor. However, the amplitude changes are more significant in the motor fibers. Multi bacillary patients showed more severe changes on EMG as compared to PB patients.[39]

In a pilot study of 10 leprosy patients, reduced conduction velocities were observed besides changes in latency and amplitude in the affected nerves. The changes in sensory nerve conduction were more pronounced and sensory latencies and amplitude changes were more severe than motor latencies and amplitude in those presenting with muscle paralysis.[47] However, a previous study had found that motor nerve conduction velocity was reduced in more patients than sensory velocity. They also found that the study of late responses was more useful in detection of early lesions of leprosy.[48]

When electrophysiological functions of ulnar and median nerves were studied in leprosy patients at different stages of disease, it was observed that the measurements show a gradual insidious deterioration of function in the affected peripheral nerve trunk. In a study where electrophysiological studies were carried out in 53 early tuberculoid leprosy patients to detect nerve damage before the onset of obvious functional deficit,[49] no statistically significant difference was observed between the nerve conduction (both motor and sensory) findings obtained from clinically thickened and nonthickened nerves, indicating that nerve thickening alone is not a reliable parameter in assessing nerve involvement in leprosy. Nonetheless, as already stated, the combination of physical palpation for nerve thickening and sensory testing with SW graded nylon filaments along with VMT is very useful, reliable and often comparable to measurement of nerve conduction in detecting nerve function impairment. In a recent study combining nerve palpation with either SW monofilament testing or VMT, increased the detection sensitivity of clinical tests by two-fold and was comparable to that detected by nerve conduction studies.[50] Many a times a direct relationship between clinical sensory deficit and electrophysiological abnormality is not always found. However, clinically observed motor power loss usually correlates well with electrophysiological abnormalities.

Nerve function assessment is important for the diagnosis of leprosy as well as early diagnosis and prevention of nerve function impairment (NFI). Simple inexpensive clinical tests are available for the assessment of nerve function in leprosy. Under field conditions, combining clinical tests, such as nerve palpation and VMT, with SW monofilament testing (described in detail in the Chapter No. 28) could prove to be a practical as well as sensitive tool for diagnosing leprosy disease and detecting nerve damage in these patients. Although electrophysiological tests may not be available or cannot be preformed in field conditions and in all leprosy clinics, they are recommended under special circumstances for further confirmation and more detailed analysis or as a research tool for nerve function assessment in leprosy.[51,52]

In conclusion, it could be stated that electrophysiological studies help in demonstrating and detecting the integrity of nerve function in leprosy. They are useful not only in assessing nerve function at the time of diagnosis but also in the follow-up study of leprosy patients and complement clinical tests[50] for nerve function assessment. Although as an individual test, nerve conduction tests proved to be more sensitive, the combination of physical palpation for nerve thickening and sensory testing with SW graded nylon filaments was closely comparable to measurement of nerve conduction in detecting nerve function impairment.

HIGH RESOLUTION ULTRASONOGRAPHY AS AN IMAGING TOOL IN LEPROSY

During the last decade, emphasis on invasive investigations such as slit skin smears, skin and nerve biopsies in the diagnosis of leprosy has reduced, one of the important reasons being the risk of acquiring HIV, Hepatitis B and HCV while doing such procedures.[53] Many clinicians, dermatologists and leprologists have been looking for alternative tools for the differential diagnosis of leprosy.[54]

Examination of skin lesions and the palpation of peripheral nerves are the two most common clinical methods used by leprosy clinicians to confirm leprosy. To assess the involvement of peripheral nerves in leprosy, clinical assessment by palpation alone has an inherent limitation of being highly subjective. Laboratory tests such as nerve conduction studies when performed as an additional tool do not provide spatial information about nerve anatomy and its surroundings.

Ultrasonography (US) and magnetic resonance imaging (MRI) is being used worldwide for the identification of structural changes of peripheral nerve trunks over the last two decades. Both were found to be very useful. Although MRI was shown to depict soft tissues with excellent resolution, it is time-consuming and may not always be as readily available compared with USG. Furthermore, MRI is expensive and the equipment is stationary. Moreover, it is difficult to follow the peripheral nerves along its superficial course for identification of pathology with MRI, which can be done easily with USG.[55] Imaging of peripheral nerves can be done with reasonable precision with high resolution ultrasonography (HRUS) and color Doppler (CD). HRUS as a tool is more sensitive, efficient, and economical when compared to MRI. This section below details the efficacy of HRUS as a tool in the diagnosis, management, follow-up and treatment of leprosy and peripheral nerve damage.

HIGH RESOLUTION ULTRASONOGRAPHY

The use of high-resolution ultrasonography (HRUS) has gained popularity in the differential diagnosis of peripheral nerve disorders and neuropathy. HRUS is a noninvasive technique and provides objective real time information that closely mirrors the pathogenic mechanisms occurring in the nerve. HRUS provides information on location and degree of nerve enlargement, alterations in nerve morphology, echo texture, vascularity and fascicular pattern that helps in understanding, interpreting, diagnosing and differentiating peripheral nerve disorders.[56-62] This noninvasive tool brings new dimension to the diagnosis of leprosy which manifest as a clinicopathological spectrum;[55] in the diagnosis of reactions/nerve damage;[63] and in the diagnosis of primary or pure neural leprosy.[55,64]

Technique of HRUS

High-frequency broadband linear array transducers, and sensitive CD technology, have improved the ability of HRUS to detect fine textural abnormalities of tender tissues as well as to identify a variety of pathological conditions. Worldwide HRUS with a broadband frequency ranging from 10–14 MHz; color Doppler (CD) with broadband frequency of 6–18 MHz and linear array transducer is being used for clinical diagnosis and imaging of peripheral nerves and neuropathy. HRUS as an imaging technique provides real-time examination of soft-tissues in static and dynamic states, which help in the assessment of parameters such as endoneural blood flow and echotexture. The improved spatial and contrast resolution of this technique has made it possible to virtually depict all nerves in the limbs and extremities with excellent details especially in the context of leprosy. There is an immediate need for the use of this noninvasive technique and training in leprosy.[65] Technical developments leading to improved image quality and reduced sizes of HRUS equipment together with a reduction in price will make it possible for HRUS to become a cost effective diagnostic tool in countries where leprosy is still endemic.

Normal peripheral nerves reveal a characteristic echotexture on HRUS which is; tubular structure with multiple hypoechoic but discontinuous linear areas separated by hyperechoic bands in longitudinal and multiple rounded hypoechoic areas in a homogenous background in transverse plane (fascicular or honeycomb pattern). (Figs 4A to C)[57,66-68] Nerve sonography can demonstrate five main pathological changes: (1) Nerve enlargement, (2) Increased hypo-echogenicity or hyperechogenicity, (3) Enlarged fascicles, (4) Increased thickness of the epineurium, and (5) Increased endo- or epineural blood flow.

In all suspected patients of leprosy, bilateral examination by HRUS of peripheral nerves such as ulnar (UN) at the elbow and proximal to epicondyle, median (MN) at wrist and forearm, lateral popliteal (LP) at the fibula head and posterior tibial (PT) at the ankle and proximal to the medial malleolus could be easily performed. Nerves can be evaluated either cross sectional or transverse and/or longitudinally (Figs 5A to H) by HRUS by changing the direction of the linear array transducer.

1. Enlargement of Peripheral Nerves

In order to demonstrate nerve enlargement, measurements should be performed and compared with a set of reference values.[69] Multiple studies have demonstrated nerve enlargement in both mono- and polyneuropathies.[56,57,63,70] The cross-sectional area (CSA) of the nerve is determined from the area within the inner margin of the hyperechoic rim (Figs 6A to H and Figs 7A to D).

2. Echogenicity of Peripheral Nerves

The echogenicity of nerves should also be evaluated at multiple sites in the transverse plane. The echo density of the nerves assessed on imaging can be graded as follows: mild = some hypo echogenicity, moderate = obvious hypoechogenicity; and severe = absence of any fascicular pattern.[63] To further standardize measurements a computerized gray-scale

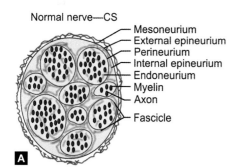
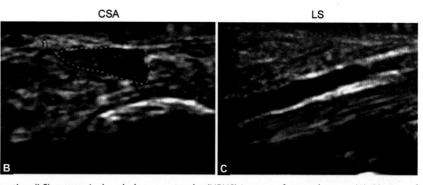

Figs 4A to C: Cross section (CS) and longitudinal section (LS) anatomical and ultrasonography (HRUS) images of normal nerve. (A) CS view of normal nerve; (B) CS view of median nerve (MN) showing CSA (6 mm²) and hypoechoic fascicles in a 'honeycomb' like pattern; (C) LS view of MN showing hyperechogenic bands in a linear pattern appearing as bundles of straw

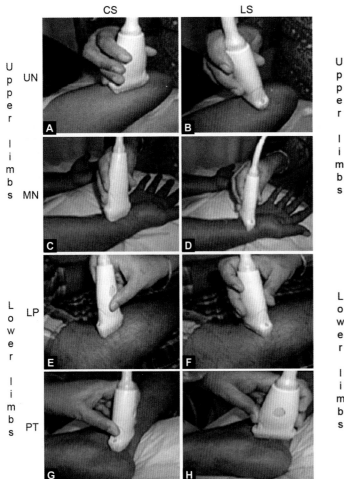

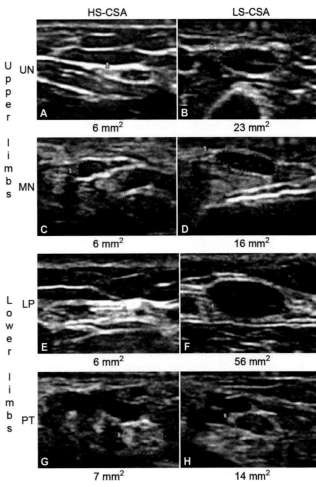

Figs 5A to H: Position of linear array transducer for HRUS imaging in upper limbs [ulnar (UN) and median (MN) nerves] and lower limbs [lateral popliteal (LP) and posterior tibial (PT) nerves]. (A and B) Position for UN at 2 cm above the elbow A: Cross section (CS), B: Longitudinal (LS); (C and D) Position for MN at wrist C: CS, D: LS; (E and F) Position for LP at head of fibula E: CS, F: LS; (G and H) Position for PT at ankle G: CS, H: LS

Figs 6A to H: HRUS comparison of cross sectional area (CSA) in healthy subjects (HS) and leprosy subjects (LS) in upper limbs [ulnar (UN) and median (MN) nerves] and lower limbs [lateral popliteal (LP) and posterior tibial (PT) nerves]. (A and B) CSA of UN A: HS-6 mm², B: LS-23 mm²; (C and D) CSA of MN C: HS-6 mm², D: LS-16 mm²; (E and F) CSA of LP E: HS-6 mm², F: LS-56 mm²; (G and H) CSA of PT G: HS-7 mm², H: LS-14 mm²

analysis can be implemented. We recently demonstrated quantitative assessment of nerve echogenicity which can reliably distinguish ulnar neuropathy in leprosy patients from healthy controls.[71] Other recent studies have shown increased hypo-echoic areas in diabetic neuropathy, carpal tunnel syndrome and ulnar neuropathy at the elbow possibly due to intraneural edema.[72,73] Therefore, nerve echogenicity is probably capable of discriminating between normal and pathological conditions of peripheral nerves (Figs 7C and F).

3. Size of Fascicles

Comparison of histological examination of nerves with nerve sonography demonstrated that the hypoechoic areas correspond with neuronal fascicles.[67] Whilst scanning along the length of nerves the size of nerve fascicles can be reliably measured in the transverse plane. Enlarged fascicles have been reported in patients with chronic inflammatory demyelinating polyneuropathy (CIDP), Charcot-Marie-Tooth (CMT) hereditary neuropathy and leprosy.[63,74,75]

4. Thickness of Epineurium

The thickness of the epineurium can also be measured in the transverse plane. HRUS has shown that the epineurium of the ulnar nerve is often strikingly thickened in leprosy patients when involved.[76]

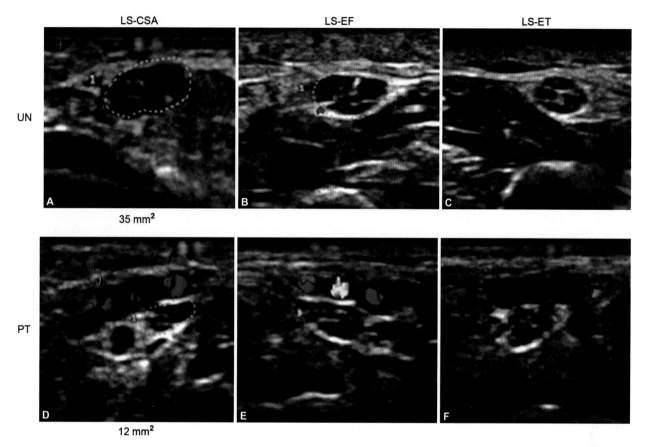

Figs 7A to F: HRUS and CD images for ulnar nerve (UN) and posterior tibial (PT) nerves in relation to cross sectional area (CSA), endoneural flow (EF) and echo texture (ET) in leprosy subjects: UN: CSA-A, EF-B, ET-C; PT: CSA-D, EF-E, ET-F

5. Vascularization of Peripheral Nerves

Peripheral nerves are supplied by a rich anastomotic system of epineural and endoneural blood vessels. The homeostasis of the epineural and endoneural microenvironment is essential for the normal nerve fiber function. To assess nerve vascularization color Doppler CD or power Doppler is used. The presence of blood flow signals in the epineural plexus or intra fascicular vessels indicates hyper vascularity of the nerve during CD imaging (Figs 7B and E).[63]

Currently, spatial resolution of color Doppler imaging is not high enough to visualize epineural or endoneural blood flow under physiological conditions. However, it is able to detect *increased* endoneural or epineural blood flow. Pathological conditions may give rise to increased blood flow due to local inflammation that is detectable with color Doppler. The local inflammation substantially contributes to nerve fiber damage in various entrapment and peripheral neuropathies and nerve abscess.[77-79] To date only few studies

have evaluated altered blood flow of peripheral nerves in pathological conditions such as carpal tunnel syndrome, ulnar neuropathy, CIDP and in patients with a type I or type II reaction in leprosy.[63,77-80] Further studies are needed to fully know their relevance and implications.

Indications and Uses of HRUS in Leprosy

Nerve thickening is one of the three cardinal signs of leprosy. With reducing case load of leprosy and integration into general health services, combined with reduction in clinical skills needed to assess the nerve thickening, it is likely that patients will be missed or misdiagnosed. However, when a patient suspected of leprosy is referred for HRUS, objective assessment of nerve thickening can be made, supporting the diagnosis of leprosy or otherwise. In addition, performing HRUS and CD during follow-up of every patient with signs and symptoms of reaction and/or suspected neuritis may help to confirm a reaction and initiate immediate intervention based on increased vascular signals and/or presence of nerve abscess. Similarly these patients can be followed up by sonography to assess improvement and prognosis.

Although no standard national or international guidelines are available as yet, it is highly beneficial to perform HRUS in following category of leprosy patients: In patients with signs and symptoms of peripheral neuropathy with no visible skin lesions (primary neuritic leprosy); in patients with skin patches with normal sensation and symptoms of peripheral neuropathy; in patients of established diagnosis of leprosy with no nerve pain or tenderness but signs of peripheral neuropathy (silent nerve paralysis); in all proven leprosy patients irrespective of presence or absence of peripheral neuropathy to assess degree of nerve thickening, and to assess the risk of impending nerve damage. In our experience we have found studying the following four nerves—ulnar (UN), median (MN), lateral popliteal (LP) and posterior tibial (PT) nerves bilaterally yields maximum results and picks up nerve involvement excellently. However, when HRUS of a particular nerve shows thickening it is important to image the regional cutaneous nerves as well to establish the extent of spread/localization.

When HRUS was performed on nerves of leprosy patients, in patients with reactions and in healthy controls, it was found that these major peripheral nerves are not only enlarged in reactions but also in leprosy patients not in reaction. This suggests that as a standard protocol all the four major peripheral nerves can be studied by sonography even in the absence of a clinical suspicion. During follow-up, only those nerves showing enlargement can be studied. Additionally, if the patient develops a clinical reaction it is advisable to again carry out sonography including CD of all of these four nerves.

Methodology

A clinician should first make the clinical assessment of UN, MN, LP and PT nerves and other nerves as necessary, bilaterally, in all leprosy patients. All these nerves and any other thickened peripheral nerves should be examined for their motor and sensory functions as well (refer to Chapter 28).

After clinical assessment the patient can undergo HRUS examination with color Doppler.[57,63,81] All peripheral nerves should be imaged using a linear array transducer with broadband frequency of at least 12 MHz, 15–18 MHz is preferable. As previously mentioned, the MN at the wrist and forearm, the UN at the elbow and proximal to the medial epicondyle, LP at the fibula head and PT nerves at the ankle and proximal to the medial malleolus (Figs 5A to H) should be examined and the length of abnormality of the nerve determined by the presence of abnormal size and echodensity

of the nerves. All nerves should be measured on transverse sections at a point where the nerve thickness is maximum in the visualized segment of the nerve. The cross-sectional area of the nerve should be determined from the area within the inner margin of the hyperechoic rim. The echodensity of the nerves is assessed on imaging and graded as: mild, moderate, and severe based on hypodensity and fascicular pattern as stated earlier. CD settings are chosen to optimize identification of weak signals from vessels with slow velocity. The presence of blood flow signals in the perineural plexus or intra fascicular vessels which indicates hyper vascularity of the nerve is observed and recorded.

Overall, the analysis and interpretation of HRUS image findings should be based on: (1) Measurement of the maximum cross-sectional area of the nerve (2) Length of nerve enlargement (3) Analysis of nerve echo texture (4) Identification of nerve compression within osteo-fibrous tunnels 5. detection of endo and epineural color flow signals. All the clinical and HRUS findings can be documented and saved in a database and recorded in a sample of proforma attached as appendix I.

Studies of HRUS in Leprosy

There are many studies that highlight the use of HRUS in leprosy.[66,82,83] It was found to be useful in imaging of all the commonly involved nerves in leprosy. In addition HRUS is also useful to assess difficult to palpate nerves such as median nerve, as well as to appreciate changes in minimally involved cutaneous nerves. The changes in the peripheral nerves which can be appreciated by imaging are, thickening of nerves, both focal and generalized, its echotexture and fascicular abnormalities, presence of nerve abscess and changes in its vascularity.

HRUS is especially useful in the confirmation of diagnosis of pure neuritic leprosy (PNL) as it not only confirms the nerve thickening but also provides information on the exact location of nerve enlargement in its course apart from other morphological alterations. This information brings a new dimension to the diagnosis of PNL.[64]

Based on their appearance on imaging a nerve was classified as normal (Group I); enlarged with fascicular abnormalities (Group II); and having no fascicular structure at all (Group III).[82] It was shown that HRUS identifies thickening of nerves even before NFI is observed clinically or even on nerve conduction studies. In a study on 21 leprosy patients, it was noted that in 3 patients, nerve conduction studies were normal, yet sonography revealed focal thickening of the ulnar nerve.[83]

Various studies have confirmed the usefulness of HRUS in identification of thickened nerves in leprosy patients. In a case control study on 20 leprosy patients HRUS demonstrated nerve enlargement of median nerve in 59%, ulnar in 44%, tibial in 33% and lateral popliteal nerve in 47% of patients.[63] Significant correlation in this study was observed between clinical parameters (grade of thickening, sensory loss and muscle weakness) and sonographic abnormalities (CSA, echotexture, endoneural flow). Studies have shown increased vascularity on CD imaging not only in the nerve trunk on the side of the inflamed skin lesions, but also in contralateral and distant nerve trunks, pointing to the more extensive involvement of nerves during reactions in leprosy compared to degree of skin involvement. The epineurium of nerves is often strikingly thickened in leprosy patients as demonstrated by HRUS, especially in those with ulnar involvement. In a recent case-control study sonographic epineural thickening demonstrated in the ulnar nerve in leprosy patients was found to be directly related to the cross sectional area of the ulnar nerve, but not with increased blood flow.[76,84]

Enlargement of the ulnar nerve at the elbow due to leprosy often has to be differentiated from that due to ulnar nerve entrapment (UNE). This can be done very effectively by HRUS. In UNE the nerve enlargement is usually at the sulcus or just above the elbow, while the ulnar nerve enlargement in leprosy is more proximal—3–4 cm above the elbow.[70]

Importance of HRUS in Leprosy

The diagnosis of leprosy involves the identification of thickened peripheral nerves by clinical palpation. Classical learning has been that the nerves are enlarged only at the sites of predilection like the elbow behind the medial epicondyle and around the head of fibula in the knee where the nerves traverse subcutaneously. However, it is now common knowledge that the nerve thickening could extend both proximally and distally from these sites where the nerve travels in a deeper plane beneath the muscle fascicles where clinical palpation is difficult. Further, wide intra and inter-observer variations have been observed in clinical palpation of nerves since it is a subjective clinical assessment. HRUS provides an objective assessment of nerve thickening where extensive lengths of the nerve can be studied even in the muscular planes or under retinacula, with no limitation to its subcutaneous course. In addition, availability of high resolution probes enables us to assess even small anatomical and morphological variations which would otherwise be impossible to ascertain by routine clinical examination.[85] With increased experience of HRUS use in leprosy, it is now becoming possible to actually visualize and study individual fascicles in more detail.

Reactions and neuritis in the nerve are known to be associated with hemodynamic changes in both the epineurium and perineurium of nerve fascicles. These changes were formally studied using invasive biopsy techniques where a sliver of suspected nerves were biopsied and studied histologically. Furthermore nerve trunk cannot be biopsied due to the danger of producing iatrogenic nerve damage. Only cutaneous nerves are biopsied and the changes are believed to mirror the changes in the bigger nerve trunk. HRUS enables us to study the nerve trunk in question and look for hemodynamic changes using color Doppler.[63,85] It may be possible with refinement of technique to be in a position to actually grade the degree of vascular change in the nerve. Studies have shown that even in the absence of clear signs and symptoms like nerve pain or tenderness, HRUS was still able to demonstrate early hemodynamic changes in the nerve progressing to develop reaction,[82] which could be useful once standardized, as an early sign to alert the physician/leprologist to start corticosteroid therapy.

Approximately, 5–10% of all leprosy patients are of PNL type, presenting with involvement of nerve(s) without skin lesions and carry the highest risk of deformity.[86-88] Therefore, in countries where leprosy occurs it can be difficult to differentiate ulnar nerve neuropathy at the elbow from PNL, and it requires a nerve biopsy or fine needle aspiration cytology for the correct diagnosis.[89,90] In such cases HRUS is very useful to confirm the diagnosis of leprosy with characteristic echotexture, endoneural flow and thickening observed in leprous neuritis.

From a Radiologist's domain, sonography is now a technological development widely used by obstetricians, gynecologists, cardiologists, neonatologists, anesthetists and neurologists as a diagnostic tool. Our experience in two HRUS training workshops conducted in recent years has been that there is a growing interest among dermatologists, neurologists and leprosy specialists to learn and apply this technique at the bed side. We have also noted that with a basic knowledge regarding nerve anatomy and course of the nerves, the technique of tracing nerves by HRUS can be learned easily by clinicians and leprologists to use it as a useful tool for leprosy diagnosis, follow-up and even to assess prognosis.[57,63]

In conclusion, HRUS is a noninvasive, cost effective tool that gives significant information on nerve structure, morphology, vascularity and real time blood flow in the nerve and this information adds a new dimension to the diagnosis of leprosy and assessment of nerve damage which can prevent disabilities. With an increasing awareness and use of HRUS it can become a routine tool in clinical practice to improve diagnosis of leprosy, in addition to being a tool to assess extent and severity of nerve involvement.

PROFORMA FOR ULTRASOUND OF PERIPHERAL NERVES

1. Name:		Serial number: Reg. No:
2. Sex:	3. Age:	4. Date of birth:
5. Occupation:		6. Date of diagnosis:
7. Duration of disease in months:		8. History of previous treatment: Yes/No
9. Clinical classification	TT/ BT/BB/BL/LL/PNL	MB/PB
10. Date of starting MDT		
11. Dose of MB. MDT completed		12. Completed in how many months:
13. Regularity	1. Regular	2. Irregular
14. Course of treatment	1. On treatment	2. RFT 3. Normal
15. Does this patient have 1. Type I reaction	2. Type II reaction	3. Neuritis alone 4. Neuritis with Type I or Type II reaction
16. Is this patient on steroid? Yes/ No		
17. How many episodes of Type I or Type II reaction? Clinical examination		
18. Lymph node enlargement: Yes/No		
19. Edema: Hands/Feet Yes/No		
20. Joints: Yes/No		
21. Skin lesion: Macules/ Papule/Infiltration/Nodules		No. of patches:
22. Appearance: Erythema/Pale; Edema/Flat; Active/Inactive		
23. No. of nerves	Trunk	Cutaneous
Investigations:		
24. Skin smear		
25. Skin biopsy		
26. Over all impression		

Appendix I

27. VMT and ST   Date:

Nerves	Ulnar		Median		LP		PT		RCN		Other cutaneous nerves	
Side	R	L	R	L	R	L	R	L	R	L	R	L
Enlargement												
Pain												
Tenderness												
VMT												

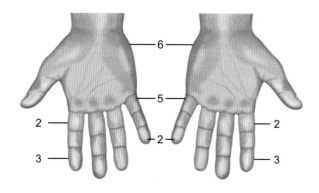

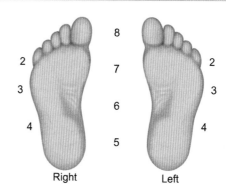

Right   Left

28. Ultrasound findings:

Nerves	Measurement of cross sectional area		Assessment of nerve structures		Endoneural color flow signals		Other findings	
	Right	Left	Right	Left	Right	Left	Right	Left
Ulnar								
Median								
LP								
PT								
RCN								
Other cutaneous nerves								

Abbreviations: RCN, regional cutaneous nerves; MDT, multidrug therapy; PNL, primary neuritic leprory; ST, skin test, VMT, voluntary muscle test, RFT, renal function test; LP, lateral plantar; PT, posterior tibial.

REFERENCES

1. Ridley DS. The structure of peripheral nerve. In: Ridley DS (Ed). Pathogenesis of Leprosy and Related Diseases. London: Wright; 1988.pp.15-9.
2. Breathnach AS. Electron microscopy of cutaneous nerves and receptors. J Invest Dermatol. 1977;69(1):8-26.
3. Boddingius J. Mechanisms of nerve damage in leprosy. In: Humber DP (Ed). Immunobiologic Aspects of Leprosy, Tuberculosis and Leishmaniasis, Excerpta Medica. London: Oxford; 1981.pp.64-73.
4. Pollard JD, Armati PJ. CIDP—the relevance of recent advances in Schwann cell/axonal neurobiology. J Peripher Nerv Syst. 2011;16(1):15-23.
5. Winkelmann RK. Cutaneous nerves. In: Zelickson AV (Ed). Ultrastructure of Normal and Abnormal Skin. Philadelphia: Lea and Febiger; 1967.pp. 203-27.
6. Kanda T. Biology of the blood-nerve barrier and its alteration in immune mediated neuropathies. J Neurol Neurosurg Psychiatry. 2013;84(2):208-12.
7. Sunderland S. The internal anatomy of nerve trunks in relation to the neural lesions of leprosy. Brain. 1973;96(4):865-88.
8. Palastanga N, Field D, Soames R. Nervous system. In: Palastanga N, Field D, Soames R (Eds). Anatomy and Human Movement. Elsevier Health Sciences; 2006.pp.5-10.
9. Sinclair DC. Normal anatomy of sensory nerves and receptors. In: Jarrett A (Ed). The Physiology and Pathophysiology of the Skin: The Nerves and Blood Vessels. Vol. 2. London: Academic Press; 1973. pp. 347-98.
10. Miller MR, Ralston HJ, Kasahara M. The pattern of the cutaneous innervations of the human hand, foot and breast. Adv Biol Skin. 1966;1:1-47.
11. Khanolkar VR. Perspectives in pathology of leprosy. Indian J Med Sci. 1955;9(Suppl 1):1-44.
12. Boddingius J. Ultrastructural changes in blood vessels of peripheral nerves in leprosy neuropathy. II. Borderline, borderline-lepromatous and lepromatous leprosy patients. Acta Neuropathol. 1977;40(1):21-39.
13. Ridley DS, Ridey MJ. Classification of nerve is modified by delayed recognition of *Mycobacterium leprae*. Int J Lepr Other Mycobact Dis. 1986;54(4):596-606.
14. Pearson JM, Ross WF. Nerve involvement in leprosy-pathology, differential diagnosis and principles of management. Lepr Rev. 1975;46(3):199-212.
15. Rea TH, Ridley DS. Lucio's phenomenon: a comparative histologic study. Int J Lepr Other Mycobact Dis. 1979;47(2): 161-6.
16. Barnetson RS, Bjune G, Pearson JM, et al. Antigenic heterogeneity in patients with reactions in borderline leprosy. Br Med J. 1975;4(5994): 435-7.

17. Boddingius J. Mechanisms of peripheral nerve damage in leprosy: electron and light microscopic studies in patients throughout the spectrum. In: Browne SG, Munzi E (Eds). Proceedings of the European Leprosy Symposium 1981. Associazione italiana "Amici di Raoul Follereau", Organizzazione per la cooperazione sanitaria internazionale; 1982.pp.65-85.

18. Teles RM, Krutzik SR, Ochoa MT, et al. Interleukin-4 regulates the expression of CD209 and subsequent uptake of *Mycobacterium leprae* by Schwann cells in human leprosy. Infect Immun. 2010;78(11):4634-43.

19. Harboe M, Aseffa A, Leekassa R. Challenges presented by nerve damage in leprosy. Lepr Rev. 2005;76(1):5-13.

20. Rambukkana A. *Mycobacterium leprae*-induced demyelination: a model for early nerve degeneration. Curr Opin Immunol. 2004;16(4):511-8.

21. Spierings E, De Boer T, Zulianello L, et al. Novel mechanisms in the immunopathogenesis of leprosy nerve damage: the role of Schwann cells, T-cells and *Mycobacterium leprae*. Immunol Cell Biol. 2000;78(4):349-55.

22. Rook GA, Lightman SL, Heijnen CJ. Can nerve damage disrupt neuroendocrine immune homeostasis? Leprosy as a case in point. Trends Immunol. 2002;23(1):18-22.

23. Shetty VP, Mistry NF, Antia NH. Current understanding of leprosy as a peripheral nerve disorder: significance of involvement of peripheral nerve in leprosy. Indian J Lepr. 2000;72(3):339-50.

24. Jacobs JM, Shetty, VP Antia NH. Teased fibre studies in leprous neuropathy. J Neurol Sci. 1987;79(3):301-13.

25. Daniel E, David A, Rao PS. Quantitative assessment of the visibility of unmyelinated corneal nerves in leprosy. Int J Lepr Other Mycobact Dis. 1994;62(3):374-9.

26. Daniel E, Thompson K. Corneal sensation in leprosy. Int J Lepr Other Mycobact Dis. 1999;67(3):298-301.

27. Jardim MR, Chimeilli L, Faria SC, et al. Clinical, electroneuromyographic and morphological studies of pure neural leprosy in Brazilian referral centre. Lepr Rev 2004;75(3):242-53.

28. Kajihara H, Parurusi IA, Saleh RM, et al. Light and electron microscopic study of peripheral nerves in patients with lepromatous leprosy (LL) and borderline lepromatous leprosy (BL). Hiroshima J Med Sci. 2000;49(1):83-92.

29. Singh N, Birdi TJ, Chandrasekhar S, et al. *In vitro* studies on extracellular matrix production by *M. leprae* infected murine neurofibroblasts. Lepr Rev. 1998;69(3):246-56.

30. Montagna NA, de Oliveira ML, Mandarim-de-Lacerda CA, et al. Leprosy: contribution of mast cells to epineurial collagenization. Clin Neuropathol. 2005;24(6):284-90.

31. Ramdan W, Mourad B, Fadel W, et al. Clinical, electrophysiological, and immunopathological study of peripheral nerves in Hansen's disease. Lepr Rev. 2001;72(1):35-49.

32. Patten J. Neurological Differential Diagnosis, 2nd edition. New Delhi: Springer (India) Ltd.; 2005.

33. Lee JH, DeLisa JA. Manual of Nerve Conduction Study and Surface Anatomy for Needle Elctromyography, 4th edition. Philadelphia: Lippincott Williams and Wilkins; 2004.

34. Hackett ER, Shipley DE, Livengood R. Motor nerve conduction velocity studies of ulnar nerve in patients with leprosy. Int J Lepr. 1968;36(3):282-87.

35. Sohi AS, Kandhari KC, Singh N. Motor nerve conduction studies in leprosy. Int J Dermatol. 1971;10(2):151-5.

36. Brown TR, Kovindha A, Wathanadilokkol U, et al. Leprosy neuropathy: Correlation of clinical and eletrophysiological tests. Indian J Lepr. 1996;68(1):1-14.

37. Ramkrishnan AG, Srinivasan TM. Electrophysiological correlates of hanseniasis. Int J Lepr Other Mycobact Dis. 1995;63(3):395-408.

38. Samant G, Shetty VP, Uplekar MW, et al. Clinical and electrophysiological evaluation of nerve function impairment, following cessation of multidrug therapy in leprosy. Lepr Rev. 1999;70(1):10-20.

39. Chaurasia RN, Garg RK, Singh MK, et al. Nerve conduction studies in paucibacillary and multibacillary leprosy: a comparative evaluation. Indian J Lepr. 2011;83(1):15-22.

40. Husain S, Malaviya GN. Early nerve damage in leprosy: an electrophysiological study of ulnar and median nerves in patients with and without clinical neural deficits. Neurol India. 2007;55(1):22-6.

41. Sebille A. Respective importance of different nerve conduction velocities in leprosy. J Neurol Sci. 1978;38(1):89-95.

42. Shetty VP, Mehta LN, Antia HN, et al. Teased fibre study of early nerve lesions in leprosy and in contacts, with electrophysiological correlates. J Neurol Neurosurg Psychiatry. 1977;40(7):708-11.

43. Marquees W, Barreira AA. Normal median nerve near potential. Braz J Med Biol Res. 1997;30:1431-5.

44. Van Brakel WH, Nicholls PG, Das L, et al. The INFIR Cohort Study: assessment of sensory and motor neuropathy in leprosy at baseline. Lepr Rev. 2005;76(4):277-95.

45. Van Brakel WH, Nicholls PG, Wilder-Smith EP, et al. Early diagnosis of neuropathy in leprosy-comparing diagnostic tests in a large prospective study (the INFIR Cohort Study). PLoS Negl Trop Dis. 2008;2(4):1-12.

46. Samant G, Shetty VP, Uplekar MW, et al. Clinical and electrophysiological evaluation of nerve function impairment following cessation of multidrug therapy in leprosy. Lepr Rev. 1999;70(1):10-20.

47. Kar S, Krishnan A, Singh N, et al. Nerve damage in leprosy: An electrophysiological evaluation of ulnar and median nerves in patients with clinical neural deficits: A pilot study. Indian Dermatol Online J. 2013;4(2):97-101.

48. Gupta BK, Kochar DK. Study of nerve conduction velocity, somatosensory evoked potential and late responses of posterior tibial nerve in leprosy. Int J Lepr Other Mycobact Dis.1994;62(4):586-93.

49. Rao SP, Bharambe MS. Electro-neuro physiological studies in early tuberculoid leprosy. Indian J Lepr. 1993;65(2):181-7.

50. Khambati FA, Shetty VP, Ghate SD, et al. Sensitivity and specificity of nerve palpation, monofilament testing and voluntary muscle testing in detecting peripheral nerve abnormality, using nerve conduction studies as gold standard; a study in 357 patients. Lepr Rev. 2009;80(1):34-50.

51. Elias J Jr, Nogueira-Barbosa MH, Feltrin LT, et al. Role of ulnar nerve sonography in leprosy neuropathy with electrophysiologic correlation. J Ultrasound Med. 2009;28(9):1201-9.

52. Capadia GD, Shetty VP, Khambati FA, et al. Effect of corticosteroid usage combined with multidrug therapy on nerve damage assessed using nerve conduction studies: a prospective cohort study of 365 untreated multibacillary leprosy patients. J Clin Neurophysiol. 2010;27(1):38-47.

53. Walker SL, Lockwood DN. The clinical and immunological features of leprosy. Br Med Bull. 2006; 77-78:103-121.
54. Kumar B, Dogra S. Leprosy: A disease with diagnostic and management challenges. Indian J Dermatol Venereol Leprol. 2009;75(2):111-5.
55. Rao PN, Jain S. Newer management options in leprosy. Indian J Dermatol. 2013;58(1):6-11.
56. Beekman R, Visser LH. Sonography in the diagnosis of carpal tunnel syndrome: a critical review of the literature. Muscle Nerve. 2003;27(1):26-33.
57. Beekman R, Visser LH. High-resolution sonography of the peripheral nervous system—a review of the literature. Eur J Neurol. 2004;11(5):305-14.
58. Chiou HJ, Chou YH, Chiou SY, et al. Peripheral nerve lesions: role of high resolution US. Radiographics. 2003;23(6):e15.
59. Bayrak AO, Bayrak IK, Turker H, et al. Ultrasonography in patients with ulnar neuropathy at the elbow: comparison of cross-sectional area and swelling ratio with electrophysiological severity. Muscle Nerve. 2010;41(5):661-6.
60. Koenig RW, Pedro MT, Heinen CP, et al. High-resolution ultrasonography in evaluating peripheral nerve entrapment and trauma. Neurosurg Focus. 2009;26(2):E13.
61. Padua L, Aprile I, Pazzaglia C, et al. Contribution of ultrasound in a neurophysiological lab in diagnosing nerve impairment: A one-year systematic assessment. Clin Neurophysiol. 2007;118 (6):1410-6.
62. Visser LH, Smidt MH, Lee ML. High-resolution sonography versus EMG in the diagnosis of carpal tunnel syndrome. J Neurol Neurosurg Psychiatry. 2008;79(1):63-7.
63. Jain S, Visser LH, Praveen TL, et al. High resolution sonography: a new technique to detect nerve damage in leprosy. PLoS Negl Trop Dis. 2009;3(8):e498.
64. Jain S, Visser LH, Yerasu MR, et al. Use of high resolution ultrasonography as an additional tool in the diagnosis of primary neuritic leprosy: a case report. Lepr Rev. 2013; 84(2):161-5.
65. Goulart IM, Goulart LR. Leprosy: diagnostic and control challenges for a worldwide disease. Arch Dermatol Res. 2008; 300(6):269-90.
66. Fornage BD. Peripheral nerves of the extremities: imaging with US. Radiology. 1988;167(1):179-82.
67. Silvestri E, Martinoli C, Derchi LE, et al. Echotexture of peripheral nerves: correlation between US and histologic findings and criteria to differentiate tendons. Radiology. 1995;197(1):291-96.
68. Boehm J, Scheidl E, Bereczki D, et al. High resolution ultrasonography of peripheral nerves: Measurements on 14 nerve segments in 56 healthy subjects and reliability assessments. Ultraschall Med. 2014 Apr 24.
69. Cartwright MS, Passmore LV, Yoon JS, et al. Cross-sectional area reference values for nerve ultrasonography. Muscle Nerve. 2008;37(5):566-71.
70. Beekman R, Visser LH, Verhagen WI. Ultrasonography in ulnar neuropathy at the elbow: a critical review. Muscle Nerve. 2011; 43(5):627-35.
71. Boom J, Visser LH. Quantitative assessment of nerve echogenicity: comparison of methods for evaluating nerve echogenicity in ulnar neuropathy at the elbow. Clin Neurophysiol. 2012;123(7):1446-53.
72. Watanabe T, Ito H, Sekine A, et al. Sonographic evaluation of the peripheral nerve in diabetic patients: the relationship between nerve conduction studies, echo intensity, and cross-sectional area. J Ultrasound Med. 2010;29(5):697-708.
73. Tagliafico A, Tagliafico G, Martinoli C. Nerve density: a new parameter to evaluate peripheral nerve pathology on ultrasound. Preliminary study. Ultrasound Med Biol. 2010;36(10):1588-93.
74. Granata G, Pazzaglia C, Caliandro P, et al. Letter to the editor referring to peripheral nerve hypertrophy in chronic inflammatory demyelinating polyradiculoneuropathy detected by ultrasonography. Intern Med. 2009;48(23):2049; author reply on 2051.
75. Martinoli C, Schenone A, Bianchi S, et al. Sonography of the median nerve in Charcot-Marie-Tooth disease. AJR Am J Roentgenol. 2002;178(6):1553-6.
76. Visser LH, Jain S, Lokesh B, et al. Morphological changes of the epineurium in leprosy: a new finding detected by high-resolution sonography. Muscle Nerve. 2012;46(1):38-41.
77. Bathala L, Kumar K, Pathapati R, et al. Ulnar neuropathy in hansen disease: clinical, high-resolution ultrasound and electrophysiologic correlations. J Clin Neurophysiol. 2012;29(2):190-3.
78. Mohammadi A, Ghasemi-Rad M, Mladkova-Suchy N, et al. Correlation between the severity of carpal tunnel syndrome and color Doppler sonography findings. AJR Am J Roentgenol. 2012;198(2):W181-4.
79. Ghasemi-Esfe AR, Khalilzadeh O, Vaziri-Bozorg SM, et al. Color and power Doppler US for diagnosing carpal tunnel syndrome and determining its severity: a quantitative image processing method. Radiology. 2011;261(2):499-506.
80. Frijlink DW, Brekelmans GJ, Visser LH. Increased nerve vascularization detected by color Doppler sonography in patients with ulnar neuropathy at the elbow indicates axonal damage. Muscle Nerve. 2013;47(2):188-93.
81. Beekman R, Schoemaker MC, van der Plas JPL, et al. The diagnostic value of high-resolution sonography in ulnar neuropathy at the elbow. Neurology. 2004;62(5):767-73.
82. Martinoli C, Derchi LE, Bertolotto M, et al. US and MR imaging of peripheral nerves in leprosy. Skeletal Radiol 2000;29(3):142-50.
83. Elias J Jr, Nogueira-Barbosa MH, Feltrin LT, et al. Role of ulnar nerve sonography in leprosy neuropathy with electrophysiologic correlation. J Ultrasound Med. 2009;28(9):1201-9.
84. Frade MA, Nogueira-Barbosa MH, Lugao HB, et al. New sonographic measures of peripheral nerves: a tool for the diagnosis of peripheral nerve involvement in leprosy. Mem Inst Oswaldo Cruz. 2013; 108(3) pii:mS0074-02762013000300257.
85. Goedee HS, Brekelmans GJF, van Asseldonk JTH, et al. High-resolution sonography in the evaluation of the peripheral nervous system in polyneuropathy—a review of the literature. Eur J Neurol. 2013;20(10):1342-51.
86. Ooi WW, Srinivasan J. Leprosy and the peripheral nervous system: basic and clinical aspects. Muscle Nerve. 2004;30(4):393-409.
87. Suneetha S, Sigamoni A, Kurian N, et al. The development of cutaneous lesions during follow-up of patients with primary neuritic leprosy. Int J Dermatol. 2005;44(3):224-9.
88. Sarkar J, Dasgupta A, Dutt D. Disability among new leprosy patients, an issue of concern: An institution based study in an endemic district for leprosy in the state of West Bengal, India. Indian J Dermatol Venereol Leprol. 2012;78(3):328-34.
89. Jacob M, Mathai R. Diagnostic efficacy of cutaneous nerve biopsy in primary neuritic leprosy. Int J Lepr Other Mycobact Dis. 1988;56(1):56-60.
90. Kumar B, Pradhan A. Fine needle aspiration cytology in diagnosis of pure neuritic leprosy. Patholog Res Int. 2011;2011:158712.

Pathomechanisms of Nerve Damage

Vanaja Prabhakar Shetty

INTRODUCTION

Leprosy is a chronic infectious disease of the peripheral nerves and other tissues, arising from aberrant, rather than protective, immune responses to *Mycobacterium leprae*. During the long course of the disease, the peripheral nerves are under additional threat from acute, subacute or chronic intraneural immune-mediated events known as 'leprosy reactions.'

Maintenance of the peripheral nervous system is the result of a complex balance between the two functions of the immune system, viz. (1) defense against infection, (2) assistance in maintenance of nerve regeneration and physiology.[1] Leprosy serves as a unique model where, due to insidious nature of the infecting organism (*M. leprae*) and its predilection for peripheral nerve Schwann cells, two functions of immune system coexists at least during initial stage. Although the earliest event/s in the encounter between the causative organism and the human body are still unclear, there is no dispute that peripheral neural involvement is inevitable once infection progresses, even before the disease manifests clinically.

In this chapter, various pathomechanisms involved in peripheral nerve damage in leprosy are discussed. In elucidating the same, as far as possible, more recent and relevant documented findings in both human and experimental models are included. Besides, some of the old documented findings that are invaluable; are also being referred to.

The broad topics presented and discussed here are:
- The general features of nerve damage
- Entry of *M. leprae* and its spread
- Significance of infection of Schwann cells by *M. leprae*
- Types of degeneration and regeneration seen in leprous nerves
- Immunological aspects of nerve damage
- Autoimmune type of nerve damage
- Role of mycobacterial antigens in nerve damage
- Role of inflammatory cytokines in nerve damage
- Insidious nerve damage
- Neuropathic pain
- Leprosy reactions and nerve damage.

GENERAL FEATURES OF NERVE DAMAGE IN LEPROSY

Infection, host response and the functional impairments of cutaneous nerve are the well-established feature of human leprosy. Some of the well-documented work of early 1980s describe how this might be taking place.

Carter, Professor of Anatomy from Grant Medical College, Mumbai, India, in a careful clinical observation and histological studies on peripheral nerves obtained at postmortem, outlined several important characteristics of the nervous system involvement by *M. leprae* like:
- The central nervous system (CNS) was unaffected
- Sensory nerve fiber involvement was an important feature
- Cutaneous and nerve trunk enlargements followed a set pattern, viz. thickening was maximal at superficial sites, ceasing when the nerve pierced the deep fascia
- Interfunicular plexuses existed within peripheral nerves, which possibly facilitated nerve damage

- 'Nuclei' (which we know today are the inflammatory cells) were present within leprous nerves viewed under the microscope.[2]

It was further postulated by Dehio in 1953 that leprous neuropathy is a centripetally ascending process, sequentially damaging the nerve structures. Motor fiber involvement resulted from lateral spread of the pathology within the mixed nerve trunk.[3] Dehio opined that infection did not descend centrifugally to the most distant intramuscular nerve terminals, but Dastur's demonstration later in 1978 of intramuscular neuritis with bacilli, belied Dehio's assertion.[4]

Extensive histological studies of the central and peripheral nervous systems by Ermakova in 1936, further confirmed that there was no pathology or bacillary invasion in the former; and that even in the later the damage was not uniform.[5] Limb nerves invaded with bacilli in their distal segments were normal at brachial and lumbosacral plexus levels, with bacilli appearing in the related dorsal root (sensory) ganglia. The uneven distribution of bacilli, inflammatory response and fiber damage along peripheral nerves was well-demonstrated in 1968 in postmortem specimens by Job and Desikan.[6] 'Ganglionitis' in the form of focal round cell infiltration was reported by Tze-Chun and Ju-Shi in 1984 from China in the autopsy material.[7] However; this study did not provide information about the neurological status of these patients. A recent study explored the involvement of CNS in 67 autopsy cases of clinically cured lepromatous leprosy (LL) patients. Paraffin sections of medulla oblongata and spinal cord were studied and vacuolar changes of motor neurons were seen in 67% of cases. Using nested polymerase chain reaction approach, *M. leprae* specific genomic DNA was detected in a large proportion (23/27, 85.2%) of cases studied. However, no acid fast bacilli were detected in any of the Fite-Faraco stained sections of these tissues. It is possible that the bacterial products may have seeped into the CNS cavity. Interestingly, presence of vacuolar changes in the spinal cord showed a good correlation with deformity of hands and feet in this study.[8]

Studies of skin lesions by Khanolkar, were among the first to focus on changes in dermal nerves and the sites of bacillary multiplication within them. He concluded that the organisms preferentially resided within axons, and were carried centripetally in the axoplasm like 'fish swimming upstream'.[9] Electron microscopic studies of leprous nerves in the 1960s by Nishiura,[10] Weddell and Palmer[11] and Lumsden[12] showed that bacillation of the Schwann cells rather than the axon was the dominant and characteristic feature. Further studies that focussed on early nerve lesions have delineated the preferential lodging of the bacilli in the nonmyelinated fiber Schwann cells, signifying its early involvement.[13] A recent clinical study using sophisticated methods also asserts that nonmyelinated or 'C' fibers are prominently involved and showed impaired function at a very early stage.[14]

Clinical and operative correlative studies on neuropathic deformities by Thomas, supported the microbiological maxim that *M. leprae* thrived in cool microenvironments, which are also the sites of nerve enlargement.[15] Measurements of nerve temperature by Sabin and associates confirmed that tissue temperatures around the ulnar nerve was lowest at the wrist and distal one-third of the arm, which are also sites of maximum bacillary invasion.[16] Brand referred to the fact that neuropathy in the limbs in leprosy usually shows a stereotyped pattern, involving the ulnar nerve around the elbow and lower arm, the median around the wrist and lower forearm, the tibial around the ankle and the common peroneal nerve around the knee and distal thigh, with sparing of the nerves supplying the girdle muscles.[17]

Motor nerve involvement occurs as a byproduct of damage to the mixed nerve, and not a primary event. It was postulated that interfunicular plexuses provided ready pathways for centripetal spread of infection from cutaneous funiculi to sensory-motor funiculi.[18] In the ulnar nerve for example, sensory and muscular branches which are in separate funiculi at the wrist, undergo regrouping and mixing in the forearm so as to form one or two large funiculi at the elbow. The development of motor symptoms in a leprous ulnar nerve, therefore, depends on the level in the forearm at which admixture of sensory and motor funiculi occurs in a particular case. A contributory factor maximizing damage at certain sites is the level-to-level change in the abundance of the investing epineurium. At the wrist, where ulnar nerve funiculi are small and numerous, compression due to intraneural inflammatory edema might be mitigated by the large amount of yielding epineurium. At the elbow on the other hand, the funiculi are few and large and the epineurium comparatively unyielding; the nerve fibers are more liable to be damaged by compression. Palande,[19] Dastur[20] and others speculated that the edematous nerve trunks themselves might be compressed as they traverse unyielding osseofibrous passages such as the carpal and cubital tunnels. A study by Carayon indicated tissue anoxia from compressed perineurial arteries as contributing factor for nerve fiber damage.[21]

Skin lesions tend to occur in areas of lowest skin temperature, e.g. extensor aspect of the forearm, elbow, hand, thigh, leg, knee, foot and on the cheeks. The corresponding cutaneous innervation arising from the ulnar, median, common peroneal, tibial and trigeminal nerves respectively, eventually implicates the nerve trunks. Weddell and Palmer pointed out that physiological processes such as cutaneous terminal axon degeneration-regeneration and Schwann cell turnover happen to be particularly marked over these regions, which might predispose these (undifferentiated) Schwann cells to the ingress by *M. leprae*.[22] *In vitro* studies using mouse dorsal root ganglion cultures also revealed vulnerability of undifferentiated Schwann cells to infection which is in consonance with the above observation.[23]

Pathological and functional characteristics of leprous nerves across the spectrum have been extensively studied and documented. Studies have shown that cellullar response to infection in the larger peripheral nerve is similar to that observed in the dermis. However, significant differences have been found between the lesions of skin and nerve mainly in the borderline region of the spectrum. The differences are quantitative, i.e. in respect of bacterial load and qualitative in respect of the nature of histopatholical responses, leading to differences in the classification.[24-26]

Cutaneous nerve fibers are affected in all types of leprosy resulting in anesthetic or hypoesthetic skin lesions.[27] In a study elucidating the evolution of nerve damage in leprosy, it has been demonstrated that the 'C' fibers are the first to show structural as well as functional changes.[28] In a large multicentric cohort study in multibacillary patients, unmyelinated C-fibers were found to be more frequently affected than small myelinated A-delta (Aδ) fibers. Nerve conduction studies (NCSs) and warm and cold threshold measurements have emerged as the most promising tool for the early detection of leprosy,[14,29] and monitoring of nerve function impairments.[30] In a study by Karanth et al. it was noted that among the 100 skin lesions studied across the spectrum, neuropeptide immunoreactivity was seen in only 14% of indeterminate leprosy specimens and was completely absent in other types of leprosy.[31] This finding highlights the diagnostic significance of early disappearance of neuropeptide immunoreactivity in leprosy lesions. Skin biopsy analysis of epidermal nerve fibers as a tool to improved diagnosis, predictive and therapeutic intervention is also picking up momentum.[32]

ENTRY OF *M. LEPRAE* INTO THE NERVES

The unique abilty of *M. leprae* to invade the peripheral nerve and spare the CNS is well-known. The question of how bacilli gain entry into the body, the nerve and the Schwann cell in particular, is important in the elucidation of pathomechanism/s of nerve damage.

All routes such as inhalation, ingestion, skin contact, and inoculation through abrasions and insect bites have been postulated over the years.[33] The current evidence implicates the nasal route as one of the important route of entry and spread in more than one way. The question of the route of entry is significant as it might also define the type of disease which develops in a susceptible individual. It has been postulated that entry of the organism through the unbroken skin or mucosa, might predispose to high cell-mediated immunity (CMI) type of response, while chance inoculation into the bloodstream via mucosal skin abrasions and wounds might promote high bacilliferous type with weak or absent CMI.[34] However, this postulation has not been conclusively proved or tested in any of the experimental models.

Entry into the peripheral nerve could essentially be the first step in the induction of neuropathy in leprosy. There are two main routes by which leprosy bacilli might enter the peripheral nerves:

1. The first is via the bloodstream into the endoneurium through the monocytes or vascular endothelial cells. Bacterial presence in the endothelial cells lining the capillaries within and around the peripheral nerve is documented in biopsies from lepromatous cases.[35] It is also established that in LL there is a continuous bacillemia[36] and that this persists for a period even after treatment.[37] This is a good evidence of the vascular spread of *M. leprae*. Recent studies on peripheral nerves in armadillos have suggested that, regardless of route of infection, bacteria-laden macrophages first aggregate around the epineurial lymphatics and blood vessels and then enter the endoneurial compartment through its blood supply.[38,39]

2. The second route of spread is via the Schwannian relay, i.e. distal sensory Schwann cells and cell to cell spread along the Schwann cell column. In humans, bacilli are seen in the terminal Schwann cells of dermal lesions throughout the Ridley-Jopling classification. Several ultrastructural studies of nerves in human leprosy across the spectrum helped in ascertaining that the Schwann cells undoubtedly are the most favored host.[13,35] Other characteristic histopathological findings namely longitudinal involvement of one or two fascicles, with sparing of others in a nerve bundle, particularly in the tuberculoid leprosy is supportive of evidence of spread of *M. leprae* along the Schwann cell columns.[40] Presence of skin lesions overlying major nerve trunks significantly puts the nerve at a greater risk for nerve function impairment, which also is an argument in line with the centripetal spread of infection.[41]

That the main bulk of infection occurs in the Schwann cells of unmyelinated fibers; was documented in a qualitative and quantitative electron microscopic study of nerve biopsies obtained from early untreated cases of leprosy by Shetty and Antia (Fig. 11.1).[42] Though it is not clear as to why there is such a preferential lodging of *M. leprae* in the Schwann cells of nonmyelinated fibers, it is reasoned that a longitudinal spread along the nonmyelinated fiber Schwann cells is facilitated by the abundance of overlapping and continuous cytoplasm. Influx of macrophages and presence of bacilli in the macrophages and endothelial cells lining the capillaries within the endoneurium occurred in the chronic and more advanced nerve lesions, whereas the cells lining the lymphatics in the epineurial area seldom showed *M. leprae*. Study of dermal lesions also showed infrequent presence in the lymphatic endothelial cells.[43] It was deduced from these findings that in man, the dissemination of infection from the nerve to other parts of the body occurs via the bloodstream.

The neural predilection of *M. leprae* is promoted by immune suppression due to low temperature, trauma to

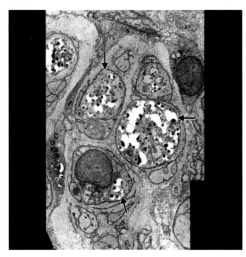

Fig. 11.1: Part of a sural nerve from an early lepromatous leprosy patient observed under electron microscope. Note the presence of large bacterial globi (arrows) in the unmyelinated fiber Schwann cells (magnification at 15,000x)

nerves causing capillary damage and bacterial stickiness.[44] Factors that protect the bacilli within the nerve are the absence of lymphatics within the endoneurial spaces and the presence of two specialized barriers namely, tight junctions of endothelial cells and of the perineural cells, which provide a higher degree of protection and seclusion from immune surveillance.[45] The barriers could also hamper the penetration of drugs into the nerve thus making the treatment less effective. The poor ability of Schwann cells to present antigens to the lymphocytes could also be one of the determinants.[46] Schwann cells are long-lived and those of nonmyelinated fibers in particular are poorly equipped with killer enzymes.[47] They thus make an ideal host for survival, multiplication and a good repository for persister *M. leprae.*[48]

INFECTION OF SCHWANN CELLS BY *M. LEPRAE*

Schwann cells unlike oligodendrocytes can dedifferentiate, proliferate and redifferentiate in response to Ras/Raf/ MEK/ ERK signaling following nerve injury.[49]

The basis of nerve damage in leprosy is the unique ability of *M. leprae* to invade, proliferate and remain inocuous within the Schwann cells. Several of the *in vitro* studies have tried to delineate the steps involved in adhesion, invasion and spread. Based on the studies utilizing murine dissociated Schwann cultures, early entry (within 6 hours) is observed with viable bacteria.[50] In another study, organized dorsal root ganglion cultures were infected with freshly harvested *M. leprae*; entry of *M. leprae* was seen only into the Schwann cells and neurofibroblasts but not into the cell body or axons. Other important findings were, the Schwann cells were more vulnerable to *M. leprae* infection in their premyelin secretory

phase. On infection with *M. leprae,* Schwann cells lost their ability to proliferate and synthesize DNA,[23] which in essence could mean a restricted proliferation of Schwann cells and defective regenerating response.

Observation that nerve biopsy of even a clinically normal nerve in leprosy patients does not result in neuroma formation, is in agreement with these findings (Antia, personal communication).

The importance of bacterial surface lipid and polysaccharide in mediating selective cytoadhesion has been demonstrated. Of relevance is the enhancement of bacterial adherence by treatment of Schwann cells with trypsin.[51]

A recent study put forth that the 'G' domain of laminin α-2 chain is a host-derived bridging molecule. It is proposed that leprosy bacilli interacts with host Schwann cells by the binding of the bridge to the α6 β4 integrin (dystroglycan) which acts as a laminin receptor on Schwann cell surface.[52] The authors suggested that presence of both α-2 laminin and a dystroglycan is responsible for restricting leprosy infection to the peripheral nervous system as these molecules are absent in the CNS. Their observations imply an almost equal predilection of *M. leprae* for Schwann cells of both myelinated and unmyelinated nerve fibers. This finding though plausible; fails to explain the well-established observations of preferential entry of *M. leprae* into the Schwann cells of unmyelinated fibers in leprosy patients. Laminin, a type IV collagen associated glycoprotein, is a component of the basal lamina in the Schwann cells of both myelinated and unmyelinated fibers *in vivo.*[53] Moreover, blocking of the dystroglycan complex could not inhibit *M. leprae*/Schwann cell adhesion completely,[54] indicating that there may be more than one molecule involved in the process.

In another set of *in vitro* and *in vivo* study using Rag-1 knockout mice, which lack mature B and T lymphocytes, the same group of workers demonstrated that myelinated Schwann cells are resistant to invasion but undergo demyelination upon bacterial attachment, whereas nonmyelinated Schwann cells engulf a large number of *M. leprae.* It was also observed that during *M. leprae*-induced demyelination, uninfected Schwann cells proliferate and generate more of nonmyelinated phenotype, which in their opinion, further facilitates propagation of *M. leprae* infection.[55]

Recent study carried out at the University of Edinburgh, by the same group headed by Anura Rambukana has found that *M. leprae* are able to change the make-up of Schwann cells in the mouse system. Using a complex set of experiments they have shown that heavily infected mouse Schwann cells *in vitro* display the property of progenitor/stem cell like cells (pSLC) of mesenchymal trait. They further provide evidence that acquisition of these properties by pSLC promotes bacterial spread by two distinct mechanisms: direct differentiation to mesenchymal tissues including skeletal and smooth muscles, and formation of granuloma like structures and subsequent release of bacteria-laden macrophages.[56] If confirmed in humans, may provide an additional angle to the way *M. leprae* disseminate in the lepromatous cases, but is of little help in understanding the pathophysiology of the disease across the spectrum and the reactional state. Moreover, *in vivo* there are two specialized barriers, viz. blood nerve and perineurial barriers that play a role in seclusion of the neural compartment.

A study by Tapinos showed that intracellullar *M. leprae* can activate ERK directly by an MEK independent and p56lck-dependent pathway whereas extracellullar *M. leprae* achieves this through the conventional Ras-Raf MEK-ERK signaling through ErbB2, a distinctive receptor tyrosine kinase belonging to the epidermal growth factor receptor family. Demyelination induced by *M. leprae* may be mediated by ErbB2 receptor tyrosine kinase signaling.[57,58] The ErbB2, a putative transporter protein may be involved only in the initial invasion by *M. leprae,* is persuasive mainly due to its apparent proximity to an evolutionarily important drug resistant domain.[59]

Nerve growth factor (NGF) plays an important role in the survival of sympathetic ganglia and is a regulator of pain sensation.[60] Downregulation of NGF in leprosy skin lesions was demonstrated by Karanth et al.[31] and Anand et al.[61] generating considerable interest in its therapeutic possibilities. Singh and coworkers studied NGF production and expression of p75 by Schwann cells and neurofibroblasts in response to *M. leprae* infection and macrophage secretory products in two strains of mice.[62] The results indicated involvement of NGF in neuroregenerative response as well as a nonsupportive role for macrophages in nerve repair in leprosy. In their opinion, different mechanism of nerve repair may be operational in Swiss White (SW) and C57BL/6 strain of mice representing lepromatous and tuberculoid spectrum of leprosy patients respectively. A recent study findings indicate that the down- regulation of NGF at the lesion sites may lead to disturbance in the mitogen-activated protein kinase (MAPK) pathway and thereby quiescent nerve damage (vide infra).

TYPE OF DEGENERATION AND REGENERATION SEEN IN LEPROUS NERVES

While the type of disease is determined on the basis of inflammatory response and bacterial load, the precise incubation period or exact duration of the disease is not always possible to determine in leprosy affected people.

The descriptions of mild, moderate or severe involvement of nerves are normally in relation to the extent of damage which varies from site to site. Various approaches have been used to assess the types of nerve involvement and nature of degenerating and regenerating changes in leprous nerves in order to understand the pathomechanisms of nerve damage

in leprosy. Qualitative and quantitative morphology using light and electron microscopy, teased nerve fiber study by itself or in combination, were used to describe the nature and severity of nerve damage along the spectrum.

In advanced leprosy lesions, some studies have shown the predominance of segmental demyelination in the lepromatous lesions and Wallerian or axonal type of degeneration in the tuberculoid type of lesions.[35,63] Some other studies have shown the predominance of demyelinating pathology along the entire spectrum of leprosy.[64] Regeneration and remyelination are also seen concomitantly. Studies on nerve biopsies from leprosy patients, using combinations of techniques, viz. morphometry and teased fiber preparation, have shown the presence of two distinct types of demyelination in leprous nerves; secondary demyelination occurring as sequel of atrophic changes in the axonal compartment (Figs 11.2A to E); and primary segmental demyelination occurring at the sites of active inflammation (Fig. 11.3).[13] The former has been linked to mitogen activated phosphokinase mediated changes in axonal cytoskeletal proteins.[65,66] The latter change was ascribed to direct myelinolytic action of the inflammatory cells, more commonly seen in borderline (BT, BB, BL) and reactional lesions in particular.[67,13]

Nerve biopsy specimens obtained from untreated, longstanding, polar LL show the presence of denervated Schwann cells that are surrounded by dense collar of connective tissue and overloaded with solidly stained (viable) bacilli (Fig. 11.4). Infiltrating cells are seldom seen in such nerve lesions which is in agreement with the immunological seclusion within the nerve. The end result is a severely involved nerve with total loss of fibers and replacement with connective tissue matrix, as has been shown in several of the studies.[13,68]

IMMUNOLOGICAL ASPECTS OF NERVE DAMAGE

"There is only one species of *M. leprae*; and the human host knows but one way to respond to it; though that way is modified greatly by the immune state of the host, a state which is liable to fluctuate with the ebb and flow of the conflict between host and invader during the long drawn saga of a leprosy infection" says Denis Ridley in his opening remark in a chapter on differential pathology of dermis and nerve in leprosy.[69]

The immune response of the host to *M. leprae* plays a pivotal role in producing the various structural and functional changes that characterize leprosy; and bacillus *per se* produces no perceptible damage.[34] CMI as well as humoral immunity (HI) are activated to varying degrees, the former predominating when bacilli are few (in tuberculoid and borderline tuberculoid forms); and the latter in the bacilliferous forms of the disease (borderline lepromatous to lepromatous forms), while combinations of CMI and

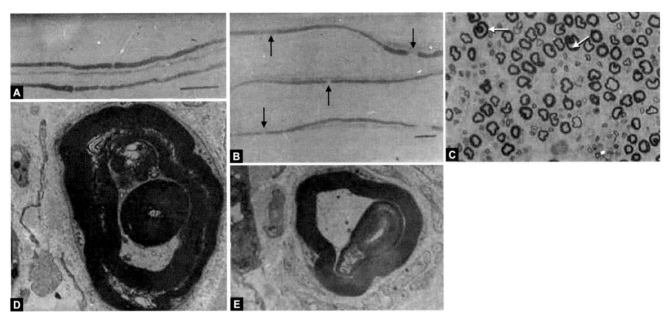

Figs 11.2A to E: Depicts various features of atrophic changes recorded in a leprous nerve viz. (A) Teased fiber preparation showing two fibers with wrinkled myelin but no widening of node; (B) A single teased fiber arranged in consecutive rows from left to right. There is widening of nodes or more extended paranodal demyelination (secondary demyelination shown by arrows) at multiple sites; (C) 1 μm thick section of sural nerve stained with toluidine blue showing several fibers with folded myelin sheath or having infolded loops of myelin within the axon (atrophic fibers shown by arrows). Several small fibers have axons which are small for the myelin sheath thickness (Magnification at 400x), (D and E) Two myelinated fibers with highly infolded myelin and normal looking axon, as seen under electron microscope (magnification at 15,000x)

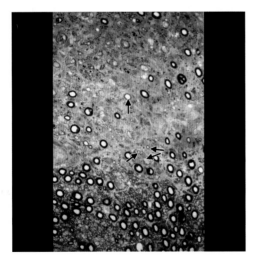

Fig. 11.3: 1 μm thick section of part of median nerve from a mid-borderline patient. Inflammatory cells including lymphocytes, macrophages, and few plasma cells are seen. Note the presence of totally denuded/demyelinated axons (primary demyelination) in the middle of inflammatory cells. Some remyelinating fibers are also seen (arrows) (magnification at 400x).

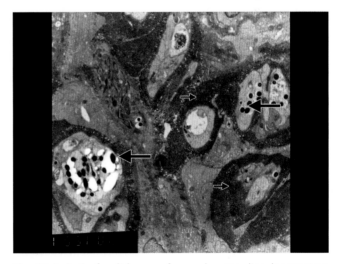

Fig. 11.4: Part of radial nerve from a longstanding lepromatous leprosy patient under electron microscope. Denervated and totally attenuated Schwann cells surrounded by dense collagen (C) (thin arrows) are seen. Large number of solidly stained bacilli are seen within the Schwann cells (thick arrows) (magnification at 15,000x)

HI responses to the bacillary antigens occur in the mixed 'borderline' type. Protective immunity in leprosy is also cell-mediated, being modulated by genes of the human leukocyte antigen (HLA) complex, particularly the HLA-DR2 loci. A major susceptibility locus has recently been mapped to chromosome 10p13 in Indian patients.[70]

AUTOIMMUNE TYPE OF DAMAGE

As early as 1964, Lumsden had suggested that nerve damage in leprosy may liberate autoantigens that can later sensitize and damage other nerve trunks in the absence of bacilli or inflammatory cells.[12] After the initial damage, myelin proteins would be expected to be released and exposed to immune system and since *M. leprae* has a powerful adjuvant activity, autosensitization to myelin proteins may be anticipated. Antibody response to peripheral nerve antigens has been investigated by several workers.

Through a functional assay, Shetty et al. demonstrated presence of demyelinating antibodies in 20% of the randomly chosen serum samples, after intraneural injection of test serum in the mouse.[71] The exact specificity of these factors was not clear. Unlike the experimental allergic neuritis (EAN) model, active participation of macrophages in myelin stripping was not seen in this study using the electron microscope. Mshana and coworkers did not find antibodies to bovine P2 protein and were unable to detect lymphocyte transformation in response to bovine P2 in lymphocytes from leprosy patients.[72,73] Eustis-Turf and coworkers demonstrated the presence of antibodies to intermediate neural proteins in the serum of some of the leprosy patients. No cross-reactivity was seen between antibodies to *M. leprae* and nerve tissue antigen. It was deduced that the antibodies were produced as an autoimmune response to nerve fiber damage and are not likely to play a primary role in nerve pathology but may aid in chronicity.[74]

Thomas and Mukherjee using the enzyme-linked immunosorbent assay (ELISA) technique reported the presence of antineural antibody directed against human peripheral nerve sonicate, in high titer and frequency along the spectrum of the disease. Their postulation was that these antibodies might be playing a role in complement-mediated cytotoxicity.[75] Similar studies by two other groups, however, have failed to consistently find antibodies against neural antigens.[76] One of the studies failed to reveal any relationship between neuropathy in leprosy and the levels of serum IgA1 and IgM antibodies against *M. leprae* derived phenolic glycolipid.[77]

A qualitative and quantitative morphological study investigating the pattern of nerve degeneration in leprous nerves along the spectrum also fails to support the hypothesis of an autoimmunological basis for nerve pathology in leprous lesions.[67,13] These studies have shown that macrophages do not take any part in the myelin stripping as is the case in EAN and Acute Inflammatory Demyelinating Polyradiculoneuropathy (AIDP). Further it was opined that a marked difference in the degree of nerve fiber involvement between adjacent fascicles,

a characteristic feature of leprous nerves particularly in the borderline spectrum, is also not consistent with an autoimmune process of the EAN type.[13]

The Schwann cell as an antigen presenting cell, has been proposed and investigated by some workers.[78,79] Studies using electron microscope failed to show Class II expression by the Schwann cells both in experimental leprous granuloma and human leprosy lesions.[80,81] A similar study by Atkinson and coworkers also revealed expression of MHC Class II antigen by endothelial and perivascular cells but not on Schwann cells in leprosy and other human peripheral neuropathies.[46]

ROLE OF MYCOBACTERIAL ANTIGENS IN NERVE DAMAGE

Leprosy is effectively treated with combination of antileprosy drugs and it has been shown using mouse foot pad method that a single dose of Rifampicin kills over 99.9% of the bacilli.[82] However, nerve damage continues to occur even after the treatment completion and killing of almost all *M. leprae*.[83]

Advances in immunohistochemistry techniques have made it possible to detect *M. leprae* by indirect methods other than acid-fast staining. Harboe et al. demonstrated antigenic cross-reactivity between Bacilleuse Calmette-Guerin (BCG) and *M. leprae* using this technique.[84,85] Several group of workers, have demonstrated the presence of mycobacterial antigens in the skin and nerve biopsies of treated tuberculoid and LL patients, in the absence of morphologically demonstrable bacilli.[48,72,86,87] A study by Shetty et al. demonstrated the presence of BCG cross-reactive antigens in 50–60% of tuberculoid nerve lesions in the absence of acid-fast organisms.[88] Experimental studies have shown that *M. leprae* antigens can evoke cell-mediated hypersensitivity.[73] This corroborates the finding of purified protein derivative (PPD) and *M. leprae* specific (T-cell) lymphocytes in granulomas of paucibacillary (PB) patients. A recent study on the other hand suggests that *M. leprae* as well as its antigens bring about deregulation of MAPK and dephosphorylation of high and medium molecular weight neurofilament proteins.[89] Thus, it is plausible that the persisting antigens may interfere with the functions of the regulatory enzymes leading to hypophosphorylation. This may explain the manner in which nerve degeneration continues to occur even after the antileprosy treatment[83] as well as corticosteroid treatment.

ROLE OF INFLAMMATORY CYTOKINES IN NERVE DAMAGE

The influx of inflammatory cells in the secondary stage of nerve damage is associated with the release of a variety of tissue damaging cytokines. Transforming growth factor beta (TGF-ß) is a potent immunosuppressive cytokine secreted by inflammatory cells such as epithelioid cells, giant cells, activated lymphocyte as well as Schwann cells. TGF-ß has the potential to influence all phases of the pathogenesis of infectious disease as an important regulator of development and modulator of inflammation, and wound healing. However, TGF-ß can also be exploited by the pathogen during entry, replication and persistence in the host. Increased levels of TGF-ß have been reported in all forms of leprosy and it increases from tuberculoid to lepromatous pole.[90] It has been suggested that TGF-ß controls the influx of inflammatory cells by downregulation of TNF-α, interferon-γ (INF-γ) as well as through inhibition of inducible nitric oxide synthase (iNOS), induction by macrophages which in turn promotes bacterial multiplication.[91]

Rook and coworkers have proposed that the nerve damage itself may interrupt normal endocrine feedback that can limit inflammation, thus enabling the local inflammation to persist.[92] In consonance with this, downregulation of gene expression for the enzymes that convert cortisone to cortisol has been observed in skin lesions at the onset of type 1 reaction where maximum damage to the nerves occurs.[93] This implies that, nerves may not only be the targets of inflammation in leprosy, directly or indirectly but their destruction may even enhance the intensity or duration of inflammatory process itself.

INSIDIOUS NERVE DAMAGE

In leprosy, neural dysfunction frequently commences and progresses so insidiously and painlessly, that the patient is unaware of the abnormality till it is quite advanced. Srinivasan et al. first drew attention to the frequency of this phenomenon, where 80% of patients reported that motor deficit had progressed 'quietly'.[94,95] In the longitudinal study by van Brakel and Khawas in Nepal, 'silent neuropathy' defined clinically as demonstrable nerve function impairment (NFI) using monofilament (MF) and voluntary muscle testing (VMT) was reported in 7% of 536 new patients, and in 21 months of follow-up, the annual incidence rate of 'silent nerve damage' was 4%, most commonly during the first year of chemotherapy.[96]

On the other hand using more sensitive test like NCS parameters, NFI was detected in 91% newly detected MB cases with no history of reaction or neuritis in the past.[97] So, it is plausible that most part of nerve damage in leprosy is insidious in nature and episodes of reaction/neuritis add more severity to the ongoing process.

The question of evolution of (when and how) the nerve damage (occurs) in leprosy has been addressed in several of the morphological and functional correlative studies in leprosy. Perhaps early detection and treatment may help in preventing further nerve damage.[98]

As early as 1980, morphological abnormalities were described in nerves, at a distance from skin lesions in lepromatous and tuberculoid type of leprosy, which were unrelated to the presence of *M. leprae* or of significant cellular infiltration.[13] It is in agreement with the insidiously occurring nerve damage discussed above. One of the frequent abnormalities recorded, in both tuberculoid and

lepromatous nerves was axonal atrophy (Figs 11.2A to E). By the same group alteration in the axonal cytoskeletal proteins in the form of hypophosphorylation was demonstrated as the cause of atrophic changes in leprous nerves.[13,66] Cytoskeletal protein metabolism was also studied in the mouse sciatic nerve model as an adjunct to human studies. It was noted that inoculation into the footpad with both viable and heat killed *M. leprae* invoked structural and biochemical changes in the axon-cytoskeletal proteins, similar to those seen in human nerves. While inoculation with heat killed *M. leprae* resulted in early onset but transient changes; but with viable bacilli, the changes though occurred later, but were persistent.[89] In leprous neuropathy, the focus always has been on Schwann cells since they are the main hosts for *M. leprae*. Results from the above studies indicate that it is the axon that is the primary target for *M. leprae* driven changes. This also gives clues as to how 'insidious' nerve damage might be occurring in leprosy. Two recent large cohort studies that applied sophisticated clinical and electrophysiological methods to detect nerve function impairment further show the magnitude of such problem and confirm that leprous neuropathy is more diffuse than envisaged.[14,97]

NEUROPATHIC PAIN

While most distinctive and characteristic feature of leprosy, skin lesion is loss of pain, a good proportion of leprosy patients experience neuropathic pain, defined as pain caused by a lesion or disease of the somatosensory system. Small diameter sensory nerves innervating the skin are responsive to noxious stimuli and an injury to these nerves is presumably related to neuropathic pain. It is estimated that 20% of leprosy patients may have symptoms and signs suggestive of neuropathic pain.[99-101] Different types of pain occur during the course of the disease. Inflammatory pain that usually occurs in skin and peripheral nerves is caused primarily by immune mediated reactions and can continue even after completion of antileprosy treatment. Inflammatory pain is typical of mostly reactional phase of disease whereas neuropathic pain may occur years after the completion of treatment. The German Research Network on Neuropathic Pain [Deutschen Forschungsverbund Neuropathischer Schmerz (DFNS)] has developed a standardized qualitative sensory testing (QST) battery that consists of seven tests measuring 13 parameters that identify changes in sensory parameters that helps to differentially identify changes in sensory parameters related to chronic neuropathic pain.[102]

LEPROSY REACTIONS AND NERVE DAMAGE

In leprosy, the peripheral nerve is damaged not only by 'silently occurring neuropathy,' but also as a result of immunologic episodes known as "leprosy reactions". Reactions may be cutaneous or neural or combined cutaneous-neural.

An acute inflammation in a pre-existing nerve lesion results in a rapid and severe nerve damage. Reactions are divided into two main types, namely; type 1 (T1R) and type 2 (T2R) on the basis of clinical and immunological characteristics, but they have shown commonalities such as their episodic nature, recurrence sometimes progressing to chronicity, induction of nerve pain/tenderness and NFI.

The relationship of lepra reactions, both T1R and T2R, to nerve damage is well-recognized, although the trigger for reaction is poorly understood.[96] High levels of inflammatory cytokines are associated with poor clinical response to steroid treatment and recurrent episodes of type 1 reaction. Manandhar et al.;[103] Sarno et al.[104] have tried to correlate nerve damage, reaction and cytokine levels. They note that MB patients with predominant nerve reactions presented with elevated serum concentrations of TNF-α. Similar observations were made in MB patients with skin reactions even in the absence of neurological complaints. Elevated levels of TNF-α were also detected in patients whose neurological grades worsened in the course of MDT. There is evidence, for example, of the expression of activation molecules as a consequence of induction of genes that are normally induced by these cytokines including intercellular cell adhesion molecule-1 (ICAM-1) and HLA DR in keratinocytes and ICAM-1 on endothelial cells. It is now widely accepted that over expression of integrins on endothelial cell surface is one of the first step in immunoinflammatory cascade. These events in association with the expression of activation molecules on the circulating leukocytes; that are also induced by the IFN-γ and TNF-α, determine at least partially the characteristics of the inflammatory cells present in the lesions. Why neutrophils are preferentially activated during T2R is not yet clear. Besides enhancing the proinflammatory activity of leukocytes and endothelial cells, TNF-α has been implicated as cytotoxic or myelinotoxic in experimental systems and diseases of the nervous system such as multiple sclerosis.[105]

A recent study addresses the issue of what triggers type 1 reaction. The study findings show that metabolically active *M. leprae* are an essential component or a prerequisite and Antigen 85 (Ag85), the secretory product may be acting as trigger for the induction of type 1 reaction in leprosy. The study findings also show that, it is the quality and not the quantity or ratio of dead to viable bacteria that play a role in the induction of T1R.[106] It is plausible then, that/since peripheral nerves are a good repository for persister bacilli,[48] it may put the patients at a higher risk of developing repeat episodes of reaction/neuritis.

CONCLUSION

Three main factors that contribute to nerve damage in leprosy are:
1. The infection.
2. Immune response of the host, and

3. Special anatomical and physiological dispositions of the nervous system. The descriptions of sequence of events and pathomechanism/s are indeed based on several sound documentations and findings in humans and are also supported by the experimental findings, but all these are nowhere near perfect to explain all events and their consequences.

It is apparent that when the infection manifests as disease there has already occurred damage to the peripheral nerves. It is the sensory compartment of the nerve that is largely affected in leprosy. The motor fiber involvement occurs as a byproduct of damage to the mixed nerve. Infection of the Schwann cells of nonmyelinated fibers in particular by *M. leprae*, is one of the characteristic features, but is not a prerequisite to the induction of the nerve damage. In the order of sequence, nonmyelinated fibers are the first to show structural as well as functional abnormality but nerve damage is not confined to the site of *M. leprae* infection, but is lot more diffuse than envisaged. How then such damage might be occurring? Though it requires further probing, most logical explanation seems to be that; through *M. leprae* induced deregulation of MAPK that produce dephosphorylation of axonal cytoskeletal proteins, it results in axonal atrophic changes and slow progressive secondary demyelination. In the pathogenesis of nerve damage, the focus always has been on the Schwann cells since they are the target cells for *M. leprae* infection. However, a careful look at the pathology of involved nerves in human leprosy clearly shows that it is the axon and not the Schwann cells, that is the primary target of *M. leprae* driven nerve damage. The process is quiescent to begin with, the inflammation, episodes of reactions and other secondary factors such as anatomical and physiological dispositions add further to the severity and magnitude of ongoing nerve damage.

ACKNOWLEDGMENTS

I am grateful to my mentor (Late) Dr NH Antia. He was always, and will remain a source of inspiration for me. I would like to thank Ms Anju Wakade for her help in organizing the manuscript and references.

REFERENCES

1. Perry VH, Andersson PB, Gordon S. Macrophages and inflammation in the central nervous system. Trends Neurosci. 1993;16:268-73.
2. Carter HV. On the symptoms and morbid anatomy of leprosy with remarks. Trans Med Phy Soc Bom. 1863;8:1-104.
3. Dehio K. On the lepra anaesthetica on the pathogenetical relation of the disease appearances. Transl. Biswas MG. Lepr India. 1952;24:78-83.
4. Dastur DK. Leprosy (an infectious and immunological disorder of the nervous system). In: Vinken PJ, Bruyn GW (Eds). Infections of the Nervous System. Amsterdam: North Holland Publishing Company; 1978: pp. 421-68.

5. Ermakova N. Studies on leprosy: the central, sympathetic and peripheral nervous systems. Int J Lepr. 1936;4:325-36.

6. Job CK, Desikan KV. Pathologic changes and their distribution in peripheral nerves in lepromatous leprosy. Int J Lepr. 1968;36:257-70.

7. Tze-chun L, Ju-shi Q. Pathological findings of peripheral nerves, lymph nodes and visceral organs of leprosy. Int J Lepr. 1984;52:377-83.

8. Aung T, Kitajma S, Nomoto M, et al. *Mycobacterium leprae* in neurons of the medulla oblongata and spinal cord in leprosy. J Neuropathol Exp Neurol. 2007;66:284-99.

9. Khanolkar VR. Studies in the histology of early lesions in Leprosy. Indian Council of Medical Research, Special Report Series No.19. New Delhi; 1951.

10. Nishiura M. The electron microscopic basis of the pathology of leprosy. Int J Lepr. 1960;28:357-400.

11. Weddell AG, Palmer E. Recent investigations into the sensory and neurohistological changes in leprosy. In: Cochrane RG, Davey TF (Eds). Leprosy in Theory and Practice. Bristol: John Wright and Sons; 1964: pp. 205-20.

12. Lumsden CE. Leprosy and the schwann cell *in vivo* and *in vitro*. In: Cochrane RG, Davey TF (Eds). Leprosy in Theory and Practice. Bristol: John Wright and Sons; 1964: pp. 221-50.

13. Shetty VP, Antia NH, Jacobs JM. The pathology of early leprous neuropathy. J Neurol Sci. 1988;88:115-31.

14. van Brakel WH, Nicholls PG, Das L, et al. The INFIR cohort study: assessment of sensory and motor neuropathy in leprosy at baseline. Lepr Rev. 2005;76:277-95.

15. Thomas RE. An investigation into paralysis in the forearm and hand in leprosy. Lepr Rev. 1954;25:11-5.

16. Sabin TD, Hackett ER, Brand PW. Temperatures along the course of certain nerves often affected in lepromatous leprosy. Int J Lepr. 1974;42:38-42.

17. Brand PW. Temperature variation and leprosy deformity. Int J Lepr. 1959;27:1-7.

18. Sunderland S. The internal anatomy of nerve trunks in relation to the neural lesions of leprosy. Observations on pathology, symptomatology, and treatment. Brain. 1973;96:865-88.

19. Palande DD. Surgery of ulnar nerve in leprosy. Lepr India. 1980;52:74-88.

20. Dastur DK, Porwal GL, Shah JS, et al. Immunological implications of necrotic cellular and vascular changes in leprous neuritis: light and electron microscopy. Lepr Rev. 1982;53:45-65.

21. Carayon A. Investigations on the physiopathology of the nerve in leprosy. Int J Lepr. 1971;39:278-94.

22. Weddell G, Palmer E. The pathogenesis of leprosy: an experimental approach. Lepr Rev. 1963;34:57-61.

23. Mukherjee R, Antia NH. Intracellular multiplication of leprosy derived mycobacteria in Schwann cells of dorsal root ganglion cultures. J Clin Microbiol. 1985;21:808-14.

24. Srinivasan H, Rao KS, Iyer CG. Discrepency in the histopathological features of leprosy lesions in the skin and peripheral nerve. Lepr India. 1982;54:275-82.

25. Nilsen R, Mshana RN, Negesse Y, et al. Immunohistochemical studies of leprous neuritis. Lepr Rev. 1986;57 (Suppl 2):177-87.

26. Ridley DS, Ridley MJ. The classification of nerves is modified by the delayed recognition of *Mycobacteium leprae*. Int J Lepr. 1986;55:99-108.

27. Chandi SM, Chacko CJ. An ultrastructural study of dermal nerves in early human leprosy. Int J lepr. 1987;55:515-20.

28. Shetty VP, Mehta LN, Irani PF, et al. Study of evolution of nerve damage in leprosy. I: Lesions of the index branch of the radial cutaneous nerve in early leprosy. II: Observations on the the the index branch of the radial cutaneous nerve in contacts of leprosy. III: Sciatic nerve lesion in mice inoculated with M. leprae with nerve conduction velocity correlates. Lepr India. 1980;52:5-47.

29. Chaurasia RN, Garg RK, Singh MK, et al. Nerve conduction studies in paucibacillary and multibacillary leprosy: a comparative evolution. Indian J Lepr. 2011;83:15-22.

30. Garbino JA, Naafs B, Ura S, et al. Neurophysiological patterns of ulnar nerve neuropathy in leprosy reactions. Lepr Rev. 2010;81:206-15.

31. Karanth SS, Springall DR, Lucas S, et al. Changes in nerves and neuropeptides in skin from 100 leprosy patients investigated by immunocytochemistry. J Pathol. 1989;157:15-26.

32. Ebenezer GJ, Hauer P, Gibbons C, et al. Assessment of epidermal nerve fibres: A new diagnostic and predictive tool for peripheral neuropathies. J Neuropathol Exp Neurol. 2007;66:1059-73.

33. Pallen MJ, McDermott RD. How might *Mycobacterium leprae* enter the body? Lepr Rev. 1986;57:289-97.

34. de Vries RR. HLA and leprosy type. In: Chatterjee BR (Ed). Leprosy: Etiobiology of Manifestations, Treatment and Control. Calcutta: Statesman Commercial Press; 1993: pp. 152-8.

35. Dastur DK, Ramamohan Y, Shah JS. Ultrastructure of lepromatous nerves–neural pathogenesis in leprosy. Int J Lepr. 1973;41:47-80.

36. Drutz DJ, Chen TS, Lu WH. The continuous bacteremia of lepromatous leprosy. New Engl J Med. 1972;287:159-64.

37. Chatterjee G, Kaur S, Sharma VK, et al. Bacillaemia in leprosy and effect of multidrug therapy. Lepr Rev. 1989;60:197-201.

38. Scollard DM, McCormick, Allen JL. Localization of *Mycobacterium leprae* to endothelial cells of epineurial and perineurial blood vessels and lymphatics. Am J Pathol. 1999;54:1611-20.

39. Scollard D M The biology of nerve injury in leprosy: a review. Lepr Rev. 2008;79:242-53.

40. Shetty VP, Antia NH. A semiquantitative analysis of bacterial load in different cell types in leprous nerves using transmission electron microscope. Indian J Lepr. 1996,68:105-8.

41. van Brakel WH, Nicholls PG, Das L, et al. The INFIR Cohort study: Investigating prediction, detection and pathogenesis of neuropathy and reactions in leprosy. Methods and baseline results of a cohort of multibacillary leprosy patients in North India. Lepr Rev. 2005;76:14-34.

42. Antia NH. The significance of nerve involvement in leprosy. Plast Reconst Surg. 1974;54:55-63.

43. Mukherjee A, Mishra RS, Meyers WM. An electronmicroscopic study of lymphatics in the dermal lesions of human leprosy. Int J Lepr. 1989;57:506-10.

44. Hastings R, Brand PW, Mansfield RE, et al. Bacterial density of the skin in lepromatous leprosy as related to temperature. Lepr Rev. 1968;39:71-4.

45. Ridley DS, Ridley MJ. Classification of nerves is modified by the delayed recognition of *Mycobacterium leprae*. Int J Lepr. 1986;54:596-606.

46. Atkinson PF, Perry ME, Hall SM, et al. Immuno-electronmicroscopical demonstration of major

Section 2: Basic Scientific Considerations and Pathology

histocompatibility class II antigen: expression on endothelial and perivascular cells but not schwann cells in human neuropathy. Neuropathol Appl Neurobiol. 1993;19:22-30.

47. Boddingius J. Mechanisms of peripheral nerve damage in leprosy: electron and light microscopic studies in patients throughout the spectrum. Quaderni Cooperations Sanitaria (Bologna)-health coop papers 1982;1:65-84.

48. Shetty VP, Suchitra K, Uplekar MW, et al. Persistence of *Mycobacterium leprae* in the peripheral nerve as compared to the skin of multidrug treated leprosy patients. Lepr Rev. 1992;63:329-36.

49. Harrisingh MC, Perez-Nadales E, Parkinson DB, et al. The Ras/Raf/ERK signalling pathway drives Schwann cell dedifferentiation. Embo J. 2004;23:3061-71.

50. Choudhary A, Mistry NF, Antia NH. Blocking of *M. leprae* adherence to dissociated Schwann cells by anti-mycobacterial antibodies. Scand J Immunol. 1988;30:505-9.

51. Itty BM, Mukherjee R, Antia NH. Adherance of *Mycobacterium leprae* to Schwann cells *in vitro*. J Med Microbiol. 1986;22:277-82.

52. Rambukkana A, Salzer JL, Yurchenco PD, et al. Neural targeting of *Mycobacterium leprae* mediated by the G domain of the laminin-α2 chain. Cell. 1997;88:811-21.

53. Save MP, Shetty VP. A critique on commentary "How *Mycobacterium leprae* infects peripheral nerves" by Freedman et al. Lepr Rev. 2001;72:102-5.

54. Rambukkana A, Yamada H, Zanazzi G, et al. Role of alpha dystroglycan as a schwann cell receptor for *Mycobacterium leprae*. Science. 1998;282:2076-79.

55. Rambukkana A, Zanazzi G, Tapinos N, et al. Contact-dependent demyelination by *Mycobacterium leprae* in the absence of immune cells. Science. 2002;296:927-31.

56. Masaki T, Qu J, Waclaw JC, et al. Reprogramming Adult Schwann cells to stem cell-like cells by leprosy bacilli promotes dissemination of infection. Cell. 2013;152:51-67.

57. Tapinos N, Rambukkana A. Insights into regulation of human Schwann cell proliferation by Erk1/2 via a MEK-independent and p56lck-dependent pathway from leprosy bacilli. Proc Natl Acad Sci USA. 2005;102:9188-93.

58. Tapinos N, Ohnishi M, Rambukkana A. ErbB2 receptor tyrosine kinase signaling mediates early demyelination induced by leprosy bacilli. Nat Med. 2006;12:961-66.

59. Eapen BR. Schwann cell invasion by M. leprae: the probable Trojan horse. Lepr Rev. 2008;79:335-37.

60. Lindsay RM, Harmar AJ. Nerve growth factor regulates expression of neuropeptide genes in adult sensory neurons. Nature. 1989;337:362-4.

61. Anand P, Pandya S, Ladiwala U, et al. Depletion of nerve growth factor in leprosy. Lancet. 1994;344:129-30.

62. Singh N, Birdi TJ, Antia NH. Nerve growth factor production and expression of p75 by schwann cells and neurofibroblasts in response to *M. leprae* infection and macrophage secretory products. Neuropathol Appl Neurobiol. 1997;23:59-67.

63. Job CK. Pathology of peripheral nerve lesions in lepromatous leprosy—a light and electron microscopic study. Int J Lepr. 1971;39:251-68.

64. Swift TR. Peripheral nerve involvement in leprosy: quantitative histologic aspects. Acta Neuropathol. 1974;29:1-8.

65. Shetty VP, Shetty KT, Save MP, et al. M. leprae-induced alterations in the neurofilament phosphorylation leads to demyelination in leprous nerves: a Hypothesis. Indian J Lepr. 1999;71:121-35.

66. Save MP, Shetty VP, Shetty KT, et al. Alterations in neurofilament protein(s) in human leprous nerves: morphology, immunochemistry and western immunoblot correlative study. Neuropath Appl Neurobiol. 2004;30:635-50.

67. Jacobs JM, Shetty VP, Antia NH, et al. Teased fibre studies in leprous neuropathy. J Neurol Sci. 1987;79:301-13.

68. Job CK. Nerve damage in leprosy. Int J Lepr. 1989;57:532-39.

69. Ridley DS. Differential pathology of dermis and nerve in leprosy. In: Antia NH, Shetty VP (Eds). The peripheral nerve in leprosy and other Neuropathies. Delhi: Oxford University Press;1997: pp. 138-50.

70. Siddiqui MR, Meisner S, Tosh K, et al. A major susceptibility locus for leprosy in India maps to chromosome 10p13. Nat Genet. 2001;27:439-41.

71. Shetty VP, Mistry NF, Antia NH, et al. Serum demyelinating factors and adjuvant-like activity of *Mycobacterium leprae* possible causes of early nerve damage in leprosy. Lepr Rev. 1985;56:221-7.

72. Mshana R, Harboe M, Stoner GL, et al. Immune responses to bovine neural antigens in leprosy patients. I. Absence of antibodes to an isolated myelin protein. Lepr Rev. 1983;54:33-40.

73. Mshana RN, Humber DP, Harboe M, et al. Immune response to bovine neural antigens in leprosy patients. II. Absence of *in vitro* lymphocyte stimulation of peripheral nerve myelin proteins. Lepr Rev. 1983;54:217-27.

74. Eustis-Turf EP, Benjamins JA, Lefford MJ. Characterization of the anti-neural antibodies in the sera of leprosy patients. J Neuroimmunol. 1986;10:313-30.

75. Thomas BM, Mukherjee R. Antineural antibodies in sera of leprosy patients. Clin Immunol Immunopathol. 1990;57:420-9.

76. Ghaswala PS, Mistry NF, Antia NH. Serum antibodies of normals and leprosy patients show equal binding to peripheral nerve. Int J Lepr. 1989;57;690-2.

77. Chujor CS, Bernheimer N, Levis WR, et al. Serum IgA and IgM antibodies against M. leprae derived phenolic glycolipid-I: A comparative study in leprosy patients and their contacts. Int J Lepr. 1991;59:441-9.

78. Wekerle H, Schwab M, Linington C, et al. Antigen presentation in the peripheral nervous system: Schwann cells present endogenous myelin auto antigens to lymphocytes. Eur J Immunol. 1986;16:1551-7.

79. Spierings E, Boer TD, Zulianello L, et al. Novel mechanisms in the immunopathogenesis of leprosy nerve damage: The role of Schwann cells, T cells and *Mycobacterium leprae*. Immunol Cell Biol. 2000;78:349-55.

80. Cowley SA, Butter C, Verghese S, et al. Nerve damage induced by mycobacterial granulomas in guinea pig sciatic nerves. Int J Lepr. 1988;56:283-90.

81. Cowley SA, Butter C, Gschmeissner SE, et al. An immunoelectron microscopical study of the expression of major histocompatibility complex (MHC) class II antigens in the guinea pig sciatic nerve following induction of intraneural mycobacterial granuloma. J Neuroimmunol. 1989;23:223-31.

82. Grosset JH. Progress in the chemotherapy in leprosy. Int J Lepr. 1994;62:268-77.

83. Croft RP, Nicholls PG, Richardus JH, et al. Incidence rates of acute nerve function impairment in leprosy: a prospective cohort analysis after 24 months. (The Bangladesh Acute Nerve Damage Study). Lepr Rev. 2000;71:18-33.

84. Harboe M, Closs O, Bjorvatn B, et al. Antibodies against BCG antigen 60 in mycobacterial infections. Brit Med J. 1977;2:430-3.

85. Harboe M, Mshana RN, Closs O, et al. Cross reactions between mycobacteria. II: Crossed electrophoretic analysis of soluble antigens of BCG and comparison with other mycobacteria. Scand J Immunol. 1979;9:115-24.

86. Barros U, Shetty VP, Antia NH. Demonstration of *M. leprae* antigen in nerves of tuberculoid leprosy. Acta Neuropathol. 1987;73:387-92.

87. Khanolkar VR, Mackenzie CD, Lucas SB, et al. Identification of *M. leprae* antigens in tissues of leprosy patients using monoclonal antobodies. Int J Lepr. 1989;57:652-8.

88. Shetty VP, Uplekar MW, Antia NH. Immunological localization of mycobacterial antigens within the peripheral nerves of treated leprosy patients and their significance to nerve damage in leprosy. Acta Neuropathol. 1994;88:300-6.

89. Save MP, Shetty VP, Shetty KT. Hypophosphorylation of NF-H and NF-M subunits of neurofilaments and the associated decrease in KSPXK kinase activity in the sciatic nerves of Swiss white mice inoculated in the foot pad with *Mycobacterium leprae*. Lepr Rev. 2009;80:388-407.

90. Khanolkar Young S, Snowdon D, et al. Immunocytochemical localization of inducible nitric oxide synthase and transforming growth factor-beta (TGF-β) in leprosy lesions. Clin Exp Immunol. 1998;113:438-42.

91. Naafs B. Treatment of reaction and nerve damage. Int J Lepr. 1996;64:S21-28.

92. Rook GA, Lightman SL, Heijnen CJ. Can nerve damage disrupt neuroendocrine immune homeostasis? leprsoy as a case in point. Trends Immunol. 2002;23:18-22.

93. Anderson AK, Atkinson SE, Khanolkar-Young S, et al. Alterations in the control-cortisone shuttle in leprosy type 1 reaction patients in Hyderabad, India. Immunol Lett. 2007;104:72-5.

94. Srinivasan H, Rao KS, Shanmugam N. Steroid therapy in recent "quiet nerve paralysis" in leprosy. Report of a study of twenty-five patients. Lepr India. 1982;54:412-19.

95. Srinivasan H, Gupte MD. Experiences from studies on quiet nerve paralysis in leprosy patients. In: Antia NH, Shetty VP (Eds). The Peripheral Nerve in Leprosy and Other Neuropathies. Delhi: Oxford University Press; 1997: pp.30-5.

96. van Brakel WH, Khawas IB, Lucas SB. Reactions in leprosy: an epidemiological study of 386 patients in West Nepal. Lepr Rev. 1994;65:190-203.

97. Khambati FA, Shetty VP, Ghate SD, et al. The effect of corticosteroid usage on the bacterial killing, clearance and nerve damage in leprosy. A prospective cohort study: Part 1-study design and baseline findings of 400 multibacillary patients. Lepr Rev. 2008;79:1-21.

98. Pai VV, Girdhar BK, Hanumanthayya K, et al. Response of patients with nerve function impairment in leprosy to low dose steriod administration: An outpatient based study. Indian J Dermatol Venereol Leprol. 2010;76:408-9.

99. Lasry-Levy E, Hietaharju A, Pai V, et al. Neuropathic pain and psychological morbidity in patients with treated leprosy : a cross sectional prevalence study in Mumbai. PLoS Negl Trop Dis. 2011;5:e981.

100. Jenson TS, Baron R, Haanpaa M, et al. A new definition of neuropathic pain. Pain. 2011;152(10):2204-5.

101. Stump PR, Baccarelli R, Marciano LH, et al. Neuropathic pain in leprosy patients. Int J Lepr. 2004;72:134-8.

102. Rolke R, Baron R, Maier C, et al. Quantitative sensory testing in the German Research Network on Neuropathic pain (DFNS): standardized protocol and reference values. Pain. 2006;123:231-43.

103. Manandhar R, Shreshtha CR, Butlin CR, et al. High levels of infalmmatory cytokins are associated with poor clinical response to steroid treatment and recurrent episodes of type 1 reactions in leprosy. Clin Exp Immunol. 2002;128:333-8.

104. Sarno EN, Sampaio EP. Role of inflammatory cytokines in the tissue injury of leprosy. Int J Lepr. 1996;64:S69-74.

105. Selmaj KW, Raine CS. Tumor necrosis factor mediates myelin and oligodendrocytes damage *in vitro*. Ann Neurol. 1988;23:339-46.

106. Shetty VP, Save M, Dighe A, et al. Viable *M. leprae* forms an essential component of reversal reaction: assessed using growth in mouse foot pad, Ag85 detection and M. leprae specific 16sr RNA. Indian J Lepr. 2012;84:78-9.

SUGGESTED READING

1. Antia NH, Shetty VP, (Eds). The Peripheral Nerve in Leprosy and Other Neuropathies. Delhi: Oxford University Press; 1997.

2. Pandya SS, Shetty VP. The neuropathy of leprosy. In: Wadia NH, (Ed). Neurological Practice: An Indian Perspective. Delhi: Elsevier; 2005.

Naturally Occurring Leprosy: *Mycobacterium leprae* and other Environmental Mycobacteria in Nature

UD Gupta, Partha Sarathi Mohanty

CHAPTER OUTLINE

INTRODUCTION

Leprosy is a chronic disease of low infectivity caused by *Mycobacterium leprae*. Leprosy is also known as Hansen's disease, after the Norwegian physician Gerhard Armauer Hansen, who first observed the bacillus under a microscope in 1873. Leprosy has affected humanity for over 4,000 years.[1] It was reported in the civilizations of ancient China, Egypt and India.[2] Leprosy was recorded in ancient India (15 century BCE), in Japan (10th century BCE) and in Egypt (16th century BCE). The first known written mention of leprosy was dated 600 BCE. Leprosy is still a serious issue in Brazil, India, Democratic Republic of Congo, Tanzania, Nepal, Mozambique, Madagascar, Angola and the Central African Republic. In India there are about 1,000 leper colonies still in existence.[3]

There are many references to leprosy in the Bible.[4]

It is primarily a granulomatous disease affecting the peripheral nerves and mucosa of the upper respiratory tract; skin lesions are the primary external sign. Leprosy results in multiple deformities, including progressive bone defects, secondary to peripheral neuropathy. Additionally, in advanced cases, *M. leprae* infection causes specific osteological deformities in the areas of the nasal aperture, anterior nasal spine and alveolar process of the premaxilla, cortical areas of the tibia and fibula, distal ends of the metatarsals, and diaphysis of the phalanges that may include both direct and reactive changes.[5]

M. leprae is a straight or slightly curved rod with parallel sides and rounded ends. The size is 1-8 μm × 0.2-0.5 μm, clubbed forms, lateral buds or branching may be observed. It is a gram-positive and acid-fast bacillus (AFB), which stains more rapidly than the tubercle bacillus. The bacilli are seen singly and in groups, intracellular or lying free outside the cells. The bacilli being bound together by a lipid like substance, the glia and occur as masses known as "globi". The parallel rows of bacilli in the globi present as a "cigar bundle" appearance.[6] The bacterium has a slow doubling time of 14 days, which is thought to be due to the restricted intake of nutrients through the pores in the large waxy walls. Mycobacteria have a unique lipid in their cell walls, called Mycolic acids that makes up their membranes, that gives them their unique characteristic. Mycolic acids are very large lipids with chains ranging from 60 to 80 carbons long.[7] Covalent bonds link these lipids to one another forming a very thick surrounding that is solid at room temperature. This large hydrophobic shell prevents polar molecules, such as germicides, commonly used in hospitals from entering the cell.

MOLECULAR BIOLOGY OF *MYCOBACTERIUM LEPRAE*

Mycobacterium leprae has the longest doubling time of all known bacteria and has thwarted every effort at culture in the laboratory.[8] Comparing the genome sequence of *M. leprae* with that of *M. tuberculosis* provides clear explanations for these properties and reveals an extreme case of reductive evolution. Less than half of the genome contains functional genes. Gene deletion and decay appear to have eliminated many important metabolic activities, including siderophore production, part of the oxidative and most of the microaerophilic and anaerobic respiratory chains, and numerous catabolic systems and their regulatory circuits.

The genome sequence of a strain of *M. leprae*, originally isolated in Tamil Nadu and designated *TN*, was completed in 2001. The genome sequence was found to contain 3,268,203 base pairs (bp) and to have an average G+C content of 57.8%, values much lower than the corresponding values for *M. tuberculosis*, which are 4,441,529 bp and 65.6% G+C. About 1,500 genes are common to both *M. leprae* and *M.*

tuberculosis. The comparative analysis suggests that both mycobacteria, probably derived from a common ancestor and at one stage, had gene pools of similar size. Downsizing from a genome of 4.42 Mbp, such as that of *M. tuberculosis*, to one of 3.27 Mbp would account for the loss of some 1,200 protein-coding sequences. It is hypothesized that many of the genes that were present in the genome of the common ancestor of *M. leprae* and *M. tuberculosis* have been lost by recombination in the *M. leprae* genome.[7]

TRANSMISSION

Throughout history, leprosy has been regarded as contagious and those affected have been secluded and barred from society. People feared that merely touching an infected person could spread the disease. Numerous studies indicate that leprosy is transmitted from person to person by close contact between an infectious patient and healthy but susceptible host. Even today, the transmission of leprosy is not clearly understood. However, theories about the possible modes of transmission, including person to person contact or contact with respiratory secretions from infected individuals, are the most probable. Various portals of entry have been hypothesized for *M. leprae,* viz., the dermal,[9,10] nasal, gastrointestinal[11,12] and transplacental routes.[13,14] The nasal and dermal routes, because of their impact on transmission, are of greatest importance.

The success of MDT is confined only to treatment and cure of the disease. The eradication of leprosy can be achieved by better understanding of the modes of transmission, potential sources of pathogen and molecular variability among the strains, so that proper intervention strategies can be used to break the transmission chain. Early detection of the pathogen from environmental sources is needed so that timely remedial action can be taken.

The question of possible extra-human sources of *M. leprae* is an important one for leprosy epidemiology and control. If nonhuman sources exist, their recognition may help to explain patterns of infection and disease in human populations. Even more importantly, they would have implications for the control of the disease, and in particular for the possibility of its "elimination" or even ultimate eradication. Though *M. leprae* is considered to be primarily a parasite of humans, there is a long history of studies, evidence and arguments which have indicated possible nonhuman sources of the agent.[15]

There have been two different sorts of observations motivating the search for extra-human sources of *M. leprae.* One is the repeated observation of clinical leprosy in individuals with no apparent history of exposure to other known cases.[16-18] The second is the observation that clinical leprosy clusters in particular areas, such as near water sources, which have led some authors to suggest that *M. leprae* may have an extra-human source in such environments.[19,20] Neither of these lines of argument, however, provides a strong case

for extra-human sources of *M. leprae.* The long incubation period of the disease, the inability to recall contacts and encounters years after the event, the fact that stigma leads to hiding of cases in many societies, and the well-recognized fact that multibacillary cases can go undetected for long periods mean that there are substantial opportunities for unrecognized, unremembered or unacknowledged source contacts. The apparent clustering of leprosy in particular environments may simply reflect that certain environments are associated with certain social groups, health conditions or behaviors which predispose to *M. leprae* transmission or the manifestation of the disease leprosy, or they may reflect environmental conditions where *M. leprae* is able to persist for extended periods outside the human body, on surfaces or even in the air.

Different authors have suggested that *M. leprae* may be harboring in soil,[21,22] in water,[23] on plants,[24,25] or in various animal species, including amoeba,[26] insects,[27,28] fish,[29-31] primates,[32] and armadillos.[33] Environmental mycobacteria (EM) are a frequent cause of opportunistic infection in human beings and livestock.[34] There is growing recognition in recent years that water is an important vehicle of transmission of EM. This is based on the fact that in the recent past, contaminated water supply systems have been responsible for several hospitals and community outbreaks of mycobacterial infections.[35-37]

Soil bacterial populations are large, diverse and are influenced by abiotic factors like climate, soil type, local vegetation and other biotic inputs. Like many other groups of bacteria, some *Mycobacterium* species are common soil and water inhabitants, and these organisms are often referred to as "EM". In contrast, the causative agents of tuberculosis (TB) and leprosy (*M. tuberculosis* and *M. leprae,* respectively) and *M. bovis,* the origin of the attenuated Bacillus Calmette-Guerin (BCG) vaccine used against TB are obligate parasites, as well as human and animal pathogens. Some EM have been implicated in human infections, particularly in immunocompromised patients, who may be exposed through inhalation, ingestion, or broken skin.

It is possible that *M. leprae* could persist within other vertebrates. However, investigators seeking to propagate *M. leprae* in the laboratory have examined a long list of experimental hosts and found only a very limited host range.[38-42] Some species of primates appear to be marginally susceptible to experimental infection and a few of them have developed spontaneous leprosy while in captivity.[43,44] However, infection among free-ranging primates has not been reported. Predilection of *M. leprae* for cool body temperatures was recognized soon after Hansen described the bacillus and, as early as 1911, Couret suggested that fish might be suitable hosts for propagating leprosy bacilli.[45] However, even with the increased use of fish as experimental laboratory animals seen in recent years, there have been no credible reports of successful infection and replication of *M. leprae* in fish. Aside from the primate infections mentioned above, the only two nonhuman environments in which *M. leprae* are known reliably to replicate are the footpad of the mouse (*Mus musculus*), and the nine-banded armadillo (*Dasypus novemcinctus*). Armadillos are a large natural reservoir for *M. leprae*, and Truman et al. have shown that wild armadillos and many patients with leprosy in the southern United States are infected with the same strain of *M. leprae* and the disease is probably a zoonosis there.[46]

Various reports have suggested that *M. leprae* can be found in the environment and may have a role in continuing transmission of the disease. The important factor which may influence transmission of disease from the environment is the viability of *M. leprae* outside human body and the likelihood that *M. leprae* might multiply in the nonhuman environment. Desikan and Sreevatsa[47] studied the viability of *M. leprae* obtained from untreated patients and subjected them to several adverse conditions. The viability was tested by the multiplication in footpads of normal mice. After drying soil samples in shade, the *M. leprae* were viable for up to 5 months. On wet soils, the viability was present up to 46 days. On exposure to direct sunlight for 3 hours a day, the bacteria survived for 7 days, while after refrigeration at −40°C bacteria could be maintained in living condition for 28 days. However, on exposure to antiseptics, like savlon* and alcohol, the bacteria were rapidly killed.

The first report on the existence of *M. leprae* in the public water resource, in the north Maluku, was reported by Matsuoka et al.[23] Using polymerase chain reaction (PCR) method, they found 21/44 of public water resources to be contaminated by *M. leprae*. Agusni et al.[48] Detected *M. leprae* in some ponds that were used as water resources by inhabitants who live in leprosy endemic area in northern coast of East Java. Interestingly, positive results were found more in the root of the water plants than in the water collected from the center of the pond. This finding lead to the suggestion that the bacilli might live and even multiply intracellularly in protozoa and amoeba, which live in the root of many water plants. Cirillo et al.[49] showed that *M. avium* can survive inside protozoa and Jadin[50] showed that *M. leprae* also could survive inside the cell of environmental protozoa. Katoch et al.[51] described the value of 16S rRNA gene for the detection of *M. leprae* using gene based probes, and also described the early diagnosis and detection of leprosy using the same technique. Lavania et al.[21] described the possible source of transmission of leprosy from soil. They detected viable *M. leprae* from soil samples by targeting mRNA of both patient and nonpatient area of Ghatampur, Uttar Pradesh (UP), India.

The most of the recent literature published on nonhuman or environmental sources of *M. leprae* have shown the evidence of *M. leprae* existence outside the human body. More studies are required to know the mechanism of survival of *M. leprae*[52] outside the human body in the form of association of other EM and other organisms or upregulation in any unknown gene for the survival.

REFERENCES

1. Holden C. (2009). Skeleton pushes back leprosy's origins. [online]. Science Now (website).. Available from news.sciencemag.org/asia/2009/05/skeleton-pushes-back-leprosys-origins. [Accessed May, 2014].
2. World Health Organization. (2014). Leprosy factsheet. [online]. Available from www.who.int/mediacentre/factsheets/fs101/en/. [Accessed May, 2014].
3. Walsh F. (2007). The hidden suffering of India's lepers. [online]. BBC News (website). Available from news.bbc.co.uk/2/hi/programmes/from_our_own_correspondent/6510503.stm. [Accessed May, 2014].
4. Dharmendra, Chatterjee SN. Examination for *Mycobacterium leprae*. In: Leprosy. Vol. 1 Dharmendra. ed. Bombay: Kothari Medical House; 1978.pp. 258-62.
5. Suzuki K, Udono T, Fujisawa M, et al. Infection during infancy and long incubation period of leprosy suggested in a case of a chimpanzee used for medical research. J Clin Microbiol. 2010;48:3432-4.
6. Paniker CK. Textbook of Microbiology. Hyderabad: University Press; 2009.
7. Cole ST, Eiglmeier K, Parkhill J, et al. Massive gene decay in the leprosy bacillus. Nature. 2001;409(6823):1007-11.
8. Truman RW, Krahenbuhl JL. Viable *M. leprae* as a research reagent. Int J Lepr Other Mycobact Dis. 2001;69(1):1-12.
9. Periaswami V. The hair follicles and the exit of *M. leprae* from the dermis. Lepr India. 1968;40:178-81.
10. Desikan KV, Iyer CG. Distribution of *M. leprae* in different structures of the skin. Lepr Rev. 1972;43(1):30-7.
11. Pedley JC. The presence of *M. leprae* in human milk. Lepr Rev. 1976;38(4):239-42.
12. Chehl SC, Job B, Hastings R. Transmission of leprosy in nude mice. Am J Trop Med Hyg. 1985;34(6):1161-6.
13. Duncan ME, Fox H, Harkness RA, et al. The placenta in leprosy. Placenta. 1984;5(3):189-98.
14. Job CK, Sanchez RM, Hastings RC. Lepromatousplacentitis and intrauterine fetal infection in lepromatous nine-banded armadillos (Dasypus novemcinctus). Lab Invest. 1986;56(1):44-8.
15. Truman R, Fine PE. 'Environmental' sources of *Mycobacterium leprae*: issues and evidence. Lepr Rev. 2010;81(2):89-95.
16. Taylor CE, Elliston EP, Gideon H. Asymptomatic infections in leprosy. Int J Lepr Other Mycobact Dis. 1965;33:716-31.
17. Fine PE. Leprosy: the epidemiology of a slow bacterium. Epidemiol Rev. 1982;4:161-87.
18. Deps PD, Alves BL, Gripp CG, et al. Contact with armadillos increases the risk of leprosy in Brazil: a case control study. Indian J Dermatol Venereol Leprol. 2008;74(4):338-42.
19. Sterne JA, Ponnighaus JM, Fine PE, et al. Geographic determinants of leprosy in Karonga District, Northern Malawi. Int J Epidemiol. 1995;24(6):1211-22.
20. Kerr-Pontes LR, Barreto ML, Evangelista CM, et al. Socioeconomic, environmental, and behavioural risk factors for leprosy in North-east Brazil: results of a case-control study. Int J Epidemiol. 2006;35(4):994-1000.

21. Lavania M, Katoch K, Katoch VM, et al. Detection of viable *Mycobacterium leprae* in soil samples: insights into possible sources of transmission of leprosy. Infect Genet Evol. 2008;8:627-31.
22. Blake LA, West BC, Lary CH, et al. Environmental non-human sources of leprosy. Rev Infect Dis. 1987;9(3):562-77.
23. Matsuoka M, Izumi S, Budiawan T, et al. *Mycobacterium leprae* DNA in daily using water as a possible source of leprosy infection. Indian J Lepr. 1999;71(1):61-7.
24. Kazda J, Irgens LM, Muller K. Isolation of non-cultivable acid-fast bacilli in sphagnum and moss vegetation by foot pad technique in mice. Int J Lepr Other Mycobact Dis. 1980;48(1):1-6.
25. Kazda J. Occurrence of non-cultivable acid-fast bacilli in the environment and their relationship to *M. leprae*. Lepr Rev. 1981; 52 Suppl 1:85-91.
26. Lahiri R, Krahenbuhl JL. The role of free-living pathogenic amoeba in the transmission of leprosy: a proof of principle. Lepr Rev. 2008;79(4):4019.
27. Saha K, Jain M, Mukherjee MK, et al. Viability of *Mycobacterium leprae* within the gut of Aedesa egypti after they feed on multibacillary lepromatous patients: a study by fluorescent and electron microscopes. Lepr Rev. 1985;56(4):279-90.
28. Sreevatsa. Leprosy and arthropods. Indian J Lepr. 1993;65(2):189-200.
29. Hutchinson J. On Leprosy and Fish-Eating. A Statement of Facts and Explanations. London: Archibald Constable and Company; 1906.pp.420.
30. Chaussinand R. Inoculation of Hansen and Stefansky bacilli in the rainbow perch Eupomotis gibbosus. Preliminary note. (Abstract). Int J Lepr Other Mycobact Dis. 1952;20:420-1.
31. Couret M. The behavior of bacillus leprae in cold-blooded animals. J Exp Med. 1911;13(5):576-89.
32. Gormus BJ, Xu K, Baskin GB, et al. Experimental leprosy in rhesus monkeys: transmission, susceptibility, clinical and immunological findings. Lepr Rev. 1998;69(3):235-45.
33. Truman RW, Shannon EJ, Hagstad HV, et al. Evaluation of the origin of *Mycobacterium leprae* infections in the wild armadillo, Dasypus novemcinctus. Am J Trop Med Hyg. 1986;35(3):588-93.
34. Falkinham JO 3rd. Nontuberculous mycobacteria in the environment. Clin Chest Med.2002;23(3):529-51.
35. Conger NG, O'Connell RJ, Laurel VL, et al. *Mycobacterium simae* outbreak associated with a hospital water supply. Infect Control Hosp Epidemiol. 2004;25(12):1050-5.
36. Wilson RW, Steingrube VA, Böttger EC, et al. *Mycobacterium immogenum* sp. nov., a novel species related to *Mycobacterium* abscessus and associated with clinical disease, pseudo-outbreaks and contaminated metalworking fland : an international cooperative study on mycobacterial taxonomy. Int J Syst Evol Microbiol. 2001;51:1751-64.
37. Winthrop KL, Abrams M, Yakrus M, et al. An outbreak of mycobacterial furunculosis associated with footbaths at a nail salon. N Engl J Med. 2002;346:1366-71.
38. Shepard CC. The experimental diseases that follows the injection of human leprosy bacilli into footpads of mice. J Exp Med. 1960;112(3):445-54.
39. Scollard DM, Adams LB, Gillis TP, et al. The continuing challenges of leprosy. Clin Microbiol Rev. 2006;19:338-81.
40. Meyers WM, Gormus BJ, Walsh GP. Experimental leprosy: leprosy. In: Hastings RC (Ed). New York: Churchill Livingstone; 1994.pp.385-408.
41. Rees RJ, Meade TW. Comparison of the modes of spread and the incidence of tuberculosis and leprosy.Lancet. 1974;7846:47-8.
42. Johnstone PA. The search for animal models of leprosy. Int J Lepr Other Mycobact Dis. 1987;55(3):535-47.
43. Meyers WM, Gormus BJ, Walsh GP. Nonhuman sources of leprosy. Int J Lepr Other Mycobact Dis. 1992;60(3):477-80.
44. Leininger JR, Donham KJ, Rubino MJ, et al. Naturally acquired leprosy in a chimpanzee. Necropsy findings and experimental transmission to other animals. Lab Invest. 1980;42:132.
45. Couret M. The behavior of bacillus leprae in cold-blooded animals. J Exp Med. 1911;13:576-89.
46. Truman RW, Singh P, Sharma R, et al. Probable zoonotic leprosy in the southern United States. New Engl J Med. 2011;364(17):1626-33.
47. Desikan KV, Sreevatsa. Extended studies on the viability of *Mycobacterium leprae* outside the human body. Lepr Rev. 1995;66(4):287-95.
48. Agusni I, Izumi S, Adriaty D, et al. Studi *Mycobacterium leprae* dari alam lingkulgan di daerah endemik kusta. Maj Kedokt Ind. 2004;54(12):491-5.
49. Cirillo JD, Falkow S, Tompkins LS, et al. Interaction of *Mycobacterium avium* with environmental amoebae enhances virulence. Infect Immun. 1997;65(9):3759-67.
50. Jadin JB. Amibes "limax" vecteurs possible des Mycobacteries et de *Mycobacterium leprae*. Acta Leprol. 1975;59-60:57-67.
51. Katoch VM, Kanaujia GV, Shivannavar CT, et al. Ribosomal RNA gene based probes for early diagnosis and epidemiology of leprosy. Quard Di Cooper Sanitor. 1992;2:163-6.
52. Wheat WH, Casali AL, Thomas V, et al. Long–term survival and virulence of *Mycobacterium leprae* in amoebal cysts. PloS Negl Trop Dis. 2014;8(12):e3405.

CHAPTER 13

Experimental Leprosy: Contributions of Animal Models to Leprosy Research

Linda B Adams, Maria T Pena, Rahul Sharma, Ramanuj Lahiri, Richard W Truman

INTRODUCTION

Although *Mycobacterium leprae,* discovered by Armauer Hansen in 1873, was one of the first microorganisms to be associated with a human infectious disease, it has yet to be cultured in axenic medium. For nearly a century, attempts by numerous investigators to cultivate the organism outside the human host, as well as develop an animal model which accurately recapitulated leprosy development and progression, were often met with frustration. Animals infected[1] included the typical laboratory animals, such as various strains of mice, rats, guinea pigs, gerbils, hamsters, rabbits and monkeys, as well as an assortment of other mammals (e.g. chimpanzees, dogs, cats, pigs, armadillos, slender loris, chinchillas, fruit bats, lemmings, voles, opossums, chipmunks and hedgehogs), birds (e.g. pigeons, chickens, paddy birds, canaries, parrots and love-birds) and cold-blooded animals (e.g. eels, fresh and salt water fish, tadpoles, frogs, turtles, snakes, lizards, and alligators). The variability in success rates for cultivation in these animals may have been due partly to the low quality of the *M. leprae* inoculum that was used, as it was largely crude patient derived biopsy material of unknown concentration and viability. In addition, early investigators used a myriad of experimental protocols which often did not take into account the prolonged growth cycle of *M. leprae* or its preference for cooler temperatures for optimum growth. The seminal reports by Charles Shepard[2] describing the reproducible cultivation and passage of *M. leprae* in the footpads (FPs) of mice, and Kirchheimer and Storrs[3] detailing the development of lepromatous leprosy (LL) in the nine-banded armadillo initiated approaches for research in leprosy that were previously unattainable. This chapter will focus on the advances and opportunities offered by the mouse and armadillo models of *M. leprae* infection.

MOUSE MODEL

Mice (*Mus musculus*) are undoubtedly the most widely used experimental animals in medical research. They are small, relatively inexpensive mammals, which are easy to house and maintain. Mice are prolific breeders and have a relatively short gestation time. There are hundreds of well-defined strains, including outbred, inbred and genetically engineered mutants, which can be purchased from several commercial vendors worldwide. Perhaps, most importantly, there is an ever-growing multitude of sophisticated biological reagents available that enable complex, and detailed examination of physiological and immunological processes.

Infection Strategies

Footpad Infection

The cultivation and passage of *M. leprae* in the footpads (FPs) of immunocompetent Carworth Farm's white mice were first reported by Charles Shepard in 1960[2] and subsequently confirmed by him and others.[4-6] The FP was chosen for infection because of its cool temperature and because other mycobacteria had been successfully cultured in this site. Shepard found that if a low number of ($\leq 10^4$) *M. leprae* were inoculated into the FP, the organisms would multiply locally with a doubling time of approximately 13 days. The growth in the FP was limited to approximately 10^6 organisms by the host immune system and after reaching this peak, the organisms were killed.[7] Inoculation with a larger number of *M. leprae* immunized the mouse. Although time-consuming and expensive, due to the long-term care and upkeep of the animals, this technique was highly reproducible, and enabled the establishment and maintenance of isolates of

M. leprae. Moreover, drug testing, detection of drug resistance, experimental vaccine evaluation, and immunological studies became feasible.

In efforts to develop murine models more representative of human LL, various investigators applied this "mouse foot-pad (MFP) assay" to immunodeficient strains. The importance of lymphocytes, especially T-cells in host defense, in leprosy was firmly established upon infection of thymectomized and irradiated mice,[8,9] congenitally athymic mice,[10-12] and severe combined immunodeficiency disease (SCID) mice.[13-15] In these immunosuppressed strains, multiplication of *M. leprae* in the FP can reach 10^{10} or more bacilli (Figs 13.1A and B). Athymic *nu/nu* mice are now routinely used for culture of large numbers of highly viable *M. leprae* for experimental use.[16]

Intranerve Infection

Because *M. leprae* does not readily infect murine Schwann cells (SCs) *in vivo*, presumably due to a lack of appropriate receptors, investigators have attempted to bypass natural infection by injecting the bacilli directly into the nerve. Shetty et al. group examined intraneural infection by inoculating 10×10^6 to 20×10^6 viable *M. leprae* into the sciatic nerve of immunocompetent and immunosuppressed mice.[17-20] When bacterial growth and viability were evaluated, however, there was little change in the number of *M. leprae* recovered over time and a striking decrease in bacterial viability upon subsequent passage of bacilli in MFP. This lack of survival and multiplication of the organism could be due to the warm temperature of the sciatic nerve. Although *M. leprae* were not observed in the SCs of either strain, a tuberculoid-type granulomatous response was elicited in normal, unsensitized, Swiss white mice, whereas unsensitized, immunosuppressed, thymectomized and irradiated mice developed a macrophage response. In later studies, upon intraneural inoculation of either live or dead *M. leprae* or whole cell wall fraction into either immunocompetent mice or *Rag1-/-* mice, which lack both T and B-cells, Rambukkana et al.[21] reported substantial demyelination compared to mice inoculated with buffer alone. Therefore, although intraneural inoculation does not represent a natural infection with *M. leprae*, these studies show that this route of administration has potential for investigation of both immunologically and nonimmunologically mediated nerve damage in leprosy.

Ear Infection

Similar to FPs, ear pinnae in mice are cooler than the rest of the body. Reports from studies with cutaneous leishmaniasis suggested interesting differences in disease development and antileishmania immune responses in FP versus ear infection.[22] Thus, intradermal inoculation of viable *M. leprae* in mice pinnae was attempted to study growth kinetics

and development of anti-*M. leprae* immune responses.[23] Mice supported limited growth of *M. leprae* in ears over 30 weeks, but the draining lymph nodes showed markedly more cellular infiltration when compared to that of FP inoculated mice. There was a general increase in the numbers of all immune cell types (CD4+/CD8+ T-cells, dendritic cells, macrophages and granulocytes) rather than any preferential infiltration of a particular cell population. There was also an increase in the numbers of IFNγ secreting CD4+ T-cells at the site of inoculation in the ears over time, suggesting a local inflammatory response. Similar cellular infiltration was seen in mice inoculated with equal numbers of heat-killed *M. leprae* in ears but the response was significantly less compared to live *M. leprae* infection. The cellular infiltration in draining lymph nodes as well as at the inoculation site was significantly reduced following rifampin treatment of mice shortly (1–3 weeks) after inoculation. Presence of different antigen presenting cell populations at these two different sites may be responsible for the observed differences in the degree of anti-*M. leprae* immune responses in FPs and ear.[24] Since cellular infiltration in the draining lymph node and at the site of infection becomes significant within 6 weeks postinoculation, unlike FP infection which may take 20–24 weeks, this ear infection model has been utilized for rapid *in vivo* screening of anti-*M. leprae* drugs or vaccine candidates using the degree of cellular infiltration, especially that of CD4+ T-cells, as a surrogate marker of efficacy.[25]

Applications of the Mouse Model

Studies of the Granuloma

The primary cell populations which respond to infection with *M. leprae* are T-cells and macrophages. However, neither the dynamics of their interactions within the microenvironment of the lesion nor their role in disease development and progression are fully understood. With a chronic disease, such as leprosy, which has an extremely slow progression and can remain asymptomatic for years between initial infection and diagnosis, it is difficult to define the early interactions of the participants in the immune response. Murine FP infection currently provides the most accessible method for the immunological investigation of the *M. leprae* induced granuloma.

Immunocompetent mice: In addition to permitting only limited growth of *M. leprae*, the histopathological changes which occur in the FP of conventional, immunocompetent mice are rather minimal.[2] The cellular infiltration into the FP is comprised largely of macrophages and epithelioid cells, which become more vacuolated as infection progresses and bacterial replication ceases, suggesting macrophage activation.[26] There are also numerous lymphocytes present but neutrophils are rare and there is no necrosis in the tissue. Nerves are not infected although there have been reports of neural damage very late (>2 years) in infection.[27] Bacilli are primarily intracellular, often in clumps and become progressively more beaded as the infection proceeds past the peak of bacterial growth.

Immunosuppressed mice: In contrast, athymic *nu/nu* mice show characteristics of LL disease. As infection progresses over the course of several months, there is an influx of macrophages into the FP to accommodate the multiplying bacilli, eventually becoming a huge "leproma" consisting of heavily infected foamy macrophages that replaces most of the normal tissue (Figs 13.1A and B).[12] These macrophages can contain hundreds of bacilli, emphasizing the nontoxic nature of this organism.[28] Bacilli are also found in striated muscle cells and eventually in perineural cells, SCs and fibroblasts. Dissemination is rather slow, but late in infection (>1 year) bacteria can be found in virtually all tissues except the central nervous system.

Genetically engineered mice: The introduction of genetically engineered mice, generated via gene transfer technology, has greatly expanded the utility of the mouse model for biological research. Hundreds of targeted gene knockout (KO) mouse strains are now commercially available, as well as strains with conditional KO, tissue-specific KO, multiple KO and knock-in mutations. Mice with defects in pathways important in host defense, especially those with deletions in specific cytokines, chemokines, cytokine and chemokine receptors, various immune modulators and cell surface markers, have been particularly useful in the study of a variety of infectious diseases. In studying a disease, such as leprosy, in which the manifestations of the spectrum are largely due to the immune response of the infected host and also perhaps to the compensatory mechanisms evoked during an inadequate response, mice with deletions at specific points of the immune

cascade have been especially enlightening for improving understanding of *M. leprae* pathogenesis. Furthermore, these murine strains have enabled immunological investigations, which had, heretofore, been problematic due to the long, protracted course of *M. leprae* infection. Finally, additional modifications can be induced in the mice. Double KO can be generated either by treating with various inhibitors or antibodies or even cross-breeding KO strains. Conversely, a KO function can be restored after infection using cytokine therapy or adoptive transfer of competent immune cells. Thus, these mouse models have been used to explore cell-mediated immunity to *M. leprae* both *in vivo* and *in vitro*, and to study the microenvironment of the granuloma in leprosy pathogenesis.

Two FP infection protocols have been utilized to examine the host response to the bacilli. The Shepard MFP assay, in which less than or equal to 10^4 freshly harvested, highly viable *M. leprae* are inoculated into each hind FP, allows bacterial growth to be monitored as well as granuloma development, both histopathologically and by immunohistochemical staining, for up to 18 months infection. An alternate higher dose infection protocol, a strategy based on the Lepromin test in humans, permits the cellular composition of the leprosy lesion to be more thoroughly explored. Mice are injected in the FP with more than 10^6 *M. leprae* and FP induration can be measured for changes throughout infection. FP tissues can be harvested at key intervals [e.g. at 4 weeks (early), 16–20 weeks (mid), and >32 weeks (late)], and examined for cytokine and chemokine expression by real-time polymerase chain reaction (RT-PCR), and for cell phenotypes by histopathological and immunohistochemical analyses. Cells can also be isolated directly from the granulomas, and analyzed by flow cytometry and ELISA for cell surface marker expression and/or cytokine production after *in vitro* culture and stimulation

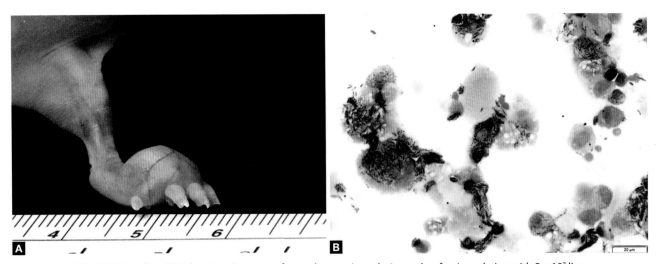

Figs 13.1A and B: (A) Athymic *nu/nu* mouse footpad approximately 6 months after inoculation with 5×10^7 live *Mycobacterium leprae*; (B) Acid-fast staining of cells obtained from such a footpad

with *M. leprae* antigens. Consequently, the long-term effects of chronic *M. leprae* infection on the granulomatous response can be evaluated.[29-31]

The host cell-mediated immune response to FP infection with *M. leprae* has been evaluated *in vivo* and *in vitro* in more than 10 KO strains of mice. Characteristics examined include growth of the bacilli, organization of the granuloma, FP induration response, T-cell and macrophage phenotype, and cytokine and chemokine generation (Table 13.1). Interestingly, when comparing the findings with intact immunocompetent control mice with high cell-mediated immunity and athymic *nu/nu* mice with virtually no cell-mediated immunity, it was found that no KO of a single cytokine, T-cell type, or antimicrobial mechanism transformed any of these strains into a totally immunocompromised model like the athymic *nu/nu* mouse. However, based on their unique characteristic profiles, most KO strains could be placed along the leprosy spectrum. These findings insinuate the presence of alternative or compensatory mechanisms of host resistance in these animals, the very mechanisms which may be occurring in borderline leprosy.

Since a strong cell-mediated immune response is important for controlling leprosy, in contrast to the humoral response, mice with deficiencies in cytokines and products important in Th1 development were first studied (Table 13.1). Compared to wild type mice, IL12/23p40 KO mice exhibited a decreased ability to control *M. leprae* growth and evidenced reduced FP induration with altered CD4+ and CD8+ T-cell composition due to the lack of protective IL-12 and proinflammatory IL-23, respectively.[31] IFNγ KO allowed augmented but not uncontrolled growth of *M. leprae*, a massive, noninvasive cellular infiltration into the FP and a Th2-type cytokine response.[32] Mice lacking TNF and LTα, two closely related cytokines, also gave very disparate responses.[33] TNF KO demonstrated extensive lymphocytic infiltration, primarily of activated CD4+ T-cells, yet growth of *M. leprae* was augmented throughout the infection period. In contrast, LTα-deficient mice were unable to recruit lymphocytes into the infected FP, develop and maintain granulomas, or optimally control the growth of *M. leprae* in the chronic

stage. Mice which have a mutation in the respiratory burst oxidase *phox91* gene exhibit responses to *M. leprae* infection, which are similar to wild type mice.[34] In contrast, NOS2 KO controlled growth of *M. leprae* similar to control mice but developed a large, destructive granulomatous response, and a concomitant strong Th1 cytokine and chemokine response.[30,35]

In addition, of great interest was the disparity in the T-cell populations between the FP granuloma and the draining lymph node.[31,34] Upon infection with *M. leprae*, the granuloma which developed in the FPs of immunocompetent mice had a very characteristic lymphocyte profile, consisting primarily of T-cells of the activated CD4+ phenotype. Lymph nodes, in contrast, generally contained more B-cells than T-cells, and equal numbers of CD4 and CD8 cells, which were of the naïve phenotype. Therefore, cell populations in the FP were distinct from those in the draining lymph node and this underscored the importance of studying the leprosy lesion itself. However, lymph node profiles were valuable in strains which yielded little granulomatous response in the FP (e.g. LTα-deficient mice).[33]

Enumeration and Viability Assays

Acid fast bacilli count versus RLEP: In the absence of growth in axenic medium, *M. leprae* until recently could only be enumerated by direct microscopic counting of acid-fast bacilli (AFB). The method, originally described by Shepard,[36] involves homogenization of infected tissues followed by spreading of an appropriately diluted aliquot onto special slides. The preparation is then fixed and stained for AFB before counting under a properly calibrated microscope. Like most other mycobacteria, *M. leprae* is prone to clumping and this may prevent uniform distribution of bacteria in tissue homogenates. In addition, tissue homogenization can be incomplete such that some bacteria may not be released from the infected tissues. Both of these drawbacks can contribute to inaccuracies in the subsequent *M. leprae* count. However, analyses of FP harvests have shown that, if done by well-trained personnel using a large number of

Table 13.1: Attributes that have been assessed to classify knockout mouse strains along the leprosy spectrum

Attribute	Mouse strain				
	B6	NOS2	P40	IFNγ	*nu/nu*
ML growth	+	+	++	++	+++
Granuloma	Minimal	Destructive	Mild	Unorganized	Leproma
FP Induration	+	+++	+/-	++	-
T-cells	CD4 > CD8	↑CD4	↑CD8	↑CD4	-
Macrophages	Epithelioid	Epithelioid	Epithelioid	↓MΦ/↑PMN	Foamy
Cytokine	Th1	↑Th1	↓Th1	Th2	Th2
Classification	Indeterminate	BT	BB	BL	LL

samples, reliable and reproducible results can be obtained.[37] Theoretically, using this method approximately 5,000 bacteria/mL of tissue homogenate can be counted but the accuracy becomes questionable when enumerating such small numbers of bacilli in infected tissues. This poses a problem in enumeration of bacteria in clinical samples where the numbers are typically below this level. Another issue is the lack of specificity in this method. There is no way to differentiate *M. leprae* from other acid-fast staining bacilli in clinical preparations during enumeration. Therefore, additional tests need to be conducted if a mixed infection is suspected clinically.

An *M. leprae*-specific real time polymerase chain reaction (PCR) based method can increase the sensitivity of *M. leprae* enumeration in tissue samples by at least 10-fold. The *M. leprae* chromosome contains a minimum of 28 copies of a dispersed repetitive sequence, RLEP, which contains an invariant 545-bp core flanked by variable structures of 100-bp at the left and 44- to 47-bp at the right.[38] The 545-bp core sequence appears to be highly specific for *M. leprae* and a TaqMan based PCR assay has been developed to amplify this region for *M. leprae* enumeration in MFPs, armadillo tissues and clinical samples.[39] This assay is highly specific for *M. leprae* and can detect as few as 300 bacteria/mL of tissue homogenate. Moreover, it is a much easier and accurate way to enumerate *M. leprae*, and is currently gaining popularity over direct counts.

Determination of M. leprae viability: The inability to culture *M. leprae* in artificial medium not only impedes the understanding of vital molecular and cellular events in the pathogenesis of leprosy, it also prevents researchers to easily and definitively distinguish between live and dead bacilli. Shepard's MFP assay was a milestone, which enabled titration of *M. leprae* suspensions in large numbers of mice to ascertain relative viability. Although this method has been used to test new antileprosy drugs, detect drug resistant strains and evaluate vaccine candidates, it is time consuming and labor intensive. Thus, researchers have been eager to bypass the MFP technique and find alternate methods to determine *M. leprae* viability.

Acid-fast staining showed that not all of the bacteria in a given sample stain uniformly; some are solid stained while others appear 'beaded'. It was postulated that the solid staining bacilli were the viable ones and a 'morphological index' for a particular sample was calculated, which essentially expressed the ratio of solid to beaded bacteria in a given sample.[40] Researchers also tried, with some success, to score for percentage of viability on the basis of *M. leprae* ultrastructure and correlating this with growth of *M. leprae* in those samples in the MFP assay.[41] However, these methods were not very reliable as they were less objective and likely dependent on variables, such as fixation and staining technique for quality. Uptake of radiolabeled purines and pyrimidines (e.g. adenosine, hypoxanthine and thymidine) can be good indicators for bacterial viability, and studies have shown some uptake of these compounds by *M. leprae* between 6–10 days of culture within macrophages. However, this method is of little value with *M. leprae* in axenic culture.[42] Determination of the Na^+/K^+ ratio in individual bacteria appears to be an indicator of *M. leprae* viability in axenic cultures[43] but requires expensive mass spectrometry set-up and has never been validated using the MFP assay or other concurrent methods. Measurement of ATP content in bioluminescence assays has been reported to have a good overall correlation with growth in MFPs by some groups.[44,45]

Among all the biochemical methods for determining *M. leprae* viability, measuring the rate of palmitic acid oxidation by a suspension of *M. leprae* is the most reliable one. In this method (radiorespirometry), ^{14}C-labeled palmitic acid is added as the sole carbon source in axenic media and the released ^{14}C-labeled carbon dioxide (CO_2), which is the end product of palmitic acid oxidation, is captured and measured daily for 7 days.[46] The cumulative seventh day count correlates extremely well with MFP data, and it is now the standard biochemical method used to determine *M. leprae* viability in axenic,[46] macrophage[47] and mouse[16] studies.

Differential staining of live and dead bacteria with fluorescent vital dyes is a simple way to score for percentage of viable *M. leprae* in a suspension. The underlying principle is to use two dyes, one of which is able to penetrate bacteria with intact membranes while the other cannot; therefore, the second dye will only stain bacteria with a damaged membrane. Assuming that bacteria with damaged membranes are not viable, one can easily score bacterial viability by differential staining. Fluorescein diacetate and ethidium bromide is one such dye combination which has been found to be satisfactory, although there have been some background staining issues.[48,49] Another dye combination that has been used extensively and validated with radiorespirometry, as well as the MFP assay, is Syto9 and propidium iodide.[50,51]

Most of the above methods suffer from a common shortcoming, which is the high number of organisms required to perform the tests. In addition, these tests must be carried out soon after acquisition of the viable bacilli. These parameters inherently compromise the sensitivity and utility of these methods for clinical studies. In theory, the most sensitive method for determination of viability of noncultivable organisms will be quantitating transcripts of target genes by reverse transcriptase-PCR (RT-PCR). Since very little is known about the expression kinetics and regulation of different genes in *M. leprae*, the challenge is to discover the right target gene(s). *sod*A message, when normalized using RLEP counts, seems to be a good indicator of *M. leprae* viability in the short-term, which makes it a suitable viability marker for *in vitro* studies.[52] A recent study by Davis et al.[51] has shown that expression levels of *esx*A and *hsp*18 are good indicators of *M. leprae* viability *in vivo*. Furthermore, these molecular viability assays can be performed on nucleic acids purified from ethanol-fixed tissues, making their adaptability to clinical and field samples plausible.

Drug Testing

The MFP assay is still the 'gold standard' for evaluation of chemotherapeutic agents against *M. leprae*. There are three different variations in which it is used in this regard, each with its advantages and limitations. (In the following discussion, the day of FP inoculation with live *M. leprae* is considered as day 0.) The most simple and straightforward among the three protocols is the 'continuous' method,[53] in which FPs of immunocompetent mice are inoculated with low numbers of live *M. leprae*, usually 5×10^3 or 1×10^4. Administration of drugs starts on day 0 or 1 and continues daily until the animals are sacrificed. Drug activity is measured by the percentage or fold inhibition of *M. leprae* multiplication in the FPs of treated mice as compared to that of placebo controls. The second and most tedious method to determine bactericidal activity of drugs against *M. leprae* is the 'proportional bactericidal' method.[54] Groups of immunocompetent mice are inoculated with serial 10-fold dilutions, starting from 5×10^3 (or 1×10^4) to 5 (or 1) *M. leprae* per FP. Drug is administered from day 0 or 1 but the length of treatment can vary anywhere from a single dose to 60 consecutive doses. Enumeration of bacteria is carried out in FPs of treated and control mice 12 months post-treatment to calculate the proportion of *M. leprae* that survived the drug treatment. The 'proportional bactericidal' method can also be used to determine the efficacy of a particular drug or treatment regimen in leprosy patients. *M. leprae* is obtained from fresh skin biopsies of patients before, during and after treatment, and serial 10-fold dilutions are inoculated into MFPs. The mice are sacrificed 12 months postinoculation (without any treatment) and *M. leprae* are enumerated to ascertain the proportion of viable *M. leprae* that were present in the inocula, which in turn will be proportional to the efficacy of the treatment.[55-57] While the 'continuous' method fails to distinguish between bactericidal and bacteriostatic activity, the 'proportional bactericidal' method cannot detect bacteriostatic activity. Thus, this shortcoming is overcome by using the 'kinetic' method[58,59] where MFPs are inoculated as in the 'continuous' method but administration of drugs does not start until day 60 when *M. leprae* are assumed to be in their logarithmic growth phase in the FPs. Depending on the protocol different drug administration regimens may be chosen, starting from a single dose to thirty or more daily doses. Efficacy of a drug is measured by the time lag between treated and control footpads in reaching 10^6 *M. leprae*/FP. In the case of a bactericidal drug, growth will not resume (or will be extremely slow) after cessation of treatment, whereas with a bacteriostatic drug *M. leprae* growth will resume giving rise to a measurable 'growth delay'. Although the 'kinetic method' can distinguish between bacteriostatic and bactericidal drugs, it may not differentiate prolonged bacteriostasis from bactericidal effects. Extended bacteriostasis may occur when the drug is retained in the host (or bacterial) system for prolonged time after completion of drug treatment, thus in effect acting as a slow release reservoir.

Recently, a variation of the kinetic method was described where athymic *nu/nu* mice were used instead of immunocompetent mice. In addition, instead of using 'growth delay' as the measure of drug efficacy, a variety of molecular and biochemical tests were used to determine *M. leprae* viability in the FPs of treated and control athymic *nu/nu* mice at 30 days after cessation of drug treatment. The argument for using athymic *nu/nu* mice is that they may be more suitable as a model for LL patients who have very little or no cell-mediated immunity against *M. leprae*. The results clearly showed that a single or even five daily doses of rifampin was not enough to achieve significant killing of *M. leprae* in athymic *nu/nu* mice unlike immunocompetent animals.[51] Studies with *M. tuberculosis* have also shown that the host immune response plays a significant role in the outcome of chemotherapy.[60,61] Reliable determination of *M. leprae* viability by these and other methods may be more rapid and objective assessments of drug efficacy in MFPs than enumeration of bacterial numbers.

Since multidrug therapy (MDT) is the only means of leprosy control available as of now, determination of emerging trends of drug resistance in leprosy endemic areas is extremely important, especially with regard to Rifampicin, which is the most important component in both MDT and Rifampicin-Ofloxacin-Minocycline (ROM) therapy. The 'continuous' method for drug evaluation can also be used for susceptibility testing on *M. leprae* obtained from patient's biopsies.[62] The major obstacle in using this method is the availability of large quantities of *M. leprae* from patient material for inoculation. Fortunately, Rifampicin resistance can be attributed to specific mutations in the *rpoB* gene of *M. leprae*, as are Dapsone and Fluoroquinolone (Ofloxacin) resistance to that of *folP* and *gyrA* genes, respectively. These mutations occur in specific regions of the target genes called drug resistance determining regions (DRDR).[63] Consequently, drug resistance can be assessed in biopsies of suspected cases by PCR amplification of the target gene DRDR followed by mutation detection by various methods.[64-66] Direct PCR sequencing of DRDRs of target genes is the method of choice for the ongoing global surveillance of drug resistance in leprosy.[63] However, the MFP assay is the only method available to ascertain resistance to such antibiotics as Clofazimine, where the mechanism of action is not yet fully understood and does not have any known target gene(s).

Evaluation of Vaccine Candidates

Charles Shepard was the first to use the MFP assay to experimentally test vaccines against *M. leprae* infection,[67] and it is still the animal model of choice to initially screen and evaluate leprosy vaccine candidates. In a typical experiment, groups of mice are vaccinated either subcutaneously or intradermally followed by a low dose (5×10^3 bacilli/FP) *M. leprae* challenge. FPs are harvested from these mice at approximately 6 months post-challenge for enumeration of AFB, and protection is calculated as a percentage or fold inhibition of *M. leprae* growth. A single intradermal injection of heat killed *M. leprae* (10^7) is used as the positive control vaccine for most protection studies.[68,69] Recently, the mouse ear pinnae infection model was also used to evaluate potential vaccine candidates.[25,69] In these studies, inhibition of cellular infiltration in the draining lymph node or infiltration of $CD4^+$ cells at the site of inoculation was taken as the end point rather than inhibition of actual growth of *M. leprae*.

Diagnostic Assays: Insights into Antigen Responsiveness

Development of a reliable laboratory diagnostic test for early or preclinical leprosy is a top priority as early treatment is essential to prevent nerve damage and deformity, and to block transmission. However, sensitivity is a problem because preclinical leprosy presents a minimum immune stimulation. Furthermore, the unknown duration since exposure and the variability in human immune responses confound results. An important advantage of the MFP assay is that it eliminates many of these issues, especially the problems of unknown length of exposure to *M. leprae* and of crossreactivity with other mycobacterial species that are common in natural hosts. Hence, MFP studies have been exploited in an effort to develop standardized protocols for immunodiagnosis. One such study involved evaluation of the cell-mediated immune response, gaged in terms of IFNγ secretion, by splenic lymphocytes from infected mice stimulated *in vitro* with *M. leprae* antigens.[70] In an attempt to model 'subclinical' or early leprosy, various doses of *M. leprae* and lengths of infection were titrated in FPs. The aim was to establish the minimum dose at the earliest time point required for the development of a measurable cell-mediated immune response. It was found that for a consistent and significant response 3 months after inoculation, a minimum dose of 1×10^5 live *M. leprae* per FP was required. Both BALB/c and C57Bl/6 mice responded similarly though the response was more robust in C57Bl/6 mice. This model was able to pick-up most, though not all, of the recombinant *M. leprae* antigens recognized by patient sera or peripheral blood mononuclear cells.[70-72] This 'early' disease model may be used to screen *M. leprae* antigens for immunodiagnostic purposes that may then be further evaluated in the natural hosts of *M. leprae*. T-cells isolated from the site of *M. leprae* infection (i.e. *M. leprae*-induced FP granuloma) are also being examined for their antigen responsiveness, and KO mice are proving increasingly useful in this regard for screening proteins for selective diagnosis.[33,34]

Limitations of the Mouse Model

Although mice are an invaluable resource, they possess some immunological differences from humans which investigators must keep in mind when using them to study immunity, especially with regard to mycobacterial diseases. For example, they lack a homologue for granulysin, a key antimycobacterial protein generated by human NK and $CD8^+$ T-cells.[73] Their repertoire of CD1 cell surface marker expression, which is important for lipid antigen recognition, is different from that of humans.[74] In addition, nitric oxide synthase 2 (NOS2) generated reactive nitrogen intermediates, which are toxic radicals of activated macrophages that have antimycobacterial properties,[75,76] are produced much more robustly by murine macrophages compared to human macrophages.[77,78] Mouse strains also vary in their ability to recognize certain mycobacterial antigens, such as CFP-10.[70,79] Finally, mice are highly resistant to infection with *M. leprae* unless they are immunosuppressed in some fashion, and they are not an ideal model for the study of nerve infection with the bacilli.

ARMADILLO MODEL

In addition to humans, nine-banded armadillos (*Dasypus novemcinctus*) are the only other natural host of *M. leprae*. Free ranging armadillos in the Southeast United States are known to harbor high rates of *M. leprae* infection and zoonotic transmission of *M. leprae* from armadillos to humans has been established.[80] Although biomarkers of *M. leprae* have been reported among armadillos at various locations in South America, the potential for zoonotic transmission of leprosy elsewhere in the Americas is only poorly understood.

Infection in the armadillo closely recapitulates many of the structural, physiological and functional aspects of leprosy seen in humans, and armadillos can be useful models for leprosy research. Because of the heavy burdens of bacilli they harbor, nine-banded armadillos have become the host-of-choice for propagating large quantities of *M. leprae* and they are advancing as an important model of the pathogenesis of leprosy nerve damage. Although they are not typically used as laboratory animals, the recently completed whole genome sequence for the nine-banded armadillo has enabled researchers to undertake more sophisticated molecular studies and to develop an array of armadillo-specific reagents. Armadillos are likely to play important roles in piloting new therapies and diagnostic regimens, and will provide new insights into the oldest known infectious neurodegenerative disorder.

Natural History and Husbandry

Armadillos are exotic looking mammals about the size of housecats. Members of the order Xenarthra, they are evolutionarily related to sloths and anteaters. Armadillos lack full dentition and have short limbs with strong claws, and a hard but flexible banded carapace protecting their body. The term "armadillo" can be applied to 21 different species in nine different genera.[81] However, the armadillo of greatest importance in leprosy research is *Dasypus novemcinctus* (i.e. the long-nosed, southern or nine-banded armadillo) (Fig. 13.2), although *Dasypus septemcinctus* (seven-banded armadillo) and *Euphractus sexcinctus* (six-banded armadillo) may also be partially susceptible to *M. leprae*.[82]

The armadillo's long lifespan (12 years) and cool body temperature (32–35°C—optimal for *M. leprae*) are the main physiological traits that first attracted the attention of leprosy researchers. Armadillos are found only in the Americas and range from northern Argentina to the central United States. They can adapt to many diverse habitats but are most abundant in low-lying and coastal areas. Their population has undergone extensive expansion in recent years;[83] however, they do not hibernate and a poor tolerance of cold temperatures is the main factor limiting their ultimate range.

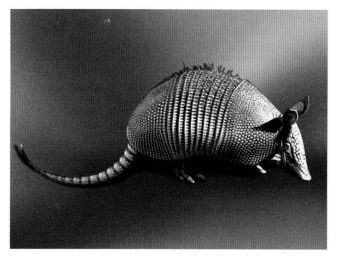

Fig. 13.2: Nine-banded armadillo, *Dasypus novemcinctus*

The reproductive cycle of the armadillo is characterized by diapausic development and polyembryony.[81] Females typically mate in the summer, but the embryos do not implant in the uterine wall until late fall, and then they divide into identical quadruplicates sharing the same hemochorial placenta. The genetically identical quadruplicates show a heritable component in the armadillo's response to *M. leprae* that can be seen among litter-mates.[84] Siblings experimentally infected with *M. leprae* show similar susceptibility and manifest similar numbers of bacilli at the time of harvest. Individual litters may be either high or low responders to infection with siblings yielding more than 10^9 *M. leprae*/g of reticuloendothelial tissue, or exhibiting nonproductive infections with either low bacillary counts ($<10^9$ *M. leprae*/g) or suffering complications from the experimentally induced infection requiring their removal from studies. Observations on human genetically identical twins with leprosy also suggest an innate predisposition for the infection and mirror the similarity in responses seen among armadillo siblings.[85] Although armadillos are not reliably bred in captivity and must be obtained from the wild for investigative purposes, gravid females taken from the wild will litter in captivity and the genetically identical offspring can be ideal models to study the role of host genetics and genomic factors on disease susceptibility.[86]

Armadillos can be maintained by any laboratory capable of housing rabbits or other medium-sized mammals. Modified rabbit cages with soft plastic flooring inserts are used to house armadillos and the animals adapt to using cat litter pans. Individual units can be ganged together with a tunnel to separate the sleeping and feeding area from the litter pan side. A small plastic trash can with shredded paper functions as a sham burrow and enriches their environment (Fig. 13.3).

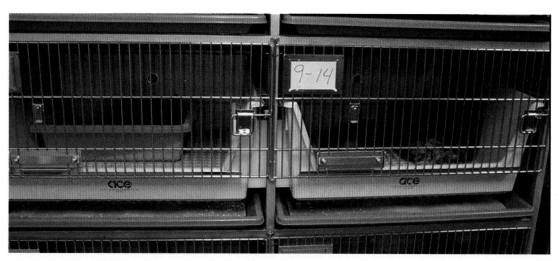

Fig. 13.3: Modified rabbit cages with soft plastic inserts are used to house armadillos

Armadillos and Zoonotic Leprosy

Natural Infection Among Wild Armadillos

Armadillos began expanding their range into the United States from Mexico only during the last century. They continue to colonize new areas and are expected to eventually roam over more than 50% of the entire geographic area of the United States. The specific factors which promoted this dramatic range expansion by armadillos are not certain, but it probably benefited from the active removal of predators by agricultural interests in the northern range, and the high carrying capacity and low competition the animals found in the northern bottomlands.[83] Armadillos in parts of Texas are reported to reach densities of up to 50/km², but much lower densities are reported among armadillos in South America.[87-92]

Pioneering armadillo populations show less genetic diversity than their counterparts elsewhere in Central and South America.[93,94] In 1975, Walsh et al.[95] discovered that free-ranging armadillos in Louisiana harbored a natural infection with *M. leprae* and subsequent investigations confirmed that the disease is widespread among North American armadillos.[96,97] Prevalence rates exceed 20% in some locations,[98] although the disease may appear to be absent in other locales.[91] The highest prevalence rates in the United States are usually reported among animals habituating low-lying poorly drained areas, especially those in the southern Mississippi river valley and other bottomlands.[98,99] These areas have high carrying capacities for insect eating armadillos, and disease prevalence rates tend to be lower in better-drained locales or other areas with lower animal densities. The origins of *M. leprae* infections among wild armadillos, its geographic range, and what risks the infection in these animals might present to humans have remained topics of interest.

Leprosy was not present in the new world during pre-Colombian times and armadillos must have acquired *M. leprae* from humans sometime in the last 300 years, and if they did so in North America, then it seems possible that armadillos also could have repeated the event at many times and in many locations over the years. Biomarkers of *M. leprae* have been reported among armadillos in Argentina,[100,101] Brazil,[102-105] Colombia[106] and Mexico.[107] In addition, epidemiological studies in Brazil have implicated environmental sources for some cases of human infection,[108] and contact with armadillos was found to be a significant risk factor for leprosy in another Brazilian study.[109]

Genotyping M. leprae from Armadillos

Recent studies also show that leprosy is a zoonosis in the southern United States and that armadillos can be involved in transmitting *M. leprae* to humans.[80] Using a combination of single nucleotide polymorphism analysis with variable number tandem repeat genotyping, a single unique *M. leprae* genotypic-strain (3I-2-v1) was found to occur among 88% of the wild armadillos sampled in a 400,000 square mile area in the southern United States. Multiple *M. leprae* genotypic-strains were identified to be circulating among human patients in the United States, an observation consistent with leprosy having been introduced here from a variety of regions. However, this unique 3I-2-v1 strain that predominates among armadillos also was found among 64% of the patient samples studied, and appeared to be the primary strain for endemic human infection in the southern United States. In addition, presentation with the 3I-2-v1 strain was significantly associated with a patient's residence history in areas where *M. leprae*-infected armadillos are found and several patients reported taking armadillos for food or having other direct contact with the animals. Where enzootic infection can be confirmed, education about armadillos as a potential risk factor for leprosy could have tremendous impact on the health of many individuals.

Manifestations of Leprosy in Armadillos

Clinical Manifestations

Armadillos exhibit few overt signs of clinical disease. A large portion of the armadillo's body is covered with armor and skin lesions are not easily seen.[110] Abrasions around the eyes, nose and feet are the most common signs but are also somewhat nonspecific. In the laboratory, plantar ulceration is common in the later stages of infection (Figs 13.4A and B). Although *M. leprae* has no toxins and is not life-threatening in man, infected armadillos develop profound anemia with compromised liver and renal functions, and eventually will succumb to secondary complications of persistent bacteremia, if not humanely sacrificed.[111] Although reticuloendothelial tissues become the most heavily burdened, nearly every major organ system will be invaded and involvement of neural tissues is demonstrable at even the earliest stages of disease.

Immunological and Histopathological Spectrum

Humans and armadillos exhibit the full immunological and histopathological spectrum of leprosy, ranging from the polar extremes of tuberculoid (TT) and LL with indistinct borderline forms in between.[112] Individual responses can be predicted by intradermal injection of *M. leprae* antigens (lepromin) in a Mitsuda reaction.[113,114] Although 70% of armadillos manifest a LL-type of response to *M. leprae*, some animals produce polar TT or borderline forms of disease.[115,116] However, the type of leprosy that each animal might manifest seems to have no relationship to their differing environmental exposures and appears to be innate. As animals with the LL form are more likely to develop heavy burdens of bacilli, they are the ones more commonly selected for *in vivo* propagation of *M. leprae* and have been the most studied.

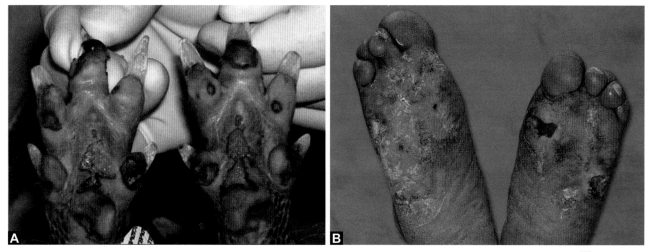

Figs 13.4A and B: Plantar ulcerations are similar in (A) Armadillos; and (B) Humans

Genetic Susceptibility

Contrary to what is seen among humans, the vast majority of armadillos appear to be susceptible to infection with *M. leprae*. However, a reliable percentage (~15–20%) of the animals readily resists challenge.[111] There is a clear genetic association for susceptibility to *M. leprae* among humans, and a number of gene sequence polymorphisms have been identified that appear to be associated with susceptibility to leprosy as well as to the type of leprosy that an individual might manifest.[85,117-119] Studies with armadillos show that quadruplet siblings and their mothers respond similarly to infection with *M. leprae*. Also, *M. leprae*-resistant armadillos share single nucleotide polymorphisms in toll-like receptors (TLR) at similar locations that were associated to leprosy resistance in humans.[31]

Neurological Involvement and Pathogenesis

Beyond sharing a unique susceptibility to *M. leprae*, the most important feature of leprosy in humans and armadillos is that they both develop extensive neurological involvement with *M. leprae*. Although known as the causative agent of leprosy for more than a century, little is known about the pathophysiology of the underlying nerve damage. It likely involves a complicated interplay of both host inflammatory and bacterial-mediated events[120,121] and a major impediment to our understanding is obtaining suitable tissues for study. Leprotic lesions are highly focal and usually distributed asymmetrically over the body.[122,123] Ethical and practical limitations make it almost impossible to biopsy affected human nerves. When fresh samples can be obtained, they rarely contain a lesion and those derived from amputated limbs are generally not suitable for detailed molecular analysis.[124] An effective animal model would greatly facilitate progress in

this area, but the most common laboratory animals (i.e. rat, rabbit, guinea pig, etc.) are naturally resistant to *M. leprae*. Although *M. leprae* does replicate when inoculated into the FPs of mice, the infection exhibits no nerve involvement. Only the nine-banded armadillo reliably exhibits extensive neurological involvement upon infection with *M. leprae*.

M. leprae manifests in armadillos as a systemically disseminated infection with similar structural and pathological changes as observed in tissues and nerves of human leprosy patients. Marked inflammation with bacilli attached to the progressively demyelinating SCs can be observed on histopathological inspection of infected armadillo nerves and a functional deficit can be demonstrated in leprotic nerves using electrophysiology.[120]

Armadillos are susceptible to experimental infection with *M. leprae* by a variety of routes, including intravenous, intradermal, percutaneous, and respiratory instillation.[111,125] In addition, many armadillo nerve trunks are sufficiently large as to permit direct inoculation of bacilli to the peripheral nerve. Regardless of the route of administration, the disease outcome in the animals depends on that particular animal's innate or pre-existing response to *M. leprae*. LL-type armadillos will eventually develop a fully disseminated infection, while the level and type of involvement will be less with animals that manifest other forms of leprosy.

The duration of infection in the armadillo is somewhat idiosyncratic but is mainly a factor of the viable challenge dose of bacilli given. Standard challenge dose is 1×10^9 highly viable *M. leprae* given intravenously. At this dose, most animals will develop a fully disseminated infection requiring humane sacrifice within 18–24 months. Prolific quantities of bacilli accumulate throughout the animal's reticuloendothelial organs and up to 10^{12} *M. leprae* can be harvested from the tissues of a single animal. Lower challenge doses require accordingly longer periods to manifest full dissemination.[39] Of course, studies addressing events of preclinical leprosy do not require fully disseminated infections and can be initiated immediately, following a challenge.

A notable advantage of the armadillo is the opportunity to examine the pathogenesis of infection at preclinical stages that have never been observed in humans and which are more likely to be effectively targeted by therapeutic intervention. Following experimental infection of armadillos, *M. leprae* populates the peripheral nerves and reticuloendothelial tissues, and slowly disseminates systemically from these early foci. The armadillo post-tibial nerve runs just beneath the skin surface of the medial aspect of the hind limb between the ankle and the knee. This nerve has a high frequency of involvement in both armadillo and human infections. It is easily accessible in the armadillo and is a useful target for studies in armadillos. Although the duration of experimental infection in armadillos (4–24 months) is highly compressed as compared to the many years involved in human infections, bacillary loads of more than or equal to 10^6 *M. leprae*/cm of the length of the post-tibial nerve are common in armadillos. Armadillo peripheral nerves are infected early in the disease process. Histopathological examination reveals characteristic interstitial neuritis with infiltration of inflammatory cells, such as macrophages and bacilli, in the perineurium, epineurium and endoneurium (Figs 13.5A and B). Quantitative estimation of bacilli in infected nerves shows higher bacterial loads and increased involvement distally. Estimates of more than 1×10^6 *M. leprae*/cm of some major nerves are not uncommon, and both sensory and motor neurons are involved.[120,126,127]

Once *M. leprae* populates the nerve, bacilli can grow to high numbers and spread to adjacent nerve trunks. Antileprosy drug therapies must have good neural penetration in order to kill bacilli sequestered in nerves.

However, even once effectively killed by the antimicrobial drugs, humans and armadillos show only slow clearance of bacilli from nerves and skin lesions. In one study, 10 *M. leprae* infected armadillos were allowed to incubate their infections for 12 months before five of them were treated with 10 mg/kg Rifampin, once monthly, for an additional 12 months. All animals and an additional five naïve controls were later sacrificed at 24 months postinfection. Although each of the treated animals showed clinical improvement in skin lesions and ulcers, as a result of the antimicrobial therapy, examination of their post-tibial nerves showed continued presence of *M. leprae*. Molecular assessment of *M. leprae* viability suggested the organisms had been effectively killed by Rifampin therapy. However, bacterial counts averaging 10^4–10^5 bacilli/cm of post-tibial nerve were still observed even after the conclusion of a full year of treatment. This heavy burden of (dead) bacilli provides a rich substrate for continued immunological interaction with the host and suggests there is insidious chronic injury to nerves involved with *M. leprae*.

Although there are no comparable human studies, armadillo nerve segments can be used effectively for gene expression profiling and analysis of cell signaling pathways. The gene expression profiles can be compared between uninfected-normal nerves, and infected-untreated or infected-Rifampin-treated armadillo post-tibial nerves with a broad array of neural specific markers. On examining the nerves described above, the gene expression profiles reflected ongoing degeneration and regeneration processes among the infected animals when compared to the naïve controls, along with evidence of persistent inflammation with enhanced expression of both IFNγ and TNF (Fig. 13.6). Though gene expression among treated animals was somewhat lower than those of the animals suffering active infection, the gene

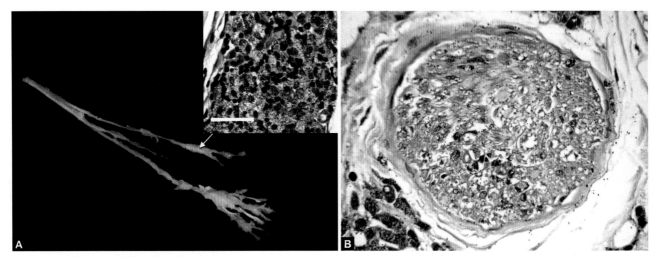

Figs 13.5A and B: (A) Invasion of armadillo nerves by *M. leprae*; (B) Histopathological examination reveals interstitial neuritis with infiltration of inflammatory cells and bacilli in the perineurium, epineurium, and endoneurium

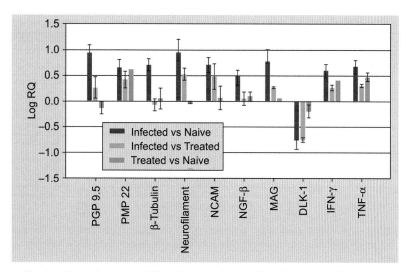

Fig. 13.6: Gene expression profiles in naïve, infected and Rifampin treated armadillos. Expression of molecular markers associated with nerve structure and function [PGP9.5 (UCHL1), PMP 22, β-tubulin, neurofilament, NCAM], growth factors (NGF-β MAG and DLK-1) and inflammation (TNF and IFNγ) was compared between armadillo post-tibial nerves harvested from 1) naïve: uninfected-normal, 2) infected untreated animals and 3) treated, infected animals that had received 12 months of Rifampin treatment. Data was normalized using GAP3DH and relative expression was computed by using the ΔΔCt method. Results represent mean ± SD from duplicate experiments on five animals in each group

expression profiles of nerve segments from Rifampin treated animals more closely resembled those of the untreated animals over the naïve controls (Fig. 13.6). The slow clearance of killed bacilli can be problematic for nerve injury. Molecular markers for neurodegeneration and regeneration, along with gene expression profile of inflammatory genes, and enumeration of the bacterial load of *M. leprae* in the nerve are useful therapeutic end-points for laboratory studies and highlight the importance of developing new therapies to enhance clearance of bacilli from the host in conjunction with antibacterial treatment in order to limit the progress of insidious neuropathy.

Electrophysiological Studies

Armadillos do not reliably respond to thermal, light or tactile nociceptive stimulants, but measurements of nerve conduction can be used effectively to assess function of armadillo motor nerves. Although their hard carapace and thick skin limit the number of nerves that can be examined, techniques have been adapted to permit assessment of conduction in both hind limbs along the post-tibial nerve that lies just beneath the skin surface between the ankle and knee, and innervates the small lumbrical and flexor muscles of each foot. Nerve conduction studies are noninvasive, and are ideal for repeated or prospective assessments studying the onset and progress of peripheral neuropathy over time in the same subject. Normal armadillos exhibit conduction profiles similar to humans [mean nerve conduction velocity (NCV) 62.09 ± 10.72 m/s, mean compound motor action potential

(CMAP) 1.55 ± 0.33 mV]. Peripheral conduction deficit among *M. leprae*-infected armadillos begins early in the course of their disease and progresses over time. Demyelination of axons results in decreased NCV measured in m/s, and loss of axons and muscular atrophy leads to a decrease in the CMAP measured in mV.[128] Conduction deficit is observed in the post-tibial nerves of 75% of all experimentally infected armadillos with onset occurring as early as 90 days postinfection. Similar to observations on humans, depressed CMAP amplitude [< 0.9 mV, mean ± 2 standard deviation (SD)] is the most common presentation, but abnormal NCV (NCV <40 m/s, mean ± 2 SD) also can be observed (Figs 13.7A to C). Most armadillos progress from normal conduction to a total conduction block by the last stages of their experimentally induced infections with *M. leprae*. Onset of conduction abnormality generally coincides with evolution of a detectable immune response to *M. leprae* [e.g. detectable phenolic glycolipid 1 (PGL1) immunoglobulin M (IgM) antibodies] and is a significant predictor of other nonspecific symptoms of neuropathy, such as foot ulcers, and nail avulsion or hypertrophy.[125] In observations of more than 175 different armadillos, nearly all of the animals that developed a conduction deficit also eventually exhibited signs of clinical neuropathy in their FPs. Increased PGL1 antibody level and decreased CMAP also were highly correlated with the clinical appearance of wounds under heavy calluses, hypertrophic nails ($p < 0.03$) and nail avulsion ($p < 0.008$, r = 0.2–0.26). In addition, the involved flexor and lumbrical muscles of infected armadillos evidenced atrophy and showed a 20% average decrease in physiological cross-sectional areas ($p < 0.02$). Unfortunately,

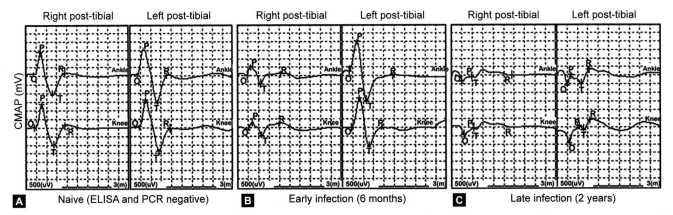

Figs 13.7A to C: Representative wave forms illustrating progressive nerve conduction deficit in compound motor action potential (CMAP; mV; y-axis) leading to complete conduction block in late infection. The upper lines show responses to stimulation at the ankle, and the lower ones to the knee

their hard carapace and thick skin limit the number of nerves that may be examined in armadillos, and sensory nerve conduction profiles have not yet been successful. However, other histopathological techniques can be substituted effectively.

Epidermal Nerve Fiber and Schwann Cell Density

The morphological and quantitative study of skin biopsy offers an alternative tool to assess thin nerve fiber structure related to the thermal sensitivity function. Immunostaining of punch skin biopsies for protein gene product 9.5 (PGP9.5), a neuronal pan axonal marker, has now been used by several investigators to visualize the intraepidermal nerve fibers, dermal nerves and SCs in lieu of nerve conduction tests which may fail to detect small nerve fiber impairment. The small fiber innervation is length dependent and robust normative data for epidermal nerve fiber densities (ENFD) in the distal limb have been developed.[129] In small fiber sensory neuropathies associated with diabetes, HIV and idiopathic small fiber sensory neuropathies, a decrease in epidermal density in the distal leg has been demonstrated.[130-133] Abnormalities have been demonstrated in cutaneous innervations, even in individuals with normal tendon reflexes at the ankles, normal sural nerve action potential amplitudes and normal quantitative sensory tests.[134] Although leprosy neuritis has been well-described clinically and histologically, the underlying mechanisms of nerve damage remain poorly understood and very little morphological work has been done to detect early damage to sensory nerves.

Quantitation of epidermal nerve fibers in skin biopsies of ears, abdomen and distal leg of naïve armadillos has shown a length dependent innervation similar to humans, and the infected animal showed a lower mean ENFD compared to naïve animals suggesting early small fiber degeneration.[135] Double staining of cutaneous axons and SCs in naïve

armadillos also mimicked the human cutaneous nerve network pattern. SCs of dermal cutaneous nerves in infected armadillos showed a trend towards increasing density and thus provide indirect evidence that during early infection SCs undergo proliferation while harboring *M. leprae*. Though this difference was not significant statistically, they affirm the feasibility of studying small fibers in the armadillo using this technique and the possibility of using it as a novel tool to test new drugs, and in therapeutic interventions.

Impairment of Muscle Architecture and Function in Infected Armadillos

A common pathological hallmark of human leprosy and *M. leprae*-infected armadillos is the involvement of extremities. In the foot, the lumbrical muscles are innervated by the medial and lateral plantar nerves and these nerves are similarly involved in some leprosy patients. Muscle paralysis can result from injury to these nerves and the pathological status of lumbrical muscles from the armadillo hind limb has been examined.

The organization of intact muscle architecture can be evaluated by labeling muscle tissues with antibodies to adult myosin, a family of adenosine triphosphate (ATP)-dependent, actin-binding and highly conserved muscle motor proteins. Antibodies specific for myosin heavy chain (HC) that react with mature myofibrils can be used to detect the myosin distribution and architecture of lumbrical muscles. Labeling of transverse sections of control armadillo muscles showed a highly organized architecture of muscle fibers with clear endomysium and perimysium, similar to human and rodent skeletal muscle.[135] In contrast lumbrical muscles from infected animals displayed a markedly disorganized pattern of muscle fibers with disorganized endomysium and perimysium. Analysis of transverse sections of lumbrical muscles with antibodies specific for basal lamina components, laminin and collagen, showed markedly disrupted and abnormal extracellular matrix expression in infected muscles as compared to control animals. Nuclear labeling revealed an increased accumulation of cells in the muscle, most likely mononuclear inflammatory cells or macrophages. In uninfected animals, nuclear labeling was found only adjacent to individual muscle fibers, which is similar to normal adult mouse and human muscles. Furthermore, the distribution of *M. leprae* within the lumbrical muscles in infected animals was studied using antibody to *M. leprae* PGL1 that specifically detects whole *M. leprae*.[136] These data revealed that *M. leprae* were predominantly localized to cells in the interstitial tissues in the perimysium, most likely within the infiltrated cells.

In agreement with these findings, functional studies also showed that the small lumbrical and flexor muscles of the armadillo foot have early involvement with *M. leprae*. Brand[137] showed that the physiological cross-sectional area (PCSA)/mass of muscles in the hands of leprosy patients could be used as a surrogate measure of grip strength and index muscle atrophy. Examining the PCSA of armadillo small (intrinsic) lumbrical and flexor muscles shows a qualitative reduction of muscle mass among infected armadillos, with PGL1 IgM positive animals having an average of 20% less muscle mass than naïve normal animals.[135] Detailed histopathological studies showed that long-term infection in the armadillo also has discernible effect on the morphological and molecular composition of skeletal muscle fibers. These features in skeletal muscles in infected armadillos resemble muscle pathology and function impairment documented in patients with LL leprosy with high bacterial load[138] suggesting the potential of using the armadillo model not only for neuropathies but also myopathies associated with human leprosy.

Diagnosis/Immunological Response

Development of early diagnostic methods is a major priority in leprosy research. However, efforts to generate new assays are complicated by the low frequency of susceptibility to leprosy in most human populations, the extraordinarily long incubation period of leprosy and our inability to discern which individuals in a population may be incubating subclinical infections. The compressed nature of *M. leprae* infection in armadillos allows both cross-sectional and prospective cohort studies, as well as a clear understanding about the actual susceptibility of the individuals under study based on known challenge results. Early serological studies using the *M. leprae*-specific PGL-1 antigen confirmed its high specificity among armadillos and showed that experimentally infected armadillos produce a detectable IgM response beginning only about 6 months postexperimental infection. These antibodies remained detectable over the course of disease and the titer generally correlated with the load of *M. leprae* in the animal's reticuloendothelial tissues.[97,139-141] More recent studies using the new leprosy Infectious Disease Research

Institute (IDRI) diagnostic (LID)-1 antigen also confirmed excellent specificity in infection among armadillos and found mainly an IgG-type response among armadillos, suggesting that a combination of the two antigens might enhance serological detection of *M. leprae* infections.[142] Similarly, IFNγ release assays have been piloted in experimentally infected armadillos. The *M. leprae*-specifc proteins ML0009, ML1601, ML2478 and ML2531 antigens induced significant IFNγ levels in PBMCs from *M. leprae* infected armadillos when compared to naïve controls.[143] These findings suggest that in addition to serological responses, even lepromatous hosts with significant exposure to *M. leprae* may have discernible cell-mediated immune responses that can be exploited for diagnostic purposes. Experimentally infected armadillos are challenged with very high numbers of bacilli for *in vivo* propagation of *M. leprae*. These artificially high challenge doses may skew some immunological responses and their immune profile may not be entirely representative of a natural infection. However, in addition to experimentally infected armadillos in the laboratory, free-ranging armadillos in some regions also are known to harbor a natural infection with *M. leprae* and they too may be exploited as population models for diagnostic development.

Limitations of the Armadillo Model

Armadillos are exotic animals and are not commonly used in laboratory studies outside of leprosy research. The primary limitation in use of armadillos is the paucity of reagents, especially antibodies, to facilitate investigations. However, with recent completion of the armadillo whole genomic sequence, investigative reagents can be generated more easily and specific antibodies and molecular probes and primers[143-145] can be designed. Of course, all of these reagents require independent development and verification of their quality.

Armadillos are not available from standard commercial vendors and must be obtained from the wild for investigative purposes. Some institutional animal care and use committees or animal facilities may not be equipped to deal with wild animals. In addition, such wild animals are highly outbred and may exhibit wide variations in response to challenge. Armadillos do not breed reliably in captivity. However, female armadillos routinely give birth to monozygotic quadruplicates and gravid females captured from the wild will litter in captivity making it possible to conduct studies on matched sets of identical twins.[110]

CONCLUSION

Effective animal models can help provide pivotal new understandings about the mechanisms involved in complex disease processes, such as those manifested in leprosy. Both the mouse and armadillo models provide large numbers of highly viable *M. leprae* for experimental use from a controlled and known infection status. Mice, with their ease of use, availability of an abundance of biological reagents, numerous genetically defined strains and readily assessable granulomatous FP lesion, are ideal for studying basic immunological parameters of infection. For many years, they have also proven useful for the evaluation of potential new antileprosy drugs and to determine experimental vaccine efficacy. With armadillos, comparative pathological studies have shown that many of the functional, physiological and structural aspects of human leprosy are closely recapitulated, but with a compressed disease duration. Other than humans, the nine-banded armadillo is the only animal that develops extensive neurological involvement with *M. leprae* and they are an abundant source of leprotic neurological fibers for basic science investigations. Rare neurological events in both normal and leprotic tissues, from time periods and in material quantities that cannot be obtained from human subjects, can be studied. Developing techniques to effectively detect, and monitor the onset and progress of leprosy neuropathy could have significant benefit to leprosy patients. Together, these models yield often complementary information and can provide insights for developing new intervention strategies.

REFERENCES

1. Johnstone PA. The search for animal models of leprosy. Int J Lepr Other Mycobact Dis. 1987;55(3):535-47.
2. Shepard CC. The experimental disease that follows the injection of human leprosy bacilli into foot-pads of mice. J Exp Med. 1960;112(3):445-54.
3. Kirchheimer WF, Storrs EE. Attempts to establish the armadillo (*Dasypus novemcinctus* Linn.) as a model for the study of leprosy. I. Report of lepromatoid leprosy in an experimentally infected armadillo. Int J Lepr Other Mycobact Dis. 1971;39(3):693-702.
4. Shepard CC. Multiplication of *Mycobacterium leprae* in the foot-pad of the mouse. Int J Lepr. 1962;30:291-306.
5. Rees RJ. Limited multiplication of acid-fast bacilli in the foot-pads of mice inoculated with *Mycobacterium leprae*. Br J Exp Pathol. 1964;45:207-18.
6. Pattyn SR. Comparative behaviour of a strain of *M. leprae* in 5 different mouse strains and in thymectomized mice. Zentralbl Bakteriol Orig. 1965;197(2):256-8.
7. Welch TM, Gelber RH, Murray LP, et al. Viability of *Mycobacterium leprae* after multiplication in mice. Infect Immun. 1980;30(2):325-8.
8. Rees RJ. Enhanced susceptibility of thymectomized and irradiated mice to infection with *Mycobacterium leprae*. Nature. 1966;211(5049):657-8.
9. Ebenezer GJ, Arumugam S, Job CK. Dosage and site of entry influence growth and dissemination of *Mycobacterium leprae* in T900r mice. Int J Lepr Other Mycobact Dis. 2002;70(4):245-9.
10. Colston MJ, Hilson GR. Growth of *Mycobacterium leprae* and *M. marinum* in congenitally athymic (nude) mice. Nature. 1976;262(5567):399-401.
11. Dawson PJ, Colston MJ, Fieldsteel AH. Infection of the congenitally athymic rat with *Mycobacterium leprae*. Int J Lepr Other Mycobact Dis. 1983;51(3):336-46.
12. Chehl S, Ruby J, Job CK, et al. The growth of *Mycobacterium leprae* in nude mice. Lepr Rev. 1983;54(4):283-304.
13. Yogi Y, Nakamura K, Inoue T, et al. Susceptibility of severe combined immunodeficient (SCID) mice to *Mycobacterium leprae*: multiplication of the bacillus and dissemination of the infection at early stage. Nihon Rai Gakkai Zasshi. 1991;60(3-4):139-45.
14. Azouaou N, Gelber RH, Abel K, et al. Reconstitution of *Mycobacterium leprae* immunity in severe combined immunodeficient mice using a T-cell line. Int J Lepr Other Mycobact Dis. 1993;61(3):398-405.
15. Ishaque M, Sticht-Groh V. Experimental transmission of human leprosy bacilli in foot pads of severe combined immunodeficient mice. Int J Lepr Other Mycobact Dis. 1994;62(4):613-4.
16. Truman RW, Krahenbuhl JL. Viable M. leprae as a research reagent. Int J Lepr Other Mycobact Dis. 2001;69(1):1-12.
17. Shetty VP. Animal model to study the mechanism of nerve damage in leprosy—a preliminary report. Int J Lepr Other Mycobact Dis. 1993;61(1):70-5.
18. Birdi TJ, Shetty VP, Antia NH. Differences in *M. leprae*-induced nerve damage in Swiss white and C57BL/6 mice. Int J Lepr Other Mycobact Dis. 1995;63(4): 573-4.
19. Shetty VP, Mistry NF, Birdi TJ, Antia NH. Effect of T-cell depletion on bacterial multiplication and pattern of nerve damage in *M. leprae*-infected mice. Indian J Lepr. 1995;67(4):363-74.
20. Shetty VP, Matharu PS, Antia NH. Sciatic nerve of normal and T200x5R Swiss white mice fails to support multiplication of intraneurally injected *M. leprae*. Int J Lepr Other Mycobact Dis. 1999;67(4):446-52.
21. Rambukkana A, Zanazzi G, Tapinos N, et al. Contact-dependent demyelination by *Mycobacterium leprae* in the absence of immune cells. Science. 2002;296(5569):927-31.
22. Baldwin TM, Elso C, Curtis J, et al. The site of leishmania major infection determines disease severity and immune responses. Infect Immun. 2003;71(12):6830-4.
23. Duthie MS, Reece ST, Lahiri R, et al. Antigen-specific cellular and humoral responses are induced by intradermal *Mycobacterium leprae* infection of the mouse ear. Infect Immun. 2007;75(11):5290-7.
24. Berman B, Chen VL, France DS, et al. Anatomical mapping of epidermal Langerhans cell densities in adults. Br J Dermatol. 1983;109(5):553-8.
25. Raman VS, O'Donnell J, Bailor HR, et al. Vaccination with the ML0276 antigen reduces local inflammation but not bacterial burden during experimental *Mycobacterium leprae* infection. Infect Immun. 2009;77(12):5623-30.
26. Evans MJ, Levy L. Ultrastructural changes in cells of the mouse footpad infected with *Mycobacterium leprae*. Infect Immun. 1972;5(2):238-47.
27. Rees RJ, Weddell AG, Palmer E, et al. Human leprosy in normal mice. Br Med J. 1969;3(5664):216-7.
28. Hagge DA, Ray NA, Krahenbuhl JL, et al. An in vitro model for the lepromatous leprosy granuloma: fate of *Mycobacterium leprae* from target macrophages after interaction with normal and activated effector macrophages. J Immunol. 2004;172(12):7771-9.
29. Krahenbuhl J, Adams LB. Exploitation of gene knockout mice models to study the pathogenesis of leprosy. Lepr Rev. 2000;71 Suppl:S170-5.

30. Cooper AM, Adams LB, Dalton DK, et al. IFN-gamma and NO in mycobacterial disease: new jobs for old hands. Trends Microbiol. 2002;10(5):221-6.

31. Adams LB, Pena MT, Sharma R, et al. Insights from animal models on the immunogenetics of leprosy: a review. Mem Inst Oswaldo Cruz. 2012;107 Suppl 1:197-208.

32. Adams LB, Scollard DM, Ray NA, et al. The study of *Mycobacterium leprae* infection in interferon-gamma gene-disrupted mice as a model to explore the immunopathologic spectrum of leprosy. J Infect Dis. 2002;185 Suppl 1:S1-8.

33. Hagge DA, Saunders BM, Ebenezer GJ, et al. Lymphotoxin-alpha and TNF have essential but independent roles in the evolution of the granulomatous response in experimental leprosy. Am J Pathol. 2009;174(4):1379-89.

34. Hagge DA, Marks VT, Ray NA, et al. Emergence of an effective adaptive cell mediated immune response to *Mycobacterium leprae* is not impaired in reactive oxygen intermediate-deficient mice. FEMS Immunol Med Microbiol. 2007;51(1):92-101.

35. Adams LB, Job CK, Krahenbuhl JL. Role of inducible nitric oxide synthase in resistance to *Mycobacterium leprae* in mice. Infect Immun. 2000;68(9):5462-5.

36. Shepard CC, McRae DH. A method for counting acid-fast bacteria. Int J Lepr Other Mycobact Dis. 1968;36(1):78-82.

37. Krushat WM, Schilling KE, Edlavitch SA, et al. Studies of the mouse foot-pad technique for cultivation of *Mycobacterium leprae*. 4. Statistical analysis of harvest data. Lepr Rev. 1976;47(4):275-86.

38. Woods SA, Cole ST. A family of dispersed repeats in *Mycobacterium leprae*. Mol Microbiol. 1990;4(10):1745-51.

39. Truman RW, Andrews PK, Robbins NY, et al. Enumeration of *Mycobacterium leprae* using real-time PCR. PLoS Negl Trop Dis. 2008;2(11):e328.

40. Ridley DS. The morphological index. Lepr Rev. 1971;42(2):75-7.

41. Silva MT, Macedo PM, Portaels F, et al. Correlation viability/morphology in *Mycobacterium leprae*. Acta Leprol. 1984;2(2-4):281-91.

42. Harshan KV, Mittal A, Prasad HK, et al. Uptake of purine and pyrimidine nucleosides by macrophage-resident *Mycobacterium leprae*: ^{3}H-adenosine as an indicator of viability and antimicrobial activity. Int J Lepr Other Mycobact Dis. 1990;58(3):526-33.

43. Wiese M, Lindner B, Seydel U. Development of an in vitro drug screening system for *Mycobacterium leprae* based on the determination of the intrabacterial sodium to potassium ratio of individual bacterial organisms. Int J Antimicrob Agents. 1994;4(4):271-9.

44. Katoch VM, Katoch K, Ramu G, et al. In vitro methods for determination of viability of mycobacteria: comparison of ATP content, morphological index and FDA-EB fluorescent staining in *Mycobacterium leprae*. Lepr Rev. 1988;59(2):137-43.

45. Gupta UD, Katoch K, Natarajan M, et al. Viability determination of M. leprae: comparison of normal mouse foot pad and bacillary ATP bioluminescence assay. Acta Leprol. 1997;10(4):209-12.

46. Franzblau SG. Oxidation of palmitic acid by *Mycobacterium leprae* in an axenic medium. J Clin Microbiol. 1988;26(1):18-21.

47. Ramasesh N, Adams LB, Franzblau SG, et al. Effects of activated macrophages on *Mycobacterium leprae*. Infect Immun. 1991;59(9):2864-9.

48. Kvach JT, Munguia G, Strand SH. Staining tissue-derived *Mycobacterium leprae* with fluorescein diacetate and ethidium bromide. Int J Lepr Other Mycobact Dis. 1984;52(2):176-82.

49. Odinsen O, Nilson T, Humber DP. Viability of *Mycobacterium leprae*: a comparison of morphological index and fluorescent staining techniques in slit-skin smears and M. leprae suspensions. Int J Lepr Other Mycobact Dis. 1986;54(3):403-8.

50. Lahiri R, Randhawa B, Krahenbuhl J. Application of a viability-staining method for *Mycobacterium leprae* derived from the athymic (nu/nu) mouse foot pad. J Med Microbiol. 2005; 54(Pt 3):235-42.

51. Davis GL, Ray NA, Lahiri R, et al. Molecular assays for determining *Mycobacterium leprae* viability in tissues of experimentally infected mice. PLoS Negl Trop Dis. 2013;7(8):e2404.

52. Martinez AN, Lahiri R, Pittman TL, et al. Molecular determination of *Mycobacterium leprae* viability by use of real-time PCR. J Clin Microbiol. 2009;47(7):2124-30.

53. Shepard CC, Chang YT. Effect of several anti-leprosy drugs on multiplication of human leprosy bacilli in footpads of mice. Proc Soc Exp Biol Med. 1962;109:636-8.

54. Colston MJ, Hilson GR, Banerjee DK. The "proportional bactericidal test": a method for assessing bactericidal activity in drugs against *Mycobacterium leprae* in mice. Lepr Rev. 1978;49(1):7-15.

55. Ji B, Jamet P, Perani EG, et al. Powerful bactericidal activities of clarithromycin and minocycline against *Mycobacterium leprae* in lepromatous leprosy. J Infect Dis. 1993;168(1):188-90.

56. Ji B, Jamet P, Perani EG, et al. Bactericidal activity of single dose of clarithromycin plus minocycline, with or without ofloxacin, against *Mycobacterium leprae* in patients. Antimicrob Agents Chemother. 1996;40(9):2137-41.

57. Ji B, Sow S, Perani E, et al. Bactericidal activity of a single-dose combination of ofloxacin plus minocycline, with or without rifampin, against *Mycobacterium leprae* in mice and in lepromatous patients. Antimicrob Agents Chemother. 1998;42(5):1115-20.

58. Shepard CC. Further experience with the kinetic method for the study of drugs against *Mycobacterium leprae* in mice. Activities of DDS, DFD, ethionamide, capreomycin and PAM 1392. Int J Lepr Other Mycobact Dis. 1969;37(4):389-97.

59. Shepard CC, Walker LL, van Landingham M, et al. Kinetic testing of drugs against *Mycobacterium leprae* in mice. Activity of cephaloridine, rifampin, streptovaricin, vadrine, and viomycin. Am J Trop Med Hyg. 1971;20(4):616-20.

60. Zhang M, Li SY, Rosenthal IM, et al. Treatment of tuberculosis with rifamycin-containing regimens in immune-deficient mice. Am J Respir Crit Care Med. 2011;183(9):1254-61.

61. Chapuis L, Ji B, Truffot-Pernot C, et al. Preventive therapy of tuberculosis with rifapentine in immunocompetent and nude mice. Am J Respir Crit Care Med. 1994;150(5 Pt 1):1355-62.

62. Shetty VP, Wakade AV, Ghate S, et al. Viability and drug susceptibility testing of M. leprae using mouse footpad in 37 relapse cases of leprosy. Int J Lepr Other Mycobact Dis. 2003;71(3):210-7.

63. Williams DL, Gillis TP. Drug-resistant leprosy: monitoring and current status. Lepr Rev. 2012;83(3):269-81.

64. Cambau E, Chauffour-Nevejans A, Tejmar-Kolar L, et al. Detection of antibiotic resistance in leprosy using genotype leprae DR, a novel ready-to-use molecular test. PLoS Negl Trop Dis. 2012;6(7):e1739.

65. da Silva Rocha A, Cunha MD, Diniz LM, et al. Drug and multidrug resistance among *Mycobacterium leprae* isolates

from Brazilian relapsed leprosy patients. J Clin Microbiol. 2012;50(6):1912-7.

66. Williams DL, Hagino T, Sharma R, et al. Primary multidrug-resistant leprosy, United States. Emerg Infect Dis. 2013;19(1):179-81.

67. Shepard CC. Vaccination against experimental infection with *Mycobacterium leprae*. Am J Epidemiol. 1965;81:150-63.

68. Ngamying M, Sawanpanyalert P, Butraporn R, et al. Effect of vaccination with refined components of the organism on infection of mice with *Mycobacterium leprae*. Infect Immun. 2003;71(3):1596-8.

69. Duthie MS, Sampaio LH, Oliveira RM, et al. Development and pre-clinical assessment of a 73kD chimeric fusion protein as a defined sub-unit vaccine for leprosy. Vaccine. 2013;31(5):813-9.

70. Lahiri R, Randhawa B, Franken KL, et al. Development of a mouse food pad model for detection of sub clinical leprosy. Lepr Rev. 2011;82(4):432-44.

71. Spencer JS, Kim HJ, Wheat WH, et al. Analysis of antibody responses to *Mycobacterium leprae* phenolic glycolipid I, lipoarabinomannan, and recombinant proteins to define disease subtype-specific antigenic profiles in leprosy. Clin Vaccine Immunol. 2011;18(2):260-7.

72. Sampaio LH, Stefani MM, Oliveira RM, et al. Immunologically reactive *M. leprae* antigens with relevance to diagnosis and vaccine development. BMC Infect Dis. 2011;11:26.

73. Liu B, Liu S, Qu X, et al. Construction of a eukaryotic expression system for granulysin and its protective effect in mice infected with *Mycobacterium tuberculosis*. J Med Microbiol. 2006;55(Pt 10):1389-93.

74. Moody DB, Besra GS, Wilson IA, et al. The molecular basis of CD1-mediated presentation of lipid antigens. Immunol Rev. 1999;172:285-96.

75. Adams LB, Franzblau SG, Vavrin Z, et al. L-arginine-dependent macrophage effector functions inhibit metabolic activity of *Mycobacterium leprae*. J Immunol. 1991;147(5):1642-6.

76. Chan J, Xing Y, Magliozzo RS, et al. Killing of virulent Mycobacterium tuberculosis by reactive nitrogen intermediates produced by activated murine macrophages. J Exp Med. 1992;175(4):1111-22.

77. Weinberg JB, Misukonis MA, Shami PJ, et al. Human mononuclear phagocyte inducible nitric oxide synthase (iNOS): analysis of iNOS mRNA, iNOS protein, biopterin, and nitric oxide production by blood monocytes and peritoneal macrophages. Blood. 1995;86(3):1184-95.

78. Jung JY, Madan-Lala R, Georgieva M, et al. The intracellular environment of human macrophages that produce nitric oxide promotes growth of mycobacteria. Infect Immun. 2013;81(9):3198-209.

79. Kamath AB, Woodworth J, Xiong X, et al. Cytolytic CD8+ T-cells recognizing CFP10 are recruited to the lung after *Mycobacterium tuberculosis* infection. J Exp Med. 2004;200(11):1479-89.

80. Truman RW, Singh P, Sharma R, et al. Probable zoonotic leprosy in the southern United States. N Engl J Med. 2011;364(17):1626-33.

81. Talmage RV, Buchanen CD. The armadillo (Dasypus novemcinctus). A review of its natural history, ecology, anatomy, and reproductive physiology. In: Monograph in Biology, Vol. 2. Houston: The Rice Institute; 1954. pp. 1-135.

82. Balina LM, Valdez RP, De-Herrera M, et al. Experimental reproduction of leprosy in dasypus-hybridus. Rev Argent Dermatol. 1985;66:7-12.

83. Taulman JF, Robbins LW. Recent range expansion and distributional limits of the nine-banded armadillo (*Dasypus novemcinctus*) in the United States. J Biogeog. 1996;23(5):635-48.

84. Storrs EE, Williams RJ. A study of monozygous quadruplet armadillos in relation to mammalian inheritance. Proc Natl Acad Sci USA. 1968;60(3):910-4.

85. Alter A, Grant A, Abel L, et al. Leprosy as a genetic disease. Mamm Genome. 2011;22(1-2):19-31.

86. Misch EA, Berrington WR, Vary JC, et al. Leprosy and the human genome. Microbiol Mol Biol Rev. 2010;74(4):589-620.

87. MacDonald DW. The encyclopedia of mammals. New York: Oxford University Press; 1985.

88. Loughry WJ, Dwyer GM. Behavioral interactions between juvenile nine-banded armadillos (*Dasypus novemcinctus*) in staged encounters. Am Midl Nat. 1998;139(1):125-32.

89. McDonough CM. Social organization of nine-banded armadillos (*Dasypus novemcinctus*) in a riparian habitat. Am Midl Nat. 2000;144(1):139-51.

90. Cullen L, Bodmer ER, Valladares-Padua C. Ecological consequences of hunting in Atlantic forest patches, São Paulo, Brazil. Oryx. 2001;35(2):137-44.

91. Timock J, Vaughan C. A census of mammal populations in Punta Leona Private Wildlife Refuge, Costa Rica. RevBiol Trop. 2002;50(3-4):1169-80.

92. Naughton-Treves L, Mena JL, Treves A, et al. Wildlife survival beyond park boundaries: the impact of slash-and-burn agriculture and hunting on mammals in Tambopata, Peru. Conserv Biol. 2003;17(4):1106-17.

93. Loughry WJ, McDonough CM. The Nine-banded Armadillo: A Natural History. Norman: University of Oklahoma Press; 2013.

94. Arteaga MC, Pinero D, Eguiarte LE, et al. Genetic structure and diversity of the nine-banded armadillo in Mexico. J Mamm. 2012;93:547-59.

95. Walsh GP, Storrs EE, Burchfield HP, et al. Leprosy-like disease occurring naturally in armadillos. J Reticuloendothel Soc. 1975;18(6):347-51.

96. Walsh GP, Meyers WM, Binford CH. Naturally acquired leprosy in the nine-banded armadillo: a decade of experience 1975-1985. J Leukoc Biol. 1986;40(5):645-56.

97. Truman RW, Shannon EJ, Hagstad HV, et al. Evaluation of the origin of *Mycobacterium leprae* infections in the wild armadillo, *Dasypus novemcinctus*. Am J Trop Med Hyg. 1986;35(3):588-93.

98. Paige CF, Scholl DT, Truman RW. Prevalence and incidence density of *Mycobacterium leprae* and *Trypanosoma cruzi* infections within a population of wild nine-banded armadillos. Am J Trop Med Hyg. 2002;67(5):528-32.

99. Truman R. Leprosy in wild armadillos. Lepr Rev. 2005;76(3):198-208.

100. Martinez AR, Resoagli EH, De Milan SG, et al. Lepra salvaje en *D. novemcinctus* (linneo 1758). Arch Argent Dermat. 1984;34:21-30.

101. Zumarraga MJ, Resoagli EH, Cicuta ME, et al. PCR-restriction fragment length polymorphism analysis (PRA) of *Mycobacterium leprae* from human lepromas and from a natural case of an armadillo of Corrientes, Argentina. Int J Lepr Other Mycobact Dis. 2001;69(1):21-25.

102. Deps PD, Santos AR, Yamashita-Tomimori J. Detection of *Mycobacterium leprae* DNA by PCR in blood sample from nine-banded armadillo: preliminary results. Int J Lepr Other Mycobact Dis. 2002;70(1):34-5.

103. Deps PD, Antunes JM, Tomimori-Yamashita J. Detection of *Mycobacterium leprae* infection in wild nine-banded armadillos (*Dasypus novemcinctus*) using the rapid ML Flow test. Rev Soc Brasil Med Trop. 2007;40(1):86-7.

104. Deps PD, Antunes JM, Faria C, et al. Research regarding anti-PGL-I antibodies by ELISA in wild armadillos from Brazil. Rev Soc Brasil Med Trop. 2008;41 Suppl 2:73-6.

105. Frota CC, Lima LN, Rocha Ada S, et al. *Mycobacterium leprae* in six-banded (*Euphractus sexcinctus*) and nine-banded armadillos (*Dasypus novemcinctus*) in Northeast Brazil. Mem Inst Oswaldo Cruz. 2012;107 Suppl 1:209-13.

106. Cardona-Castro N, Beltran JC, Ortiz-Bernal A, et al. Detection of *Mycobacterium leprae* DNA in nine-banded armadillos (*Dasypus novemcinctus*) from the Andean region of Colombia. Lepr Rev. 2009;80(4):424-31.

107. Amezcua ME, Escobar-Gutierrez A, Storrs EE, et al. Wild Mexican armadillo with leprosy-like infection. Int J Lepr Other Mycobact Dis. 1984;52(2):254-5.

108. Kerr-Pontes LR, Barreto ML, Evangelista CM, et al. Socioeconomic, environmental, and behavioural risk factors for leprosy in North-east Brazil: results of a case-control study. Int J Epidemiol. 2006;35(4):994-1000.

109. Deps PD, Alves BL, Gripp CG, et al. Contact with armadillos increases the risk of leprosy in Brazil: a case control study. Indian J Dermatol Venereol Leprol. 2008;74(4):338-42.

110. Truman R. Armadillos as a source of infection for leprosy. South Med J. 2008;101(6):581-2.

111. Truman RW, Sanchez RM. Armadillos: Models for leprosy. Lab Anim. 1993;22:28-32.

112. Ridley DS, Jopling WH. Classification of leprosy according to immunity. A five-group system. Int J Lepr Other Mycobact Dis. 1966;34(3):255-73.

113. Mitsuda K. On the value of skin reaction with emulsion of leproma. Jpn J Dermatol Urol. 1949;19:697-708.

114. Krotoski WA, Mroczkowski TF, Rea TH, et al. Lepromin skin testing in the classification of Hansen's disease in the United States. Am J Med Sci. 1993;305(1):18-24.

115. Job CK, Kirchheimer WF, Sanchez RM. Variable lepromin response to *Mycobacterium leprae* in resistant armadillos. Int J Lepr Other Mycobact Dis. 1983;51(3):347-53.

116. Job CK, Truman RW. Comparative study of Mitsuda reaction to nude mouse and armadillo lepromin preparations using nine-banded armadillos. Int J Lepr Other Mycobact Dis. 2000;68(1):18-22.

117. Abel L, Sanchez FO, Oberti J, et al. Susceptibility to leprosy is linked to the human *NRAMP1* gene. J Infect Dis. 1998;177(1):133-45.

118. Mira MT, Alcais A, Nguyen VT, et al. Susceptibility to leprosy is associated with *PARK2* and *PACRG*. Nature. 2004;427(6975):636-40.

119. Cardoso CC, Pereira AC, de Sales Marques C, et al. Leprosy susceptibility: genetic variations regulate innate and adaptive immunity, and disease outcome. Future Microbiol. 2011;6(5):533-49.

120. Scollard DM. The biology of nerve injury in leprosy. Lepr Rev. 2008;79(3):242-53.

121. Wilder-Smith EP, Van Brakel WH. Nerve damage in leprosy and its management. Nature Clin Prac Neurol. 2008;4(12):656-63.

122. Nations SP, Barohn RJ. Peripheral neuropathy due to leprosy. Curr Treat Opt Neurol. 2002;4(3):189-96.

123. Rodrigues LC, Lockwood DN. Leprosy now: epidemiology, progress, challenges, and research gaps. Lancet Infect Dis. 2011;11(6):464-70.

124. Antunes SL, Chimelli LM, Rabello ET, et al. An immunohistochemical, clinical and electroneuromyographic correlative study of the neural markers in the neuritic form of leprosy. Brazil J Med Biol Res. 2006;39:1071-81.

125. Sharma R, Lahiri R, Scollard DM, et al. The armadillo: a model for the neuropathy of leprosy and potentially other neurodegenerative diseases. Dis Models Mech. 2013;6(1):19-24.

126. Scollard DM, Lathrop GW, Truman RW. Infection of distal peripheral nerves by M. leprae in infected armadillos; an experimental model of nerve involvement in leprosy. Int J Lepr Other Mycobact Dis. 1996;64(2):146-51.

127. Scollard DM, Truman RW. The armadillo leprosy model with particular reference to lepromatous neuritis. In: Zak O, Sande M (Eds). Handbook of Animal Models of Infection. New York: Academic Press; 1999.pp.331-5.

128. Franssen H. Electrophysiology in demyelinating polyneuropathies. Exp Rev Neurotherapeut. 2008; 8(3): 417-31.

129. McArthur JC, Stocks EA, Hauer P, et al. Epidermal nerve fiber density: normative reference range and diagnostic efficiency. Arch Neurol. 1998;55(12):1513-20.

130. Holland NR, Stocks A, Hauer P, et al. Intraepidermal nerve fiber density in patients with painful sensory neuropathy. Neurol. 1997;48(3):708-11.

131. Periquet MI, Novak V, Collins MP, et al. Painful sensory neuropathy: prospective evaluation using skin biopsy. Neurol. 1999;53(8):1641-7.

132. Polydefkis M, Hauer P, Sheth S, et al. The time course of epidermal nerve fibre regeneration: studies in normal controls and in people with diabetes, with and without neuropathy. Brain. 2004;127(Pt 7):1606-15.

133. Goransson LG, Brun JG, Harboe E, et al. Intraepidermal nerve fiber densities in chronic inflammatory autoimmune diseases. Arch Neurol. 2006; 63(10):1410-3.

134. Gibbons CH, Griffin JW, Polydefkis M, et al. The utility of skin biopsy for prediction of progression in suspected small fiber neuropathy. Neurol. 2006;66(2):256-8.

135. Truman R, Ebenezer G, Pena M, et al. The armadillo as a model for peripheral neuropathy in leprosy. Inst Lab Anim Res. 2013:54(3):306-16.

136. Masaki T, Qu J, Cholewa-Waclaw J, et al. Reprogramming adult Schwann cells to stem cell-like cells by leprosy bacilli promotes dissemination of infection. Cell. 2013;152(1-2):51-67.

137. Brand PW, Beach RB, Thompson DE. Relative tension and potential excursion of muscles in the forearm and hand. J Hand Surg Am.1981;6(3):209-19.

138. Werneck LC, Teive HA, Scola RH. Muscle involvement in leprosy. Study of the anterior tibial muscle in 40 patients. Arqu Neuro-psiquiat,1999; 57(3B): 723-734.

139. Truman RW, Morales MJ, Shannon EJ, et al. Evaluation of monitoring antibodies to PGL-I in armadillos experimentally infected with M. leprae. Int J Lepr Other Mycobact Dis. 1986;54(4):556-9.

140. Job CK, Drain V, Truman RW, et al. Early infection with *M. leprae* and antibodies to phenolic glycolipid-I in the nine-banded armadillo. Indian J Lepr. 1990;62(2):193-201.

141. Job CK, Drain V, Williams DL, et al. Comparison of polymerase chain reaction technique with other methods for detection of *Mycobacterium leprae* in tissues of wild nine-banded armadillos. Lepr Rev. 1991;62(4):362-73.

142. Duthie MS, Truman RW, Goto W, et al. Insight toward early diagnosis of leprosy through analysis of the developing antibody responses of *Mycobacterium leprae*-infected armadillos. Clin Vaccine Immunol. 2011;18(2):254-9.

143. Pena M, Geluk A, Van Der Ploeg-Van Schip JJ, et al. Cytokine responses to Mycobacterium leprae unique proteins differentiate between *Mycobacterium leprae* infected and naive armadillos. Lepr Rev. 2011;82(4):422-31.

144. Adams JE, Pena MT, Gillis TP, et al. Expression of nine-banded armadillo (*Dasypus novemcinctus*) interleukin-2 in E. coli. Cytokine. 2005;32(5):219-25.

145. Pena MT, Adams JE, Adams LB, et al. Expression and characterization of recombinant interferon gamma (IFN-gamma) from the nine-banded armadillo (*Dasypus novemcinctus*) and its effect on Mycobacterium leprae-infected macrophages. Cytokine. 2008;43(2):124-31.

Clinical, Laboratory Diagnosis and Differential Diagnosis

14

CHAPTER

History Taking and Clinical Examination

Aparna Palit, Ragunatha S, Arun C Inamadar

INTRODUCTION

Leprosy is a chronic inflammatory disease caused by *Mycobacterium leprae*, primarily affecting the peripheral nerves and skin. The clinical presentation of leprosy mainly depends on the ability of the host to induce cell-mediated immunity (CMI) against *M. leprae*. The type of immune response, which varies from person to person, determines the manifestations of the disease in various clinicopathological patterns. In the spectrum of leprosy, the patient presents with a combination of different types of skin lesions and nerve function impairments, simulating a wide variety of dermatological and neurological diseases. Early and accurate diagnosis of leprosy is crucial because late recognition may give rise to permanent deformity resulting from the disease.

Apart from the host and agent factors, geographic, sociocultural and economic factors also play a role in the outcome of the disease and its complications. Hence, history taking and clinical examination in leprosy should address all these aspects, which ultimately help in decision-making regarding chemotherapy, prevention of disability, health planning and community-based rehabilitation (CBR).

HISTORY TAKING

Primary goal of history taking is to establish the diagnosis by excluding other conditions simulating leprosy. History should be taken according to the following steps, mostly like any other medical history:
- Personal identification and demographic data
- Presenting complaints
- History of present illness
- Past history
- Family history
- Personal history.

In the following section, the importance and relevance of eliciting specific history from the patients suffering from leprosy will be discussed.

Identification and Demographic Data

In any leprosy control program, the main focus is on early diagnosis and treatment. The demographic factors determine the attitude of the patient toward the disease, compliance to treatment, risk of deformities and rehabilitation. Apart from medical management, the knowledge of demographic factors helps in formulating policies and logistics for eradication of leprosy.

Name

Addressing the patients by name helps in gaining their confidence and building good rapport with them. It is also important for identification or recording of the patient.

Age

Though leprosy occurs at all ages, children are more susceptible. However, clinical leprosy is more commonly observed in adults. Paucibacillary disease is more common in children and the incidence of reactions is lower in this age group. Epidemiologically, childhood leprosy is an index of transmission of the disease in a population and helps in detection of the source of infection.[1]

Sex

There exists a gender inequality in leprosy. Though it affects both the sexes, male predominance is observed in adults but in children, the gender distribution is nearly equal.

The disease is more severe in males, but the sociocultural impact of the disease is more in females.[2] Women are at higher risk of development of reactions. However, the deformities are less common in females.[3]

During pregnancy, the patient may be at increased risk of development of the disease, relapse and reactions. Postpartum period is temporally associated with occurrence of reversal reaction due to recovery of CMI. While treating a woman of child-bearing age with thalidomide, due precaution must be taken to avoid teratogenicity.[3]

Address

Residential address is necessary for follow-up and surveillance. Distance between home and the health center is one of the factors for delay in coming for follow-up, increased incidence of deformities and default of treatment.[4] In nonendemic states or countries, specific enquiry should be made to know whether the patient originally belongs to that region or had migrated or traveled from a state or country endemic for leprosy, for occupational or some other reasons. The important differential diagnosis of leprosy, like leishmaniasis (cutaneous, mucocutaneous and visceral), onchocerciasis, etc., are to be considered in certain geographical regions, where these diseases are prevalent.[5]

Occupation

Occupation is one of the factors determining susceptibility of the already diagnosed leprosy patients to develop deformities. Such patients should be identified for advice, either to use protective measures or change of occupation. In manual laborers, the peripheral nerves are usually prominent and due care should be undertaken while interpreting nerve enlargement in the absence of nerve function impairment (NFI).[6]

Socioeconomic Status

Low socioeconomic status, poor housing, overcrowding and rural inhabitation are associated with increased incidence of leprosy. Alternatively, the diagnosis of leprosy carries a stigma and may worsen the socioeconomic status of a patient. Type of occupation, housing status and number of dependents are the key socioeconomic indices. Identification of these factors and early socioeconomic rehabilitation decreases the risk of disability.[6]

Marital Status

The diagnosis of leprosy has a profound effect on marriage. Leprosy has been a reason for rejection of bride or bridegroom and divorce in many communities.[3] Unfortunately, leprosy was a ground for divorce in the Indian law, till recently.

Presenting Complaints

Patients with leprosy may present with varied clinical manifestations (Table 14.1). The symptoms suggestive of peripheral nerve involvement with or without skin lesions should direct the history taking and clinical examination toward diagnosis, differential diagnosis and complications, which the individual patients might have.

Table 14.1: Various presenting features of leprosy	
In absence of reaction	• Skin lesions: hypopigmented/erythematous, hypoesthetic patches, skin-colored/erythematous papules, plaques, nodules, which may be waxy ± umbilication • Hypoesthesia along distribution of peripheral nerves/glove and stocking hypoesthesia • Spontaneous blisters and ulcers on the hands and/or feet • Trophic changes; dryness, ichthyosis, fissuring/trophic ulcer • Diffuse swelling of hands and feet (early sign of lepromatous leprosy/leprosy reactions) • Nasal stuffiness, epistaxis (early sign of lepromatous leprosy) • Irregular thickening of ear and nodules on face (lepromatous leprosy)
While in reaction	• Tingling and numbness of hands and/or feet • Sudden weakness of hands and/or feet or inability to close eyelids • Sudden redness, swelling and pain of existing lesions and/or appearance of new lesions with or without constitutional symptoms (type 1 reaction) • Sudden appearance of crops of evanescent, erythematous, painful nodules on apparently normal looking skin with or without constitutional symptoms (erythema nodosum leprosum/type 2 reaction) • Painful swelling on the dorsal aspect of wrists (tenosynovitis) • Acute scrotal pain (epididymo-orchitis) • Pain in and around eyes, redness, photophobia or diminished vision (iridocyclitis)
In presence of deformity	• Inability to use hands for precision works; e.g. button a shirt, eating rice with hands, typing, etc. • Inability to make a power-grip; e.g. holding a rod, carrying utensils • Inability to wear slipper (all these are indicative of peripheral anesthesia and poor functioning of small muscles of hands and feet)

History of Present Illness

Any question asked from the patient or information collected should be interpreted in relation to the diagnosis, differential diagnosis, management, prevention of disability and rehabilitation. In addition, these observations should also guide the examiner regarding further questioning. The following points should be asked to get clues about the disease.

Duration

The duration of the presenting complaints has both diagnostic and prognostic importance. Hypopigmented patches present since birth or of few days duration are unlikely to be due to leprosy. The former is suggestive of nevus anemicus or nevus depigmentosus.[7] NFI of less than 6 months duration responds better to systemic corticosteroid therapy than that of more than 6 months. The delay in presentation (>6 months) is one of the risk factors for development of deformities.[8] Multibacillary disease of duration more than 10 years is a risk factor for ocular complications.[9]

Mode of Onset

Skin lesions and NFI in leprosy usually have insidious onset. Sudden appearance of skin lesions and NFI is indicative of leprosy reactions. Eruption of new lesions may suggest ENL or reversal reaction. However, the ENL lesions are evanescent, appear in crops and last for few days; whereas the lesions are persistent in reversal reactions.[7]

Progression and Evolution

The hypopigmented patches and NFI in nonreactional leprosy undergo a gradual, continuous course. Increase in the size of lesion and/or appearance of new lesions in a patient with apparently stable disease indicates persistent activity, downward progression of disease or relapse. History of rapid nerve function deterioration resulting in paralysis is due to lepra reaction resulting in neuritis. Rarely, the ENL lesions may develop bullae and undergo ulceration, which is seldom seen in erythema nodosum.[7]

The trophic ulcer evolves initially from a trauma/deep fissure/callosity or there may be tenderness over pressure-bearing areas of palms and soles. The area breaks down into a frank painless ulcer discharging serosanguineous fluid.[10]

Nerve function impairment in leprosy is mostly localized, asymmetrical and distal, unlike the NFI secondary to toxic, nutritional, metabolic or hereditary causes which are more diffuse, symmetrical and involve both proximal and distal areas of limbs.[11]

The hypopigmented lesions of nevus anemicus increase in size proportional to the body growth. Postinflammatory hypopigmentation remains stationary and regresses in few weeks. The lesions of pityriasis alba may be persistent, recurrent and respond to topical therapy.[7]

Symptoms

As such, skin lesions in leprosy are asymptomatic. The presence of itching may help in differentiating urticaria from red papules and nodules of lepromatous leprosy (LL) or ENL. Pain is a common feature of both type 1 reaction (T1R) and ENL.[7]

Patients may complain of spontaneous blistering after a long walk. Painful trophic ulcer indicates presence of secondary infection or involvement of underlying structures like bone.[10] The presence of pain along with paresthesia and impaired sensation differentiates diabetic and alcoholic neuropathy from leprosy.[5] Constitutional symptoms, like fever, malaise, joint pain, etc. usually accompany reactions and infected trophic ulcer.[7,10]

Distribution of Lesions

The hypopigmented patches in tuberculoid spectrum are usually localized and few in number; whereas these are generalized and wide spread in the lepromatous spectrum.[7]

Involvement of three or more body areas is one of the risk factors for NFI and reversal reaction.[12] Patches over major nerve trunks and face are associated with increased risk of underlying nerve damage and reactions.[13] Sensory impairment is difficult to elicit if the patches are present over the face because of its overlapping nerve supply. The ENL lesions commonly occur on face and extensor aspects of extremities.[7] Lesions of erythema nodosum are usually localized to legs.

The interpretation of the presenting complaints leads to further enquiry into the disease depending upon the spectrum of leprosy and reactional states. For example, if the history is suggestive of lepromatous spectrum, the symptoms related to visceral involvement should be asked for. If the history is suggestive of type 2 reaction (T2R) apart from symptoms of systemic involvement, precipitating factors, if any, should also be elicited.

Visceral Involvement and Complications

Usually clinical manifestations of leprosy are limited to the skin and peripheral nervous system. However, other organs can also be affected mainly in patients with LL and T2R. Only few organs present with symptoms suggestive of their involvement and specific questions can be asked to detect these (Table 14.2).[9,14]

Precipitating Factors

If history is suggestive of reaction, precipitating factors should be searched for:[7]
- Any recent infection? (sore throat/frequency of urination/ loose motions)

Table 14.2: Looking for other organ involvement in leprosy[9,14]	
Organ	*Specific questions to be asked*
Eye	• Difficulty in eye closure? (Lagophthalmos) • Red eye with pain, watering and sticky discharge? (Corneal ulceration) • Red eye with pain, photophobia and diminished vision? (Iridocyclitis) • Localized redness, severe radiating pain to temporal region, normal/slightly reduced vision? (Scleritis) • Localized redness, mild pain, normal vision? (Episcleritis)
Upper respiratory tract	• Unable to perceive smell of food and scented materials? (Anosmia) • Nose is blocked with occasional bleeding? • Change of voice, chronic cough, and occasional breathlessness? (Laryngeal involvement) • Any episode of acute respiratory distress? (Laryngeal edema)
Cardiovascular system*	• Palpitation? • Dyspnea on exertion? • Swelling of feet?
Adrenal glands**	• Features of adrenal insufficiency? For example, hypotension, asthenia, prostration
Male reproductive system	• Normal/diminished libido? (Testicular atrophy) • Enlarging male breasts? (Testicular atrophy) • If married, whether having children? (Sterility)

*Cardiovascular involvement in leprosy is very rare and rarely gives rise to symptoms. Involvement of peripheral blood vessels, though frequent, is rarely symptomatic.
**Adrenal suppression is very rare in leprosy. However, it may occur rarely during an episode of T2R.

• Physical and mental stress? [overwork, familial dispute/ marital disharmony/employment status (whether recent loss of job), etc.]
• Recent vaccination?
• Recent surgical procedures?
• Pregnancy/recent child birth?

In case of trophic ulcers, history of trauma, penetrating injury, barefoot walking or ill-fitting footwear should be noted.[10]

Associated Diseases

Certain diseases are commonly associated with leprosy and influence the course of the disease. Tuberculosis is common in leprosy patients; moreover different therapeutic regimen has to be used to treat this coinfection in order to prevent Rifampicin resistant tuberculosis.[14] Concomitant HIV infection is associated with increased risk of recurrent T1R, T2R and immune reconstitution inflammatory syndrome (IRIS), especially after the institution of antiretroviral therapy (ART).[15]

Treatment Taken for Presenting Complaints

Leprosy patients may have tried many topical and systemic medications before consulting or being referred to the specialists, with misdiagnosis of the hypopigmented patches as pityriasis versicolor, dry eczema or dermatophytic infection. A persistent, asymptomatic, hypopigmented patch not responding to topical therapy should arouse the suspicion of leprosy.

Past History

The factors that influence the course, classification, prognosis and management of leprosy may become more clear from the past history. If the patient had been diagnosed as having leprosy before, following details should be elicited:
• Predominant clinical features; skin lesions and/or area of loss of sensation, diagnosis made in the past (type of the disease).
• History of spontaneous disappearance of a skin patch, persistence of nerve thickening and area of sensory loss pose a difficulty in confirming diagnosis of primary neuritic leprosy.
• Any deformities developed.
• If treatment taken earlier, the treatment schedule, its duration and side effects? (Multibacillary leprosy with high BI is associated with increased chances of relapse). If the patient is a defaulter, reason for default should be asked.
• In case of history suggestive of reaction:
  – Its duration.
  – Number of episodes.
  – Any precipitating factor(s).
  – How the reaction was managed earlier? (If the patient is educated, try to elicit the history of treatment taken

with duration, doses of steroids or other antireactional drugs administered, and any side effects thereof).
- Relationship of reaction with starting of multidrug therapy (MDT).

Type 1 reaction often occurs after initiation of MDT. The interval between initiation of therapy and onset of reaction will be shorter at tuberculoid pole and longer at the lepromatous pole. It may occur before MDT starts in borderline tuberculoid (BT) leprosy or may also occur after completion of MDT, especially in borderline lepromatous (BL) and subpolar LL. In the absence of therapy, the course of the disease or T1R is more likely to be downgrading. Downgrading of the disease while on MDT suggests either delayed initiation of therapy, inadequate therapy, treatment default, development of resistance to drugs, immunological deterioration or instability. Similarly T2R may occur before or after initiation of MDT. However, it is more common after initiation of therapy because of increased antigenic load following the killing of bacilli.[7] It has been observed that T2R develops after a course of antibiotics effective against *M. leprae* when given to these patients for other infections including urinary tract infection (UTI).

- History of any chronic illness like diabetes mellitus, jaundice, HIV infection, etc.

Diabetes mellitus also causes peripheral neuropathy and it is one of the differential diagnoses for neuritis and hypoesthesia.[5] Rifampicin, a microsomal enzyme inducer, is known to decrease the plasma levels of oral hypoglycemic agents.[16] Leprosy reactions do not seem to be a primary cause of hepatitis, but may worsen underlying liver disease.[14] Treatment with antiretrovirals in presence of coinfection with HIV may result in IRIS, and in untreated patients reactions may be more frequent.

Any history of drug hypersensitivity syndrome induced by Sulfonamides should be asked for, as cross reactivity may occur with dapsone.[17]

Family History

Household contacts are at an increased risk of contracting leprosy. History of leprosy in the family and examination of other family members is vital, especially if the patient is a child.[18] Number of dependents in a family is one of the indices of socioeconomic factors. History of any drug reaction (especially with Sulfonamides) in a family member or any close relative should be specifically asked for as it may be predictive of an increased risk of the same in the patient.[17]

Personal History

Daily routine of the patient is asked with regards to:
- Diet (though not specifically associated, concomitant malnutrition may slow the recovery).[19]

- Appetite; poor appetite should lead the clinician to search for a cause beyond anemia and malnutrition.
- Sleep (adequate sleep is necessary in patients with reaction).
- Bowel and bladder function.
- Hobbies and habits; alcoholic neuropathy is one of the differential diagnoses and may occur together with leprosy.[5] Chronic alcoholism and liver damage are associated with increased incidence of severe hepatotoxicity; when Rifampicin is given alone or concurrently with other hepatotoxic drugs.[16] Chronic smokers may have pre-existing vascular compromise and may be more susceptible to develop blistering and ulceration.

History gives clues to the spectrum of leprosy, complications and associated risk factors. Based on these historical findings, the clinical examination should be conducted. For example, if the patient is suffering from lepromatous spectrum of disease or is in T2R, apart from cutaneous and peripheral nerve examination, thorough systemic examination should be done to detect the underlying organ system involved, if any.

CLINICAL EXAMINATION

An adequate history taking is followed by a thorough clinical examination of the patient. This is imperative in all cases of leprosy, as it is a disease with wide variations in the clinical presentation. Moreover, morphological details of the skin lesions, extent of peripheral nerve involvement, areas of sensory loss and systemic involvement allow the clinician to assess the disease spectrum the patient belongs to. This in turn helps in individualizing the therapeutic schedules for patients and assessing the chances of complications, the patient may face during the course of illness and/or treatment.

Clinical examination involves the following steps:
- General physical examination.
- Cutaneous examination.
- Mucosal examination.
- Ocular examination.
- Palpation of peripheral nerves and testing for sensory impairment.
- Examination of musculoskeletal system.
- Examination of external genitalia.
- Other systemic examination, wherever indicated.

General Physical Examination

Overall nutritional status of the patient should be assessed, as patients with long-standing lepromatous disease may develop malnutrition. Thorough general physical examination should be performed with special search for pallor, edema and lymphadenopathy. These may be a part of lepromatous disease or may be associated with leprosy reactions. If a patient on dapsone therapy shows profound pallor of sudden onset, evidence of hemolysis and jaundice should be looked for.

Pulse and blood pressure of all patients should be recorded at presentation and followed up thereafter during every visit. Tachycardia may be noted in patients with leprosy reactions. Hypertension in patients with leprosy may result from chronic renal impairment due to repeated T2R or renal amyloidosis.

Bilateral pedal edema, often involving the dorsa of hands also (Fig. 14.1), is seen in lepromatous patients. Generalized edema may be reactive, resulting from autonomic neuropathy affecting the small blood vessels; or it may be indicative of acute glomerulonephritis associated with T2R or severe hypoproteinemia, common among the leprosy patients. Widespread tender lymphadenopathy is suggestive of T2R.[7]

If the patient is acutely ill with fever, arthralgia and prostration, possibility of T2R or severe T1R should be considered and cutaneous examination should be directed to confirm it.

Cutaneous Examination

A quick general cutaneous survey should be done followed by examination of individual skin lesions. Prior explanation to the patient along with gaining his or her confidence is of immense importance in achieving patient cooperation. Cutaneous examination should be done in adequate day-light, following proper exposure and ensuring privacy. The patient should face the source of light (e.g. window) with the examiner sitting against it.[19] The skin lesions are better appreciated in an oblique light (especially the ill-defined macules of LL disease), initially from a distance, thereafter close examination is done.[19]

Widespread infiltration, evident by shiny skin, sparse body hair, prominent follicular openings and mild thickening appreciable by gentle pinching of the skin, is suggestive of lepromatous disease (Fig. 14.2). Infiltrated face with thick skin folds and nodularity (leonine facies) (Fig. 14.3), depressed nasal bridge, sparse beard and moustache (Fig. 14.4) are all indicative of advanced LL.

Sagging or loose facial skin (rather than infiltration) (Fig. 14.5) and enlarged, pendulous ear lobules (Buddha ears) (Fig. 14.6) are seen in treated lepromatous cases, as well as in patients with long-standing or burnt-out disease.

Unilateral or bilateral gynecomastia in males (Fig.14.7) suggests impairment of testicular function in LL.

An overall brownish pigmentation involving skin, conjunctiva (Figs 14.8A and B) and oral mucosa indicates treatment with Clofazimine, either currently or in the recent past.

In an institutional set-up, individual skin lesions should preferably be documented on a body charting printed proforma (Fig. 14.9).[20] This allows a proper follow-up of the patients with respect to the course of nerve and existing skin lesions, appearance of new lesions or fresh peripheral nerve involvement during the course of the disease.

Examination of Individual Skin Lesion

While examining individual skin lesions, the following points should be noted:

Total Number

Single, 1–5, above 5 (multiple) or innumerable. Fewer the number of the lesion, lower the bacillary load, the higher level of resistance to disease and *vice versa*. Counting the number of skin and nerve lesions enable the clinician to categorize the disease as paucibacillary or multibacillary.

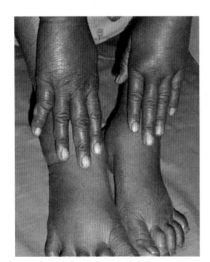

Fig. 14.1: Edema of hands and feet in a patient with untreated lepromatous leprosy

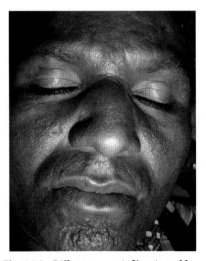

Fig. 14.2: Diffuse, coarse infiltration of face

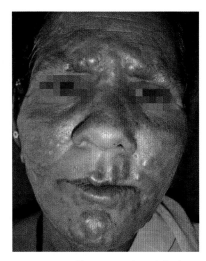

Fig. 14.3: More severe infiltration with nodular lesions (Leonine facies) with few papular lesions and plaques on chin

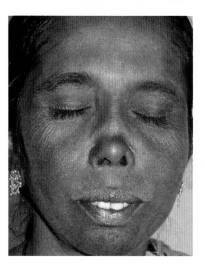

Fig. 14.5: Loose facial skin in a treated case of LL following regression of skin infiltration

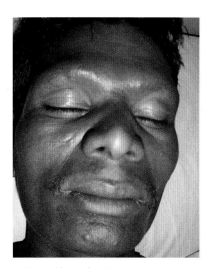

Fig. 14.4: Bilateral loss of eyebrows, moustache and beard

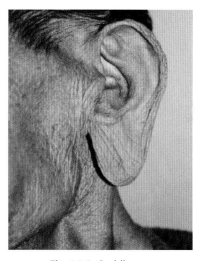

Fig. 14.6: Buddha ear

Distribution
Trunk, extremities, face; protected sites like, scalp,[21] axillae, groin, perineum, genitalia,[22] palms and soles[23] may also be involved and should be searched for lesions. Covered body sites like genitalia[24] (Fig. 14.10) or buttocks may be the only site of initial skin lesions and should never be overlooked.

Bilateral symmetrical distribution indicates lowest spectrum (LL), and asymmetry in distribution indicates borderline spectrum of the disease.

Shape
Regular (round/oval), irregular/bizarre, annular.

Size
A lesion may occupy an entire limb or a quadrant of trunk [tuberculoid leprosy (TT), BT] (Fig. 14.11) or they may be small and multiple (BL, LL) (Fig. 14.12). Widespread, monomorphic, coalescent macules are suggestive of LL disease.

Morphology
Patch/papules/plaque/nodule/vesicle/bulla. Lesions should be examined for:
• Color (hypopigmented/hyperpigmented, skin-colored, erythematous, coppery).

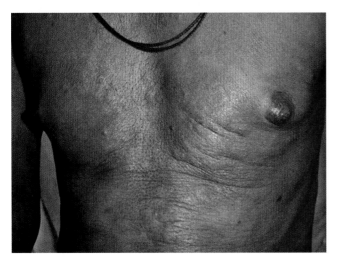

Fig. 14.7: Bilateral gynecomastia in a patient with untreated LL

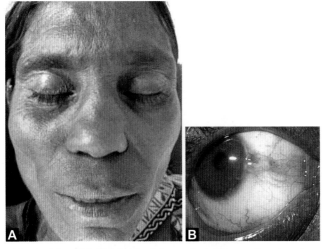

Figs 14.8A and B: Brownish pigmentation of face and conjunctiva following MDT due to Clofazimine

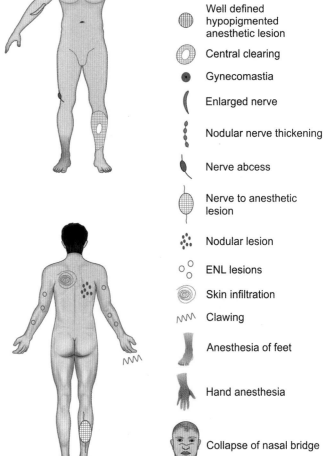

≡	Hypopigmentation
‖‖	Area of anesthesia
▦	Hypopigmented anesthetic patch
⊕	Well defined hypopigmented anesthetic lesion
◯	Central clearing
◉	Gynecomastia
(	Enlarged nerve
⸭	Nodular nerve thickening
⸙	Nerve abcess
⊘	Nerve to anesthetic lesion
⸫	Nodular lesion
○○	ENL lesions
◎	Skin infiltration
ᶺᶺᶺ	Clawing
	Anesthesia of feet
	Hand anesthesia
	Collapse of nasal bridge

Fig. 14.9: Diagrammatic charting of skin lesions, nerves and areas of sensory changes in patients with leprosy to be used for keeping records (Modified from Thangaraj RH)[20]

- Surface (no change, dry/scaly/smooth and shiny/ edematous/ulcerated).
- Border [well/ill-defined, raised/flat, sloping (in or outward), punched-out]. Well-defined border of a lesion is indicative of tuberculoid pole of the disease. The border may be incomplete or complete or broken at places. There may be slight extension of the border to form pseudopodia and in the periphery of some lesions there may be small, discrete, satellite lesions.
- Presence/absence/sparseness of hair (Fig. 14.13).
- Lesional tenderness.

An ill-defined, hypopigmented, flat, imperceptible lesion without surface changes (preserved skin markings) may be an indeterminate leprosy patch (Fig. 14.14).

Thick, elevated margin of a lesion with or without granularity is suggestive of TT/BT lesion (Fig. 14.15). In annular lesions, both inner and outer margins are to be palpated. A better-defined inner border with outer border sloping into the surrounding skin giving a "punched-out" appearance (inverted saucer-shaped) is suggestive of a BB lesion (Fig. 14.16).[25] The type with inner sloping border and well-defined outer border indicates a TT lesion.

Presence of pseudopodia and satellite lesions along the margins of large lesions are suggestive of a BT lesion.[25] New satellite lesions may also appear, when such a patient is in reaction or the disease is downgrading (Fig. 14.17). A "feeding nerve to the lesion" can be detected by gentle rolling of a finger along the borders mostly in TT or BT spectrum (Fig. 14.18).

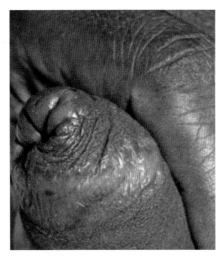

Fig. 14.10: Annular lesion of BT leprosy over the prepuce

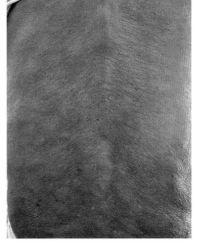

Fig. 14.12: Multiple small, ill-defined, symmetrical skin lesions in LL leprosy

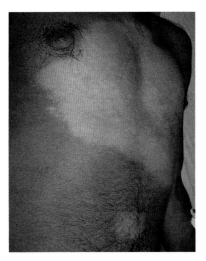

Fig. 14.11: Large lesion of BT leprosy on the chest

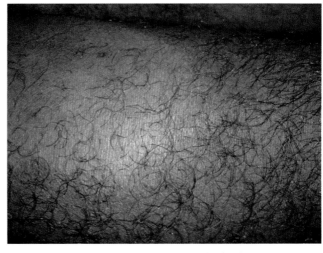

Fig. 14.13: Sparse hair on a patch of BT leprosy

In case of single or few large BT lesions, the entire border should be inspected thoroughly to see whether it is well-defined all around or ill-defined and vague at places (partially defined), indicative of downgrading of a particular lesion. Morphology of nodules should be studied carefully:

- Persistent, asymptomatic erythematous/coppery/normal skin-colored nodules, firm on palpation, of variable size, with sloping edges on to the surrounding infiltrated skin (Fig. 14.19) are seen in lepromatous spectrum of the disease (BL/LL).
- Well-defined, succulent, hemispherical glistening nodules, with or without umbilication, present on apparently normal-appearing skin may suggest histoid

leprosy (Fig. 14.20). These lesions are in various stages of evolution, starting as pin-point to pin-head sized papules, fully formed nodules and finally nodules with ulcerated surface.

- Recurrent, erythematous, evanescent, tender, nodules on the skin, commonly distributed over face, arms and thighs, unrelated to pre-existing skin lesions and healing with postinflammatory hyperpigmentation are suggestive of erythema nodosum leprosum (ENL), a feature of type 2 leprosy reaction (Fig. 14.21).

Rarely, few ulcerated lesions may be present in patients with untreated LL leprosy, histoid leprosy and ENL lesions or over the lesions of T1R. Such ulcers are usually present

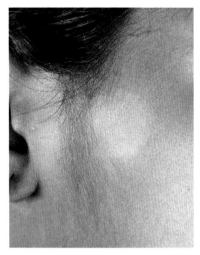

Fig. 14.14: Ill-defined patch of indeterminate leprosy

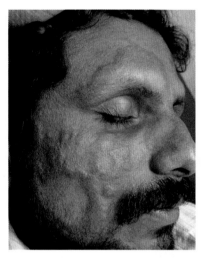

Fig. 14.16: Annular BB lesion with punched-out inner border and outer border sloping down to the surrounding skin

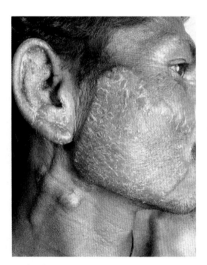
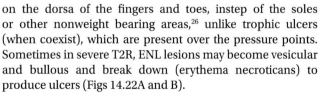

Fig. 14.15: Well-defined, raised outer border of a TT lesion ending abruptly; while the inner margin is ill-defined, sloping and waning toward the center. Enlarged, nodular great auricular nerve and involvement of ear is noted

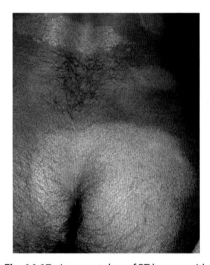

Fig. 14.17: Large patches of BT leprosy with pseudopodia and satellite lesions

on the dorsa of the fingers and toes, instep of the soles or other nonweight bearing areas,[26] unlike trophic ulcers (when coexist), which are present over the pressure points. Sometimes in severe T2R, ENL lesions may become vesicular and bullous and break down (erythema necroticans) to produce ulcers (Figs 14.22A and B).

Sudden onset of lesional erythema, edema (lesions may stand out clearly from the surrounding skin) and tenderness are suggestive of T1R (Fig. 14.23). Ulceration of such a lesion indicates increased severity of the reaction. Presence of scaling or wrinkling in a patch or plaque suggests subsiding T1R (Fig. 14.24).

Showers of small, new lesions while the patient is in reaction may indicate downgrading (Fig. 14.25).

Patients may have a combination of lesions characteristic of different spectra of the disease, e.g. large, hypoesthetic, dry patch of BT, annular plaque of BB and numerous macular or papular lesions of BL, indicative of a downgrading course.

Testing Sensations

Lesional sensation should be tested for
- Temperature (hot/cold water in test-tubes).
- Touch (wisp of cotton-wool or nylon monofilaments for objective sensory testing).

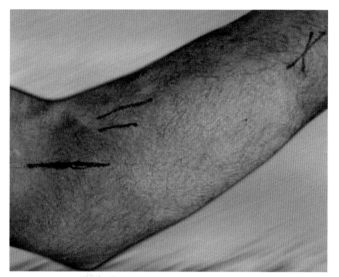

Fig. 14.18: Feeding nerve-twigs along the border of a TT lesion

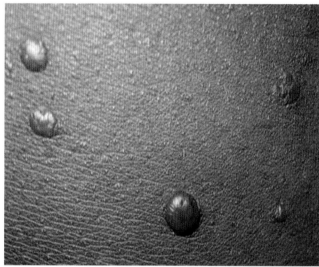

Fig. 14.20: Skin-colored, dome-shaped, shiny nodules of histoid leprosy, located on normal-looking skin

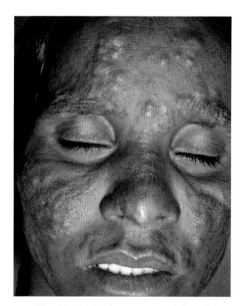

Fig. 14.19: Erythematous nodules of LL leprosy located on infiltrated skin

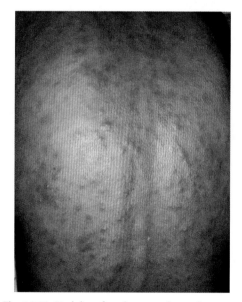

Fig. 14.21 Nodules of erythema nodosum leprosum

- Pain (pin-prick; the pin should be discarded after use on each patient).

Before starting the sensory testing, the patient should be explained the procedure in colloquial language and a trial of the method is conducted with eyes of the patient open. He or she is asked to count loudly each time the stimulus is felt or to locate the area tested with finger. Once followed it correctly, the patient is instructed to close the eyes, and the test is repeated to interpret.

While testing sensation, the examiner should proceed from uninvolved to the involved skin. All the sensations should be tested gently, only once at one site, for a short while, not pressing the test object too hard or brushing it on patient's skin.[7,19] The clinician may obtain an approximate idea by prior application of the test object on his or her own skin to assess the pressure and duration of contact required to elicit a normal sensory response. Even with adequate explanation and prior demonstration, the patient may not be

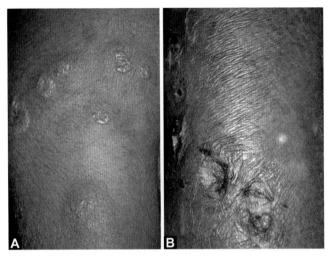

Figs 14.22A and B: Vesicular lesions of ENL and erythema necroticans

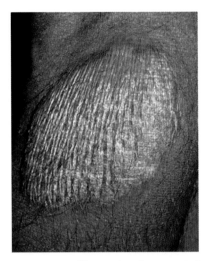

Fig. 14.24: Wrinkling and scaling, suggestive of subsiding T1R

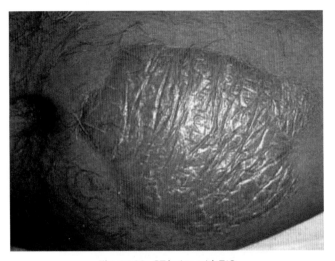

Fig. 14.23: BT lesion with T1R

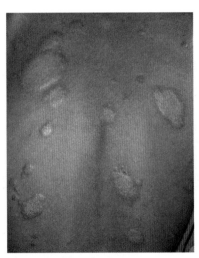

Fig. 14.25: Untreated BT leprosy with downgrading T1R, and showers of small new lesions

able to point the exact location of the application of stimulus (misreference), which may be an early sign of hypoesthesia.[7] The permissible limits of misreference on hands are 1 cm, on face, 2 cm and on back it is up to 7 cm.[7]

In regions with thicker skin (palms and soles) touch sensation can be tested with the tip of a ball-point pen gently, so as not to produce an indentation deeper than 2 mm.[27] Testing with Semmes-Weinstein monofilaments helps in detecting early hypoesthesia.

The examiner should keep in mind the following facts while interpreting sensory impairment in a patient with leprosy:

- The degree of sensory loss may be variable in different lesions (indeterminate +/–, TT and BT ++, LL +/–, or normal) and different parts of a large lesion (center/periphery).

- Lesions on face may not show expected degree of hypoesthesia.
- A patient in reaction may not be able to appreciate lesional sensory loss and such lesions may show hyperalgesia.[7]
- Testing sensations and interpretation of the findings in a child could be difficult at times. Younger children may be tested for lesional sensation while asleep and watched for withdrawal response, which is indicative of intact sensation.

Extremities should be examined for "gloves and stockings" hypoesthesia, demonstrable in lepromatous pole of the disease. Though named so, it may be patchy and asymmetrical in contrast to other causes of predominantly sensory peripheral neuropathy.[11]

Some sites should specifically be tested even when definite hypoesthesia is not demonstrable in skin lesions or along the distribution of a peripheral nerve. These sites of early cutaneous sensory loss in disease of lower spectrum are as follows:[11]
- Dorsa of the hands and feet.
- Dorso-medial aspect of forearm.
- Anterolateral aspect of legs.

The WHO recommended sensory testing sites on palms and soles (10 sites on each side) for disability grading have been presented in Figure 14.26.[28] Brandsma et al. have suggested lesser number of testing sites for this purpose, as follows:[28]
- *Hands*: *Ulnar nerve*; distal pulp and proximal phalanx of little finger and hypothenar eminence. *Median nerve*; distal pulp of thumb and index fingers and thenar eminence.
- *Feet*: Big toe, metatarsal heads (first, fifth), mid-lateral border of foot.

Trophic Changes

Asymptomatic, deep, nonhealing fissures on hands and feet (Figs 14.27A and B) may be observed in people who walk bare foot and agricultural or manual workers suffering from leprosy. Callosities may be present on both palms and soles or other bony prominences (pressure points) over anesthetic limbs, like lateral malleolus (Fig. 14.28), knuckles, point of elbows, etc.

Multiple, spontaneous and asymptomatic blisters on hands (Fig. 14.29) and feet (which might have gone unrecognized by the patient) are indicative of anesthetic hands and feet.

Vulnerable pressure points on palms, soles and bony pressure points like lateral malleoli, heel of the hand (pisiform bone) and point of the elbow should be inspected for trophic ulcers.[26]

Some sites of predilection for plantar ulcers are as follows:[26]
- Head of first metatarsal.
- Mid-portion of plantar surface of big toe.
- Mid-lateral border of the foot at the base of fifth metatarsal.
- Heel.
- Over the knuckles in presence of claw hand and tips of the clawed toes in presence of claw feet. The clinician should aim at identifying a trophic ulcer at an early stage. Some subtle clinical clues to a "threatened ulcer" on feet are as follows:[26]
  - Mild edema and warmth on the dorsum of fore-foot.
  - Slight splaying of the adjacent toes (Fig. 14.30).
  - Deep tenderness over plantar surface of metatarsal head or base of proximal phalanx.

Presence of a blister at pressure points may represent a 'concealed ulcer' which, when ruptures, forms the

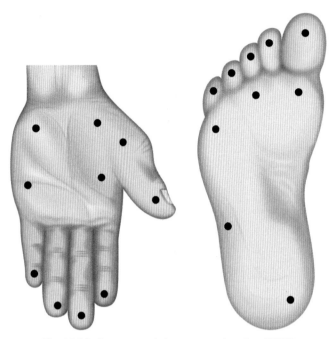

Fig. 14.26: Recommended sensory testing sites (WHO) on palms and soles

'manifest ulcer', with a hyperkeratotic rim around it (Fig. 14.31).[26]

Each trophic ulcer should be examined carefully for evidence of secondary bacterial infections (foul smell, dirty slough, discharge). Constant discharge of pus, in spite of adequate wound care, suggests involvement of deeper structures like pulp space, synovial sheath, tendon, capsule or bone.[29] Absence of discharge, sloping edge of the ulcer and bluish epithelium covering the granulation tissue at the floor are the signs of healing.[26]

Ichthyosis

Widespread dryness indicates lack of sweat and sebum secretion (autonomic neuropathy).[7] Large areas of ichthyosis may be present over extremities (Fig. 14.32). Brownish discoloration of the ichthyotic scales indicates that the patient is receiving or has received treatment with Clofazimine.

Sweating

A dry lesion (TT/BT) indicates focal loss of sweating. In case of doubtful lesions, anhidrosis can be detected by pilocarpine test[25] or the noninvasive ninhydrin test.[30]

Compensatory hyperhidrosis, especially involving face, trunk and axillae, is present in some patients.

Mucosal Examination

Mucosal involvement is indicative of an untreated disease of long duration and should be examined with as equal care as skin. Following findings should be looked for:[31,32]

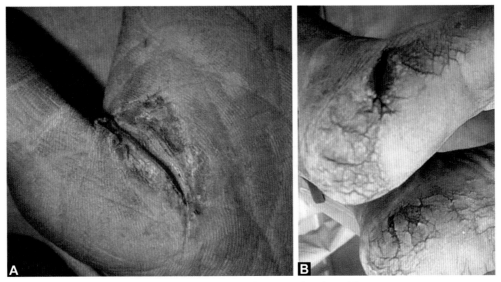

Figs 14.27A and B: Deep fissures on hands and feet

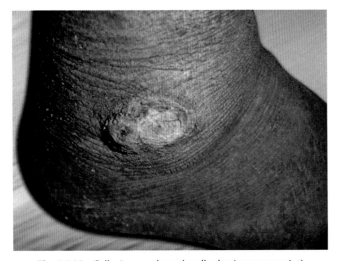

Fig. 14.28: Callosity over lateral malleolus (pressure point)

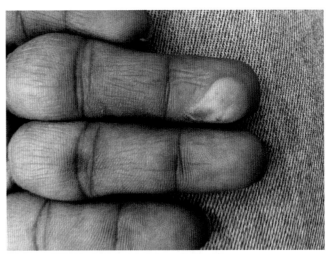

Fig. 14.29: Spontaneous blister on finger

Lips and Oral Mucosa

- Diffuse enlargement of lips or macrocheilia may be part of infiltration in lepromatous disease or T1R involving a BT lesion overlying lips and surrounding areas.[33]
- Nodular infiltration (reddish/reddish-yellow, sessile/pedunculated lesions) of lip (Fig. 14.33), tongue, palate (may be ulcerated/perforated) and uvula may be seen in patients with lepromatous disease. Fissuring of tongue may be present in florid LL disease.[7,34]
- Uvula; intact or partial/complete destruction. Uvular movement normal or restricted (fibrosis).

Nasal Mucosa

Nasal mucosal examination should be performed in suspected lepromatous disease with an artificial light source and nasal speculum. Mouth-breathing and foul-smell may indicate presence of nasal crusts. Removal of crusts facilitates better visualization of the mucosa, which is insensitive, pale, thickened and irregular with destruction of inferior turbinates. Presence of bleeding and septal perforation should be looked for. Neglected patients may harbor maggots in the nasal cavity.[7]

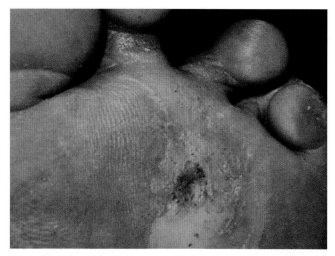

Fig. 14.30: Splaying of adjacent toes around a threatened ulcer

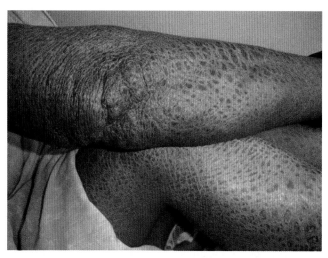

Fig. 14.32: Secondary ichthyosis in lepromatous leprosy with brownish discoloration of the scales due to Clofazimine

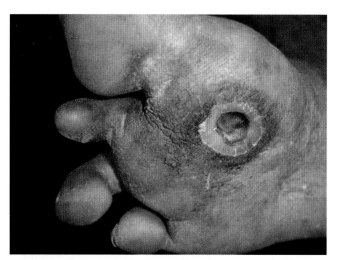

Fig. 14.31: Trophic ulcer

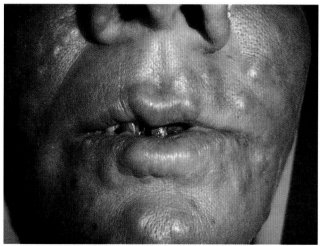

Fig. 14.33: Nodular infiltration of lip in LL leprosy

Ocular Examination

Patient's face should be inspected closely for:
- Any skin lesion involving the periocular area.
- Frequency of blinking, blink-interval and blink-completeness should be observed. A regular blinking (normally 6/minute) is indicative of preserved protective corneal sensation.[35]
- Width of palpebral fissure, while the patient gazes straight at a distant object.
- Photophobia, redness of eyes, watering and any other obvious ocular abnormalities.

Ocular examination is done with a well-focused torch and preferably with a corneal loupe.[25] Opinion of the ophthalmologist should be sought for in situations difficult to reach a conclusion. Intraocular pressure is assessed by gentle palpation of the closed eyes with both index fingers; and ocular tenderness should be noted at the same time by looking at patient's face. Raised intraocular tension may be indicative of glaucoma. Presence or absence of following features should also be noted.

Eyebrows and Eyelashes

Superciliary (loss of/sparse eyebrow) and ciliary (loss of eyelashes) madarosis are features of advanced LL (Fig. 14.34). Look for inwardly directed eyelashes (trichiasis).

Eyelids

In all cases of facial BT lesion, patient should be examined for lagophthalmos at an early stage. Normally, while the gaze is fixed straight at a distant object, the upper lid covers the upper 2 mm of the cornea and the lower lid is at the level of lower border of limbus, so that sclera is not visible above or below cornea.[35] Visible thin strip of white sclera above or below cornea, in this position, is suggestive of lid retraction or lagophthalmos.[35]

If lagophthalmos is not obvious, patient is asked to close the eyes gently. Faulty eye-closure with visible Bell's phenomenon is due to improper approximation of the eyelids. Mild lag or ectropion of only lower eyelid with pooled tear-film suggests selective involvement of the zygomatic branch of the facial nerve, which may result from an overlying BT lesion, with or without T1R.[25] It may rarely be bilateral due to large BT lesion involving eyelids on both sides.[36] Bilateral lagophthalmos may be a feature of widespread pure neuritic disease[37] or untreated advanced LL disease (Fig. 14.35). Lagophthalmos is of sudden onset and severe in borderline disease (mostly related to T1R), whereas, more gradual in onset and milder in LL disease.[35]

Pterygium

If pterygium is present, it usually harbors bacilli, and indicates high ocular bacillary load.[9]

Redness of Eyes

A perilimbal redness is indicative of iridocyclitis, which may be a part of LL disease or associated with type 2 lepra reaction (Fig. 14.36). Redness of the entire conjunctiva is suggestive of conjunctivitis.[25]

Cornea

Corneal surface is looked for xerosis and/or abrasions or obvious corneal ulcer. Xerosis of eyes can be detected by Schirmer test[38] and staining the tear-film with 1% fluorescein dye (with the help of a glass rod), helps in detecting corneal abrasions.[35]

Corneal sensation is tested (following proper cleaning of hand) with a clean wisp of cotton-wool, rolled into a point on one end. The examiner approaches the patient from one side and the cornea is touched gently, 2 mm inside the limbus at the 6 o'clock position while the patient looks straight (Fig. 14.37).[35] Normally there should be a brisk blink response.

Unilateral loss of corneal reflex may result from the involvement of ophthalmic nerve (trigeminal) due to a same

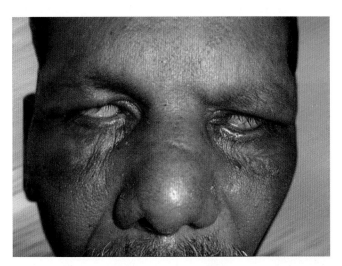

Fig. 14.35: Untreated lapromatous leprosy with bilateral lagophthalmos

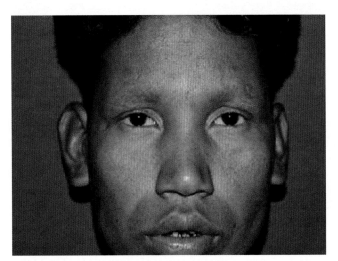

Fig. 14.34: Loss of eyebrows and eyelashes, diffuse infiltration of face, earlobes and lips in a patient with LL leprosy. Bacteriological Index was 6+ in this case

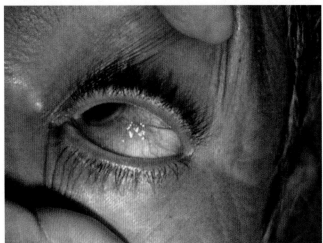

Fig. 14.36: Perilimbal redness of eye, suggestive of iridocyclitis in a patient with LL leprosy and T2R

sided periocular BT lesion. Bilateral absence of corneal reflex indicates damage to corneal nerves due to advanced LL disease.[7] Testing for corneal sensation is not recommended during field survey for safety reasons.[28]

Pupil

Small, irregular pupil, nonreactive to light is indicative of iridocyclitis, or adhesions of iris.

Visual Acuity

Visual acuity of the patient should be assessed by finger-count test and thereafter using Snellen's chart; it may be impaired due to large corneal opacity, cataract or glaucoma.

Palpation of Peripheral Nerves

Clinician should be well aware of the specific sites or bony landmarks along which the peripheral nerves commonly involved in leprosy are to be palpated, as well as the area of distribution of sensory nerves. Method of palpation of some peripheral nerves has been presented in Tables 14.3A and B (Figs 14.38 to 14.43).[39,40]

Nerve palpation should be gentle (using pulps of fingers rather than tips) to avoid causing pain to an inflamed nerve (neuritis).[19,20] Each nerve should be palpated on both sides for comparison, even if the involvement is felt to be asymmetric.

It is prudent to remember that interpretation of palpation of peripheral nerves is subjective in nature (may vary from examiner to examiner).[41,42] Moreover, peripheral nerve trunks may be palpable normally, especially in thin-built individuals and manual workers. Hence while interpreting nerve thickening in doubtful cases, associated loss of sensation

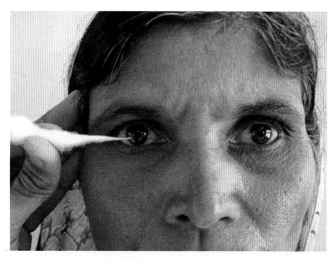

Fig. 14.37: Testing corneal sensation

in its distribution (one of the cardinal features of leprosy) and/or weakness of the muscles supplied by the affected nerve should be looked for.[42] Comparison of nerves on both sides helps in appreciating unilateral nerve enlargement. It should be remembered also that the ulnar nerve on the dominant (working) side is comparatively slightly thicker than on the opposite side.

Following features should be assessed while palpating a peripheral nerve:
- Palpable or not? Large peripheral nerve trunks are usually not palpable in indeterminate and TT disease.
- Is the nerve compressible? (Lack of compressibility indicates a fibrosed nerve, which may appear even thinner and cord-like).
- Unilateral or bilateral? If enlarged bilaterally, assess the difference between two sides, if any. Asymmetric nerve enlargement is a feature of borderline disease.
- Extent of the nerve palpable in its course (ulnar, lateral popliteal, etc.).
- Presence of nodularity or abscess (diffuse, fusiform swelling).
- Nerve tenderness (indicative of neuritis); look at patient's face for a wince.

The aim is to detect early neuritis or nerve thickening. Sometimes, there may be very little or no demonstrable nerve tenderness. Such cases should be examined with due care, as demonstration of an increase in the "area of anesthesia" or in "weakness of the muscles supplied by the nerve trunk" may suggest silent neuritis.[7] Neuritis is much more severe in T1R as compared to that in T2R.

Hypoesthesia or anesthesia along the course of a peripheral nerve may be the chief complaint in pure neuritic disease. However, unlike other causes of peripheral neuropathy, sensory impairment in leprosy may not strictly follow the distribution of a peripheral nerve or nerve root.[11]

The areas of sensory distribution by cutaneous branches of major nerve trunks on hands and feet are given in Figure 14.44.

Among cranial nerves, peripheral branches of trigeminal (supratrochlear, supraorbital) and facial nerves (zygomaticotemporal, buccal, marginal mandibular, cervical) may be palpable in presence of facial lesions or as part of pure neuritic leprosy.[37,43] These nerves should be looked for in presence of facial lesions. The anatomical location of the terminal branches of facial nerve has been shown in Figure 14.45. Involvement of other cranial nerves (glossopharyngeal, vagus, hypoglossal) in leprosy has been reported rarely,[44] and this may be the cause of nasal regurgitation, complained by some patients. However, routine examination of these nerves is not done, unless specific clinical features, not attributable to other causes, are present.

Features like postural hypotension and asymmetric pupil may indicate presence of advanced autonomic neuropathy.[7]

Table 14.3A: Methods of palpating different peripheral nerves (head, neck and upper extremity)[39,40]

Nerve	Site/bony landmark	Patient position	Method
Head and Neck			
Supraorbital	Supraorbital notch at the junction of medial one-third and lateral two-thirds of supraorbital ridge	Sitting/standing with head kept straight	Palpate with both thumbs on both sides (Fig. 14.38)
Supratrochlear	Medial to the supraorbital nerve	Same as above	Same as above
Infraorbital	Infraorbital foramen, just below the medial part of inferior orbital margin	Same as above	Same as above
Branches of facial nerve: Zygomatic and temporal	Zygomatic arch	Same as above	Same as above
Great auricular	Lateral side of neck, crosses sternomastoid muscle, from lateral side to infra-auricular area	Sitting/standing with head turned completely to opposite side	Easily visible, crossing sternomastoid obliquely. May be palpated with 2 fingers
Clavicular (3 sets)	Shaft of clavicle	Sitting/standing straight	Fingers rolled along the shafts of both clavicles
Upper Extremity			
Radial	Spiral groove on humerus, posterior to the deltoid insertion	Sitting/standing with elbow flexed at 90° Examiner's right hand holds patient's right hand in shaking-hand manner and *vice versa*	Examiner's left fingers roll the nerve in the radial groove
Ulnar	Ulnar groove on medial epicondyle of humerus, medial to the point of elbow	Same as above (Both the nerves may be palpated simultaneously for better comparison)	Examiner's left little finger locate the nerve in the groove; other fingers palpate the nerve upward along medial aspect of arm (Fig. 14.39)
Radial cutaneous	Lateral border of radius, just proximal to the wrist; thereafter along the proximal part of extensor pollicis longus tendon, which stands out prominently on ulnar side of the anatomical snuff box	Same as above Patient is asked to extend the thumb to visualize the anatomical snuff box	Examiner's left fingers roll the nerve against radius (Fig. 14.40). It can be further traced and rolled from side to side on extensor pollicis longus tendon and dorsum of hand
Median	Proximal to the flexor aspect of wrist joint (proximal to flexor retinaculum), between the tendons of palmaris longus and flexor carpi radialis	Sitting/standing with elbow flexed at 90°, and wrist in supination. Examiner's left hand stabilizes patient's right hand and *vice versa*	Examiner's right fingers palpate the nerve deep between the tendons

Examination of Musculoskeletal System

Inspection of the patient as a whole provides clues to the involvement of musculoskeletal system. Detailed examination can be done thereafter.

Face

Look for the contour of the nose:
- Collapse of the bridge (destruction of anterior nasal spine) (Fig. 14.46).
- Destruction of ala nasi.
- Columella, rarely may be destroyed.[45]

Teeth should be inspected for the loosening or loss of upper incisors. Nasal and dental changes, in association with flat cheeks and thin upper lip constitute the 'facies leprosa', as seen in patients with advanced lepromatous disease.[7,25]

Facial muscle paralysis in TT mostly involves the upper face (orbicularis oculi) in contrast to other common causes of lower motor neuron facial palsy (e.g., Bell's palsy), where both upper and lower parts of the face are involved (Fig. 14.47). Mask-like facies may be a feature of advanced LL disease and indicates paralysis of muscles of facial expression (involvement of terminal branches of facial nerve in their superficial course).[11] Usually such paralysis is asymmetric and

Table 14.3B: Methods of palpating different peripheral nerves (lower extremity)[39,40]

Nerve	Site/bony landmark	Patient position	Method
Ant. Cut. nerves of thigh (3 sets)	Anterior aspect of thigh	Sitting; Standing upright may help to visualize the nerves better	Fingers rolled on the anterior aspect of both thighs
Lateral popliteal	Just below the lateral aspect of knee, along neck of fibula	Sitting with legs dangling freely	Knee stabilized by placing the thumbs on upper border of patella on both sides and the nerve rolled with fingers, against neck of fibula (Fig. 14.41)
Sural	Posterior aspect of leg, between the two bellies of gastrocnemius above and tendo Achilles below	Standing/lying prone	Palpated on both sides with fingers (Fig. 14.42)
Anterior tibial	On the dorsum of foot, lateral to the tendon of extensor hallucis longus and dorsalis pedis artery	Patient sitting on bed with legs straight and is asked to extend the great toe to make the extensor hallucis longus tendon stand out	Palpated by rolling of fingers
Posterior tibial	Medial aspect of ankle (deep to flexor retinaculum) between medial malleolus and tendo Achilles	Sitting on bed with knee flexed/standing	Palpated by rolling of fingers (Fig. 14.43)

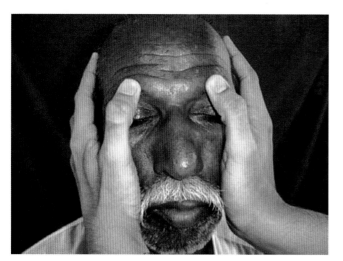

Fig. 14.38: Palpation of supraorbital nerve with the thumbs; fingers are used to stabilize the head

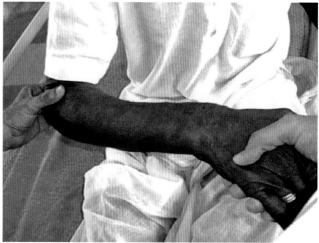

Fig. 14.39: Palpation of ulnar nerve

patchy. Careful examination may reveal following unusual deformities at the initial stages:
- Out-pouching of the lips at the angle of the mouth (weakness/paralysis of orbicularis oris muscle).
- 'V'-like configuration of lateral part of forehead wrinkles on attempt to raise eyebrows (medial part of frontalis muscle, which is paralyzed earlier than the lateral part).
- Concentric creases extending from corners of mouth (buccinator smile; superficial facial muscles forming the nasolabial fold are paralyzed, but action of buccinator is retained).

Upper Extremity

Look for:
- Obvious deformities like wrist drop or claw hand (partial/complete) (Fig. 14.48).
- Compare thenar and hypothenar eminences of patient's palm with opposite normal side or with examiner's hand to detect wasting.
- Guttering of the interosseous spaces, suggestive of wasting of the interossei and lumbricals (Fig. 14.49).
- Normal bulging contour of medial aspect of forearm; flattened due to wasting of flexor carpi ulnaris (high ulnar paralysis) (Fig. 14.50).

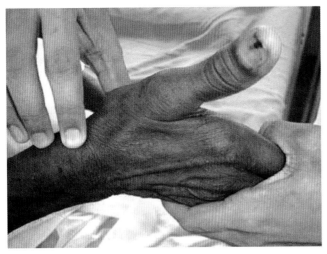

Fig. 14.40: Palpation of radial cutaneous nerve

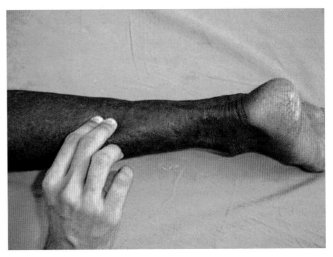

Fig. 14.42: Palpation of sural nerve

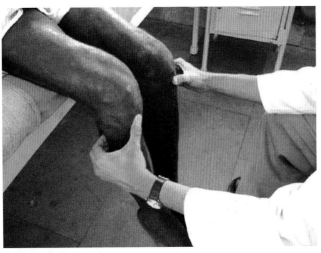

Fig. 14.41: Palpation of lateral popliteal nerve

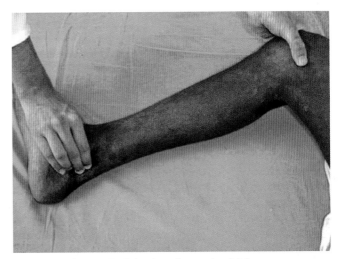

Fig. 14.43: Palpation of posterior tibial nerve

- Swelling (fusiform/sausage-shaped) of fingers with or without tenderness, suggestive of dactylitis (Figs 14.51A and B).
- Test patient's grip; whether pinch grip (holding small objects with tips of fingers) and power grip (holding a rod firmly) are possible; or only hook grip (holding a bucket by handle) is retained, suggestive of both ulnar and median nerve palsy.[46]
- Secondary deformities due to nerve palsy:[47]
  - *Hooding*; contracture of the fingers due to attenuation of central extensor tendons of fingers in long-standing claw hand.
  - *Z-thumb*; hyperextension of metacarpophalangeal (MCP) joint and hyperflexion of interphalangeal (IP) joints of thumb, loss of primary flexion of MCP joint due to ulnar nerve palsy (Fig. 14.52).
- Shortening of fingers indicative of resorption of terminal phalanges, e.g. paddle hand, mitten hand (severe shortening of digits).[47]
- Frozen hand (nonfunctional hand, flexed at wrist with stiff, twisted fingers at odd directions, dorsal skin is hyperpigmented, leathery and tethered to deeper tissue) indicates repeated lepra reactions in the past.[46]
- Soft silky hand (loss of normal resilient feel of palms due to lepromatous infiltration and destruction of the fibrous septa attaching palmar skin to the palmar fascia).[23]

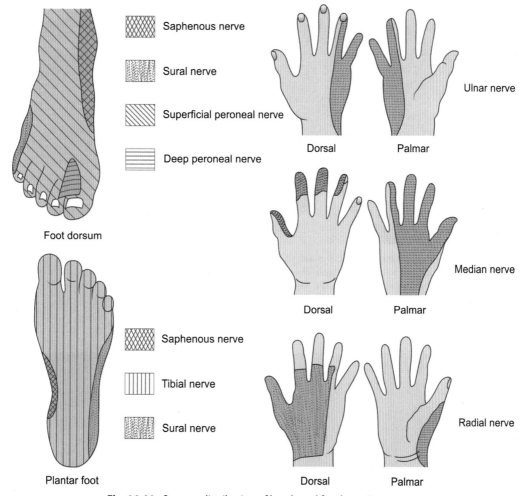

Saphenous nerve

Sural nerve

Superficial peroneal nerve

Deep peroneal nerve

Foot dorsum

Saphenous nerve

Tibial nerve

Sural nerve

Plantar foot

Dorsal   Palmar   Ulnar nerve

Dorsal   Palmar   Median nerve

Dorsal   Palmar   Radial nerve

Fig. 14.44: Sensory distribution of hands and feet by various nerves

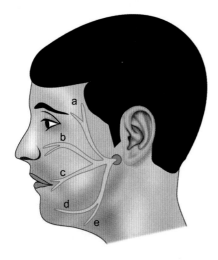

Fig. 14.45: Terminal branches of facial nerve
a - Temporal; b - Zygomatic; c - Buccal;
d - Marginal mandibular; e - Cervical

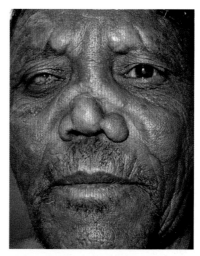

Fig. 14.46: Collapse of the bridge of the nose and
right sided corneal opacity

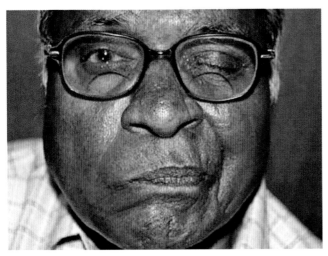

Fig. 14.47: A case of Bell's palsy (right side). The facial paralysis in leprosy involves upper part of face (due to selective involvement of zygomatic branch of facial nerve by a leprosy lesion in the vicinity). In Bell's palsy, the involvement of facial nerve is higher up due to edematous compression in facial canal, affecting all branches, leading to paralysis of both upper and lower parts of face

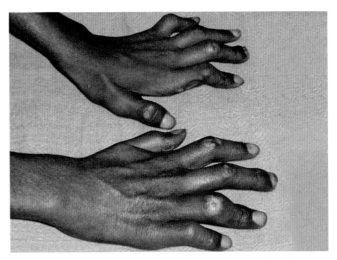

Fig. 14.49: Bilateral complete claw hands with guttering of dorsal interosseous spaces and callosities on interphalangeal joints

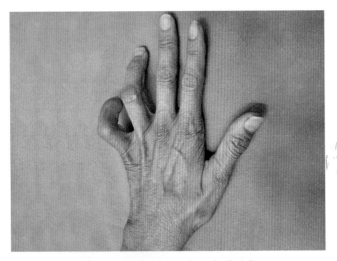

Fig. 14.48: Partial or ulnar clawhand

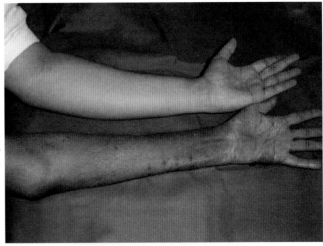

Fig. 14.50: Flattening of normal bulging contour of medial aspect of forearm; high ulnar nerve palsy

Lower Extremity

Look for:
- Gait abnormality (high-stepping gait) and obvious deformities like foot drop or claw toes (Fig. 14.53).
- Collapsed arch(es) of the foot or feet.
- Guttering of the interosseous spaces, wasting of interossei and lumbricals.
- Dactylitis involving toes.
- Shortening of toes indicative of resorption of phalanges (Fig. 14.54).
- Wasting of peronei muscles in lateral compartment of leg (supplied by superficial peroneal branch of lateral popliteal nerve).

Deep tendon reflexes are usually preserved in patients with leprosy, or there may even be hyperreflexia. Functions of the muscles of the forearm, hand, leg and feet are assessed by certain tests like voluntary muscle testing (VMT). Various methods of VMT have been presented in Tables 14.4A and B (Figs 14.55 to 14.59).[7,19,20,25,39,40,48] The six grades for VMT [Medical Research Council (MRC) scale] are as follows:[49]
- *Grade 5*: Normal power (with full resistance).
- *Grade 4*: Muscle contraction against slight resistance but power subnormal.
- *Grade 3*: Movement possible without resistance.
- *Grade 2*: Active movement when gravity is eliminated.

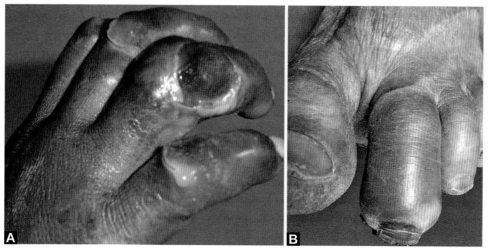

Figs 14.51A and B: Dactylitis involving fingers (A) and toe (B). Note the blistering and ulceration of the skin on fingers

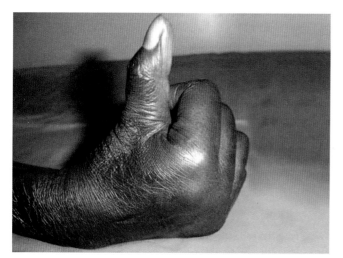

Fig. 14.52: 'Z' thumb deformity

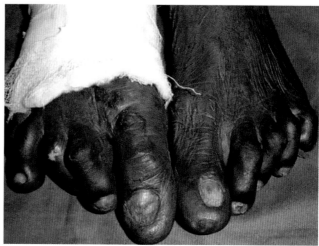

Fig. 14.53: Claw toes

- *Grade 1*: Flicker of movement.
- *Grade 0*: No movement.

Before starting VMT, the power of the muscle is assessed approximately by noting the range of movement the patient can perform (active and passive) with the affected limb or digit. If it is apparently normal, muscle power testing can be started directly against resistance. For testing small muscles of hands and feet, effect of gravity is negligible.[50]

Some simple, quick and easy methods of muscle testing, appropriate for field workers, suggested by different authors have been presented in Table 14.5.[51-53]

Claw hands should be tested for mobility. Passive flexion (by examiner) of the hyperextended MCP joint enables the patient to extend the flexed proximal IP joints (mobile claw hands/toes), indicating early stage of deformity which may be amenable to physiotherapy or corrective surgery.[39] Fixed

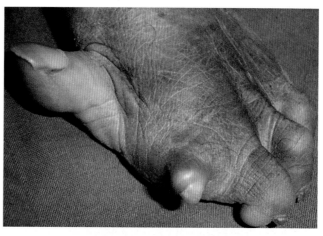

Fig. 14.54: Resorption of digits

Table 14.4A: Examination of muscles of face and upper extremities[7,19,20,25,39,40,48]

Muscle to be tested	Nerve supply	Test	Interpretation	Deformity/disability
Face				
Orbicularis oculi	Zygomatic and temporal branches of facial nerve	Patient asked to close the eyes forcefully and examiner tries to separate the eyelids	In normal eye, separation of the eyelids is quite difficult. Ability to open the eyelids indicates weakness of the muscle	Lagophthalmos (*vide* text for details)
Upper Extremity				
Extensors of wrist joint	Postinterosseous branch of radial	Close fist and dorsiflex the wrist against resistance	Weakness: radial nerve involvement	Inability to extend wrist and fingers Wrist drop
Flexor digitorum superficialis and profundus (lateral part)	Median nerve at or above elbow	Patient asked to clasp both hands **(Ochsner's clasping test)** (Fig. 14.55)	Index finger of affected side does not flex and remains straight	**Pointing index/Benediction sign.**[48] Outstretched index finger with flexion of other fingers
Abductor pollicis brevis	Median nerve	Patient's hand is laid flat (palmar surface up) on a table and asked to touch a pen held slightly higher, by moving the thumb vertically up (abduction) **(Pen test)** (Fig.14.56)	Inability to touch the pen, loss of abduction movement of thumb	Thumb lies flat in the same plane of hand (adducted, hyperextended and rotated at carpometacarpal joint and flexed at MCP and IP joints. **Ape-thumb deformity**
Opponens pollicis	Median nerve	Examiner stabilizes patient's hand with own and patient is asked to swing the thumb across the palm (the thumb-nail lying parallel to palm) to touch the tips of other fingers, while examiner resisting this action with his index finger	Inability to perform the action against resistance indicates weakness of opponens pollicis	
1st palmar interossei and adductor pollicis	Deep branch of ulnar nerve	Patient asked to hold a book between two hands by keeping the adducted thumbs straight on its upper surface. Examiner tries to pull the book in opposite direction **(Book test)** (Fig. 14.57)	Flexion of the distal IP joint of thumb **(Froment's sign)** with hyperextension of MCP joint on affected side indicates weakness of these two muscles and action of flexor pollicis longus (median nerve)	Guttering of 1st interosseous space
Lumbricals + interossei	1st and 2nd: median nerve; 3rd and 4th: deep branch of ulnar nerve Interossei: deep branch of ulnar nerve	Patient asked to flex the fingers at MCP joints against resistance	Inability indicates weakness of these two groups of muscles	**Claw hand**; hyperextension at MCP and flexion at IP joints *Partial* (1st, 2nd, 3rd or 4th and 5th fingers): only median nerve or only ulnar nerve involvement; *Complete* (all fingers): both median and ulnar nerve involvement Difficulty in grasping
Palmar interossei	Deep branch of ulnar nerve	Patient asked to keep fingers extended as well as adducted. A firm paper-card is inserted in each web-space serially and patient is instructed to grasp it tightly while the examiner tries to pull it out **(Card test)** (Fig. 14.58)	Inability to hold the card tightly indicates weakness of palmar interossei	Subtle abducted position of little finger **(Wartberg's sign)**[29] earliest sign of ulnar nerve involvement (Fig. 14.59) Mild guttering of interosseous spaces Inability to bring fingers together Difficulty in eating rice with hands and holding small objects like coin[46]
Dorsal interossei	Deep branch of ulnar nerve	Patient asked to spread out fingers against resistance by examiner's hand	Inability indicates weakness of dorsal interossei	Guttering of interosseous spaces Reduced finger span Function like typing is difficult[46]

Abbreviations: IP, interphalangeal; MCP, metacarpophalangeal.

Table 14.4B: Examination of muscles of lower extremities[7,19,20,25,39,40,48]

Muscles to be tested	Nerve supply	Test	Interpretation	Deformity/disability
Dorsiflexors of ankle Extensor hallucis longus Peronei longus and brevis	Common peroneal nerve	Patient asked to perform following movements against resistance by examiner's hand: • Dorsiflexion at ankle • Extension of great toe • Eversion of foot	Inability indicates weakness of these muscles	**Foot drop** In long-standing cases, foot is fixed at plantar-flexed and inverted position (late stage, rigid equinovarus deformity
Intrinsic muscles of feet	Medial and lateral plantar branches of tibial nerve	Patient asked to adduct/abduct toes against resistance	Inability indicates weakness of these muscles	Collapse of arch of foot Guttering of inter-tarsal spaces Clawing of toes (ground is touched by the tip of toes rather than the pad) Inability to squeeze the toes together or spread them Inability to use regular foot wears and requires special one

Abbreviations: IP, interphalangeal; MCP, metacarpophalangeal.

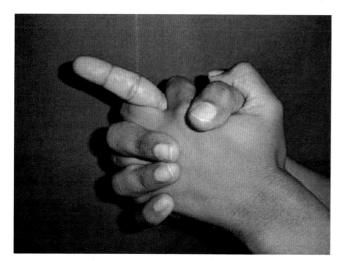

Fig. 14.55: Ochsner's clasping test with pointing index

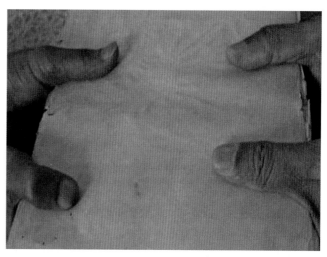

Fig. 14.57: Book test with positive Froment's sign (right side)

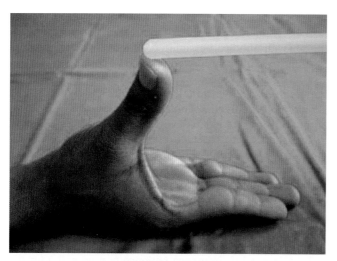

Fig. 14.56: Pen test

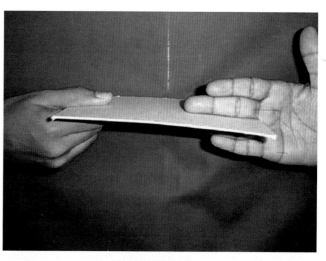

Fig. 14.58: Card test

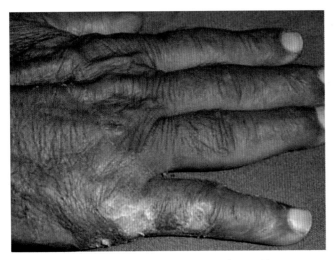

Fig. 14.59: Positive Wartberg's sign: earliest evidence of ulnar nerve palsy

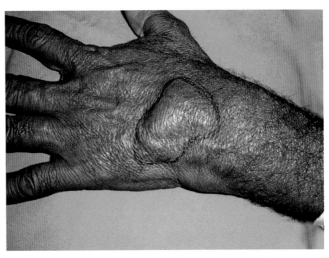

Fig. 14.60: Globular, cystic swelling around wrist joint following T1R suggestive of tenosynovitis

flexion along middle finger creases suggests long-term neglected claw hand.[39]

Acute-onset, symmetric, peripheral polyarthralgia may be an accompaniment of both T1R and T2R[34] and has to be differentiated from rheumatoid arthritis by ancillary clinical findings.

Presence of globular, cystic, tender swelling, usually on the dorsal surface of wrist joint, following an episode of T1R in borderline disease is indicative of tenosynovitis (Fig. 14.60). Individual joint effusion or bursitis may be present.[34]

Examination of External Genitalia

Though a protected site, lesions of the external genitalia are not uncommon in leprosy. Hence genitalia of both male and female patients should be inspected for presence of skin lesions. In addition, in male patients, testicles should be palpated gently to see for:[34]

Size and consistency: Whether the testicles are firm, resilient and of appropriate size or small and soft (sequel of advanced disease and/or repeated T2R).

Testicular sensation: If absent, indicates fibrosis resulting from repeated episodes of epididymo-orchitis (T2R).

Tenderness: Acute testicular pain indicates epididymo-orchitis, a part of T2R and this may be the presenting feature of T2R.

While examining for testicular sensation and tenderness, the examiner should observe the patient's face.

Other Systemic Examination

Upper respiratory tract is the most common site of involvement. Though several other organs are involved in LL and also during T2R, clinical manifestations of such involvement are unusual and are recognized only during histopathological examination or autopsy.[14]

A hoarse voice, dry, hacking cough and occasional breathlessness are indicative of laryngeal involvement and/or uvular dysfunction; features of LL leprosy. Acute respiratory distress during an episode of T2R may be a pointer to the rapidly developing laryngeal edema. Lower respiratory tract should be examined for evidence of bronchopneumonia which is a common sequel of laryngeal dysfunction. Pulmonary tuberculosis may be an accompaniment in leprosy patients (2.4–13.3%, Indian study 7.7%);[54] hence clinical evidence of pulmonary tuberculosis has to be ruled out in each patient as such cases need alteration in the treatment schedule for leprosy, to avoid rifampicin resistance.

Clinical features of renal dysfunction may be evident in patients with long-standing disease (renal amyloidosis), or patients suffering from recurrent episodes of ENL which may lead to glomerulonephritis. If untreated patients with LL present with jaundice, possibility of leprous hepatic granuloma resulting in hepatic dysfunction should be considered.

During an episode of severe T2R, sudden drop of body temperature, hypotension, hypoglycemia and hyperkalemia should alert the treating clinician of the possibility of acute adrenal crisis and sudden death.

In patients with repeated episodes of leprosy reactions, any focus of infection should be sought for (caries teeth, pharyngitis, tonsillitis, UTI, chronic amoebiasis, etc.), which might precipitate the recurrence.

Patient's mental status should also be assessed as depression is commonly associated, especially in patients with recurrent reactions.[55]

Examination of a patient suffering from leprosy is an art indeed. It requires immense patience and empathy for the

Table 14.5: Some tests for quick examination of muscle power/nerve paralysis in the field[51-53]

Nerve	Test	Interpretation
Upper Extremity		
Median nerve	Affected palm facing up or both palms facing each other the patient is asked to abduct the thumb/thumbs and maintain it in that position for 30 seconds[51]	If tip of the thumb points to the roof at the end of 30 seconds, it is normal. If points anteriorly, it indicates weakness of median nerve
	Tip-to-tip thumb opposition to the 4th finger:[52] Patient asked to oppose the thumb to touch tip of 4th finger, with slight flexion of thumb IP joint and nails of both thumb and 4th finger lying in the same plane, so as to form an 'O' and maintain this position	The angle between long axis of both the nails measured approximately: <100°: evident median nerve function loss <150° but >120°: minimal median nerve function loss >150°: Normal nerve function
	Detection of hidden/latent clawing of index and middle finger (performed when clawing is not evident): Patient asked to grasp and squeeze examiner's forearm[53]	Digging of examiner's forearm by the tips of index and middle fingers of patient due to hyperflexion of IP joints and limited flexion of MCP joint
Ulnar nerve	Flap-flexion of fingers: Wrist of the patient kept in neutral position, and asked to perform flexion and extension of MCP joints few times keeping the fingers straight (like a flap). Thereafter the hand is held in this position (MCP joints flexed and IP joints extended, fingers straight) for few seconds[52]	Normal person is able to keep the fingers straight. Flexion of the fingers at IP joints indicates clawing
Radial nerve	The person is asked to stretch both the arms and forearms anteriorly, keeping the wrists dorsiflexed and fingers extended and maintain this position for 30 seconds	Inability to maintain this position indicates weakness of radial nerve and helps to detect radial palsy early
Assessment of combined functions of radial, ulnar and median nerves	Beak test: Patient is instructed to dorsiflex the wrist and straighten all the fingers to join the fingertips simulating head and beak of a bird and maintain this position for 30 seconds	Normal person is able to maintain this position. In radial nerve palsy, patient is unable to dorsiflex the wrist, and in ulnar and median nerve palsies, little finger and thumb stands out respectively
Lower Extremity		
Common peroneal	Patient is asked to stand on both heels and keep all the toes lifted[51]	Normal persons are able to maintain this position for few seconds. Inability indicates weakness of dorsiflexors
Tibial nerve	Patient is asked to retract/pull back the toes by keeping the feet firmly on ground[51]	Curling of the toes, rather than retraction indicates weakness of intrinsic muscles of feet

Abbreviations: IP, interphalangeal; MCP, metacarpophalangeal.

patient. A searching eye and an eager mind is imperative to scan the patient as a whole, in a brief span of time to detect as many clinical findings as possible.

REFERENCES

1. Mahajan S, Sardana K, Bhushan P, et al. A study of leprosy in children from a tertiary pediatric hospital in India. Lepr Rev. 2006;77(2):100-2.
2. Pfaltzgraff RE. What is the actual male/female ratio in leprosy patients? Lepr Rev. 2003;74(2):180-1.
3. Shale MJ. Women with leprosy. A woman with leprosy is in jeopardy. Lepr Rev. 2000;71(1):5-17.
4. Heynders ML, Meijs JJ, Anderson AM. Towards an understanding of non compliance. An assessment of risk factors for defaulting from leprosy treatment. Lepr Rev. 2000;71(3):369-76.
5. Nunzi E, Fiallo P. Differential diagnosis. In: Hastings RC, Diltor VAO (Eds). Leprosy, 2nd edition. Edinburgh: Chuchill Livingstone; 1994.pp.291-315.
6. Withington SG, Joha S, Baird D, et al. Assessing socio-economic factors in relation to stigmatization, impairment status and selection of socio-economic rehabilitation: a 1 year cohort of new leprosy cases in north Bangladesh. Lepr Rev. 2003;74(2):120-32.
7. Pfaltzgraff RE, Ramu G. Clinical leprosy. In: Hastings RC, Diltor VAO (Eds). Leprosy, 2nd edition. Edinburgh: Chuchill Livingstone; 1994.pp.237-86.

8. WHO Expert Committee on leprosy, 7th report. WHO Technical Report Series No 874. Geneva: World Health Organization; 1998.pp.1-43.

9. Thompson K, Daniel E. Management of ocular problems in leprosy. Indian J Lepr. 1998;70(3):295-315.

10. Bryceson ADM, Pfaltzgraff RE. Complications due to nerve damage. In: Bryceson ADM, Pfaltzgraff RE (Eds). Leprosy, 3rd edition. Edinburgh: Chuchill Livingstone; 1990:pp.133-52.

11. Sabin TD, Swift TR, Jacobson RR. Leprosy. In: Dyck PJ, Thomas P (Eds). Peripheral neuropathy, 4th edition. Philadelphia: Saunders; 2005.pp.1354-80.

12. van Brakel WH, Khawas IB. Nerve damage in leprosy: an epidemiological and clinical study of 396 patients in west Nepal. Part 1. Definition, methods and frequencies. Lepr Rev. 1994;65(3):204-21.

13. van Brakel WH, Nicholls PG, Das L, et al. The INFIR cohort study: investigating prediction, detection and pathogenesis of neuropathy and reaction in leprosy. Methods and baseline results of a cohort of multibacillary leprosy patients in north India. Lepr Rev. 2005;76(1):14-34.

14. Klioze AM, Ramos-Caro FA. Visceral leprosy. Int J Dermatol. 2000;39(9):641-58.

15. Trindade MA, Manini MI, Masetti JH, et al. Leprosy and HIV co-infection in five patients. Lepr Rev. 2005;76(2):162-6.

16. Petri WA. Chemotherapy of tuberculosis, mycobacterium avium complex disease and leprosy. In: Brunton LL, Lazo JS, Parker KL (Eds). Goodman and Gillman's The Pharmacological Basis of Therapeutics. 11th edition. New York: McGraw Hill; 2006.pp.1203-41.

17. Knowels SR, Shear NH. Cutaneous drug reactions with systemic features. In: Wolverton SE (Ed). Comprehensive Dermatologic Drug Therapy, 2nd edition. Philadelphia: Saunders; 2007. pp.977-90.

18. Krishnamoorthy KV, Desikan KV. Indeterminate leprosy in an infant. Lepr Rev. 2006;77:377-80.

19. Bryceson ADM, Pfaltzgraff RE. Symptoms and signs. In: Bryceson ADM, Pfaltzgraff RE (Eds). Leprosy, 3rd edition. Edinburgh: Churchill Livingstone; 1990.pp.25-54.

20. Thangaraj RH. Clinical examination. In: Thangaraj RH (Ed). A manual of leprosy, 4th edition. New Delhi: The Leprosy Mission, Southern Asia; 1985.pp.78-87.

21. Shaw IN, Ebenezer G, Babu B, et al. Borderline tuberculoid leprosy of the scalp. Lepr Rev. 2001;72(3):357-61.

22. Kumar B, Kaur I, Rai R, et al. Involvement of male genitalia in leprosy. Lepr Rev. 2001;72(1):70-7.

23. Indira D, Kaur I, Sharma VK, et al. Palmoplantar lesions in leprosy. Indian J Lepr. 1999;71(2):167-72.

24. Ghorpade A, Ramanan C. Primary penile tuberculoid leprosy. Indian J Lepr. 2000;72(4):499-500.

25. Jopling WH, McDougall AC. The disease. In: Jopling WH, McDougall AC (Eds). Handbook of leprosy, 5th edition. Delhi: CBS Publishers and Distributors; 1996.pp.10-53.

26. Srinivasan H, Dharmendra. Treatment of ulcers in leprosy patients. In: Dharmendra (Ed). Leprosy. Bombay: Kothari Medical Publishing House; 1978.pp.599-616.

27. Owen BM, Stratford CJ. Assessment of the methods available for testing sensations in leprosy patients in a rural setting. Lepr Rev. 1995;66(1):55-62.

28. Brandsma JW, Van Brakel WH. WHO disability grading: operational definitions. Lepr Rev. 2003;74(4):366-73.

29. Virmond M. Indications for surgery in leprosy. Lepr Rev. 1998;69(3):297-304.

30. Markendeya N, Srinivas CR. Ninhydrin sweat test in leprosy. Indian J Lepr. 2004;76(4):299-304.

31. Girdhar BK, Desikan KV. A clinical study of the mouth in untreated lepromatous patients. Lepr Rev. 1979;50(1):25-35.

32. Costa A, Nery J, Oliveira M, et al. Oral lesions in leprosy. Indian J Dermatol Venereol Leprol. 2003;69(6):381-5.

33. Singh G, Nagaraja, Prabhu S. Leprosy presenting as macrocheilia. Indian J Lepr. 1999;71(3):341-2.

34. Kumar B, Rai R, Kaur I. Systemic involvement in leprosy and its significance. Indian J Lepr. 2000;72(1):123-42.

35. Daniel E. Lagophthalmos in leprosy. Indian J Lepr. 1998;70(1):39-47.

36. Inamadar AC, Palit A. Bilateral facial palsy in Hansen's disease. Lepr Rev. 2003;74(4):383-5.

37. Khan A, Sardana K, Koranne RV, et al. Bilateral seventh nerve palsy—a manifestation of polyneuritic leprosy. Indian J Lepr. 2005;77(2):140-7.

38. Passerotti S, Salotti RA, Vieth H. Assessment and treatment of the dry eye in leprosy. Indian J Lepr. 1998;70:103-8.

39. Yawalkar SJ. Deformities and their management. In: Yawalkar SJ (Ed). Leprosy for medical practitioners and paramedical workers, 6th edition. Basle: Ciba Geigy Ltd; 1994.pp.92-133.

40. Das S. Examination of peripheral nerve lesions. In: Das S (Ed). A manual on clinical surgery, 6th edition. Calcutta: Dr. S.Das; 2007.pp.90-105.

41. Brown TR, Kovindha A, Wathanadilokkol U, et al. Leprosy neuropathy: correlation of clinical and electrophysiological tests. Indian J Lepr. 1996;68:1-14.

42. McDougall AC. The clinical examination of peripheral nerves in leprosy. Indian J Lepr. 1996;68(4):378-9.

43. Desikan KV, Anbalagan J, Maheshwari PK. Pure neuritic leprosy of supraorbital nerve as unusual presentation. Indian J Lepr. 2001;73(1):47-50.

44. Dhar S, Sharma VK, Kaur S. Facial, glossopharyngeal, vagus and hypoglossal nerve palsy in a case of lepromatous leprosy. Indian J Lepr. 1993;65(3):333-6.

45. Siddappa K, Inamadar AC, Reddy LS. Destruction of ala nasi and loss of columella in borderline tuberculoid leprosy—a case report. Indian J Lepr. 1989;61(1):113-4.

46. Srinivasan H, Dharmendra. Deformities of hands. In: Dharmendra (Ed). Leprosy. Bombay: Kothari Medical Publishing House; 1978.pp.205-17.

47. Schwarz RJ, Brandsma JW. Re-enablement of the neurologically impaired hand—2: Surgical correction. Report of a Surgical Workshop held at Green Pastures Hospital and Rehabilitation Centre, November 2004, Pokhara, Nepal. Lepr Rev. 2006;77(4):326-42.

48. Lumley JSP. Peripheral nerve injuries. Hamilton Bailey's physical signs. Demonstration of Physical Signs in Clinical Surgery. 18th edition. Oxford: Butterworth-Heinemann; 2000.pp.411-8.

49. Pearson JMH, The evaluation of nerve damage in leprosy. Lepr Rev. 1982;53(2):119-30.

50. Brandsma JW. Monitoring motor nerve function in leprosy patients. Lepr Rev. 2000;71(3):258-67.

51. Srinivasan H. Guidelines for implementing disability prevention programme in the field. National Leprosy Elimination Programme (NLEP). Indian J Lepr. 1999;71(4):539-612.
52. Bourrel P. Two objective 'Archivable' tests for voluntary muscle testing in ulnar and median nerve paralysis. Indian J Lepr. 1997;69(1):13-23.
53. Brandsma JW, Schwarz RJ. Re-enablement of the neurologically impaired hand—1: terminology, applied anatomy and assessment. Report of a Surgical Workshop held at Green Pastures Hospital and Rehabilitation Centre, November 2004, Pokhara, Nepal. Lepr Rev. 2006;77(4):317-25.
54. Kumar B, Kaur S, Kataria S, et al. Concomitant occurrence of leprosy and tuberculosis. A clinical, bacteriological and radiological evaluation. Lep India. 1982;54(4):671-6.
55. Nishida M, Nakamura Y, Aosaki N. Prevalence and characteristics of depression in a Japanese leprosarium from the view points of social stigma and ageing. A preliminary report. Lepr Rev. 2006;77(3):203-9.

Case Definition and Clinical Types of Leprosy

Bhushan Kumar, Sunil Dogra

CHAPTER OUTLINE

INTRODUCTION

Leprosy is a slowly progressive, mildly infectious disease caused by *Mycobacterium leprae* complicated by potential intermittent hypersensitivity reactions (lepra reactions) in its rather placid course. It is a disease which primarily affects the skin and nerves, and in highly bacillated state, internal organs also. The damage to peripheral nerves results in sensory and motor impairment with characteristic hideous deformities and disabilities so deeply associated with stigmatization of the disease. Stigma remains a major obstacle to the social management of leprosy despite good leprosy control as a result of advances in bacteriology, chemotherapy and epidemiology. Early diagnosis and therapy are most important for the control of disease and prevention of disabilities. Diagnosis and classification of leprosy have been based primarily on the clinical features. Skin smears and histopathology are also considered contributory when facilities are available.

CASE DEFINITION

As per the eighth meeting of the WHO Expert Committee on Leprosy in 2010,[1] a case of leprosy is defined as an individual who has not completed the course of treatment and has one or more of the three cardinal signs:

1. Hypopigmented or erythematous skin lesion(s) with definite loss/impairment of sensation,
2. Involvement of the peripheral nerves, as demonstrated by definite thickening with sensory impairment,
3. Skin smear positive for acid-fast bacilli (AFB).

Any one of these signs has been regarded as sufficient for the diagnosis of leprosy in majority of the cases, so the sensitivity is high. Each sign is also quite specific in itself so the specificity is also high. The most important potential source of error is the reliability of the examination of an individual patient and reading of the skin smears, referred to as interobserver variation.[2] The WHO Expert Committee recommended monitoring of the quality of diagnosis, as part of regular technical supervision. If there are indications of substantial overdiagnosis, a validation exercise on a representative sample of cases can be conducted to determine the magnitude of the problem.

Clinical Problems with Cardinal Signs

It is very pertinent to highlight that diagnosis of leprosy should be made after very careful and detailed clinical consideration. A useful maxim which should not be forgotten, especially when dealing with children is "when in doubt, never diagnose leprosy." The statement like "you have suspicious signs of leprosy," should be avoided as the outlook of the society towards leprosy has not changed radically even in the 21st century. The psychological and emotional distress caused to patients by diagnosis of leprosy should be kept in mind. When a diagnosis is certain, encourage the patient to adopt a responsible attitude towards the disease and its management by taking treatment regularly. Even the cardinal signs (vide supra) which are quite sensitive and specific, are not infallible in certain situations when the signs are borderline, the intra-observer variation is wide and in situations where leprosy is very rare and likely to be a diagnosis at the bottom of the list.[3] Details are provided about the occurrence of lesions which may closely mimic the situation in leprosy due to nerve involvement or presence of similar looking skin lesions (*See* Chapter-22 on Differential Diagnosis of Neurological and Other Disorders in Relation to Leprosy).

Given below are the details of the sensitivity and specificity of the cardinal signs in the different conditions—dermatological and nondermatological.

Skin Lesions with Sensory Impairment

Hypopigmented or erythematous patches/plaques are often the first clinical sign of the disease in many newly diagnosed leprosy patients. Since many other conditions produce similar lesions, accompaniment of definite sensory loss is a must to be specific for leprosy. Requirement of presence of both the signs together greatly reduces the sensitivity of this feature, especially in multibacillary (MB) cases where lesions are less distinct and less likely to be anesthetic.

In a most rigorous study carried out in Malawi, sensory examination was done in histopathologically proven paucibacillary (PB) lesions.[4] The sensitivity of the loss of touch sensation in a lesion as a diagnostic test was 48.5% and the specificity 72%. Other published studies gave higher figures for the sensitivity of this test among PB patients, figures of 93% from India,[5] 92% from Bangladesh[6] and 86% from Ethiopia[7] have been reported. It is likely that the mixture of cases in different stages of evolution and stage of the disease at which they were examined account for some of these differences. However, specificity was not calculated in these studies. Hypoesthesia in some of the lesions is occasionally seen in conditions other than leprosy such as chronic dermatitis producing thick lichenified skin, which may lead to over diagnosis in some situations.

Very few studies have examined anesthesia as a marker in lesions of MB cases, because there is less perceived difficulty in the diagnosis using the traditional cardinal signs, including skin smears. Published figures for the sensitivity of anesthesia in skin lesions in MB patients are almost similar to the figures for PB disease, i.e. 49% from Bangladesh[6] and 54% from Ethiopia.[7]

In Ethiopia, the sensitivity of this single criterion was 70% for all patients. A large proportion (74%) of those whose lesions were not anesthetic were smear-positive, and therefore, represented potential source of *M. leprae* in the community.[7] In other words, employing anesthesia over the skin patches as the single criterion, almost 30% of leprosy patients may be missed and most of them are likely to be smear positive.

Other lesions without sensory loss can also be confused with some common dermatoses resulting in misdiagnosis. In the field conditions, erythematous plaque lesions of leprosy may be labelled as tinea, psoriasis, lupus vulgaris, etc. and hypopigmented patches are often confused with postinflammatory hypopigmentation, pityriasis alba, pityriasis versicolor, and vitiligo, etc. or vice-versa when a leprosy lesion can be diagnosed as a benign dermatological disease.

The specificity of the diagnosis based on the presence of anesthetic and hypopigmented or erythematous macular/papular lesions is still more reduced in MB cases because the lesions can be less distinct and less anesthetic. Consequently, presence of macular anesthetic lesions as a single diagnostic criterion for MB disease has resulted in up to 30% of patients being missed; this contrasts with distinct maculoanesthetic lesions of PB disease, which are reportedly diagnostic in 90% of cases. In Ethiopia where all three cardinal signs were used, the diagnostic sensitivity was 97%.[7]

Peripheral Nerve Trunk Enlargement

Peripheral nerve enlargement usually appears later than the skin lesions. The most commonly involved nerves are the ulnar and common peroneal. The presence of one or more enlarged nerves is seen more commonly in PB disease, however in late stages of the disease, thickened nerves are more common in MB than among PB patients. Nerve enlargement was found in a greater proportion of new cases in Ethiopia (ulnar nerve in 68%),[7] where the patients typically present late, than in India (ulnar nerve in 23%),[8] where detection is generally much earlier. Reported figures for nerve enlargement in MB and PB patients from Bangladesh are 96% and 86% respectively,[6] whereas in Ethiopia, the corresponding figures were 91% and 76%.[7] In a study of early PB patients from India, only 20% patients had enlarged nerves.[5]

The reproducibility and specificity of the examination for nerve enlargement has been questioned.[9] A study from India found only moderate reproducibility among eight experienced paramedical workers.[8] False positive findings may occur because of poor examination technique or because of nonspecific enlargement of a nerve seen in some heavy manual workers. On the other hand, some diseases and conditions with nerve thickening (hereditary sensory motor neuropathy, Dejerine-Sotta syndrome, amyloidosis, and neurofibromatosis) or without nerve thickening (diabetic, alcoholic neuropathy, lead/arsenic toxicity, and vitamin B deficiency) may simulate leprosy like sensory loss with or without deformities, paralysis, trophic ulcers, etc.

To improve certainty of the diagnosis of leprosy, a balanced approach to the diagnosis is strongly recommended, and it would be the presence of a thickened nerve and one other diagnostic sign such as: typical hypopigmented or erythematous skin lesions with or without sensory loss or typical nerve-function impairment such as loss of sensation in the area supplied by the involved nerve. Also, simple modalities for assessing nerve function impairment such as monofilament testing and voluntary muscle testing, can be combined with nerve palpation to give a two-fold improvement in the sensitivity for evaluating nerve damage at field level.[10]

Neuritic leprosy presents as peripheral neuropathy in which there are no skin lesions suggesting leprosy. The diagnosis depends on finding definite nerve enlargement with nerve function impairment.[11] In Ethiopia, the diagnosis was made in 0.5% of newly detected cases;[12] whereas in India 4.6% of newly detected cases exhibit this form of disease.[13] In Nepal, 8.7% of new patients in the field were found to have neuritic leprosy.[14] These patients would be diagnosed by the classical cardinal sign of peripheral nerve enlargement but not by the single criterion of an anesthetic skin patch.

Slit-Skin Smears

Skin smears have traditionally represented one of the cardinal signs of leprosy with specificity of 100%. However, the sensitivity of this examination alone is low, because smear-positive patients represent 10–50% of all patients as reported in various studies. Skin smears identify MB cases who are the most infectious, and the bacteriological index (BI) calculated as a measure of the bacillary load, aids in the classification of the disease. Repeated assessment of BI during the course of treatment helps to monitor the progress and identify those patients who are experiencing bacteriological relapse.[15] Differentiating between viable (solid staining acid-fast rods) and dead bacilli (irregularly stained or fragmented) to measure the morphological index (MI) is also a valuable pointer to the effect of treatment. The inherent problems of skin smears are the logistics and the reliability of the technique of taking, staining, and interpreting the smears. Measurement of BI and MI is particularly subject to interobserver variations and is therefore not always reliable.

CLASSIFICATION OF DISEASE

Ridley and Jopling (1966) defined five groups on the basis of clinical, bacteriological, histological and immunological features (Table 15.1): (1) tuberculoid leprosy (TT), (2) borderline tuberculoid (BT), (3) borderline borderline (BB), (4) borderline lepromatous (BL), and (5) lepromatous leprosy (LL).[16] This is a very useful classification for research purposes but often not feasible in field conditions and primary health centers. This classification does not include indeterminate and pure neuritic types of leprosy. In general, PB disease is equivalent to indeterminate (I), TT and BT, and MB is equated with BB, BL and LL disease. In view of the restricted availability of laboratory facilities for slit-skin smear (SSS) or histopathology in an endemic country like India, and the presently uncertain state of polymerase chain reaction (PCR) technology, the WHO Expert Committee on Leprosy, recommended that diagnosis of most cases of leprosy in the field will continue to be based on clinical evidence alone.[1] However, inaccessibility to laboratory facilities not only leads to misdiagnosis, commonly PB instead of MB disease, but also leads to over diagnosis of leprosy.[17,18] Hence, present scenario portends to be less than ideal, especially when the disease incidence is declining and where more sensitive diagnostic tools and procedures are the need of the hour to ensure that all cases that need treatment are correctly diagnosed and cured.[19]

Table 15.1: Characteristics of Ridley-Jopling classification*

Observation	TT	BT	BB	BL	LL
Number of lesions	Usually single (up to 3)	Few (up to 10)	Several (10–30)	Many, asymmetrical (>30)	Innumerable, symmetrical
Size of lesions	Variable, usually large	Variable, some are large	Variable	Small, some can be large†	Small
Surface	Very dry, scaly, lesions look turgid	Dry, scaly, lesions look bright and infiltrated	Dull/slightly shiny	Shiny	Shiny
Sensations in lesions	Absent	Markedly diminished	Moderately diminished	Slightly diminished	Minimally diminished, not affected
Hair growth in lesions	Absent	Markedly diminished	Moderately diminished	Slightly diminished	Not affected initially§
AFB in lesions	Nil	Nil or scanty	Moderate in number	Many	Plenty, including globi
Lepromin reactivity	Strongly positive (+++)	Weakly positive (+ or ++)	Negative/weakly positive	Negative	Negative

Abbreviations: TT, tuberculoid; BT, borderline tuberculoid; BB, borderline borderline; BL, borderline lepromatous; LL, lepromatous; AFB, acid-fast bacilli.
* Compartmentalization of the features is not very stringent. All these features occur in various combinations as the disease progresses.
† Presence of large lesions indicates downgrading of the disease from higher spectrum.
§ In disease of long standing—almost all body hair are lost.

Table 15.2: Current WHO classification	
	Criteria
MB	≥ 6 skin lesions, or positive bacterial index
PB	≤ 5 skin lesions and negative bacterial index

Abbreviations: MB; multibacillary; PB, paucibacillary.

For field workers, WHO has classified leprosy based on number of skin lesions for treatment purposes (Table 15.2).[1] The sensitivity and specificity of this operational classification, tested using SSS and skin biopsy results as the gold standard was found to be 63% and 85%, respectively. The sensitivity has been shown to increase to 98.5% on addition of two other clinical criteria, i.e. number of body areas affected and size of the largest skin lesion.[20]

The report of 8th WHO expert committee on leprosy excluded single lesion paucibacillary type (SLPB).

- Current NLEP classification also includes nerve involvement as follows:
    - Paucibacillary leprosy: Single nerve involved
    - Multibacillary leprosy: Two or more nerves involved.

CLINICAL FEATURES

Clinical features of leprosy reflect the pathology, which is dependent upon the balance between bacillary multiplication and the host cell-mediated immune response. Leprosy affects skin, nerves and produces systemic involvement in lepromatous disease. Patients commonly present with skin lesions, weakness of hands or feet or numbness caused by a peripheral-nerve trunk involvement, deformities, resorption of fingers and toes or a burn or ulcer in an anesthetic hand or foot. Sometime patients may present in reaction with nerve pain, sudden palsy, new skin lesions, painful red eye, or a systemic febrile illness. The severity of disease in a given patient may vary from the presence of an insignificant hypopigmented anesthetic skin patch to widespread damage to peripheral nerves and signs and symptoms suggestive of systemic involvement. Leprosy is unique as an infectious disease for the width of the spectrum of signs and symptoms that it exhibits. Clinical features of the disease are more often the result of the host response to the presence of bacilli rather than of direct damage due to bacillary invasion.[21]

Inspection of the whole body in good light is important because otherwise lesions with faint erythema or slight hypopigmentation, more often on covered areas in borderline disease, might be missed. Skin lesions should be examined for hypoesthesia to light touch, temperature and for anhidrosis.

Early Lesions and Presenting Symptoms

The common presenting symptom is an area of variable sensory loss on the skin or a visible hypopigmented/ erythematous, anesthetic/hypoesthetic skin lesion. The most common skin lesion(s) are one or few hypopigmented macules of indeterminate leprosy. These lesions have no distinctive diagnostic features and are often not reported to the physician. Early tuberculoid lesions are more or less well-defined hypopigmented and often erythematous anesthetic plaques. Early lepromatous lesions are vague, ill-defined coppery or hypopigmented, minimally infiltrated macules which are often missed, and the disease remains unnoticed until the skin lesion becomes infiltrated or gross neurological deficit sets in. Rarely nasal stuffiness and epistaxis may be the initial symptoms in lepromatous patients. In some patients, neurological symptoms draw attention towards the disease, with presenting complaint of sensory loss with or without muscular weakness of the hand or foot, but without any apparent skin lesions noticed by the patient. This could be due to early nerve function impairment, while a small proportion of such cases may have pure neuritic leprosy. Rare presenting complaints may be a result of reactions, like fever, joint pains, painful erythematous tender skin lesions, edema of hands and feet and neuritic pains.[3,22] Hence, patients with presence or development of such symptoms need to be kept under regular follow-up, especially in field conditions so as to avoid the preventable delay in the diagnosis and initiation of treatment. This was shown by a cohort study carried out in hyperendemic Gadchiroli district of Maharashtra, India. At 1-year follow-up visit, their study team detected a large number of new cases among those suspects who did not seek treatment earlier, mainly because of fear of stigma, ignorance about leprosy or preference for faith healers.[23]

The clinical features of the various presentations of leprosy and also as given in the Ridley-Jopling classification are described further in this chapter.

Indeterminate Leprosy

It is contended that though most workers consider these lesions under the title "indeterminate," this is not an appropriate designation because most of them have definite clinical and certain histopathological features which are in the process of evolution. The first lesion to appear is not infrequently a small to medium sized hypopigmented patch usually 1–5 cm in diameter, often situated on the external aspect of the thigh, face, extensor aspects of limbs with rather vague edges and some loss of tactile and thermal sensations (Figs 15.1A to C). With the progression of disease, similar patches may appear over other parts of body. The edges of the larger macules are usually fairly definite, whereas the periphery of the smaller macules is indefinite and fades imperceptibly into the surrounding skin. Great majority of these lesions are small with somewhat hazy edges. Hair growth and nerve functions are usually not affected. These lesions may be slightly dry than the normal adjacent skin and occasionally present with a creased or wrinkled appearance.

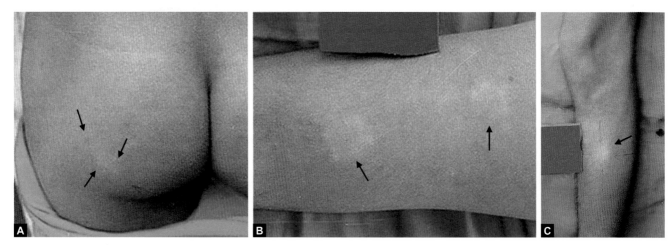

Figs 15.1A to C: Examples of indeterminate leprosy; the patches are faintly visible, with not very clear sensory impairment. The diagnosis usually requires histopathological evaluation, besides clinical criteria
Courtesy: Dr Pankaj Sharma, PGIMER, Dr RML Hospital, New Delhi.

There may be a suggestion of hypoesthesia. Usually there is no definite morphological change except for a slight change in skin color.[24,25]

The diagnosis of indeterminate leprosy can only be confirmed when a biopsy has shown the presence of bacilli or typical neural infiltration, or when there is definite impairment of sensations. Biopsy may show perineurovascular infiltrate, however AFB are mostly not demonstrable albeit sometimes by newer molecular diagnostic methods, like PCR which is of definite value in such cases.[26]A striking feature of all these cases is the variability of the lepromin reaction. It is seldom strongly positive, may be weakly positive or negative and in some instances a negative reaction has been reported to transform to a positive one. Indeterminate leprosy is the first sign of the disease in 20–80% of patients.[24]When populations are regularly examined, or patients come forward early, it is by far the most common presentation. Many patients, however, do not notice such lesions and present only with characteristic determinant lesions at some point.

Many minor childhood skin ailments like pityriasis alba may be mistaken for indeterminate leprosy.[27] Movement into the tuberculoid pole of the spectrum is indicated by lesions exhibiting increasingly defined margins, increased hypopigmentation or erythema/infiltration and anesthesia. Perhaps three out of four indeterminate lesions undergo self-healing and the rest become determinate and enter the clinical spectrum.[28] Prognosis with treatment is excellent; lesions clear without any reactional or neurological sequelae. When the clinical diagnosis of indeterminate leprosy is doubtful and histology is not available or inconclusive, it is appropriate to keep a given patient in close supervision for few months to observe its course rather than to label a patient having leprosy and make him/her suffer the stigma. If the lesion still persists for more than 6 months of monitoring

and further diagnostic facilities are limited especially in field conditions, then treatment can be considered.

Tuberculoid Leprosy

Tuberculoid leprosy is a benign form, relatively stable, infrequently positive on bacteriological examination, and presents as erythematous, elevated, well-defined lesions. Sequelae of peripheral nerve involvement appear only in a limited proportion of cases. Nerve involvement occurs as a result of extension from or through cutaneous nerve branches rather than through systemic dissemination of lepra bacilli, and so the nerve damage is patchy, asymmetrical and often unilateral.

Skin lesions are single or up to three in number and seldom measure more than 10 cm in diameter. The typical lesion is a well-defined erythematous plaque with raised and clear-cut edges sloping inward (Figs 15.2A and B). Many times the center is rather flattened and even hypopigmented acquiring an annular configuration. Dark skins may not show the erythema clearly. The surface is dry, hairless, anesthetic and usually scaly. Sensory impairment may be difficult to demonstrate on the face because of the generous supply of sensory nerve endings. Autonomic nerve damage within the lesions is often severe, surface is dry and sweating is lost. Skin texture is rough, creases are exaggerated and the lesion has scanty hair which may even be completely lost. Tuberculoid skin lesions may appear at any site on the skin, though there may be a predilection for body parts not covered by clothing.[29] Usually a solitary peripheral nerve trunk may be thickened in the vicinity of a TT lesion; for example, a thickened ulnar nerve if the lesion is on the forearm. On SSS examination, often no AFB are found. Lepromin test is strongly positive, signifying good host immunity that is capable of anchoring

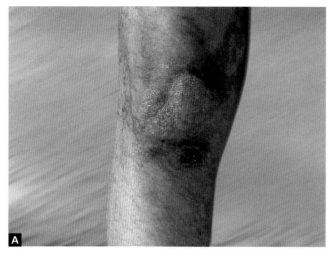
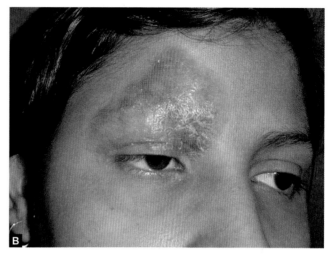

Figs 15.2A and B: (A) Tuberculoid leprosy plaque on the elbow; (B) A single patch of TT leprosy with reversal reaction. Note the erythema and scaling in the patch which had sensory impairment
Courtesy: Dr HK Kar, PGIMER, Dr RML Hospital, New Delhi.

the infection within limited lesions. Tuberculoid disease has also been subdivided into minor and major tuberculoid forms.[30,31]

- *Minor tuberculoid*: Skin lesions are usually hypopigmented, only slightly to moderately elevated, often only at the margin or even in a part of the margin and mostly have an irregular surface. Loss of sensation to touch and temperature is common, but presence of AFB on SSS is very rare. Enlarged cutaneous nerve in vicinity of the lesion is infrequently found.
- *Major tuberculoid*: In general characteristics, there is little difference between major and minor lesions. This division is arbitrary and for convenience; the difference is seen in the degree and not the nature of change. Major tuberculoid lesions manifest in individuals in whom there is an active, severe immune response in the skin and nerves to the presence of *M. leprae*. Lesions are well-defined, erythematous, grossly infiltrated plaques which are very large, with loss of touch, temperature and pain sensations. The lesions are frequently seen on the face and dorsolateral aspect of extremities. Larger lesions when more in number, (although less than five) have now been considered as indicative of MB disease. Interestingly, major tuberculoid lesions tend to invade certain "immune zones" like axilla, lumbosacral area, palms, etc. In lesions with marked erythema, AFBs may be seen on routine methods of examination. Frequently the small cutaneous nerves may become enlarged and the thickened nerve can usually be traced to an erythematous infiltrated lesion. Thickened nerve may persist long after the patch has regressed.

True TT is expected to heal itself in majority of the patients even without treatment.[32] Since skin lesions of TT seldom lead to significant peripheral nerve damage, or related disability, the prognosis can be stated to be good. Only if a large nerve trunk is involved it leads to gross deformity. When the lesions are located on the face or on the fingers, some damage can occur indirectly due to anesthesia.

Borderline Leprosy

Borderline leprosy spans the spectrum between the tuberculoid and lepromatous poles. It is the most important part of the spectrum in terms of number of patients, frequency and severity of reactions and nerve damage. Patients with borderline disease suffer most of the disabilities and deformities seen in leprosy.

In this spectrum (also known as dimorphous leprosy in the Madrid classification), it is often possible to find features suggestive of two forms of leprosy in a single patient. These dimorphous appearances reflect the instability of borderline disease. Histology is often necessary to appreciate how far the disease may have shifted from its starting point on the spectrum. If histology is unavailable, the BI obtained from a SSS is useful. For accurate classification within the borderline part of the spectrum, careful consideration should be given to various characteristics like the number, distribution and symmetry of the skin lesions, type of borders, sensory impairment, sweating and hair growth; distribution, extent and nature of peripheral nerve damage; mucosal and systemic involvement and results of SSS.[33]

Patients who are untreated, or inadequately treated or who have relapsed, may downgrade toward the lepromatous pole, and may finally lose all cell-mediated immunity (CMI) responses to *M. leprae*, and become subpolar lepromatous, but some clinical features such as skin lesions of different morphologies, thickened, asymmetrical nerves give a clue to their former state in a higher spectrum. While in most other patients the spectrum does not shift considerably and the clinical features remain characteristic of BT or BL form. In BT, cell-mediated hypersensitivity underlies most of the clinical features, whereas in BL, bacillary positivity, grossly impaired cell mediated immunity (CMI) and its sequelae are more important for the clinical manifestations. In borderline disease, lepromin test is positive near the tuberculoid spectrum and negative in BB and BL. Variation in lepromin reaction may be seen in an individual patient also, with variation in clinical activity resulting in a shift in the spectrum of the disease.

While BB disease is rare, the ratio of BT to BL patients shows an interesting geographical pattern. BT disease predominates in Africans, while BL disease is mostly seen in Asians. This difference presumably reflects a genetic difference in the ability to express CMI to *M. leprae*. Some patients (not necessarily as a result of treatment) may reverse or upgrade, their disease becoming more towards tuberculoid in nature but downgrading occurs more often. Downgrading and upgrading may occur silently but is often associated with type 1 reactions. Even on treatment, downgrading in the form of appearance of new lesions or subclinical lesions becoming clinically overt is known to occur as a part of type 1 reaction or relapse. These events are of great significance for their influence on classification and therapy of leprosy, as it might call for a change of label from PB to MB, if the total number of skin lesions increase to more than five.[34]

Borderline Tuberculoid

The skin lesions resemble those of tuberculoid leprosy, but there is evidence of the disease not being contained. Individual lesions do not show the well-defined margins and the border in part may start sloping outward and even fade imperceptibly into the normal skin (Figs 15.3 and 15.4A to D). There may be small extension of the lesion at one edge (pseudopodium) or there may even be satellite lesions. The number of lesions may vary from three to 10 and they show variation in size and contour. The size of lesions tends to be larger and at times it may cover the whole limb. Loss of sensations is less intense than in the lesions of TT. Dryness, scaling and erythema or hypopigmentation of the lesions are also less conspicuous than in TT.

Several of the peripheral nerves are likely to be enlarged in an asymmetrical pattern. Nerve damage is an important characteristic of BT leprosy and anesthesia or motor deficit is often found at the time of presentation. Even when treated with antileprosy drugs, nerve damage may progress to produce extensive anesthesia with destruction and deformities, unless the patient is closely supervised and appropriate preventive/therapeutic measures are taken.

Borderline leprosy with large pale macules and nerve involvement is often called maculoanesthetic or low-resistant TT (macular tuberculoid). These may present as single or a few lesions. Lesions tend to be large and asymmetrical in their distribution, and are more commonly found on the face, lateral aspects of the extremities, buttocks and scapulae. The lesions are hypopigmented, and not depigmented, with rather well-defined edges which show a clear demarcation between affected and healthy skin, but are not raised. The macules especially over the extremities usually feel dry to touch and show some degree of loss of sweating. The main differentiating features from other types of macular lesions in leprosy are, clear definition of the edge of the lesion, limited number of macules, asymmetry of their distribution; and finally, they show a dry and somewhat rough surface, and the loss of sensation to light touch or temperature is clearly demonstrable. In addition, there may also be areas of sensory loss on the extremities which follow the course of large cutaneous nerves.[35]

One of the most striking features of BT leprosy is the susceptibility to type I reactions in either skin lesions or nerves or both. Often it is the onset of type 1 reaction that causes a patient with longstanding BT leprosy especially with macular lesions, to seek medical help. Such a patient should be carefully examined for nerve tenderness and early evidence of weakness or anesthesia of hands or feet requiring immediate intervention. If left untreated, BT leprosy may continue even for many years with recurrent bouts of reactions, leading to progressive nerve damage, paralysis and deformity. Few patients with repeated reactions tend to deteriorate and the disease downgrades across the spectrum to BL or LL, with an increasing BI.

Borderline Borderline

Mid-borderline disease is unstable and mostly "downgrades" toward the lepromatous pole especially if untreated. Presence of dimorphous type of lesions is the

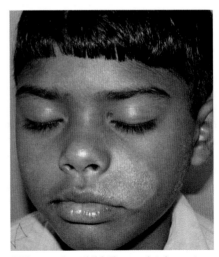

Fig. 15.3: BT leprosy in a child. The patch is hypopigmented, dry, scaly, with erythema and well-defined margin

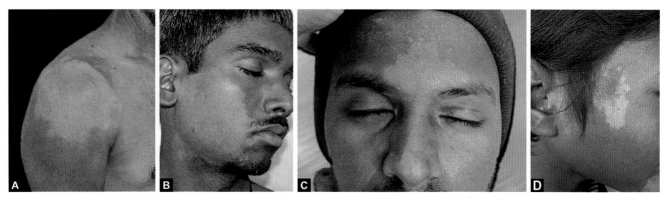

Figs 15.4A to D: (A and B) BT leprosy in two patients, the lesions are hypopigmented, dry, with definite sensory loss. The lesions are not raised (maculo-anesthetic type) (C) Borderline tuberculoid—well-defined plaque on forehead with satellite lesions; (D) Well-defined hypopigmented patch of BT leprosy on face

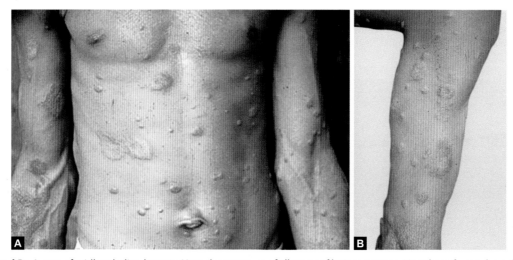

Figs 15.5A and B: A case of midborderline leprosy. Note the presence of all types of lesions representing those from tuberculoid (plaques) and lepromatous (papules and nodules), and the annular lesions (characteristic of borderline leprosy)
Courtesy: Dr HK Kar, PGIMER, Dr RML Hospital, New Delhi.

rule. There are multiple skin lesions with a tendency to symmetry. The lesions are of all shapes and sizes including papules, plaques, circinate lesions and rarely even nodules. Characteristic skin lesions are annular where the inner edge is well demarcated "punched out" and the outer edge is ill-defined and slopes toward normal skin. Clinically, normal looking skin within such plaques gives a "Swiss cheese" appearance (Figs 15.5A and B, Figs 15.6 and 15.7).

Face may show infiltration with occasional nodules over ears and chin. Because of immunological instability, the BB state is short-lived, such patients are evidently rarely seen and the disease rapidly changes its spectrum, rarely to BT but more often to BL. Many nerves are involved, though not symmetrically as in LL.

Nerve damage is variable in BB disease. If the patient is downgrading from BT, many nerves may be enlarged but asymmetrically. In a patient upgrading from BL, often as a result of treatment, the peripheral nerves will be affected but there may not be much neurological deficit until a type 1 reaction precipitates the loss. Peripheral sensory loss in a symmetrical fashion in BB is unusual.

Skin smears show moderate number of AFBs in majority of the lesions.

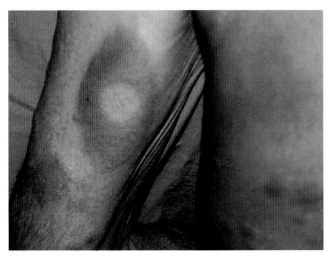

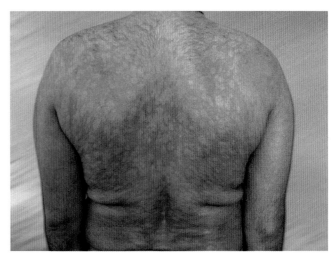

Fig. 15.6: Annular (punched out) lesion, the hallmark of borderline leprosy. It has sharp abrupt ending inner margin while the outer margin is sloping outwards into the surrounding skin. Also note the other types of lesions, i.e. papules, plaques over the trunk
Courtesy: Dr HK Kar, PGIMER, Dr RML Hospital, New Delhi.

Fig. 15.8: Downgrading of unstable disease to BL leprosy. The lesions are small numerous papules and plaques with erythema and in bilateral symmetrical distribution. There was no history of antileprosy treatment

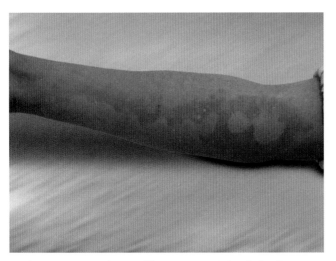

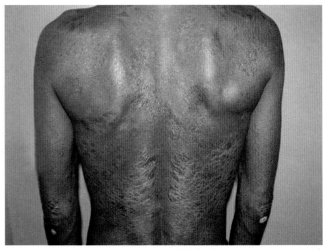

Fig. 15.7: Inverted saucer like appearance in borderline leprosy

Fig. 15.9: BL leprosy, the lesions are ill-defined, showing tendency to bilateral symmetry, some of them with coppery hue. In between the diffuse infiltration; some ichthyosis can be observed which can occur as a result of disease itself (due to dryness of skin as a result of autonomic neuropathy) or due to treatment with clofazimine component of MDT

Borderline Lepromatous

There are numerous skin lesions, classically distinct but not so well-defined. They occur as slightly infiltrated macules with coppery hue, round or oval, of about 2–3 cm in diameter, in not so symmetrical distribution with areas of apparently normal skin in between. With disease progression, papules, nodules and plaques may develop, with sloping margins which merge imperceptibly into the normal skin (Figs 15.8 to 15.10). Infiltration takes place within the initial macules, creating a plaque like appearance, especially on the face and ears.

Signs of nerve damage within the lesion such as loss of sensation, decreased sweating and hair growth start sooner in BL than in LL. Associated large lesions (and of variable morphology) indicate downgrading of disease from a higher spectrum. However, the real place of the disease in the spectrum may be suspected from the extent, number and small size of majority of the skin lesions and the fact that the infiltration is central rather than peripheral, especially in the newer lesions.

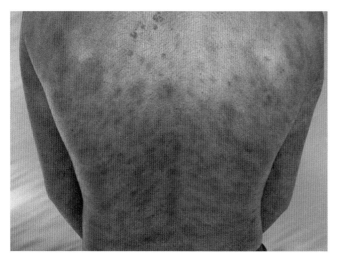

Fig. 15.10: Borderline lepromatous—multiple small papules and plaques on the back

Peripheral nerve trunks become thickened at the sites of predilection but lack symmetry with corresponding anesthesia and paresis. Nerves get damaged not as quickly as in BB and BT leprosy but sooner than in LL. Eyebrows are either not involved or are lost partially. Symmetrical anesthesia involving hands and feet does not develop till late in the disease and usually there are no symptoms pertaining to oral cavity or eyes. The testes are normal in size and texture on palpation. BL patients are more prone to develop type 2 reactions [erythema nodosum leprosum (ENL)] than those in BB spectrum. Type 1 reactions in skin lesions and nerves, though uncommon, also add to morbidity of the disease.

The prognosis in BL is very variable. If the disease began as BL and it is diagnosed and treated before further downgrading, then the prognosis should be good. With careful supervision and management for type 1 reactions, which are likely to occur during the chemotherapy, there should be little disability. Patients downgrading from BT to BL may already have significant nerve damage and lepra reactions (as may be expected during chemotherapy), which further complicates neuritis and aggravates disabilities. Patients who downgrade to subpolar LL, face the additional complications of further extension of cutaneous lesions and nerve involvement and type 2 reactions during or after chemotherapy.[33,35]

Lepromatous Leprosy

Multiplication and universal spread of *M. leprae* and almost no resistance mounted by the host, account for many of the features of the disease at the lepromatous pole. Early lesions of LL are small macules, innumerable in number, widely disseminated and distributed symmetrically. Although the infiltration is clinically not very obvious, on careful examination, these macules are found to be slightly infiltrated.

Their edges are indistinct, merging imperceptibly into the normal skin and their surface is shiny and erythematous, rather than hypopigmented. Unlike macules of BT, the early macules of LL are not anesthetic, show no change in skin texture, hair growth or sweating, and have in addition, a slightly shiny appearance. The inconspicuous edge and lack of significant tissue reaction result in minimal color contrast between affected and the normal skin. Owing to erythema, these lesions are better seen in an oblique light as shiny waxy macules. Insidious onset and steady progression may allow the disease to advance for years before the patient or his associates recognize a shiny, waxy appearance. Though all lepromatous macules are infiltrated, but it is not of a sufficient degree to alter the grossly macular nature of the lesions.

Lepromatous leprosy with infiltrated lesions presents as three distinct forms: (1) diffuse, (2) infiltrated, and (3) nodular forms.

Diffuse Lepromatous Leprosy

It is believed that this is a true subtype of LL, but many workers are of the opinion that diffuse LL is usually the result of gradual coalescing of the numerous vague macular lesions of LL. These cases in the initial stages are often missed since no actual lesions are discernible. The skin has a shiny look with slight infiltration which is better appreciated by touch rather than by sight. This infiltration is more easily appreciated by pinching the skin of the patient between the fingers. Thickness of the skin is most marked over the face especially the forehead, earlobes, eyebrows, nose and malar surfaces (Figs 15.11A and B). The ear-lobes are usually thickened and shiny in nodular LL (Figs 15.12A to C). Thickening and nodulation of the ear lobes is best appreciated by standing behind the patient.

Eyebrows may show some thinning or loss of hair, but it must be remembered, however, that loss of eyebrows is often a late sign of LL.

Infiltrated Lepromatous Leprosy

Lepromatous leprosy may be detected clinically at the stage of macules, diffuse infiltration or as areas of marked infiltration or nodules. Infiltrated leprosy is merely a more advanced stage of macular LL with easily visible infiltration which may be a sign of advancement of diffuse LL disease. It must be emphasized, that even when infiltration appears, the gross characteristics of the lepromatous lesion remain the same. The edges, while raised, do not stand out as in TT. Lesions are often shiny and succulent in consistency but color may vary in different ethnic populations.

Nodular Lepromatous Leprosy

Nodular leprosy is the result of progressive deterioration of the macular, diffuse or infiltrated forms of LL. In the early stage,

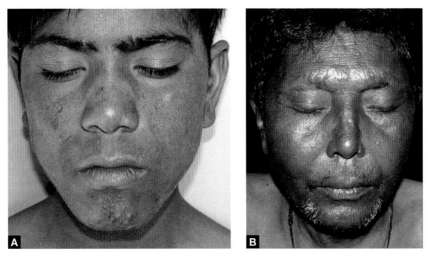

Figs 15.11A and B: Diffuse LL (A) and infiltrated LL (B). In both the cases the slit-skin smears were highly positive (6+ with globi)

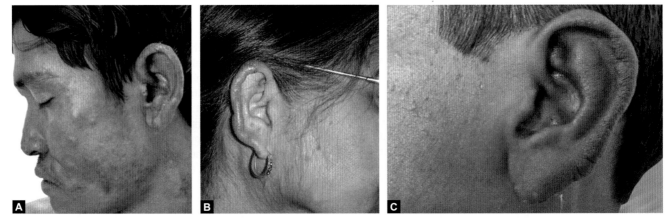

Figs 15.12A to C: (A and B) Nodular LL. The nodular lesions over ears are prominent in both cases shown. The slit skin smears are highly positive. (C) Infiltrated earlobe in a patient of lepromatous leprosy

nodules appear first on the ears, (Figs 15.12A to C) and as the disease advances they may appear anywhere on the body and are commonly seen over the buttocks and extremities especially the elbows, fingers (Fig. 15.13), over the joints and sometimes on the genitals. Diagnosis is never in doubt when disease has reached to such a nodular stage. The infiltrated plaques accentuate the skinfolds producing the classical leonine facies (Figs 15.14A and B). Nodules, even plaques on the face and other areas of body may follow. At first many of such nodules tend to be adherent to the skin and are movable in the subcutaneous tissues, but later they become fixed and are liable to ulcerate.

By this time the peripheral anesthesia is extensive and is accompanied by anhidrosis with compensatory hyperhidrosis of the face, trunk and axillae. The sensory loss is symmetrical and is first detected over the extensors of forearms, legs, hands and feet, which gradually results in the typical glove and stocking distribution. The nail growth may be disturbed late in the course of the disease and nail plates become lustureless, ridged and curved. This perfectly symmetrical, diffuse infiltrative type of leprosy typifies the relatively uncommon patient whose disease has been pure lepromatous (polar LL) from the start of the illness. In many patients, however the disease has downgraded from borderline spectrum, in that the disease may not be so symmetrical and other evidences of variable sized lesions, asymmetrical nerve thickening may be present indicating downgrading (subpolar LL).

Despite the gradual appearance of sensory and autonomic nerve damage, it may be difficult to find a clinical sign of damage to the large peripheral nerves until the disease is

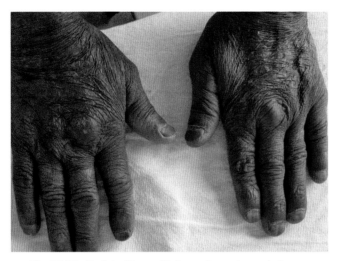

Fig. 15.13: Nodular LL—multiple small papules and plaques on the dorsum of hands

well-advanced especially in polar LL. Sensory fibers are usually damaged first. The nerves are often not palpably enlarged and nerve conduction studies may be near normal early in the disease. As the disease progresses the peripheral nerves first become thickened, firm and then fibrosed, at the sites of predilection where nerve trunks are close to cooler skin surface (like radial groove, behind medial epicondyle of ulna, neck of fibula). Weakness usually starts early in the intrinsic muscles of hands and feet, possibly because the muscles of hand and feet are affected by direct bacillary invasion as well as through the peripheral nerves.

In lepromatous disease, the hands and feet take on a characteristic appearance with swollen digits tending to taper towards the tips (fusiform swelling). Before the stage of anesthesia, hands and feet may be hypersensitive, so that small knocks or even walking causes feelings like electric shocks or (neuralgic) pain. Frequently the joints become swollen and later angulated. Digits may shorten due to resorption of the phalanges, even though there have been no ulceration and secondary infection. When significant anesthesia has developed, the hands and feet are liable to trauma and pressure necrosis of soft tissue, which leads to ulceration and secondary infection with clinical signs of cellulitis and osteomyelitis. Deformity from bony destruction may then proceed rapidly.

Involvement of the upper respiratory tract mucosa is found in about 80% of new LL cases. It may be noted that involvement of lower respiratory tract below the level of larynx, has not been seen in leprosy. It causes (not invariably the first symptom) a stuffy or blocked nose like that in coryza, often followed by epistaxis. There may be anosmia, crusting or bleeding and nasal septal perforation in up to 40% of LL patients. The septal perforation in leprosy is due to bacillary destruction of the bony portion of the nasal bridge, i.e. nasal spine, leading to the typical saddle nose deformity, commonly seen in advanced lepromatous cases. Just to recall for academic interest, in syphilis, the destruction of nasal septum involves only cartilaginous portion (chondritis) wherein the bony shape of the nose is preserved. Oral mucosa may be involved in the form of nodules and plaques involving tongue and palate. In severe cases, involvement of larynx can cause hoarseness of voice and stridor. Early eye involvement includes corneal anesthesia due to bacillary infiltration of

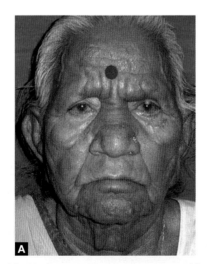 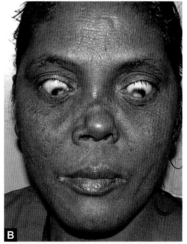

Figs 15.14A and B: LL, the typical leonine facies in an elderly female (A). An advanced LL case with diffuse infiltration, saddle nose and eye involvement (B). Skin smears were 6+ in both cases

corneal nerves and later from damage to the ophthalmic division of the trigeminal nerve. Other ocular manifestations include lagophthalmos, uveitis, corneal ulceration, perforation and opacity and blindness.

Lepromatous leprosy does not remit naturally, though in few patients it does burn out itself. Before the days of effective treatment, the disease continued its relentless course. The patient's downhill course was accelerated by bouts of acute inflammation in nerves and systemic illness (type 2 reactions). Death supervenes due to secondary infection, (particularly pneumonia and tuberculosis), amyloidosis and renal failure. If patients are treated properly with effective antileprosy drugs (multidrug therapy), given the benefit of anti-inflammatory drugs when indicated, with sustained efforts for prevention of disabilities—even LL disease does have a much better prognosis and quality of life.[33,35]

RARE VARIANTS OF LEPROSY

Few unusual forms or expressions of leprosy do not fit into the standard classification of disease. Rarely these presentations may pose a difficulty in diagnosis.

Lucio Leprosy

Lucio leprosy (LuLp) is a pure, primitive and diffuse form of LL, commonly seen in Mexico (23%) and Costa Rica, not infrequent in the Gulf coast, but quite rare in the rest of the world. There is not yet an appropriate definition, and its nosological status, underlying pathomechanisms, and reasons for its restricted global distribution are far from clear. Only recently in 2008, a new species, namely *Mycobacterium*

lepromatosis, was isolated from two patients of Mexican origin with diffuse LL, who died of the disease.[36] Further PCR-based species-specific assays have concluded that this strain is probably more prevalent than *M. leprae* in Mexico. It specifically causes a diffuse form of LL apart from causing dual infections with *M. leprae* in other clinical forms of LL.[37]

Lucio leprosy presents as slowly progressive diffuse infiltration of skin of face and most of the body without any previous evidence of discrete lesions. The skin looks waxy and has shiny appearance (lepra bonita, beautiful leprosy) with obvious diffuse infiltration of the ear lobes and forehead, loss of eyebrows and sometimes eyelashes, and not infrequently all body hair. There may be hoarseness of voice, numbness and edema of hands and feet mimicking myxedema. The appearance is that of a sheet of clear and just perceptible infiltration.[38] The disease is often unmasked by a specific severe reactional state, the Lucio's phenomenon (LP). The so called "lepra manchada" (denominated years later as Lucio leprosy-LuLp) was first described by Lucio and Alvarado in Mexico in 1852, and further elaborated on by Latapi and Zamora in 1948. Although LP peculiarly develops in the untreated diffuse form of leprosy in the Mexican region, it is clinically indistinguishable when seen in other parts of the world or when it rarely develops the classic nodular form of LL.[39-41]

Clinically, LP presents as multiple, well-defined, angular, jagged purpuric lesions evolving into massive ulcerations, spreading in a characteristic ascending fashion over the extremities and healing with atrophic scarring (Figs 15.15A and B). There are no nodules, or lymph node enlargement or arthritis, as in ENL.

Bacteriological and morphological indices show high positivity. Endothelial cell injury is the main event in the

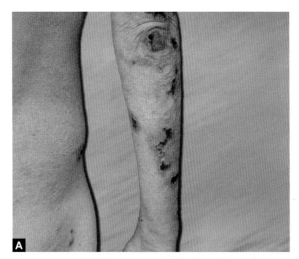 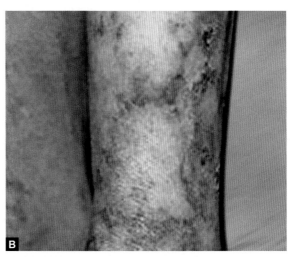

Figs 15.15A and B: (A) Lucio phenomenon—healed lesions with atrophic scarring; (B) Well-defined angular lesions with ulceration
Courtesy: Prof Luna Azulay, Rio De Janeiro, Brazil.

pathogenesis. Once *M. leprae* has entered the endothelial cell, the microorganism damages the blood vessels, leading to specific patterns affecting all cutaneous vessels:

- Colonization of endothelial cells by AFB
- Endothelial proliferation and marked thickening of vessel walls to the point of obliteration
- Angiogenesis
- Vascular ectasia
- Thrombosis.[42,43]

Histologically, there is necrosis of the epidermis and dermis, a histiocytic and neutrophilic infiltrate in and around nerve fibers, blood vessels and adnexa, thickening of the vessel walls with obliteration and thrombosis can be observed in some cases. Although it is not entirely clear, it seems that pathogenesis of LP involves uninhibited multiplication of bacilli leading to diffuse infiltration of the integument in an anergic background. LP usually begins in untreated leprosy, and treatment with antileprosy regimens containing rifampicin is quite effective. High-dose corticosteroids, thalidomide and clofazimine are much less effective compared with their efficacy in ENL. In the literature, cases of LP are treated generally with MDT and immunosuppressants. There are reports of the efficacy of MDT alone, as the pathogenesis is considered by some authors not as a leukocytoclastic vasculitis but thrombotic, on account of *M. leprae* in the vessel wall. The necrotic lesions of LP are similar to those of the cutaneous manifestations of antiphospholipid antibody syndrome (APS). LP could probably be considered as APS secondary to LuLp, a high bacterial load, anergy and/or an exaggerated humoral response. This phenomenon is not well-understood because only a small number of cases have been reported in the literature.

The necrotizing variant of ENL has a similar clinical picture, but the absence of fever and constitutional symptoms and the presence of large areas of ulceration and of AFB in the vascular endothelium favor the diagnosis of LP.[44,45] For management of LP (*See* Chapter-32 on Management of Leprosy Reactions).

Pure Neuritic Leprosy (Also see Chapter on Classification of Leprosy)

It is characterized by an area of sensory loss along the distribution of an involved nerve trunk with or without motor deficit, in the absence of any skin patch. The host CMI is able to contain the infection within one or more nerves, without evidence of skin involvement, wherein it is known as "pure" or "primary" neuritic leprosy. "Secondary" neuritic leprosy refers to leprous neuropathy, accompanied by skin lesions. Suneetha et al.[46] detected histopathological evidence of leprosy in apparently normal skin in one-third of patients with primary neuritic leprosy and 38% of these later developed skin lesions, thereby implying that a neuritic phase often precedes the development of cutaneous lesions. (*See* Chapter-16 on classification).

Neuritic leprosy is seen most frequently, but not exclusively, in India and Nepal, where it accounts for 5–10% of all patients with leprosy. Although not included in the Ridley-Jopling classification, pure neuritic leprosy can display almost the complete spectrum, with BT being the most frequently observed finding. For practical purposes, it is classified as PB or MB leprosy on the basis of presence of AFB in nerve biopsy sections or the number of thickened nerves.

The nerves are often grossly thickened in TT and less so in borderline groups. The presence of a nerve abscess indicates tuberculoid spectrum. Nerve conduction studies that can detect alteration in the nerve amplitude and speed of conduction, sensory and motor functions, have been shown to be a sensitive marker to assess early neural damage.[47] A nerve biopsy may be necessary to establish the diagnosis, which is usually undertaken from sensory nerves of less functional importance. Histology of a cutaneous nerve usually reveals an infiltrate, characteristic of leprosy, although diagnostic intraneural epithelioid granulomas are seen only in a few cases.[11] Lepromin test aids in classification, as being strongly positive in TT, weakly positive in BT and negative in others.

Histoid Leprosy

Histoid leprosy first described in 1960, is now a well-recognized but rarely reported entity.[48] Controversy still remains whether to consider histoid leprosy as a separate entity or as part of the general spectrum of leprosy. It was thought that this type of disease occurs as a consequence of dapsone monotherapy or inadequate therapy but now it is recognized that it does occur *de novo* more often. Clinically the histoid lesions commonly appear as smooth, shiny, hemispherical, dome-shaped, nontender soft to firm nodules which may be superficial, subcutaneous or fixed deeply under the skin and plaques or pads appearing on otherwise normal-looking skin (Figs 15.16A to C). In a given patient, the number of lesions may vary from few to a hundred (Fig. 15.17). The lesions are usually located on the face, back, buttocks and extremities and over bony prominences, especially around the elbows and knees. Histopathologically, the striking feature is predominance of spindle shaped cells and unusually large numbers of AFB.[49,50] (*See* Chapter-18 on Histoid Leprosy).

Lazarine Leprosy

An unusual expression of BT leprosy is spontaneous ulceration of skin lesions. This is presumably the result of exaggerated hypersensitivity in type 1 reactions. Rarely this occurs without any history or evidence of pre-existing skin lesions or coexistent nerve pathology. Histopathology shows necrosis due to extreme cellular hypersensitivity. Systemic corticosteroids are necessary for the treatment in addition to antileprosy drugs. If the disease remains undiagnosed and

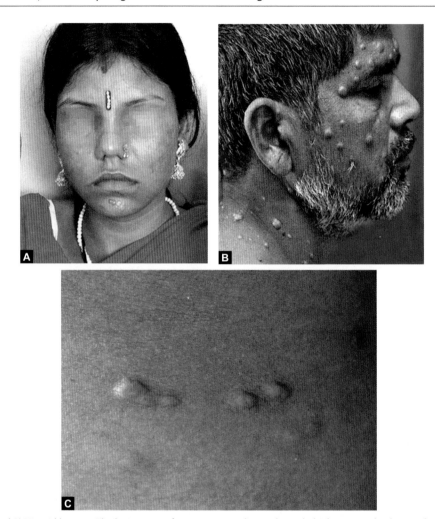

Figs 15.16A to C: (A and B) Histoid leprosy. The lesions over face present as dome-shaped, thick, nontender, hemispherical shiny papules and nodules. Slit skin smear show innumerable *M. leprae* with globi; (C) Histoid Hansen—discrete nodules on normal appearing skin

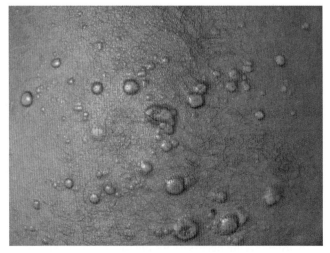

Fig. 15.17: Molluscum like lesions of histoid leprosy

untreated, patients subsequently manifest with typical skin lesions and nerve involvement.[51-53]

Inoculation Leprosy

The term "inoculation leprosy" includes leprosy following scarification/tattooing, vaccination, needle stick injury or trauma. First reported by Lowe and Chatterjee in 1939,[54] inoculation has been regarded as a rare, yet important mode of transmission of leprosy, as seen in other mycobacterial diseases like tuberculosis. Once the lepra bacilli are introduced into the skin through unsterile needles or abrasions, they may initially remain dormant for a few days to many years, until the formation of a clinically evident lesion at or around the site of trauma.

The exposed areas of the upper and lower extremities are primarily affected. It manifests mainly in the form of

TT or BT lesions and rarely of the lepromatous spectrum.[55] Type 1 reversal reaction has also been observed in a tattoo inoculation BT lesion, with the tattoo becoming edematous.[56] Histopathology usually reveals a compact tuberculoid granuloma formed by large number of epithelioid cells, a few lymphocytes, and several Langhans giant cells in addition to clumps of dermal tattoo pigment. Some lymphocytes may be found abutting the epidermis (epidermal erosion). Acid-fast lepra bacilli are difficult to demonstrate.[55]

Inoculation leprosy should be differentiated from that of cutaneous sarcoidal reaction to tattoo pigments. Even inoculation tuberculosis (lupus vulgaris) might need histological exclusion. Inoculation leprosy should be treated by the standard regimen according to the clinical spectrum.

The "Immune Zones" (Relatively Spared Zones) in Leprosy[57]

The distribution of leprosy lesions, affecting predominantly the skin, nasal mucosa and peripheral nerves, particularly more superficial ones is the evidence for suggesting that *M. leprae* prefers a growth temperature of less than 37°C. Certain anatomical sites like scalp, groin, axillae, perineum and a transverse strip of skin over lumbosacral region were considered immune or relatively immune to the development of leprosy by many workers. The term "immune zones" (relatively spared zones) is used in a nonimmunological sense and it does not pertain to local immunity but only to relative sparing of certain anatomical sites of leprosy lesions. The "immunity" is attributed to the relative warmth of these regions. Palms and soles are also included in the relatively

"immune zones" by some workers. The thick epidermis of palms and soles along with the good amount of fibro-fatty tissue provides an insulating property and hence a high nerve bed temperature, which renders the palmoplantar localization of *M. leprae* less likely. However, some studies have cast doubts on the existence of "immune zones" especially in LL. In the clinical practice, it appears that practically no area on the surface of skin is immune to leprosy. However, as the incidence of lesions and AFBs in these regions is relatively less, these areas can be considered as relatively spared zones, but not completely resistant to development of lesions of leprosy (Fig. 15.18).

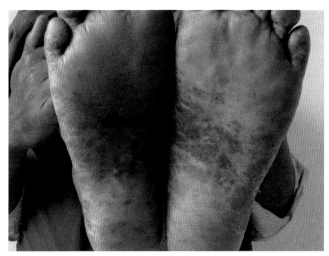

Fig. 15.18: Lepromatous leprosy with involvement of the soles

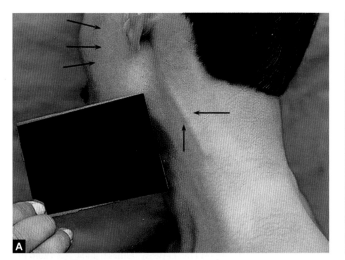

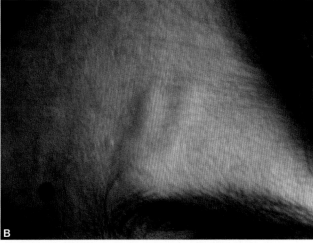

Figs 15.19A and B: (A) Enlargement of great auricular nerve (between the arrows over neck). Also note the tuberculoid patch over left side of cheek (arrows at the lesion margin). This nerve is usually better appreciated by inspection, than palpation (*Courtesy*: Dr Pankaj Sharma, PGIMER, Dr RML Hospital, New Delhi); (B) Thickened supraorbital nerve (*Courtesy*: Prof PN Rao, Hyderabad)

NERVE INVOLVEMENT

Nerve damage occurs in two settings—peripheral nerve trunks and small dermal nerves. Small dermal sensory and autonomic nerves are affected in the early part of disease establishment producing hypoesthesia and anhidrosis within skin lesions. Of the nerve trunks, ulnar nerve is the most commonly affected, followed by the median, lateral popliteal, and facial nerves. Involvement of these nerves produces enlargement, with or without tenderness, and regional sensory and also motor loss. Thickening of greater auricular nerve is better seen than felt (Figs 15.19A and B). Rarely nerve abscess is encountered in the thickened peripheral nerve trunks primarily in the TT and BT spectrum, mostly in the ulnar and lateral popliteal nerves. The mutilations, morbidity and disability associated with leprosy are secondary to nerve damage which is hastened by reactions. About 25% of leprosy patients have some degree of disability, which is seen early in the course of BT disease with nerve involvement and later in neglected BL and LL disease. Early recognition and treatment is crucial to the prevention of deformities.[58-60] (See Chapter-11 on Pathomechanisms of Nerve Damage).

SYSTEMIC INVOLVEMENT

Features of systemic involvement occur usually in a long standing disease and are mainly seen in patients near the lepromatous pole due to bacillary deposits and associated granulomatous infiltration affecting various organs especially nasal mucosa, larynx, eyes, bones, testes, kidneys, lymph nodes, liver and spleen. Besides the disease, systemic manifestations in the form of constitutional symptoms like fever, malaise, joint pains and acute inflammation of eyes, joints, reticuloendothelial system, etc. can occur as a part of type 2 lepra reaction.[61] (See Chapter-23 on Systemic Involvement in Leprosy).

ACKNOWLEDGMENT

We are grateful to Professor Luna Azulay from Brazil, for her inputs in improving the component of the chapter on Lucio leprosy and Lucio phenomenon.

REFERENCES

1. World Health Organization. (2012) WHO expert committee on leprosy, 8th report. [online] Available from http://www.searo.who.int/entity/global_leprosy_programme/publications/8th_expert_comm_2012.pdf. [Accessed May, 2014].
2. Georgiev GD, McDougall AC. Skin smears and the bacterial index (BI) in multiple drug therapy leprosy control programs: an unsatisfactory and potentially hazardous state of affairs. Int J Lepr Other Mycobact Dis. 1988;56:101-4.
3. Kumar B, Dogra S. Leprosy: a disease with diagnostic and management challenges! Indian J Dermatol Venereol Leprol. 2009;75:111-5.
4. Ponnighaus JM, Fine PE. A comparison of sensory loss tests and histopathology in the diagnosis of leprosy. Lepr Rev. 1989;60:20-7.
5. Sirumban P, Kumar A, Durai V, et al. Diagnostic value of cardinal signs/symptoms in paucibacillary leprosy. Indian J Lepr. 1988;60:207-14.
6. Groenen G, Saha NG, Rashid MA, et al. Classification of leprosy cases under field conditions in Bangladesh. II. Reliability of clinical criteria. Lepr Rev. 1995;66:134-43.
7. Saunderson P, Groenen G. Which physical signs help most in the diagnosis of leprosy? A proposal based on experience in the AMFES project, ALERT, Ethiopia. Lepr Rev. 2000;71:34-42.
8. Kolappan C, Selvaraj R, Khudoos A, et al. Repeatability of nerve thickness assessment in the clinical examination for leprosy. Lepr Rev. 1995;66:224-8.
9. McDougall AC. The clinical examination of peripheral nerves in leprosy. Indian J Lepr. 1996;68:378-80.
10. Khambati FA, Shetty VP, Ghate SD, et al. Sensitivity and specificity of nerve palpation, monofilament testing and voluntary muscle testing in detecting peripheral nerve abnormality, using nerve conduction studies as gold standard; a study in 357 patients. Lepr Rev. 2009;80:34-50.
11. Kumar B, Kaur I, Dogra S, et al. Pure neuritic leprosy in India: an appraisal. Int J Lepr Other Mycobact Dis. 2004;72:284-90.
12. Saunderson PR, Gebre S, Desta K, et al. The ALERT MDT Field Evaluation Study (AMFES): a descriptive study of leprosy in Ethiopia. Patients, methods and baseline characteristics. Lepr Rev. 2000;71:273-84.
13. Mahajan PM, Jogaikar DG, Mehta JM. A study of pure neuritic leprosy: clinical experience. Indian J Lepr. 1996;68:137-41.
14. van Brakel WH, de Soldenhoff R, McDougall AC. The allocation of leprosy patients into paucibacillary and multibacillary groups for multidrug therapy, taking into account the number of body areas affected by skin, or skin and nerve lesions. Lepr Rev. 1992;63:231-46.
15. Porichha D. A plea to revive skin smear examination. Int J Lepr Other Mycobact Dis. 2001;69:116-9.
16. Kundu SK. Features of Ridley-Jopling classification and its application in the clinical field. Int J Lepr Other Mycobact Dis. 1979;47:64-5.
17. Hagge DA, Thappa P, Shrestha IR, et al. Is counting lesions enough: the significance of slit skin smears and biopsy histopathology in the clinical diagnosis, treatment and classification of leprosy patients. 18th International Leprosy Congress, Brussels, September 16-19, 2013. p. 39.
18. Gelber R, Pardillo FE, Fajardo TT, et al. Counting lesions in the Philippines often misclassifies patients as PB that are MB by earlier criteria. 18th International Leprosy Congress, Brussels, September 16-19, 2013. p. 39.
19. Pannikar VK. Defining a case of leprosy. Lepr Rev. 1992;63:61-5.
20. Gupta R, Kar HK, Bharadwaj M. Revalidation of various clinical criteria for the classification of leprosy-a clinic-pathological study. Lepr Rev. 2012;83:354-62.
21. Abulafia J, Vignale RI. Leprosy: pathogenesis updated. Int J Dermatol. 1999;38:321-34.
22. Britton WJ, Lockwood DN. Leprosy. Lancet. 2004;363:1209-19.
23. Shetty VP, Pandya SS. One year follow up of a cohort of suspected leprosy cases: findings from a leprosy 'Selective Special Drive' in Gadchiroli district, Maharashtra, India. Lepr Rev. 2012;83:64-70.

24. Cardama JE. Early lesions (indeterminate forms). In: Latapi F, Saul A, Rodriguez O, Malacara M, Browne SG (Eds). Leprosy. Proceedings of the XI International Leprosy Congress, Mexico City, November 13-18, 1978. Amsterdam: Excerpta Medica. 1980. pp. 68-74.

25. Gomez L. The question of the initial lesion of leprosy. J Philippine Islands Med Assoc. 1923;3:227-9.

26. Banerjee S, Biswas N, Kanti Das N, et al. Diagnosing leprosy: revisiting the role of the slit-skin smear with critical analysis of the applicability of polymerase chain reaction in diagnosis. Int J Dermatol. 2011;50:1522-7.

27. Pettit JH. Should indeterminate leprosy ever be diagnosed? Int J Lepr Other Mycobact Dis. 1981;49:95-6.

28. Lara CB. Leprosy in children. General considerations: initial and early stages. Acta Leprol. 1970;38:29-60.

29. Imbiriba EB, Hurtado-Guerrero JC, Garnelo L. Epidemiological profile of leprosy in children under 15 in Manaus (Northern Brazil), 1998-2005. Rev Saude Publica. 2008;42:1021-6.

30. Ramanujam K. Findings of a nineteen year follow-up of children with untreated leprosy. In: Latapi F, Saul A, Rodriguez O, Ma'lacara M, Browne SG (Eds). Leprosy. Proceedings of the XI International Leprosy Congress, Mexico City, November 13-18, 1978. Amsterdam: ExcerptaMedica. 1980. pp. 75-79.

31. Ekambaram V, Sithambaram M. Self-healing in non-lepromatous leprosy in the area of ELEP leprosy control project Dharmapuri (Tamil Nadu). Lepr India. 1977;49:387-92.

32. Noordecn SK. Evolution of tuberculoid leprosy in a community. Lepr India. 1975;47:85-93.

33. Moschella SL. An update on the diagnosis and treatment of leprosy. J Am Acad Dermatol. 2004;51:417-26.

34. Rao PN, Suneetha S, Pratap DV. Changes in the size and number of skin lesions in PB leprosy on treatment and follow-up. Lepr Rev. 2011;82:244-52.

35. Pfaltzgraff RE, Bryceson A. Clinical leprosy. In: Hastings RC (Ed). Leprosy. New York: Churchill Livingstone; 1989. pp. 134-76.

36. Han XY, Seo YH, Sizer KC, et al. A new *Mycobacterium* species causing diffuse lepromatous leprosy. Am J Clin Pathol. 2008;130:856-64.

37. Han XY, Sizer KC, Velarde-Félix JS, et al. The leprosy agents *Mycobacterium lepromatosis* and *Mycobacterium* leprae in Mexico. Int J Dermatol. 2012;51:952-9.

38. Latapi F, Zamora AC. The spotted leprosy of Lucio: an introduction to its clinical and histopathological study. Int J Lepr Other Mycobact Dis. 1948;16:421-9.

39. Quismorio FP Jr, Rea TH, Chandor S, et al. Lucio's phenomenon: an immune complex deposition syndrome in lepromatous leprosy. Clin Immunol Immunopathol. 1978;9:184-93.

40. Saoji V, Salodkar A. Lucio leprosy with Lucio phenomenon. Indian J Lepr. 2001;73:267-72.

41. Kumari R, Thappa DM, Basu D. A fatal case of Lucio phenomenon from India. Dermatol Online J. 2008;14:10.

42. Vargas-Ocampo F. Diffuse leprosy of Lucio and Latapí: a histologic study. Lepr Rev. 2007;78:248-60.

43. Azulay-Abulafia L, Pereira Spinelli L, Hardmann D, et al. Lucio-Phänomen: Vaskulitis oder okklusive Vaskulopathie? Hautarzt. 2006;57:1101-5.

44. Kaur C, Thami GP, Mohan H. Lucio phenomenon and Lucio leprosy. Clin Exp Dermatol. 2005;30:525-7.

45. Sehgal VN. Lucio's phenomenon/erythema necroticans. Int J Dermatol. 2005;44:602-5.

46. Suneetha S, Sigamoni A, Kurian N, et al. The development of cutaneous lesions during follow-up of patients with primary neuritic leprosy. Int J Dermatol. 2005;44:224-9.

47. Rodriguez G, Pinto R, Gomez Y, et al. Pure neuritic leprosy in patients from a high endemic region of Colombia. Lepr Rev. 2013;84:41-50.

48. Wade HW. The histoid variety of lepromatous leprosy. Int J Lepr Other Mycobact Dis. 1963;31:129-42.

49. Sehgal VN, Srivastava G. Histoid leprosy: a prospective diagnostic study in 38 patients. Dermatologica. 1988;177:212-7.

50. Kaur I, Dogra S, De D, et al. Histoid leprosy: a retrospective study of 40 cases from India. Br J Dermatol. 2009;160:305-10.

51. Nanda S, Bansal S, Grover C, et al. Lazarine leprosy--revisited? Indian J Lepr. 2004;76:351-4.

52. Thappa DM. What is lazarine leprosy? Is it a separate entity? Indian J Lepr. 2005;77:179-81.

53. Skinsnes LK, Higa LH. The role of protein malnutrition in the pathogenesis of ulcerative "Lazarine" leprosy. Int J Lepr Other Mycobact Dis. 1976;44:346-58.

54. Lowe J, Chatterjee SN. Scarification, tattooing etc. in relation to leprous lesions of skin. Lepr India. 1939;11:14-8.

55. Ghorpade A. Inoculation (tattoo) leprosy: a report of 31 cases. J Eur Acad Dermatol Venereol. 2002;16:494-9.

56. Ghorpade A. Reactional tattoo inoculation borderline tuberculoid leprosy with oedematous tattoos. Lepr Rev. 2004;75:91-4.

57. Kaur I, Indira D, Dogra S, et al. "Relatively spared zones" in leprosy: a clinicopathological study of 500 patients. Int J Lepr Other Mycobact Dis. 2003;71:227-3.

58. Spierings E, De Boer T, Zulianello L, et al. The role of Schwann cells, T-cells and *Mycobacterium leprae* in the immunopathogenesis of nerve damage in leprosy. Lepr Rev. 2000;71:121-9.

59. Shetty VP, Mistry NF, Antia NH. Current understanding of leprosy as a peripheral nerve disorder: significance of involvement of peripheral nerve in leprosy. Indian J Lepr. 2000;72:339-50.

60. Ooi WW, Srinivasan J. Leprosy and the peripheral nervous system: basic and clinical aspects. Muscle Nerve. 2004;30:393-409.

61. Kumar B, Rai R, Kaur I. Systemic involvement in leprosy and its significance. Lepr Rev. 2000;72:123-42.

16
CHAPTER

Classification

Radhey Shyam Misra, Joginder Kumar Kataria

INTRODUCTION

Leprosy is a chronic disease with the manifestations as varied as the single cutaneous/nerve lesion to the involvement of whole of the integument and systemic organs. The disease can present with predominantly neural symptoms or mainly with cutaneous involvement. In ancient India, the disease had been called '*vat rakta*' denoting the cases with neural component while '*arunkushta*' represented the cutaneous form of leprosy.[1] This categorization was almost similar to the classification prevalent elsewhere dividing leprosy into the nodular and anesthetic groups.[2] This simplicity of classification was also seen even in the 20th century when Leonard Wood Memorial in Manila in 1931 evolved an international system of classification for the first time.[3] In this classification, the disease had been categorized into cutaneous, neural and mixed types. This Manila classification formed the basis of future classifications and underwent several transformations that finally culminated in the so called International or Madrid classification in 1953, which became the official classification of international bodies.[4] In the following period, the terminology changed with various modifications. The term cutaneous was replaced by lepromatous that represented a widespread involvement of the skin and the term neural got replaced by tuberculoid that represented raised lesions with neural deficit. These terms—tuberculoid (tuberculosis like histopathology) and lepromatous (foam cell histopathology) had initially depicted the pathological changes but later acquired the clinical dimensions representing specific clinical and morphological lesions. Throughout the evolution of classification while there was no conflict over the specific and definite entities namely the tuberculoid and lepromatous which came to be regarded as polar types, a widespread discontentment among the leprologists had been simmering over maculoanesthetic lesions and pure neuritic cases. The confusion over placement of the maculoanesthetic lesions and pure neuritic types became so obvious at the Tokyo International Leprosy Conference in 1958 that the decision to categorize these cases was left to the individual leprologist.[5]

Since long, the Indian leprologists regarded the maculoanesthetic and pure neuritic forms as distinct entities and to remove the confusion surrounding these categories the Indian classification was drafted in 1953, just a little before the Madrid classification came into existence. The Indian classification had been proposed by Dharmendra and Chatterjee on behalf of Indian Association of Leprologists (IAL). It was almost similar to the Madrid classification and was officially accepted and adopted by the IAL in 1955.[6]

In 1962, the spectral classification was advanced by Ridley and Jopling calling it a classification for research purposes.[7] This five-group classification was detailed further in 1966,[8] and later on called Ridley-Jopling classification. It failed to excite leprologists initially but slowly gained global acceptance. The high point of this classification was its precision and stress upon the disease as a spectrum, dictated by the immunological response of the patients.

In the year 1982, to give a momentum to the leprosy control, the WHO gave definitiveness to the treatment of leprosy by introducing the concept of fixed-duration multidrug therapy (FD-MDT). For FD-MDT, the disease was categorized into paucibacillary (PB) and multibacillary (MB) on the basis of lesional bacterial density as estimated by bacterial index (BI) in slit-skin smears.[9] To overcome the operational difficulties, especially at the field worker level, the necessity of slit skin smear was done away with in 1998 and a clinical criterion in the form of number of skin lesions was added to this categorization.[10] Henceforth, all the patients with six or more skin lesions were also to be classified as MB without any reference to the slit-skin smears. This newer classification as such or with some minor modifications (vide infra) is now being followed in the leprosy eradication program in India as well as all over the world.

At present, the most common classifications in use the world over are the WHO classification for treatment purposes, and Ridley-Jopling classification for academic and research purposes.

NEED FOR CLASSIFICATION

The wide variation in the disease presentation, its course, prognosis and complications forces one to consider these variants as distinct entities making the classification a contentious issue. The classification becomes important to thread these entities as a single disease yet maintaining the distinctiveness of each one of these.

With the WHO guidelines for leprosy control programs, the classification assumes utmost importance to decide the line of treatment. The correct classification not only helps to decide upon the treatment options, but the clinician can visualize beyond the present stage of the disease also. He can envisage the nature, progression and prognosis of the disease with the relative risk to development of deformities and response to the therapy. The frequency and the type of leprosy reaction that the patient is likely to undergo also become clear. The clinician can educate the patient and plan for the future to prevent the deformities. The infectivity of a case and its epidemiological importance can also be determined.

The comparison of clinical, histopathological, bacterio logical and immunological parameters among the classified groups helps to understand the finer nuances of the disease. A uniform classification helps in communication with the other workers, sharing the ideas on a common platform and the comparison of data becomes more clear and realistic.

CLASSIFICATION CRITERIA

For a clinician, the issues pertaining to the treatment are vital while an epidemiologist or a research worker has different perceptions altogether. A single classification to meet everyone's expectation though desirable may be very difficult to arrive at. Defining the criteria for any type of categorization is crucial, for the specific groups of workers may lay more stress upon certain specific parameters more useful or helpful to them. Leprosy may be classified based upon bacteriological, immunological, clinical or histopathological parameters individually or by using a correlated combination of these.

Bacteriological Criteria

The BI is a measure of the density of the organisms in the lesional tissue and is estimated by slit-skin smear technique or in a biopsy specimen. The latter is more sensitive,[11] but technically is not feasible universally. The skin smears are easier to perform and their specifications and grading criteria have been standardized. They are regarded as the gold standard for the bacteriology based WHO classification for treatment purposes.

Infective (Open) and Noninfective Categorization

In this epidemiologically valuable classification, the patient is classified as an open and infective case if his routine slit-skin smears or nasal scrapings demonstrate bacilli.[12]

Immunological Criteria

The basic immunological aberration in leprosy, the specific deficiency of cell-mediated immunity (CMI) against *M. leprae*, is measured indirectly by lepromin testing and the patients classified as lepromin positive (good immunity) to lepromin negative (poor immunity) on a standard scale. The categorization into immune and nonimmune status may be perceived as a predictor of the course of the disease better than any other criterion. The test is also very useful in classifying the "difficult to classify cases" (i.e. the indeterminate and pure neuritic leprosy) into lepromatous or nonlepromatous categories.

Histopathological Criteria

The histopathological observations reflect the actual processes going on inside the body in the form of tissue reactions to the injury or insult. The varied lesions of leprosy have distinct histopathological pictures which form a good ground for the classification. The histopathological features have been precisely defined and can be described as the most definitive criteria for defining the different entities. The interpretations are not influenced by external factors, are less prone to the subjective errors and are less likely to be erratic as the clinical judgment at times tends to be. However, histological studies are tedious to perform and it is not practicable to apply them universally over a large leprosy population.

Clinical Criteria

A classification based on the clinical features is the easiest to apply and the most desirable because the clinician has the advantage of examining the patient in entirety rather than looking at a selected presented material. Clinical features can be identified with some training by even a health worker in the field. Typical morphological descriptions may be used (macular, nodular, etc.) or the classification can have a well-defined terminology denoting clinical picture (tuberculoid, lepromatous, etc.).

The presently used WHO classification for leprosy control is entirely based on clinical features. All other classifications in practice have used a combination of these parameters.

The well-accepted classifications include Madrid, Indian, new IAL, Ridley-Jopling, and WHO classification for leprosy control.

MADRID CLASSIFICATION[4] (BOX 16.1)

Conceived and adopted at the International Leprosy Congress held at Madrid in 1953, this classification was regarded as a major improvement over the preceding ones.[4] Often referred to as The International Classification, it included 'two types' and 'two groups'. The term 'type' denoted definite and typical clinical entities while the 'groups' were less distinct nontypical entities. The two types were lepromatous (L) and tuberculoid (T); while the two groups were indeterminate (I) and borderline or dimorphous (B). The morphological subtypes with descriptive nomenclature had been added up under each of these entities and were called the varieties. Under tuberculoid type the difference between minor and major varieties was the degree of infiltration. The former had mild or a patchy infiltration with pebbly appearance over the lesions (sometimes infiltration of only of a part of the lesion or part of the margin) while in the latter the infiltration was marked and tended to be diffuse though at times broad infiltration at the periphery made it appear as an annular lesion. This classification was exhaustive, yet the pre-existing objections could not be done away with entirely. Many a leprologist earlier tended to regard pure neuritic leprosy as a homogenous clinical entity and its placement under different categories was not considered to be justified. However, in the present perspective of better understanding, the so called splitting of pure neuritic cases under different types appears to be more appropriate. The pure neuritic type under lepromatous group and that under tuberculoid group are likely to differ in their course and prognosis and would also be treated on different lines. It is a different matter altogether that the existence of pure neuritic variety under lepromatous group is still doubtful.

Box 16.1: The Madrid classification (1953)

Lepromatous Type (L)
- Macular
- Diffuse
- Infiltrated
- Nodular
- Neuritic, pure (?)

Tuberculoid Type (T)
- Macular (Tm)
- Minor tuberculoid (micropapuloid) (Tt)
- Major tuberculoid (plaques, annular lesions, etc.) (TT)
- Neuritic, Pure (Tn)

Indeterminate Group (I)
- Macular (Im)
- Neuritic type (In)

Borderline (Dimorphous) Group (B)
- Infiltrated
- (Others ?)

Box 16.2: The Indian classification (1955)

- Lepromatous (L)
- Tuberculoid (T)
- Maculoanesthetic (MA)
- Polyneuritic (P)
- Borderline (B)
- Indeterminate (I)

INDIAN CLASSIFICATION[6] (BOX 16.2)

The Indian classification was drafted on behalf of the IAL at almost the same time as the Madrid classification (1953) but was accepted and adopted in 1955. The Indian leprologists were not satisfied with the earlier international classifications (prior to Madrid classification). The main objection was that the classification criteria were not entirely clinical and their applicability and usefulness at all levels of leprosy workers was doubtful. There was much confusion regarding the categorization of maculoanesthetic and pure neuritic leprosy which were thought to be separate entities. The maculoanesthetic was said to be a separate category because of the flat lesions in contrast to the raised lesions of the tuberculoid type.[13]

The Indian classification recognized six groups that included maculoanesthetic and pure neuritic as separate categories. The classification was kept flexible for workability at various levels, i.e. for field workers it was made to be a three-group classification comprising: (1) nonlepromatous (N) that collectively included tuberculoid, maculoanesthetic and polyneuritic, (2) lepromatous (L) and (3) intermediate

(N?L) group. The latter entity (N?L) was applicable to doubtful classification cases. On the other hand, the research workers could go further than the simple six groups mentioned and could classify even up to varieties or subtypes (i.e. nodular, macular, etc.). The slit-skin smear studies, if possible, could be used as an additional criteria and the positivity denoted by putting a sign of + after the disease entity, i.e. T+ or I+.

NEW IAL CLASSIFICATION[14] (BOX 16.3)

A modification in the Indian classification had been adopted in 1981 by the IAL wherein the maculoanesthetic (MA) leprosy was merged with tuberculoid (T) leprosy. The resultant five-group classification was called the New IAL Classification of Leprosy.

RIDLEY-JOPLING CLASSIFICATION[7,8] (BOX 16.4)

Also referred to as the immunological classification, the Ridley-Jopling classification is based upon the fact that bacteriological, immunological, histopathological and clinical features of leprosy are intrinsically interwoven. After bacteriological invasion, the immunological factors come to play in the form of CMI and delayed type of hypersensitivity (DTH) determining the tissue reactions and the resultant clinical picture. In effect, this is the classification based upon the correlation of all these parameters. Most important aspect is the emphasis on the spectral concept of leprosy.

It is essentially a five-group classification with two polar forms: tuberculoid (TT) and lepromatous (LL) at the two extremes which are more or less immunologically stable. Between these two polar forms lies a big immunologically unstable borderline group which has been subdivided into three categories: (1) borderline tuberculoid (BT), (2) mid-borderline or borderline borderline (BB), and (3) borderline lepromatous (BL). BB is the most unstable form of the leprosy. All these entities form a continuous spectrum with

---

Box 16.3: The new Indian Association of Leprologists classification (1981)

- Lepromatous (L)
- Tuberculoid (T)
- Polyneuritic (P)
- Borderline (B)
- Indeterminate (I)

Box 16.4: Ridley-Jopling classification (1966)

- Tuberculoid leprosy (TT)
- Borderline tuberculoid leprosy (BT)
- Mid-borderline leprosy (BB)
- Borderline lepromatous leprosy (BL)
- Lepromatous leprosy (LL)

---

frequent transformation of one form into another-especially among the borderline group by the process of the so-called upgrading or downgrading. The clinical, histopathological, bacteriological and immunological features show slow but continuous changes from one pole to the other pole. For example, the immunity decreases while the lesional bacterial density increases from TT to LL pole. The immunological variation also manifests as lepromin positivity in tuberculoid and negativity in the lepromatous type. The spectral concept helps to understand all these entities as denominations of a single disease in spite of their diverse course and prognosis. One can predict the course, outcome and complications of a patient's disease depending upon its place in the spectrum. It also helps us to understand leprosy reactions in their true perspective.

The advantages of Ridley-Jopling classification are that not only it is easier to comprehend, but also helps to understand the disease and its nuances in a better way. It also strengthens the polar and spectral concept. It is based on the foundation of correlationship among the various parameters that describe the entities more precisely. For these reasons, this classification has now been widely accepted. Initially suggested as classification for research purposes, this classification has almost replaced the other classifications even for the clinical purposes (with inclusion of indeterminate as a separate entity by some workers).

The main drawback of Ridley-Jopling classification is that there is no specific place for the indeterminate and pure neuritic leprosy in the spectrum. The indeterminate leprosy had been regarded as the incipient stage of leprosy that has not yet fully evolved to be classifiable in the spectrum as the features are rather vague.[15] Though it is not part of the spectrum yet it can be placed near tuberculoid or near lepromatous end of the spectrum, depending upon the lepromin testing and slit-skin smear results. The pure neuritic leprosy is said to have evolved in a similar pathogenetic mechanism, through the same immunologic interactions as that of the skin lesions and hence needed to be classified within the TT-LL spectrum in the similar manner, and on the same criteria.[16] Hence, the pure neuritic cases have to be categorized into any of the types on the basis of histopathology of the affected nerve. However, one must be cautioned that the histopathology of nerve lesions may not reflect the actual category of the disease as in many patients with non-pure neuritic leprosy (with coexistent skin and nerve involvement) the nerve histopathology confirmed to that of the lower type (toward LL) as compared to the skin lesions.[17,18]

In general, the bacteriological and immunological parameters do not present any problem in correlating them with the various subtypes; rather it is the clinicohisto pathological discordance that may cause confusion. The histopathological concordance with the clinical features has been reported to be about 50% to almost 100%.[19-24] In a large series of 2,696 leprosy biopsies, the histopathological picture coincided with the clinical diagnosis in 98%, 97%, 95%, 89% and 87% in LL, TT, BT, BB and BL disease respectively, which appears to be quite satisfactory.[24] However, in another large series from north India the overall clinicohistopathological concordance was an unsatisfactory low of only 49.5% with corresponding figures for BT, BB, BL and LL being 61.2%, 20%, 35.7% and 56.7% respectively.[19] The studies also reflect that the concordance tends to be low in the borderline group while it increases toward the polar forms. It must be remembered that any change in pathological picture may be reflected clinically only after 2–3 months and some degree of discordance may be observed which can be explained on this basis, especially discordance of one step higher or lower.[15] Discordance may also be there as the histopathological changes evolve slowly and could be in the phase of transition at the time of examination while the clinical presentation is clearly defined and more stable. Moreover, the clinical diagnosis is more prone to error depending upon the clinician's alertness and expertise, while histopathological interpretations do not show much subjective variations. Here again, it should be remembered that the biopsy sample sent for the histopathological evaluation, may also have missed the granuloma, which may reflect in discordant clinical and histopathological observations.

The suitability of this classification for the field level worker is open to discussion.

Concept of Polar and Subpolar Forms

The LL group at the pole appears to be heterogeneous and includes two subgroups named polar LL (LLp) and subpolar LL (LLs). The LLp is immunologically stable and starts as lepromatous and remains the same throughout without any downgrading while LLs, (earlier called LI or leproma indefinite),[25] is immunologically unstable and originates from downgrading of borderline group. It may even upgrade afterward. The LLs may still have some lesions of its predecessor borderline leprosy as the evidence of having downgraded from it and also has lesser foamy changes histologically.[26] It has somewhat higher immunity and occupies the place between LLp and BL in the spectrum. During an upgrading reaction, LLs may regain its lost CMI.[27] On the tuberculoid end of the spectrum, a similar subclassification has been predicted in the form of primary/polar (TTp) and secondary/subpolar (TTs) types.[28] The TTp originates as polar tuberculoid never having gone through a borderline phase while TTs is said to arise by upgrading from borderline leprosy or can downgrade to borderline leprosy. However, the immunological behavior of TTp and TTs does not equate to that of LLp and LLs.

WORLD HEALTH ORGANIZATION CLASSIFICATION (1988) FOR LEPROSY CONTROL PROGRAMS[9,10,29] (BOX 16.5)

This happens to be the most important categorization of the disease for any treating leprologist. The patients are categorized into PB or MB leprosy depending upon whether the slit-skin smears demonstrate any bacilli or not. The concept was conceived and implemented in 1982.[9] Earlier the cases with a BI of 2 or less had been categorized as PB[9] but later on, for feasibility and operational difficulties, all the patients with demonstrable bacilli in slit skin smear without any reference to BI were to be categorized as MB.[29]

The pure neuritic leprosy deserved special comments. While most of these cases were said to belong to the PB group, the correct classification was considered difficult. Lepromin testing, number of nerves involved and nerve biopsy were thought to be some useful parameters toward classification of these pure neuritic cases.

This strategic WHO classification for control programs was necessitated to streamline and optimize the limited resources and to improve logistics. Large number of patients and operational difficulties had to be kept in mind. The basis of this categorization had been the observation that PB patients have the bacillary count of less than 10^6 log and hence the drug resistant mutants are unlikely to originate.[9] In MB forms, the number is likely to exceed 10^6 log and the chances of at least one mutation leading to drug resistant organisms is strong. The classification was established once the field trials and studies justified segregation of these two groups for treatment purposes as the less bacillated patients could be treated with lesser number of drugs for shorter period; while to control the heavily bacillated cases, one needed additional drugs for longer periods.

Box 16.5: WHO classification (1988)

- **Paucibacillary leprosy**
It includes only smear negative cases belonging to:
  - Indeterminate (I), tuberculoid (TT), and borderline tuberculoid (BT) cases as classified under Ridley-Jopling classification, and
  - Indeterminate (I), and tuberculoid (T) cases under Madrid classification
- **Multibacillary leprosy**
Includes all
  - Mid-borderline (BB), borderline lepromatous (BL), and lepromatous (LL) under Ridley-Jopling classification, and
  - Borderline (B) and lepromatous (L) cases under the Madrid classification
  - Any other smear positive case

(*Note*: Though there is no indeterminate in Ridley-Jopling Classification, it has been included here by WHO as some workers use it simultaneously with Ridley-Jopling Classification.)

WORLD HEALTH ORGANIZATION CLASSIFICATION (1998) (BOX 16.6)

Application of slit skin smears universally and to maintain their quality control emerged as the biggest hurdle in the implementation of control programs.[30,31] The operational problems led to the suggestion of doing away with the skin smear, if it is not practicable and also to the new criterion of PB and MB categorization, proposed in 1998 by WHO which was based upon the total number of leprosy lesions in the patient.[10] This is a corollary to the fact that PB patients have good immunity and present with only a limited number of lesions. Furthermore, the single lesion leprosy was also segregated on the ground that this can be treated with the limited amount of chemotherapy. For the sake of practicality and its utility in the field the WHO expert committee formed the new classification based on the number of lesions.

It should be emphasized that the classification based on the number of lesions is not intended to replace the previously defined PB and MB definitions. Wherever skin smears are practiced, any patient with positive smear should be placed in MB type irrespective of the number of lesions. Skin smears remain the gold standard for the classification. Presently the single lesion leprosy has been merged with the PB type thus making it essentially a two-group classification consisting of a PB and an MB group.[32]

The main objection to this solely operational classification is the wrong categorization of some MB cases into PB that may result in under treatment, hence the increased possibility of relapse and emergence of drug resistance. The apprehension may not be totally unfounded.[33-36] However, on operational side, since 1985 more than 14 million leprosy cases have been treated using multidrug therapy (MDT) with only very few relapses and hence its performance appears to be satisfactory.[37] It is the success of MDT-based control programs that gave an impetus to the activities making the target of leprosy eradication achievable. The sensitivity and specificity of this classification has been reported to be about 90%.[38,39] Moreover, a good clinical examination by an experienced clinician may further increase its sensitivity.[38] Inclusion of the number of involved nerves (not included in the WHO 1998 classification) as an additional criterion, may add up on the sensitivity of this classification.[36,39] Later on, National Leprosy Eradication Program (NLEP) of Government of India in collaboration with Global Alliance for Leprosy Elimination and WHO; prepared a document on classification of leprosy wherein, the nerve involvement was kept as a factor to classifying leprosy into PB and MB forms.[40]

CLASSIFICATION PRESENTLY USED IN INDIA FOR TREATMENT PURPOSES (WHO CLASSIFICATION AS MODIFIED UNDER NLEP) (TABLE 16.1)

Presently in India, the number of nerves involved is also taken into consideration along with the skin lesion count while categorizing the patients into PB and MB types as per the criteria laid down under the NLEP of Government of India[41] which are similar to those of the International Federation of Antileprosy Associations (ILEP).[42] Inclusion of the factor of nerve involvement becomes important especially in pure neuritic leprosy which constitutes about 4–5% of all leprosy cases in our country,[43-45] with more than one nerve involvement in over 60% of these.[44] Henceforth, an MB case has been defined as the one having six or more lesions and/or more than one nerve involvement and/or a positive skin smear from any site.

MISCELLANEOUS CRITERIA IN USE FOR CLASSIFICATION INTO PB AND MB

The skin lesion count at times can be ambiguous or erroneous because of presence of some nonspecific looking lesions or due to some hidden lesions. Therefore, some workers have tried using other parameters to classify the cases on PB/MB scale either alone or in combination with WHO lesion count classification. These parameters include:

1. *The number of body areas involved*: The rationale is that the occurrence of lesions on different body areas indicates dissemination and should be classified as MB irrespective

---

Box 16.6: WHO classification based on the number of lesions (1998)

- Paucibacillary single lesion leprosy (SLPB);
- Paucibacillary leprosy (two to five skin lesions) (PB);
- Multibacillary leprosy—six or more skin lesions and also, all smear-positive cases (MB).

Note: Later the SLPB was merged with PB making it a two group classification.

Table 16.1: Classification under NLEP, India (2009)		
Characteristics	*PB*	*MB*
Skin lesions	One to five lesions (including single nerve lesion if present)	Six and above
Peripheral nerve involvement	No nerve/only one nerve with or without one to five lesions	More than one nerve irrespective of the number of skin lesions
Skin smears	Negative at all sites	Positive at any site

Abbreviations: PB, paucibacillary; MB, multibacillary.

Note: If skin smear is positive, irrespective of number of skin and nerve lesions, the disease is classified as MB leprosy; but if skin smear is negative it is classified on the basis of the number of skin and nerve lesions.

of number of lesions. This categorization of PB and MB has not been yet standardized as in one study MB case corresponded to more than one body area involvement[46] while in other, it was occurrence on more than two body areas.[47]

2. *Size of the biggest lesion*: Basis of this categorization is that while the skin lesion count may be erroneous because of the small/faint/ill-defined lesions, a large lesion is unlikely to be missed. A size of 5 cm or more corresponded to MB in one study.[46]

3. *Serology based*: The presence of antibodies against *M. leprae* specific antigens [phenolic glycolipid 1 (PGL-1)] have been found to correlate with the bacterial load of leprosy patients. Hence, the detection of these antibodies can be used for categorization of patients into MB cases. The methodology used may be ELISA-based tests or more recently developed ML flow test which is an immunochromatic flow test and measures the IgM antibodies against PGL-1 antigen of *M. leprae*.[48,49] The ML flow test is said to be fast and easy to perform. It was found to be positive in almost all smear-positive cases and had also been found to be positive even in some of the cases classified PB under WHO classification.[49]

Another immunological marker to differentiate PB from MB leprosy especially at its incipient stage, includes cytokine profile. The preliminary studies have shown that secretion of antigen-specific interferon-gamma (IFN-γ) indicates a disease that is progressing toward tuberculoid pole (PB) while IL-4 or IL-5 favored progression toward lepromatous pole (MB).[50]

CLASSIFICATION: PRESENT GLOBAL PERSPECTIVE

Presently almost all over the world, the treatment guidelines based on skin/nerve lesion count as proposed by WHO (with or without some modifications) are being used. A plan for uniform MDT (U-MDT) is already under trial by WHO[51] and if it succeeds, soon the present WHO classification will lose its relevance. On the other hand, Ridley-Jopling classification is being used successfully for academic and research purposes.

CORRELATION AMONG VARIOUS CLASSIFICATIONS

There is not much difference in the Madrid and Indian classifications. Tuberculoid, lepromatous, borderline and indeterminate remain the same entities in both these classifications. The maculoanesthetic of Indian classification corresponds to the macular variety of tuberculoid under Madrid classification while the neuritic leprosy of Indian classification represents a heterogeneous group that has been split and placed separately as varieties under tuberculoid, lepromatous and indeterminate in the Madrid classification.

The borderline group is very broad in both these classifications and includes all three subtypes of borderline in Ridley-Jopling classification. Under Ridley-Jopling classification, the maculoanesthetic type of Indian classification has been included in the tuberculoid or borderline tuberculoid while the indeterminate has been left unclassified. Similarly, the pure neuritic of Madrid and Indian classifications has not been separated as a distinct entity in Ridley-Jopling system, but is to be classified under the TT-LL groups on the basis of lepromin and histopathology. In WHO classification also, the pure neuritic leprosy does not find any place as such but can be classified as MB or PB on the basis of number of nerve involvement, lepromin testing and nerve biopsy findings. Any type of leprosy under Ridley-Jopling classification or Madrid classification or Indian classification with less than six skin/one nerve lesions (without positivity in slit-skin smear examination, if done) qualifies for PB categorization under WHO classification of 1998 (based on number of lesions). However, as a rough correlation TT and BT of Ridley-Jopling classification and I and T of Madrid classification confirmed to PB leprosy while BB, BL and LL of Ridley-Jopling and B and L of Madrid classification is classifiable as MB (Box 16.5). The indeterminate of Indian classification is almost same as macular indeterminate of Madrid classification and hence is classified as PB along with its T and MA types. However, it must be remembered that indeterminate type at times evolves into MB leprosy.

In conclusion, it can be said that a consensus classification that can be applied at all levels of leprosy work has not yet been worked out. Presently, the WHO classification, based on skin/nerve lesion count, is simple to understand and practical to follow and is extensively in practice for treatment purposes globally. Ridley-Jopling classification remains the sheet anchor for academic and research purposes.

REFERENCES

1. Kunjlal K. English translation of Sushruta Samhita in 3 volumes, 1907, 1911 and 1916. In: Dharmendra. Classification of Leprosy. Calcutta.
2. Danielssen DC, Boeck CW. Traite de la Specalsked ou elephantiasis de grecs. Bailliere. Paris; 1848.
3. Leonard Wood Memorial Conference on Leprosy. Round Table Conference in Manila. Philippine J Science. 1931;44:449.
4. International Congress of Leprosy, Madrid. Report of the committee on classification. Int J Lepr. 1953;21:504-16.
5. International Congress of Leprosy, Tokyo. Report of the Committee on Classification. Int J Lepr. 1958;26:379.
6. All India Leprosy Workers Conference 1955. Classification of leprosy adopted by the Indian Association of Leprologists. Lepr India. 1955;27:93-5.
7. Ridley DS, Jopling WH. A classification of leprosy for research purposes. Lepr Rev. 1962;33:119-28.
8. Ridley DS, Jopling WH. Classification of leprosy according to immunity. A five-group system. Int J Lepr. 1966;34(3):255-73.

9. WHO Study Group. Chemotherapy of leprosy for control programmes. Geneva: World Health Organization; 1982. Report No.: 675.
10. WHO Expert Committee on Leprosy, 7th report, Geneva: World Health Organization; 1998. Report No.: 874.
11. Bhushan P, Sardana K, Koranne RV, et al. Diagnosing multibacillary leprosy: A comparative evaluation of diagnostic accuracy of slit-akin smear, bacterial index of granuloma and WHO operational classification. Indian J Dermatol Venereol Leprol. 2008;74:322-6.
12. Dharmendra, Chatterjee SN. Examination for *Mycobacterium leprae*. In: Dharmendra (Ed). Leprosy, Vol 1. Bombay: Kothari Medical Publishing House; 1978.pp. 258-62.
13. Dharmendra. The International Classification. In: Dharmendra (Ed). Leprosy, Vol 1. Bombay: Kothari Medical Publishing House; 1978: pp. 326-9.
14. Clinical, Histopathological, and immunological features of the five type classification approved by the Indian Association of Leprologists. Lepr India. 1982;54:22-32.
15. Ridley DS. Classification. In: Chatterjee BR (Ed). Leprosy-Aetiobiology of Manifestations, Treatment and Control. Calcutta: Leprosy Field Research Unit, Jhalda, West Bengal. pp. 280-93.
16. Ridley DS. The R-J classification re-viewed: Classification of leprosy- origin and outcome. In: Chatterjee BR (Ed). Leprosy-Etiobiology of manifestations, treatment and control. Calcutta: Leprosy Field Research Unit, Jhalda, West Bengal. pp. 295-7.
17. Mukherjee A, Misra RS. Comparative histology of skin and nerve granulomas in leprosy patients. Lepr Rev. 1988;59:177-80.
18. Srinivasan H, Rao KS, Iyer CG. Discrepancy in the histological features of leprosy lesions in the skin and peripheral nerves. Lepr India. 1982;54:275-82.
19. Dogra S, Kumaran MS, Narang T, et al. Clinical characteristics and outcome in multibacillary (MB) leprosy patients treated with 12 months WHO MDT-MBR: a retrospective analysis of 730 patients from a leprosy clinic at a tertiary care hospital of Northern India. Lepr Rev. 2013;84:65-75.
20. Bhatia AS, Katoch K, Narayanan RB, et al. Clinical and histopathological correlation in the classification of leprosy. Int J Lepr. 1993;61:433-8.
21. Sehgal VN, Rege VL, Reys M. Correlation between clinical and histopathological classification in leprosy. Int J Lepr. 1977;45:278-80.
22. Narayan NP, Ramu G, Desikan KV, et al. Correlation of clinical, histological and immunological features across the leprosy spectrum. Indian J Lepr. 2001;73:329-42.
23. McDougall AC, Ponnighaus JM, Fine PE. Histopathological examination of skin biopsies from an epidemiological study of leprosy in northern Malawi. Int J Lepr. 1987;55:88-98.
24. Nadkarni NS, Rege VL. Significance of histopathological classification in leprosy. Indian J Lepr. 1999;71:325-32.
25. Ridley DS, Waters MFR. Significance of variations within the lepromatous group. Lepr Rev. 1969;40:143-52.
26. Ridley DS. Histological classification and the immunological spectrum of leprosy. Bull WHO. 1974;51:451-65.
27. Jopling WH, McDougall AC. The Disease: Handbook of Leprosy, 5th edition. New Delhi: CBS Publishers and Distributors; 2005: pp.10-53.
28. Ridley DS. The pathogenesis and classification of polar tuberculoid leprosy. Lepr Rev. 1982;53:19-26.

29. WHO Expert Committee on Leprosy. 6th report. Geneva: World Health Organization. 1988. Tech Rep Ser 768.
30. Georgiev GD, McDougall AC. Skin smears and Bacteriological Index (BI) in multiple drug therapy control program: an unsatisfactory and potential hazardous state of affairs. Int J Lepr. 1988;56:101-4.
31. Vetton L, Pritze S. Reliability of skin smear results: experience with quality control of skin smears in different routine services in leprosy control programs. Lepr Rev. 1989;60:187-97.
32. World Health Organization. (2012). WHO expert committee on leprosy, 8th report. WHO 2012; No.968. [online] Available from: http://www.searo.who.int/entity/global_leprosy_programme/publications/8th_expert_comm_2012.pdf. [Accessed May, 2014].
33. Dasananjali K, Schreuder PA, Pirayavaraporn C. A study on the effectiveness and the safety of the WHO/MDT regimen in the Northeast of Thailand. A prospective study. 1984-1996. Int J Lepr Other Mycobact Dis. 1997;65:28-36.
34. Fleury RN, Aranda CM. Detection of AFB in tuberculoid biopsies. Int J Lepr. 1995;63:103.
35. Pardillo FE, Fajardo TT, Abalos RM, et al. Methods for the classification of leprosy for treatment purposes. Clin Infect Dis. 2007;44:1096-9.
36. Chandna R, Patnaik A, John O, et al. Does nerve examination improve diagnostic efficacy of the WHO classification of leprosy? Indian J Dermatol Venereol Leprol. 2008;74:327-30.
37. Global strategy for further reducing the leprosy burden and sustaining leprosy control activities. (Plan period 2006-2010). World Health Organization, 2005.
38. Croft RP, Smith WC, Nicholls P, et al. Sensitivity and specificity of methods of classification of leprosy without use of skin-smear examination. Int J Lepr Other Mycobact Dis. 1998;66:445-50.
39. Norman G, Joseph G, Richard J. Validity of the WHO operational classification and value of other clinical signs in the classification of leprosy. Int J Lepr Other Mycobact Dis. 2004;72:278-83.
40. World Health Organisation, Leprosy Elimination Group. (2000). [online] Guide to eliminate leprosy as a public health problem; WHO/CDS/CPE/CEE/2000.14. Available from http://whqlibdoc.who.int/hq/2000/WHO_CDS_CPE_CEE_2000.14.pdf [Accessed May, 2014].
41. Training manual for medical officers: NLEP. Chapter 7. Classification and management of leprosy. Directorate of Health Services, Ministry of Health and Family Welfare, Nirman Bhavan, New Delhi. Available on internet: http://nlep.nic.in/training.html (last accessed on 18-02-2009). pp. 54-65.
42. Learning material on leprosy for capacity building of District Nucleus Staff and Medical officers working in Hospital/PHC/CHC and dispensaries. Govt. of India and International Federation of Anti-leprosy Associations (ILEP). Directorate General of Health Services. Min of Health and Family Welfare (leprosy division) 2005. (also available at http://ilepindia.org/)
43. Mahajan PM, Jogaikar DG, Mehta JM. A study of pure neuritic leprosy: clinical experience. Indian J Lepr. 1996;68:137-41.
44. Kumar B, Kaur I, Dogra S, et al. Pure neuritic leprosy in India: an appraisal. Int J Lepr Other Mycobact Dis. 2004;72:284-90.
45. Arora M, Katoch K, Natrajan M, et al. Changing profile of disease in leprosy patients diagnosed in a tertiary care centre during years 1995-2000. Indian J Lepr. 2008;80:257-65.

46. Gupta R, Kar HK, Bhardwaj M. Revalidation of various clinical criteria for the classification of leprosy- a clinic-pathological study. Lepr Rev. 2012;83:354-62.

47. Rao PN, Sujai S, Srinivas D, et al. Comparison of two systems of classification of leprosy based on number of skin lesions and number of body areas involved-a clinicopathological concordance study. Indian J Dermatol Venereol Leprol. 2005;71:14-9.

48. Buhrer-Sekula S, Smits HL, Gussenhoven GC, et al. Simple and fast lateral flow test for classification of leprosy patients and identification of contacts with high risk of developing leprosy. J Clin Microbiol. 2003;41:1991-5.

49. Contin LA, Alves CJ, Fogagnolo L, et al. Use of ML-Flow test as a tool in classifying and treating leprosy. Ann Bras Dermatol. 2011;86:91-5.

50. Sampaio LH, Sousa AL, Barcelos MC, et al. Evaluation of various cytokines elicited during antigen-specific recall as potential risk indicators for the differential development of leprosy. Euro J Clin Microbiol Infect Dis. 2012;31:1443-51.

51. Report of the 8th meeting of WHO Technical advisory group on leprosy control held at Aberdeen, Scotland, April 2006. Published by WHO regional office, New Delhi, 2006.

17

CHAPTER

Methods of Nerve Examination

BK Girdhar

INTRODUCTION

Leprosy is considered to be primarily a disease of the nerves and it is the Schwann cell which plays host to *Mycobacterium leprae.* In leprosy, the nerve damage is largely limited to the peripheral nerves and it is because of damage to the nerves that disabilities, deformities and stigma results. All the three functions of the nerves, viz. sensory, motor and autonomic, can get affected. Damage to the nerves (due to inflammatory response and/or bacilli) results in varying degrees of sensory and motor deficit in the region supplied by the affected nerve/s. Because of nerve damage, secondary manifestations such as blisters, ulcers, trophic changes and deformities, etc. are seen on the body.

Despite being a generalized infection, not all the nerves get affected in leprosy. Only the peripheral nerves bear the brunt of damage and this in turn appears to be limited to certain segments of the nerve that are close to the joints. It has been observed that the so-called 'sites of predilection' of nerve damage correspond to the sites where the nerves are most superficial, without the cover of the muscle mass and hence cooler. This is possibly due to the localization of *M. leprae* in these segments having relatively lower temperature. Another possible reason for nerve damage at these sites is that here, the nerves lie near or across the joints and hence prone to frequent microtrauma due to stretching. Further, at these sites, the nerves pass through tough fibro-osseous tunnels. Any inflammation here, presses upon the blood supply and increased pressure on both affected (damaged) and unaffected nerve fibers to result in nerve ischemia and damage. Consequent to invasion of nerve by *M. leprae*, local inflammation results in nerve thickening. Sudden increase in inflammation and inflammatory edema in the nerve may give rise to varying degrees of pain and/or nerve tenderness on palpation, and if the process is acute,

it may result in further and even permanent damage to the nerve.

Thus thickening of nerves, with or without pain and tenderness on palpation, is an important clinical feature of leprosy. Indeed, nerve thickening is one of the three cardinal signs for diagnosis of leprosy. Therefore in leprosy examination of commonly affected nerves, as also their functional assessment is extremely important for diagnosis, classification, type of leprosy and the line of treatment. This is more so in pure neuritic leprosy, where the diagnosis is totally based on finding of thickened nerves and nerve function deficit. Equally important is the examination of nerves for classification of leprosy patients into paucibacillary (PB) or multibacillary (MB) groups, as also in assessing the risk of reactions, deformities and planning preventive measures.

NERVE EXAMINATION

Before one starts nerve examination, it is essential to have some knowledge of the surface anatomy of peripheral nerves, where these are superficial. Figure 17.1 gives a rough location of commonly examined nerve segments in leprosy. All cadres of medical and paramedical workers, involved in leprosy work are expected to know where and how to palpate greater auricular, ulnar, radial, median, common peroneal (lateral popliteal), superficial peroneal and posterior tibial nerves. In addition to above, the medical officers working in leprosy are required to know the status of other important nerves. These include supratrochlear and supraorbital nerves in the forehead, facial nerve and its zygomatic branch on the side of face, supraclavicular nerves over the clavicle, radial cutaneous and dorsal cutaneous branch of ulnar at the wrist, three antebrachial cutaneous nerves in the upper limb, the three cutaneous nerves in the thigh, infrapatellar nerve at the knee and the sural nerve in the lower leg posteriorly.

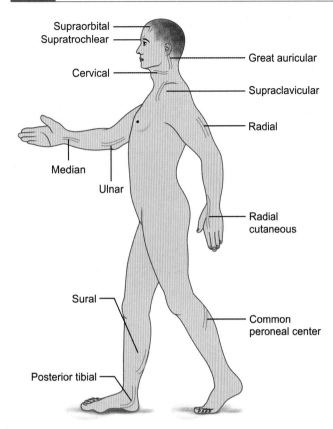

Fig. 17.1: Surface marking of nerves commonly affected in leprosy

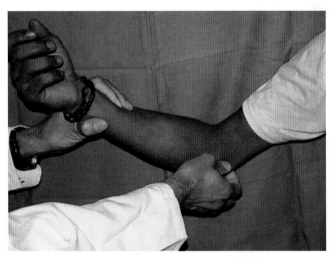

Fig. 17.2: Examination of ulnar nerve

Apart from the above named nerves, areas around and in particular, proximal to the patch or loss of sensation, must be examined for any thickened named or unnamed cutaneous nerves.

For ease of nerve examination, the patient should preferably be seated on a stool. Nerve palpation should be done with pulp of fingers and not by the tip of the digits. The two sides should be compared to detect any difference and abnormality. Initially a gentle palpation is done, if no tenderness is observed, mild pressure could be applied on the nerves. While palpating the nerves, following points are noted:

- *Tenderness*: If present, its severity
- *Thickness*: Whether normal or thickened, if thickened, the degree of thickness
- *Consistency*: Soft, normal, firm or hard
- *Regularity*: Smooth or regular. If swelling is present its extent, nature—uniform, sausage shaped or beaded, whether the swelling is solid or fluctuant.

PALPATION OF NERVE TRUNKS

Ulnar Nerve

A majority of leprosy patients have thickening of ulnar nerve. This is particularly the case if there is lesion/s in the distribution of the nerve. To palpate ulnar nerve, the elbow is flexed at 70–80°. For palpating the right ulnar nerve, holding the patient's hand/wrist in the left hand, right hand is placed above the elbow and with the fingers coming from below, medial epicondyle of the humerus is located with little and ring finger. Palpation of ulnar nerve can be made, in line above the epicondyle with the remaining fingers (Fig. 17.2). For left ulnar nerve, patient's hand is held in the right hand and palpation made as above with the left hand. In our experience, palpating the ulnar nerve is easier from the medial side. However, some workers find it more convenient to palpate the nerve with their fingers coming from the lateral side of elbow.

Median Nerve

In leprosy, the median nerve may also get inflamed and thickened. This occurs little above or at the wrist. To examine the nerve, palmaris longus tendon is located by asking the patient to flex the wrist against resistance. Median nerve lies slightly medial and deeper to above tendon (Fig. 17.3). As this muscle is absent in almost 30% of the individuals, nerve can be located in line with the ring finger just above the creases of the wrist. Tingling or tenderness can be used in confirming palpation of the nerve.

Radial Nerve

With elbow partially flexed and the arm held in position with shoulder internally rotated, radial groove at the insertion of deltoid muscle is identified. For right radial nerve, fixing the flexor muscle mass with left thumb, the pulp of the fingers is pressed deep in the radial groove to palpate the radial nerve (Fig. 17.4). The left radial nerve is palpated with the right hand in the similar manner. Tingling down the course or local tenderness can be taken as guide.

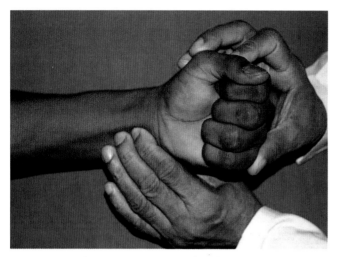

Fig. 17.3: Examination of median nerve

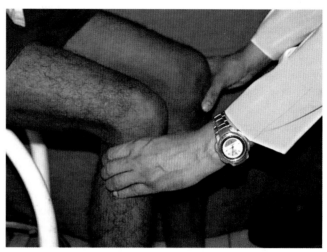

Fig. 17.5: Examination of common peroneal nerve

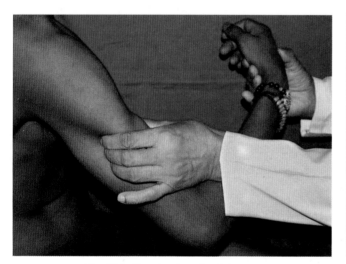

Fig. 17.4: Examination of radial nerve

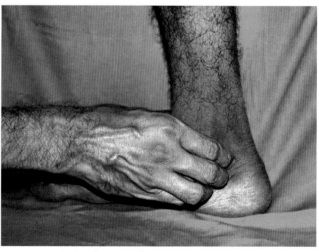

Fig. 17.6: Examination of posterior tibial nerve

Common Peroneal (Lateral Popliteal) Nerve

With patient sitting on the stool and knees bent or standing with knees slightly bent, both the nerves can be simultaneously palpated by the examiner sitting in front of him. The thumbs are placed on the tibial tuberosities and the fingers on the lateral aspects of the knees. Fibular head is located and the nerves are palpated just below it both posteriorly and winding round the insertion of biceps femoris muscle on the neck of the bone (Fig. 17.5).

Posterior Tibial Nerve

With the ankle in the neutral position, the nerve can be palpated at the mid-point between medial malleolus and the tuberosity of calcaneus, i.e. point of heel (Fig. 17.6).

Facial Nerve and its Zygomatic Branch

The facial nerve can be palpated just below and front of the ear lobule. On pressing the site, tenderness of the nerve is felt by the patient, if the nerve is affected and enlarged. The zygomatic branch can be palpated over the middle of the zygomatic bone of the cheek. An easy way is to put both the thumbs on the side of the nose and the index fingers in front of the ear lobule and bring the fingers anteriorly across the zygoma. Thread like structures in the middle of arch and a twitching of corresponding eyelid confirms the nerve.

PALPATION OF CUTANEOUS NERVES

Superficial cutaneous nerve/s often get thickened especially if there is a lesion in the distribution/region of their sensory supply. Thickening of one or more cutaneous nerves may be the only confirmatory sign of leprosy. In general, when thickened, the nerves are visible and/or palpable especially when the skin over them is stretched or tightened. Occasionally, the normal or not thickened nerve/s may also be visible in muscular individuals, e.g. in sportsmen and laborers.

Great Auricular Nerve

To assess the status of this nerve, the head is turned to the opposite side, as much as comfortably possible, to stretch the sternomastoid muscle (Fig. 17.7). The nerve is seen to cross the upper-third of the muscle. In thin individuals and those with very little fat, the nerve is visible as such. The nerve may also be visible in healthy muscular individuals.

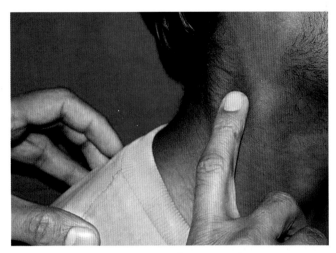

Fig. 17.7: Examination of great auricular nerve

Supratrochlear, Supraorbital and Infraorbital Nerves

These branches of trigeminal nerve provide sensory supply to the forehead and the frontal region of the scalp, and area below the eyes (Fig. 17.8). The nerves can be palpated running vertically up from the junction of medial one third and lateral two-third of the eyebrows (supratrochlear, at the supratrochlear notch) and at the junction of medial two-third and lateral one-third (supraorbital). The infraorbital nerve can be palpated below the eyes, lateral to the nose (Fig. 17.9). Most often, their thickening is associated with lesion/s in the forehead region or on the cheeks. When significantly thickened, these nerves are mostly visible.

Supraclavicular Nerves

The three supraclavicular nerves or branches, when thickened can be seen and/or palpated going down the medial, middle and the lateral third of the clavicle on to the pectoral area of the chest.

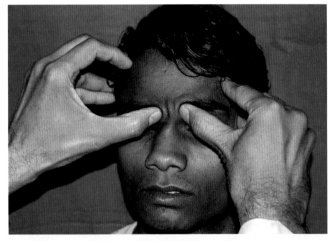

Fig. 17.8: Examination of supratrochlear nerve medially over eyebrows. Similarly supraorbital nerve can be palpated laterally

Cutaneous Nerves of the Forearm

The three cutaneous nerves of the forearm: (1) the medial, (2) posterior, and (3) the lateral cutaneous nerves, when thickened are visible and/or palpable in borderline (BT) patients especially when there are lesions in the forearm or hands. The medial cutaneous nerve is seen or palpated running down from the medial side of insertion of biceps toward the middle of the forearm, often branching and leading into the lesion, if present. The posterior cutaneous starting almost from the same point, immediately winds round posteriorly. The lateral cutaneous nerve on the other hand is seen or felt right down the lateral border from mid-arm to the mid-forearm.

Radial Cutaneous Nerve

This terminal sensory branch of the radial nerve that carries sensations from lateral half of dorsa of hand lies at the mount

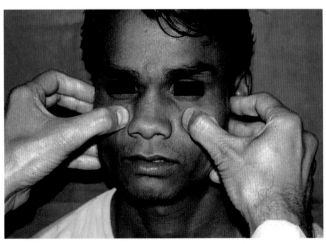

Fig. 17.9: Examination of infraorbital nerve

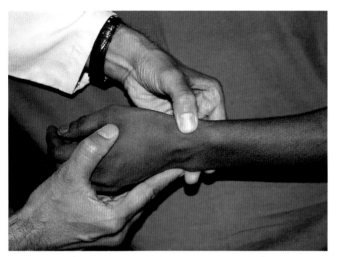

Fig. 17.10: Examination of radial cutaneous nerve

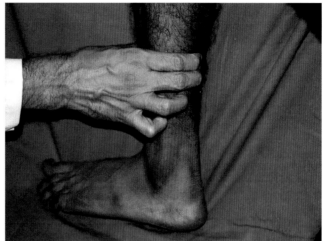

Fig. 17.12: Examination of sural nerve

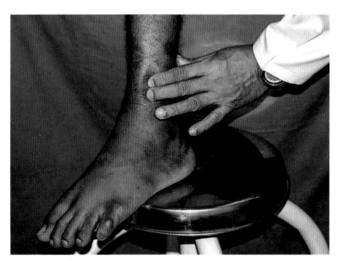

Fig. 17.11: Examination of musculocutaneous nerve (superficial peroneal) nerve. Note the prominent TT leprosy patch in front of ankle and the foot drop

of the wrist. The nerve can be palpated easily just above the anatomical snuff box when the hand is held in slight flexion and the forearm in semiprone position (Fig. 17.10).

Cutaneous Branch of the Ulnar Nerve

This cutaneous nerve lies at the base of the fifth metacarpal, just below the styloid process of the ulna as it comes from medial to the lateral side and supplies medial half of the dorsum of hand.

Cutaneous Nerves (Medial, Anterior and Lateral) of the Thigh

When thickened, the nerves can be palpated in front of the thigh starting 5–7 cm below the inguinal ligament and running vertically down on the inner side of the thigh, middle of the thigh and anterolateral aspect of the thigh, respectively. These nerves are often thickened in borderline (especially BT) patients with lesions on the thigh.

Superficial Peroneal Nerve (Musculocutaneous Nerve)

This nerve carries sensations from greater part of the dorsum of the foot (with the exception of the adjoining area between the first and second toe, which is supplied by medial branch of the deep peroneal nerve from below). When thickened, the nerve can be seen and palpated in front of ankle coming toward the second and third toe. Gently medially rotating and plantar flexing the foot makes the nerve stand out when thickened, especially in nonobese patients with lesion/s on the dorsum of the foot (Fig. 17.11).

Sural Nerve

This cutaneous nerve provides sensory supply to the lateral side of the foot and the heel. The nerve may get thickened if there is lesion in this area. With patient sitting straight or standing, the nerve can be palpated between the two bellies of the gastrocnemius muscle above, running along the lower quarter of Achilles tendon on the back of the leg (Fig. 17.12).

ACKNOWLEDGMENTS

The above methods of nerve examination were the consensus arrived at a workshop held at National JALMA Institute of Leprosy and other Mycobacterial Diseases. The author gratefully acknowledges contribution of each and every member who participated in the deliberations. The author thankfully acknowledges the gesture of department of Dermatology, Venereology and Leprology, Dr Ram Manohar Lohia Hospital, New Delhi, for adding the clinical photographs in this chapter.

18
CHAPTER

Histoid Leprosy

Virendra N Sehgal

INTRODUCTION

Histoid leprosy (HL) is a well-recognized clinical entity, and is anexpression of multibacillary (MB) leprosy. It is characterized by typical cutaneous and/or subcutaneous nodules and plaques over an apparently normal skin with unique histopathology and characteristic bacterial morphology.[1-4] Spontaneous appearance of multiple asymptomatic papules and/or nodules over an apparently normal skin of the trunk may herald the onset of the disease.[5] It usually manifests itself in patients on diaminodiphenylsulfone (DDS) for a long time, reflecting initial improvement followed by a relapse. Irregular and inadequate therapy may further compound its occurrence. Some workers believe that it is due to the development of drug resistance to DDS,[6,7] while others postulate that mutant organisms, that emerge from a predominantly sulfone susceptible bacterial population, may be responsible.[8,9] However, it is now well-known that the disease may occur *de novo* in patients who have never been exposed to any antileprosy therapy.

Apart from its occurrence in lepromatous leprosy (LL), histoid lesions may occasionally be seen in borderline[10,11] and indeterminate leprosy.[12]

Ever since the description of HL by Wade,[4] an emphasis was laid on its retrospective histological diagnosis.[13] However, it is diagnosed with certainty, relying only on its clinical features[2,14] a fact reiterated by Professor Moschella,[15] while reviewing a report on this entity in the Year Book of Dermatology, 1988.[16]

HISTORICAL LANDMARKS

The term histoid was originally coined in the year 1960 by Wade.[12] Since then many reports have documented the entity.[2-4,6-14] Although some authors,[2,15,17] regard it as a distinct clinicopathological entity; others[4,6-8,11] consider it as a variant of LL. Initially, the entity was recorded in MB leprosy, on irregular, and inadequate dapsone monotherapy, later *de novo*[2,14] cases were also encountered.

Despite sporadic reporting, HL was not given a serious thought, until Sehgal et al.[18] documented for the first time the immunological profile of this unique expression of MB leprosy.

DEFINITION

Histoid leprosy is an expression of MB leprosy, characterized by the occurrence of nodules and/or plaques on the skin and/ or the subcutaneous tissues. Well-demarcated, cutaneous nodule is its cardinal feature. The lesions are present over an apparently normal skin.[10] Reactional episodes are seldom recorded.[2,4]

EPIDEMIOLOGY

Sehgal and Srivastava[2,14] diagnosed 50 patients of HL among a total of 1,551 fresh leprosy patients, thus giving its incidence as 3.2%. Rodriquez[8] found that of the 72 relapsed LL patients, 28 (39%) ultimately developed histoid lesions. The data thus far available, therefore, indicates that its incidence is significant in MB leprosy *per se* or in relapsed patients taking irregular antileprosy drugs.[2,14] Kalla et al. from northwest Rajasthan, recorded 25 biopsy proven HL patients among a total of 893 new leprosy patients, thus giving an incidence of 2.8%.[19]

Histoid leprosy has rarely been reported in children.[11] However, histoid lesions have been recorded to occur at an age as early as 10 years and as late as 84 years.[6] Sehgal and Srivastava[14] reported that 58% of their patients were between the age of 20 years and 39 years.

CLINICAL FEATURES

Histoid lesions have variously been classified as:[2-4,14,20]
- Subcutaneous nodules
- Deeply fixed cutaneous nodules
- Superficially placed cutaneous nodules
- Soft nodules, and (Figs 18.1A to E)
- Plaques or pads.

In a single patient,[2,4,11] three to more than 50 such lesions may be seen. The lesions are usually located on the back, buttocks, face, extremities and over bony prominences, especially, around the elbows, and the knees.[2,11,14,21]

The cutaneous histoid lepromas that arise directly in the dermis may promptly become elevated and protuberant, and even pedunculated. Typical young lesions are firm, reddish, or skin colored, dome-shaped or oval papules, regular in contour with shiny and stretched overlying skin. At times, there is constriction around their bases. The skin surrounding the lesion is apparently normal.

Subcutaneous Nodules

Subcutaneous nodules[2,4] may vary in size but usually are not larger than 5 cm in diameter (Figs 18.2 to 18.4). The smaller

nodules are soft and on scraping the cut surface is abundantly pulpy. The older larger nodules are relatively, but secondarily fibrotic, and so the cut surface is likely to be pale and tough.

Cutaneous Plaques/Pads

Cutaneous plaque[2] is the another form of histoid lesion(s). They are non-nodular and of a different growth pattern, but of a similar nature cytologically as well as bacteriologically.[4,8] These are sharply delineated, thick scaly pads, which in some cases may develop on pressure points, especially on the elbows.[2,4,22] It is generally believed that HL patients do not undergo erythema nodosum leprosum (ENL) type of reaction.[22] However, some patients do develop ENL only after the institution of therapy.[6,8,10,23,24]

Histoid facies[14] is its classical presentation and it is identified either as:
- *First type*: Old, wrinkled, atrophic facial skin, relics of a burnt out LL, with scanty eyebrows, and sometimes with depressed nasal bridge and eye changes. They have scanty histoid lesions on their face.
- *Second type*: It is an apparently normal facial skin without any manifestation of leprosy. Histoid lesions, however, are regularly present over the face (Figs 18.5A and B).

A noticeable feature in majority of histoid patients is the persistence of eyebrows.[6] Nasal mucosa is usually spared. Even after years of uncontrolled disease, the nasal cartilage remains unaffected.[6,8] Histoid patients usually are in good general health and they tend to remain so.[6]

BACTERIOLOGY

Slit-skin smears,[2,3,14,25] prepared from these lesions, always reveal an abundance of organisms occurring singly, sometimes in clusters or as globi. Majority of the organisms

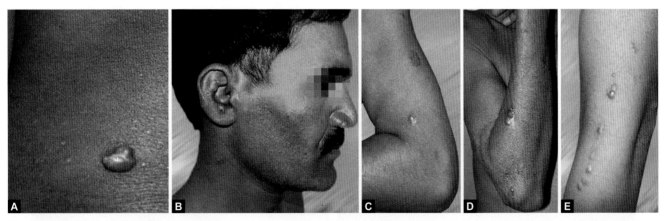

Figs 18.1A to E: Histoid leprosy. The characteristic lesions are papulonodular, firm, erythematous or copper-colored, hemispherical, dome shaped, glistening shiny, present over apparently normal looking skin. (A) The common sites are face, ears; (B) limbs and trunk; (C to E) Note the development of new lesions as a result of scratching; (Koebner's phenomenon) in picture marked E.
Courtesy: Dr Inderjeet Kaur and Dr Sunil Dogra, PGIMER, Chandigarh, India.

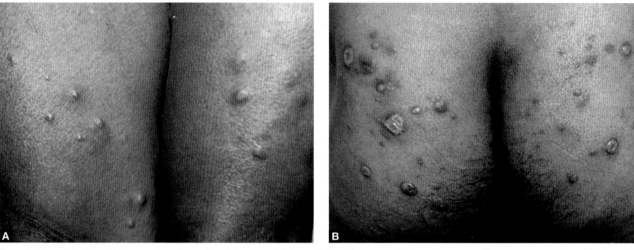

Figs 18.2A and B: Histoid leprosy. Papules and nodules over thighs and gluteal regions. The lesions are usually present over normal looking skin.
Courtesy: Dr Inderjeet Kaur and Dr Sunil Dogra, PGIMER, Chandigarh, India.

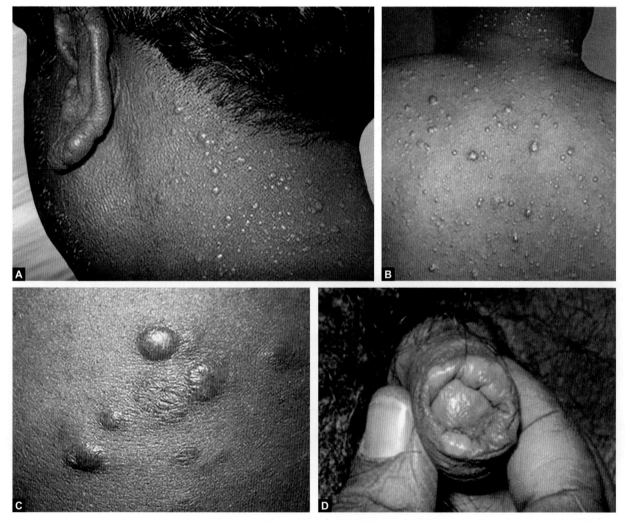

Figs 18.3A to D: Histoid leprosy, shiny hemispherical nodules over ear, nape of the neck, trunk regions, histoid nodules on the prepuce
Courtesy: Dr Aparna Palit and Dr AC Inamadar, BLDEA'S SBMP Medical College, Hospital and Research Center, Bijapur, Karnataka, India.

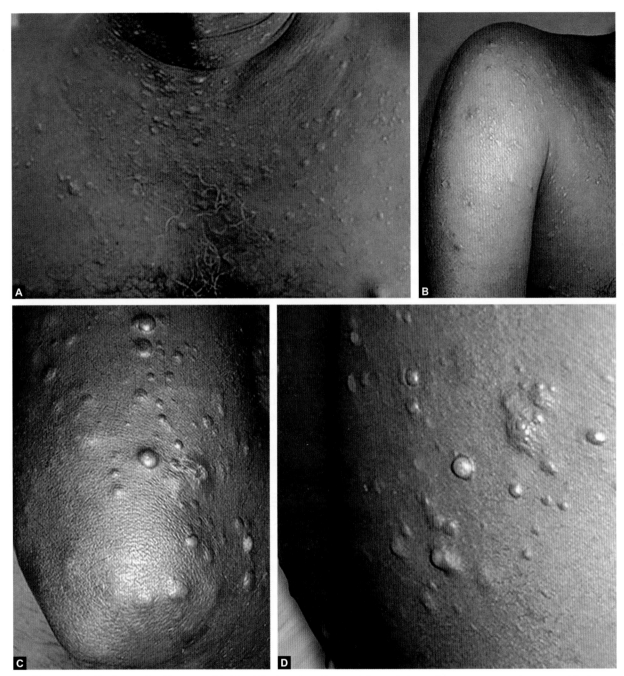

Figs 18.4A to D: Generalized innumerable histoid lesions (papules, nodules and plaques) present over trunk areas and limbs
Courtesy: Dr Aparna Palit and Dr AC Inamadar, BLDEA'S SBMP Medical College, Hospital and Research Center, Bijapur, Karnataka, India.

are solid staining bacilli. They are well-preserved and appear as uniformly stained, long rods with tapering ends, distinctly longer than the (ordinary) leprosy bacilli.[2,14]

HISTOPATHOLOGY

Histoid leprosy has several striking histopathological connotations, which are relevant in contemporary context.[13]

Its most prominent feature being the well-circumscribed nature of the lesion, the predominance of spindle-shaped cells and/or polygonal cells. Unusually, large numbers of acid-fast bacilli are seen in young active lesions. They are also found in both subcutaneous and cutaneous nodules. Histoid lepromas, unlike ordinary lepromatous lesions, grow in an expansible rather than an infiltrative fashion.[2,4,5] The epidermis overlying the lesion is usually stretched, and atrophic due to

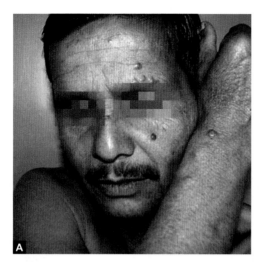 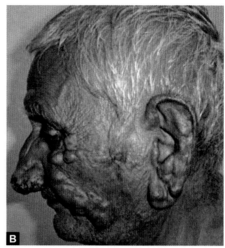

Figs 18.5A and B: (A) Hemispherical nodules on the face; (B) Grossly enlarged nodules and plaques over face and ears
Courtesy: Dr Inderjeet Kaur and Dr Sunil Dogra, PGIMER, Chandigarh, India.

expanding lesion in the dermis. Sanchez[26] however, reported mild acanthosis and flattening of rete ridges in the epidermis in some of his patients. In most cases, a free subepidermal grenz zone (band of Unna) is present.[3,4,9,14]

The lesion is usually located in the dermis, subcutis or both. A pseudocapsule is often seen surrounding the lesion, formed by the compression of the adjacent tissue due to the expanding nature of the lesion, but it may not be well-appreciated in specimens from plaques. The circumscribed nature of lesion is one of the most cardinal features of the histoid lepromas[3,27] by virtue of which, it resembles a tissue forming process rather than a granuloma.[4]

The most striking and classical feature is the presence of numerous, thin, spindle-shaped histiocytes forming interlacing bands, whorls and at times tight curlicules.[2-4,14] The constituent spindle-shaped cells have a moderate amount of cytoplasm, with oval and lightly stained nuclei.[3,9] A higher magnification of the cells may reveal slight vacuolation of their cytoplasm, but this never assumes marked cytoplasmic vacuolation of typical lepra cells in their full stage of development.[7] An admixture of spindle-shaped histiocytes and polygonal cells in various proportions may be found within the histoid lepromas. Their presence signifies the aging of the lesions.[7,8]

Histoid lesions can also have lymphocytes and occasionally, polymorphonuclear leukocytes, especially at the periphery of the nodule.[9] Plasma cells can also be observed in some sections.[6] Deposition of collagen is not present in early stages, but as the lesion grows older, the amount of collagen increases, and the lesion may even turn fibrotic.

The bacilli in the histoid lesions constitute one of the most distinctive, and interesting feature. The acid-fast bacilli are described as measurably longer than the ordinary leprosy bacilli.[2,4,14] In the spindle-shaped histiocytes, they

are arranged in groups or parallel bundles aligned along the long axis of the cell, described as histoid habitus. Isolated bacilli are scattered throughout the lesion.[27] Often a relatively large number of bacilli within the histoid lesions are solid-staining.[2,4,14] Wade found the characteristic absence of globus formation in histoid lesions, which he attributed to the lack of production of gloea, the essential matrix substance secreted by metabolism of such bacilli. However, presence of few globi is not unusual on slit-skin smear as well as histopathological examination.

TUBERCULOID CONTAMINATION

Tuberculoid contamination, a peculiar phenomenon may be seen in subcutaneous histoid lepromas. This is the occurrence of definite foci of epithelioid cells, located within the lesion substance or in the encircling fibrous tissue encapsulation.[3,14,28,29] No satisfactory explanation of this occurrence is postulated,[28] but it is likely that the epithelioid cells represent the tuberculoid component of the earlier borderline phase of the disease. We possibly can make this supposition only if most patients with subcutaneous lepromas had evidence of downgrading.

ULTRASTRUCTURE

The appearance of cells of histoid lesions varies widely within the granuloma. In the center of the lesions, the cells are either polygonal or of classical type, i.e. thin, spindle-shaped histiocytes. At the periphery, on the other hand, the histiocytes are elongated or spindle-shaped, especially in the area adjoining the capsule.[17] The main cell type in the lesion is a macrophage[30] of which three variants are seen.[17,30] The first variant is a rounded cell with a very large, oval nucleus and sparse cytoplasm, containing a few mitochondria and a little rough endoplasmic reticulum. It thus resembles a monocyte. A few cells of this type, which usually contain bacilli as single, solid organisms form the second category. The third variant is a more mature cell of the same size with uniformly granular nucleus, and the cytoplasm containing bacilli, which are solid.

An abundance of bacilli is seen in histoid lesions.[16,30-32] Most of them are solid in appearance. Unlike the usual lepromatous lesions, the cross-sections of most of the organisms show uniformly electron-dense cytoplasm.[31] Usually, the bacilli are scattered singly, but globi can also be seen. Sometimes, several cross-divisions of bacilli can be noted.[16] An electron-transparent zone is always seen around single bacillus or globi.[16,30,31]

One of the most significant differences of histoid lesions from lepromatous lesions, is the absence of large amount of electron-transparent substance (ETS) or foam in the former, which could be due to the rapidity of the development of the lesion.[31] It is believed that ETS interferes with bacterial metabolism, and causes their death. Its absence might help preserve the bacilli within cells.

IMMUNOPROFILE

Sehgal et al.[8] were the first to study the immunological profile of HL patients, and comparison thereof with the nonhistoid active lepromatous as well as healthy controls. The observations could be summarized as follows:

A diminished cell-mediated immunity (CMI) response was observed in HL patients when compared with healthy controls. This was evident by the lowered percentage of early as well as total T-lymphocytes, and negative early (Fernandez) and late (Mitsuda) lepromin test. The CMI, however, was found to be relatively better, when compared with active lepromatous patients. This may well be explained by the attempted localization of the lesions, to limited regions of the body in HL.[2,18]

The humoral immunity was found to be considerably augmented, as revealed through their increased percentage, as well as absolute count of B-lymphocytes and the raised levels of immunoglobulins IgG, IgA and IgM.

The levels of the complement C3 were significantly lowered in the patients while the total concentration of circulating immune complexes (CIC) was grossly raised. Cryoglobulins were also detected in majority of the patients.

The pathogenesis of this rare and unusual variant of leprosy still remains unresolved. The interplay of genetic factors, immune response, and treatment received in a given patient seems to influence the manifestations of HL. Though HL is considered to be a variant of LL, there exists an enhanced immune response against *M. leprae* in these patients compared to LL with respect to both CMI and humoral immunity.[18] An indication in favor of an augmented local CMI is the presence of necrosis and ulceration as observed in some histoid lesions

that might be considered as a localized effort to combat *M. leprae*.[24] Immunohistochemical correlations of increased CMI include increased CD36 expression by the keratinocytes, predominance of CD4 lymphocyte over CD8 lymphocytes, and high numbers of activated lymphocytes and macrophages in the lesions.[23] Despite the presence of adequate numbers of macrophages, it has been claimed that they lack the functional property to kill bacilli that exist in high numbers in histoid lesions.[23] It is possible that under the influence of *M. leprae* antigens, they lose their bacteriolytic property or produce "suppressor" cytokines, such as IL-10, that adversely inhibit T-cell mediated responses to *M. leprae*.[24,33]

DIAGNOSIS

The diagnosis of this entity is fairly easy if the classical clinical features are carefully looked for. It is imperative to 'suspect' this entity in MB leprosy, *per se* or on treatment.

History

The natural history should include the details of treatment, namely; the nature of drug(s), duration of treatment, the regularity, dose and its frequency.

Clinical Features

The clinical peculiarities of histoid lepromas are characteristic enough to delineate this entity with certainty in most patients. The facial appearance often gives a clue toward the development of histoid lesions, and thus may aptly be designated as 'histoid facies'.

Microscopic Examination

Slit-skin smears reveal an abundance of uniformly stained acid-fast bacilli. In contrast, there is relative paucity of them in the surrounding normal-looking skin, a feature helpful in distinguishing histoid from lepromatous nodules. Moreover, the morphology of 'histoid' bacilli is striking, for they are long, strongly and uniformly stained throughout their length, and rarely form globi.[14]

DIFFERENTIAL DIAGNOSIS

Clinically, cutaneous histoid lesions may simulate either conventional lepromatous nodules, ENL, von Recklinghausen's disease[10,11,34,35] and/or molluscum contagiosum.[8,10] However, there are certain distinguishing features with regard to cutaneous histoids. Unlike the resilient von Recklinghausen nodules, they are firm on palpation, and also histoid lesions generally lack umbilication so typical of molluscum contagiosum. Some histoid lesions do show central depression (Fig. 18.2B).

Cutaneous plaques can sometimes be confused with keloids. However, they are less firm, skin-slit smears show the presence of numerous acid-fast bacilli. Other disorders that can mimic HL include multiple subcutaneous lipomatosus,[35] post-kala-azar dermal leishmaniasis[36,37] and cutaneous sarcoidosis (Table 18.1).[38-40]

Histologically, histoid lesions may mimic nodular subepidermal fibrosis,[41] dermatofibroma and similar skin tumors, on routine hematoxylin-eosin stains. Staining for acid-fast bacilli may however, easily differentiate histoid from such tumors.

TREATMENT

The effect of drug therapy is variable in HL patients. Wade remarked on the resistance of these patients to

Table 18.1: Differential diagnosis

Disease	Clinical	Histopathology	Others
Histoid leprosy[1]	Superficial cutaneous or deep subcutaneous nodules are most common findings. Also seen are plaques or pads. Typical lesions are firm, reddish/skin colored, regular in contour with shiny and stretched overlying skin. Constriction around the base of the lesion (if present) is typical	Circumscribed lesion with spindle-shaped cells and unusually large number of bacilli. Grenz zone is mostly present. Interlacing bands, whorls and tight curlicules formed by numerous, thin, spindle-shaped histiocytes	1. Negative lepromin test 2. Raised immunoglobulins 3. Lowered complement component (C3)
Lepromatous leprosy[20]	Disseminated nodules and/or plaques, typical sensory loss (glove and stocking anesthesia) and trophic changes, ulcerations	Epidermal atrophy, clear subepidermal zone (Grenz zone) and foamy histiocytes, laden with lepra bacilli, granulomas are characteristic	1. Strongly positive Ziehl Neelsen and Fite-Faraco stain 2. Negative lepromin test
Post-kala-azar dermal leishmaniasis[36,37]	May appear as hypopigmented macules or micropapular or macropapular eruptions, nodules, plaques during or shortly after treatment (African—early) even after up to 10 years (Indian—late). Face is commonly affected	Granuloma comprises mainly of lymphocytes, macrophages and plasma cells in the dermis. LD bodies are rare in macules but are commonly seen in nodules	LD bodies are difficult to demonstrate. Positive immunofluorescence antibody test, enzyme-linked immunosorbent assay test, and fast agglutination screening test is a rapid test
Neurofibromatosis type 1, 3, 4	Multiple well-circumscribed, skin colored/ brown papulonodular lesions, Café au lait spots, intertriginous freckling (Crowe sign). On application of pressure the nodules may sink in a pit like depression, the Button-hole sign	Circumscribed lesions composed of Schwann cells, fibroblasts, mast cells in an admixture of collagen and extracellular matrix	1. Cerebellar hamartomas, unidentified bright objects on magnetic resonance imaging 2. Lisch nodules (iris hamartomas) on slit-lamp examination
Sarcoidosis[38-40]	Firm, mobile nodules without epidermal involvement. Plaques and papules may also be found. Subcutaneous nodules, lupus pernio, erythema multiforme are some of the other nonspecific manifestations. Systemic involvement in form of hilar lymphadenopathy, pulmonary fibrosis may be encountered	A noncaseating naked (without the peripheral rim of lymphocytes) granuloma is cardinal. A reactive process without granuloma is a nonspecific finding	1. Hypercalcemia 2. CD4/CD8 ratio > 3.5 3. Abnormal chest radiogram
Dermatofibroma[42]	Firm, minimally elevated, dome-shaped with central hyperpigmentation. Isolated small lesions. Pinching the lesion leads to an apparent downward movement, the dimple sign	Nodular dermal proliferations of predominantly spindle-shaped fibroblasts and myofibroblasts arranged as short intersecting fascicles	Positive immunohistochemical reactions for vimentin, muscle-specific actin

Abbreviation: LD, Leishman-Donovan.

Table 18.2: The recommended dosage schedule for histoid leprosy[1]		
Drug	**Dose**	**Duration**
Rifampicin	600 mg once a month, supervised	All the three drugs for at least 2 years; preferably till smear negativity
Clofazimine	300 mg, once a month, supervised and 50 mg daily, self-administered	
Diaminodiphenylsulfone (Dapsone, DDS)	100 mg daily, self-administered	

treatment.[32] Price and Fitzherbert[6] observed an adequate response to treatment in some of their patients by using sulforthomidine after they had unsuccessfully tried sulfone, thiambutosine, sulfamethoxypyridazine and ditophal, singly or in combination, for 1–5 years. A few investigators report the occurrence of ENL during treatment,[6,23,24] but this resolves with adequate treatment for reaction.

The recommended schedule of treatment of HL as practiced is outlined in Table 18.2. It is very similar to the earlier recommendations of WHO for the treatment of MB leprosy for 2 years, preferably till skin smear negativity.

With the advent of more effective treatment modalities for the treatment of MB leprosy, the same regimens can be applied to HL. Various workers have tried pefloxacin and ofloxacin[43,44] in the treatment of HL.

The role of immunotherapy in HL has not been evaluated.

SIGNIFICANCE OF HISTOID LEPROMAS

Only a few studies have so far been done to elucidate the significance of HL.[2,4,14] The presence of elongated, well-preserved, peculiarly arranged acid-fast bacilli, invariable absence of globi formation and sometimes the resistance to sulfone treatment, suggest that one is probably dealing with sulfone-resistant mutant organisms. Mouse footpad sensitivity tests have shown that the bacilli present in histoid lesions are often resistant to DDS. Many workers do not believe Dapsone resistance to be the principle cause for the development of histoid nodules or even an important factor in the epidemiology of this variant of leprosy.

The immunohistochemical expression of these lesions indicates an augmented CMI. These lesions remain well-circumscribed tumorous collections of spindle-shaped histiocytes trapping the 'mutant' histoid bacilli.[2,14] The appearance of histoid lesions certainly indicates a highly active lepromatous process. The morphology of the lesion striking histologic features, which mimics a neoplasm, would suggest a possible cellular alteration. Presence of enormous number of bacilli in the lesion and a paucity in its neighboring areas would indicate an alteration of an immunologic mechanism or the presence of other factors resulting in uninhibited multiplication of bacilli in limited areas.[2,9]

Although structurally resembling a neoplasm, they are essentially an inflammatory condition as shown by the presence of large number of AFB and response to antileprosy treatment.[6,10,11]

In a recent appraisal of clinical, bacteriological, histopathological and immunological features, it was postulated by Sehgal and Srivastava[2,14] that HL is a relatively stable component of MB leprosy. It has its unique status in the leprosy spectrum with its fairly delineated characteristics:[15]

- The lesions are cutaneous and/or subcutaneous nodules and less frequently plaques
- They most frequently occur on the lower back and buttocks. They also involve the limbs and the face
- There are usually six to 50 lesions. Majority of patients have fewer than 30
- The patients seldom develop ENL[45]
- On histopathologic examination, one sees large number of spindle-shaped cells with enormous number of bacilli, especially in the spindle cells. Few globi are present
- There is augmented CMI in HL compared to that in active LL. The humoral immunity is also considerably enhanced.

Its importance in National Leprosy Eradication Program cannot be overemphasized. Hence, the details about the entity should be well known to all those working in institutions and the field.[46]

Changing Scenario

It is worthwhile to recall five-group classification of Ridley and Jopling,[47] i.e. tuberculoid (TT), borderline tuberculoid (BT), borderline borderline (BB), borderline lepromatous (BL), and LL, which subsequently was expanded to a seven-group classification[48] by the inclusion of indeterminate (I) and primary neuritic leprosy (PNL).[49] The indeterminate leprosy has been termed as a pivot from where the other well-established clinical groups of leprosy (other than the polar forms at the two extremes of the disease spectrum, TT(p) and LL(p), which are believed to arise *de novo*, and not as a result of upgrading or downgrading of disease). The conversion of indeterminate leprosy into histoid form *per se* has recently been demonstrated, thus establishing HL as one of the groups (8th) on a continuous leprosy spectrum.[50] It is, therefore, envisaged that HL may have MB or PB variants.[13,51]

REFERENCES

1. Sehgal VN, Srivastava G. Manual of Histoid Leprosy. New Delhi: Jaypee Brothers Medical Publishers (P) Ltd; 2013.
2. Sehgal VN, Srivastava G. Status of histoid leprosy–a clinical, bacteriological, histopathological, and immunological appraisal. J Dermatol (Tokyo). 1987;14:38-42.
3. Sehgal VN, Srivastava G, Beohar PC. Histoid leprosy—a histopathological reappraisal. Acta Leprol. 1987;5:125-31.
4. Wade HW. The histoid variety of lepromatous leprosy. Int J Lepr. 1963;31:129-42.
5. Sehgal VN, Singh N, Prasad PV, et al. Spontaneous appearance of multiple asymptomatic papules and/or nodules over an apparently normal skin of the trunk. Int J Dermatol. 2013;52:395-7.
6. Price EW, Fitzhebert H. Histoid variety of lepromatous leprosy. Int J Lepr. 1966;34:367-74.
7. Mansfield R. Histoid leprosy. Arch Pathol. 1969;87:580-5.
8. Rodriguez JN. The histoid leproma, its characteristics and significance. Int J Lepr. 1969;37:1-21.
9. Desikan KV, Iyer CG. Histoid variety of lepromatous leprosy: A histopathologic study. Int J Lepr. 1972;40:149-56.
10. Ramanujam K, Ramu G. Wade's histoid lepromatous leprosy. Report of a clinical study. Lepr India. 1969;41:293-7.
11. Bhutani LK, Bedi TR, Malhotra YK, et al. Histoid leprosy in north India. Int J Lepr. 1974;42:174-81.
12. Ramanujam K, Ramu G. Histoid transformation from unstable forms of leprosy. Abstract of Congress Papers 17/335. Int J Lepr. 1973;41:685.
13. Sehgal VN, Srivastava G, Singh N. Histoid leprosy: histopathological connotations' relevance in contemporary context. Am J Dermotopathol. 2009;31:268-71.
14. Sehgal VN, Srivastava G. Histoid leprosy a prospective diagnostic study in 38 patients. Dermatologica. 1988;177:212-7.
15. Moschella SL. Status of histoid leprosy—a clinical, bacteriological, histopathological, and immunological appraisal. Arthur J, Sober, Fitzpatric B (Eds). Year Book of Dermatology. Chicago: Year Book Medical Publisher; 1988: pp. 177-83.
16. Liu J, Kong QY, Ye GY, et al. Observations on ultra-structure of histoid leproma. Int J Lepr Other Mycobact Dis. 1982;50:471-6.
17. Sehgal VN, Srivastava G, Saha K. Immunological status of histoid leprosy. Lepr Rev. 1985;56:27-33.
18. Kalla G, Purohit S, Vyas MC. Histoid, a clinical variant of multibacillary leprosy: report from so-called non-endemic areas. Int J Lepr Other Mycobact Dis. 2000;68:267-71.
19. Kaur I, Dogra S, De D,. Histoid leprosy: a retrospective study of 40 cases from India. Br J Dermatol. 2009;160:305-10.
20. Sehgal VN. Textbook of Clinical Leprosy, 5th edition. New Delhi: Jaypee Brothers Medical Publishers (P) Ltd; 2005: pp. 43-6.
21. Chaudhary DS, Chaudhary M, Armah K. Histoid variety of lepromatous leprosy. Lepr Rev. 1971;42:203-7.
22. Sehgal VN, Srivastava G, Gautam RK, et al. Erythema nodosum leprosum (ENL) in histoid leprosy. Indian J Lepr. 1985;57:346-9.
23. Sehgal VN, Chaudhary A, Mahajan DM, et al. Type II (ENL) reaction in histoid leprosy in a child. Lepr Rev. 1991;62:431-7.
24. Sehgal VN, Joginder. Slit-skin smear in leprosy. Int J Dermatol. 1990;29:9-16.
25. Sanchez J. Lepromatous leprosy with lesions resembling nodular subepidermal fibrosis. Int J Lepr. 1965;33:179-85.
26. Sehgal VN, Srivastava G, Sharma VK. Simultaneous occurrence of upgrading and downgrading type 1 (lepra) reaction. Int J Dermatol. 1990;29:356-7.
27. Srivastava G. Epithelioid cells in histoid histology. Indian J Lepr. 1988;60:136.
28. Porichha D, Bhatia VN. Epithelioid and Polygonal cells in histoid leprosy. Indian J Lepr. 1987;59:191-3.
29. Ridley MJ, Ridley DS. Histoid leprosy. An ultrastructural observation. Int J Lepr Other Mycobact Dis. 1980;48:135-9.
30. Job CK, Chacko CJ, Taylor PM. Electromicroscopic study of histoid leprosy with special reference to its histogenesis. Lepr India. 1977;49:467-71.
31. Liu JH, Liw Z, Yang LH, et al. Further observations on ultra-structure of histoid leprosy. Abstract of XII International Leprosy Congress Papers. Int J Lepr. 1984;52:755-6.
32. Misra RC. Leprous histiocytoma. Lepr India. 1980;52:582-5.
33. Sehgal VN, Oberai R, Venkatesh P, et al. Plexiform neurofibroma affecting the upper parietal scalp, with cerebellar hamartoma: role of histopathology, colour Doppler imaging and magnetic resonance imaging. Clin Exp Dermatol. 2013;38:285-8.
34. Sehgal VN, Verma P, Chatterji K. Von Recklinghausen's disease (neurofibromatosis type-1): an overview. Cutis. 2013 (Forthcoming).
35. Kumaravel S. Multiple subcutaneous lipomatosis in a case of relapsed lepromatous leprosy masquerading as histoid leprosy. Indian J Lepr. 1995;67:187-90.
36. Chakrabarti A, Kumar B, Das A, et al. Atypical post kala-azar dermal leishmaniasis resembling histoid leprosy. Lepr Rev. 1997;68:247-51.
37. Napier EL, Das Gupta CR. A clinical study of post kala-azar demal leishmaniasis. Indian Medical Gazette. 1930;65:249-59.
38. Sehgal VN, Bhattacharya SN, Sardana K, et al. Cutaneous (papulo-nodular) sarcoidosis following hilar lymphadenopathy: an intriguing manifestation. Skinmed. 2003;2:131-3.
39. English JC 3rd, Patel PJ, Greer KE. Sarcoidosis. J Am Acad Dermatol. 2001;44:725-43.
40. Sehgal VN, Riyaz N, Chatterjee K, et al. Sarcoidosis as a systemic disease. Clin Dermatol. 2014;32(3):351-63.
41. Pfaltgraff RE, Bryceson A. Clinical Leprosy, 3rd edition. New York: Churchill Livingstone; 1990.
42. Chen TC, Kuo T, Chan HL: Dermatofibroma is a clonal proliferative disease. J Cutan Pathol. 2000;27:36-9.
43. Vora NS, Vora VN, Mukhopadhyay AK, et al. A case of histoid leprosy responding to ofloxacin along with standard MDT. Indian J Lepr. 1995;67:183-6.
44. Mahajan PM, Jadhav VH, Mehta JM. Pefloxacin in histoid leprosy. Int J Lepr Other Mycobact Dis. 1994;62:297-8.
45. Sehgal VN, Srivastava G, Gautam RK, et al. ENL in histoid leprosy. Int J Lepr Other Mycobact Dis. 1984;52:543-4.
46. Sehgal VN, Aggarwal A, Srivastava G, et al. Evolution of histoid leprosy (de novo) in lepromatous (multibacillary) leprosy. Int J Dermatol. 2005;44:576-8.

47. Ridley DS, Jopling WH. Classification of leprosy according to immunity. Int J Lepr. 1966;34:255-73.

48. Sehgal VN. A seven group classification for institutional and field work. Lepr Rev. 1989;60:75

49. Sehgal VN, Sardana K. "Intriguing" repercussions of primary neuritic leprosy in evolution of leprosy across the leprosy spectrum. Int J Dermatol. 2006;45:1121-3.

50. Sehgal VN. Spontaneous appearances of papules, nodules, and/or plaques: A prelude to abacillary, paucibacillary, or multibacillary histoid leprosy. Skinmed. 2006;5:139-41.

51. Sehgal VN, Srivastava G, Singh N, et al. Histoid leprosy: the impact of the entity on post-global leprosy elimination era. Int J Dermatol. 2009;48:603-10.

19
CHAPTER

Laboratory Diagnosis

Joyce Ponnaiya

INTRODUCTION

The laboratory has an important role in the diagnosis and documentation of leprosy. With the decline in the number of new cases, restructuring of leprosy services, and the integration of leprosy services with general health services in the field, it is likely that there will be loss of expertise. Although the clinical picture of leprosy varies widely from a small area of hypopigmented skin, to extensive damage to peripheral nerves and its consequences; it is generally accepted that an expert leprologist can identify most patients by clinical examination alone. However, in a general practice setting, there is a real danger of delays in diagnosis, especially in cases with atypical presentations. This can prove costly as new cases are now frequently diagnosed after the onset of disability. Laboratory has an important role in early diagnosis as well as in monitoring the response to treatment. Contacts of multibacillary (MB) leprosy patients also require screening for early and subclinical infections.

Leprosy is a chronic disease and patients can continue to have reactions well after the completion of antileprosy treatment. Distinguishing reactions from active leprosy or relapse so as to institute appropriate treatment is dependent on accurate laboratory diagnosis.

Expertise in the laboratory diagnosis of leprosy is now restricted to a few large centers. In expert hands, the specificity and sensitivity of diagnostic tests has greatly increased. There is scope for these centers to offer short training modules to both pathologists and technicians in the techniques and reporting of skin smears and biopsies.

SLIT-SKIN SMEAR EXAMINATION

Slit-skin smear technique was first developed by Wade and Rodriguez in 1927, described by Wade in 1935, standardized by Cochrane in 1947, and International Federation of Antileprosy Associations (ILEP) has described it in great details.[1] Of all the laboratory tests in leprosy service, slit-skin smear examination is the most simple and valuable.

SLIT-SKIN SMEAR—ITS ROLE AND INDICATIONS

Role of Slit-Skin Smear Examination

Demonstration of acid-fast bacilli (AFB) in smear examination serves several purposes:
- To confirm the diagnosis of leprosy
- To classify the disease
- To determine the disease activity in a patient
- To assess progress of the disease
- To follow-up patients on treatment.

Indications for Slit-Skin Smear Examination

- Diffuse skin infiltration without any sensory impairment or with vague sensory impairment
- Numerous, bilaterally symmetrical, ill-defined macular lesions without any (or vague) sensory impairment
- Papules, plaques and nodules on the earlobes, face, trunk back and extensor aspects of limbs, without any (or vague) sensory impairment

- A clinical situation where it is unclear whether the patient is suffering from paucibacillary (PB) or MB leprosy
- At the time of release from therapy (RFT) of all MB patients, for reference baseline data for the diagnosis of relapse, if at all, it occurs later
- A leprosy patient presenting with fresh lesions after RFT
- Any other with a diagnostic difficulty in a patient with chronic granulomatous lesions
- Any chronic ulcerative lesion showing no tendency to heal, where there is possibility of malignant change.

Sites for Slit-skin Smear

When the technique was introduced, smears were obtained from multiple sites which included both ear lobes, both cheeks, forehead, chin, both buttocks and additional six suspicious sites. The number of sites is now brought down to four without compromising the value of the test, at present the suggested routine sites are: (1) right earlobe, (2) forehead, (3) chin, and (4) left buttock in men and left upper thigh in women.[2] However, other active or suspicious lesions must be included, especially if the disease spectrum is closer to the PB side.

In borderline leprosy, the bacterial load in different sites may vary considerably and it is recommended that in such cases smears may be obtained from eight sites to include four active lesions in addition to the four routine sites.

Technique of Slit-skin Smear

Equipment Used

- Microscopic glass slides
- Disposable surgical gloves
- Surgical scalpel with detachable sterile blades
- Cotton swabs soaked in methyl alcohol
- Tincture benzoin
- Methyl alcohol
- Spirit lamp or a gas burner.

Method of Taking Slit-skin Smears

Clean glass slides free of grease, are prepared as follows:
- The slides are boiled in water with a detergent or soap for 30 minutes and washed in running water. They are then kept in dichromate solution overnight, washed again in running water, rinsed in distilled water and stored in methyl alcohol. Just before use, the slides are taken out using forceps and cleaned with a soft cloth.
- Using a diamond glass marking pencil write the patient's identification number on the extreme left side of the glass slide.
- Just before taking the smear, clean the skin site using sterile cotton wool soaked in methyl alcohol. Let the area become dry.

- Pinch the fold of skin tightly using the thumb and index finger till it blanches.
- Using a surgical scalpel with a detachable sterile blade (Bard Parker No. 15), make a cut on the skin fold 5 mm long and 2 mm deep just to expose the subepithelial tissue. Ordinarily there should be no bleeding, if there is, wipe off the blood with a sterile swab.
- Turn the blade at 90° and scrape out fragments of tissue and fluid from the bottom and side of the cut.
- Place the material thus obtained on the clean slide and spread evenly to make a smear about 8–10 mm in diameter.
- Flame the blade and place it on its stand.
- The skin cut may be sealed with a small piece of cotton wool dipped in Tincture of benzoin.
- Using a second blade make the smear from the next site. The cooled first blade is used to make the smear from the third site. Repeat the procedure until all the smears are taken. About four to five smears can well be made on a single slide.
- Allow smears to dry at room temperature.
- Fix the smear by moving the slide briefly over a flame; from a methyl alcohol lamp or a gas burner (alternatively the smears can be fixed by keeping in formalin fumes for 10 minutes). They are now ready for staining. Remember, the heating of slides should be gentle as excess heat will likely destroy the smear tissue.
- Slides used once should never be used again.

Preparation of Dichromate Solution

Dichromate solution is prepared by dissolving 25 gm of potassium dichromate in 25 mL of distilled water and then adding 50 mL concentrated sulfuric acid slowly with stirring (always add acid to water). Cool the solution and store it in a glass bottle. Discard when it turns green.

Staining of Slides: Ziehl-Neelsen Method

Chemicals required:
- Basic fuchsin
- Decolorizing agent
- Methylene blue (counter stain).

Preparation of Reagents

Carbol fuchsin (To make 200 mL):
- Basic fuchsin: 2 gm
- Phenol-melted : 10 mL
- Absolute alcohol (95%): 20 mL
- Distilled water: 170 mL.

In a large conical flask take 2 gm of basic fuchsin and then add 10 mL of melted phenol and mix well. Then add 20 mL of 95% absolute alcohol and mix well. Finally add 170 mL of distilled water and shake until the dye is dissolved. Filter the solution (using Whatman filter paper No. 40) every time before use.

Decolorizing Agent

Sulfuric acid (5%) (To make 200 mL):
- 1-N Concentrated sulfuric acid: 10 mL
- Distilled water: 190 mL.

Take 190 mL of distilled water in a large conical flask and add to it (slowly down the side of the flask) 10 mL of concentrated sulfuric acid. Rotate the flask and shake as you pour the acid.

Caution: Never pour water into the acid, always acid into the water.

Hydrochloric acid (1%) in 70% absolute alcohol (To make 100 mL):
- Concentrated hydrochloric acid: 1 mL
- Absolute alcohol (70%): 99 mL.

Counter Stain

Methylene blue (0.2%) (To make 200 mL):
- Methylene blue powder: 0.4 gm
- Distilled water : 200 mL.

Method of Staining

- The slides with the fixed smears are stained individually.
- They are placed separately on staining rods over a sink.
- Flood the slides with freshly prepared and filtered carbol fuchsin (or filtered if made previously) and keep the stain for 20 minutes. Alternatively, the slides may be gently heated using a gas flame or a methyl alcohol lamp, under the slide, just to produce steam to rise from all parts of the slide, but boiling must be avoided. The lamp should not be kept static at any area under the slide; it should be kept moving from side to side. Keep the stain for 10–15 minutes without any further heating.
- Wash the slides gently in running water.
- Destain the slide by using either 5% sulfuric acid for 10 minutes, or by using 1% hydrochloric acid in 70% absolute alcohol for 3–5 seconds.
- Wash the slides gently in running water.
- Flood the slides with counter stain 0.2% methylene blue and keep it for 1 minute.
- Wash the slides gently with running water.
- Stand the slide inclined on its narrow side on a blotting paper until it is dry.

Examination of the Smear

Skin smears are examined using a light microscope under an oil immersion objective. To make the examination easier a binocular microscope is preferred. Binocular microscopes should have clean lenses and uniformly lighted objectives, preferably with an artificial lamp for proper study of the slide. The number of AFB in each field is counted and graded as described further in this chapter.[3] In addition, the morphology of the bacilli is carefully examined to find out whether the AFB present are live or killed; if they are undergoing granularity and fragmentation. It is believed that the solid staining organisms are probably live and viable; whereas the granular, broken and fragmented ones are dead and nonviable.[4]

BACTERIAL INDEX

The universally accepted standard method for assessment of the mycobacterial load in a leprosy patient is the assessment of bacterial index (BI) as defined by Ridley (1958), based on a logarithmic scale and is a modification of Cochrane's index. The bacterial load is graded as detailed below:
- 6+: Over 1,000 bacilli and globi in an average microscopic field (Fig. 19.1)
- 5+: Over 100 bacilli but less than 1,000 in an average miscroscopic field
- 4+: Over 10 bacilli but less than 100 in an average microscopic field (Fig. 19.2)
- 3+: 1–10 bacilli in an average field
- 2+: 1–10 bacilli in 10 microscopic fields
- 1+: 1–10 bacilli in 100 microscopic fields
- Zero: No bacilli observed after searching at least 100 microscopic fields.

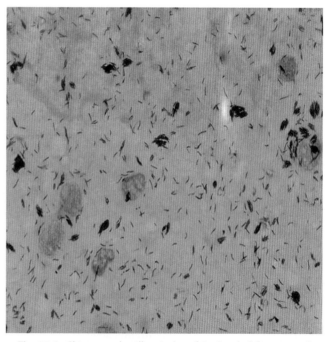

Fig. 19.1: Skin smear bacillary index of 6+. Beaded, fragmented and few solid bacilli are seen

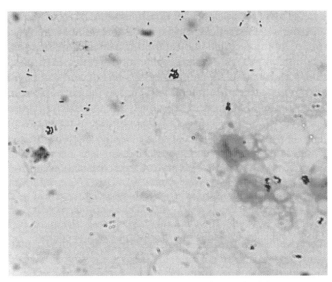

Fig. 19.2: Skin smear with a BI of 4+ with globi and mainly solid bacilli

The BI is arrived at by adding the values from all the skin sites examined (usually four) and by dividing the total by the number of sites.

Example:

Right ear	5+
Forehead	4+
Chin	3+
Buttock	3+

Bacterial index (BI):	$15 \div 4 = 3.75$

It is recommended that where the count varies significantly between sites, the highest count should be taken in labeling and classifying the disease.

MORPHOLOGICAL INDEX

Morphological index (MI) is the percentage of solid stained bacilli, calculated after examining 200 bacilli lying singly. If less than 100 organisms are available, the percentage is calculated according to the number of bacilli available for examination. Bacilli are considered solid staining if the organisms satisfy the following criteria:
- The entire organism must be uniformly stained
- The longitudinal sides are parallel
- Both ends are rounded
- The length is five times its width.

Slit-skin smear technique and the assessment of BI and MI should be carried out by well-trained technicians with meticulous care. Any compromise or short cut in any of the steps, namely taking of smears, numbering of the slides, staining and examining the slides to measure the

bacteriological indices, will result in disastrous consequences in the diagnosis and management of leprosy. Some of the possible (and common) errors, which must be avoided, include:
- If the skin-cut is not deep enough to reach the granuloma and scraping of the cut surface is not done properly, an adequate sample of the tissue containing enough bacilli may not be obtained.
- If the material obtained is not spread properly and evenly on the slide, the count of the bacilli may be erroneous.
- If the specimen obtained is not immediately fixed, the bacilli will degenerate and are lost in the count.
- If the light source of the microscope is inadequate and not with uniform illumination, the identification of solid staining bacilli will be erroneous.

When technicians are not well-trained, there can be wide inter-observer variation.

The poor quality of work in the slit-skin smear studies reported from laboratories attached to the Leprosy Control Programs had resulted in the abandonment of skin smear studies altogether. Instead, steps should have been taken to improve the work by offering periodic refresher courses to technicians, strict supervision of laboratories, and introducing quality control measures. With widespread implementation of multidrug therapy (MDT) during the past two decades the disease load has been brought down considerably and the disease declared eliminated. In the foreseeable future, the hope of eradicating the disease is bright. It is during this critical period, that there should be increased efficiency in our efforts to diagnose, assess, and manage the disease in its early stages, when the diagnosis offers many hurdles. Establishment of referral centers with experts to offer supervision and quality control to peripheral laboratories, and reintroduction of the slit smear test as a routine procedure, is imperative to help in hastening the eradication of the disease.

NASAL MUCOSAL SMEARS

In lepromatous leprosy, the involvement of the nasal mucosa is almost 100%.[5] Nasal mucosal epithelial lining is thin and is easily ulcerated and therefore, is the most common site from where *M. leprae* are disseminated into the environment. It has been reported that in a lepromatous patient about 10 million bacilli per day can be collected from the nasal secretions.[6] Following antileprosy therapy, the nasal ulcers heal fast and therefore, examination of smears obtained from the nasal mucosa and nasal secretion is very helpful in assessing the response of a patient to treatment and his infectivity. For a period nasal smears were discontinued because of the belief that the presence of acid fast saprophytes present in the nose may vitiate the findings. Now with careful staining these artefacts can be avoided.

It has been found that the material collected from nasal blows first thing in the morning, especially before the patient has cleared his nose, contains enough AFB shed from the ulcerated mucosa to evaluate the bacterial load in a lepromatous patient.

Method of Taking Nasal Mucosal Smears

To obtain nasal smears, a nasal mucosal scraper specially prepared for the purpose is used. A bicycle spoke 2 mm thick and 15 cm long is obtained; one end of it is beaten to a width of 4 mm to make a blade 1 cm long and 4 mm broad. One side of this blade is filed to make it blunt and the other side is sharpened. However, this simple manufactured surgical instrument should always be sterilized (either in the autoclave or in boiling water) before use.

The collection of specimen is done very gently and only under direct vision of the nasal cavity with good illumination. A nasal speculum may be used for adequately viewing the nasal mucosa. The smears are obtained either from the anterior end of inferior turbinate or from the septum. The mucosa is not cut but scraped with the blade. Bleeding is avoided as far as possible. The material thus obtained including the tissue fragments, is smeared on to a glass slide and processed in a similar manner as for skin smears. If crusts are present in the nasal mucosa, they are softened with irrigation using normal saline. Only after removing the crusts the smears are taken. After taking the smear a small ball of cotton is pressed into the nostril to stop the bleeding, if there is any.

Method of Collecting Nasal Blows

The patient is given a small thin cellophane bag with a 6 inches wide opening on one side and is asked to blow his nose into it. It is preferable to obtain the specimen early in the morning soon after he gets up from the bed, even before he washes his face, mouth and nose. A smear is made on a slide from the specimen in the cellophane bag using a cotton swab mounted on a stick, then processed just as skin smears.

In evaluating the specimens obtained from nasal smear or nasal blow, it is important to remember that nose may harbor acid fast saprophytes. Therefore, the decolorization of the smears from the nose should always be done with an acid-alcohol decolorizing solution. Finding of a rare and a single organism in a nasal smear should be interpreted carefully, with much scrutiny and meticulous study of the clinical picture and other relevant factors.

SKIN BIOPSY

Under ideal circumstances, every patient of leprosy should undergo skin biopsy examination to confirm the diagnosis and type of leprosy, to identify the complications like reactions, and to help in the management of the disease. In some countries where medical facilities are adequate and leprosy patients are few, this is strictly followed. In countries where there are large number of patients, and adequate funds and trained medical personnel are not readily available, a thorough and detailed clinical examination and all required laboratory tests are not done as a routine. Now, when there is worldwide reduction of number of patients, and more and more, early and difficult to diagnose patients are seen, it is essential that the patients are given the benefit of these laboratory studies. Further, following the integration of leprosy with general medical services, more patients will be cared for by primary care physicians, then by paramedical workers and hopefully, the efficiency in the care of leprosy patients will improve.

Site of Skin Biopsy

If the presenting sign is a small hypopigmented patch suspected to be indeterminate leprosy, the biopsy should be taken from the middle of the lesion where the disease is active.[7] Where there are multiple lesions, the most active lesion should be chosen. In such patients, the active infiltrated edge should be chosen for the biopsy and no normal skin need to be included. If there are numerous skin lesions with different morphology, more than one biopsy is required for proper evaluation. In many patients reporting at early stage, the lesions are usually vague. When the skin is infiltrated with local anesthetic for the biopsy procedure, the vague skin lesion may become obscure and not be easily identifiable. Therefore, it is better to mark the biopsy site with a skin marking pencil before local anesthetic is administered.

Size of the Biopsy

The biopsy size may vary, depending on the clinical picture and the purpose for which the biopsy is done. In early lesions where diagnosis of the disease is in question, and the histopathologic changes pesent in the skin are minimal, (as in indeterminate leprosy), a fairly large sample of the skin lesion should be obtained to allow proper evaluation. The biopsy should be an elliptical piece of skin 1.5 cm long, 0.6 cm wide and deep enough to include the full depth of the dermis and subcutaneous tissue, so that the nerves in the deep dermis and possibly in the subcutaneous region are available for study. For assessment of clinically well-established lesions, for repeat biopsies for follow-up studies and management of the disease, a 5 mm punch biopsy sample is adequate. When the lesion is on the face (especially in a child or a female patient) care should be taken to reduce the size to the minimum necessary (3 mm punch) so that only a very small scar is left behind.

Biopsy Procedure

The lesion and the surrounding areas are cleaned with spirit and covered with a sterile towel which has a small square cut-out at the center. One mL of 2% lignocaine is drawn into a syringe. After injecting a small quantity of local anesthetic intradermally, the needle is inserted into the skin downward in stages, injecting lignocaine. Then the skin piece should be excised with a cold knife or a 5 mm punch. While taking out the skin piece great care should be exercised so that the tissue is not crushed with the forceps. If the biopsy specimen has to be held, while removing it, only the edge of biopsy should be held by forceps. Once the biopsy specimen is crushed the cells that form the tissue are also destroyed beyond recognition. Soon after removal, the skin biopsy is spread on a small piece of blotting paper (or filter paper) so that it will not curl upon itself. Immediately the biopsy piece sticking to the blotting paper is immersed into the fixative. Any delay in transferring the tissue into the fixative will cause autolysis of cells and make it unsuitable for histopathologic study.

A busy clinician taking time to do the biopsy should also spend a little more time to check and see that the biopsied skin piece is transferred into the fixative immediately after removal and the bottle with the fixative and specimen is properly labeled.

FIXATIVES

Neutral Formalin (Universal Fixative) (To Make 1 L)

- Formaldehyde solution (40%) : 100 mL
- $NaH_2PO_4.2H_2O$: 3.5 gm
- $Na_2HPO_4.2H_2O$: 6.5 gm
- Distilled water : 900 mL.

Neutral formalin 10% is a universal fixative and can be easily and routinely used in a busy out-patient clinic. AFB stain also works well in tissues fixed in formalin. However, it has certain drawbacks, there is some shrinkage of collagen which pulls apart the tissue and the granuloma and blurs the cytological details. The use of pure 40% formalin as fixative is best avoided, as it causes distortion of granuloma.

Lowy's Fixative

Lowy's fixative [formaldehyde, mercuric chloride, acetic acid (FMA)]:
- Formaldehyde solution (40%) : 100 mL
- Mercuric chloride: 20 gm
- Glacial acetic acid: 30 mL
- Distilled water : 1,000 mL.

First dissolve mercuric chloride in water with gentle heat and then add the other reagents.

Formaldehyde, mercuric chloride, acetic acid fixative should be freshly prepared every 3 months. After 2 hours of fixation in this solution, the tissue must be transferred to 70% ethyl alcohol in which it can be stored for any length of time. If the tissue is kept in FMA fixative longer than 2 hours it gets hardened and further processing of the tissue is hampered.

If properly used, this fixative offers very good preservation of cellular details without any shrinkage of collagen. After the biopsies have undergone fixation they may be transferred to 70% alcohol and transported to properly equipped histopathology laboratory. It is advisable to use this fixative for research studies but only, if properly trained technical personnel are available.

The skin biopsies are processed for paraffin sectioning and the sections are made of 4–5 μm thickness. Several staining procedures are now available to allow detailed study of the biopsies, especially for early lesions; and to differentiate a leprosy lesion from that of other granulomatous conditions.

The following stains may be done depending on the nature of the study:
- Hematoxylin-eosin stain (H&E) for routine histopathologic examination
- Job-Chacko modification of Fite-Faraco stain for *M. leprae*[8]
- Gomori's-Grocott methenamine silver stain to demonstrate remnants of degenerating *M. leprae*[9]
- Fluorescent microscopy to detect *M. leprae*[10]
- Immunochemical staining using mycobacterial antibodies to detect products of *M. leprae* in tissues[11-13]
- *In situ* hybridization and polymerase chain reaction (PCR) in the early diagnosis of leprosy[14-15]
- S-100 stain, to selectively bring out neural fragments from a destroyed nerve.[16-18]

Of all these above listed staining procedures, the H&E stain and the Fite-Faraco stain for *M. leprae* are done as a routine on all biopsies, which will be described in detail. The other four staining procedures mentioned require well-equipped laboratories and specially trained technicians, and are done only when a specific problem arises or for research studies.

HEMATOXYLIN-EOSIN STAIN

- Paraffin sections 5 μm in thickness, are mounted on clean glass slides
- Deparaffinize using two changes of xylene for 5 minutes each
- Bring ultimately to tap water using graded alcohol.

If the sections are from FMA fixative, treat them with 1% alcohol-iodine solution for 10–15 minutes. Wash with tap water. Treat with sodium thiosulfate for 5 minutes. Wash well with water, before staining with hematoxylin.
- Stain with Harris hematoxylin for 10 minutes
- Rinse in tap water to remove excess stain
- Decolorize by quickly dipping the stained slides into 1% hydrochloric acid two or three times
- Wash in running water for 10 minutes
- Dip in lithium carbonate solution if blueing is not sufficient
- Counter stain with 1% Eosin for 1 minute
- Wash in running water for 10 minutes
- Dehydrate in graded alcohol

- Clear using two changes of xylene for 1–2 minutes
- Mount the section in DPX medium.

Preparation of Solutions

Harris Hematoxylin

- Hematoxylin: 5 gm
- Absolute alcohol: 50 mL
- Potassium alum: 100 gm
- Mercuric oxide: 2.5 gm
- Glacial acetic acid: 25 mL
- Distilled water : 1,000 mL.

Dissolve hematoxylin powder in absolute alcohol. Separately dissolve potassium alum in warm distilled water. Mix the two solutions and heat to boiling point. Then slowly add mercuric oxide. Cool the stain rapidly in ice or cold water. When it is cool, add glacial acetic acid.

Eosin Stain

- Eosin: 1 gm
- Phloxin B (aqueous): 100 mg
- Glacial acetic acid: 4 mL
- Distilled water : 100 mL
- Absolute alcohol: 890 mL.

Dissolve 1 gm of eosin in 100 mL of distilled water. Add 10 mL of aqueous solution of 100 mg phloxin B. Add absolute alcohol to make up to 1,000 mL. Finally add 4 mL of glacial acetic acid.

Alcohol Iodine Solution

- Iodine crystals : 1 gm
- Alcohol 95%: 100 mL.

Sodium Thiosulfate Solution

Sodium thiosulfate: 5 gm
- Distilled water : 100 mL.

Lithium Carbonate Solution

- Lithium carbonate: 5 gm
- Distilled water : 500 mL.

JOB-CHACKO MODIFICATION OF FITE-FARACO STAIN FOR *M. LEPRAE*

Staining Procedure: Each Slide is Stained Separately

- Deparaffinize sections in a mixture of xylene and peanut oil (2 parts of xylene, 1 part peanut oil), two changes of 6 minutes each

- Drain, wipe off excess oil and blot with filter paper
- Wash in running tap water for 4 minutes
- Stain in Ziehl-Neelsen carbol fuchsin solution for 30 minutes at room temperature
- Wash in tap water for 2 minutes
- Decolorize slides in 5% sulfuric acid in 25% alcohol for two changes of 1.5 minutes each
- Wash in running tap water for 5 minutes
- Counter stain with Harris hematoxylin for 5 seconds
- Wash in running tap water for 5 minutes
- Drain the excess water, blot with filter paper and air dry the section at room temperature. Do not use alcohol to dehydrate.
- Clear in two changes of xylene and mount.

This staining procedure has two modifications from the routine Fite-Faraco stain for *M. leprae*. Use of alcohol is minimized to prevent over-decolorization of already stained *M. leprae* especially in biopsies from indeterminate patients. The other change is in the use of counter stain. Instead of methylene blue, hematoxylin is used. The nuclei are well-stained and therefore the cells and the tissue structures are clearly identified in relation to the presence of AFB. Fite-Faraco stain also clearly identifies mast cells in addition to AFBs.[18] Finding of AFB in any one of the following sites such as, the subepidermal region of the skin, inside Schwann cells, endothelial cells and arrectoris pilorum muscle cells, will confirm the diagnosis of leprosy.

GOMORI-GROCOTT METHENAMINE SILVER STAIN

This staining procedure is ordinarily used for staining fungi in tissue sections. It has been found that *Mycobacteria* also take up the silver stain and appear black. Since the lipid coat of AFB is stained, even dead, fragmented and granular *M. leprae* (which usually do not take up the Fite's stain) can be visualized by using this method. Since the organisms appear black, they are easily identified under the microscope. The acid-fast stain fades in course of time and it is difficult to preserve AFB stained slides for any length of time. The Gomori-Grocott method retains the stain for many years.

Silver stains the fibrous connective tissue and elastic tissue, therefore, selective staining of *M. leprae* especially in a tissue like skin, with abundant fibrous connective tissue and elastic fiber, is not possible and therefore the specificity is poor, although the sensitivity is high. Thus, it is not ordinarily used in routine skin biopsy studies. In the internal organs such as lymph nodes, liver, spleen, bone marrow, and adrenals, where fragmented *M. leprae* may persist for many years inside small clumps of foamy macrophages, this stain is very useful to identify the presence of remnants of *M. leprae*. Also in healed skin lesions of patients in the lepromatous spectrum, where remnants of *M. leprae* may not be demonstrable using routine stains for AFB, Gomori's stain will help to identify them.

FLUORESCENT MICROSCOPY TO DETECT *M. LEPRAE*

Finding of *M. leprae* during histopathologic examinations of early lesions is an important criterion in the diagnosis of leprosy. Routine acid fast stains are not so sensitive because of the variability in the destaining procedures using acid alcohol. In the search for more sensitive staining procedures, fluorescent method of staining *M. leprae* has been found to be useful.

In a study of 56 skin biopsies from early leprosy lesions, using a slight modification of Kuper and May's method to obtain optimum fluorescence, 39 biopsies showed *M. leprae* as compared to only 25 in sections stained by the Fite-Faraco stain.[10] Although fluorescent staining has found a place in detection of *Mycobacterium tuberculosis*, it has not been widely used to detect *M. leprae*.

IMMUNOCHEMICAL STAINING TO DEMONSTRATE MYCOBACTERIAL ANTIGENS

It has been reported that the identification of early lesions of leprosy using histopathologic techniques is very much enhanced by using immunochemical staining procedures to demonstrate the presence of antigens of *M. leprae*.[11-13] In a study of 51 skin biopsies from patients suspected of early leprosy, only in nine patients (17.6%) AFBs were found using routine AFB staining technique, whereas in 24 patients (47.1%) the diagnosis of leprosy was confirmed by finding mycobacterial antigens by immunostaining using polyclonal Bacillus Calmette-Guerin (BCG) antibodies.[11] If in a skin biopsy there are histopathologic changes of early leprosy, such as perivascular, peri- and intraneural inflammation; and if the antigenic components of *M. leprae* are demonstrated inside nerves and macrophages using immunohistochemical techniques, it is reasonable to make a diagnosis of leprosy.

In a recent study using *in situ* hybridization procedure for *M. leprae*, 25 patients each from early leprosy and suspected leprosy were studied. The positivity rates for demonstrating the presence of *M. leprae* using *in situ* hybridization procedures were considerably higher than those with routine Fite-Faraco stain.[14] *In situ* PCR studies also appear to improve rates of detection of early cases.[15]

S-100 STAIN FOR SCHWANN CELLS

In skin biopsies from tuberculoid (polar and subpolar) and borderline tuberculoid leprosy patients, AFBs are not ordinarily demonstrable. Therefore, a firm diagnosis depends on demonstration of active invasion and destruction of dermal and cutaneous nerves by the granulomas. In several patients these nerves are destroyed beyond recognition on routine histopathology. Only remnants of these nerves (composed of Schwann cell clumps) are left behind in the granulomas. In such instances, the spindle shaped Schwann-cell-clumps may not be easily distinguished from the collections of epithelioid cells. S-100 stain which selectively stains Schwann cells, may be used to bring out the remnants of the destroyed nerves lying in tuberculoid granulomas. Several publications[16-19] have clearly brought out the usefulness of this stain in the diagnosis of tuberculoid leprosy and differentiating it from other tuberculoid granulomas of the skin such as tuberculosis, deep fungal infections and sarcoidosis.

It should be noted that S-100 stain also stains melanocytes, dendritic cells and the cells lining the sweat ducts. But they can be easily identified and differentiated from Schwann cells by the morphological appearances.

NERVE BIOPSY

Nerve biopsy is a procedure which should not be undertaken lightly and should ideally be done by either a neurologist or a neurosurgeon. Since such highly qualified experts are not readily available, a physician, or a surgeon well-trained, may perform the nerve biopsies. A thickened sensory nerve is selected for biopsy. The suitable nerves include supraorbital branch of the fifth cranial nerve, supraclavicular nerve, great auricular nerve in the neck, radial cutaneous nerve at the wrist, a cutaneous nerve of the forearm or thigh, sural nerve at the back of the leg or superficial peroneal nerve on the dorsum of the foot.

The nerves usually chosen for biopsy are a branch of sural nerve at the level just above the ankle, or a branch of radial cutaneous nerve at the wrist region. In the tuberculoid spectrum, cutaneous nerves adjacent to a skin lesion, may be enlarged and in such cases that nerve may be chosen for biopsy. The nerve deficit resulting from these procedures is usually minimal.[20]

After proper sterilization of the area, small amount of 2% lignocaine is injected around the nerve and after waiting for 5 minutes, a transverse skin incision is made. The nerve is separated by blunt dissection. A small nick is made in the nerve, to divide one or two fasciculi, which are then picked up and stripped from the nerve bundle. Since in tuberculoid and borderline leprosy the involvement of nerve is longitudinal, a 2 cm long nerve twig may be dissected out using fine iris forceps and scissors. The nerve tissue is then laid on a blotting paper or a filter paper to keep its longitudinal orientation preserved and immediately transferred to a fixative. The common fixative used for nerve biopsies is 10% neutral formalin.

Nerve biopsies are done usually to confirm the diagnosis of leprosy, especially in patients who present with pure neural leprosy where there are no skin lesions. The biopsies are processed for paraffin sections and 5 μm thick sections are cut. The following staining procedures are available for study:
- Hematoxylin-eosin stain
- Job-Chacko modification of Fite-Faraco stain for AFB[8]

- Luxol fast blue stain for myelin[21]
- Bodian stain for axons.[22]

During histopathological examination when acid fast organisms are demonstrated inside nerves; or when granulomatous inflammation destroying the nerve parenchyma is seen, the diagnosis of leprosy is easily made. There is also patchy demyelination seen in Luxol fast blue stain and fragmentation of axons in the Bodian stain. When these diagnostic evidences are absent, other neurological diseases should be considered and further detailed studies may be done to identify specific changes due to the other neuropathies listed below:

Neuropathies are broadly classified into four groups:
1. Disorders with thickened nerves
2. Disorders with patchy areas of cutaneous hypoesthesia
3. Polyneuropathy
4. Spinal cord disease

A detailed description of these diseases is beyond the purview of this chapter. The reader is referred to the chapter in this textbook, on differential diagnosis of neurological conditions.

In a rare patient, there is total fibrous replacement of the nerve parenchyma and fibrosis of the perineurium. The intraneural fibrous tissue may show extensive hyalinization. No acid fast organisms or inflammatory granuloma or caseous necrosis is observed. The end stage of leprous neuritis may only show a totally hyalinized nerve and cannot be differentiated from the end stage of some of the other neuropathies. Fortunately, this appearance is almost always present in healed leprosy lesions only.

HISTAMINE TEST

There are few other diagnostic tests which should be mentioned although they are not ordinarily done in routine practice.

The Principle of Flare Histamine Test[23,24]

The response in the skin to histamine depends on the integrity of nerves of the autonomic nervous system. The autonomic nerves are nonmyelinated nerve fibers sheathed only by Schwann cells and are distributed along with the small dermal blood vessels. In early leprosy, which manifests as localized skin patches, the Schwann cells are parasitized by *M. leprae*. There is perivascular and perineural inflammation and the functions of sympathetic nerves of the skin supplying the blood vessels are impaired, even before the sensory nerves are affected.

Histamine elicits two reactions in normal skin in which the sympathetic nervous system is intact: a flare, caused by dilation of small blood vessels of the skin and a weal, due to local injury to the skin. In the skin affected by leprosy, flare may be impaired or absent, due to malfunctioning of the sympathetic nervous system and only a weal is seen.

Method of Doing the Test

Two drops of histamine hydrochloride solution 0.1% (1 mg in 1 mL) are placed, one each on the normal skin and the other on the suspected patch. With a sharp sterile needle a prick is made through the drops on both sites deep enough to penetrate the epidermis. The histamine solution is wiped off and the area is watched for 5 minutes. In the normal skin, a weal at the site of prick and a flare of 2 cm diameter surrounding the weal would be seen (test labeled as positive). The flare disappears in 10 minutes. In the patch of leprosy the flare is impaired or absent and only a weal is seen (test negative). The flare is feeble and delayed in indeterminate and borderline leprosy, and absent in a tuberculoid lesion.

The test is useful only to differentiate hypopigmented macules of leprosy from those of other skin diseases. There will be a normal flare (positive test) in other hypopigmented macules due to nonleprosy conditions like vitiligo, pityriasis alba, fungal infections, etc. Further, the histamine test will also be negative in patients without any skin changes but only with areas of nerve deficit due to other peripheral neuropathies. Also, in patients with dark skin this test may not be useful because the flare is not easily visible.

THE SWEAT TEST

The Principle of Sweat Test[25,26]

Similar to histamine test, sweat test also evaluates the function of autonomic nerves which appear to be impaired much earlier than the sensory nerves. The sweat glands are activated by parasympathetic nerves and the substances that act upon these nerves will increase sweating. Pilocarpine nitrate, methacholine chloride, acetyl choline, and carbaminoyal choline are some of the chemicals injected into the skin to demonstrate increase of sweating. In tropical countries, the use of drugs may be avoided and the part of the skin to be tested may be exposed to the sun for a short period. The common drugs used are pilocarpine nitrate and acetyl choline. Acetyl choline acts faster and its effects do not cause long lasting discomfort.

Method of Performing the Test

The hypopigmented patch in the skin to be tested and the adjoining area of normal skin are thoroughly cleaned with methylated alcohol, and painted with tincture iodine. Wait till the area dries and then paint the area with starch. An aqueous solution of 0.05 mL of 0.1% of acetyl choline is injected intradermally into the hypopigmented lesion and also into the adjoining normal skin which acts as control. Examine the areas 5–10 minutes later. The area turns blue if there is sweating. Instead of acetyl choline, 0.2 mL of 0.1% solution (1 in 1,000) of pilocarpine nitrate or 0.1 mL of 1% solution of methacholine chloride may also be used.

66. Plikaytis BB, Gelber RH, Shinnick TM. Rapid and sensitive detection of *Mycobacterium leprae* using a nested-primer gene amplification assay. J Clin Microbiol. 1990;28:1913-7.

67. Cox RA, Kempsell K, Fairclough L, et al. The 16S ribosomal RNA of *Mycobacterium leprae* contains a unique sequence which can be used for identification by the polymerase chain reaction. J Med Microbiol. 1991;35:284-90.

68. Pattyn SR, Ursi D, Ieven M, et al. Polymerase chain reaction amplifying DNA coding for species-specific rRNA of *Mycobacterium leprae*. Int J Lepr Other Mycobact Dis. 1992;60:234-43.

69. Misra N, Ramesh V, Misra RS, et al. Clinical utility of LSR/A15 gene for *Mycobacterium leprae* detection in leprosy tissues using the polymerase chain reaction. Int J Lepr Other Mycobact Dis. 1995;63:35-41.

70. Donoghue HD, Holton J, Spigelman M. PCR primers that can detect low levels of *Mycobacterium leprae* DNA. J Med Microbiol. 2001;50:177-82.

71. Jadhav RS, Kamble RR, Shinde VS, et al. Use of reverse transcription polymerase chain reaction for the detection of *Mycobacterium leprae* in the slit-skin smears of leprosy patients. Indian J Lepr. 2005;77:116-27.

72. Phetsuksiri B, Rudeeaneksin J, Supapkul P, et al. A simplified reverse transcriptase PCR for rapid detection of in skin specimens. FEMS Immunol Med Microbiol. 2006;48:319-28.

73. Sharma RK, Katoch K, Shivannavar CT, et al. Detection of M. leprae by gene amplification; combined ethidium-bromide staining and probe hybridization. Int J Lepr Other Mycobact Dis. 1996;64:409-16.

74. Banerjee S, Sarkar K, Gupta S, et al. Multiplex PCR technique could be an alternative approach for early detection of leprosy among close contacts—a pilot study from India. BMC Infect Dis. 2010;10:252.

75. Banerjee S, Biswas N, Kanti Das N, et al. Diagnosing leprosy: revisiting the role of the slit-skin smear with critical analysis of the applicability of polymerase chain reaction in diagnosis. Int J Dermatol. 2011;50:1522-7.

76. Cruz AF, Furini RB, Roselino AM. Comparison between microsatellites and Ml MntH gene as targets to identify *Mycobacterium leprae* by PCR in leprosy. Anais Brasileiros de Dermatologia. 2011;86:651-6.

77. Gupta UD, Katoch K, Sharma RK, et al. Analysis of quantitative relationship between viability determination in leprosy by MFP, ATP bioluminescence and gene amplification assay. Int J Lepr Other Mycobact Dis. 2001;69:328-34.

78. Singh HB, Katoch K, Natrajan M, et al. Effect of treatment on PCR positivity in multibacillary leprosy patients treated with conventional and newer drugs ofloxacin and minocycline. Acta Leprol. 1999;11:179-82.

79. Katoch K, Katoch VM, Natarajan M, et al. Long term follow-up results of 1 year MDT in MB leprosy patients treated with standard MDT + once a month Minocycline and Ofloxacin. Indian J Lepr. 2008;80:331-44.

80. Das SN. Examination for *Mycobacterium leprae*. Dharmendra (Ed). Bombay: Kothari Medical Publishing House;1978.

81. Ridley DS. Bacterial Indices. In: Cochrane RG (Ed). Bristol: John Wright and Sons;1964.

82. Dayal R, Singh SP, Mathur PP, et al. Diagnostic value of in situ polymerase chain reaction in leprosy. Indian J Pediatr. 2005;72:1043-6.

83. Singh HB, Katoch VM, Natrajan M, et al. Improved protocol for PCR detection of *Mycobacterium leprae* in buffered formalin-fixed skin biopsies. Int J Lepr Other Mycobact Dis. 2004;72:175-8.

84. Kramme S, Bretzel G, Panning M, et al. Detection and quantification of *Mycobacterium leprae* in tissue samples by real-time PCR. Med Microbiol Immunol. 2004;193:189-93.

85. Martinez AN, Britto CF, Nery JA, et al. Evaluation of real-time and conventional PCR targeting complex 85 genes for detection of *Mycobacterium leprae* DNA in skin biopsy samples from patients diagnosed with leprosy. J Clin Microbiol. 2006;44:3154-9.

86. Sharma R, Lavania M, Katoch K, et al. Development and evaluation of real-time RT-PCR assay for quantitative estimation of viable *Mycobacterium leprae* in clinical samples. Indian J Lepr. 2008;80:315-21.

87. Shepard CC. The experimental disease that follows the injection of human leprosy bacilli into foot-pads of mice. J Exp Med. 1960;112:445-54.

88. Musser JM. Antimicrobial agent resistance in mycobacteria: molecular genetic insights. Clin Microbiol Rev. 1995;8:496-514.

89. Honore N, Roche PW, Grosset JH, et al. A method for rapid detection of rifampicin-resistant isolates of *Mycobacterium leprae*. Lepr Rev. 2001;72:441-8.

90. Williams DL, Spring L, Harris E, et al. Dihydropteroate synthase of *Mycobacterium leprae* and dapsone resistance. Antimicrob Agents Chemother. 2000;44:1530-7.

91. Cambau E, Carthagena L, Chauffour A, et al. Dihydropteroate synthase mutations in the folP1 gene predict dapsone resistance in relapsed cases of leprosy. Clin Infect Dis. 2006 42:238-41.

92. Williams DL, Waguespack C, Eisenach K, et al. Characterization of rifampin-resistance in pathogenic mycobacteria. Antimicrob Agents Chemother. 1994;38:2380-6.

93. Zhang L, Namisato M, Matsuoka M. A mutation at codon 516 in the *rpoB* gene of *Mycobacterium leprae* confers resistance to rifampin. Int J Lepr Other Mycobact Dis. 2004;72:468-72.

94. Sapkota BR, Ranjit C, Macdonald M. Reverse line probe assay for the rapid detection of rifampicin resistance in *Mycobacterium leprae*. Nepal Medical College J: NMCJ. 2006;8:122-7.

95. Li W, Matsuoka M, Kai M, et al. Real-time PCR and high-resolution melt analysis for rapid detection of *Mycobacterium leprae* drug resistance mutations and strain types. J Clin Microbiol. 2012;50:742-53.

96. Drlica K, Xu C, Wang JY, et al. Fluoroquinolone action in mycobacteria: similarity with effects in *Escherichia coli* and detection by cell lysate viscosity. Antimicrob Agents Chemother. 1996;40:1594-9.

97. Takiff HE, Salazar L, Guerrero C, et al. Cloning and nucleotide sequence of *Mycobacterium tuberculosis gyrA* and *gyrB* genes and detection of quinolone resistance mutations. Antimicrob Agents Chemother. 1994;38:773-80.

98. Kim SK, Lee SB, Kang TJ, et al. Detection of gene mutations related with drug resistance in *Mycobacterium leprae* from leprosy patients using Touch-Down (TD) PCR. FEMS Immunol Med Microbiol. 2003;36:27-32.

99. Cardona-Castro NM, Restrepo-Jaramillo S, Gil de la Ossa M, et al. Infection by *Mycobacterium leprae* of household contacts of lepromatous leprosy patients from a post-elimination leprosy region of Colombia. Mem Inst Oswaldo Cruz. 2005;100:703-7.

100. Geluk A, Spencer JS, Bobosha K, et al. From genome-based in silico predictions to ex vivo verification of leprosy diagnosis. Clin Vaccine Immunol. 2009;16:352-9.

21
CHAPTER

Differential Diagnosis of Dermatological Disorders in Relation to Leprosy

NL Sharma, Vikram Mahajan

INTRODUCTION

The clinical presentation of leprosy is highly variable and, in all its stages, it can mimic a great variety of lesions present in other diseases. The diagnosis can be made easily, as in the case of lepromatous leprosy, as soon as the patient enters the clinic, while on the other extreme there are few cases so subtle that even a most experienced clinician may get confounded. If the clinical diagnosis is in doubt, the lesion is perhaps too early as in case of indeterminate leprosy, or it is not leprosy. The benefit of doubt for the diagnosis in such cases may go in favor of a period of strict observation before making sure of the diagnosis, as stigma for leprosy is still important. The differential diagnosis of cutaneous lesions is so wide that one has to exclude a variety of dermatological conditions before making the diagnosis of leprosy. Similarly, neurological symptoms of leprosy can simulate a number of neurological disorders. The leprosy reactions too need to be differentiated from a number of systemic illnesses. However, along with characteristic skin lesions, the presence of other cardinal signs of leprosy, viz., anesthesia (lesional or in glove and stocking distribution), thickened nerve trunks (at the sites of predilection) and acid-fast bacilli in slit skin smears, are most useful in diagnosing leprosy.

The high index of clinical suspicion for leprosy is always rewarding, especially if the lesions are nonpruritic, evolving slowly, mostly asymptomatic and nonresponsive to routine treatment. A combination of skin lesions and neural involvement should always arouse a strong suspicion for leprosy. The diagnosis becomes more certain if there is sensory impairment, decreased sweating and reduced hair growth. Occasionally, in the absence of frank skin lesions, patient may present with edema of the legs, nasal stuffiness, crusting and epistaxis. Madarosis, i.e., absence of eyebrows or eyelashes may add to the index of suspicion. Erythema nodosum leprosum (ENL) cases often land up with general practitioners or physicians for complaints of fever, malaise, arthralgia, etc. A thorough examination of morphology of lesions and nerves may clinch the diagnosis.

Leprosy shows lesions of varied morphologies: macules (erythematous or hypopigmented), infiltrated lesions, plaques, nodules, noduloplaques and subsequent to autonomic neuropathy, there occurs scaliness and dryness over the lesions. Infiltrative lesions produce destruction of hair follicles and sweat glands leading to loss of hair and dryness of skin. Dryness of skin can be more generalized due to widespread disease or the administration of antileprosy drugs. Acute inflammatory lesions occur and edema of the limbs gets accentuated in leprosy reactions. So, the differential diagnosis would include many diverse diseases which can mimic lesions of leprosy.

Tables 21.1 to 21.6 give the list of differential diagnosis of majority of the cutaneous lesions which need to be differentiated from the lesions of leprosy.

The exhaustive list of diseases given in the tables (some may still have been left out) is indicative of a wide array of skin lesions that need to be differentiated from those of leprosy. The more common are described in details.

	Table 21.1: Differential diagnosis of hypopigmented macular lesions	
1.	Pityriasis alba	Hypopigmented asymptomatic scaly patches usually over the face of children. No sensory changes/nerve thickening (Fig. 21.1)
2.	Vitiligo	Almost milky white macules of variable size and shape (Fig. 21.2). Only loss of pigment without any skin/hair/sensory changes. Early lesions which are not completely white may be misleading
3.	Progressive macular hypomelanosis	Affects young adults mainly women and seen in all races with ill defined, nummular, hypopigmented, nonscaly macules over trunk
4.	Idiopathic guttate hypomelanosis	Acquired leukoderma, discrete, round or oval porcelain-white macules of approximately 2–5 mm, increase in number with aging
5.	Albinism/Albinoidism	Hereditary generalized absence of skin/iris pigment, photophobia, no hypoesthesia/nerve thickening
6.	Lichen sclerosus	Initially presents as pruritic, erythematous patch which evolves into depigmented atrophic plaque with a dirty white appearance
7.	Localized scleroderma/Morphea	Sclerotic or atrophic plaque without sensory changes (Fig. 21.3)
8.	Achromic onchocerciasis	Depigmentation or leopard skin is one of the commonly seen manifestations. The patches symmetrically distributed, typically appear over the shins
9.	Tinea corporis	Annular, scaly, erythematous plaque with definitive active border (Figs 21.4 to 21.7). Demonstration of fungus in KOH is diagnostic
10.	PKDL	History of past febrile episodes of kala-azar, hypopigmented macules, noduloplaques, papular or nodular infiltrations. Giemsa stained slit-skin smears show amastigotes (LD bodies), no acid-fast bacilli on ZN stain
11.	Acquired hypomelanosis (postinflammatory)	Usually preceding history of primary dermatosis, no hypoesthesia, nerve thickening, or acid-fast bacilli in slit-skin smears
12.	Incontinentia pigmenti achromicus	Hereditary disorder having blashkoid (whorled) pattern of hypomelanosis without sensory changes
13.	Seborrheic dermatitis	Erythemato-scaly plaque, mostly involving scalp (dandruff), may spread around hairline, postauricular area and on to the trunk. Isolated facial lesion might arouse suspicion of leprosy but typical changes may be seen involving eyebrows, scalp. Sensory changes of leprosy will be absent
14.	Pityriasis versicolor	The lesions are usually small and numerous, hypopigmented, covered with fine powdery scales. Scrapping from the lesion will show *Malassezia furfur* in characteristic "meatball and spaghetti" appearance in KOH mounts
15.	Leukoderma syphiliticum	Depigmented spots on a background of hyperpigmentation over back/sides of neck in secondary syphilis. Lymphadenopathy and reactive VDRL serology are significant findings

Abbreviations: PKDL, post-kala-azar dermal leishmaniasis; ZN, Ziehl-Neelsen's; VDRL, venereal disease research laboratory; KOH, potassium hydroxide; LD, Leishman Donovan.

PITYRIASIS ALBA

This entity is commonly seen in children and resembles indeterminate leprosy to a great extent. The lesions vary from single to many in number and occur usually over face or occasionally on upper trunk. The lesions are hypopigmented or occasionally erythematous, ill defined, round to oval, slightly scaly patches (Fig. 21.1). They often show seasonal variation and self-resolution. The lesions do not show loss of sensation, impairment of sweating or hair growth, or peripheral/lesional nerve thickening. Biopsy is rarely required which will show changes of spongiotic dermatitis. Treatment with emollients or mild steroids will resolve the condition. It is likely to recur.

POLYMORPHIC LIGHT ERUPTION

This photodermatosis presents as hypopigmented lesions, which may be asymptomatic or slightly itchy, mainly located over exposed parts. The hypopigmented lesions, especially over face may be confused with indeterminate leprosy (Fig. 21.8).

VITILIGO

Another common dermatosis that may be confused with leprosy is vitiligo. Although complete loss of pigment, as in vitiligo, is never due to leprosy, the lesions of vitiligo will show hypopigmentation when they are in the incipient stage

	Table 21.2: Differential diagnosis of papuloplaque lesions with or without annular configuration	
1.	Granuloma faciale	Primarily facial, asymptomatic, nodular lesions with smooth orange peel like surface. Leukocytoclastic vasculitis histopathology is characteristic
2.	Lymphocytoma cutis	Asymptomatic, erythematous/violaceous nodules or plaques on face/head/ears. Biopsy essential
3.	Follicular mucinosis	Follicular boggy pruritic papules or plaques over face/scalp without sensory changes. Histopathology will show fenestrations, mucin deposits, no granulomatous inflammation or acid fast bacilli
4.	Kaposi sarcoma	Commonly arises on hands and feet, the lesions bleed easily, if injured. Classical histology and absence of acid fast bacilli excludes leprosy
5.	Cellulitis/Erysipelas	Acute inflammation following pyococcal infection, characterized by erythematous, warm, painful, tender swelling. Pyrexia, malaise may be associated in severe cases. Needs differentiation from lesions of leprosy reaction. Cardinal signs of leprosy are absent
6.	Mycosis fungoides	Cutaneous T-cell lymphoma is characterized by persistent, infiltrated plaques in tumor stage; early stage may show scaling, erythema, annular plaques with active margins. Lesions are mostly asymptomatic (Fig. 21.9). Lymphadenopathy may occur. Cardinal signs of leprosy are absent
7.	Urticaria	Severely pruritic, evanescent, erythematous, edematous plaques are characteristic. Cardinal signs of leprosy are absent
8.	Erythema multiforme	Erythematous, minimally infiltrated, target-like lesions may have a vesicle/bulla in the center of the lesion. Mostly occur over acral parts or face following *Herpes simplex virus* infection or as an adverse drug rash. The eruptions are sudden with no sensory deficit
9.	Sweet syndrome	Plum colored erythematous, warm, tender noduloplaque lesions (Fig. 21.10) with pseudovesiculation over neck and hands, associated with fever, malaise, headache, conjunctival congestion and peripheral polymorphocytosis. Histological evidence of neutrophilic infiltrate and edema in the upper dermis, without evidence of leukocytoclastic vasculitis, like fibrin deposition, neutrophils within the vessel walls. However, there may be swollen endothelial cells, dilated blood vessels and fragmented neutrophil nuclei. No change in epidermis
10.	Syphilis	Secondary syphilis manifesting as asymptomatic, erythematous, infiltrated, papular, papulosquamous (Figs 21.11 and 21.12) or papuloplaques with annular configuration, mainly over forehead (corona venereum) and upper trunk. Positive Buschke-Ollendorff sign, lymphadenopathy and reactive VDRL serology are diagnostic findings
11.	Angiofibroma	Firm, discrete, brownish-red, telangiectatic papules over face, associated other features of tuberous sclerosis complex (Fig. 21.13). Histopathology is characteristic
12.	Lichen myxedematosus	Very uncommon disease. Numerous small firm papules often arranged in linear configuration against the background of erythema and thickening of skin
13.	Granuloma annulare	Usually skin colored beaded papules, often arranged in annular pattern, over dorsa of hands (Figs 21.14 to 21.16). Frequent association with diabetes mellitus
14.	Lichen planus	Polygonal, purple, flat topped papules over flexures, often with Wickham's striae. Annular lichen planus plaques have atrophic pigmented center and active bluish lichenoid margin. May appear similar to a tuberculoid leprosy lesion. Lesions are usually pruritic as against those of leprosy
15.	Nummular eczema	Discoid plaque of papulovesicles, scaling and crusting, intensely itchy (Fig. 21.17). Recurrent nature
16.	Necrobiosis lipoidica	Yellowish red edematous plaque, mostly over shins, no sensory loss. Frequent association with diabetes mellitus
17.	Cutaneous sarcoidosis	To be distinguished from lesions of tuberculoid leprosy. Lesions are granulomatous infiltrated papuloplaques. Scalp lesions may attain annular/arcuate shape, no sensory loss. Additionally, signs of systemic sarcoidosis or erythema nodosum may be present. Histologically, compact, naked epithelioid granulomas without caseation necrosis are characteristic
18.	EAC	Arcuate/circinate lesions, advancing red border, trailing scales (Fig. 21.18) usually on trunk. Few lesions attain large size
19.	Granuloma multiforme	Small noduloplaques or circinate lesions of varying size, few with fine infiltrated borders, slightly erythematous or skin colored, rarely hypopigmented. Usually affect adults, lesions mostly distributed over face, trunk and arms. The lesions do not show impairment of sensation or sweating, and heal slowly and spontaneously

(Contd...)

(Contd...)

20.	Psoriasis	Erythemato-scaly plaques of variable size and shape, may have annular shape, present over extensors or trauma prone sites. Individual lesion may mimic tuberculoid leprosy or subsiding type 1 reaction. Positive Auspitz sign and absence of cardinal signs of leprosy are differentiating features
21.	Lupus vulgaris	Common over face, has variable morphology and has to be differentiated from tuberculoid leprosy. Characterized by chronic reddish-brown granulomatous plaque, causing significant tissue destruction and scarring. Lesions tend to heal at one edge and spread from another
22.	Tuberculids	A heterogeneous group of cutaneous eruptions secondary to an internal focus of tuberculosis in an individual with a moderate to high degree of immunity to *Mycobacterium tuberculosis*. Papulonecrotic tuberculid, the most common form of tuberculid occurs as recurrent crops of asymptomatic or itchy, symmetric, firm, erythematous papulonodular lesions with central crusting which heal spontaneously leaving hyperpigmentation. The lesions can be differentiated from papulonodular leprosy lesions by the absence of cardinal signs of leprosy
23.	DLE	Erythematous infiltrated lesions with adherent scales and scarring, discoid lesions may simulate tuberculoid leprosy lesions
24.	Malignant atrophic papulosus	Crops of pink/red 2–5 mm necrotic/umblicated papules with central white porcelain like scar, usually on the dorsal aspects of lower limbs
25.	Onchocerciasis	Characterized by lichenified dermatitis, hypopigmentation, atrophy and infiltration. Skin biopsy required
26.	Pityriasis rosea	An acute self-limiting disease, probably infective in origin affecting mainly children and young adults, characterized by annular erythemato-squamous lesions mainly over trunk and proximal parts of limbs (Fig. 21.19)

Abbreviations: EAC, erythema annulare centrifugum; DLE, discoid lupus erythematosus.

	Table 21.3: Differential diagnosis of acquired ichthyotic lesions	
1.	Nutritional/malabsorption ichthyosis	Lipid and vitamin deficiency leads to ichthyotic lesions, other signs of deficiency present
2.	Ichthyosis secondary to malignancies	Most common with Hodgkin's lymphomas, others are hypothyroidism, sarcoidosis. Look for other signs of the disease
3.	Drug-induced ichthyosis	Clofazimine, cholesterol lowering drugs, INH can produce ichthyotic skin. Elicit history of long-term drug intake

Abbreviation: INH, isoniazid.

	Table 21.4: Differential diagnosis of infiltrated lesions	
1.	PKDL	Infiltration associated with hypopigmented macules, nodules, plaques (Figs 21.20 to 21.24). Giemsa slit-skin smear is diagnostic showing amastigotes (LD bodies). Past history of kala-azar, absence of cardinal signs of leprosy, are helpful clues
2.	Rosacea	Diffuse erythema and thickening of skin, telangiectases, papules and pustules over central area of face
3.	Reticulohistiocytosis	Firm brown or yellow papules/plaques over extensors, face scalp hands with mutilating shortening of fingers due to arthritis. Biopsy is confirmatory
4.	Sarcoidosis	Papulonodules, diffuse facial papular eruption, plaques, diffuse or patchy ichthyotic lesions. All of these may mimic leprosy (Figs 21.25 to 21.32). Biopsy will show sarcoid granulomas
5.	Disseminated cutaneous leishmaniasis	Not seen often. Widespread plaques, papules, nodules on face, extensor limbs. Resembles lepromatous leprosy. Slit-skin smear and biopsy helpful
6.	Lipoid proteinosis	Uncommon disease. Beaded papules or yellow-brown nodules, loss of eyelashes, hoarseness of voice. Histology helps in diagnosis

	Table 21.5: Differential diagnosis of madarosis	
1.	Hypothyroidism	Loss of lateral third of eyebrows, associated with puffiness of face, yellowish thickening of skin. Hormone assays are essential
2.	Follicular mucinosis	Follicular boggy pruritic papules or plaques over face/scalp/eyebrow with hair loss. Biopsy confirmatory
3.	Alopecia areata	Involvement of eyebrows and eyelashes simulate madarosis of leprosy (Fig. 21.33). Alopecia areata lesions over scalp, beard, etc. Presence of "exclamation sign" hair in the patches and absence of cardinal signs of leprosy are differentiating features

	Table 21.6: Differential diagnosis of erythema nodosum leprosum lesions	
1.	Cutaneous polyarteritis nodosa	A rare dermatosis may closely mimic ENL, lesions are dermal/subcutaneous tender nodules located on lower legs/ankles or other areas, associated with constitutional symptoms/nerve involvement, rarely ulcerate. Detailed history, clinical examination and biopsy help in the diagnosis
2.	Erythema nodosum	Sudden onset painful erythematous warm nodules and plaques. Mostly limited to shins, knees and ankles. Other signs of leprosy absent, lesions here are deeper than ENL
3.	Nodular vasculitis/erythema induratum	Indolent deep-seated ill-defined nodular lesions over back of legs, usually in middle aged obese women. Other signs of leprosy absent
4.	Erythema multiforme	Relatively superficial cutaneous dull red slightly raised maculopapular target lesions with cyanotic center over distal extremities, resolve in 2–3 weeks. No nerve thickening or other signs of leprosy
5.	Cutaneous small vessel vasculitis	Usually a crop of papules, nodules, vesicles plaques with bullae pustules and palpable purpura, or necrosis over lower legs/ankles (Fig. 21.34). Detailed workup for exclusion of other conditions. Cardinal signs of leprosy absent
6.	Papular urticaria/prurigo nodularis	This group comprises of erythematous/pigmented/urticarial/papular or nodular lesions often on legs and arms. Signs of excoriation present. Mostly pruritic lesions with other signs of leprosy absent

Abbreviation: ENL, erythema nodosum leprosum.

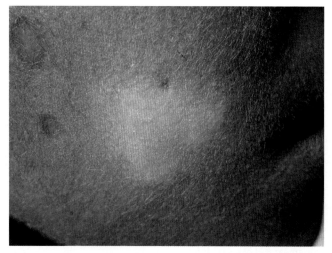

Fig. 21.1: Pityriasis alba: Often confused with indeterminate leprosy

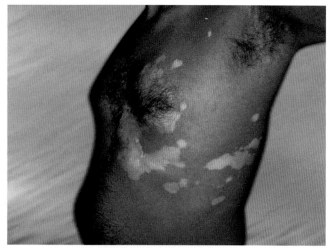

Fig. 21.2: Vitiligo—the hypopigmented lesions. No sensory impairment
Courtesy: Dr Pankaj Sharma, PGIMER, Dr RML Hospital, New Delhi.

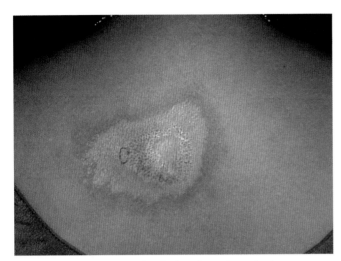

Fig. 21.3: Localized scleroderma (morphea)
Courtesy: Dr Pankaj Sharma, PGIMER, Dr RML Hospital, New Delhi.

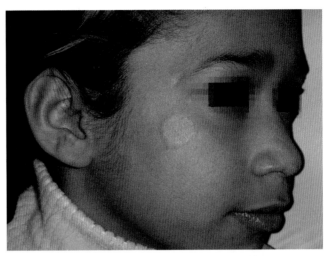

Fig. 21.6: Tinea faciei resembling tuberculoid leprosy
Courtesy: Dr HK Kar, PGIMER, Dr RML Hospital, New Delhi.

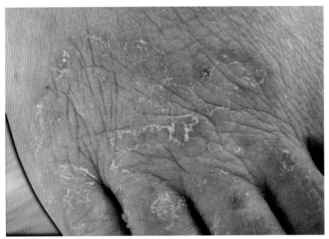

Fig. 21.4: Tinea lesion over foot-central hypopigmentation, scaling and peripheral erythema

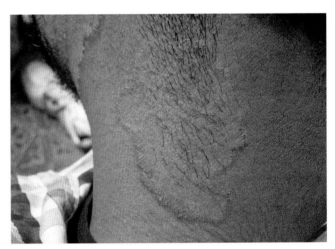

Fig. 21.7: Tinea lesion: Side of neck

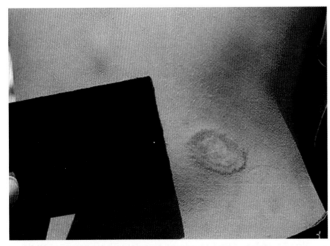

Fig. 21.5: Tinea corporis resembling tuberculoid leprosy
Courtesy: Dr Pankaj Sharma, PGIMER, Dr RML Hospital, New Delhi.

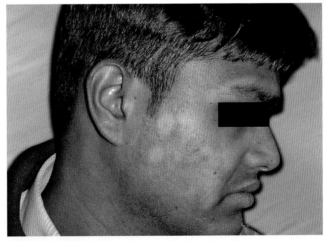

Fig. 21.8: Polymorphic light eruption—hypopigmented lesions, usually over sun exposed areas, may be slightly itchy. No sensory impairment. Mimics indeterminate leprosy

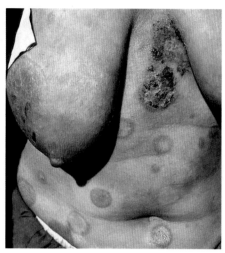

Fig. 21.9: Mycosis fungoides: Annular plaques of variable morphology resembling borderline leprosy

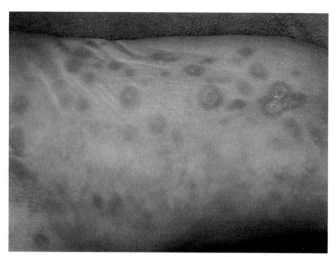

Fig. 21.12: Secondary syphilis: Papulosquamous rash on sole

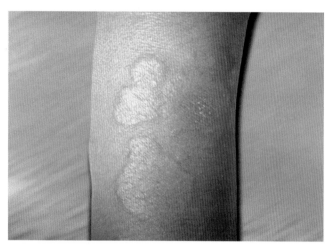

Fig. 21.10: Sweet's syndrome: Targetoid plaques resembling borderline leprosy

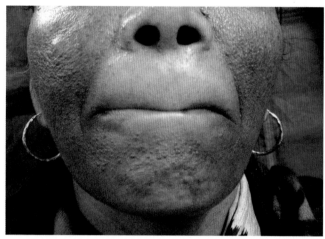

Fig. 21.13: Angiofibromas over face (tuberous sclerosis) mimicking lepromatous leprosy

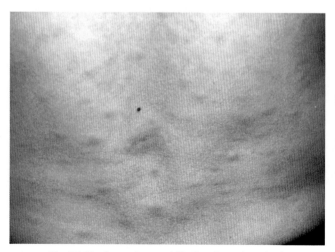

Fig. 21.11: Secondary syphilis: Papular rash on back

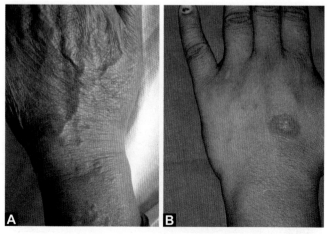

Figs 21.14A and B: Granuloma annulare: These asymptomatic lesions look like tuberculoid leprosy
Courtesy: Dr HK Kar, PGIMER, Dr RML Hospital, New Delhi.

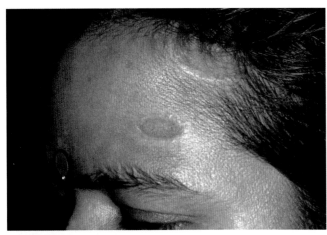

Fig. 21.15: Granuloma annulare: Two lesions over face
Note: The half of upper lesion is lying over hairy area.
Courtesy: Dr HK Kar, PGIMER, Dr RML Hospital, New Delhi.

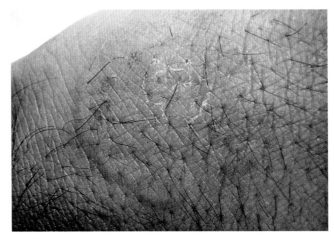

Fig. 21.18: Erythema annulare centrifugum

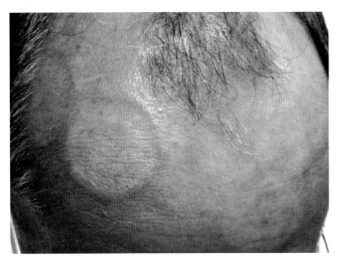

Fig. 21.16: Granuloma annulare—forehead

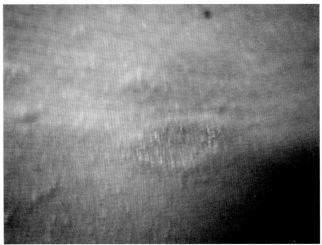

Fig. 21.19: Pityriasis rosea: Herald patch

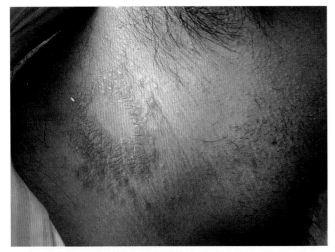

Fig. 21.17: Nummular eczema: Annular lesion, side of neck

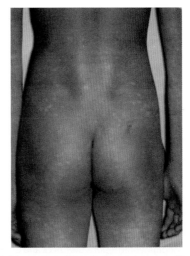

Fig. 21.20: Leishmaniasis: Macular hypopigmented lesions of PKDL
Courtesy: Dr HK Kar, PGIMER, Dr RML Hospital, New Delhi.

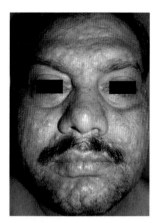

Fig. 21.21: Papulonodular lesions of post-kala-azar dermal leishmaniasis over face. Mimics nodular lesions of lepromatous leprosy
Courtesy: Dr V Ramesh, VM Medical College and Safdarjung Hospital, New Delhi.

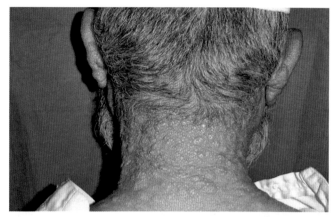

Fig. 21.24: Post-kala-azar dermal leishmaniasis: Papules and nodules over nape of the neck. Note the earlobe infiltrations, overall picture mimicking lepromatous leprosy
Courtesy: Dr HK Kar, PGIMER, Dr RML Hospital, New Delhi.

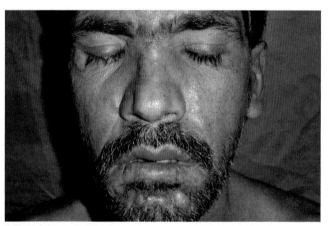

Fig. 21.22: Papulonodular lesions of post-kala-azar dermal leishmaniasis over face
Courtesy: Dr HK Kar, PGIMER, Dr RML Hospital, New Delhi.

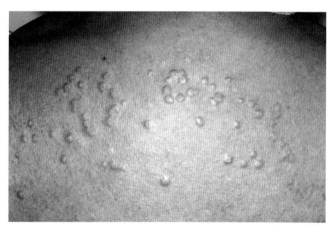

Fig. 21.25: Sarcoidosis: Papular lesions

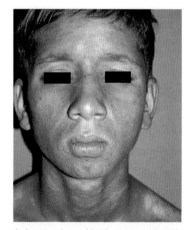

Fig. 21.23: Post-kala-azar dermal leishmaniasis: Papules and infiltration over face; and hypopigmented lesions over neck and upper chest
Courtesy: Dr V Ramesh, VM Medical College and Safdarjung Hospital, New Delhi.

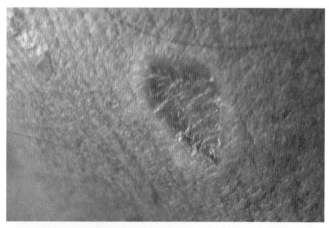

Fig. 21.26: Sarcoidosis: Atrophic plaque mimics tuberculoid leprosy

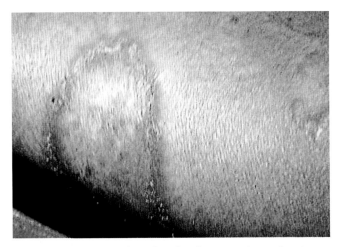

Fig. 21.27: Sarcoidosis: Annular plaque may be confused with tuberculoid leprosy

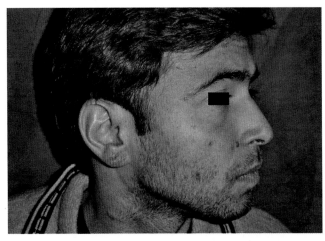

Fig. 21.30: Sarcoidosis: Erythematous infiltrated papules and plaques, note the earlobe infiltration
Courtesy: Dr HK Kar, PGIMER, Dr RML Hospital, New Delhi.

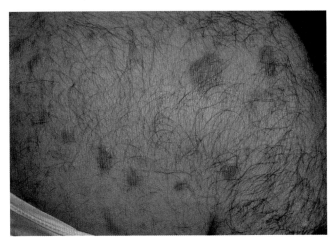

Fig. 21.28: Sarcoidosis: Multiple erythematous papules and plaques with tendency towards symmetry, can be confused with borderline lepromatous leprosy

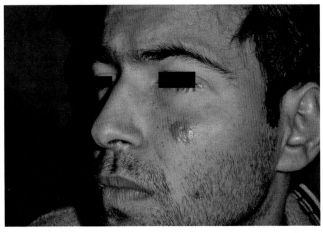

Fig. 21.31: Sarcoidosis: Erythematous infiltrated papules and plaques over face

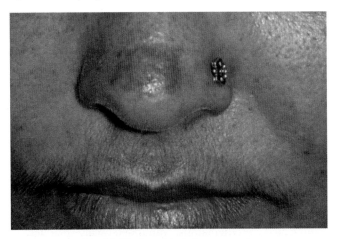

Fig. 21.29: Sarcoidosis: Lupus pernio
Courtesy: Dr HK Kar, PGIMER, Dr RML Hospital, New Delhi.

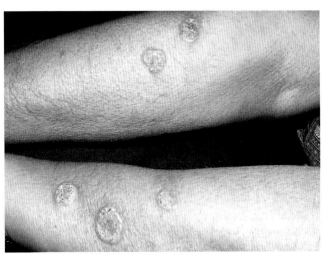

Fig. 21.32: Sarcoidosis—annular lesions

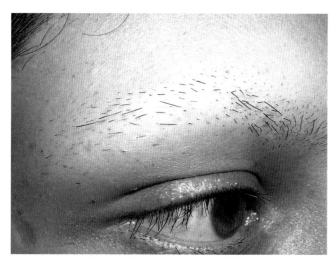

Fig. 21.33: Alopecia alreata: Loss of eyebrow

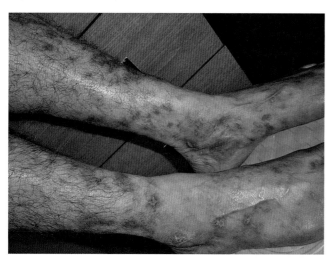

Fig. 21.34: Small vessel vasculitis lower legs

or being treated (Fig. 21.2). However, in such a scenario, the lesions will not show sensory impairment, hair loss or decreased sweating. Similarly, the skin texture in vitiligo lesion will be normal except for some of the lesions which have been partially treated and the surface may show atrophy or thickening depending upon nature of the treatment. History, absence of cardinal features of leprosy help in differentiating these cases. Rarely skin biopsy may be required.

NEVUS ACHROMICUS/NEVUS ANEMICUS

Nevus achromicus is a circumscribed area of hypomelanosis usually present at birth, sometimes have bizarre shapes and show a variable degree of hypopigmentation. The lesion is usually single or occasionally multiple and has feathery, serrated well-defined borders (Fig. 21.35). The texture

and character of the skin is otherwise normal. It does not disappear on diascopy.

Nevus anemicus on the other hand is a vascular anomaly where the vasculature in a circumscribed area is pharmacologically abnormal and produces a hypopigmented area. The lesion of nevus anemicus disappears on diascopy. Some of these birth marks may fade slowly over years, but unlike leprosy, characteristically they do not change their appearance or extent.

ACQUIRED HYPOMELANOSIS

There are numerous causes of acquired hypomelanosis. Endocrinal abnormalities, nutritional and chemical factors may produce hypopigmented lesions. Frequently, hypomelanotic lesions may follow some inflammatory conditions (Fig. 21.36) like psoriasis (Fig. 21.37), eczema (Figs 21.38 to 21.40) syphilis, pinta, yaws, lichen planus, lupus erythematosus (Fig. 21.41) or sarcoidosis. Long-term use of potent topical corticosteroids or their intralesional administration (Fig. 21.42) can sometimes produce cutaneous hypomelanosis and atrophy. A careful history and morphology of lesions may elicit their origin.

CONTACT LEUKODERMA

A number of chemicals can produce hypopigmented to depigmented lesions, which may mimic leprosy lesions. Chemicals often used in rubbers, footwears, cosmetics or apparels may produce hypopigmentation or depigmentation called contact leukoderma that may occasionally simulate leprosy lesions. However, in contact leukoderma distribution of the lesions depends upon the site and type of contact with the chemical, for instance, they are on the hands in occupational leukoderma due to latex gloves, and on feet in case of footwear contact leukoderma, and on the forehead in case of "Bindi", or vermilion contact leukoderma.

PITYRIASIS VERSICOLOR

The lesions in pityriasis versicolor are small, smaller than leprosy macules, hypopigmented and show fawn colored fine scaling. Lesions are asymptomatic and individual lesions are discrete, but often fuse to form large lesions mimicking leprosy. However, they do not show any impairment of sensations or hair loss. A potassium hydroxide (KOH) mount from scales will reveal short, unbranched hyphae and spores in characteristic arrangement.

PSORIASIS

Chronic plaque psoriasis is characterized clinically by well-demarcated, erythematous, infiltrated scaly plaques of variable size and shape which may mimic leprosy lesions,

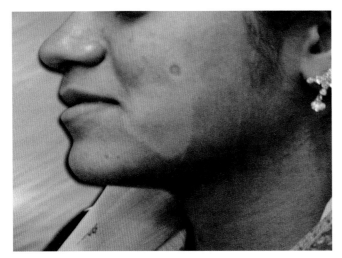

Fig. 21.35: Nevus dyschromicus
Courtesy: Dr HK Kar, PGIMER, Dr RML Hospital, New Delhi.

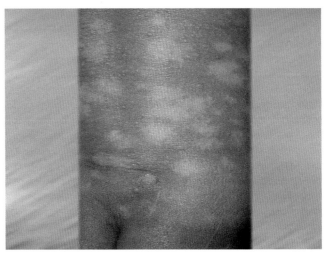

Fig. 21.38: Postinflammatory hypopigmentation (PIH): After healing of lesions of atopic dermatitis in a child

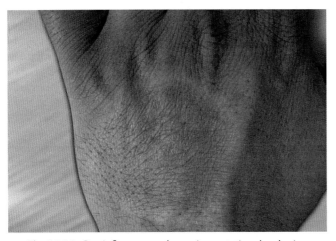

Fig. 21.36: Postinflammatory hypopigmentation developing after healing at trauma site

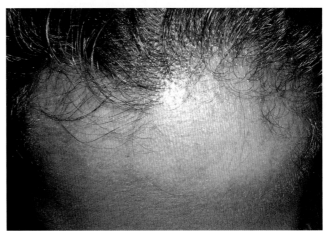

Fig. 21.39: Seborrheic dermatitis—hypopigmented lesions over forehead

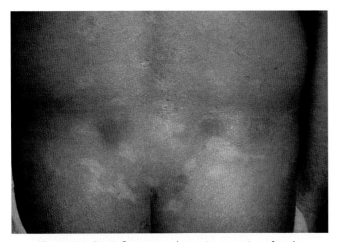

Fig. 21.37: Postinflammatory hypopigmentation after the healed lesions of psoriasis
Courtesy: Dr HK Kar, PGIMER, Dr RML Hospital, New Delhi.

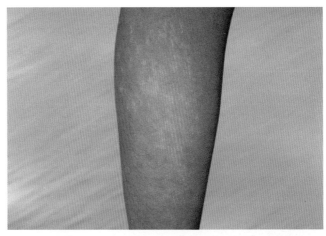

Fig. 21.40: Lichen striatus—hypopigmented lesions over leg

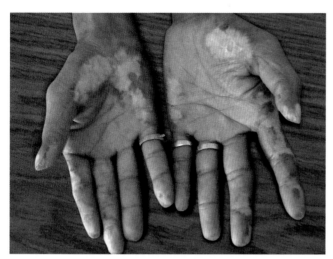

Fig. 21.41: Discoid lupus erythematosus

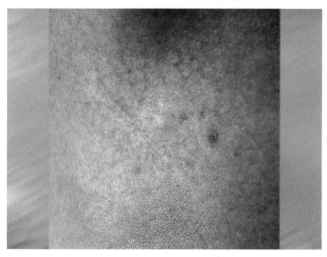

Fig. 21.42: Postinflammatory hypopigmentation at the site of infiltration with corticosteroids

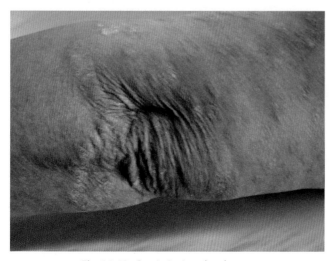

Fig. 21.43: Psoriasis: Annular plaques

especially when in reaction (Figs 21.43 to 21.45). Following therapy or otherwise resolving psoriasis lesion may leave hypopigmentation in a patchy pattern (Fig. 21.42) which may also be confused with hypopigmented leprosy lesions. The lesions of psoriasis will have characteristic silvery scales which can be scrapped off with ease unmasking fine bleeding papillae (Auspitz sign), normal sensations, normal hair, no nerve thickening or acid fast bacilli in slit-skin smears. The erythrodermic psoriasis can sometimes lead to hair loss, which may lead to confusion with hair loss of leprosy, i.e. madarosis (Fig. 21.46).

CUTANEOUS SARCOIDOSIS

It is a chronic multisystem disease of unknown etiology characterized by variability of presenting lesions (Figs 21.25 to 21.32), viz. papules, (Fig. 21.25), plaques (Figs 21.26 to 21.31), nodules, ichthyotic, psoriasiform and keloidal lesions, some lesions taking annular (Figs 21.27 and 21.32) or polycyclic shapes. The disease may affect skin, eyes, heart, lungs and nervous system. The lesions of sarcoidosis have almost similar morphology to that of leprosy lesions. They are chronic, mostly asymptomatic, and of granulomatous nature. Papules or plaques forming annular or polycyclic shapes closely resemble tuberculoid or borderline leprosy. Ichthyotic sarcoidosis may closely mimic similar skin changes seen in leprosy. However, there is no loss of sensations or nerve thickening. Skin-slit smear examination will show no acid-fast bacilli and histology shows compact well-circumscribed granulomas, devoid of lymphocytic rim (naked granuloma) and absence of central caseation.

GRANULOMA ANNULARE

It is a disease of unknown etiology that is characterized by a ring of small, smooth flesh colored papules. It commonly occurs in young adults. The most common variant is seen over dorsa of hands as asymptomatic, skin colored, nonscaly, annular plaque with beaded margins and centrifugal extension. (Figs 21.14 to 21.16). The disseminated variety has multiple such lesions. Localized annular variant needs differentiation from the tuberculoid or borderline tuberculoid leprosy; and the generalized variant from lepromatous leprosy. There is no sensory deficit or nerve thickening. Biopsy will help in making the diagnosis.

LEISHMANIASIS

Leishmaniasis is a chronic protozoal parasitic disease with a wide spectrum of presentation. Immunity of the individual as well as the nature of infecting parasite decides the morphology and course of the disease. There are numerous forms of leishmaniasis which can present real difficult situations in differentiating leprosy. Some countries have prevalence of both the diseases and similar epidemiological distribution.

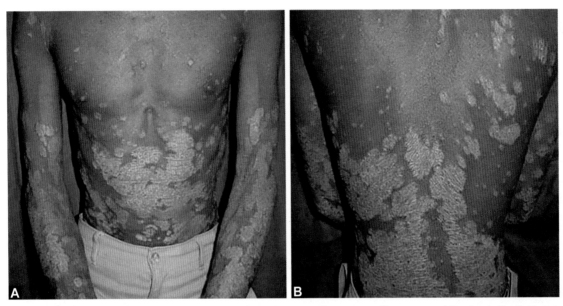

Figs 21.44A and B: Psoriasis: Erythematous scaly papules and plaque, some confluent; some discrete, resembling borderline lepromatous leprosy
Courtesy: Dr HK Kar, PGIMER, Dr RML Hospital, New Delhi.

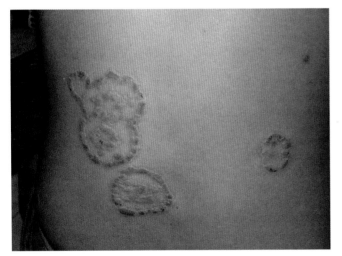

Fig. 21.45: Psoriasis—annular lesions

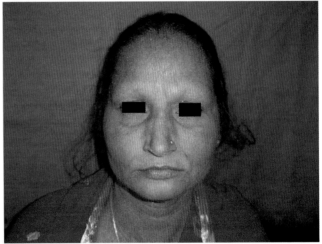

Fig. 21.46: Psoriasis: Madarosis in a case of psoriatic erythroderma, mimicking lepromatous leprosy
Courtesy: Dr Pankaj Sharma, PGIMER, Dr RML Hospital, New Delhi.

Cutaneous leishmaniasis may be of localized or disseminated variety. In localized form there are slowly progressive chronic granulomatous lesions. Morphology may be furuncle-like, atrophic plaque-like or infiltrated plaques over face and ear lobes. Nodular or noduloulcerative lesions (Figs 21.21 and 21.22), lupoid (Fig. 21.47) or crateriform (Fig. 21.48) lesions may be seen. The crateriform lesions have to be differentiated from the tuberculoid or borderline tuberculoid forms. The lesions of leishmaniasis do not show any abnormality of sensation or nerve thickening. Giemsa stained slit-skin smears will show amastigotes [Leishman Donovan (LD) bodies].

Disseminated cutaneous form of leishmaniasis will show nodular or plaque lesions and may even produce leonine facies. History of visiting endemic area, absence of nerve thickening or impairment of cutaneous sensitivity and demonstration of amastigotes in smears will help differentiation.

Post-kala-azar dermal leishmaniasis (PKDL), a late complication of visceral form of leishmaniasis is seen in

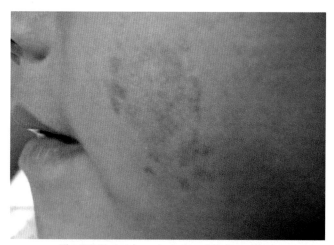

Fig. 21.47: Leishmaniasis: Lupoid lesions (face)

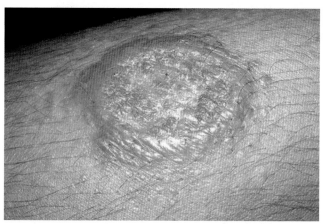

Fig. 21.48: Crateriform cutaneous leishmaniasis

India and Africa, where leprosy is also endemic. It has hypopigmented macules (Fig. 21.20) over trunk, noduloplaque lesions or diffuse infiltration of face and other body parts and even nodulation of pinna of ear (Fig. 21.21 to 21.24) closely simulating or even being wrongly treated as lepromatous leprosy. However, lesions in PKDL are mostly distributed towards midline and commonly involve orogenital mucous membranes. Cardinal signs of leprosy will help differentiation in most cases.

CUTANEOUS TUBERCULOSIS

Lupus vulgaris is a form of post-primary tuberculosis of variable morphology that occurs in patients with high degree of immunity. Usually starts as reddish-brown papule or nodule, which tend to heal at one edge and spread from another evolving into a plaque which may attain annular shape (Fig. 21.49). Tissue destruction and atrophic scarring

are the hallmarks of this disease. Such lesions may closely resemble the tuberculoid or borderline tuberculoid forms of leprosy. Absence of nerve involvement and impairment of sensations helps in differentiating the two conditions.

Tuberculids represent immunologic reactions to degenerated *Mycobacterium tuberculosis* or antigenic fragments deposited in the skin and subcutaneous tissue. The cutaneous lesions are a heterogeneous group and comprise true tuberculid where *M. tuberculosis* play significant role, viz., papulonecrotic tuberculid, lichen scrofulosorum and facultative tuberculid, i.e. erythema induratum of Bazin, which has the bacillus as one of the trigger. The papulonecrotic tuberculid lesions are asymptomatic or itchy, firm, erythematous, papulonodules occurring in crops and have central adherent crust. There are usually no systemic symptoms and it subsides spontaneously with hyperpigmentation and varioliform scar. Histopathology usually shows leukocytoclastic vasculitis, lymphocytic or granulomatous vasculitis with or without fibrinoid necrosis. Papulonodular lesions of lepromatous leprosy or ENL may sometimes mimic papulonecrotic tuberculids. Absence of cardinal signs of leprosy, histology showing vasculitis, response to antituberculosis treatment are the differentiating features.

LUPUS MILIARIS DISSEMINATIVE FACIEI

Lupus miliaris disseminative faciei (LMDF) is an uncommon, chronic, inflammatory dermatosis characterized by red, yellow or brown papules over the face (Fig. 21.50), particularly on and around the eyelids. The lesions may occur singly or in crops. Once considered a tuberculid because of the histology, many authors now consider LMDF to be a variant of granulomatous rosacea. Others believe it is a distinct entity because of its characteristic histopathology and occasional involvement of noncentral facial areas. The lesions can sometimes cause confusion with lepromatous leprosy or ENL lesions.

DISCOID LUPUS ERYTHEMATOSUS

Early lesions of discoid lupus erythematosus (DLE) over face can resemble tuberculoid leprosy plaque, especially before atrophy and scarring appears, but unlike leprosy DLE lesions have follicular plugging. Cardinal signs of leprosy will also be absent. Subacute cutaneous lupus erythematosus may attain polycyclic configuration resembling leprosy (Figs 21.41 and 21.51).

MALIGNANCIES

The malignant conditions like leukemias and lymphomas can sometime present with nodular infiltrated cutaneous lesions, which are difficult to differentiate from nodular lesions of

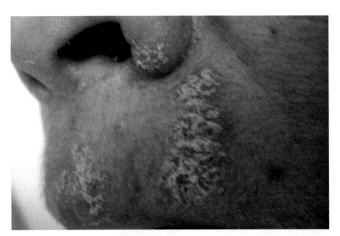

Fig. 21.49: Lupus vulgaris: Annular plaque with central atrophy

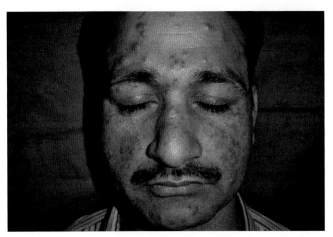

Fig. 21.50: Lupus miliaris disseminatus faciei. The papules and nodules over face mimic lesions of lepromatous leprosy, and also those of erythema nodosum leprosum (ENL)
Courtesy: Dr HK Kar, PGIMER, Dr RML Hospital, New Delhi.

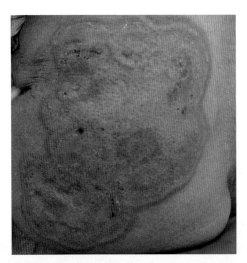

Fig. 21.51: Subacute cutaneous lupus erythematosus: Annular and polycyclic plaques

leprosy (Figs 21.9 and 21.52). General physical examination, hepatosplenomegaly, lymphadenopathy, or hematological findings would help arriving at the diagnosis. Cardinal signs of leprosy would be absent.

MISCELLANEOUS RARE CONDITIONS

Pseudochondritis has rarely been reported in leprosy. Thus, all the causes of chondrodermatitis must be kept in mind in the differential diagnosis of leprosy. Similarly bullous lesions are occasionally seen in leprosy. Although they may not occur as an isolated finding, but still clinician must be aware of this situation, especially if the disease is in reaction. Granulomatous swelling of lips in Melkersson Rosenthal syndrome may mimic as infiltration and may rarely cause confusion, especially if it is associated with facial nerve palsy. Nodular histiocytosis may mimic nodules of leprosy (Figs 21.53A and B). Lupoid sycosis barbae (Fig. 21.54) may simulate a patch of tuberculoid leprosy.

Interestingly, zoster like presentation of lepromatous leprosy in the form of erythematous nodules, and plaques over chest and abdomen in segmental distribution has been seen. This case compels to keep other zosteriform lesions in mind while dealing with leprosy. An unusual presentation of borderline tuberculoid leprosy with abnormal lip swelling resembling cheilitis granulomatosa has been reported.

Apart from dermatological conditions, a word needs to be mentioned about polyarthritis, an important differential diagnosis of leprosy. Salvi and Chopra (2013) from Pune reported two cases who presented with acute onset polyarthritis, skin rash and mild sensory neurodeficit to rheumatology clinic and were diagnosed as borderline lepromatous leprosy in type 1 reaction. They also refer to 19 cases in a database of 35,000 cases to highlight the missed diagnosis of Hansen's disease and its unusual association with rheumatoid arthritis.

SOME GENERAL POINTS TO REMEMBER

To avoid misdiagnosis, the clinicians also need to be familiar with normal range of skin color (erythema may not be very obvious in dark skin), local customs to treat skin diseases (cauterization of skin lesions can cause ulcers/scarring), local occupations (manual labor causes calluses or thickening of palmer skin) and social attitudes (social ostracism of leprosy patients often leads people to hide the disease) as all these may be altering the clinical picture and increase the difficulty in diagnosing leprosy or prevent patients from seeking treatment.

Two or more diseases presenting together may also pose diagnostic problem, e.g. patients with cutaneous leishmaniasis may also get leprosy and the skin lesions at

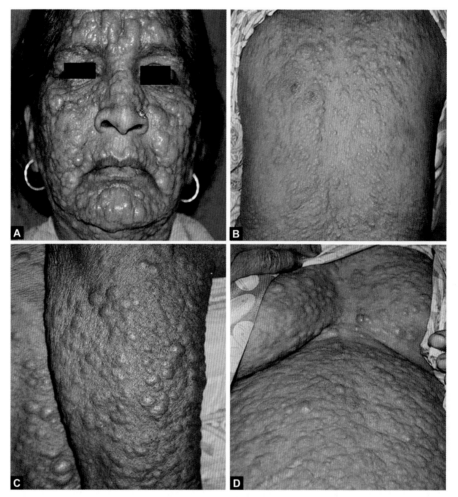

Figs 21.52 A to D: Acute myeloid leukemia: Multiple generalized nodular lesions involving face, limbs and trunk regions. The extensive infiltrated lesions over the face producing the "leonine facies" and can be confused with lepromatous leprosy. This patient died of the disease within 2 weeks of the diagnosis
Courtesy: Dr HK Kar, PGIMER, Dr RML Hospital, New Delhi.

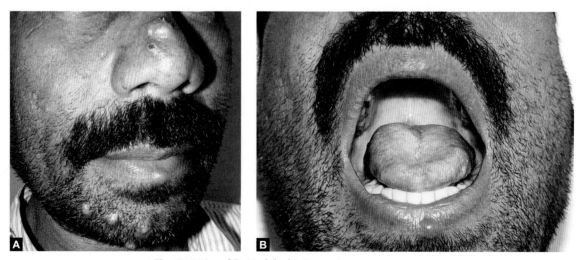

Figs 21.53A and B: Nodular histiocytosis

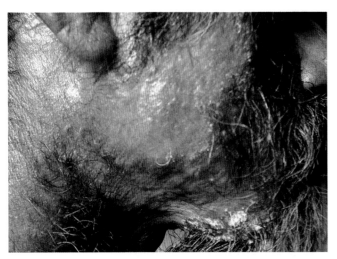

Fig. 21.54: Lupoid sycosis barbae

first look may appear confusing. It will be prudent to wait and watch in doubtful cases instead of treating for leprosy. A wrong diagnosis may cause social problems and difficulty in rehabilitation of these patients.

BIBLIOGRAPHY

1. Barman KD, Goel K, Agarwal P, et al. Lepromatous leprosy with an uncommon presentation: A case report. Indian J Lepr. 2013;85:27-31.
2. Burns T, Breathnach S, Cox N, Griffiths C. Rook's Textbook of Dermatology, 7th edition. Massachusetts: Blackwell Publishing Company; 2004.
3. Hastings RC, Opromolla DV. Leprosy, 2nd edition. Edinburgh: Churchill Livingstone; 1994.
4. Liu D, Li G, Huang W, et al. Analysis of newly detected leprosy cases and misdiagnosis in Wuhan. Lepr Rev. 2009;80:410-5.
5. Maroja MF, Lima LL, Pereira PM, et al. Zoster-like segmental presentation of lepromatous. Lep Rev. 2010;81:224-7.
6. Moulick A, Jana A, Sarkar N, et al. Non pitting edema, arthiritis and ichthyosis; presenting manifestation of leprosy. Indian J Lepr. 2013;85:83-6.
7. Rao R, Kaur GJ, Rao AC, et al. Borderline leprosy masquerading as cheilitis granulomatosa: A case report. Lepr Rev. 2013; 84:95-9.
8. Salvi S, Chopra A. Leprosy in a rheumatology setting: a challenging mimic to expose. Clin Rheumatol. 2013;32:1557-63.
9. Subbarao NT, Jaiswal AK. A case of leprosy with multiple cranial neuropathy mimicking Melkerson Rosenthal syndrome. Indian J Lepr. 2011;83:101-2.
10. Yawalkar SJ. Leprosy for Medical Practitioners, 5th edition. Basle: Ciba Geigy Limited; 1992.

Differential Diagnosis of Neurological Disorders in Relation to Leprosy

Bela J Shah

INTRODUCTION

Peripheral neuropathy is one of the manifestations of a number of disorders in which there is damage to the peripheral nerves (not involving the brain or the spinal cord). It can be due to host of different causes like nutritional, toxic, metabolic, trauma, etc. but in few cases, the cause remains unknown. The most common cause is diabetes mellitus in India. Of the infectious causes, leprosy is the most common of treatable neuropathies. The job of the dermatologists should not be restricted to simply rule out Hansen's disease, but it should be much more. Very often, patients with neuropathy are referred by the physicians; hence we must possess a thorough knowledge and skill so that we can differentiate other disorders which may present with similar features.

Neuropathies are broadly divided into two types:
1. *Affecting the sensory component*: Patient presents with loss or alteration of the sensations
2. *Affecting the motor component*: Patient presents with weakness or paralysis.

Other types are:
- *Mixed type*: Patient presents with both sensory and motor component
- *Areflexic or hyporeflexic neuropathy*: Patient has normal sensory and motor functions but loses the reflex action
- *Autonomic type (dysautonomia)*: Classically presents as postural hypotension, may also present with sphincter abnormalities and impotence.

PATTERNS OF NEUROPATHY

The four patterns of peripheral neuropathy are:
1. *Polyneuropathy*: Involvement of multiple nerves, often symmetric, seen mostly affecting extremities as seen in diabetic polyneuropathy
2. *Mononeuropathy*: Involvement of a single nerve as seen in carpal tunnel syndrome
3. *Mononeuritis multiplex*: It is also known as polyneuritis multiplexa, defined as the simultaneous and asynchronous involvement of more than one nerves in disparate body areas as in vasculitic neuropathy.
4. *Autonomic neuropathy*: Involvement of nerves that supply the body viscera via sympathetic and parasympathetic supply, as in amyloid and hereditary sensory and autonomic neuropathy (HSAN).

Among these, the most common form is (symmetrical) peripheral polyneuropathy, mainly referred to as the "glove and stocking" neuropathy (Fig. 22.1).

Another classification of the pattern of neuropathy depends on the size of the nerve fibers involved:
- *Large fiber peripheral neuropathy*: Leprosy, chronic inflammatory demyelinating polyradiculoneuropathy (CIDP), acromegaly, entrapment neuropathy, etc.
- *Small fiber peripheral neuropathy*: Most common cause is diabetes mellitus.[1] Other causes include human immunodeficiency virus (HIV) neuropathy, alcoholic neuropathy, etc.

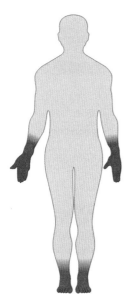

Fig. 22.1: Depicting glove and stocking distribution of neuropathy

Neuropathy may also be classified on the basis of the onset of symptoms:

- Acute neuropathy, as seen in trauma, Bell's palsy, *Guillain-Barré syndrome (GBS)*, porphyrias or toxic neuropathies due to poisoning, etc.
- Chronic neuropathy, e.g. diabetes mellitus, leprosy, sarcoidosis, familial polyneuropathies, nutritional, or neuropathy associated with malignancy, etc.

EPIDEMIOLOGY

The incidence of peripheral neuropathy is not known, but it is a common feature of many systemic diseases. Diabetes mellitus (27%) and alcoholism are the most common etiologies of peripheral neuropathy in adults. The most common worldwide cause of treatable neuropathy is leprosy.[2] The number of peripheral neuropathies for which an etiology cannot be found despite extensive evaluation ranges from 13% to 22%.[3,4] The population prevalence worldwide is about 2,400/100,000 (2.4%), rising with age to 8,000/100,000 (8%) in adults above 55 years.[5]

BASIC ANATOMY

Nerves are composed of different types of axons:
- Large, myelinated axons include motor axons and the sensory axons responsible for vibration sense, proprioception and light touch.
- Small myelinated axons are composed of autonomic fibers and sensory axons which are responsible for light touch, pain and temperature.

- Small, unmyelinated axons are also sensory and help in pain and temperature perception.

So to differentiate clinically large-fiber neuropathies from small-fiber neuropathies one has to remember that large fibers carry "sensation for vibration and proprioception," while small fibers carry "sensation for pain and temperature." Sensation for light touch is carried by both large and small nerve fibers.

PATHOPHYSIOLOGY

Although there are multiple etiologies for neural damage, but only three types of mechanisms are recognized:

1. *Wallerian degeneration (also known as anterograde or orthograde degeneration)*: Wallerian degeneration is a process that occurs on cutting or crushing of a nerve (Box 22.1), wherein distal to the injury the axonal part separated from the cell body of the neuron degenerates. This process begins within 24–36 hours.[6] It has been postulated that it is the failure to deliver sufficient quantities of the essential axonal protein NMNAT2 which is a key initiating event.[7] The axonal degeneration is followed by degradation of the myelin sheath and infiltration by macrophages which clear the debris. The neurolemma does not degenerate and remains as a hollow tube (Fig. 22.2).

2. *Axonal degeneration—dying back neuropathy*: It is the most common response of neurons to metabolic or toxic disturbances. The most distal portions of axons are usually the first to degenerate and axonal atrophy advances slowly

---

Box 22.1: Peripheral nerve injury classification (Figs 22.2 and 22.3)

Neuropraxia: This is the least severe form of nerve injury, where complete recovery occurs. In this case, the actual structure of the nerve remains intact, but there is an interruption in conduction of the impulse down the nerve fiber. Most commonly, this involves compression of the nerve or disruption to the blood supply (ischemia). There is a temporary loss of function which is reversible within hours to months of the injury (the average is 6–9 weeks). Wallerian degeneration does not occur, so recovery does not involve actual regeneration.

Axonotmesis: This is a more severe nerve injury with disruption of the neuronal axon, but with maintenance of the myelin sheath. If the force creating the nerve damage is removed in a timely fashion, the axon may regenerate, leading to recovery.

Neurotmesis: Neurotmesis is the most severe lesion with least potential of recovering. It occurs on severe contusion, stretch, laceration, or local anesthetic toxicity, not only to the axon, but the encapsulating connective tissue also, in their continuity. If the nerve has been completely divided, axonal regeneration causes a neuroma to form in the proximal stump.

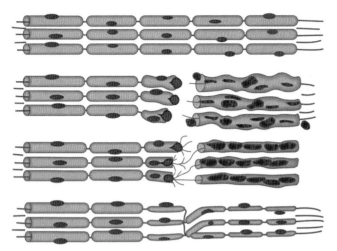

Fig. 22.2: Normal nerve. On transaction, Wallerian degeneration begins followed by sprouting of proximal nerve terminals followed by neurogenic arrangement to restore the nerve function

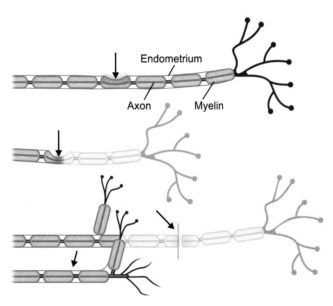

Fig. 22.3: Top part of figure shows neuropraxia wherein the actual structure of the nerve is intact and only the conduction is impaired due to an external pressure (arrow). The middle part shows axonotmesis with axonal disruption as well (arrow). The bottom part shows neurotmesis where there is total discontinuity in the nerve (arrow)

toward the cell body of the nerve (Fig. 22.4). If the cause is removed, regeneration is possible, though the prognosis depends on the duration and severity of the stimulus.

3. *Demyelination*: Also known as myelinopathy or "demyelinating polyneuropathy," is due to a loss of myelin. This demyelination slows down or completely blocks the conduction of action potentials through the axon of the nerve cell. The most common cause is acute inflammatory

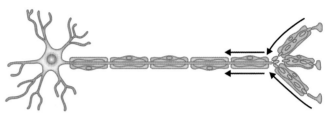

Fig. 22.4: Axonal degeneration—dying back neuropathy

demyelinating polyneuropathy; others may be infections, autoimmune or iatrogenic.

BASIC TERMINOLOGY[8]

- *Allodynia*: Pain sensation induced by nonpainful stimulus, further classified as dynamic (brush evoked) or static (pressure evoked).
- *Dysesthesias*: An abnormal or unpleasant sensation, whether spontaneous or evoked.
- *Hyperesthesia*: An increased pain response to a stimulus which is normally painful.
- *Paresthesias*: An abnormal, although not unpleasant sensation, whether spontaneous or evoked.

DIAGNOSTIC APPROACH[9,10]

A structured diagnostic approach can increase the diagnostic yield. The following algorithm can be of great help to come to a diagnosis (Flow chart 22.1):

HISTORY[8-10]

The course of a neuropathy varies, based on the etiology. Hence, the first step to reach the diagnosis is to ask the onset, duration and progression of symptoms as with trauma or ischemic infarction, the onset will be acute, with most severe symptoms at onset, whereas in inflammatory and metabolic neuropathies there is a subacute course extending over days to weeks. A chronic course over weeks to months is the hallmark of most of the toxic and metabolic neuropathies. A chronic, slowly progressive neuropathy over many years occurs with diabetes mellitus connective tissue disorders, nutritional deficiencies, most hereditary neuropathies and with CIDP. Neuropathies with a relapsing and remitting course include GBS.

The symptoms and signs of neuropathy not only suggest the presence and pattern of neuropathy but may also indicate the type of axons involved and its possible etiology as indicated below:

Neuropathies Predominant in Upper Limbs

- Guillain-Barré syndrome
- Diabetes mellitus
- Porphyrias

Flow chart 22.1: Diagnostic approach to peripheral neuropathy

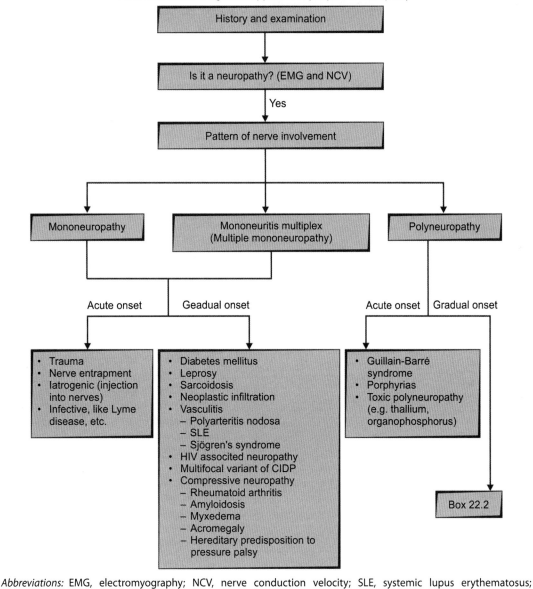

Abbreviations: EMG, electromyography; NCV, nerve conduction velocity; SLE, systemic lupus erythematosus; HIV, human immunodeficiency; CIDP, chronic inflammatory demyelinating polyneuropathy.

- Hereditary sensory neuropathy
- Vitamin B_{12} deficiency
- Hereditary amyloid neuropathy type II
- Lead neuropathy.

Clues to the Diagnosis

- With significant pain:
    - Diabetes mellitus
    - Vasculitis

- Amyloidosis
- HIV-related distal symmetric polyneuropathy
- Alcohol neuropathy
- Toxic neuropathy
- Idiopathic distal small-fiber neuropathy
- Predominantly sensory:
    - Cisplatin toxicity
    - Sjögren's syndrome
    - Paraproteinemia
    - Leprosy

Box 22.2: Polyneuropathies with gradual onset

- Endocrine disorders
  - Diabetes mellitus
  - Hypothyroidism
  - Acromegaly
- Nutritional disorders
  - Alcoholism, thiamine deficiency
  - B_{12} deficiency
  - Folate deficiency
  - Whipple's disease, postgastrectomy syndrome
  - Phosphate deficiency
- Malignancy
  - Lymphomas, multiple myeloma, Waldenstrom macroglobulinemia
- Connective tissue diseases
  - Rheumatoid arthritis
  - Polyarteritis nodosa
  - Systemic lupus erythematosus
  - Churg-strauss vasculitis
  - Cryoglobulinemic vasculitis
- Metabolic anomalies
  - Amyloidosis
  - Gouty neuropathy
- Infectious diseases
  - Leprosy
  - HIV
  - Lyme disease
  - Diphtheria
  - Tabes dorsalis
- Toxic neuropathy
  - Acrylamide
  - Ethylene oxide
  - Carbon monoxide
  - Glue sniffing
  - Heavy metals like arsenic, mercury, gold, thallium
  - Organophosphorus poisoning
- Iatrogenic[11]
  - Vincristine
  - Paclitaxel
  - Nitrous oxide
  - Colchicine
  - Isoniazid
  - Hydralazine
  - Metronidazole
  - Pyridoxine
  - Didanosine
  - Lithium
  - Interferon alpha
  - Dapsone
  - Phenytoin
  - Cimetidine
  - Disulfiram
  - Chloroquine
  - Ethambutol
  - Amiodarone
  - Amitriptyline
  - Gold
  - Thalidomide
  - Cisplastin
- Familial polyneuropathy

- Predominantly motor:
  - GBS
  - CIDP
  - HMSN
  - Porphyria
  - Vincristine
  - Dapsone, etc.
- Involving autonomic nervous system
  - Diabetes mellitus
  - Amyloidosis
  - GBS
  - Porphyria
- Cranial nerves involved:
  - Diabetes mellitus
  - GBS
  - HIV
  - Lyme disease
  - Sjögren's syndrome
  - Sarcoidosis

Ischemic neuropathies often have pain as a prominent feature. Small-fiber neuropathies often present with burning pain, lightning-like or lancinating pain, aching, or uncomfortable paresthesias (dysesthesias). Patients may complain of pain with innocuous stimuli such as sheets rubbing over their feet (allodynia). They may also describe a tight, band-like sensation around the ankles or wrists. Sensory symptoms include tingling or paresthesias, hyperesthesia and numbness or reduced sensation. Proximal muscle involvement should be checked by asking for any difficulty in climbing stairs, getting out of a chair, lifting or combing hair. This helps to rule out myopathies wherein the deficit is usually proximal.

The clinical assessment should also include a careful past medical history, looking for systemic diseases that can be associated with neuropathy, such as diabetes or hypothyroidism. Any use of medications that can cause a peripheral neuropathy should be thoroughly enquired. Detailed enquiries about drug and alcohol use, as well as exposure to heavy metals and solvents, should be asked. All patients should be questioned regarding HIV risk factors, diet and the possibility of a tick bite (Lyme disease).

The specific points which indicate the presence of Hansen's disease have to be enquired like history of skin lesions, epistaxis, pedal edema, reactional episodes, any deformity or disability and if there is any history of contact in the family or outside.

PHYSICAL EXAMINATION

- Peripheral and cranial nerve examination should always be carried out as cranial nerve involvement can be seen in leprosy, diabetes mellitus, GBS, HIV/AIDS neuropathy, Lyme disease, sarcoidosis, and diphtheria, etc.
- Fundoscopic examination may show abnormalities such as optic pallor, which can be present in leukodystrophies and vitamin B_{12} deficiency.

- Testing of muscle power enervated by cranial nerves V, VII, IX/X, XI and XII is important, as mild bilateral weakness can be missed by observation only.
- All the peripheral sensations, viz. pain, temperature, touch, vibration sense and proprioception should be checked.
- The motor examination includes testing for tone, bulk, power, a search for fasciculations or cramps, and the pattern of weakness: symmetric or asymmetric, distal or proximal, and confined to a particular nerve, plexus or root level.
- Deep tendon reflexes must always be elicited
- Any trophic changes:
  Radiographic examination of limbs may show loss of bone density, thinning of phalanges, pathologic fractures or neuropathic arthropathy. Trophic changes are most prominent in leprosy, diabetes, amyloid neuropathy, hereditary motor sensory neuropathy (HMSN) with prominent sensory involvement, and hereditary sensory neuropathy.
- Nerve thickening is found in leprosy, HMSN type 1, amyloid neuropathy, neurofibromatosis and Dejerine-Sottas syndrome (familial hypertrophic peripheral neuropathy).
- Last but not the least, a complete spine and foot examination is a must to look for pes cavus, spina bifida, etc.

General physical examination can provide evidence of orthostatic hypotension without a compensatory rise in heart rate when autonomic fibers are involved. Respiratory rate and vital capacity should be evaluated in GBS to assess for respiratory compromise. The presence of lymphadenopathy, hepatomegaly or splenomegaly, and skin lesions may provide evidence of a systemic disease. Pale transverse bands in the nail beds, parallel to the lunula (Mees' lines), suggest arsenic poisoning.

LABORATORY TESTING

- Complete blood count
- Liver and kidney function tests
- Erythrocyte sedimentation rate
- Fasting blood glucose level, HbA1c or glucose tolerance test
- Thyroid-stimulating hormone level
- Vitamin B_{12} and folate level
- Hepatitis virus panel
- HIV serology
- Urine for heavy metal toxicity
- Antinuclear antibodies, perinuclear antineutrophil cytoplasmic antibody (P-ANCA), cytoplasmic antineutrophil cytoplasmic antibody (C-ANCA), Rh-factor
- *Nerve biopsy*: Indicated in asymmetric polyneuropathy, abnormal nerve conduction study (NCS).

VARIOUS NEUROPATHIC DISORDERS

Mononeuropathies

Carpal Tunnel Syndrome

Median nerve passes through a narrow passageway at the wrist. Pressure on this nerve causes pain and abnormal sensations in lateral three fingers, the radial side of palmar aspect of hand and wrist, and is relieved by hanging the arm down and shaking the hand. In long standing cases, there is wasting of the thenar eminence and weakness of abductor pollicis brevis and opponens pollicis muscles (Figs 22.5 and 22.6).

Ulnar Nerve Palsy (Figs 22.7 and 22.8)

Ulnar nerve a mixed nerve passes through the groove between the medial epicondyle and the olecranon process close to the surface of the skin at the elbow. The aponeurosis between the olecranon and medial epicondyle forms the roof of an osseofibrous canal (the cubital tunnel). The nerve is easily damaged by repeatedly leaning on the elbow resulting into tingling, pins-and-needles sensation in the little and ring fingers. Ulnar nerve palsy that results from more severe injury makes the nerve in the hand weak, ulnar nerve is the most common to be involved in leprosy. Severe, chronic ulnar nerve palsy can cause muscles to waste away (atrophy), resulting in a claw hand deformity. Avoiding pressure on the elbow is recommended.

Radial Nerve Palsy

Radial nerve, a mixed nerve, passes between the long and medial heads of the triceps and then through the spiral groove of the humerus. Radial nerve is not very often involved in

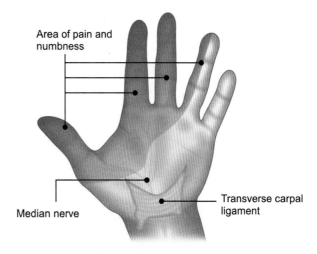

Fig. 22.5: Involvement of lateral three fingers in carpal tunnel syndrome

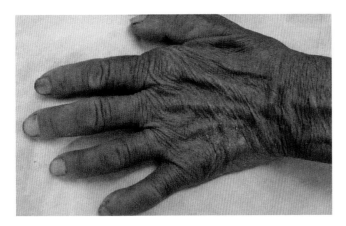

Fig. 22.6: Wasting of muscles in carpal tunnel syndrome

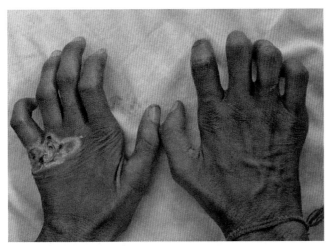

Fig. 22.7: Clawing of hand due to ulnar nerve palsy

leprosy, but distally the radial cutaneous nerve is more often involved. Prolonged pressure on this nerve results in radial nerve palsy. This disorder is sometimes called "Saturday night palsy" because it occurs in people who drink heavily (often during weekends) and then sleep soundly with an arm draped over the back of a chair or under their partner's head. If crutches fit incorrectly and press on the inside of the arm near the armpit, they can cause this disorder. The nerve damage weakens the wrist and fingers so that the wrist may flop into a bent position with the fingers curved known as wrist drop (Fig. 22.9). Occasionally, sensations are lost on the back of the hand. Usually, the palsy resolves once the pressure is relieved.

Peroneal Nerve Palsy

Peroneal nerve rounds the head of the fibula, passes close to the surface of the skin on the outer, lower part of the knee before entering the substance of the peroneous longus muscle. Pressure on this nerve results in peroneal nerve palsy. This disorder weakens the muscles that lift the foot, so the foot cannot be flexed upward, resulting in foot drop (Fig. 22.10). It is most common among thin people who are confined to bed, people who are incorrectly strapped into a wheelchair, and people who habitually cross their legs for long periods of time. Avoiding pressure on the nerve, for example, by avoiding crossing the legs—usually relieves the symptoms.

Sural Nerve

The sural (short saphenous nerve) a sensory nerve, is formed by the junction of the medial sural cutaneous with the peroneal anastomotic branch of the lateral sural cutaneous nerve. It passes downward near the lateral margin of the tendo calcaneus, lying close to the small saphenous vein, to the interval between the lateral malleolus and

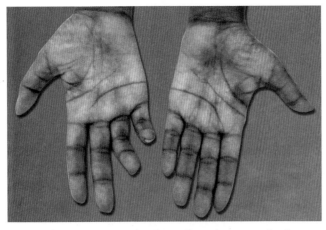

Fig. 22.8: Clawing and wasting of hypothenar muscles due to ulnar nerve palsy

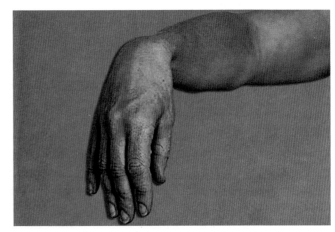

Fig. 22.9: The wrist drop due to radial nerve palsy

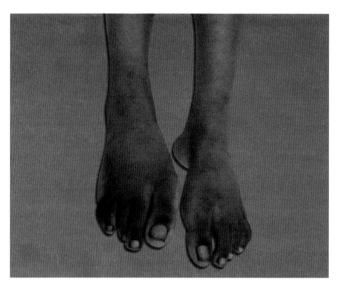

Fig. 22.10: Bilateral foot drop due to peroneal nerve involvement

the calcaneus. Removal or inflammation results in only a relatively trivial sensory deficit on most occasions, but may sometimes present with chronic pain in the posterior aspect of the leg, usually exacerbated with physical exertion.

Facial Nerve

It is the seventh cranial nerve and is known as the nerve of facial expression. Its important functions include innervations of muscles of facial expression, carrying the taste sensations of the anterior two-thirds of the tongue and supplying parasympathetic preganglionic fibers to various head and neck glands. The nerve emerges from brainstem between pons and medulla and enters the petrous temporal bone via the internal auditory meatus and then runs a tortuous course through the facial canal emerging from the stylomastoid foramen and passes through the parotid gland, where it divides into five major branches (Fig. 22.11). Bell's palsy, a type of acute idiopathic facial nerve palsy is the most common cause (>80%) of facial nerve paralysis (Fig. 22.12). Other causes include herpes zoster of the facial nerve (Ramsay-Hunt syndrome), stroke, tumors, trauma, multiple sclerosis, etc. The patient may present with inability to raise eyebrows, lagophthalmos, inability to whistle or blow, hyperacusis and loss of taste sensation from the anterior two-third of the tongue.

Supratochlear Nerve and Supraorbital Nerve

They are branches of frontal nerve which is a branch of ophthalmic division of fifth cranial nerve. The supratrochlear supplies the conjunctiva, medial upper lid, forehead and side of the nose. Supraorbital branch supplies the upper lid, conjunctiva, the forehead and the scalp. These are very commonly involved in patients of leprosy giving rise to a cord like thickening when palpated above the eyebrows.

Mononeuritis Multiplex

Mononeuritis multiplex is asymmetrical, asynchronous sensory and motor peripheral neuropathy involving isolated damage to at least two separate nerve areas. The neuritis sometimes is a painful condition. Common diseases causing mononeuritis multiplex are:
- Polyarteritis nodosa
- Diabetes mellitus
- Connective tissue diseases such as rheumatoid arthritis or SLE (the most common cause in children)
- Amyloidosis
- Paraneoplastic syndromes

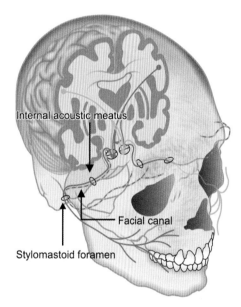

Fig. 22.11: Pathway of the facial nerve

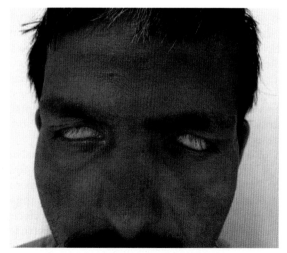

Fig. 22.12: Face of a patient suffering from facial nerve paralysis

- Blood disorders (such as hypereosinophilia and cryoglobulinemia)
- Lyme disease
- Leprosy
- Sarcoidosis
- Symptoms will depend on the specific nerves involved, and may include:
  - Loss of bladder or bowel control
  - Loss of sensation in one or more areas of the body
  - Paralysis in one or more areas of the body
  - Tingling, burning, pain, or other abnormal sensations in one or more areas of the body. One important example of that is meralgia paraesthetica where due to involvement of the lateral cutaneous nerve of thigh, there is numbness or pain in the outer thigh
  - Weakness in one or more areas of the body.

Polyneuropathies

Brief has been given at the beginning.

Leprosy

Leprosy is the most common treatable cause of neuropathy in the world.[1] The pattern of leprosy neuropathy is classified under polyneuropathy. It starts as a demyelinating process and evolves to axonal damage. All three components of the peripheral nervous system are affected: (1) sensory, (2) motor and (3) autonomic. Sensory functions are most severely affected.

- Sensory loss causes anesthesia, analgesia, and inability to discriminate hot and cold.
- Motor deficit causes muscle weakness, paralysis, and atrophy. However, tendon jerks may be preserved till late.
- Damage to autonomic nerve fibers impairs sweating and causes dry skin.

Nerve damage directly caused by *M. leprae* is called primary impairment. The complications that result from nerve damage, e.g., ulcers, contractures, bone destruction, and shortening of fingers and toes, are called secondary impairments and may lead to a variety of disabilities and handicaps. When detected and treated early, primary impairments may be reversible. However, 11–51% of patients do not recover.[12] In addition, 33–56% of newly registered patients already have clinically detectable impairments.

Leprosy often has an insidious protracted course and may not be recognized early.

- In tuberculoid leprosy, involvement of small dermal nerves supplying the corresponding areas of the skin produces sensory loss over the patch or patches. Pain, temperature, touch and pressure sensations are typically impaired in affected skin areas. Vibration and proprioceptive sensations are spared until later, when finally nerve trunks are affected.

- In lepromatous leprosy, there is widespread symmetrical glove and stocking type of sensory loss due to involvement of peripheral nerve trunks. Patients with advanced lepromatous leprosy (both polar and subpolar) may have progressive symmetrical, distal peripheral polyneuropathy or damage to disparate nerve trunks and may produce a picture like mononeuritis multiplex.[13]
- Borderline leprosy has a propensity to involve nerve trunks, producing a picture of multiple mononeuropathies or mononeuritis multiplex. The most frequently affected peripheral nerves are peroneal and posterior tibial nerves in the lower extremities and ulnar nerve in the upper extremity. Patients with borderline leprosy have an unstable immune balance between the host's cell-mediated immunity and bacterial replication and can progress unpredictably to either pole.[14] A shift toward lepromatous pole (a downgrading), allows extensive proliferation of bacilli. Subsequent shift to the tuberculoid pole (an upgrading or reversal reaction), evokes an intense inflammatory response, resulting in extensive damage to the nerve trunks.[15]

During leprosy reactions, acute neuritis leads to pain, tenderness, and loss of nerve function. The main risk factor for the development of neuropathy is the presence of skin lesions overlying nerve trunks. Skin lesions overlying the nerve increase the risk of sensory or motor impairment by three to four times. Reactional signs in the cutaneous lesions further increase this risk to six to eight times. Therefore, patients with skin lesions overlying peripheral nerve trunks should be carefully monitored for development of sensory or motor impairment.

Silent neuropathy/quiet nerve paralysis is a clinical term used for slowly progressive neuropathy in leprosy wherein sensory or motor impairment occurs without signs of reaction, without nerve pain or tenderness (burning or shooting pain), paresthesia or numbness.[16] The patient is unaware of neuropathy until late. Ultimately, due to low grade inflammation, it results in fibrosis of the neural tissue. Occasionally, even in mild reversal reactions, nerve damage may be asymptomatic, and damage may progress silently for prolonged periods. Although it has been observed across the spectrum of leprosy, it is more common in the borderline group.

Patients with leprosy may also suffer from chronic neuropathic pain. Pain usually affects the distribution of one or more major nerves and may even have a symmetrical glove and stocking distribution. Anticonvulsants and tricyclic antidepressants are effective in reducing chronic neuropathic pain.[17]

Thickened peripheral nerve trunks are one of the cardinal manifestations of leprosy. As a general rule one should be cautious about accepting nerve thickening alone, without sensory loss, muscle weakness or skin changes, as a reliable sign of leprosy. In most of the patients, the ulnar nerve is the first to be affected and that too may be apparent only in the later stages of the disease. Nerve thickening may be uniform or it may have a beaded appearance. Unilateral peripheral nerve thickening may also be observed physiologically in patients with lean body mass and doing physical activities as in laborers and body builders but here there is no loss of sensation accompanying the nerve thickening. Other causes of nerve thickening are enumerated in Box 22.3.

Nerves which can be affected are:

Supraorbital nerve	Above the eyebrows
Greater auricular nerve	Winds around sternocleidomastoid
Supraclavicular nerve	Across the clavicle
Ulnar nerve	Behind medical epicondyle
Radial cutaneous nerve	Lower end of radius at wrist
Lateral popliteal nerve	Neck of fibula
Superficial peroneal nerve	Front of ankle
Posterior tibial nerve	Below medial malleolus

Nerve abscesses may occur in peripheral nerves in patients with leprosy. Caseation may occur in microscopic foci within the granulomas, or areas of necrosis may coalesce, forming a cold abscess, particularly when the immunity is high. Cold abscesses occur more frequently in the tuberculoid form, especially in India.[18] Once the nerve abscess has been detected, it has to be incised and drained without affecting the continuity of the nerve trunk; otherwise, it may rupture and drain through the skin.

Delayed peripheral nerve dysfunction can be seen long after the completion of multidrug therapy (MDT). Several patients have been described with progressive, symmetrical, predominantly sensory neuropathy and acute or subacute multiple mononeuropathy developing approximately 10 years after MDT. These patients with delayed neuropathy show limited response to corticosteroids.[19] Pathogenesis of delayed nerve impairment is not properly understood. Antigens from dead bacilli can provoke immunological reactions and late manifestations.

Among cranial nerves, facial and trigeminal nerves are the most frequently affected.[20] Facial skin lesions are associated with a 10-fold increase in the risk of facial nerve involvement.

Box 22.3: Differential diagnosis of peripheral nerve thickening include

- Diabetes mellitus
- Neurofibromatosis
- Refsum's disease
- Amyloidosis
- Acromegaly
- HSMN Type I (Charcot-Marie-Tooth disease): (Greater auricular nerve mostly)
- Autosomal dominant hypertrophic neuropathy

In leprosy facial nerve involvement is common and can be bilateral.[20,21] Involvement of zygomatic and temporal branches of facial nerve may result in lagophthalmos. Involvement of the ophthalmic division of trigeminal nerve may result in corneal and conjunctival sensory loss. With presence of lagophthalmos and a dry and insensitive cornea, there is an increased risk of corneal trauma, ulcerations, and eventually blindness. Among the risk factors, facial nerve involvement is associated with facial patches and also the type-1 leprosy reaction.

Motor involvement is less common than sensory involvement. Atrophy, weakness, and claw hand deformity are the most frequent motor complications seen in leprosy. In the lower extremities, unilateral or bilateral foot drop may occur secondary to involvement of superficial peroneal nerves around neck of the fibula. Posterior tibial nerve involvement may result in weakness and atrophy of intrinsic foot muscles.

Diabetes Mellitus

Diabetes is the most common cause of polyneuropathy in most countries. It is also by far the most common polyneuropathy to be associated with bowel, bladder, and erectile dysfunction.[22] Diabetes mellitus gives rise to a variety of peripheral neuropathies, but the most frequent is polyneuropathy.[22] Severity and manifestations are highly variable from being completely asymptomatic to a severe disabling neuropathy with marked wasting and weakness and impaired gait and hand function. Fortunately, severe neuropathies are relatively uncommon. Diabetic autonomic neuropathy is a frequent accompaniment of severe diabetic polyneuropathy. It is important to note that this can be restricted to certain organs or functions, or may be widespread, involving most or all of the autonomic nervous system.

Neurosarcoidosis

Sarcoidosis is a chronic, inflammatory, granulomatous disorder affecting the lungs most commonly, but may also present as a small fiber neuropathy. It occurs in patients having substantial systemic involvement with noncaseating granulomas in lymph nodes and various organs. Most patients present in fourth to fifth decade with complaints of multifocal peripheral hyperalgesia and allodynia. Cranial nerve involvement is also seen frequently with facial nerve being the most common nerve involved.[23] When facial neuropathy is associated with uveitis, fever and parotid gland enlargement, it is known as Heerfordt's Syndrome.

Amyloid Neuropathy

Amyloid is a proteinaceous substance, deposited in various tissues in certain disease states or as the result of a gene abnormality. There are various types of amyloidosis, but those manifesting as somatic and autonomic neuropathy are:

- Immunoglobulin amyloidosis
- Certain types of familial amyloidosis.

Immunoglobulin amyloidosis (now called AL, after the light chain proteins that constitute the amyloid) occurs either as a primary disorder, or associated with multiple myeloma, Waldenstrom's macroglobulinemia or non-Hodgkin's lymphoma. Polyneuropathy is initially of the "small fiber type". Painful paresthesiasis are, therefore, prominent, and examination shows a peripheral loss predominantly of pain and temperature sensations. There is involvement of motor functions later on. Carpal tunnel syndrome occurs in about a quarter of the patients.[24] The clinical course is relentless progression resulting in death within 5 years of the diagnosis due to renal, cardiac or gastrointestinal involvement by amyloid.

Porphyria

Porphyrias are hereditary disorders affecting hepatic heme metabolism. The four types with neurological manifestations are:

1. Acute intermittent porphyria
2. Variegate porphyria
3. Hereditary coproporphyria
4. δ-amino levulinic acid dehydratase deficiency.

Patients can have acute attacks of predominantly motor and often proximal neuropathy, in conjunction with psychiatric features and abdominal pain. Latter features often precede the neuropathy. Constipation, intestinal stasis and dilatation, micturition difficulties, orthostatic hypotension, paroxysmal hypertension and tachycardia may all be concurrent findings.

Guillain-Barré Syndrome

Also known as acute inflammatory demyelinating polyneuropathy (AIDP), patient presents with recent history of diarrhea or respiratory tract infection following which patient starts developing ascending paralysis, beginning in the feet and hand and migrating toward the trunk. Autonomic nervous system is frequently involved. Major fluctuations in blood pressure are common, consisting of both hypertension and hypotension. A variety of cardiac arrhythmias can occur, and may be responsible for sudden death in some patients. Anhidrosis occurs over the extremities. One should carefully watch for development of respiratory and pharyngeal muscle weakness, which necessitates admission in intensive care unit (ICU).

Syringomyelia

There is a cyst or a "syrinx" formation within the spinal cord which gradually enlarges to produce damage to the neural structures. The symptoms depend on the site and size of the syrinx. A classical presentation of "cape like" dissociated sensory loss with loss of pain and temperature over the back and arms is described but is not diagnostic. Although it develops gradually over time, acute development of symptoms is known with forceful coughing and straining. Syringomyelia may be congenitally present as seen with Arnold-Chiari malformations or may be acquired due to trauma, tumor, hemorrhage or arachnoiditis. A spinal computed tomography (CT) or magnetic resonance imaging (MRI) is required for diagnosis.

HEREDITARY NEUROPATHY

- Hereditary sensorimotor neuropathy
  - HSMN type I (peroneal muscle atrophy or Charcot-Marie-Tooth disease-type I)
  - HSMN type II (Charcot-Marie-Tooth disease axonal form)
  - HSMN type III (Dejerine Sotta's disease or Charcot-Marie–Tooth disease type III)
  - HSMN type IV (Refsum's syndrome)
- Hereditary sensory and autonomic neuropathy
  - HSAN type I (perforating foot ulcer disease, mutilating acropathy, insensitive foot disease)
  - HSAN type II (congenital sensory neuropathy, congenital absence of pain)
  - HSAN type III (dysautonomia or Riley-Day syndrome).

KEY POINTS

- Peripheral neuropathy has a variety of systemic, metabolic, infective and toxic causes. The most common treatable causes include Hansen's disease, diabetes mellitus, hypothyroidism, and nutritional deficiencies.
- The diagnosis requires careful clinical assessment, judicious laboratory testing, electrodiagnostic studies or biopsy.
- A systematic approach begins with localization of the lesion to the peripheral nerves, identification of the underlying etiology, and exclusion of potentially treatable causes.
- Initial blood tests should include a complete blood count, comprehensive metabolic profile, and measurement of erythrocyte sedimentation rate and fasting blood glucose, vitamin B_{12}, and thyroid-stimulating hormone levels; specialized tests should be ordered if clinically indicated.
- Lumbar puncture and cerebrospinal fluid analysis may be helpful in the diagnosis of GBS and chronic inflammatory demyelinating neuropathy.
- Electrodiagnostic studies, including nerve conduction studies and electromyography, can help in the differentiation of axonal versus demyelinating or mixed neuropathy.
- Treatment should address the underlying disease process, correct any nutritional deficiencies, and provide symptomatic treatment.

REFERENCES

1. Polydefkis M, Griffin JW, McArthur J. New insights into diabetic polyneuropathy. JAMA. 2003;290:1371-6.
2. Sabin TD, Swift TR, Jacobson RR. Leprosy. In: Dyck PJ, Thomas PK (Eds). Peripheral Neuropathy. Philadelphia: Saunders. 1993.pp.1354-79.
3. Asbury AK, Gilliatt RW. The clinical approach to neuropathy. In: Asbury AK, Gilliatt RW (Eds). Peripheral Nerve Disorders: A Practical Approach. London: Butterworths; 1984. pp. 1-20.
4. McLeod JG, Tuck RR, Pollard JD, et al. Chronic polyneuropathy of undetermined cause. J Neurol Neurosurg Psychiat. 1984;47:530-5.
5. Martyn CN, Hughes RAC. Epidemiology of peripheral neuropathy. J Neurol Neurosurg Psychiat. 1997;62:310-8.
6. Coleman MP, Freeman MR. Wallerian degeneration, wld(s), and nmnat. Annual Rev Neurosci. 2010;33:245-67.
7. Gilley J1, Coleman MP. Endogenous Nmnat2 is an essential survival factor for maintenance of healthy axons. PLoS Biol. 2010 Jan 26;8(1):e1000300.
8. International association for the study of pain taxonomy. http://www.iasp-pain.org/Education/Content.aspx?ItemNumber=1698.
9. Donofrio PD, Albers JW. AAEM minimonograph #34. Polyneuropathy: classification by nerve conduction studies and electromyography. Muscle Nerve. 1990;13:889-903.
10. Thomas PK, Ochoa J. Symptomatology and differential diagnosis of peripheral neuropathy. In: Dyck PJ, Thomas PK (Eds). Peripheral neuropathy. Philadelphia: Saunders. 1993. pp.749-74.
11. Weimer LH, Sachdev N. Update on medication-induced peripheral neuropathy. Curr Neurol Neurosci Rep. 2009;9:69-75.
12. Van Brakel WH. Peripheral neuropathy in leprosy and its consequences. Lepr Rev. 2000;71 (Suppl):S146-53.
13. Polston DW, Dyck PJ, Litchy WJ, et al. A 46-year-old man with numbness and shock-like sensations in hands, feet, and jaw. Lancet Neurol. 2004;3:63-7.
14. Boggild AK, Keystone JS, Kain KC. Leprosy: a primer for Canadian physicians. CMAJ. 2004;170:71-8.
15. Chad DA, Hedley-Whyte ET. Case records of the Massachusetts General Hospital. Weekly clinicopathological exercises. Case 1-2004. A 49-year-old woman with asymmetric painful neuropathy. N Engl J Med. 2004;350:166-76.
16. Srinivasan H, Rao KS. Steroid therapy in quiet nerve paralysis in leprosy. Indian J Lepr. 1982;54:412-9.
17. Haanpaa M, Lockwood DN, Hietaharju A. Neuropathic pain in leprosy. Lepr Rev. 2004;75:7-18.
18. Char G, Cross JN. Ulnar nerve abscess in Hansen's disease. West Indian Med J. 1986;35:66-8.
19. Rosenberg NR, Faber WR, Vermeulen M. Unexplained delayed nerve impairment in leprosy after treatment. Lepr Rev. 2003;74:357-65.
20. Gopinath DV, Thappa DM, Jaishankar TJ. A clinical study of the involvement of cranial nerves in leprosy. Indian J Lepr. 2004;76:1-9.
21. Inamdar AC, Palit A. Bilateral facial palsy in Hansen's disease. Lepr Rev. 2003;74:383-5.
22. Ewing DJ, Campbell IW, Clarke BF. The natural history of diabetic autonomic neuropathy. Q J Med. 1980;193:95-108.
23. Said G, Lacroix C, Plante-Bordeneuve V. Nerve granulomas and vasculitis in sarcoid peripheral neuropathy. Brain. 2002;125 (Pt 2): 264-75.
24. Benson M, Kincaid J. The molecular biology and clinical features of amyloid neuropathy. Muscle Nerve. 2007;36:411-23.

Systemic Involvement and Special Situations of Leprosy

CHAPTERS

23
CHAPTER

Systemic Involvement in Leprosy

V Ramesh, Joginder Kumar Kataria

CHAPTER OUTLINE

- Bacillemia in Leprosy
- Bones, Joints and Muscles
- Nail Involvement
- Eyes
- Upper Respiratory Tract (Nose, Paranasal Sinuses, Oral Cavity, Oropharynx, and Larynx)
- Lower Respiratory Tract
- Gastrointestinal Tract

- Reproductive System
- Kidneys
- Endocrine Glands
- Lymph Nodes, Bone Marrow, and Spleen
- Central Nervous System
- Cardiovascular System
- Hematology and Serology

INTRODUCTION

Leprosy is predominantly a disease of the skin and peripheral nerves. Conventional workbooks and manuals avoid discussing the systemic components of the infection. This does not mean that *Mycobacterium leprae* does not spread to other areas of the body. It does happen but the smouldering nature of the infection and lack of symptoms mask these occurrences. Consequently, systemic involvement has often been relegated to the pathologists in research institutions; or as a part of some academic work. In recent times, the effective use of multidrug therapy (MDT) has also rendered it redundant.

Systemic manifestations occur mostly toward the lepromatous pole of the spectrum and the number of such patients is very small. Moreover, the early institution of therapy halts the progression of systemic involvement. Nonetheless, awareness of systemic disease is important because apart from the paralytic deformities, some organs, like the eyes and bones, which bear the brunt of systemic infection can be damaged early, greatly impairing the quality of life. Patients of multibacillary leprosy, which include the borderline borderline, borderline lepromatous and lepromatous forms in the Ridley-Jopling classification in whom this could happen, will continue to be seen till eradication of the disease occurs and one should remain alert to these systemic manifestations. The patient rarely ever presents with symptoms pertaining exclusively to the involvement of internal organs though

most of them are found to be affected at autopsy/necropsy in lepromatous leprosy. The organisms disseminate to the internal organs through hematogenous route during the phase of bacillemia.

BACILLEMIA IN LEPROSY

Taking nasopharyngeal route as the main gateway to acquiring infection through inhalation,[1] the bacilli quickly migrate to cooler areas of the body with temperature lesser than 37°C, accounting for skin and peripheral nerves as the predominant sites of disease manifestations.[2] In multibacillary disease, the bacilli seem to override this preference and occupy the warmer sites too. In most individuals, the disease is arrested at a relatively early stage of entry of the bacilli into the axoplasm of the sensory nerves in the skin where the histiocytes transform into epithelioid cells and engulf the lepra bacilli, but in some patients with low resistance the infection progresses where histiocytes convert to lepra cells. Unchecked without treatment it becomes a systemic disease, and the organisms (either in the body of the histiocytes or flowing freely in the blood or lymph stream) are rapidly transported to distant parts of the body.[3] As many as 5×10^8 lepra bacilli circulate at any point of time in an untreated lepromatous leprosy patient and can be grown from blood inoculated in the footpads of mice.[4] Yet the remarkable silent nature of the infection is maintained as the bacilli do not secrete any toxins and so infection by lepra bacilli differs from other septicemic conditions which are characterized by fever, chills and coagulation anomalies.[5] Lepra bacilli, though less often, have also been demonstrated in the blood in indeterminate and tuberculoid forms too.[6] The frequency of bacillemia observed by some authors appears to be similar in both borderline and lepromatous forms of the disease, with the maximum number of bacilli seen at the lepromatous end of the spectrum.[7,8] The degree of bacillemia does not correlate well with the bacterial load in the skin and often has been detected in patients with negative slit-skin smears.

Histopathological studies demonstrating the presence of bacilli within or between the epithelial cells of the nasal mucosa suggest this to be a possible site for the entry of bacilli into the bloodstream.[9] An important pathological observation in lepromatous leprosy is the invasion of endothelium of blood vessels and lymphatics by *Mycobacterium leprae* which accounts for further spread of infection.[10] The study of *M. leprae* genome has led to identification of surface proteins called *adhesins* that appear to play a prominent role in their dissemination by helping attachment of bacilli to Schwann cells and endothelial cells. The bacilli disseminate to involve almost every part of the body (Fig. 23.1).[11] Apart from the skin and peripheral nerves, the tissues that show significant infiltration resulting in clinical manifestations include the bones, eyes, upper respiratory tissues, kidneys, liver and testes (Table 23.1).[12]

BONES, JOINTS AND MUSCLES

The lesions of the skeletal system are very important for they lead to the most dreaded facet of leprosy—deformities and disabilities. The bony lesions in the anthropological excavations have revealed the presence of leprosy many centuries ago in India, as well as in many other countries. The bone changes may be specific or nonspecific.[13]

- *Specific*: When they occur due to direct invasion by *M. leprae*.
- *Nonspecific*: When they are affected indirectly.

The nonspecific involvement is much more common and includes osteomyelitis, osteoporosis, atrophy and absorption of the bones. They result from the impairment of sensations, repeated trauma, trophic changes and restricted movement of the muscles. Inability to use a limb or a part thereof due to paralysis or weakness of the muscles causes disuse atrophy and osteoporosis. The altered biomechanical forces acting on the bones and joints due to asymmetrical muscular involvement may lead to deformities and disabilities, and contribute significantly to the disuse atrophy. The compromised nerve function and impaired blood supply caused by infiltrating granuloma are other contributory factors. In males, the deficient testosterone production due to leprous testicular atrophy hastens and aggravates the disuse osteoporosis.[14]

In the hands, slow resorption and atrophy start from the distal end of the terminal phalanx, and proceed proximally to involve the middle and proximal phalanges. The metacarpals and carpals usually remain uninvolved. However, in the feet, both the tarsals and metatarsals are also affected in addition to phalanges. The metatarsals become thinned out distally, a change referred to as 'penciling' or a 'sucked candy stick' and the tarsals disintegrate. Foot models have shown that when osteomyelitis and unsightly trophic ulcers develop, the progression of bone lesions is due to the combined effect of high vertical stresses and osteoporosis.[15] Concentric resorption of phalanges has also been seen quite frequently.[16] The muscle weakness/paralysis also results in the realignment of muscle actions and redistribution of pressure and traction forces, and may contribute to the deformity and the formation of calluses and corns. At times, one can see a rare manifestation in the form of dactylitis presenting as a fusiform swelling confined to the finger only, often of the right hand (Fig. 23.2).

It is important to realize that nonspecific changes can occur even after the institution of treatment, usually due to neglect in the care of insensitive hands and feet. As the control of leprosy improves and proper education is given to such persons to take good care of the extremities, the incidence of deformities is expected to come down.

The specific changes due to bacillary deposits in the bones and their feeding vessels are less common and are seen as osteitis, periosteitis, lytic lesions, erosions and bone cysts in phalangeal bones.[17] *M. leprae* specific osteomyelitis has also been described.[18,19]

Specific bone lesions have been seen in 5% of hospitalized patients in one study and have been said to occur more often due to contiguous spread of infection from overlying tissues than via circulation.[20] Radiologically, islands of dense areas within the bones of hands, feet and rarely long bones have been seen in bacilliferous patients indicating reparative activity in response to the damage due to presence of lepra bacilli.[21]

The facial changes (obviously due to damage to facial bones) are the ones that carry the imprint of leprosy. The full description by the Danish physician Moller-Christensen constitutes 'facies leprosa' which includes a triad of lesions considered characteristic of leprosy, namely (i) atrophy of the anterior nasal spine, (ii) atrophy and recession of the maxillary alveolar processes, and (iii) endonasal inflammatory change.[22] These lesions are not individually diagnostic of leprosy but together they constitute a reliable marker of leprosy in the study of ancient skull remnants. Atrophy of anterior nasal spine is the commoner bone involvement and contributes to the nasal collapse. The atrophy of the maxillary alveolar processes results in the loss of grip on the teeth, which then become loose.[23] The central incisors are maximally affected and are often lost due to total loss of bone around them.

The joints involvement in leprosy has been under estimated by leprologists as the symptoms are not severe enough to warrant specific treatment, except in cases of lepra reactions. An incidence of up to about 75% has

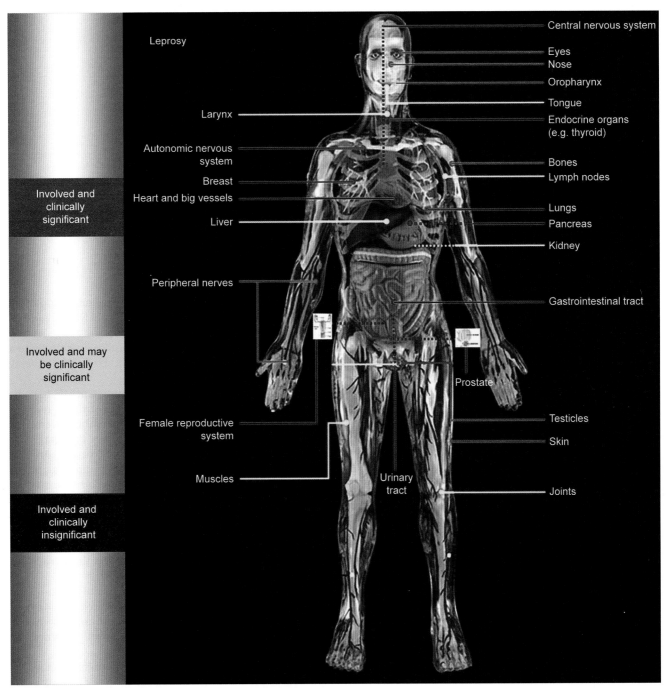

Fig. 23.1: Sites affected in leprosy

been recorded in some of the leprosy clinics.[24-26] The joint involvement is seen across the whole spectrum of leprosy. The functional incapabilities do not arise except during reactionary episodes. The diagnosis rests on the presence of other features of leprosy. However, occasionally the leprous rheumatic involvement can occur without any skin lesion.[27,28] The patients are known to have sought initial consultation in rheumatology clinics and later diagnosed as leprosy.[24,29]

Three types of joint involvement have been noted: (1) A chronic insidious onset arthritis, (2) an acute arthritis seen during reactionary episodes, and (3) neuropathic or Charcot's arthropathy. The reactionary episodes probably contribute maximum towards occurrence of arthritis.[30]

Table 23.1: Sites affected in relation to clinical significance in multibacillary leprosy

Clinically significant	May be clinically significant	Clinically insignificant
Skin	Joints	Autonomic nerve dysfunction of cardiac and respiratory systems
Peripheral nerves	Kidneys	Breasts
Bones	Larynx	Central nervous system
Eyes	Liver	Endocrine organs
Nose	Lymph nodes	Female reproductive system
Oropharynx	Muscles of face and limbs	Gastrointestinal tract
Testicles	Tongue	Heart and big vessels
		Lungs
		Pancreas
		Prostate
		Urinary tract (ureters, bladder and urethra)

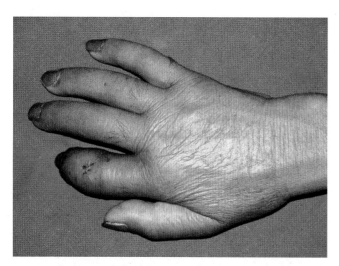

Fig. 23.2: Dactylitis in a woman who had faint macules on trunk on examination

The insidious arthritis occurs without any reactionary episode and tends to involve multiple peripheral joints, especially the small joints of hands and feet in a symmetrical manner. The other joints including knees and elbows can be involved. Sacroiliitis can occur.[31] Axial involvement has been reported recently as spondylodiscitis of cervical spine in a treated case of Hansen's where polymerase chain reaction (PCR) for *M. leprae* was positive from the involved site.[32] Histopathologically the synovium shows nonspecific granuloma, epithelioid cells and sometimes *M. leprae*. The polyarthritic symmetrical small joint arthritis of leprosy can easily be confused with that of rheumatoid arthritis.[24,33] The juxta-articular erosions seen in rheumatoid arthritis at times can be seen in leprosy radiologically.[34,35] The often positive immunological markers, i.e. rheumatoid (RA) factor and antinuclear antibodies (ANA), in lepromatous leprosy further

complicate the diagnosis. The distinction becomes important as therapy with tumor necrosis factor-alpha (TNF-α) has been followed by leprosy lesions even in countries where leprosy is nonendemic.[36,37] Detection of the anticyclic citrullinated peptide (anti-CCP) antibodies in the blood is helpful in being specific for rheumatoid arthritis.[38]

The lepra reactions, both type I and type II, may be associated with the development of acute arthritis and the joint pain can be a presenting complaint of the patient. The pain may be very severe and some degrees of impairment in functional capabilities are usually there. The arthritis appears to have an immunological basis and is usually associated with constitutional symptoms or other features of reactionary episodes. Clinically, the arthritis is polyarticular and symmetrical, very often resembling the rheumatoid arthritis. The timely intervention (please see chapter on Treatment of Reactions) in addition to antileprosy treatment is of paramount importance in preventing the permanent damage to the tissues.

The Charcot's arthropathy develops insidiously without any obvious symptoms. It is related to impaired sensations of joints and the surrounding tissues. The arthropathy usually involves the weight bearing joints though other joints, like wrist, has been reported to be affected.[39]

Skeletal muscle involvement is rare which clinically presents as pea sized nodules inside the muscle mass of the extremities or sometimes as myositis.[40,41] Myositis may present with pain in the affected muscle while the nodules do not interfere with the function of the muscle. The histopathological specimens may reveal lepromatous granulomas between muscle fibers and connective tissue coverings of the muscle. The fibers surrounding the granuloma are degenerated. Acid-fast bacillus (AFB) can be seen in the macrophages, lepra cells and even lying freely between the muscle fibers. In various other studies changes like loss of striations, hyaline, fatty and sarcolemmal changes, necrosis, fibrosis and endomysial thickening have been described.[42]

Involvement of the musculoskeletal system involving the limbs may have serious repercussions for the patient due to subsequent deformities and permanent disability robbing one of daily livelihood. Whenever the facilities are available, the advice of an orthopedician/rehabilitation expert/ physiotherapist should be sought. However, when such help is not available, the clinician should teach the patient some active and assisted exercises, and educate on the importance of self-care and avoiding trauma to the insensitive part.

NAIL INVOLVEMENT

Nail changes in leprosy are generally nonspecific and nails may appear dystrophic. The changes are seen in both paucibacillary and multibacillary disease, but are much more frequent and extensive in the latter.[43] Both the finger as well as toe nails undergo such changes. The affection of nails has been attributed to many factors that include neuropathy, trauma, vascular changes and infections.[43,44] The changes have been related to the long duration of the disease. In a large series of 300 patients, the changes noted were longitudinal melanonychia, longitudinal ridging and subungual hyperkeratosis.[43] The nonspecific nail changes of chronic disease, such as striae, pitting, leukonychia, *Beau's* lines, and in the advanced disease with the absorption of fingers, anonychia can be seen.[45] Observation of recurrent dermatophytic skin infections in some patients of leprosy has been attributed to pre-existing nail infection (onychomycosis) that hitherto had remained unsuspected.[46]

EYES

Prior to availability of effective antileprosy therapy the eyes were the common sites of affection. The outer structures of the eye as well as the eye ball tissues can be involved. Madarosis or the loss of eyebrows usually involves the outer third but there can be complete loss of eyebrows. In tuberculoid leprosy, it may be unilateral and occurs only if there is a patch over that area; while lepromatous infiltration destroys the hair roots and loss of eyebrows is usually bilateral giving a striking look to the face. Eyelashes may be lost in a similar manner. The heavy infiltration of the eyelids may result in its drooping (upper eyelid) or ectropion (lower eyelid) because of tissue weight.

Involvement of the eyes can also occur indirectly. Considerable damage may also take place during reactionary episodes. The indirect mode of involvement is the one seen more frequently[47,48] and it is not due to the spread of bacilli to the ophthalmic structures but results from involvement of nerves supplying the ophthalmic area, namely the trigeminal (fifth cranial nerve) and facial (seventh cranial nerve) nerves. The trigeminal nerve is responsible for sensory innervations to cornea, conjunctiva and ocular adnexae; while the

facial nerve supplies the orbicularis oculi muscles. In the affliction of the former, the corneal reflex is impaired and there is conjunctival/corneal anesthesia or hypoesthesia; while involvement of the latter affects lid closure. In both the instances, there is a grave danger of corneal ulceration resulting from exposure keratitis, which becomes much greater when both the nerves are affected concurrently. The corneal ulceration may lead to iritis or iridocyclitis with their associated potentially disastrous consequences. Conjunctivitis can also occur in a manner similar to exposure keratitis. The conjunctivitis is usually restricted to the area corresponding to the palpebral fissure and is more intense near sclerocorneal junction.

Direct spread results from lodgement of the lepra bacilli in the eyes and occurs only in multibacillary leprosy. The bacilli reach the ocular tissue through the blood stream. The structures in the relatively cooler anterior compartment are usually involved. Here the cornea, ciliary body, part of the choroid and the walls of blood vessels are infiltrated by heavily bacillated macrophages. The posterior part of the eye is usually spared though nodules in the retina have been occasionally observed.[49]

Beading and opacification of the corneal nerves is an early indication and is seen universally in almost all lepromatous leprosy patients. It is due to multiplication of bacilli in or adjacent to the nerves and is best seen with slit lamp broad beam.[50] Whitish dots appear over the cornea giving rise to leprotic punctuate keratitis. These dots are miliary lepromata and represent the microaggregates of *M. leprae* lying between the epithelium and Bowman's membrane. This is then followed by pannus which forms all around the cornea and eventually leads to sclerosing keratitis, which resembles arcus senilis. An important manifestation is chronic iridocyclitis, which can be so insidious that there is no redness and minimal ocular discomfort. Just like quiescent ("silent") nerve paralysis, this too can lead to blindness if left undiagnosed. Leprous iridocyclitis is less common in India as compared to the other endemic countries.[48] With slit-lamp examination, the lepromata are seen as iris "pearls". These are located at the sites of autonomic nerve plexuses that supply the muscles of iris. Initially they are seen near the pupillary margin as creamy spheres less than 0.5 mm but later may appear elsewhere on the iris and coalesce to form larger lesions. The iridocyclitis runs a protracted course and extensive iris atrophy may take place.

Secondary cataracts, glaucoma and ciliary body herniation can also occur. The acute form of iridiocyclitis is usually encountered during reactions. Ocular defects are seen mostly in smear positive persons with long standing disease, which is often associated with other deformities.[50] Lagophthalmos, pterygium, impaired corneal sensation, dry eye syndrome and cataracts are some of the common complications seen in newly diagnosed lepromatous and near lepromatous cases.[51] In lepromatous leprosy, lagophthalmos is generally bilateral, while in tuberculoid it is ipsilateral. In contravention of the common assertion that the lower lid is affected due to preferential involvement of zygomatic branch of the facial nerve as it courses over the zygomatic process, some observers feel that the upper and lower facial muscles are affected in the same proportion.[52] Lagophthalmos in paucibacillary leprosy depends on the location of the patches, the large patches also involving other branches of the facial nerve. In lepromatous leprosy, lagophthalmos is due to diffuse infiltration of not only the nerve but also of the muscles. Chronic uveitis should be suspected in those with small pupils and poor pupillary reaction.

High-risk factors that can lead to loss of vision may be present even after release from treatment. A recent study found corneal causes to be the major sight threatening factors which were related to the longer duration of disease.[53] To prevent blindness or visual impairment, it is essential to examine the patient for visual acuity, lagophthalmos at monthly visits and check for any signs of reaction on the face.[54] Care of the eyes is essential, like that of anesthetic hands and feet, and is something that the patient should be well educated about and clearly instructed to adhere, during and well after completion of therapy (See Chapter 27 on Ocular Leprosy).

UPPER RESPIRATORY TRACT (NOSE, PARANASAL SINUSES, ORAL CAVITY, OROPHARYNX, AND LARYNX)

Leprosy confines itself mainly to the upper part of the respiratory tract while the lower respiratory tract and lungs appear to escape. The nose is the portal of entry for *M. leprae* and is the earliest site of involvement in lepromatous leprosy. It becomes heavily bacillated remaining a potential source for the exit of *M. leprae* from the body. Edema and mucosal thickening are the main findings seen commonly in the anterior aspect of the inferior turbinate and nasal septum.[55] Chronic rhinitis can occur. Though not discernible during examination, in a study, a standardized test for odor showed lower scores for smell as compared to controls, indicating leprous affection of the first cranial nerve, which could be reversed by therapy.[56] An important clinical clue is to ask for a history of epistaxis, which is often passed off by the patients as an unrelated occurrence. Many times this history would be in the form of brownish crusts which can be brought out by the patient. On examination, when these crusts are cleared, one may be able to even see septal perforation in advanced cases by shining a torch through the other nostril. The combination of anterior nasal spine collapse and septal destruction causes total collapse of the nose. The paranasal sinuses are also involved along with in majority of the patients with lepromatous leprosy.[57] Exophytic lesions of leprosy affecting the anterior nasal septum in absence of lesions, elsewhere, have been observed.[58] This observation must be carefully interpreted since majority of the patients have mild diffuse infiltration of the nasal mucosa, usually missed on routine examination, but can be unmasked by doing a nasal scrape or slit skin smear to reveal AFB.

Oral cavity and oropharyngeal lesions have been commonly recorded in lepromatous patients.[59] They include involvement and ulceration of tongue, pharynx, hard and soft palate, tonsillar pillars, and the uvula. Later, perforation of the palate can occur.[60,61] Perforations of the palate and nasal septum have been seen even in burnt out cases. Patients with bilateral blindness, destruction of facial bones and perforations in the oral cavity giving a grotesque appearance are still being seen.[18] Histopathologically, granulomas consisting of epithelioid cells, plasma cells and lymphocytes are seen in subepithelial zone around blood vessels, nerves and muscle bundles.[62,63] The AFBs are seen not only in histiocytes, nerves, connective tissue, muscles and mucosal epithelial cells; but also in the salivary duct epithelium. The absence of clear submucosal zone and the presence of AFB in epithelium is said to allow the shedding of large number of bacilli even from intact mucosa. Reactions can give rise to palatal palsy presenting with nasal regurgitation of food.[64] About 75–80% of the multibacillary patients have shown dental caries and periodontal disease.[65] Alveolar bone loss involves maxilla as well as mandible, and may lead to loosening and sometimes loss of teeth. The gingival and periodontal changes appear to be due to lack of oral hygiene, severe plaque and calculus formation, mouth breathing, and also because of specific granulomatous infiltrations.[66] *M. leprae* have been demonstrated in the material from dental pulp and dental tubuli.[67] Instructions regarding taking care of oral hygiene may be useful in reducing the gingival and periodontal disease.

Involvement of paranasal sinuses is very important in MB leprosy patients for the sinuses form a big reservoir of *M. leprae* and the nasal discharge of these patients can be highly bacilliferous. Endoscopic and radiological [computed tomography (CT)] studies have revealed the involvement of all paranasal sinuses with ethmoid sinuses being most frequently affected, followed by maxillary sinus while frontal and sphenoid sinuses are least affected.[68,69] The evidence of their involvement was seen even in those lepromatous patients who had been treated with Dapsone, Rifampicin and Clofazimine for over 2 years.[69] Involvement may be unilateral or bilateral and can be co-related with the positivity of nasal blow smears.[70] The radiological studies reveal localized or diffuse thickening of mucosa and opacity of the sinus. Endoscopically, the inflamed mucosa, ulcerations and granulomatous lesions can be seen.[71] Histologically, the findings include histiocytic infiltration, granuloma formation and findings consistent with lepromatous leprosy. AFBs are usually demonstrable in the biopsy specimen.

Laryngeal involvement is a late phenomenon and may present as ulceration, nodules and thickening, which results in fibrosis later. The leprotic lesions are found in the epiglottis, arytenoid, false and true vocal cords, and subglottic space.[72]

With the impaired mobility of the vocal cords, the resultant hoarseness of the voice is the manifest symptom in all these conditions. Such patients are quite often very poor, and in the past their croaking sobs for alms have deeply moved the travellers and writers alike.[73] Impairment of laryngeal sensations may insidiously result in aspiration of food and secretions into the lungs leading to fatal pneumonia.[74]

Granulomas have been seen most frequently in the vocal cords and sometimes even in epiglottis. Bronchial hyporeactivity and impaired cough reflexes due to involvement of postganglionic vagal fibers have been documented.[75]

LOWER RESPIRATORY TRACT

Various degrees of tracheobronchial involvement have been described and *M. leprae* have been demonstrated in the bronchial washings. However, the trachea, bronchi and lungs have not been known to be directly involved.[76-78]

GASTROINTESTINAL TRACT

Apart from affection of oral and oropharyngeal structures, rest of the gastrointestinal tract is uninvolved. The esophagus, stomach, small and large intestines have been found to be free of disease, and so are the pancreas, gall bladder and biliary tract.[76-78]

Involvement of the liver is through hematogenous spread and has been noted in both tuberculoid and lepromatous leprosy.[79] The involvement is dependent upon severity of the lesions on skin, and the frequency and intensity of bacteremia.[80] Leprous granulomata are found throughout the parenchyma and are heavily bacillated in lepromatous leprosy. They do not have any specific distribution pattern in relation to the portal triad or central vein. Steatosis and Kupffer cell hyperplasia have been noted.[81] Hepatic dysfunction can also occur.[82] Jaundice occurring in erythema nodosum leprosum (ENL) reaction and prolonged jaundice in lepromatous leprosy has been reported.[83] The metabolism of drugs can be altered.[84] Hepatic involvement has been related to the oxidative stress.[85]

REPRODUCTIVE SYSTEM

Male Reproductive System: Testes

The testicular involvement occurs to variable degrees in a large proportion of lepromatous patients, particularly in those experiencing repeated attacks of epididymo-orchitis during type 2 reaction. *M. leprae* are present in the testes in almost all multibacillary patients and in many of them oligospermia is demonstrable.[86] The initial presentation is of testicular pain and swelling, gradually changing to typical picture of chronic epididymo-orchitis with testes feeling firm

to hard. However, more often they feel soft, reduced in volume and finally turn atrophic in the late stage. There is significant lowering of fertility.[87] During type 2 reaction, edema and acute inflammatory exudates suddenly appear in those foci, resulting in testicular hypofunction. Both the seminiferous tubules (exocrine part) and the interstitial cells (endocrine part) are involved. The seminiferous tubules are involved first by the disease; these are obliterated by hyaline deposition on Leydig cells and the final stage is one of complete fibrosis. The atrophy of the exocrine portion results in aspermatogenesis, leading to sterility, with no loss of sexual potency. The atrophy of the interstitial cells (Leydig cells) which occurs late, affects the production of testosterone, causing impotence. The testicular involvement is commonly bilateral and when marked, is associated first with azoospermia, and later with impotence. Initially, endocrine functions are affected with marked reduction in male sex hormones (testosterone) resulting in impotence, reduced testicular volume, altered hair pattern, lack of testicular sensation and gynecomastia.[88,89] Mean blood levels of gonadotropic hormones [follicle stimulating hormone (FSH), luteinizing hormone (LH)] are raised, while that of testosterone is reduced. The hormonal aberrations co-relate well with the duration of disease. In reactional states, repeated attacks of epididymo-orchitis hasten testicular atrophy.

The epididymis also shows leprous granulomata but the prostate and seminal vesicles have not been found to be involved.[77,78]

Female Reproductive System

In contrast to the universal involvement of testes in males in multibacillary disease, the female reproductive organs are not significantly involved in leprosy. Necropsy studies did not reveal any evidence of leprosy in these organs; neither in tuberculoid nor in lepromatous leprosy.[76] The biopsy findings from endometrium did not reveal any involvement.[90] The menstrual fluid was found to be free of leprosy bacilli, even in patients having bacillemia. The menarche, menstruation and fertility remain unaffected. The bacilli have been found occasionally in breast milk[91] and possibly can cross the placental barrier.[92]

KIDNEYS

Renal involvement in leprosy is quite a frequent finding. The exact histopathological lesions in the kidneys and their nature are not clearly defined. A wide variety of histological changes in varying incidence have been reported from different geographic areas. Almost all types of glomerulonephritis have been observed in lepromatous leprosy and they have been thought to have an immunological basis, particularly during reactions.[93,94] Functional abnormalities have been found to be more common than the histopathological changes. These include proteinuria, microscopic hematuria, granular, hyaline and red blood cell casts; and the biochemical aberrations, like increased serum urea, serum creatinine, altered distal tubular functions and reduced glomerular filtration rate. Renal amyloidosis has been seen to vary in Indian patients from 0–15%. A higher incidence of amyloidosis (up to 31%), has been reported in Latin American countries.[95] and has been found to be a leading cause of death due to renal failure, in the absence of routine investigations.[96] The low incidence of renal amyloidosis in India is attributed to dietary factors like vegetarian food habits.[97] The involvement of kidneys, though occurring less frequently as compared to the other organs, should never be ignored.[98] Acute renal failure can occur during reactional states when all measures should be taken to restore normal kidney functions to ward off the critical situation. Long-standing renal disease, like glomerulonephritis or amyloidosis, can cause chronic renal failure necessitating hemodialysis.[99]

The ureters, urinary bladder and urethra have not been found to be involved.[78]

ENDOCRINE GLANDS

Adrenal glands have been found to be histologically involved though no functional deficit manifests clinically. However, there is some evidence to suggest a functional insufficiency of the adrenals during reactions in leprosy, and the function returning to normal on the subsidence of acute reactional state.[100] In severe cases of type 2 reactions, a fall in temperature and blood pressure below basal levels, along with hypoglycemia and increased serum potassium levels, should be viewed with caution, as it indicates an adrenal crisis, which is one of the causes of sudden death in type 2 reactions. This calls for prompt treatment with corticosteroids in adequate doses, which may require lifelong maintenance.[101,102] The postmortem studies have shown adrenal involvement in lepromatous leprosy in the form of granulomas in the cortex as well as medulla, mainly in and around the corticomedullary zone. Amyloid deposits may also be detected.

The other endocrine glands, i.e. parathyroid, pancreas and pituitary glands, remain free of disease. Data about involvement and dysfunction of thyroid is scanty. Increased uptake of radioactive iodine and high prevalence of thyroid autoantibodies in leprosy has been reported, the significance of which is not clear because no functional abnormality has been observed.[103]

LYMPH NODES, BONE MARROW, AND SPLEEN

Experimental studies have suggested that reticuloendothelial system gets involved early in the course of the disease. In experimental leprous inoculation in armadillos, the bacilli initially reached the regional lymph nodes, followed by colonization of other groups of lymph nodes, liver, spleen and finally the other organs.[104]

Lymph Nodes

Clinically appreciable enlargement of lymph nodes is uncommon in leprosy, except during reactions. The histopathologic findings of biopsy[105] and autopsy specimens,[72,78] however, suggest involvement of these nodes throughout the leprosy spectrum from tuberculoid to lepromatous forms of the disease, including indeterminate leprosy, but is often significant only in multibacillary disease. The involvement is seen in the form of mild to moderate enlargement of the regional lymph nodes which do not show any matting or suppuration. In tuberculoid leprosy, only the regional lymph nodes draining the affected cutaneous area are involved, while in lepromatous leprosy the involvement is more widespread and generalized affecting, even the visceral nodes, if the concerned organ has leprous involvement, e.g. hepatic lymph nodes and splenic hilar lymph nodes, in hepatic and splenic affection, respectively. The size of the glands was found to be proportional to the duration of the disease.[105]

In tuberculoid leprosy, the lymph glands show leprous lesions with foci of epithelioid cells and formation of granulomata. AFB can also be detected in some cases.[106] Patchy fibrosis, without any caseation, can take place replacing the normal tissue.[105] The aspirates of lymph nodes in lepromatous leprosy demonstrate lepra cells in a reactive lymphoid background[81] while the biopsy specimens reveal involvement of both the cortex and the medulla by the bacilli laden foamy macrophages. Well-formed typical lepromatous granulomas may be seen.

Bone Marrow

Bone marrow aspirates from lepromatous leprosy patients invariably reveal presence of lepra cells and there may be a relative increase of plasma cells.[81] Ziehl-Neelson staining for AFBs show their presence within foamy macrophages, as well as lying freely in the interstitium.[107] Bone marrow aspiration done to evaluate anemia in old treated patients may sometimes reveal AFB.[108] Leukopenia secondary to bone marrow infiltration by *M. leprae* has been reported.[109] The bone marrow may continue to show organisms even when the skin smears have turned negative after treatment, indicating late clearance from this site.[110] This fact may have some bearing in cases of relapse.

Spleen

The spleen is usually not palpable, either in tuberculoid or in lepromatous leprosy. In the latter, the microscopy of splenic tissue shows diffuse infiltration of sinusoids with foamy macrophages and lepromas in the red and white pulp. *M. leprae* are present within the macrophages, lying freely in the sinusoids and within the cells lining the sinusoids. There may be thickening of the walls of medium and small sized arteries due to amyloidosis. Amyloid deposits can also be seen in the centers of Malphigian corpuscles and elsewhere in the pulp.[75,76]

CENTRAL NERVOUS SYSTEM

Affections of V and VII cranial nerves in leprosy are well known but the brain and spinal cord are said to escape the infection. However, some recent studies refute this. Using brainstem auditory evoked potentials (BAEPs) and visual evoked potentials (VEPs), abnormal conduction of auditory and visual pathways have been demonstrated.[111] Perceptive deafness of cochlear type has also been reported.[112] Subclinical phrenic nerve involvement has been documented.[113] Autopsies conducted on some treated lepromatous leprosy patients have shown vacuolar changes of motor neurons of medulla oblongata and spinal cord.[114] These vacuolated areas were found to be PGL-1 positive and PCR could detect *M. leprae* specific genomic DNA in many of these cases. Dementia attributable to leprosy has also been reported.[115]

CARDIOVASCULAR SYSTEM

Leproma of the heart has been reported[116] though many studies could not establish such an involvement conclusively.[76,78] Autonomic neural supply to the heart may be affected[117] and may lead to dysautonomia.[118] Aorta and other major vessels do not appear to be involved.[78]

Involvement of smaller vessels has been confirmed by many studies.[119] The vessels get infiltrated by *M. leprae* during the phase of bacillemia. Use of special stains has demonstrated the presence of these organisms in all the three layers of the vessel wall.[120] All types of vessels, including arteries, veins and capillaries, in the dermis, as well as subcutaneous tissues have shown infiltration. The histopathological changes are observed throughout the thickness of the vessel wall, which includes homogenization of the vessel wall and fibrosis. Well-developed lepromatous *granulomata* in the intima of the veins may distort the lumen.[121] Leprous phlebitis of external jugular vein showing extensive fibrosis, tuberculoid granulomas with AFB positivity have been reported.[122] In addition, the vasa nervorum also show mycobacteria. Experimental studies in armadillos have demonstrated that the infection of the endothelial cells of epineural blood vessels precedes the infection of endoneurial lining, raising the possibility that the neural involvement in leprosy could be routed through the nutrient vessels of the nerve.[120,123] Vascular involvement may help in the dissemination of disease and could also be a contributing factor for trophic changes seen in leprosy. The smooth muscle of the media of blood vessels may remain a protected site for the microorganism.[120]

HEMATOLOGY AND SEROLOGY

With time, the usually observed changes in other chronic diseases make their appearance in leprosy also. Lower levels of hemoglobin, a raised erythrocyte sedimentation rate (ESR), low serum iron levels and lower levels of serum albumin are often observed.[6,124] These abnormalities (not usually severe enough to warrant any special attention) are seen more commonly towards the lepromatous pole of the spectrum. The chronicity of lepromatous leprosy and formation of immune complexes result in development of many autoantibodies. Lepromatous leprosy since long has been described as a cause for false positivity of anticardiolipin antibodies based serological tests for syphilis [venereal disease research laboratory (VDRL), Wasserman test (WR), rapid plasma reagin (RPR), etc.]. Lupus erythematosus (LE) cells can also be seen in some cases. Antispermatozoal antibodies are often present in the blood of lepromatous leprosy patients.[125] Other autoantibodies detected in lepromatous leprosy include antimitochondrial antibodies, RA factor, ANA, anti-single stranded DNA antibodies, antineutrophil cytoplasmic antibodies (more commonly c-ANCA, and also p-ANCA and atypical ANCA), lupus anticoagulant antiphospholipid antibodies, anti-β-2 glycoprotein and antiprothrombin antibodies.[126-129] Serum complement levels may also be raised.[130]

Taken individually, it is seen that almost every system is involved in multibacillary forms of leprosy, though in practice, the classification and treatment of disease is based on a thorough examination of the skin and peripheral nerves. The importance of systemic evaluation assumes significance in reactional states when many systems can be noticeably affected. Some of these can have very atypical presentations, simulating other immune-complex diseases, like systemic LE, characterized by malar flush, alopecia, skin eruptions, fever and joint pains (Figs 23.3A and B). Such patients may have ANA; anti-single stranded DNA, antineutrophil cytoplasmic antibodies and positive RA factor,[127] but are negative for anti-double stranded DNA antibodies.[131] They are thought to result from stimulation of B-cells by antigenic complexes of *M. leprae* plus autologous tissue.[132]

Leprosy is not a fatal disease, but it is a chronic and crippling disease, if not diagnosed and treated early. Most of the systemic complications and their disfiguring sequelae can be prevented by early diagnosis and treatment.[133] In the past, severe reactions accounted for high morbidity. A relatively better understanding of the reactions and their treatment using corticosteroids, as well as access to thalidomide and its availability in the open market has improved the scene. Recurrent reactions and prolonged use of corticosteroids can increase susceptibility to infections, and their judicious use has helped in keeping the mortality well below acceptable levels.

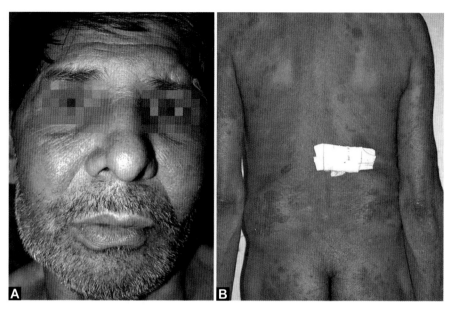

Figs 23.3A and B: Fever, fatigue and arthralgias in a man admitted to medical ward as lupus erythematosus with positive antinuclear antibodies, (A) showing malar erythema and (B) eruptions that appeared a week later; slit-skin smear revealed acid-fast bacillus 3+ and history disclosed incomplete antileprosy therapy 5 years ago

REFERENCES

1. Rees RJ, McDougall AC. Airborne infection with *Mycobacterium leprae* in mice. J Med Microbiol. 1977;10:63-8.
2. Shepard CC. Stability of *Mycobacterium leprae* and temperature optimum for growth. Int J Lepr. 1965;33:159-64.
3. Khanolkar VR. Pathology of leprosy. In: Cochrane RG, Davey TF (Eds). Leprosy in theory and practice, 2nd edition. Bristol: John Wright; 1964.pp.125-51.
4. Lane JE, Balagon MV, Dela Cruz EC, et al. *Mycobacterium leprae* in untreated lepromatous leprosy: more than skin deep. Clin Exp Dermatol. 2006;31:469-70.
5. Drutz DJ, Chen TS, Lu WH. The continuous bacteremia of lepromatous leprosy. N Eng J Med. 1972; 287:159-64.
6. Karat AB, Rao PS. Haematological profile in leprosy. Part I—general findings. Lepr India. 1977; 49:187-96.
7. Raval SN, Sen Gupta U, Ramu G, et al. A study of continuous bacillaemia in borderline and lepromatous leprosy. Lepr India. 1982;54:623-33.
8. Desikan KV. Bacteraemia in leprosy. In: Dharmendra (Ed). Leprosy. Bombay: Samant and Co.; 1985.p. 78.
9. McDougall AC, Rees RJ, Weddell AG, et al. The histopathology of lepromatous leprosy in the nose. J Pathol. 1975;115:215-26.
10. Pessolani MC, Marques de Melo MA, Reddy VM, et al. Systemic dissemination in tuberculosis and leprosy: do mycobacterial adhesins play a role? Microbes Infect. 2003;5:677-84.
11. Klioze AM, Ramos-Caro AF. Visceral leprosy. Int J Dermatol. 2000;39:641-58.
12. Kumar B, Rai R, Kaur I. Systemic involvement in leprosy and its significance. Indian J Lepr. 2000;72:123-42.
13. Choudhuri H, Thappa DM, Kumar RH, et al. Bone changes in leprosy patients with disabilities/deformities (a clinico-radiological correlation). Indian J Lepr. 1999;71:203-15.
14. Ishikawa S, Mizushima M, Furuta M, et al. Leydig cell hyperplasia and maintenance of bone volume: bone histomorphometry and testicular histopathology in 29 male leprosy autopsy cases. Int J Lepr Other Mycobact Dis. 2000;68:258-66.
15. Patil KM, Jacob S. Mechanics of tarsal disintegration and plantar ulcers in leprosy by stress analysis in three dimensional foot models. Indian J Lepr. 2000;72:69-86.
16. Thappa DM, Sharma VK, Kaur S, et al. Radiological changes in hands and feet in disabled leprosy patients: a clinico-radiological correlation. Indian J Lepr. 1992;64:58-66.
17. Dave S, Nori AV, Thappa DM, et al. Leprous osteitis presenting as bone cyst and erosions. Dermatol Online J. 2004;10:17.
18. Job CK. Pathology of leprous osteomyelitis. Int J Lepr. 1963;31:L26-33.
19. Moller-Christensen V. New knowledge of leprosy through paleopathology. Int J Lepr. 1965;33:603-10.
20. Kustner-Chimenos E, Pascual-Cruz M, Dansis-Pinol C, et al. Lepromatous leprosy: A review and case report. Med Oral Pathol Oral Cir Buc. 2006;11:E474-9.
21. Carpintero P, Garcia-Frasquet A, Tarradas E, et al. Bone island and leprosy. Skeletal Radiol. 1998;27:330-3.
22. Moller-Christensen V, Bakke SN, Melson RS, et al. Changes in the anterior nasal spine of the alveolar process of the maxillary bone in leprosy. Int J Lepr. 1952;20:335-40.
23. Blau S, Yagodin V. Osteoarchaeological evidence for leprosy from western Central Asia. Am J Phys Anthropol. 2005;126:150-8.
24. Mandal SK, Sarkar RN, Sarkar P, et al. Rheumatological manifestations of leprosy. J Indian Med Assoc. 2008;106:165-6.
25. Vengdakrishnan K, Sarasvat PK, Mathur PC. A study of rhematological manifestations of leprosy. Indian J Dermatol Venereol Leprol. 2004;70:76-8.
26. Alcocer J, Herrera CL, Guidino J, et al. Inflammatory arthropathy in leprosy. Arthritis Rheum. 1979;22:587.

27. Agarwal V, Wakhlu A, Aggarwal A, et al. Tenosynovitis as the presenting manifestation of leprosy. J Indian Rheumatol Assoc. 2002;10:69-70.

28. Haroon N, Agarwal V, Aggarwal A, et al. Arthritis as presenting manifestation of pure neuritic leprosy—a rheumatologist's dilemma. Rheumatology. 2007;46:653-6.

29. Ker KJ, Pan JY, Lui NL, et al. An under-recognized cause of polyarthritis: Leprosy. Ann Acad of Med. 2013;42:366-7.

30. Pereira HL, Ribeiro SL, Pennini SN, et al. Leprosy-related joint involvement. Clin Rheumatol. 2009;28:79-84.

31. Cossermelli-Messina W, Festa Neto C, Cossermelli W. Articular inflammatory manifestations in patients with different forms of leprosy. J Rheumatol. 1998;25:111-9.

32. Kim SJ, Lee TH, Shin JJ, et al. Leprotic cervical spondylodiscities. Eur Spine J. 2010;19 (suppl 2):S211-5.

33. Gibson T. Bacterial infections: the arthritis of leprosy. Baillieres Clin Rheumatol. 1995;9:179-91.

34. Chauhan S, Wakhlu A, Agarwal V. Arthritis in leprosy. Rheumatology. 2010;49:2237-42.

35. Modi TH, Lele RD. Acute joint manifestations in leprosy. J Assoc Physicians India. 1969;17:247-54.

36. Freitas DS, Machado N, Andriqueti FV, et al. Lepromatous leprosy associated with the use of anti TNF-alpha therapy: case report. Rev Bras Reumatol. 2010;50:333-9.

37. Scollard DM, Joyce MP, Gillis TP. Development of leprosy and type 1 leprosy reactions after treatment with infliximab: A report of 2 cases. Clin Infect Dis. 2006;43:e19-22.

38. Riberio SL, Pereira HL, Silva NP, et al. Anticyclic cirtullinated peptide antibodies and RF in leprosy patients with articular involvement. Braz J Med Biol Res. 2008;41:1005-10.

39. Carpintero P, Garcia-Frasquet A, Pradilla P, et al. Wrist involvement in Hansen's disease. J Bone Joint Surg Br. 1997;79:753-7.

40. Convit J, Arnelo JJ, Mensoza S. Lepromatous myositis. Int J Lepr. 1960;28:417-22.

41. Gupta S, Mehta A, Lakhtakia R, et al. An unusual presentation of lepromatous leprosy. MJAFI. 2006;62:392-3.

42. Kaur S, Malik AK, Kumar B. Pathologic changes in striated muscles in leprosy. Lepr India. 1981;51:52-6.

43. Kaur I, Chakrabarti A, Dogra S, et al. Nail involvement in leprosy: A study of 300 patients. Int J Lepr Other Mycobact Dis. 2003;71:320-7.

44. Patki AH, Baran R. Significance of nail changes in leprosy: a clinical review of 357 cases. Semin Dermatol. 1991;10:77-81.

45. Romero IB, Rincón RJ, Rabell RF. Nail involvement in leprosy. Acta Dermosifiliogr. 2012;103:276-84.

46. Ramesh V, Misra RS. Nail changes in leprosy and recognition of fungal nail infections. Indian J Lepr. 1987;59:360-1.

47. Gopinath DV, Thappa DM, Jaishankar TJ. A clinical study of the involvement of cranial nerves in leprosy. Indian J Lepr. 2004;76:1-9.

48. Samanta SK, Das D. Recent advances in ocular leprosy. Indian J Lepr 2007;79:135-50.

49. Ebenezer GJ, Daniel E. Pathology of a lepromatous eye. Int J Lepr Other Mycobact Dis. 2000;68:23-6.

50. Kim EC. Hansen Disease. e-article updated June 22, 2006 (www.medscape.com).

51. Daniel E, Koshy S, Rao GS, et al. Ocular complications in newly diagnosed borderline lepromatous and lepromatous leprosy patients: baseline profile of the Indian cohort. Br J Opththalmol. 2002;86:1336-40.

52. Lubbers WJ, Schipper A, Hogeweg M, et al. Paralysis of facial muscles in leprosy patients with lagophthalmos. Int J Lepr Other Mycobact Dis. 1994;62:220-4.

53. Rohatgi J, Dhaliwal U, Singal A. Factors associated with sight threatening lesions of leprosy in patients on multidrug therapy. J Indian Med Assoc. 2004;102:297-8, 300, 302-3.

54. Thompson KJ, Allardice GM, Babu GR, et al. Patterns of ocular morbidity and blindness in leprosy—a three centre study in Eastern India. Lepr Rev. 2006;77:130-40.

55. Editorial: The nose and leprosy. Lancet. 1976;1:1062.

56. Mishra A, Saito K, Barbash SE, et al. Olfactory dysfunction in leprosy. Laryngoscope. 2006;116:413-6.

57. Sharma VK, Bapuraj JR, Mann SB, et al. Computed tomographic study of paranasal sinuses in leprosy. Int J Lepr. 1998;66:201-7.

58. Gupta A, Seiden AM. Nasal leprosy: case study. Otolaryngol Head Neck Surg. 2003;129:608-10.

59. Scollard DM, Skinsnes OK. Oropharyngeal leprosy in art, history, and medicine. Oral Surg Oral Med Oral Pathol Oral Radiol Endod. 1999;87:463-70.

60. Rao AG, Konda C, Jhamnani K. Palatal involvement in lepromatous leprosy. Indian J Dermatol Venereol Leprol. 2008;74:161-2.

61. Sharma VK, Kumar B, Kaur S, et al. Involvement of tongue in leprosy. Indian J Lepr. 1985;57:841-4.

62. Kumar B, Yande R, Kaur I, et al. Involvement of palate and cheek in leprosy. Indian J Lepr. 1988;60:280-4.

63. Motta AC, Komesu MC, Silva CH, et al. Leprosy specific oral lesions: a report of three cases. Med Oral Pathol Oral Cir Bucal. 2008;13:479-82.

64. Pavithran K. Palatal palsy in a case of lepromatous leprosy. Lepr Rev. 1994;65:248-52.

65. Rawlani SM, Rawlani S, Degwekar S, et al. Oral health status and alveolar bone loss in treated leprosy patients of central India. Indian J Lepr. 2011;83:215-24.

66. Hideo Arai. Oral disease in leprosy. In: Makino M, Matsuoka M, Goto M, Hatano K (Eds) Leprosy: Science working towards dignity. Tokyo: Tokai University Press; 2011.pp.216–26.

67. Garrington GE, Crump MC. Pulp death in a patient with lepromatous leprosy. Oral Surg Oral Med Oral Pathol. 1968;25:427-34.

68. Srinivasan S, Nehru VI, Bapuraj JR, et al. CT findings in involvement of the paranasal sinuses by lepromatous leprosy. Br J Radiol. 1999;72:271-3.

69. Kiris A, Karlidag T, Kocakoc E, et al. Paransal sinus computed tomography findings in patients treated for lepromatous leprosy. J Laryngol Otol. 2007;121:15-8.

70. Barton RP, McDougall AC. The paranasal sinuses in lepromatous leprosy. Lepr India. 1979;51:481-5.

71. Hauhnar CZ, Mann SB, Sharma VK, et al. Maxillary antrum involvement in multibacillary leprosy: a radiologic, sinuscopic and histologic assessment. Int J Lepr Other Mycobact Dis. 1992;60:390-5.

72. Sakamoto K. Otorhinolaryngological findings of leprosy. In: Makino M, Matsuoka M, Goto M, Hatano K (Eds) Leprosy: Science working towards dignity. Tokyo: Tokai University Press; 2011.pp.209-15.

73. Mehta V. Reflections: "Gaze of Lazarus", In: Portrait of India. New York: Farrar, Straus and Giroux; 1970.pp. 437-41.

74. Bretan O, De Souza LB, Lastoria JC. Laryngeal lesion in leprosy and the risk of aspiration. Lepr Rev. 2007;78:80-1.

75. D'souza GA, Jindal SK, Malik SK, et al. Airway response to aerosol inhalation in leprosy. Indian J Med Res. 1988;87:190-3.

76. Powell CS, Swan II. Leprosy: pathologic changes observed in fifty consecutive necropsies. Am J Pathol. 1955;31;1131-47.

77. Desikan KV, Job CK. A review of post-mortem findings in 37 cases of leprosy. Int J Lepr. 1968;36:377-83.

78. Liu TC, Qiu JS. Pathological findings on peripheral nerves, lymph nodes and visceral organs of leprosy. Int J Lepr. 1984;52:377-83.

79. Kaur S, Chakravarti RN, Wahi PL. Liver pathology in leprosy. Lepr India. 1974;46:222.

80. Chen TS, Drutz DJ, Whelan GE. Hepatic granulomas in leprosy. Their relation to bacteraemia. Arch Pathol Lab Med. 1976;100:182-5.

81. Singh N, Bhatia A, Lakra A, et al. Comparative cytomorphology of skin, lymph node, liver and bone marrow in patients with lepromatous leprosy. Cytopathology. 2006;17:257-61.

82. Nigam PK, Gupta GB, Khare A. Hepatic involvement and hepatitis B surface antigen (HbsAg) in leprosy. Indian J Dermatol Venereol Leprol. 2003;69:32-4.

83. Kumar B, Koshy A, Kaur S, et al. Leprosy, liver and jaundice. Indian J Lepr. 1987;59:194-202.

84. Kumar B, Narang AP, Koshy A, et al. *In vivo* an *in vitro* drug metabolism in patients with leprosy. Lepr India. 1982;54:75-81.

85. Naumov V, Mesniankina O, Aprishkina M. Metabolic disorder in subsided cases of multibacillary types of leprosy. Presented at: 18th International Leprosy Conference, Hidden challenges; 2013 Sept 16 – Sept 19; Brussels, Belgium.

86. Singh N, Arora VK, Jain A, et al. Cytology of testicular changes in leprosy. Acta Cytol. 2002;46:659-63.

87. Kumar B, Raina A, Kaur S, et al. Clinico-pathological study of testicular involvement in leprosy. Lepr India. 1982;54:48-55.

88. Abraham A, Sharma VK, Kaur S. Assessment of testicular volume in bacilliferous leprosy: correlation with clinical parameters. Indian J Lepr. 1990;62:310-5.

89. Saporta L, Yuksle A. Androgenic status in patients with lepromatous leprosy. Br J Urol. 1994;74:221-4.

90. Sharma SC, Kumar B, Dhall K, et al. Leprosy and female reproductive organs. Int J Lepr. 1981;49:177-9.

91. Girdhar A, Girdhar BK, Ramu G, et al. Discharge of *M. leprae* in milk of leprosy patients. Lepr India. 1981;53:390-4.

92. Survey RB, Hardas UD, Chakravarti D. Leprosy complicating pregnancy and puerperium. Lepr India. 1974;46:234-7.

93. Kaur S. Renal manifestations of leprosy. Indian J Lepr. 1990;62:273-80.

94. Kirsztajn GM, Nishida SK, Silva MS, et al. Renal abnormalities in leprosy. Nephron. 1993;65:381-4.

95. Nakayama EE, Ura S, Fleury RN, et al. Renal lesions in leprosy: a retrospective study of 199 autopsies. Am J Kidney Dis. 2001;38:26-30.

96. da Silva Junior GB, Daher Ede F. Renal involvement in leprosy: retrospective analysis of 461 cases in Brazil. Braz J Infect Dis. 2006;10:107-12.

97. Gupta JC, Panda PK. Amyloidosis in leprosy. Lepr India. 1980;52:260-6.

98. Gupta JC, Diwakar R, Singh S, et al. A histopathologic study of renal biopsies in fifty cases of leprosy. Int J Lepr Other Mycobact Dis. 1977;45:167-70.

99. Lomonte C, Chiaruli G, Cazzato F, et al. End-stage renal disease in leprosy. J Nephrol. 2004;17:302-5.

100. Dash RJ, Sriprakash ML, Kumar B, et al. Adrenal cortical reserve in leprosy. Indian J Med Res. 1985;82:388-92.

101. Ramanaujam K, Dharmendra. Management of reactions in leprosy. In: Dharmendra (Ed). Leprosy. Bombay: Kothari Medical.1978.pp.512-34.

102. Jopling WH, McDougall AC. Other aspects of treatment. In: Handbook of Leprosy, 5th edition. New Delhi: CBS Publishers; 1996.pp. 118-34.

103. Yumnam IS, Kaur S, Kumar B, et al. Evaluation of thyroid functions in leprosy. Lepr India. 1977;49:485-91.

104. Job CK, Drain B, Truman R, et al. The pathogenesis of leprosy in the nine-banded armadillos and the significance of IgM antibodies to PGL-1. Indian J Lepr, 1992;64:137-51.

105. Kar HK, Mohanty HC, Mohanty GN, et al. Clinico-pathological study of lymph node involvement in leprosy. Lepr India. 1983:55:725-31.

106. Apte DC, Zawar M, Mehta MC, et al. Regional lymph node involvement in tuberculoid leprosy. Lepr India. 1983;55:680-5.

107. González-Villarreal MG, Gómez-Almaguer D, Salazar-Riojas R, et al. Bone marrow involvement in leprosy. Rev Invest Clin. 1991;43:192-4.

108. Suster S, Cabello-Inchausti B, Robinson MJ. Nongranulomatous involvement of the bone marrow in lepromatous leprosy. Am J Clin Pathol. 1989;92:797-801.

109. Brooks FJ, Alvarez S, Yoder L. Leukopenia secondary to mycobacterium leprae. J La State Med Soc. 1990;142:35-6.

110. Sen R, Sehgal PK, Singh U, et al. Bacillaemia and bone marrow involvement in leprosy. Indian J Lepr. 1989;61:445-52.

111. Kocher DK, Gupta DV, Sandeep C, et al. Study of brain stem auditory-evoked potentials (BAEPs) and visual-evoked potentials (VEPs) in leprosy. Int J Lepr. 1997;65:157-65.

112. Mann SB, Kumar B, Yande R, et al. Eighth nerve evaluation in leprosy. Indian J Lepr. 1987;59:20-5.

113. Dhand UK, Kumar B, Dhand R, et al. Phrenic nerve conduction in leprosy. Int J Lepr Other Mycobact Dis. 1988;56:389-93.

114. Aung T, Kitajima S, Nimoto M, et al. *Mycobacterium leprae* in neurons of the medulla oblongata and spinal cord in leprosy. J Neuropathol Exp Neurol. 2007;66:284-94.

115. Goto M, Kimura T, Hagio S, et al. Neuropathological analysis of dementia in a Japanese leprosarium. Dementia. 1995;6:157-61.

116. Holla VV, Zawar PB, Deshmuckh SD, et al. Leproma of the heart. A case report. Indian Heart J. 1983;35:111-3.

117. Ramachandran A, Neelan PN. Autonomic neuropathy in leprosy. Indian J Lepr. 1987;59:277-85.

118. Khattri HN, Radhakrishanan K, Kaur S, et al. Cardiac dysautonomia in leprosy. Int J Lepr Other Mycobact Dis. 1978;46:172-4.

119. Chopra JS, Kaur S, Murthy JM, et al. Vascular changes in leprosy and its role in the pathogenesis of leprous neuritis. Lepr India. 1981;53:443-53.

120. Coruh G, McDougall AC. Untreated lepromatous leprosy-histopathological findings in cutaneous blood vessels. Int J Lepr. 1979;47:500-11.

121. Mukherji A, Girdhar BK, Malviya GN, et al. Involvement of subcutaneous veins in lepromatous leprosy. Int J Lepr. 1983;51:1-5.

122. Thompson AM, Lynn AA, Robson K, et al. Lepromatous phlebitis of the external jugular vein. J Am Acad Dermatol. 2003;49:1180-2.

123. Scollard DM, McCormick G, Allen JL. Localization of *Mycobacterium leprae* to endothelial cells of epineurial and perineurial blood vessels and lymphatics. Am J Pathol. 1999;154:1611-20.

124. Kumar B, Sehgal S, Ganguly NK. Total and differential serum proteins and globulins in leprosy. Lepr India. 1982;54:263-9.

125. Gupta SC, Chhabra B, Mehrotra TN, et al. A study of antispermatozoal antibodies in leprosy. Int J Lepr. 1982;50:43-6.

126. Guedes Barbosa LS, Gilbrut B, Shoenfeld Y, et al. Autoantibodies in leprosy sera. Clin Rheumatol. 1996;15:26-8.

127. Pradhan V, Badakere SS, Shankar KU. Increased incidence of cytoplasmic ANCA (cANCA) and other autoantibodies in leprosy patients from western India. Lepr Rev. 2004;75:50-6.

128. deLarrañaga GF, Forastiero RR, Martinuzzo ME, et al. High prevalence of antiphospholipid antibodies in leprosy. Lupus. 2000;9:594-600.

129. Sehgal S, Kumar B. Circulating and tissue immune complexes in leprosy. Int J Lepr. 1981;49:294-301.

130. Kumar B, Ganguly NK, Kaur S, et al. Complement profile in leprosy. Lepr India. 1980;52:217-22.

131. Danda D, Cherian AM. Rheumatological manifestations of leprosy and lepra reaction. Indian J Lepr. 2001;73:58-60.

132. Azulay RD. Auto aggressive Hanseniasis. J Am Acad Dermatol. 1987;17:1042-6.

133. Chatterjee G, Kaur S, Sharma VK, et al. Bacillaemia in leprosy and effect of multidrug therapy. Lepr Rev. 1989;60:197-201.

CHAPTER 24

Leprosy and Human Immunodeficiency Virus Coinfection

Archana Singal

Leprosy continues to be a significant public health problem in India. Most endemic countries for leprosy also have a high prevalence of human immunodeficiency virus-1 (HIV-1) infection, thereby increasing the possibility of HIV-leprosy coinfection. HIV coinfection has a major effect on the natural history of many infectious diseases, notably tuberculosis (TB) and other mycobacterial diseases. Therefore, it was imperative to expect similar outcome in leprosy patients coinfected with HIV. Immunosuppressive effect of HIV on the prevalence and clinical manifestations of leprosy has been the subject of much speculation and epidemiological investigations. However, studies on epidemiological and clinical aspect of leprosy suggest that unlike other mycobacterial diseases the course of leprosy is not markedly modified by the HIV pandemic.[1]

There are conflicting reports regarding the clinical presentation, rate of reactions and relapse and disease management outcomes in patients with coinfection. HIV coinfection may impact following aspects of leprosy:

- Prevalence and diagnosis
- Predominance of multibacillary (MB) or paucibacillary (PB), and clinical features
- Complications, reactions, relapse and outcome of the disease
- Response to treatment (antileprosy treatment and treatment of reactions).

Impact of leprosy on HIV disease, progression and antiretroviral therapy.

In addition, a specific condition immune reconstitution inflammatory syndrome (IRIS) following initiation of highly active antiretroviral therapy (HAART) has been reported to develop in patients with Leprosy-HIV coinfection due to restored immunity.

PREVALENCE AND DIAGNOSIS

The relationship between leprosy and HIV coinfection is not fully understood as little is known about the natural history of the coinfected patients. It is a matter of debate whether HIV infection increases the risk of acquiring leprosy. It is difficult to carry out case-control or prospective cohort studies on the incidence of leprosy in HIV positive patients and HIV negative controls due to long incubation period and low incidence of leprosy. Studies in Malawi,[2] south India[3] and Brazil[4] found no association between HIV infection and leprosy. However, few studies have demonstrated small increase in HIV seroprevalence among leprosy patients.[5-7] This increase is substantially lower than that present in tuberculosis or diseases due to *Mycobacterium avium complex* (MAC). However, there are major drawbacks in these studies such as small number of coinfected patients; nonconsideration of immunosuppression (blood CD4 counts) and other confounding factors like age, sex, sexual behavior, urban/rural set-up and socioeconomic status. There are also concerns regarding the reliability of HIV diagnoses in some of these studies. Leprosy might affect the specificity or sensitivity of some serological assays for diagnosis of HIV because patients with lepromatous leprosy have a polyclonal hypergammaglobulinemia that can give rise to false positive results. Leprosy patients also produce antibodies to mycobacterial cell wall antigens, which may cross react with HIV-1 *pol* and *gag* proteins in certain assays.

In a study from India, western blot (WB) analysis revealed that sera samples from HIV negative leprosy patients across the spectrum showed high reactivity with *p18, Gp41* and *p55* resulting in high frequency of false positive results.[8] So, there is a need for caution in reporting HIV infection among leprosy patients. Newer serological assays are more reliable and indeterminate or nonconfirmed results should be assessed by PCR or other techniques. Conversely, HIV infection causing false positive serological assays for leprosy has also been reported, though diagnosis of leprosy depends mainly on clinical, bacteriological and histological indices.

PREDOMINANCE OF MULTIBACILLARY OR PAUCIBACILLARY TYPE AND CLINICAL FEATURES

Though HIV-1 infection has been shown to be strongly associated with the development of active tuberculosis[9,10] and diseases caused by other mycobacteria;[11] its association with leprosy is much less clear. As the cell-mediated immune response of an individual determines the type of leprosy that will develop, theoretically predominance of multibacillary (MB) leprosy and a faster clinical evolution is expected in patients with dual infection, because of reduced cell-mediated immunity in HIV-1 positive individuals. Several case reports and case series published to determine this association document that all types of leprosy occur in coinfected patients. A weak association between HIV positivity and MB leprosy has been suggested by few reports from East Africa.[5,12] A case control study conducted in Tanzania observed that HIV prevalence was higher with MB cases (5/28, 18%), as compared to PB cases (4/65, 6%).[5] Further, the clinical presentation and disability grade of HIV-1 infected patients was similar to that of patients without HIV infection.[5] A positive association of HIV infection with leprosy was claimed in a subsequent study from Tanzania itself (odds ratio 2.5; 95% CI 2.0–3.2) but the authors have not commented on the differential association with MB and PB disease in leprosy patients. This data also suggested that the protective effect of BCG vaccination against leprosy is lessened by HIV infection.[7] On the contrary, a study from Brazil demonstrated predominance (78%) of paucibacillary disease among HIV positive individuals.[13] Another study from Ethiopia did not find any significant difference between the ratios of lepromatous and tuberculoid leprosy in HIV coinfected patients.[14] In 23 HIV and leprosy coinfected patients from Ethiopia, all types of leprosy was seen, with higher number of BT cases despite HIV infection. There were higher rates of reaction with more steroid resistant reactions in the coinfected group.[15]

No definite conclusions can be reached based on this limited and contradictory data. It has been postulated that relatively long incubation periods for leprosy (2–5 years for tuberculoid and 5–15 years for lepromatous disease) might bias towards tuberculoid disease, since patients might die of AIDS related complications before manifesting lepromatous disease.

Spectrum of skin lesions ranging from hypopigmented tuberculoid lesions to nodular lepromatous lesions have been described in HIV-infected patients. Worsening of nerve damage might be expected in patients with dual infection as HIV may alter the immune response in nerves to *M. leprae*. HIV is itself neuropathic, so it could also act synergistically with *M. leprae*. However, conclusive evidence to support this hypothesis is lacking.

COMPLICATIONS, REACTIONS, RELAPSE AND OUTCOMES

Many authors have evaluated HIV positivity as a risk factor for various complications of leprosy. A study from Uganda demonstrated significant increase in the incidence of type 1 reactions in HIV seropositive MB patients as compared to HIV seronegative MB patients (9/12 vs. 8/40, $p < 0.0005$). Further development of acute neuritis was observed in significantly more number of HIV seropositives as compared to seronegative MB population (8/9 vs 3/8, $p < 0.0005\%$).[16] However, no significant difference was observed in the incidence of these complications in seropositive and seronegative PB patients.[16] Vreeberg reported early onset severe neuritis in patients with dual infection along with many severe episodes of intercurrent infections that proved fatal in two patients, probably as a result of long established HIV-1 infection with advanced immunological disturbances.[17] Though reversal reactions and neuritis, both acute and chronic, were not significantly influenced by HIV status, a possible increase in recurrent reversal reactions in HIV positive cases has been reported.[14] In a cohort study, Talhari et al. observed upward shifting of all clinical forms of leprosy after initiation of HAART and multidrug therapy.[18] On the other hand, neuritis was not found to be more severe or different in character in HIV positive cases and no association existed between HIV positivity and degree of impairment at the start of treatment, after completion or 5 years follow-up thereafter.[14] Three untreated borderline leprosy patients with HIV-1 infection developed reversal reaction with neuritis and not downgrading reaction towards lepromatous pole.[19] Further, the current situation concerning continued new leprosy case detection and HIV infection in India emphasizes the importance of monitoring the occurrence of coinfections. A longer duration of surveillance is advisable after fixed duration therapy for the detection of early relapse. Moreover, the impact of immune restoration in coinfected patients receiving antiretroviral therapy is commonly observed in cases with borderline leprosy.[20]

Erythema nodosum leprosum (ENL) reactions were not reported in HIV positive individuals until recently and it has been suggested that HIV infection may decrease the risk of this complication.[21] However, of late case reports of ENL in HIV positive leprosy patients have started to appear albeit infrequently. In one study, HIV positive individuals were reported to have a higher risk of ENL reactions (relative risk 5.2: 95% CI 1.7–15.9)[14] though Nery et al. observed no enhanced risk of ENL among their patients.[22]

Reversal reactions and acute neuritis in leprosy occur as a result of cell mediated, delayed type hypersensitivity, so the reactions may be expected to be reduced in HIV positive cases. Likewise, ENL reactions occur due to circulating immune complexes and their increased prevalence—if it actually occurs in HIV positive cases should be a paradox. Increased death rate among leprosy patients with HIV coinfection has been reported,[23] particularly in those who developed recurrent reversal reaction as a result of advanced immunosuppression.[14]

Relapse in a case of BB leprosy with HIV coinfection has been reported by Rath and Kar. They described three HIV-positive leprosy cases; two BT with CD4+ counts of 482 and 540 cells/μL and one BB case with CD4+ counts 240 cells/μL; with antileprosy therapeutic response. Both BT cases responded well to conventional WHO MDT (PB) for 6 months; whereas the BB case relapsed 3 months after completion of MDT (MB) for one year. However, the disease became inactive again following a further one-year course of MDT (MB).[24]

RESPONSE TO TREATMENT

Management of a coinfected patient is a challenge for want of clear cut guidelines or uniform consensus and is further confounded by the lack of information on the natural course of dual infection.

Antileprosy Treatment

It was postulated that HIV infection might affect the efficacy of multidrug therapy for leprosy with HIV-positive patients potentially taking longer to clear mycobacteria from the lesions or experience a higher relapse rate. However, coinfected patients treated with standard duration of WHO-MDT regimen seem to respond adequately and experience similar side effect profile.[16,19] The clinical evolution and response to treatment with MDT is reported to be similar in both HIV positive and HIV negative leprosy patients.[25] Therefore, it has been recommended that HIV/leprosy coinfected patients should be treated with standard MDT together with HAART.[26] As the relapse rates are rare after multidrug therapy both in tuberculoid as well as lepromatous patients, assessment of HIV infection as an important cofactor in slight increase in relapse rate may be difficult unless mandatory HIV testing is included in the sentinel surveillance of all patients relapsing after MDT. However, the Sarno study observed a 3.4% relapse rate in coinfected patients on ART compared to 1.0% relapse rate in HIV negative patients[13] suggesting that patients with coinfection should be monitored more closely for relapse after treatment.

Treatment of Reactions

Patients with borderline leprosy and coexistent HIV-1 infection developing reversal reaction have been reported to respond adequately to steroid therapy.[19] No difference has been reported in the response to steroid therapy among seropositive and seronegative leprosy patients in the management of acute neuritis or reversal reaction.[13,14] On the other hand, poorer outcome to steroid therapy has been reported by others.[17]

Thalidomide has been used traditionally for the management of ENL in immune competent leprosy patients. It has been used with success in the management of severe, recurrent ENL, refractory to high doses of daily steroid therapy in a patient with coexistent HIV infection.[27] Recently it has also been reported to produce an antiretroviral effect without any negative effect on immune competence,[28] possibly through inhibition of TNF production and by blocking TNF stimulated HIV replication.[29] Due to these properties, it appears to be the drug of choice for treating ENL in HIV positive leprosy patients. However, the drug has to be used with caution in view of a report of increased viral counts caused by thalidomide.[30]

Recently, an interesting case of refractory type 2 reaction occurring in a HIV positive patient with normal CD4 has been reported that responded favorably to the institution of HAART.[31]

IMPACT OF LEPROSY ON HIV PROGRESSION AND ANTIRETROVIRAL THERAPY

Tuberculosis is known to accelerate the decline of immune functions in HIV-positive individuals by augmenting the rate of HIV replication, resulting most likely from marked proinflammatory cytokine drive in tuberculosis patients. This issue has not been addressed in relation to leprosy as this cytokine drive is not present in leprosy patients except during severe ENL reaction.

Early institution of highly active antiretroviral therapy (HAART) is reported to provide an edge in improving therapeutic outcome in a patient with dual infection. In the management of reactions, addition of HAART not only improves the therapeutic response to lower doses of steroids but also helps in their complete withdrawal, subsequently.[27] However, since most of the clinical signs of leprosy are dependent on cell-mediated immunity, it has been postulated that when HIV infected patients with latent leprosy receive HAART, their immune system recovers and *M.leprae* antigens are recognized with subsequent development of clinical leprosy and exacerbation of existing leprosy lesions. Talhari et al. reported two such AIDS patients with very low CD4 count (71 and 6 cells per μL) on HAART for 1–2 months, who developed skin lesions of borderline lepromatous leprosy (BL).[32] MB MDT was instituted in addition to HAART. About 2–3 months later, their CD4 counts increased, and both patients presented with swollen lesions of BT with type 1 reaction which was documented histologically and treated with systemic steroids. These cases represent unusual presentation of occurrence of BL leprosy as a result of augmented immunity following HAART therapy and subsequent shifting of BL to BT as IRIS after institution of MB MDT in addition to HAART.

IMMUNOLOGY AND HISTOLOGY IN LEPROSY-HIV COINFECTION

Leprosy is characterized by a wide spectrum of clinical and histological features that depend on the specific host immunity. Patients with tuberculoid leprosy have adequate cell-mediated immune response to *M. leprae* resulting in few skin lesions, which histologically have well organized, lymphocyte (CD68+, CD3+, CD8+, CD4+)-rich granulomas with predominantly CD4+ T-cells. *In vivo* these patients exhibit strongly positive lepromin test and *in vitro* cells from these patients respond strongly to *M. leprae* in the lymphocyte proliferation assay. In contrast, patients with lepromatous disease have a strong humoral response but poor or absent cell-mediated immunity, resulting in uncontrolled growth of bacilli and disseminated skin lesions. Histology reveals loose infiltrate comprising of macrophages and small number of almost exclusively CD8+ T-cells. *In vitro*, cells from these patients do not respond to *M. leprae*, but produce high titers of *M. leprae* specific antibodies. Immunologically driven inflammation is also responsible for much of the clinically apparent nerve injury. Nerve function impairment is more rapid and severe in patient with aggressive cellular immune response, i.e. in tuberculoid disease and during reactional states especially type 1 reaction. As HIV principally affects cell-mediated immune responses, these pathogens may have potentially interesting immunologic interactions in the human host.

Unlike tuberculosis where HIV infection affects granuloma formation depending upon the degree of immune suppression as reflected by blood CD4+ counts, host granulomatous response to *M. leprae* is preserved among individuals with HIV.[33] Sampaio et al.[34] described 11 patients, three borderline lepromatous (BL) and eight borderline tuberculoid (BT) patients with HIV coinfection and low blood CD4+ counts. They found that biopsy of skin lesions in patients with BT revealed well-formed granulomas that on immunostaining demonstrated normal numbers of CD4+ lymphocytes while BL patients revealed relatively higher number of CD8+ lymphocytes. This observation is intriguing since the predominant cell type towards tuberculoid end of clinical spectrum is CD4+ T lymphocyte, which is also the target cell for HIV. They also demonstrated expression of human leukocyte antigen (HLA)-DR by dermal cells adjacent to granulomas as an evidence of local interferon-γ production. Absence of bacilli in the lesion indicated good immunity. In

addition, HIV infection did not alter the lack of response to *M. leprae* antigens either *in vitro* or *in vivo* in lepromatous leprosy.

Similar observations have been reported by Pereira et al.[35] on histopathological analysis and immunostaining on nine MDT-naive (BT 6, TT 2 ad LL 1) patients with HIV coinfection. BT lesions were characterized by less circumscribed epithelioid granulomas and a few Langerhans CD68+ cells in the center surrounded by CD3+ lymphocytes, a few of them with the CD8+ phenotype. Nerve damage was observed in the histopathologic examination of five of six BT lesions and two were AFB positive. The TT leprosy lesions had well-formed granulomas with CD68+, epithelioid, multinucleated Langerhans cells and macrophages in the center surrounded by a lymphocytic mantle of CD3+ T-cells and few CD8+ T-cells. The TT lesions were AFB negative and nerves were not visualized. The only leprosy skin lesion categorized as LL had a diffuse CD68+, vacuolated, histiocytic cell infiltrate with few CD3+ lymphocytes, a high (3+) AFB positivity, and nerve damage. In all histopathologic categories, few NK CD57+ cells were observed. Similar characteristics on histopathology and immunostaining were observed on seven skin lesions (TT = 3, BT = 3, and indeterminate [I] = 1) collected from coinfected patients on MDT, except for a lower level of cellularity. Thus, histological architecture and cell phenotypes within the leprosy skin lesions are not much changed by HIV. In this cohort of dually infected 22 patients, regardless of the clinical form of leprosy (MB or PB), histopathologic classification, AFB positivity in lesions and MDT status, none including one lepromatous case, had detectable IgM antibodies specific for *M. leprae* PGL I. This finding is consistent with low sensitivity of anti-PGL1 serology in patients with PB leprosy,[35] but not expected in a LL case, as 90% of LL patients without HIV show positivity to antibody. However, as it was a single case, studies on larger number of HIV coinfected LL patients are desirable to provide conclusive results. On the other hand, divergent finding in the form of absent CD4+ cells in the biopsy specimens of all 10 subjects of BT leprosy has been reported in a recent cohort study.[16]

Recently Carvalho et al. explored cellular immunity in patients coinfected with HIV-1 and *M. leprae*.[36] Twenty-eight individuals were studied, comprising four groups: healthy controls, HIV-1 and *M. leprae* coinfection, HIV-1 monoinfection, and *M. leprae* monoinfection. Peripheral blood mononuclear cells (PBMC) were analyzed to evaluate T-cell subpopulations and their activation status, dendritic cell (DC) distribution phenotypes and expression of IL-4 by T-cells. The coinfected group exhibited lower CD4: CD8 ratios, higher levels of CD8+ T-cell activation, increased Vδ1 : Vδ2 T-cell ratios and decreased percentages of plasmacytoid DC, compared with HIV-1 monoinfected subjects. Across infected groups, IL-4 production by CD4+ T lymphocytes was positively correlated with the percentage of effector memory CD4+ T-cells, suggesting antigenically driven differentiation of this population of T-cells

Table 24.1: Summary of impact of HIV-1 on leprosy: expected versus actual[37]

		Theory	*In practice*
Epidemiological	Incidence	Increase in leprosy	No change
Clinical	Lepromatous leprosy	Increase	No change
	Treatment response	Less than expected	No change
	Type 1 reactions	Fewer	Increased
	Neuritis	More frequent and severe	?
	Novel findings	Presentation as IRIS	
Histological	Granuloma formation	Decreased	No change
	Bacterial index	Increased	No change

in both HIV-1 and *M. leprae* infections. Coinfection with *M. leprae* may exacerbate the immunopathology of HIV-1 disease. A T helper 2 (Th2) bias in the CD4+ T-cell response was evident in both HIV-1 infection and leprosy, but no additive effect was apparent in coinfected patients.

The exact immune-pathophysiological mechanism underlying the possible increase in frequency of leprosy reactions is not clear. Dysregulation of the immune system and the heightened state of immune activation in HIV infection may be responsible. In addition, delayed clearance of *M.leprae* antigen due to impaired phagocytic function of macrophages has also been implicated.[33]

Table 24.1 summarizes the impact of HIV-1 on leprosy: expected versus actual.[37]

IMMUNE RECONSTITUTION INFLAMMATORY SYNDROME

The immune reconstitution inflammatory syndrome (IRIS) in HIV-infected/AIDS patients results from restored immunity to specific infectious or noninfectious antigens following initiation of highly active antiretroviral therapy (HAART) and presents with the manifestation or unmasking of a previously subclinical coinfection or the symptomatic deterioration of an opportunistic infection that had been responding to the treatment.[38] Such reactions typically occur during the first 4 months of treatment with HAART; the most rapid phase of immune recovery. The prevalence of IRIS in cohort studies of HIV patients ranges from 3% to over 50% and is dependent on the underlying AIDS defining illness.[39] Risk factors for the development of IRIS include advanced HIV disease with CD4 cell count under 50 cells/µL, unrecognized opportunistic infection or high microbial burden and the number and presence of prior opportunistic infections.[40] IRIS was initially observed in cases of coinfection with mycobacteria (*Mycbacterium avium complex and Mycbacterium tuberculosis*) in 1998.[41] Subsequently, association with viral (*cytomegalovirus, herpes simplex, varicella zoster, human papilloma virus* and *hepatitis B* and

Table 24.2: Proposed criteria for the diagnosis of IRIS[43]

- HIV positive
- Receiving HAART
  - Decrease in HIV-1 RNA level from baseline
  - Increase in CD4+ cells from baseline (may lag HIV-1 RNA decrease)
- Clinical symptoms consistent with inflammatory process
- Clinical course not consistent with
  - Expected course of previously diagnosed opportunistic infection
  - Expected course of newly diagnosed opportunistic infection
  - Drug toxicity

C virus), fungal (*Cryptococcus neoformans, Histoplasma capsulatum)*, and protozoal infections (*Toxoplasma gondii, Leishmania donovani* and *Pneumocystis jerovecii*) have been reported.[40] In some cases, IRIS appears in the absence of oppurtunistic pathogens and manifests itself as an autoimmune or granulomatous disease, of which sarcoidosis is the most frequent.[42] Diagnostic criteria of IRIS as described by Shelburne et al.[43] has been given in Table 24.2.

After initiation of HAART, there is numerical increase in circulatory CD4+ cells. Of these, activated memory cells (CD4+, CD45RO+) account for the early incremental phase of CD4+ cell recovery. Recovery of lost responses to specific antigens also occurs during this early phase, probably because of cellular redistribution rather than a *denovo* specific CD4+ cell proliferation. IRIS has been thought to be a result of several factors: response to a high antigen burden, an excessive response by the recovering immune system, exacerbated production of pro-inflammatory cytokines or a lack of immune regulation due to inability to produce regulatory cytokines. Disease susceptibility genes for specific subset of IRIS have been identified, e.g. TNFA-308*2 for mycobacterial disease and HLA-B44 for herpes virus related IRIS. In addition, a CD4+ cells subset (known as T-regulatory cells) (CD4+, CD25+ Fox P3+) has an intrinsic ability to downregulate the immune response and may play a role in the pathogenesis of IRIS. These T-regulatory cells are susceptible to HIV infection and their numbers also decrease in AIDS.[43]

IRIS in association with leprosy was first described by Lawn et al. in 2003 in a 37-year old seropositive male patient (CD4+ count of 10/µL) from Uganda.[44] Since then 23 reports of patients developing IRIS have been published mostly from the parts of world which are considered endemic for both HIV/AIDS and leprosy, and where ART is more readily available, so 70% were from South America (58% from Brazil) and 20% from India (Table 24.3).[37,44-55] Most of the reported cases belong to borderline tuberculoid (BT) leprosy except one case of IRIS described by Singal in a patient with borderline lepromatous (BL) leprosy.[51] Clinically leprosy as IRIS usually presents as type 1 reaction with the development of erythematous, odematous skin lesions which may develop unusual ulceration and neuritis with nerve paresis/paralysis.

All these cases fulfilled the *case definition* for leprosy associated IRIS, that has been proposed to facilitate correct identification of cases based on the clinical presentation, evidence of immune restoration and timing of onset and include the following: (1) leprosy and/or leprosy reactions presenting within 6 months of starting HAART; (2) advanced HIV infection; (3) a low CD4 count before starting HAART; (4) CD4 count increasing after institution of HAART.[56]

Using this data, *four types of presentation of IRIS* have been identified:[57]

1. *Unmasking*: When patients develop leprosy or type 1 reaction after starting HAART. They were not diagnosed to have leprosy, probably incubating the disease which

manifest after the immune restoration occurs. This is the most common occurrence. A slightly different presentation has been reported recently when a HIV positive patient manifested histoid leprosy rather than reversal reaction or other features of IRIS, 7.5 months after the initiation of HAART.[58]

2. *Overlap of immune restoration*: When leprosy has been diagnosed before starting HAART. When MDT and HAART are started, type 1 reaction occur as a paradoxical reaction within 3 months.

3. Undiagnosed leprosy or previously treated leprosy recurs at least 6 months before HAART. Type 1 reaction occurs when HAART is introduced.

4. *Unmasking followed by overlap of immune restoration after HAART and MDT*: When leprosy has been diagnosed within 6 months of starting HAART and MDT. The patient develops reaction later.

Treatment of IRIS Associated Reaction

Leprosy patient even if HIV positive, need immune-suppression for treating leprosy reactions and neuritis. Patient being treated with steroids need careful monitoring to ensure early detection and management of opportunistic infections. Anti-inflammatory drugs and specific antimicrobial agents may be required along with the continuation of HAART.[59]

As access to HAART is increasing in leprosy endemic countries including India, the numbers of IRIS cases due to leprosy are likely to increase in future. Recognition of leprosy as an IRIS-associated entity is important in order to institute timely intervention.

Table 24.3: Leprosy cases in HIV positive patients presenting with IRIS

Author, Reference	Age and sex	Clinical presentation	CD4 count/µL before/after	Time interval
Lawn SD et al. 2003[44]	37 M	BT-Type 1 Reaction	10/70	1 month
Couppié P et al. 2004[46]	54 M	BT-Type 1 Reaction	87/257	2 months
	40 M	TT-Type 1 Reaction	130/278	5 months
	39 F	TT-Type 1 Reaction	31/171	3 months
Pignataro P et al. 2004[47]	48 M	TT-Type 1 Reaction	147/499	3 months
	34 F	Reversal Reaction	37/200	1 month
Visco-Comandini U et al. 2004[48]	32 M	TT-Type 1 Reaction	7/90	2 months
Pereira GAS et al. 2004[49]	38 F	BT-Type 1 Reaction	73/270	2 months
	25 M	BT-Type 1 Reaction	35/100	6 months
*Narang T et al. 2005[50]	28 M	BT-Type 1 Reaction	125/280	2 months
*Singal A et al. 2006[51]	32 M	BL-Type 1 Reaction	108/224	3 months
*Kharkar V et al. 2007[52]	35 M	BT-Type 1 Reaction	299/504	3 months
	42 M	BT-Type 1 Reaction	114/ 184	2 months
Talhari C et al. 2007[53]	35 M	BT-Type 1 Reaction	92/426	3 months
Batista MD et al. 2008[54]	32 M	BT-Type 1 Reaction	14/172	2 months
	53 M	BT-Type 1 Reaction	104/235	2 months
*Kulkarni V et al. 2009[55]	27 M	PB-Type 1 Reaction	174/436	5 months
	30 M	PB-Type 1 Reaction	31/144	4 months

REFERENCES

1. Massone C, Talhari C, Ribeiro-Rodrigues R, et al. Leprosy and HIV coinfection : a critical approach. Expert Rev Anti Infect Ther. 2011;9(6):701-10.
2. Pönnighaus JM, Mwanjasi LJ, Fine PE, et al. Is HIV infection a risk factor for leprosy? Int J Lepr Other Mycobact Dis. 1991;59:221-8.
3. Sekar B, Jayasheela M, Chattopadhya D, et al. Prevalence of HIV infection and high-risk characteristics among leprosy patients of south India; a case-control study. Int J Lepr Other Mycobact Dis. 1994;62:527-31.
4. Andrade VL, Avelleira JC, Marques A, et al. Leprosy as cause of false-positive results in serological assays for the detection of antibodies to HIV-1. Int J Lepr Other Mycobact Dis. 1991;59:125-6.
5. Borgdorff MW, van den Broek J, Chum HJ. HIV-1 infection as a risk factor for leprosy; a case-control study in Tanzania. Int J Lepr Other Mycobact Dis. 1993;61:556-62.
6. Meeran K. Prevalence of HIV infectionamon patients with leprosy and tuberculosis in rural Zambia. BMJ. 1989;298:364-65.
7. van den Broek J, Chum HJ, Swai R, et al. Association between leprosy and HIV infection in Tanzania. Int J Lepr Other Mycobact Dis. 1997;65:203-10.
8. Hussain T, Sinha S, Katoch K, et al. Serum samples from patients with mycobacterial infections cross-react with HIV structural proteins Gp41, p55 and p18. Lepr Rev. 2007;78(2):137-47.
9. Long R, Scalcini M, Manfreda J et al. Impact of human immunodeficiency virus type 1 on tuberculosis in rural Haiti. Am Rev Respir Dis. 1991;143:69-73.
10. Selwyn PA, Hartel D, Lewis VA, et al. A prospective study of the risk of tuberculosis among intravenous drug users with human immunodeficiency virus infection. N Engl J Med. 1989;320:545-50.
11. Pitchenik AE. The treatment and prevention of mycobacterial disease in patients with HIV infection. AIDS. 1988;2 (Suppl 1):S177-82.
12. Orege PA, Fine PE, Lucas SB, et al. A case control study on human immunodeficiency virus-1 (HIV-1) infection as a risk factor for tuberculosis and leprosy in western Kenya. Tuber Lung Dis. 1993;74:377-81.
13. Sarno EN, Illarramendi X, Nery JA, et al. HIV-M. leprae interaction: can HAART modify the course of leprosy? Public Health Rep. 2008;123:206-12.
14. Gebre S, Saunderson P, Messele T, et al. The effect of HIV status on the clinical picture of leprosy: a prospective study in Ethiopia. Lepr Rev. 2000;71:338-43.
15. Lockwood D, Lambert SM, Nicholls P, et al. Leprosy HIV Co-infection observational study in Ethiopia. Presented at: International Leprosy Congress; 2013 Sept 16 – Sept 19; Brussels, Belgium.
16. Bwire R, Kawuma HJ. Type 1 reactions in leprosy, neuritis and steroid therapy: the impact of the human immunodeficiency virus. Trans R Soc Trop Med Hyg. 1994;88:315-6.
17. Vreeburg AE. Clinical observations on leprosy patients with HIV1-infection in Zambia. Lepr Rev. 1992;63:134-40.
18. Talhari C, Mira MT, Massone C, et al. Leprosy and HIV coinfection: a clinical pathological immunological and therapeutic study of a cohort from a Brazilian referral center for infectious diseases. J infect Dis. 2010;202:345-54.

19. Arunthathi S, Ebenezer L, Kumuda C. Reversal reaction, nerve damage and steroid therapy in three multibacillary HIV positive patients. Lepr Rev. 1998;69:173-7.
20. Kar HK, Sharma P. Does concomitant HIV infection has any epidemiological, clinical, immunopathological and therapeutic relevance in leprosy? Indian J Lepr. 2007;79:45-60.
21. Miller RA. Leprosy and AIDS: a review of the literature and speculations on the impact of CD4+ lymphocyte depletion on immunity to Mycobacterium leprae. Int J Lepr Other Mycobact Dis. 1991;59:639-44.
22. Nery JA, Sampaio EP, Galhardo MC, et al. M. leprae-HIV co-infection: pattern of immune response in vivo and in vitro. Indian J Lepr. 2000;72:155-67.
23. Lewis DE, Yang L, Luo W, et al. HIV-specific cytotoxic T lymphocyte precursors exist in a CD28-CD8+ T cell subset and increase with loss of CD4 T cells. AIDS. 1999;13:1029-33.
24. Rath N, Kar HK. Leprosy in HIV infection: A study of three cases. Indian J Lepr. 2003;75:355-59.
25. Jacob M, George S, Pulimood S, et al. Short-term follow up of patients with multibacillary leprosy and HIV infection. Int J Lepr. 1996;64:391-95.
26. Trindade MA, Manini MI, Masetti JH, et al. Leprosy and HIV co-infection in five patients. Lepr Rev. 2005;76:162-6.
27. Sharma NL, Mahajan VK, Sharma VC, et al. Erythema nodosum leprosum and HIV infection: A therapeutic experience. Int J Lepr Other Mycobact Dis. 2005;73:189-93.
28. Stirling DI. Thalidomide and its impact in dermatology. Semin Cutan Med Surg. 1998;17:231-42.
29. Ravot E, Lisziewicz J, Lori F. New uses for old drugs in HIV infection: the role of hydroxyurea, cyclosporin and thalidomide. Drugs. 1999;58:953-63.
30. Radomsky CL, Levine N. Thalidomide. Dermatol Clin. 2001; 19:87-103.
31. Sachdeva S, Amin SS, Qaisar S. Type 2 lepra reaction with HIV1 co-infection: a case report with interesting management implications. Indian J Lepr. 2011;83:103-6.
32. Talhari C, Ferreira LC, Araújo JR, et al. Immune reconstitution inflammatory syndrome or upgrading type 1 reaction? Report of two AIDS patients presenting a shifting from borderline lepromatous leprosy to borderline tuberculoid leprosy. Lepr Rev. 2008;79:429-35.
33. Ustianowski AP, Lawn SD, Lockwood DN. Interactions between HIV infection and leprosy: a paradox. Lancet Infect Dis. 2006;6:350-60.
34. Sampaio EP, Caneshi JR, Nery JA et al. Cellular immune response to Mycobacterium leprae infection in human immunodeficiency virus-infected individuals. Infect Immun. 1995;63:1848-54.
35. Pereira GA, Stefani MM, Araújo Filho JA, et al. Human immunodeficiency virus type 1 (HIV-1) and Mycobacterium leprae co-infection: HIV-1 subtypes and clinical, immunologic, and histopathologic profiles in a Brazilian cohort. Am J Trop Med Hyg. 2004;71:679-84.
36. Carvalho KI, Maeda S, Marti L, et al. Immune cellular parameters of leprosy and human immunodeficiency virus-1 co-infected subjects. Immunology. 2008;124:206-14.
37. Lockwood DJ, Lambert SM. Leprosy and HIV, where are we at? Lepr Rev. 2010;81:169-75.
38. Murdoch DM, Venter WD, Van Rie A, et al. Immune reconstitution inflammatory syndrome (IRIS): review of

common infectious manifestations and treatment options. AIDS Res Ther. 2007;4:9.

39. Müller M, Wandel S, Colebunders R, et al. Immune reconstitution inflammatory syndrome in patients starting antiretroviral therapy for HIV infection: a systematic review and meta-analysis. Lancet Infect Dis. 2010;10:251-61.

40. Shelburne SA, Visnegarwala F, Darcourt J, et al. Incidence and risk factors for immune reconstitution inflammatory syndrome during highly active antiretroviral therapy. AIDS. 2005;19:399-406.

41. Race EM, Adelson-Mitty J, Kriegel GR, et al. Focal mycobacterial lymphadenitis following initiation of protease-inhibitor therapy in patients with advanced HIV-1 disease. Lancet. 1998:351:252-5.

42. Blanche P, Passeron A, Gombert B, et al. Sarcoidosis and HIV infection: Influence of highly active antiretroviral therapy. Br J Dermatol. 1999:140:1185.

43. Shelburne SA III, Hamill RJ, Rodriguez-Barradas MC, et al. Immune reconstitution inflammatory syndrome: emergence of a unique syndrome during highly active antiretroviral therapy. Medicine (Baltimore). 2002;81:213-27.

44. Lawn SD, Wood C, Lockwood DN. Borderline tuberculoid leprosy: an immune reconstitution phenomenon in a human immunodeficiency virus-infected person. Clin Infect Dis. 2003;36:e5-6.

45. Sanghi S, Grewal RS, Vasudevan B, et al. Immune reconstitution inflammatory syndrome in leprosy. Indian J Lepr. 2011;83:61-70.

46. Couppié P, Abel S, Voinchet H, et al. Immune reconstitution inflammatory syndrome associated with HIV and leprosy. Arch Dermatol. 2004;140:997-1000.

47. Pignataro P, Rocha AS, Nery JA, et al. Leprosy and AIDS: two cases of increasing inflammatory reactions at the start of highly active antiretroviral therapy. Eur J Clin Microbiol Infect Dis. 2004;23:408-11.

48. Visco-Comandini U, Longo B, Cuzzi T, et al. Tuberculoid leprosy in a patient with AIDS: a manifestation of immune restoration syndrome. Scand J Infect Dis. 2004;36:881-3.

49. Pereira GAS, Stefani MMA, Araujo Filho JA, et al. Human immunodeficiency virus type 1 (HIV-1) and *Mycobacterium leprae* coinfection: HIV-1 subtypes and clinical, immunologic, and histopathologic profiles in a Brazilian cohort. Am J Trop Med Hyg. 2004;71:679-84.

50. Narang T, Dogra S, Kaur I. Borderline tuberculoid leprosy with type 1 reaction in an HIV patient-a phenomenon of immune reconstitution. Int J Lepr Other Mycobact Dis. 2005; 73:203-5.

51. Singal A, Mehta S, Pandhi D. Immune reconstitution inflammatory syndrome in an HIV positive leprosy patient. Lepr Rev. 2006;77:76-80.

52. Kharkar V, Bhor UH, Mahajan S, et al. Type 1 lepra reaction presenting as immune reconstitution inflammatory syndrome. Indian J Dermatol Venereol Leprol. 2007;73:253-6.

53. Talhari C, Machado PRL, Ferreira LC, et al. Shifting of the clinical spectrum of leprosy in an HIV-positive patient: a manifestation of immune reconstitution inflammatory syndrome? Lepr Rev. 2007;78:151-4.

54. Batista MD, Porro AM, Maeda SM, et al. Leprosy Reversal Reaction as Immune Reconstitution Inflammatory Syndrome in Patients with AIDS. Clinical Infectious Diseases. 2008;46: e56–e60.

55. Kulkarni V, Joshi S, Gupte N, et al. Human immunodeficiency virus and leprosy co-infection in Pune, India. J Clin Microb. 2009;47:2998-99.

56. Deps PD, Lockwood DN. Leprosy occurring as immune reconstitution syndrome. Trans R Soc Trop Med Hyg. 2008;102:966-8.

57. Deps P, Lockwood DN. Leprosy presenting as immune reconstitution inflammatory syndrome: proposed definitions and classification. Lepr Rev. 2010;81:59-68.

58. Bumb RA, Ghiya BC, Jakhar R, Prasad N. Histoid leprosy in an HIV positive patient taking cART. Lepr Rev. 2010;81:221-3.

59. Shelburne SA, Montes M, Hamill J. Immune reconstitution inflammatory syndrome: more answers, more questions. J Clin Microbiol. 2006;57:167-70.

Leprosy and Pregnancy

Neena Khanna

INTRODUCTION

Leprosy, though predominantly a disease of the skin and peripheral nerves, does spread to other organs of the body, mostly in the highly bacillated lepromatous leprosy (LL) patients. The dissemination of *Mycobacterium leprae* is assisted by surface proteins called 'adhesins' which facilitate attachment to the endothelial cells (of blood vessels and lymphatics) and Schwann cells. The organs which show significant infiltration resulting in clinical manifestations include liver, lymph nodes, testes, bones, eyes, upper respiratory tract, kidneys, adrenals and bone marrow.[1] However, the number of such patients is dwindling because of the early institution of multidrug therapy (MDT).

In contrast to the universal involvement of testes in multibacillary (MB) disease, the female reproductive organs are not significantly involved in leprosy.

The present chapter discusses the involvement of the female reproductive system by leprosy, the effect of pregnancy on the course of leprosy, and episodes of leprosy reactions as also effect of leprosy on maternal and perinatal outcome.

EFFECT OF LEPROSY ON FEMALE REPRODUCTIVE SYSTEM

Mitsuda described the presence of lepra cells in the endometrium, Fallopian tubes and capillaries of vaginal mucosa, but was emphatic that leprosy in women does not result in sterility.[2,3] In contrast, Leger et al.[4] found that 54% of females with leprosy were infertile and similarly, King and Marks[5] also reported gross menstrual abnormalities in women with leprosy. In neither of the two studies was the hormonal profile evaluated. Bogush[6] reported menstrual dysfunction

in their patients with leprosy which could be prevented by early institution of therapy. He, however, did not comment on the fertility status of these patients. Hardas et al.[7] noted that although obstetric events could alter the course of the disease, leprosy itself had no effect on events like menstrual cycle or fertility. Interestingly, in only 18% of their patients, the endometrial biopsy taken in the premenstrual period showed secretory phase, indicating that though fertility was not affected, there was some hormonal imbalance. Sharma et al.[8] in a study of 35 adult female patients with MB leprosy, found that the infection had no direct effect on menarche, menstrual cycle, fertility and menopause. The biopsy findings from endometrium did not reveal any involvement, and the menstrual fluid was found to be free of leprosy bacilli even in patients having bacillemia.[8] Significantly three (8.6%) of their lepromatous patients had never conceived. Khanna et al.[9] in a study of 86 women with MB leprosy in the reproductive age group, reported irregularity of periods in more than a third of them with the irregularity postdating the onset of leprosy in 30% of the patients. Of the 24 married women with irregular periods, 50% were infertile and about 30% of these patients had elevated levels of follicle-stimulating hormone (FSH) and luteinizing hormone (LH) almost reaching the castration levels. The mean levels of LH, FSH, and prolactin were all significantly elevated in patients with MB leprosy *vis-à-vis* controls. Similar findings suggesting a primary ovarian failure have been reported by Arora et al.[10]

The exact mechanism of ovarian failure in patients with MB leprosy really needs to be further explored, but it could be due to autoimmunity since both cell-mediated and humoral immune responses do play an important role in premature ovarian failure and autoimmune oophoritis, which manifest as irregularity of menstrual cycle and infertility.[11,12] Autoantibodies to granulosa and theca cells, zona pellucida of the oocyte as well as antibodies to adrenal and ovarian steroidogenic enzymes have been demonstrated in these women, indicating an important pathogenic role of autoimmunity in causation of infertility.[11,12] Similarly, the cellular infiltrate in the ovaries results in low estradiol levels with a compensatory increase in FSH levels. Interestingly, the infiltrate spares the granulosa cells resulting in normal to high levels of inhibin A and B.[13] Since MB leprosy is itself associated with increased production of a host of autoantibodies [antineural antibodies,[14] antinuclear antibodies,[15] atypical antineutrophil cytoplasm antibodies (A-ANCA),[16] antimitochondrial antibodies[17] and antispermatozoa antibodies[18]] it may be postulated that the ovarian failure in leprosy is due to formation of autoantibodies against some components of the ovary.

EFFECT OF PREGNANCY ON LEPROSY

Cause of Altered Course of Leprosy in Pregnancy

Several diseases, including infections and autoimmune disorders, have an altered course during pregnancy and puerperium because of:
- Altered immunological response
- Nutritional changes
- Altered secretion of steroids.

Altered Immunological Response

Pregnancy and puerperium are associated with biphasic alterations in both, the humoral and cell-mediated immunity (CMI).[19]

Cell-Mediated Immunity

Pregnancy and puerperium are associated with a biphasic alteration of CMI,[20] which is mediated through an interaction of Th2 (which are protective for pregnancy) and Th1 cytokines (which are associated with failure of pregnancy). Hence pregnancy is associated with downregulation of Th1 response resulting in decreased production of both Th1-associated [interleukin-1 (IL-1), IL-2 and interferon gamma] and other proinflammatory [tumor necrosis factor alpha and (IL-12)] cytokines and an increased production of Th2-associated (IL-4 and IL-10) cytokines.[20]

The pathogenesis of the depressed CMI in pregnancy may be influenced by neuroendocrine factors which are powerful modulators of cytokine expression.[21] Two plasma proteins: pregnancy zone protein (PZP) and placental protein-14 also known as glycodelin-A, which increase dramatically during pregnancy, have been found individually and synergistically to inhibit T-cell activation, in a dose-dependent manner without affecting production of Th2 cytokine, IL-4. This

activity appears to be independent of the PZP receptor (CD91) or PZP's antiproteinase activity.[22]

Due to a shift to Th2 type immune response during pregnancy, diseases pathogenically associated with a predominance of a Th1 immune response like rheumatic diseases clinically improve.[23] Similarly, due to a depressed CMI, pregnant women are more susceptible to infections in which a Th1 protective response is important (viral infections and toxoplasmosis).[24] The same should also hold true for leprosy, but unfortunately there is a paucity of data, especially from the era of MDT on the course of leprosy in pregnancy.[25]

Humoral Immunity

Pregnancy is also associated with a biphasic alteration of humoral response, with a heightened humoral response during pregnancy. Though the exact mechanism of this has not been clearly elucidated, but pregnancy is associated with shift from a Th1 to Th2 response probably influenced by elevated levels of estrogen and progesterone during pregnancy with a reversal in puerperium.[26] This may be partially responsible for aggravation of antibody mediated disorders like systemic lupus erythematosus in pregnancy and their improvement in postpartum period.[27]

Nutritional Changes

An optimum state of nutrition with an adequate intake of vitamins and minerals results in a proinflammatory Th1 cytokine-mediated response which is necessary for effective protective immunity while malnutrition (due to an inadequate intake of vitamins and minerals) results in an anti-inflammatory Th2 mediated immune response which is associated with an increased risk/worsening of infections. Supplementation with micronutrients reverses the Th2 response to a proinflammatory Th1 response with enhanced innate immunity.[28] A state of malnutrition can cause worsening of leprosy as demonstrated by observations on inmates with leprosy in Sungei Buloh Leper Hospital under Japanese occupation, where several patients had a downhill course of their leprosy under conditions of near starvation.[29]

Pregnancy is a state of relative (because of increased demand of pregnancy) and absolute malnutrition including deficiency of protein, vitamins, iron and other minerals. Malnutrition, which is known to inhibit rosette forming T-lymphocytes, may partly be responsible for the depression of CMI seen in pregnancy.[30]

Altered Secretion of Steroids

Levels of free cortisol and 17-hydroxycorticosteroid increase during pregnancy may partly be responsible for the depression of CMI in pregnancy.[31] The depressed CMI results in improvement of rheumatoid arthritis and ulcerative colitis (both of which are mediated through cellular immunity).[31] The increased levels of steroids may partially be responsible for the exacerbation of tuberculosis and leprosy during pregnancy. Though the specific influence of steroids on *M. leprae* is not known, Shepherd et al.[32] have demonstrated that in mice fed with hydrocortisone, the viability of *M. leprae* in the mouse foot pad improved, even though the rate of multiplication of bacteria did not.

PRESENTATION OF LEPROSY IN PREGNANT WOMEN

Clinical Features of Leprosy in Pregnancy

Twenty to 30% women develop signs and symptoms of leprosy for the first time in pregnancy (due to depression of CMI and resultant multiplication of *M. leprae)* or shortly thereafter (due to recovery of CMI, resulting in reversal reaction).[25] In a study from the presulfone era, Tajiri[33] reported that more than a fifth of their cohort of 240 Japanese females presented with leprosy for the first time during pregnancy. Similarly King and Marks[5] reported about 35% of their women patients presented with leprosy for the first time either during pregnancy or shortly thereafter. In a study from India, Hardas et al. observed that about 10% of their 68 patients, first noticed lesions of leprosy in pregnancy and more than 50% in puerperium.[7] Duncan et al. in a study from Ethiopia, reported a new case detection rate of 3% in women attending antenatal clinic in contrast to 0.1% in the nonpregnant women.[34] Though there are no controlled studies/reports from the MDT era, Lyde in 1997, reported two women from the US, who developed symptoms and signs of leprosy for the first time during pregnancy.[35]

Activity of Leprosy in Pregnancy

Due to suppression of CMI during pregnancy and its recovery during puerperium, leprosy aggravates or downgrades in pregnancy and upgrades during lactation. This has been supported by several observational studies. In the presulfone era, King and Marks[5] and Tajiri[33] noted aggravation of leprosy in 48% and 78% of pregnancies respectively. Unfortunately, in both these studies 'aggravation of leprosy' was not defined. However, subsequent studies have clearly demonstrated a disease progression toward lepromatous end of spectrum [appearance of new skin lesions and progressive nerve function impairment (NFI)] during pregnancy and reversal reaction (RR) in the postpartum period.[36] In a prospective study of 114 Ethiopian pregnant women with leprosy, almost half (48.2%) showed worsening of their leprosy status during pregnancy with more than a quarter (27.2%) developing the downhill trend during the third trimester of pregnancy.[37]

Load of *M. leprae* in Pregnancy

There is an increase in the bacillary load during pregnancy, due to suppression of CMI and this is compounded by the reluctance of women to take medication during pregnancy.[25] In the era of dapsone monotherapy, Duncan et al.[34] reported an increase in bacteriological index (BI) in about a quarter of paucibacillary (PB) patients (BI converted from negativity to positivity) and the increase of BI in about half of MB patients. The increase in the BI occurred both in patients on antileprosy therapy (ALT) as well as those not on therapy. In 38% of these patients, the increased bacterial load was due to multiplication of dapsone resistant *M. leprae*,[38] a reflection of the primary low-grade dapsone resistance already existing in the community in Ethiopia.[39] The increased BI is maximum in the third trimester of pregnancy and fortunately in about 50% of patients the increase in BI is temporary, declining to the prepregnancy levels during lactation, as CMI is restored.[34]

Relapse of Leprosy in Pregnancy

Pregnancy-associated relapse is due to suppressed CMI which allows multiplication of persisters especially during the third trimester.[40] In the era of dapsone monotherapy, Duncan et al.[37] observed a relapse rate of 36% in pregnant women with PB leprosy, 3–36 months after release from treatment (RFT) with about a third harboring dapsone resistant *M. leprae*.[38] Though most of the reports on relapse of leprosy in pregnancy belong to era of dapsone monotherapy, there are anecdotal reports of relapse in pregnancy even in patients treated with MDT. Lyde reported a case of lepromatous relapse in a pregnant patient who had taken 20 months of daily rifampicin and dapsone.[35] But the problem of relapse in pregnancy after MDT requires systematic evaluation with particular attention to factors which predispose to it and its relationship to the trimester of pregnancy and to lactation.[25]

Pregnancy and Reactions

Reactions in leprosy are acute immunologically mediated episodes in the chronic course of the disease. They are broadly classified as:

- *Type 1 reaction (T1R)*: T1R is due to alteration (improvement or deterioration) of CMI, occurs in borderline leprosy and is characterized by erythema and edema of pre-existing skin lesions, appearance of new lesions as well as neuritis which may additionally manifest with motor and sensory deficits. Constitutional symptoms are minimal or absent.
- *Type 2 reaction (T2R)*: T2R is due to immune complex deposition (due to antigen antibody excess) occurs in MB leprosy and manifests as ENL, neuritis and with constitutional symptoms.

Since the immunological changes are different during pregnancy and puerperium, the impact of pregnancy and lactation on the two types of reactions is discussed separately.

Type 1 Reaction

Type 1 reaction, also known as RR, pathogenically due to improvement in CMI, are less frequent during pregnancy (due to decreased CMI) and more frequent in lactation (due to improved CMI). A prospective cohort study of 114 pregnant Ethiopian women with leprosy,[37] reported that 40% of RRs occurred during pregnancy and 60% during lactation. However, the controls in this study were nonleprosy pregnant women, so it is not possible to ascertain whether there was a true decrease of RRs during pregnancy (and an increase during lactation) or not. Patients with BL and subpolar LL are at the greatest risk of developing RRs.[39]

When RRs occur in pregnancy and early postpartum period, cutaneous manifestations are more frequent and conspicuous than the neuritis. However, even when lesional erythema or edema is seen, it is relatively subdued in comparison to those of nonpregnant/nonpuerperal state except in women in whom ALT has recently been instituted (Fig. 25.1).[40] The differential clinical picture in pregnancy and puerperium has been attributed to the varied antigenic expression of *M. leprae* due to fluctuations in the host CMI.[41,42] In pregnancy, when the CMI is low only surface antigens of *M. leprae* multiplying in the skin are exposed, resulting in predominantly cutaneous lesions.

Type 2 Reaction

Unlike T1R, T2Rs do not have a clear temporal association with pregnancy and lactation.[25] They are more frequent in patients with higher antigenic load (BI ≥ 4), untreated patients and those harboring drug resistant *M. leprae*. ENL may be severe (Fig. 25.2) and recurrent,[25,35] neuritis (including motor and sensory deficits) is frequent (in 70% of women) during pregnancy. Systemic symptoms are less marked in pregnancy but conspicuous in lactation.[43]

Duncan and Pearson[44] in a prospective study of 76 Ethiopian women with MB leprosy (LL; BL) followed through pregnancy and lactation, observed that 38% developed ENL during the study period (LL, 59%; BL, 22%). The first episode of ENL could occur as early as the first trimester or as late as 15 months postpartum. In a retrospective multicentric analysis from USA, Maurus reported that 32% of the 26 women with leprosy on treatment followed through 62 pregnancies had episodes of ENL.[45] Interestingly, more than 65% of the women with a BI of greater than or equal to 4+ experienced ENL during pregnancy. However, there was no information on the clinical features, the temporal relation of these episodes with pregnancy or parturition, or presence of previous episodes of ENL.

Lyde reported that 70% of women who developed ENL during pregnancy had neuritis,[35] as compared with 30% in the non-ENL group. Lucio phenomenon has also been reported from Brazil in a pregnant woman with BL disease. The reaction responded to systemic steroids and had little impact on the outcome of pregnancy.[46]

Effect on Leprosy Neuritis[47]

Pathogenically nerve involvement can be due to:[48]
- Disease progression
- Reactions (T1R or T2R)
- Occasionally a combination of T1R and T2R.

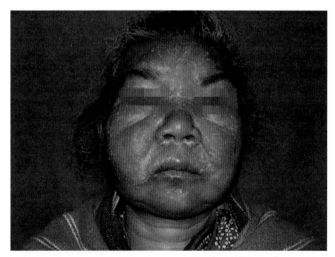

Fig. 25.1: Lesional erythema and edema (type 1 reaction) in postpartum period in a patient with borderline leprosy (BL) in whom antileprosy treatment has recently been instituted

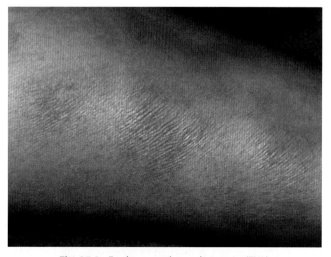

Fig. 25.2: Erythema nodosum leprosum (ENL) in a patient in postpartum period

Women with leprosy (both PB and MB) irrespective of the status of treatment are at a risk of developing neuritis during pregnancy, with the nerve function deteriorating in about 50% of the women.[47]

Neuropathy of Disease Progression

Due to pregnancy related immunosuppression, there is an increased load of *M. leprae* which results in a spreading granuloma in the nerve resulting in damage to the nerve and its function.[49]

Neuritis in T1R (RR)

Women with BL developed neuritis mostly during treatment period, but neuritis may also be seen in newly diagnosed patients and relapsed PB patients. In contrast, in BT/TT cases, neuritis was less common and did not show any relationship to pregnancy or lactation.

Neuritis in T2R

Neuritis of T2R can occur in any trimester of pregnancy (most frequently, first and third) or during lactation and is due to development of ENL lesions in the nerves. It is more severe in highly bacillated (BL/LL) patients, in untreated patients or in the presence of drug resistant *M. leprae.*

EFFECT OF LEPROSY ON PREGNANCY

Transplacental Infection

There is evidence of transplacental transmission of *M. leprae* in animal models. Job et al.[50] reported lepromatous placentitis in three pregnant nine-banded armadillos (*Dasypus novemcintus*) as shown by the presence of *M. leprae* in decidual tissue and trophoblastic cells of the chorionic villi of placenta. They also demonstrated acid fast bacilli (AFB) in spleens of three of four fetuses born to infected armadillos.

Unlike in armadillos, evidence of transplacental transmission of leprosy in humans is more tenuous, being largely based on presence of IgA (in 30%) and IgM (in 50%) antibodies to *M. leprae* in the cord blood of babies born to mothers with LL but not in babies born to women with tuberculoid leprosy. This probably indicates intrauterine immunologic stimulation due to transplacental transmission of *M. leprae.*[50] Further, at 3–6 months there was a significant increase of anti-*M. leprae* IgA and IgM antibodies in babies born to lepromatous mothers as compared to mothers with tuberculoid disease. In contrast to the persistently elevated levels of IgA and IgM antibodies, the levels of anti-*M. leprae* IgG antibodies showed a continuous and marked decline in sera of all babies, at 3–6, 6–9 and 15–24 months after birth.[51]

Impact on Fetus

Though, the early leprosarium based study,[45] reported several complications including prematurity (22%) and fetal loss (17%) in 26 women with leprosy followed through 62 pregnancies, subsequent studies from Ethiopia have not confirmed such obstetric complications in women with leprosy.[52] However, babies born to mothers with LL weigh significantly less at birth than babies born to mothers with tuberculoid leprosy as well as normal healthy controls.[53] Intrauterine growth retardation has been attributed to fetoplacental inadequacy in pregnant women with LL based on lower mean estrogen excretion[54] (an index of fetoplacental function)[55] between 32–40 weeks of gestation, compared to controls.[58] Though the definite cause of fetoplacental dysfunction is not known, it is probably due to decreased uteroplacental perfusion.[56]

Impact on Placenta

Though the morphology and immunohistology of placenta in women with leprosy (even LL) is normal,[57] the placental weight and placental coefficient (ratio of baby weight to placental weight) is lower in women with leprosy and this is mostly marked in women with LL disease.[52,54] The small placental size of women with leprosy is due to a decrease in size of cells of placenta and not due to reduced number of cells. Though there is no morphological evidence of infection of the placenta with *M. leprae*, a few AFB have been demonstrated in a small number of patients.[57]

POSTPARTUM PERIOD

Postpartum Clinical Manifestations in Mother

In puerperium, when CMI improves, bacilli in the nerves are destroyed, exposing cytoplasmic antigens resulting predominantly in neuritis. The late RRs which are observed in puerperium are probably due to release of sensitized lymphocytes during this period, which were trapped in the spleen during pregnancy.[17]

Due to recovery of CMI during puerperium and lactation, there is increase in occurrence of RRs.

The peak incidence of new RRs occurs 3–16 weeks after delivery, but recurrent episodes may continue even late into lactation (late RRs).[40]

In the postpartum period, RRs, neuritis and NFI including sudden and severe motor damage like claw hand (Fig. 25.3) and foot drop are seen more frequently (in up to 90% of patients) and the skin may not even be involved.[43] Neuritis is more frequently seen during the first 6 months of lactation as compared to the pregnant state. Systemic symptoms of T2R are more frequent during lactation.

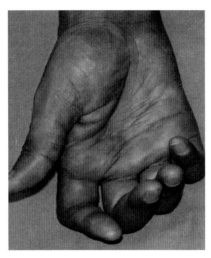

Fig. 25.3: Claw hand in a woman who delivered recently

IMPACTS ON INFANT AND LACTATING MOTHER

There are anecdotal reports of leprosy in infants probably indicating intrauterine transmission of leprosy in humans. Duncan et al. reported that of the 38 bacillated pregnant leprosy women who delivered, two children were diagnosed to have leprosy at the age of 9–17 months.[58] The proof of suspected intrauterine infection lay in the continued presence of IgA and IgM type of anti-*M. leprae* antibodies in the cord sera associated with an early and significant increase in these antibodies after birth. A decrease in serum IgG anti-*M. leprae* antibody was demonstrated in one of the babies after complete response to treatment.

Eighty percent of the babies born to LL mothers have been found to be severely underweight (Boston standards) even at 12 months of age.[52] These infants, especially those born to mothers with LL, had a higher incidence of respiratory problems,[54] more serious childhood infections and a higher infant mortality rate as compared to children of nonleprosy mothers.[56] The newborns of mothers on MDT may present with exfoliative dermatitis in the first hours of life due to dapsone and brownish discoloration of skin due to impregnation of clofazimine in the skin.[25]

The pubertal skeletal growth spurt, and in girls menarche was delayed in children born to mothers with LL as compared to healthy controls, but the growth curve of these children eventually caught up with controls by late teens.[59] It is difficult to explain the delay in growth in adolescent children of mothers with LL.

Impact of Leprosy on Lactating Mother

Though *M. leprae* is secreted in breast milk, more so in patients with MB leprosy[60] the protective effect of breast milk of women with LL is similar to that of normal controls as the levels of secretory IgA, lactoferrin, albumin and total protein in colostrum and breast milk samples in patients with LL were comparable to that of normal controls.[59] Many of the antileprosy drugs are secreted in breast milk and may affect the breast fed infants.

Lacunae in the Studies

Though some studies on pregnancy and leprosy have been published, there are several lacunae in the available information:[25]

Lack of appropriate studies:
- *Inappropriate study design*: Most studies are retrospective or case reports, so the data provided is often incomplete and sketchy.
- *Inappropriate controls in studies*: In many studies, healthy contacts of patients were recruited as controls when ideally, women with leprosy but without pregnancy should have been recruited, because the use of such controls would have permitted the calculation of the relative risk of developing T1R and T2R in pregnancy and lactation.[25]
- *Paucity of data from MDT era*: Information on course of leprosy in pregnant women is available from presulfone and sulfone era[5,33] and the early 1980s (the 'bridge period' between the era of dapsone monotherapy and MDT).[25] Data from MDT era is scanty (only as anecdotal reports).[61,62] It may be difficult to extrapolate the data from these studies to the present day MDT treated leprosy patients because:
  - Clofazimine present in MB MDT regimen protects women against T2R especially severe recurrent ENL as has been reported in the Ethiopian studies.[25] Similarly, the bactericidal effect of rifampicin (even after the first dose) by preventing further increase in the number (rather reduction in bacillary load) of *M. leprae*, may nullify (even if partially), the effect of depressed CMI, thereby reducing severity and incidence of ENL, both of which occur more frequently in highly bacillated patients.
- *Geographical localization of studies*: Most studies are from Ethiopia and it may not always be possible to extrapolate the findings of these studies to populations in Asia, Latin America or even other parts of Africa.[25] The lack of good studies from India is surprising, particularly given the high load of patients and the existence of an effective leprosy control program, which could have easily accumulated and analyzed this useful data.

With these deficiencies in the available data on the interaction of leprosy and pregnancy, it is important that a cohort of women with leprosy on treatment with MDT or those RFT, be followed to find out the course of leprosy in pregnancy and postpartum period.

PRACTICAL TIPS

- Leprosy is not a contraindication for pregnancy
- All pregnant leprosy patients need to be started on MDT irrespective of the trimester. MDT is to be continued during pregnancy and lactation
- Oral corticosteroids are the preferred anti-reaction drugs in pregnancy
- Antireactional drugs like thalidomide, methotrexate, cyclosporine, azathioprine are contraindicated in pregnancy
- Early detection and treatment of reactions is important to prevent complications
- Breast feeding must be continued even with the ongoing MDT
- Regular follow-up of the mother and child is necessary during the postpartum period.

Abbreviation: MDT, multidrug therapy.

CONCLUSION

The association between leprosy and pregnancy is uncommon, may be due to underreporting of cases and lack of any large studies. The pregnant women with leprosy need a close medical care due to immunological, hormonal and metabolic alterations in pregnancy. Such changes bring various alterations in the normal course of leprosy which also predisposes them to leprosy reactions. A regular follow-up after delivery is essential to detect any reversal reactions early and prevent the irreversible nerve damage. Antileprosy and antireactional drugs need to be selected appropriately keeping in mind the adverse effect profile like teratogenicity and at the same time effectiveness in controlling the bacillary load. Though the risk of leprosy transmission to the fetus is minimal, it also needs periodic examinations. In contrast to plethora of studies on effect of leprosy on gonads and gonadal function in males, there is a paucity of literature on the involvement of gonads and gonadal functions in females with leprosy. More studies are required for a better understanding of the clinicoimmunological relationship of this uncommon association.

REFERENCES

1. Kumar B, Rai R, Kaur I. Systemic involvement in leprosy and its significance. Indian J Lepr. 2000;72:123-42.
2. Mitsuda K. The significance of the vacuole in the Virchow lepra cells and the distribution of lepra cells in certain organs. Int J Lepr. 1936;4:491-8.
3. Mitsuda K, Ogawa M. A study of 150 autopsies on cases of leprosy. Int J Lepr. 1937;5: 53-60.
4. Leger J, Biric B, Prica S. Importance of leprosy in gynaecology and midwifery. Trop Dis Bull. 1963;60:446-7.
5. King JA, Marks RA. Pregnancy and leprosy; a review of 52 pregnancies in 26 patients with leprosy. Am J Obstet Gynecol. 1958;76:438-42.
6. Bogush TG. The question of the menstrual function in women with lepromatous leprosy before pubescence. Sci Works Lepr Res Institute. 1979;9:116-8.
7. Hardas U, Survey R, Chakravarty D. Leprosy in gynaecology and obstetrics. Int J Lepr. 1972;40:399-400.
8. Sharma SC, Kumar B, Dhall K, et al. Leprosy and female reproductive organs. Int J Lepr Other Mycobact Dis. 1981;49:177-9.
9. Khanna N, Ammini AC, Singh M, et al. Ovarian function in female patients with multibacillary leprosy. Int J Lepr Other Mycobact Dis. 2003;71:101-5.
10. Arora M, Katoch K, Natrajan M, et al. Study of hormonal profile in female leprosy patients. Indian J Lepr. 2008;80:89.
11. Nelson LM, Covington SN, Rebar RW. An update: spontaneous premature ovarian failure is not an early menopause. Fertil Steril. 2005;83:1327-32.
12. Nandedkar TD, Wadia P. Autoimmune disorders of the ovary. Indian J Exp Biol. 1998;36:433-6.
13. Welt CK. Autoimmune oophoritis in the adolescent. Ann N Y Acad Sci. 2008;1135:118-22.
14. Park JY, Cho SN, Youn JK, et al. Detection of antibodies to human nerve antigens in sera from leprosy patients by ELISA. Clin Exp Immunol. 1992;87:368-72.
15. Garcia-De La Torre I. Autoimmune phenomena in leprosy, particularly antinuclear antibodies and rheumatoid factor. J Rheumatol. 1993;20:900-3.
16. Freire BF, Ferraz AA, Nakayama E, et al. Anti-neutrophil cytoplasmic antibodies (ANCA) in the clinical forms of leprosy. Int J Lepr Other Mycobact Dis. 1998;66:475-82.
17. Guedes Barbosa LS, Gilbrut B, Shoenfeld Y, et al. Autoantibodies in leprosy sera. Clin Rheumatol. 1996;15:26-8.
18. Saha K, Gupta I. Immunologic aspects of leprosy with special reference to the circulating antispermatozoal antibodies. Int J Lepr Other Mycobact Dis. 1977;45:28-37.
19. Priddy KD. Immunologic adaptations during pregnancy. J Obstet Gynecol Neonatal Nurs. 1997;26:388-94.
20. Wegmann TG, Lin H, Guilbert L, et al. Bidirectional cytokine interactions in the maternal-fetal relationship: is successful pregnancy a TH2 phenomenon? Immunol Today. 1993;14:353-6.
21. Ostensen M, Forger F, Villiger PM. Cytokines and pregnancy in rheumatic disease. Ann N Y Acad Sci. 2006;1069:353-63.
22. Skornicka EL, Kiyatkina N, Weber MC, et al. Pregnancy zone protein is a carrier and modulator of placental protein-14 in T-cell growth and cytokine production. Cell Immunol. 2004;232:144-56.
23. Da Silva JA, Spector TD. The role of pregnancy in the course and aetiology of rheumatoid arthritis. Clin Rheumatol. 1992;11:189-94.
24. Luft BJ, Remington JS. Effect of pregnancy on resistance to Listeria monocytogenes and Toxoplasma gondii infections in mice. Infect Immun. 1982;38:1164-71.
25. Lockwood DN, Sinha HH. Pregnancy and leprosy: a comprehensive literature review. Int J Lepr Other Mycobact Dis. 1999;67:6-12.
26. Canellada A, Alvarez I, Berod L, et al. Estrogen and progesterone regulate the IL-6 signal transduction pathway in antibody secreting cells. J Steroid Biochem Mol Biol. 2008;111:255-61.
27. Varner MW. Autoimmune disorders and pregnancy. Semin Perinatol. 1991;15:238-50.
28. Wintergerst ES, Maggini S, Hornig DH. Contribution of selected vitamins and trace elements to immune function. Ann Nutr Metab. 2007;51:301-23.

29. Ryrie GA. Some impressions of Sungei Buloh Leper Hospital under Japanese occupation. Lepr Rev. 1947;18:10-7.
30. Chandra RK. Rosette-forming T lymphocytes and cell-mediated immunity in malnutrition. Br Med J. 1974;3:608-9.
31. Scott JS. Immunological diseases in pregnancy. Prog Allergy. 1977;23:321-66.
32. Shepard CC, McRae DH. Mycobacterium leprae in mice: minimal infectious dose, relationship between staining quality and infectivity, and effect of cortisone. J Bacteriol. 1965;89:365-72.
33. Tajiri I. Leprosy and childbirth. Int J Lepr. 1936;4:189-94.
34. Duncan ME, Melsom R, Pearson JM, et al. The association of pregnancy and leprosy. I. New cases, relapse of cured patients and deterioration in patients on treatment during pregnancy and lactation–results of a prospective study of 154 pregnancies in 147 Ethiopian women. Lepr Rev. 1981;52:245-62.
35. Lyde CB. Pregnancy in patients with Hansen disease. Arch Dermatol. 1997;133:623-7.
36. Duncan ME. An historical and clinical review of the interaction of leprosy and pregnancy: a cycle to be broken. Soc Sci Med. 1993;37:457-72.
37. Duncan ME, Pearson JM, Ridley DS, et al. Pregnancy and leprosy: the consequences of alterations of cell-mediated and humoral immunity during pregnancy and lactation. Int J Lepr Other Mycobact Dis. 1982;50:425-35.
38. Duncan ME, Pearson JM, Rees RJ. The association of pregnancy and leprosy. II. Pregnancy in dapsone-resistant leprosy. Lepr Rev. 1981;52:263-70.
39. Pearson JM, Haile GS, Rees RJ. Primary dapsone-resistant leprosy. Lepr Rev. 1977;48:129-32.
40. Rose P, McDougall C. Adverse reactions following pregnancy in patients with borderline (dimorphous) leprosy. Lepr Rev. 1975;46:109-14.
41. Duncan ME, Pearson JM. Neuritis in pregnancy and lactation. Int J Lepr Other Mycobact Dis. 1982;50:31-8.
42. Lopes VG, Sarno EN. Hanseníase e gravidez. Rev Ass Med Brasil. 1994;40:195-201.
43. Weddell AG, Pearson JM. Leprosy histopathological aspects on nerve involvement. In: Hornbrook RK (Ed). Topics in Tropical Neurology. Philadelphia; 1975. pp. 17-28.
44. Duncan ME, Pearson JM. The association of pregnancy and leprosy-III. Erythema nodosum leprosum in pregnancy and lactation. Lepr Rev. 1984;55:129-42.
45. Maurus JN. Hansen's disease in pregnancy. Obstet Gynecol. 1978;52:22-5.
46. Heliner KA, Fleischfrasser I, Kucharski-Esmanhota LD, et al. The Lucio's phenomenon (necrotizing erythema) in pregnancy. Ann Bras Dermatol. 2004;79:205-10.
47. Duncan ME. Pregnancy and leprosy neuropathy. Indian J Lepr. 1996;68:23-34.
48. Antia NH, Shetty VP, Mehta LN. Study of evolution of nerve damage in leprosy. Part IV-An assessment. Lepr India. 1980;52:48-52.
49. Shetty VP, Suchitra K, Uplekar MW, et al. Higher incidence of viable Mycobacterium leprae within the nerve as compared to skin among multibacillary leprosy patients released from multidrug therapy. Lepr Rev. 1997;68:131-8.
50. Job CK, Sanchez RM, Hastings RC. Lepromatous placentitis and intrauterine fetal infection in lepromatous nine-banded armadillos (Dasypus novemcinctus). Lab Invest. 1987;56:44-8.
51. Melsom R, Harboe M, Duncan ME. IgA, IgM and IgG anti-M. leprae antibodies in babies of leprosy mothers during the first 2 years of life. Clin Exp Immunol. 1982;49:532-42.
52. Duncan ME. Babies of mothers with leprosy have small placentae, low birth weights and grow slowly. Br J Obstet Gynaecol. 1980;87:471-9.
53. Duncan ME, Melsom R, Pearson JM, et al. A clinical and immunological study of four babies of mothers with lepromatous leprosy, two of whom developed leprosy in infancy. Int J Lepr Other Mycobact Dis. 1983;51:7-17.
54. Morrison A. A woman with leprosy is in double jeopardy. Lepr Rev. 2000;71:128-43.
55. Bhansali KG, Eugere EJ. Quantitative determination of 17 beta-estradiol and progesterone in cellular fractions of term placentae of normal and hypertensive patients. Res Commun Chem Pathol Pharmacol. 1992;77:161-9.
56. Duncan ME, Oakey RE. Estrogen excretion in pregnant women with leprosy: evidence of diminished fetoplacental function. Obstet Gynecol. 1982;60:82-6.
57. Duncan ME, Fox H, Harkness RA, et al. The placenta in leprosy. Placenta. 1984;5:189-98.
58. Melsom R, Harboe M, Duncan ME, et al. IgA and IgM antibodies against Mycobacterium leprae in cord sera and in patients with leprosy: an indicator of intrauterine infection in leprosy. Scand J Immunol. 1981;14:343-52.
59. Duncan ME, Miko T, Howe R, et al. Growth and development of children of mothers with leprosy and healthy controls. Ethiop Med J. 2007;45 (Suppl 1):9-23.
60. Girdhar A, Girdhar BK, Ramu G, et al. Discharge of M. leprae in milk of leprosy patients. Lepr India. 1981;53:390-4.
61. Boddinghaus BK, Ludwig RJ, Kaufmann R, et al. Leprosy in a pregnant woman. Infection. 2007;35:37-9.
62. Gimovsky AC, Macri CJ. Leprosy in pregnant woman, United States. Emerg Infect Dis. 2013;19:1693-4.

Childhood Leprosy

Archana Singal, Namrata Chhabra

CHAPTER OUTLINE

- Epidemiology
- Transmission
- Classification
- Clinical Presentation

- Diagnosis
- Treatment
- Prevention

INTRODUCTION

Leprosy has been a major public-health problem in many developing countries for centuries. Children are believed to be the most vulnerable group to infection with *Mycobacterium leprae* given their nascent immunity and possible intra-familial contact.[1] Leprosy in children has a significantly unique aspect because of its potential to cause progressive physical deformity with serious consequent psychosocial impact on both the child and the family. Epidemiologically, childhood leprosy is an index of transmission of disease in the population[2] and allows identification of index case.[3] In the postelimination era, incidence of leprosy amongst young children indicates active foci of transmission in the community, making it a robust epidemiological indicator to assess the progress of leprosy control programs.

EPIDEMIOLOGY

Global Scenario

The number of new cases detected during the year 2013, as reported by 103 countries, was 215656 and India topped the list with its contribution of 126913 (58.8%) to the pool. Three countries namely India, Brazil and Indonesia together contributed 81% of the new cases in 2013, with their individual contribution of 58.8%, 14.2% and 8% respectively. India and Brazil had a very slow decline in new case detection since 2006 and 2007. On the contrary, Indonesia, after attaining a plateau in 2006, had a significant increase in 2011 followed by appreciable decrease again in 2013.[4]

The proportion of children among newly detected cases of leprosy is a strong indicator of disease transmission in the community. Globally, this ratio has shown a considerable variation within different regions, e.g. in Africa, the childhood proportion has ranged from as high as 38.25% in Comoros to as low as 1.12% in Burundi. Similarly, this proportion varied from 12.34% in the Dominican Republic to 0.59% in Argentina in the Americas Regions; from 12.25% in Indonesia to 6.43% in Thailand in the South East Asia Region, from 10.78% in South Sudan to 2.27% in the Eastern Mediterranean Region and from 39.66% in Marshall Islands to 2.53% in China in the Western Pacific Region.[4]

Indian Scenario

According to the National Leprosy Eradication Programme report of March 2013, a total of 13,387 child cases were recorded in 2012–13 in India, which gives an annual new case detection rate (ANCDR) of childhood leprosy as 9.93%. Proportion of child cases was more than 10% of new cases detected in 12 States/UTs namely, Andhra Pradesh (11.34%), Maharashtra (12.51%), Bihar (15.88%), Tamil Nadu (10.76%), Puducherry (10.53%) Dadar & Nagar Haveli (26.09%), Arunachal Pradesh (25.00%), Karnataka (15.63%), Kerala (12.86%), Manipur (12.50%), Meghalaya and Sikkim (15.79%).

The demographic characteristics of the children affected by leprosy have been evaluated in many studies in India either by school surveys or hospital based studies with contact assessment. A substantial variation in the prevalence rates of childhood leprosy of 4–34% has been observed in these studies conducted in different parts of the Indian subcontinent (Table 26.1).[5-7] Variation in the upper age limit for childhood case definition (ranging from < 14 years to < 19 years) in different studies might have contributed to this statistical disparity.

Age and Sex Distribution

Leprosy is known to occur at all ages ranging from early infancy to old age. Amongst children, the disease tends to occur with highest frequency in children of 5–14 years age group and only 5.8–6% cases are below 5 years of age. This may be due to the relatively long incubation period of leprosy and delayed diagnosis of indeterminate lesions in children.[3,7-10] However, the youngest patient diagnosed to have leprosy was only 3 weeks old from Martinique, a small island near West Indies.[11] Results from a review of literature, information from pathology files and correspondence survey conducted in 1985 revealed 91 infants under one year of age with diagnosed leprosy proving a mistaken belief that leprosy is exceedingly rare or non-existent in the very young. The youngest infant was 2–3 months old and had no known familial contact.[12]

Among children, boys are more commonly affected than girls.[7,9,13] This may be due to greater mobility and increased opportunities for contact in male child.[3,14] Moreover, detection in girls may possibly be lower than boys due to neglect of the female child.

Contact History

It is known that children form a high risk group in families of leprosy patients. Familial contacts are known to have a significant role in the development of childhood leprosy.[8] The risk of developing leprosy in a person is four times when there is a neighborhood contact. However, this risk increases to nine times when the contact is intra-familial. Further, the risk gets higher if contact has multibacillary (MB) form of the disease (Fig. 26.1).[15] The attack rate reportedly increases when the index case is mother.[8] Analysis of published data on childhood leprosy from India showed that the history of

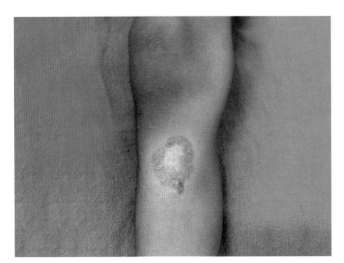

Fig. 26.1: Single annular, erythematous plaque of BT leprosy on the lower limb of a 6-year-old child whose father (index case) was a diagnosed case of LL

familial contact was present in 0.66–47% cases.[16] In a cross sectional study involving examination of all the children from 100 families with proven leprosy and 100 nonleprous families (control group) residing in the same area, it was found that the prevalence of childhood leprosy was 14.2 times higher in leprous families in comparison to the control group.[17] Further, the prevalence rate was still higher in families where family contact had either the lepromatous disease or had more than one lesion. The common clinical types were tuberculoid, indeterminate, borderline and pure neuritic in decreasing order. This indicates that a case of childhood leprosy may provide an opportunity to detect the index case, usually within the family. The prevalence of familial contact in childhood leprosy has ranged from 10 to 36% as observed in different studies (Table 26.1).

TRANSMISSION

The mode of transmission of leprosy is still not conclusively proven although infection by nasal droplets is believed to be the main route.[18] Other factors that may influence transmission include genetic susceptibility, extent of exposure and the environmental conditions. There is also epidemiologic evidence to suggest that leprosy may be transmissible from mothers to offsprings via placenta.[19] The report of child developing leprosy at the age of 3 weeks is an example where the infection could have been intrauterine.[11] Although *M. leprae* are known to be present in the breast milk of mothers suffering from lepromatous leprosy, the risk of acquiring leprosy infection in the breastfed infant via the gastrointestinal tract remains uncertain.[20]

There are numerous observations from Africa of a first patch of leprosy on the forehead or cheek of a baby, carried on the naked back of lepromatous mother. The first lesions were also observed on the bare buttocks of toddlers, acquired possibly from sitting on contaminated soil suggesting that the skin is at least one of the most important routes of transmission of the disease, particularly from patients with the lepromatous disease.[21]

Inoculation leprosy is defined as transmission of *M. leprae* through the broken skin after trauma of various kinds like thorn prick, tattooing and road side injury etc.[22-24] The abraded skin has been proposed as an entry point for *M. leprae*.

CLASSIFICATION

A five group clinicohistological classification based on immunological status described by Ridley and Jopling is still the most widely accepted.[25] The revised Indian classification by IAL in 1981 divided leprosy into five broad groups viz. indeterminate, borderline, tuberculoid, lepromatous and polyneuritic. A simplified classification based on the number of lesions was given by WHO in 1998; up to 5 lesions (paucibacillary-PB) and 6 or more lesions (multibacillary-MB).[26]

Table 26.1: Prevalence of important epidemiological data of childhood leprosy

Authors and Ref/ Study period	n/ % age of total leprosy cases	Age group (years)	Positive family history (%)	% age of BT cases	% age of PB cases	AFB Positivity on SSS (%)	Clinicohistological concordance (%)	% age of cases with reaction	% of cases with deformity
Singal et al.[29]/ 2000-2009	172/9.6	0–14	14.5	70.3	48.3	19.8	86.1	18.6	12.8
Santos et al.[50]/ 2001-2010	77/0.14	0–14	–	–	42.9	–	–	–	–
Rao[42]/2004-2009	32/11.43	0–18	18	68	81.2	25	37.5	6.24	3.12
Shetty et al.[10]/2007	68/34.1	0–14	–	58.1	73.5	8	93	0	4.4
Horo et al.[51]/2004-2006	151/–	0–14	–	42.4	67	30	–	4.6	16
Mahajan et al.[31]/1992-2003	86/7.71	0–15	26.7	73	63	28	60	2.3	13
Burman et al.[7]/1998-2002	20/4.45	0–14	10	55	50	30	–	–	20
Grover et al.[14]/1997-2002	137/7.06	0–14	21.9	70.8	71	22.6	–	2	24
Kumar et al.[43]/ 1990-1999	61/4.5	0–14	–	78.7	–	–	60.6	–	–
Jain et al.[8]/ 1990-1999	306/9.8	0–14	36.9	66.3	83	9.4	–	29.7	–
Selvasekar et al.[9]/1990-1995	794/31.3	0–14	29.8	60.5	98	2	–	4.1	0.5
Kaur et al.[3]/ 1982-1989	132/12.4	0–19	16.7	59	–	17.4	–	7.6	6.8

Abbreviations: n, sample size; AFB, Acid-fast bacilli; BT, Borderline tuberculoid; PB, Pauci-bacillary; SSS, Slit skin smear; –, Information not available.

Leprosy in children presents predominantly as PB disease.[3,8,9,27] It is a paradox that children who have poor cell-mediated immunity rarely present with MB disease. In most children, when diagnosed early, the spectrum of leprosy is reported to be incomplete and largely confined to tuberculoid (TT), borderline tuberculoid (BT), mid-borderline (BB), and indeterminate forms.[12,14] Lepromatous leprosy (LL) seems to be rare during the first year of life. BT leprosy is the most common clinical type (Fig. 26.2) with the prevalence ranging from 42–78% of all childhood cases in different studies (Table 26.1). The indeterminate form is an early presentation of leprosy and it may either resolve spontaneously or develop into one of the subpolar forms.[10] Pure neuritic leprosy occurs infrequently in children than adults. Histoid leprosy is extremely rare in children.

CLINICAL PRESENTATION

The data on clinical presentation and disease spectrum in childhood leprosy is mostly derived from hospital

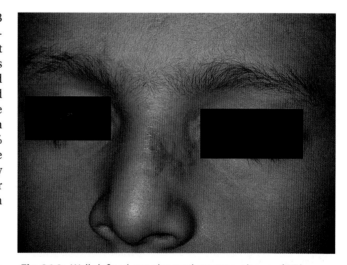

Fig. 26.2: Well-defined, annular, erythematous plaque of BT leprosy on the face of an 8-year-old boy

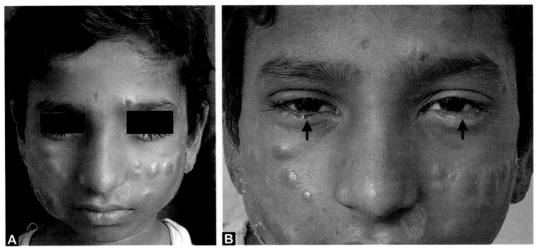

Figs 26.3A and B: BL leprosy: Multiple erythematous lesions (nodules and plaques) on face with infiltrated eyelids in a young boy

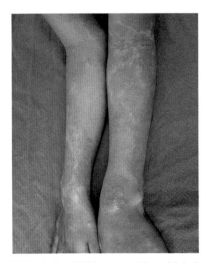

Fig. 26.4: Mid-borderline (BB) leprosy with multiple, large, annular, erythematous plaques over both upper limbs of a 7-year-old boy

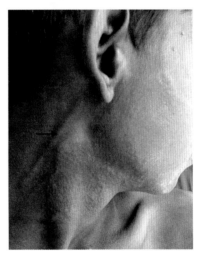

Fig. 26.5: Thickened greater auricular nerve in the vicinity of a large erythematous plaque on the neck

based studies. The disease usually manifests as a single hypopigmented patch with normal or impaired sensation.[27,28] predominantly involving the exposed body parts.[3,9,29] On the contrary, few studies have reported a very low rate of single skin lesions.[7,8] The clinical presentation in the form of bilateral and symmetrical ill defined macular hypoesthetic lesions, diffuse infiltration of the face and ear lobes, or nerve thickening are less commonly observed because of the rarity of BB, BL and LL leprosy in children (Figs 26.3 to 26.7). When LL develops in children, the lesions seem to be confined to the head and the extremities, i.e. the colder parts of the body.

Indeterminate Leprosy

Indeterminate leprosy (IL) is an early and transitory stage of leprosy found in persons whose immunological status is not yet fully defined. Subsequently, it may resolve spontaneously in most cases or progress to one of the other determinate forms of the disease in about 30%, more often towards the lepromatous end.[30] It usually presents with macular lesions with fairly well-defined edges and slight or no loss of sensations, usually over covered area of the body (Fig. 26.8). This clinical ambiguity in the diagnosis of IL is further compounded by negative slit skin smears for AFB and the non specific histology of the lesion. There are many common

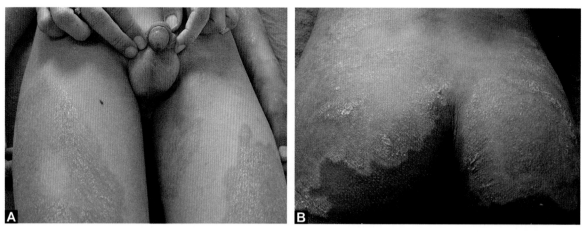

Figs 26.6A and 6B: Large annular plaques of BB leprosy involving both thighs, unusual genital lesions in a 7-year-old boy, and buttocks

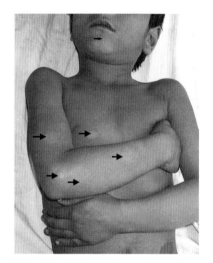

Fig. 26.7: A girl with multiple erythematous and hypopigmented papules and plaques of BL leprosy

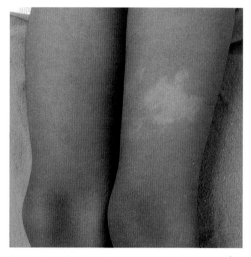

Fig. 26.8: Indeterminate leprosy: Hypopigmented macule with well-defined, irregular margins present over anterior aspect of thigh in a 4-year-old girl, the index case being father with LL

benign dermatological conditions which can be confused with the lesions of IL.[31] Therefore, one has to be very careful while giving a diagnostic label of leprosy in a child for obvious psychological trauma to the family and the child. Table 26.2 gives a list of common dermatological conditions with their characteristic differentiating features. In addition, one has to remember that in contrast to leprosy lesions, these conditions have no impairment of sensation. However, testing for sensory impairment can be a problem in young children, in particular on the facial lesions.

Nodular Leprosy of Childhood

Nodular leprosy of childhood (NL) has been described as a benign clinical variant of tuberculoid leprosy that affects breast-feeding infants and young children inhabiting a highly infected environment. The lesions tend to undergo complete resolution. The lesions are usually localized on areas such as cheeks, arms, buttocks, and limbs and may result from the intimate skin contact with lepromatous parents or relatives. On histopathology, NL lesions are characterized by dense granulomatous inflammatory reaction associated with neural compromise, with a greater number of confluent tubercles in comparison to the classical tuberculoid lesions. No difference was demonstrated in the tissue reaction, frequency of mycobacterial antigen, the lymphocyte subsets (CD45RO+, CD4+, CD8+, B, NK), dendritic cells (epidermal CD1a+ cells and S100+ dermal dendrocytes), and macrophages in skin lesions of NL group when compared with lesions of classical tuberculoid leprosy in children and adult. NL, thus, has been

Table 26.2: Differential diagnoses of hypopigmented lesions in children

Clinical conditions	Important differentiating features
Pityriasis alba	Usually multiple lesions Principally affects face
Pityriasis versicolor	Fine brawny scaling Fungal hyphae in skin scales on KOH examination
Vitiligo	Depigmentation rather than hypopigmentation Usually multiple lesions/ leucotrichia/ perifollicular pigmentation
Morphea	Indurated skin lesions Absent hair growth and sweating Violaceous margins
Post-kala-azar dermal leishmaniasis (PKDL)	In addition to macules, papules and nodules may be present on face Facial erythema with a 'butterfly' distribution Leishman-Donovan (LD) bodies in skin biopsy
Nevus depigmentosus	Well defined, irregular margins Present at birth or early childhood

Note: In all these conditions, sensations are well preserved in the lesions, which is a very helpful sign in older children. However, testing of sensations is difficult in small children.

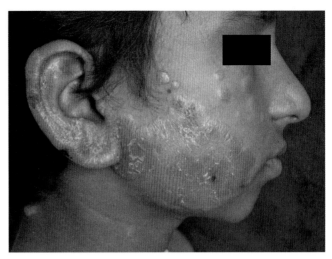

Fig. 26.9: BL leprosy with type 1 reaction

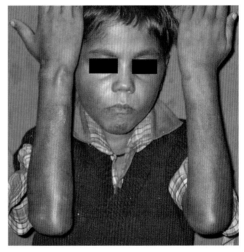

Fig. 26.10: BL leprosy with type 2 reaction

regarded as a manifestation of hypersensitivity and congenital immunity to *M. leprae*. Strong stimulation of cell mediated immunity against *M. leprae* evoked by the inoculation of bacilli into the skin has been thought to be responsible for the high resistance, stability, and auto-resolution of nodular leprosy of childhood.[32]

Reactions

In childhood leprosy, reactional episodes and disabilities are less frequently seen (Figs 26.9 and 26.10). However, when present, they tend to occur in older children, due to their relatively well developed immunological status.[8,9,33-35] Recently, a higher incidence of reactional episodes, both type 1 and 2 (erythema nodosum leprosum or ENL) occurring with or without neuritis in children have been observed, mostly in hospital based studies (Table 26.1).[7,8,28,32,36] Enlarged nerves may show nodularity at times (Fig. 26.11). In general, children with MB disease are at higher risk for reversal reactions.

Deformities and Disability

Children with irreversible deformity and disability face many difficulties in education, social life, and day to day activities, which differ to some extent from their adult counterparts.

Prevalence of deformities associated with childhood leprosy in India varies from 0.5–24% (Table 26.1). Majority of these deformities involve upper limbs and only 10% occur in lower limbs.[37] Various factors responsible for increased risk of deformities in childhood leprosy have been identified. Presence of neuritis significantly increases the risk of deformities, especially in older children with multibacillary disease.[29] It was observed that children with thickened nerve trunks are at 6.1 times higher risk of developing deformities compared to those who did not have nerve enlargement.[37] Other factors contributing to the development of deformities include; delay in accessing health care, multiple skin lesions, multiple nerve involvement, reaction at the time of presentation and smear positivity. Children with the aforesaid risk factors should be followed up more diligently

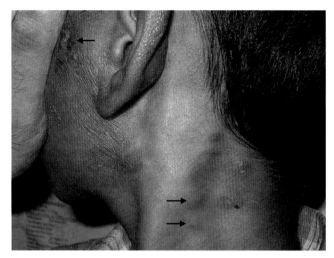

Fig. 26.11: Thickened and nodular left great auricular nerve (arrows) and facial lesion with type 1 reaction

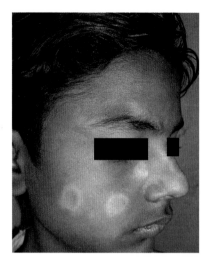

Fig. 26.12: Pityriasis alba: Multiple hypopigmented, mildly scaly lesions over the face of a 9-year-old boy with atopy

so as to detect the onset of any deformity as early as possible. These findings overemphasize the significance of careful neurological examination at the time of diagnosis and during follow-up in these patients.

Disease Evolution

The course of childhood leprosy is unpredictable. Progression or regression of lesions is common. In children, spontaneous regression may occur in 33–75% of cases. IL in children tends to heal spontaneously in a significant proportion and only about 30% progress to a determinate type, more often towards the lepromatous pole of the spectrum.[30]

DIAGNOSIS

Accurate diagnosis is important in children but it can be very difficult at times. For instance, single hypopigmented patch on the face in children has high risk of misdiagnosis, since there are numerous common causes of hypopigmented patches (Table 26.2) in this age group (Figs 26.12 and 26.13).[31] Secondly, eliciting sensory impairment may be quite difficult in children on the facial lesions as well as otherwise. Further, the evidence that indeterminate leprosy may be a precursor of LL,[38] emphasizes the need for greater caution in ruling out leprosy among younger children. It also suggests that there is a need for less invasive diagnostic tests since demonstration of classical histological features of leprosy or AFB in cutaneous lesions of IL is difficult.

Slit-skin Smear Examination

Slit-skin smears from the suspected case of leprosy, are stained for AFB is the standard technique to estimate the

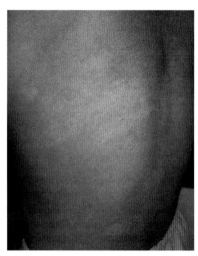

Fig. 26.13: Nevus depigmentosus: Hypopigmented macule with well-defined feathery margins present over back of a 12-year-old boy

number of *M. leprae* when present, [Bacillary Index, (BI)] and the proportion of viable bacilli [Morphological Index (MI)]. Smears are positive in LL, BL and some BT cases. However, a large proportion of early cases of childhood leprosy remain AFB negative because most of them are TT, BT, or indeterminate. Positive skin smears have been reported in less than 10% cases in many previous studies.[8,27,28,39] Some of the recent studies have reported higher smear positivity rates ranging from 17.4% to 30% (Table 26.1).[3,7,14] The skin smear positivity has been shown to increase with age.[40]

Histopathology

In children, histological diagnosis is often required in combination with the clinical evidence, since the common

Table 26.3: Dosage of MDT for children with paucibacillary leprosy

PB-MDT		
Age group (years)	Rifampicin: monthly dose, supervised (mg)	Dapsone: daily dose, unsupervised (mg)
3–5	150–300	25
6–14	300–450	50–100
15 or above	600	100

Duration: 6 months

Table 26.4: Dosage of MDT for children with multibacillary leprosy

MB-MDT				
Age group (years)	Rifampicin Monthly supervised dose (mg)	Dapsone Daily unsupervised dose (mg)	Clofazimine	
			Unsupervised dose (mg)	Monthly supervised dose (mg)
3–5	150–300	25	100 once weekly	100
6–14	300–450	50–100	150 once weekly	150–200
15 or above	600	100	50 daily	300

Duration: 12 months

forms seen (BT, IL) can pose diagnostic dilemma. The clinico-pathological correlation in childhood leprosy is low, at 37–63%.[3,27,40-42] which could be due to multiple reasons. The non-specific histological features in childhood cases may be due to the poor immune system in children.[43] It has also been suggested that selection of the site of the biopsy plays an important role in the histopathological diagnosis and clinically dissimilar lesions biopsied from the same patient can show different types of histopathology.[28] However, a higher rate of clinico-histopathological concordance has been reported in recent studies.[10,29]

Newer Methods

In situ PCR on slit skin smear can be a useful method to diagnose cases when skin smears are negative for AFB and in those cases where skin biopsy cannot be done because of unusual location of lesions, or because of sensitive age of the patient.[44] Estimation of serum beta glucuronidase (a lysosomal enzyme) levels may be another parameter to assess the activity and extent of pathogenesis in leprosy.[45] Hybridization with gene probes targeting 16SrRNA or 16S rDNA are the potential useful methods for confirming active MB disease in children, and it may also be used for monitoring treatment.[44]

TREATMENT

The disease in children is eminently responsive to treatment.[46] Multidrug therapy (MDT) is the mainstay of the leprosy

elimination strategy as it cures patients, reduces the reservoir of infection and interrupts its transmission.[47] The dosage regimen, of both paucibacillary and multibacillary MDT for children, according to the different age groups, has been shown in Tables 26.3 and 26.4. Fortunately, tolerance to standard antileprosy drugs is good in children. A small quantity of these drugs is excreted in the breast milk but no systemic adverse effects have been reported in the breastfed babies except for a mild skin discoloration resulting from clofazimine.[48]

There is not enough data regarding safety of newer anti-leprosy drugs in children. Minocycline is generally contraindicated in early childhood. Quinolones, such as ofloxacin have been shown to cause arthropathy (degenerative changes in weight bearing joints) in young *animals,* so have to be used with caution in children and adolescents. However, field trial using single dose regime of minocycline and ofloxacin in children for the treatment of single lesion paucibacillary leprosy did not show significant adverse effects.[48]

Treatment of reactions: Children with reversal reactions require prompt use of steroids for the prevention of nerve damage and deformity. Systemic steroids remain the mainstay of treatment for type 2 reactions as well. Rehabilitative measures such as physiotherapy and corrective surgeries should also be offered to selected patients.

PREVENTION

For every new case of childhood leprosy, leprosy control program should ensure household and extended contact surveys to detect the likely source of infection. Evidence suggests that chemoprophylaxis of close contacts of newly diagnosed cases with single dose rifampicin reduce clinical leprosy by 57%; the effect being substantial in 10–14 years age group and in those who have received BCG in the past. In addition, ongoing trials are in favor of second dose of BCG vaccination after the age of 5 years, to enhance existing BCG induced immunity in endemic countries.[49]

CONCLUSION

Leprosy in children is a strong indicator of recent transmission of disease by active sources of infection and suggests that population is being exposed to cases not yet diagnosed by health care personnel. This problem gets compounded by the fact that the diagnosis of leprosy in infants and young children may frequently be missed and disregarded. Hence, effective planning to bring down the incidence of leprosy and its complications in children should become a top priority. It is important to take detailed contact history and screen family members of the affected child to search for index case so as to break the chain of transmission by timely institution of appropriate treatment. Reactions, deformities and MDT intolerance are fortunately uncommon in children. Fear of social ostracism may dissuade children or their families from seeking medical care at an early stage. So, children will have a low frequency of voluntary reporting for leprosy care, unless there are serious consequences. Regular school surveys and annual contact surveys for early detection of cases is therefore an important tool in achieving the goal of elimination of leprosy.

REFERENCES

1. Noussitou FM. Lepra Infantil. WHO, Geneva. 1999.
2. Norman G, Joseph GA, Udaysuriyan P, et al. Leprosy case detection using school children. Lepr Rev. 2004;75:34-9.
3. Kaur I, Kaur S, Sharma VK, Kumar B. Childhood leprosy in northern India. Pediatr Dermatol, 1991;8:21-4.
4. World Health Organization. Global leprosy situation, 2013. Weekly Epidemiological Record; 2013, 88(35):365-80.
5. Bhavsar BS, Mehta NR. An epidemiological study of leprosy through school survey in Surat District (South Gujarat). Lepr India. 1980;52:548-56.
6. Naik SS. Repeat leprosy survey after 7 years in night high schools in greater Bombay. Indian J Lepr. 1996;68:377-8.
7. Burman KD, Rijall A, Agrawal S, et al. Childhood leprosy in eastern Nepal: a hospital-based study. Indian J Lepr, 2003;75: 47-52.
8. Jain S, Reddy RG, Osmani SN, et al. Childhood leprosy in an urban clinic, Hyderabad, India: clinical presentation and the role of household contacts. Lepr Rev. 2002;73:248-53.
9. Selvasekar A, Geetha J, Nisha K et al. Childhood leprosy in an endemic area. Lepr Rev. 1999;70:21-7.
10. Shetty VP, Ghate SD, Wakade AV et al. Clinical, bacteriological, and histopathological characteristics of newly detected children with leprosy: a population based study in a defined rural and urban area of Maharashtra, Western India. Indian J Dermatol Venereol Leprol. 2013;79:512-7.
11. Montestruc E, Berdonneau R. Two new cases of leprosy in infants in Martinique (in French). Bull Socpathol Exot Filiales. 1954;47:781-3.
12. Brubaker ML, Meyers WM, Bourland J. Leprosy in children one year of age and under. Int J Lepr Other Mycobact Dis. 1985; 53:517-23.
13. Sehgal VN, Rege VL, Mascarenhas MF et al. The prevalence and pattern of leprosy in a school survey. Int J Lepr Other Mycobact Dis. 1977;45:360-3.
14. Grover C, Nanda S, Garg VK et al. An epidemiologic study of childhood leprosy from Delhi. Pediatr Dermatol. 2005;22: 489-90.
15. Van Beers SM, Hatta M, Klatser PR. Patient contact is the major determinant in incident leprosy: implications for future control. Int J Lepr Other Mycobact Dis. 1999;67:119-28.
16. Palit A, Inamadar AC. Childhood leprosy in India over the past two decades. Lepr Rev. 2014;85(2):93-9.
17. Dave DS, Agrawal SK. Prevalence of leprosy in children of leprosy parents. Indian J Lepr. 1984;56:615-21.
18. Rodrigues LC, Lockwood DNJ. Leprosy now: epidemiology, progress, challenges, and research gaps. Lancet Infect Dis. 2011;11:464-70.
19. Duncan ME, Melsom R, Pearson JM et al. A clinical and immunological study of four babies of mothers with lepromatous leprosy, two of whom developed leprosy in infancy. Int J Lepr Other Mycobact Dis. 1983;51:7-17.
20. Jopling WH, McDougall AC. The Disease: Handbook of Leprosy, 5th edn (International). New Delhi, India. CBS Publishers and distributors; 2005 (reprinted).pp.1-9.
21. Girdhar BK. Skin to skin transmission of leprosy. Indian J Dermatol Venereol Leprol. 2005;71:223-5.
22. Mittal RR, Singla A, Gupta R. Inoculation leprosy after tattooing. Indian J Dermatol Venereol Leprol. 2002;68:116.
23. Brandsma JW, Yoder L, MacDonald M. Leprosy acquired by inoculation from a knee injury. Lepr Rev. 2005;76:175-9.
24. Ghorpade A. Inoculation (tattoo) leprosy: a report of 31 cases. J Eur Acad Dermatol Venereol. 2002;16:494-9.
25. Ridley DS, Jopling WH. Classification of leprosy according to immunity–a five group system. Int J Lepr. 1966;34:255-73.
26. WHO Expert Committee on Leprosy. Seventh report. Geneva: World Health Organization. Tech Rep Ser. 1998.p.874.
27. Sehgal VN, Joginder. Leprosy in children: correlation of clinical, histopathological, bacteriological and immunological parameters. Lepr Rev. 1989;60:202-5.
28. Nadkarni NJ, Grugni A, Kini MS, et al. Childhood leprosy in Bombay: a clinico-epidemiological study. Indian J Lepr. 1988; 60:173-88.
29. Singal A, Sonthalia S, Pandhi D. Childhood leprosy in a tertiary-care hospital in Delhi, India: A reappraisal in the post-elimination era. Lepr Rev. 2011;82:259-69.
30. Price J. E. BCG vaccination in leprosy. Int J Leprosy. 1982;50: 205-12.
31. Mahajan S, Sardana K, Bhushan P, Koranne RV, Mendiratta V. A study of leprosy in children, from a tertiary pediatric hospital in India. Lepr Rev. 2006;77:160-2.
32. Fakhouri R, Sotto MN, Manini MI, et al. Nodular leprosy of childhood and tuberculoid leprosy: a comparative, morphologic, immunopathologic and quantitative study of skin tissue reaction. Int J Lepr Other Mycobact Dis. 2003;71: 218-26.

33. Chen XS, Li WZ, Jiang C, et al. Leprosy in children: a retrospective study in China, 1986-1997. J Trop Pediatr. 2000;46:207-11.

34. Pandhi D, Mehta S, Agrawal S, et al. Erythema nodosum leprosum necroticans in a child- an unusual manifestation. Int J Lepr Other Mycobact Dis. 2005;73:122-6.

35. Gupta R, Singal A, Pandhi D. Genital Involvement and type I reaction in childhood leprosy. Lepr Rev. 2005;76;253-7.

36. Imbiriba EB, Hurtado-Guerrero JC, Garnelo L, et al. Epidemiological profile of leprosy in children under 15 in Manaus (Northern Brazil), 1998-2005. Rev Saude Publica. 2008; 42:1021-6.

37. Kar BR, Job CK. Visible deformity in childhood leprosy—a 10-year study. Int J Lepr Other Mycobact Dis. 2005;73:243-8.

38. Job CK, Baskaran B, Jayakumar J, Aschhoff M. Histopathologic evidence to show that indeterminate leprosy may be a primary lesion of the disease. Int J Lepr Other Mycobact Dis. 1997;65(4):443-9.

39. Kumar V, Baruah MC, Garg BR. Childhood leprosy-a clinico-epidemiological study from Pondicherry. Indian J Dermatol Venereol Leprol. 1989;55:301-4.

40. Keeler R, Deen RD. Leprosy in children aged 0-14 years. A case report of 11 years control programme. Lepr Rev. 1985;56: 239-48.

41. Lucas SB, Ridley DS. The use of histopathology in leprosy diagnosis and research. Lepr Rev. 1989;60:257-62.

42. Rao AG. Study of leprosy in children. Indian J Lepr. 2009; 81:195-7.

43. Kumar B, Rai R, Kaur I. Childhood leprosy in Chandigarh; clinico-histopathological correlation. Int J Lepr Other Mycobact Dis. 2000;68:330-1.

44. Kamal R, Dayal R, Katoch VM, et al. Analysis of gene probes and gene amplification techniques for diagnosis and monitoring of treatment in childhood leprosy. Lepr Rev. 2006;77:141-6.

45. Nandan D, Venkatesan K, Katoch K, et al. Serum beta-glucuronidase levels in children with leprosy. Lepr Rev. 2007;78:243-7.

46. Mani RS. Importance of systematic school survey in urban leprosy control. Lepr India. 1976;48(4 Suppl):813-8.

47. WHO. Chemotherapy of Leprosy for control programme. Technical Report Series 675, WHO, Geneva, 1982.

48. WHO Model Prescribing Information. Drugs used in Leprosy, 1998

49. Butlin CR, Saunderson P. Children with leprosy. Lepr Rev. 2014;85(2):69-73.

50. Santos MJ, Ferrari CK, de Toledo OR, et al. Leprosy among children and adolescents under 15 years-old in a city of Legal Amazon, Brazil. Indian J Lepr. 2012;84:265-9.

51. Horo I, Rao PS, Nanda NK, et al. Childhood leprosy: profiles from a leprosy referral hospital in West Bengal, India. Indian J Lepr. 2010;82:33-7.

Ocular Leprosy

Ebenezer Daniel

INTRODUCTION

Blindness is a catastrophic event, and in leprosy there exist several mechanisms that can lead up to this event. Good vision is critical especially to a person who has lost sensory function in the hands and feet, developed visible deformities, and because of the stigma attached to the disease can ill-afford to be dependent on anyone. The magnitude of ocular morbidity and blindness is to a large extent influenced by the clinical, demographic, psychological and social dimensions associated with the disease.

A longitudinal study of ocular leprosy from India, Philippines and Ethiopia (longitudinal study of ocular leprosy) was conducted on a cohort of newly diagnosed multibacillary (MB) leprosy patients who received treatment with multidrug therapy (MDT) for 2 years and who were followed up for 5 years after completion of MDT. These patients were seen by ophthalmologists in a well-equipped eye clinic of a tertiary leprosy institution and underwent comprehensive standardized ophthalmic examinations every 6 months. Patients were recruited through active case finding. Although the results of the study cannot be generalized for the whole country or the world leprosy population, it does give a glimpse of the nature and severity of ocular problems encountered in the later part of the 20th and the early part of the 21st century, which are different from what was observed during the early 20th century.

The study showed that 11% of patients already had potentially blinding leprosy related ocular pathology (PBLROP) at enrollment.[1] A further 9% of patients developed PBLROP during their 2-year treatment with MDT.[2] Therefore, one in five patients who have completed MDT is likely to have ocular complications. The study also showed that each year

after the completion of MDT, 4% of patients continued to develop PBLROP.[3] The longitudinal study clearly showed that patients can develop ocular complications while on treatment with MDT but more importantly, complications continue to occur long after the patient had obtained bacteriological cure. Complications can persist and progress, leading to blindness.[4]

Several significant changes have occurred in the leprosy field since the results of the longitudinal study of ocular leprosy were published. India adopted a policy of integrating leprosy services into the general health system removing the need for active case finding in the field. The integrated system encourages leprosy patients to present and self-report at the primary health centers and district hospitals. The post-integration trend among patients in the same area of the study showed an increase in the mean age of patients registering in the outpatient department, increase in MB leprosy patients and those with grade 2 disabilities.[5] A shift toward increasing incidence of MB patients compared to paucibacillary (PB) patients in many areas of the world makes the results of this longitudinal study on ocular complications in MB patients more pertinent for the coming decade. MB patients have more than twice the amount of ocular complications than PB patients. It is also reasonable to assume that an increasing number of patients would not present themselves at the primary clinics until they are in a relatively late stage of the disease, possibly with more deformities. An important result from the longitudinal study of ocular leprosy was that patients with more severe hand and leg deformities had more ocular complications, some of them not likely to be recognized by a cursory examination in the field. Patients in the integrated leprosy system are also likely to be examined by physicians with varying amounts of knowledge of the disease unlike ophthalmologists with expertise in leprosy in the longitudinal study of ocular leprosy. Therefore, the number of patients presenting and developing ocular complications may be an underestimation relative to what is actually taking place in the population, emphasizing the need for more skills and knowledge on ocular leprosy at the primary health centers as well as regular and consistent ocular care of patients with severe deformities.[6-9]

The evolution of better and shorter treatments for leprosy during the past few decades has produced an apparent reduction in its morbidity among newly diagnosed leprosy patients. Ocular complications that were common three or four decades ago are now observed less frequently among patients who access treatment early in their disease. However, the large pool of aging bacteriologically cured leprosy patients who have lived through the decades of dapsone monotherapy and who continue to have substantial leprosy related ocular problems are of public health importance and concern. Certain leprosy complications of the eye, should they occur or progress, pose a grave threat to the patients and it is important that those associated with the care of leprosy patients are well-acquainted with the prevention, presentation and treatment of these ocular complications.[10] In view of these considerations, this chapter will address the key ocular complications related to leprosy, briefly mention older and rarer ones and give some suggestions for future research.

OCULAR INVOLVEMENT

Mycobacterium leprae survive and proliferate in parts of the body that have relatively low temperatures. The bacilli enter the ocular tissues through hematological spread and proliferate mostly in the lids, the adnexa and the anterior parts of the eyeball. This presentation can vary in animals where the bacilli are found in almost all the ocular tissues.[11,12] In humans, although they have been demonstrated in the choroid, they are rarely seen to extend beyond the equator of the eyeball.[13] Therefore, most ocular complications, particularly the ones that result from the host reactions to the bacilli, can easily be observed without the aid of specialized ophthalmic equipment or the presence of an experienced ophthalmologist. However, to confirm the findings of the screening examinations done by health workers in the field and to initiate and sustain appropriate ocular therapy, it will be necessary for an ophthalmologist to examine the patient in a clinical setting.

CLINICAL EXAMINATION OF THE EYE IN LEPROSY

Ocular complications can occur during any phase of the disease in relation to MDT; before, during and after treatment, and therefore regular systematic ocular examinations in all leprosy patients are important. In most instances, preliminary

ocular screening examinations take only a few minutes and can be done by trained paramedical personnel or health workers who can then refer patients with ocular complications to an ophthalmologist for a more comprehensive examination. Quick screening examinations in the field should include recording visual acuity, checking for lagophthalmos and redness in the eye and need not be exhaustive. Traditionally, before the integration of leprosy services into general health services occurred, leprosy field personnel were trained to look only for leprosy related ocular complications when screening a patient or a patient suspect, but the postintegration period requires a more comprehensive ophthalmic examination, diagnosing ocular complications that might be unrelated to leprosy.

History

A detailed history must first be recorded at the patient's initial visit. It should include key demographic characteristics such as age and sex; leprosy characteristics such as type, duration of the disease, treatment, reactions and skin smear/ biopsy results; ocular history of face patches, lagophthalmos, corneal ulcers, corneal opacity, scleritis, iridocyclitis, cataract and glaucoma; comorbid infections such as tuberculosis, human immunodeficiency virus (HIV) and syphilis as well as systemic noninfectious diseases such as diabetes mellitus and hypertension.

Visual Acuity

An ophthalmic examination should always begin with an accurate assessment of visual acuity in both eyes. Documenting the visual acuity at the first visit and every subsequent visit will reveal the status of vision and the extent of vision loss or gain over time. There are excellent treatises that deal with the art of taking and recording visual acuity and the reader is recommended to read one of these for a comprehensive understanding on the subject.[14] In the field, whenever possible, the examiner should use a Snellen's chart, at a distance of 6 meters or 20 feet, in a well-lit area for evaluating visual acuity of both eyes independently and binocularly. If a patient cannot see the largest letter on the Snellen chart, visual acuity should be measured by the following methods, listed in order of decreasing visual function:

1. Counting fingers, the patient can count fingers displayed between 1 foot and 5 feet away from the eyes.
2. Hand movements, the patient can distinguish horizontal from vertical hand motions at 1 foot.
3. Light perception, the patient can tell if a bright light is shined directly into the eye.
4. No light perception, the patient cannot tell if a bright light is shined into the eye. Patients already wearing glasses should have their visual acuity taken with and without the

spectacles. In patients over 40 years of age recording near vision should not be neglected.

A "systematic ophthalmic examination" should follow the visual acuity assessment. Examine the eyes from the outside to the inside: face, eyebrow, eyelid, nasolacrimal duct, conjunctiva, sclera, cornea, anterior chamber, iris and pupil, lens, and finally a crude measure of intraocular pressure (IOP).

Face

Facial Palsy

Examine the face carefully for any inequality between both sides. Signs of facial nerve palsy may include loss of forehead wrinkling, difficulty in closing the eye and the drawing of the mouth to one side. Bell's palsy, which is an acute form of facial palsy without detectable cause, occurs in around 0.3% of the general population and therefore could occur in a leprosy patient. The distinguishing features of Bell's palsy are its sudden appearance, unilaterality, lower motor neuron type (complete paralysis) of palsy followed by a rapid and complete natural recovery in more than 70% of affected people.[15] In contrast, the facial nerve palsy caused by leprosy is usually gradual, although it could occur rapidly with a type 1 reaction [reversal reaction (RR)] on the face, can be bilateral, is almost never complete (only some parts of the face are involved) and recovery is dependent upon early recognition and treatment with oral corticosteroids.

Face Patches

Skin patches on the face may be hypopigmented, erythematous or hypoesthetic or various combinations of all three. These patches especially ones that involve the zygomatic/malar area or the eyelids are known risk factors for lagophthalmos.[16,17]

Face Nodules

Nodules on the face and lids should be noted and may be a sign of histoid leprosy. Facial pigmentation is sometimes seen prominently in patients receiving clofazimine.

Eyebrows

Madarosis

Loss of eyebrows is called superciliary madarosis and the loss of eyelashes, ciliary madarosis. Madarosis usually occurs in lepromatous leprosy (LL) but can occur in the tuberculoid form of leprosy if associated with a face patch. In LL, the hair loss of the eyebrows starts laterally and progresses medially, presumably because the lateral side is cooler than the center of the face.

Eyelids

Orbicularis Oculi Muscle Weakness

Muscle strength of the orbicularis oculi is tested by asking the patient to close the eyes tightly with the examiner trying to pry open the lids gently with the thumb and index finger. Normal strength of the muscle will easily counter this effort and the eyelids cannot be pried open easily whereas in weakness of the orbicularis oculi muscle the lids will pry open easily.

Lagophthalmos

It is the inability to close the eyelids (Fig. 27.1). Watering or itching can be symptoms but often lagophthalmos occurs without obvious symptoms and early lagophthalmos can easily be missed if not looked for specifically. Every patient who is being examined must be asked to close the eyes and any gap between the lids must be recorded.

Visibility of Upper Sclera

Normally the superior sclera is hidden under the upper eyelid and is not visualized but if upper eyelid retraction is present it may be exposed even in normal distant gaze. If present, visibility of the upper sclera should be documented.[18]

Measurements in Lagophthalmos

Lagophthalmos, if present, should have three measurements of the palpebral fissure taken at each visit. Palpebral fissure is the area between the upper and lower lids. Measurement is done on the widest area of the palpebral fissure using a transparent millimeter scale; when the patient gazes at a distant object (normal straight gaze without any attempt at

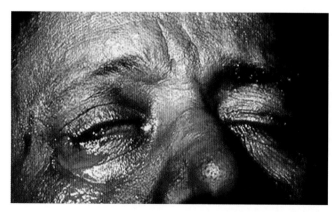

Fig. 27.1: Lepromatous leprosy patient with lagophthalmos. On gentle closure there is a gap in the right eye while the left eye closes normally. Bell's phenomenon is present in the affected eye with the cornea being drawn up during attempted closure of the lids. Mucus collection at the medial canthus of the right eye should raise suspicion of blocked nasolacrimal duct

closure); when the eyes are closed gently (gentle closure) and when the eyes are closed tightly (forced closure). These recordings are critical during follow-up and for deciding appropriate treatment (Figs 27.2A to C).[18]

Blink Rate

Record the involuntary blink rate per minute. Note, if complete closure occurs with blinking.

Bell's Phenomenon

The presence or absence of Bell's phenomenon should be noted. The eyes roll up on attempted closure of the lids and it is a defense mechanism that is absent in 25% of the population. In patients with lagophthalmos and/or impaired corneal sensation without this reflex, the cornea is at increased risk of sustaining injury.

Nodules on the Lid

Presence of nodules on the lid may or may not be related to leprosy. Histoid leprosy may present with multiple nodules all over the body including the lids.

Ectropion

In ectropion, the lids are turned outward and the inner conjunctival layer is exposed. It is most commonly seen in the lower lid, and in leprosy is usually associated with lagophthalmos. The amount of ectropion should be measured.

Entropion

Entropion is turning in of the eyelids or in-rolling of the eyelids, usually the lower lid. The lid margins or the lashes brush against the cornea. In addition to the unpleasant sensation of irritation in the eyes, there may be excessive mucus discharge and eyelid crusting.

Trichiasis

Trichiasis exists when the eyelashes are turned inward and rub against the cornea. The eyelashes must be examined with the eye positioned in the normal distance gaze and the presence and number of these malpositioned eyelashes should be noted.

Examination of Adnexa

Nasolacrimal duct patency and mucocele: The tears drain through the papillae near the medial end of eyelid margin and enter the nasal mucosa through the nasolacrimal duct from where they are absorbed. Blockage of the nasolacrimal duct can cause excessive tearing and delayed healing of infected corneal ulcers. To check for patency, gentle pressure should be applied over the nasolacrimal area and if there is efflux of material through the papillae a block may be present. If there is a provision, syringing must be done to check the patency of the nasolacrimal sac. A small amount of fluid is forced into the lower papillae using a syringe and a blunt needle and the patient instructed to confirm if the flow of fluid can be felt in the nose or throat. A mucocele is often easily noticed as a visible painless swelling in the area over the nasolacrimal sac (Fig. 27.3).

Conjunctiva

Conjunctival Redness

Conjunctival redness could result because of exposure, corneal ulcer, episcleritis, scleritis or iridocyclitis. Viral and bacterial conjunctivitis which are common causes of redness in the general population should be differentiated from the redness caused by these serious conditions. Depending on the severity of bacterial or viral conjunctivitis, there may be mucus or watery discharge but visual acuity is not affected. Redness with lowered visual acuity should be referred to an ophthalmologist as soon as possible.

Conjunctival nodules may be seen in the histoid type of leprosy.

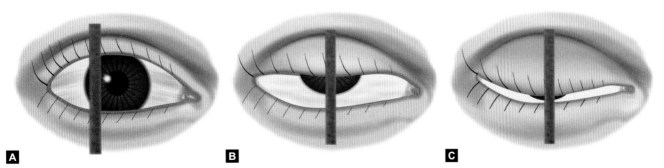

Figs 27.2A to C: Measurements to be recorded in a case of lagophthalmos at every visit. (A) Measure in millimeters with transparent scale the widest gap on normal gaze; (B) Measure the widest gap on gentle closure; (C) Measure the widest gap on forced closure

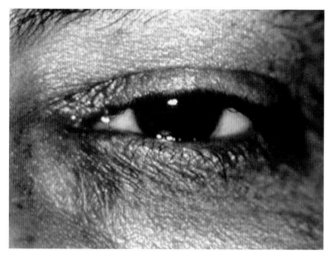

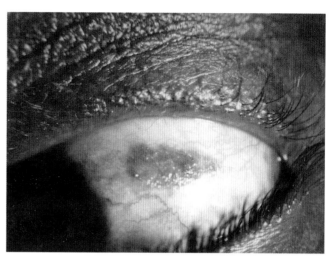

Fig. 27.3: Mucocele, a painless swelling of the nasolacrimal sac due to blockage in the nasolacrimal duct. If a corneal ulcer occurs in the eye it can be unresponsive to therapy as the sac can harbor pathogens that reflux into the tear film and produce recurrent secondary infections

Fig. 27.4: Clofazamine pigmentation in the conjunctiva seen prominently in an area of Bitot spot in a patient receiving MDT. The pigmentation disappeared in a few weeks after completion of MDT

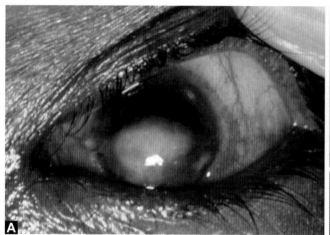

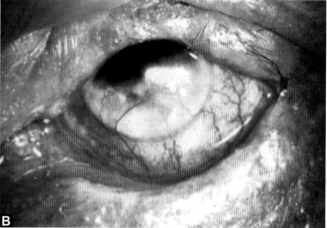

Figs 27.5A and B: (A) A dense corneal opacity after healing of a corneal ulcer; (B) Exposure keratitis in a patient with lagophthalmos. Repeated punctate injury to the cornea leads to opacification and vascularization of the exposed cornea

Clofazimine Pigmentation

Clofazimine or B663 used as a systemic drug in conjunction with MDT or used alone can cause dark pigmentation on the conjunctival surface especially in areas where there has been previous injury (e.g. Bitot spots) (Fig. 27.4). This pigmentation gradually disappears after the clofazimine therapy is completed. Clofazimine crystals can sometimes be observed as shiny reflective objects in the conjunctiva and cornea in some patients receiving B663 therapy. These are visualized better on a slit lamp with high magnification. Vision is not usually affected.

Cornea

The cornea is normally transparent. Corneal opacities can occur anywhere in the cornea (Fig. 27.5A). In exposure keratitis, they usually occur in the lower half where they are maximally exposed to the atmosphere in a patient with lagophthalmos (Fig. 27.5B). In dry eye, they can occur anywhere but usually are in the mid-region of the cornea. They can also present as small multiple opacities near the limbus (the corneoscleral junction).

Corneal Ulcer

These can be small, large or secondarily infected. Small punctate ulcers are called superficial punctate keratitis and are usually the result of exposure. Abrasions especially in corneas having reduced sensation can become secondarily infected with bacteria or fungus and cause severe inflammatory reaction producing a hypopyon, which is sterile pus in the anterior chamber. To differentiate between an active corneal ulcer and a healed opacity, a drop of fluorescein is applied to the tears. Corneal opacities will not stain with the fluorescein dye, but the corneal ulcer will stain readily and will appear green and the dye will persist for a few minutes. Pooling of the fluorescein dye in a large scar can occur which can mimic staining (Figs 27.6A and B).

Corneal Pannus

Corneal pannus presents as thin blood vessels growing into the corneal surface. Pannus usually occurs in the anterior layers of the cornea in the peripheral region near the limbus (the area where the cornea joins the sclera) (Fig. 27.7).

Interstitial Keratitis

Interstitial keratitis is characterized by cellular infiltration and vascularization of the corneal stroma with minimal involvement of the corneal epithelium or endothelium. It is situated deeper than a pannus.

Corneal Sensation

Loss of sensation is the hallmark of leprosy and decreased corneal sensation should be tested in a clinic. The traditional

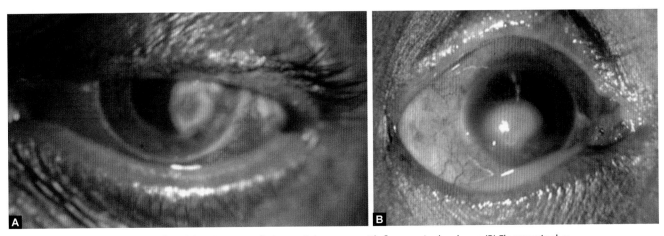

Figs 27.6A and B: (A) Active corneal ulcer staining green with fluorescein dye drops; (B) Fluorescein dye does not stain the opacity where an active ulcer is absent

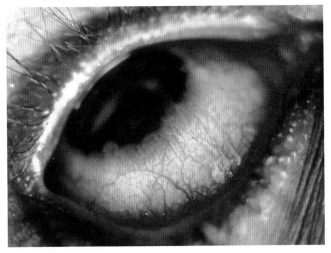

Fig. 27.7: Corneal pannus where vessels and infiltration are seen to invade the superficial cornea near the limbus

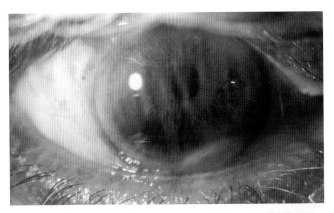

Fig. 27.8: A lepromatous leprosy patient with longstanding disease, and impaired corneal sensation. Etchings on the corneal epithelium that the patient was unaware of were a result of the patient rubbing the eye with a cloth. These corneal abrasions can become corneal ulcers if they become secondarily infected

testing of corneal sensation with a cotton wisp in the field must be avoided. Corneal hypoesthesia is present in long-standing LL. Foreign bodies can be embedded in these corneas without any symptoms and corneal abrasions may not present with pain (Fig. 27.8). A careful examination of the cornea should be an important part of the examination of the eye to exclude these foreign bodies. A standardized method of measuring corneal sensation can be performed by using the Cochet and Bonnet esthesiometer. However, the esthesiometer is expensive and it takes a long time to complete an examination with this instrument.

Corneal Nerve Enlargement and Beading

When the cornea is examined under magnification with a slit lamp, thickening, beading or enlargement of corneal nerves can be observed sometimes in LL patients. These nerve beadings are believed to be due to calcified collections of large amounts of *M. leprae* on the fine nerves that traverse the corneal stroma. They can be missed on perfunctory biomicroscopy.

Chalky White Corneal Precipitates

LL patients with high bacillary counts can also present with chalky white precipitates on the surface of the cornea, usually in the superior outer quadrant (Fig. 27.9).

Corneal Dellen

These are small, saucer-like excavations at the margin of the cornea adjacent to a perilimbal elevation such as a pterygium. A pterygium is a triangular, vascular, fleshy growth that originates on the conjunctiva and that can spread to the corneal limbus and into the cornea. *M. leprae* has been shown in pterygium.[19]

Climatic droplet keratopathy: It is a degenerative condition characterized by the accumulation of translucent material in the superficial corneal stroma within the interpalpebral area, beginning peripherally and spreading centrally. They resemble droplets of oil and can be primary or secondary to a disease. Old lepromatous corneas may show signs of this degenerative condition (Fig. 27.10).[20]

Band-shaped Keratopathy

Deposition of calcium phosphate salts in the interpalpebral region of the cornea can be seen in old LL patients with long-standing exposure or uveitis (Fig. 27.11).

Sclera

Episcleritis

Patchy redness in the episcleral tissues (just beneath the conjunctival tissue), typically without pain or tenderness (Fig. 27.12).

Scleritis

Deeper redness that can be patchy, nodular or necrotizing and is usually accompanied by pain and tenderness. Thinning of the sclera can occur after severe and recurrent scleritis (Figs 27.13A to C).

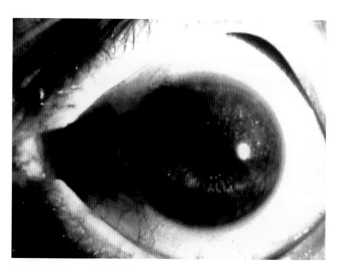

Fig. 27.9: Corneal chalky white precipitates seen in the upper temporal quadrant of the cornea. Three small iris pearls can also be seen at 5 o'clock at the pupillary margin. These manifestations, when present are pathognomonic of lepromatous leprosy with large bacterial loads

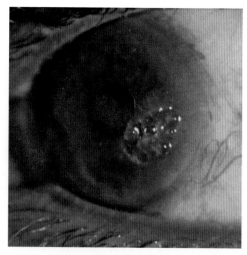

Fig. 27.10: Climatic droplet keratopathy. Oil droplet like degeneration seen in the cornea of a lepromatous leprosy patient

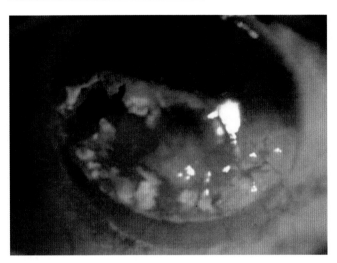

Fig. 27.11: Band-shaped keratopathy in an LL patient

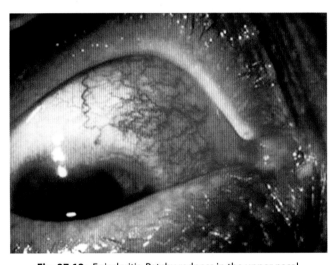

Fig. 27.12: Episcleritis. Patchy redness in the upper nasal quadrant with little or no symptoms

Iris

Iridocyclitis (Uveitis, Anterior Uveitis, Iritis)

It is more common among LL and borderline lepromatous (BL) patients. A common perception is that iridocyclitis occurs in leprosy as part of erythema nodosum leprosum (ENL) or type 2 reaction, but more often than not iridocyclitis occurs independent of other signs of ENL.[21] Symptoms include decreased vision, photophobia, pain and conjunctival redness. Signs include redness especially around the limbal area (circumcorneal congestion), keratic precipitates, flare and cells in the anterior chamber, small sluggishly reacting pupil and irregular pupil (Figs 27.14A to C).

Iris Atrophy

Prolonged overt or chronic subclinical uveal inflammation can lead to iris atrophy. Areas of iris are seen to be hypopigmented and in severe forms through and through holes can be seen, termed polycoria (Fig. 27.15).

Iris Pearls

These are small rounded white pearl like structures found stuck to the iris in longstanding lepromatous patients, signifying large quantities of bacilli. They are simply a presentation with no association with loss of vision (Fig. 27.9).

Nodules on the Iris

Lepromatous nodules can sometimes be observed on the anterior surface of the iris.[22]

Cataract

Cataract is opacity of the lens. It can be cortical, nuclear or subcapsular. It is seen as a whitish opacity on the lens on oblique illumination. It is common among patients who are older and those who have had episodes of intraocular inflammation (Figs 27.14 to 27.16).

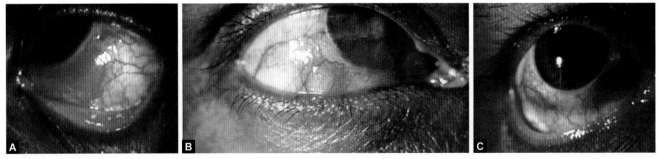

Figs 27.13A to C: Scleritis. (A) Intense redness with pain and tenderness that is patchy; (B) Scleritis presenting as a nodular type; (C) Scleral thinning in the eye of a patient after repeated episodes of scleritis. Pale blue areas in the inferior sclera denote the thinning. An irregular pupil with posterior synechia is also present

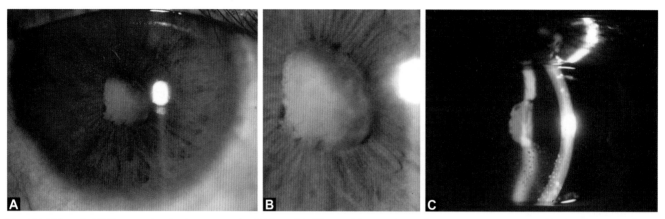

Figs 27.14A to C: (A) Cataract developing as a result of iridocyclitis. The pupil is irregular and a cataract can be seen in the pupillary area; (B) The enlarged pupillary area shows the iris stuck to the anterior surface of the cataractous lens; (C) Slit lamp beam showing keratic precipitates which are small circular adhesions at the back of the cornea

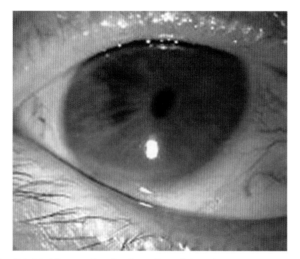

Fig. 27.15: Iris atrophy. Small oval pupil in a lepromatous patient showing varying degrees of iris atrophy with a small area that has full thickness iris atrophy

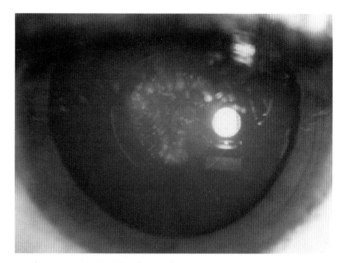

Fig. 27.16: Posterior subcapsular cataract in a patient who had received large amounts of oral corticosteroid treatment for neuritis

Intraocular Tension

In the clinic, IOP is measured using a Goldman applanation tonometer that is usually fixed to a slit lamp. Increased pressure of over 20 mm Hg may be indicative of ocular hypertension or glaucoma. These patients require a fundus examination and a field examination. Conversely hypotony, which is pressure below 5 mm Hg can occur in patients with longstanding uveitis. In the field, with no equipment, a rough estimation of IOP can be made out by the fingers applied over the lid gently to gauge the relative hardness of the globe.

Table 27.1 gives an overview of possible ocular complications seen in leprosy.

LAGOPHTHALMOS AND OTHER LID DEFORMITIES

Lagophthalmos, from the Greek word for "hare," describes a condition where a patient loses the ability to completely close the eyes due to loss of function in the eyelids. It is due to facial nerve palsy affecting the orbicularis oculi muscle and is a common ocular complication in both MB and PB leprosy patients. The eyelid plays a crucial role in protecting and providing nourishment for the surface of eye and when eyelid closure function is lost, the health of the eye is at risk. Lagophthalmos can lead to several other ocular complications such as dry eye, exposure keratitis and corneal ulceration. It can occur before, during and after MDT.

Table 27.1: An overview of the ophthalmic manifestations of leprosy

Face	Seventh nerve palsy
	Hypopigmented/erythematous patches
	Nodules around the eyes
Eyebrows	Superciliary madarosis
Lids	Ciliary madarosis
	Lagophthalmos
	Ectropion
	Entropion
	Trichiasis
	Nodule on the eyelids
Nasolacrimal duct	Blockage of nasolacrimal duct
	Mucocele
Conjunctiva	Exposure conjunctivitis
	Subconjunctival fibrosis
	Conjunctival nodules
	Clofazimine crystals
	Clofazimine pigmentation
Cornea	Enlarged and visible corneal nerves
	Corneal nerve beading
	Corneal pannus
	Corneal ulcer
	Corneal opacity
	Corneal hypoesthesia
	Punctate epithelial keratopathy
	Exposure keratitis
	Interstitial keratitis
	Dellen
	Climatic droplet keratopathy
	Chalky white precipitates
	Band-shaped keratopathy
Anterior chamber	Hypopyon
	Flare and cells
Sclera	Scleral nodule
	Episcleritis
	Scleritis
	Scleral thinning
	Anterior staphyloma
Iris	Keratic precipitates
	Anterior synechia and peripheral anterior synechia
	Irregular pupil
	Iris nodules
	Iris atrophy and polycoria
	Iris pearls
Lens	Posterior subcapsular cataract
	Nuclear cataract
Intraocular pressure	Glaucoma and ocular hypertension
	Hypotony

Risk Factors for Developing Lagophthalmos

Several risk factors for developing lagophthalmos have been described:

1. Face patches: Hypopigmented, erythematous or hypoesthetic areas in the area supplied by the zygomatic branch of the seventh cranial nerve.
2. Initial months of MDT possibly by initiating a type 1 reaction (RR).
3. Borderline forms of leprosy (which is more unstable in the spectrum).
4. Grade 2 deformities in the hands and feet.

Recognition of these risk factors should lead to careful and frequent ocular examinations to detect and treat lagophthalmos at its earliest presentation.

Management of Lagophthalmos

Lagophthalmos is the result of inflammation and damage to the branches of the seventh cranial nerve innervating eyelid muscles. The initial step in the management of lagophthalmos involves diagnosing the condition early and starting effective treatment to reduce the inflammation. Diagnosing lagophthalmos early involves regular frequent examination of patients with known risk factors and educating patients to recognize the symptoms and report when they occur. Patient education must include but not be limited to recognizing that common symptoms such as tearing and irritation of the eyes may be the initial presenting symptoms of lagophthalmos. A regular daily practice of testing for gaps on gentle closure of the lids in front of a mirror should be encouraged. All clinical examinations of leprosy patients must never exclude the simple test of asking the patient to gently close the eyes.

The presentation of lagophthalmos is usually rapid during or after type 1 reaction. This does not preclude lagophthalmos occurring in patients without obvious reactions or face patches. In polar lepromatous patients, the presentation and progression of lagophthalmos is gradual resulting from a low-grade persistent chronic inflammation in the superficial branches of the facial nerve.

Early lagophthalmos has been arbitrarily defined as one that is of less than 6 months duration. Unless treated early and rigorously, lagophthalmos is likely to become permanent. Oral steroid therapy is the mainstay of treatment and is similar to treating other neuritis in leprosy. In an average adult patient, Prednisolone 60 mg daily is given and tapered by 5 mg every 2 weeks. The dosage is adjusted according to weight in younger patients and for those with diabetes and hypertension. Although a smaller dose steroid regimen has been shown to be effective in treating early lagophthalmos,[23] the intention must be to bring down the inflammation in the nerve as rapidly as possible. It is therefore, desirable to start therapy with a higher dose and gradually reduce the dosage as the inflammation comes down. The steroid treatment should be accompanied by adequate protection of the exposed corneal surface that can develop dry eye and corneal damage.

Substitute/Artificial Tear Drops

There are a number of artificial tear drops available in the market. Methyl cellulose or hydroxylpropyl methylcellulose (0.25–1% concentrations) are cellulose ethers that are commonly used as tear substitutes because they are cheap and effective. Patients should instill these eyedrops three times a day or more frequently depending upon the symptoms. Polyvinyl alcohol is a vinyl derivative and the next most commonly used tear substitute, but is less viscous and more expensive than methyl cellulose. Sodium hyaluronate is used in many intraocular surgeries and sometimes has been prescribed for dry eye, but for any long-term treatment they are very expensive.

For protecting the exposed cornea during daytime, dark goggles can be worn. To some extent, this also decreases the evaporation of tears. The eyes must also be protected at night during sleep, usually with the application of liberal quantities of sterile paraffin in the interpalpebral region and by covering the eye with a light cloth.

In leprosy, the superficial branches of the facial nerve are involved in a patchy and scattered distribution and this affects the muscles supplied by the nerve to varying degrees.[24] Paralysis of orbicularis oculi presents with various grades of severity and unlike a lower motor neuron type of paralysis, some muscle fibers retain their function and this forms the basis for blinking exercises and physiotherapy. Blinking exercises must be taught to the patient and it essentially involves taking time daily to try and to shut the eyelids by voluntarily contracting the orbicularis oculi—developing a routine to do this exercise consistently is extremely important.

While treating the patient with steroids, tear substitute drops or exercises, the patient must be examined at regular intervals for any increase in symptoms, damage to the corneal surface and increase or decrease in the width of palpebral fissure measurements on gentle and forced closure.

Surgery for Lagophthalmos

The indications for surgery in lagophthalmos are poorly defined and inconsistent. The primary aim of the surgery should be to help close the eyelids and prevent corneal dryness and injury. Surgery is often undertaken when medical therapy has failed, when symptoms of lagophthalmos increase in severity, and/or when the health of the cornea is threatened. The health of the cornea includes health of the tear film (decreased tear breakup time), presence of punctate keratitis, filamentary keratitis or exposure keratitis, extensive areas of conjunctiva that stain with Lissamine green dye and corneal epithelial abrasions. Surgery is advocated to help heal a corneal ulcer when it has already occurred and also when there is a 5 mm or more gap on gentle closure of the eye which is a good quantitative measure.

Retrospective studies have shown that eyes with reduced corneal sensation if associated with lagophthalmos have more pathology. There are a variety of surgeries for lagophthalmos and the decision to choose the type of surgery should be left to the patient after adequate explanation. In certain countries and in certain situations some of these decisions are limited by resources, by available surgical expertise and the difficulty in following up patients with eye examinations.

In instances where there is improvement of the lagophthalmos due to ongoing steroid therapy and lid exercises but the health of the cornea is threatened then temporary measures such as taping the lids can be performed.

Temporary Tarsorrhaphy

When recovery of the eyelid closure is expected within a few weeks, a temporary tarsorrhaphy can be performed suturing together the upper lid and the lower lid without creating raw areas on the lid margins. The cornea can be protected adequately by suturing the lateral one-third of the eyelids together. Once the lagophthalmos has recovered, the suture can be removed (Figs 27.17A and B).

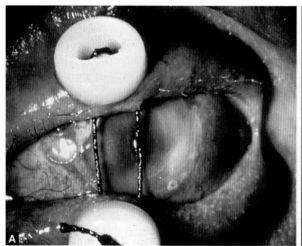 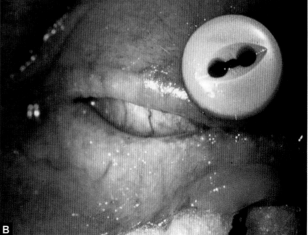

Figs 27.17A and B: Temporary tarsorrhaphy. Sutures passing through sterile buttons and lids can be removed after lagophthalmos improves or if a more permanent surgery is planned

Permanent Tarsorrhaphy

When the lagophthalmos is not expected to improve and longer duration of protection is needed a permanent tarsorrhaphy can be performed by creating a raw area on the eyelid margins at the site of the sutures to create intermarginal adhesions. The sutures are removed after about 10 days. If the patient regains useful function of the orbicularis oculi muscle, the adhesions can be incised and separated. Lateral tarsorrhaphy is the most common surgery for leprosy lagophthalmos. It is a simple surgery and does not require as much expertise as some of the other surgeries. It may be cosmetically unacceptable to patients and can limit peripheral vision. Medial tarsorrhaphy is used only if the medial part of the cornea is affected and cannot be effectively covered by a lateral tarsorrhaphy. It is cosmetically more disfiguring than lateral tarsorrhaphy. Complications of tarsorrhaphy include loosening of the sutures, inadequate lid coverage of the cornea and trichiasis (Fig. 27.18).

Temporalis Muscle Transfer

Temporalis muscle transfer (TMT) surgery described by Gillies and Anderson is a dynamic and cosmetically acceptable surgery for lagophthalmos (Figs 27.19A and B).[25] The temporalis muscle is used for chewing and has a compartmentalized innervation by the mandibular branch of the trigeminal nerve which is not usually affected in leprosy.[26] Surgery is done by detaching a tendon of the muscle, splitting it into two halves and rerouting each by tunneling through the upper and lower eyelids near their margins and attaching it to the medial palpebral tendon. TMT requires expertise and the surgery is usually performed by an orthopedician or a plastic surgeon and rarely by an ophthalmologist. It needs to be combined with intense physical therapy before and after

surgery. Retrospective studies on the effectiveness of TMT have described favorable outcomes in closure of the lids, in reducing the damage to the corneal surface and in reducing symptoms.[27,28] Complications that can occur with TMT include ectropion and ptosis.[29] Ectropion occurs when the tendon intended to be at the lid margin either is misplaced or slips away from the original position near the lid margin (Fig. 27.20). The ectropion is corrected by replacing the tendon

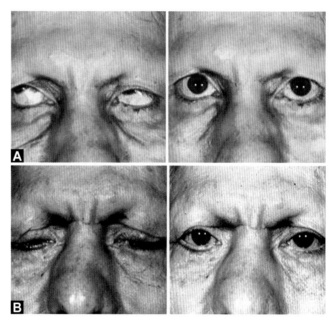

Figs 27.19A and B: (A) Bilateral lagophthalmos in a lepromatous leprosy patient. Gentle closure reveals a large gap in both eyes with Bell's phenomenon pulling the cornea up under the protective cover of the upper eye lid; (B) The eyes of the same patient as in Fig. 27.19 A after temporalis muscle transfer (TMT) surgery had been done. There is complete eyelid closure in the left and almost complete closure in the right eye with a good cosmetic outcome

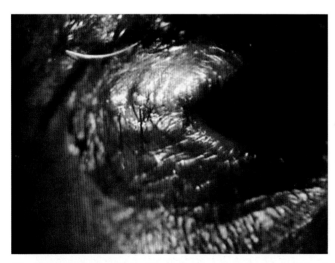

Fig. 27.18: Permanent lateral tarsorrhaphy where the lids are joined together permanently in the lateral one-third of the eye

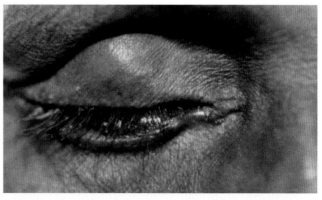

Fig. 27.20: Ectropion developing as an unwanted result after TMT surgery. The tendon at the lower eye lid margin had been displaced posteriorly. The ectropion was corrected surgically

in its correct position and buttressing it with nonabsorbable sutures. Ptosis is due to over correction and tightness of the encircling tendon. These complications are less likely in experienced hands.

Other surgical procedures used for lagophthalmos include various forms of lower lid tightening procedures and levator recession surgeries that have variable success rates. Lagophthalmos could also be treated with gold weights, magnets, silicon slings and autogenous facial slings but the results of these have not been extensively reported in leprosy literature. Gold implants that act by gravity in pulling the upper eyelid down by its weight have been shown to be not very effective in leprosy lagophthalmos, having a high extrusion rate and chronic inflammation of the lids,[30] but steel weights in one study have claimed better results.[31]

It is not clear whether all patients with permanent lagophthalmos need to be surgically treated and whether surgery will benefit all.[32] One study found that only half of those patients with lagophthalmos had surgery, and among those who had an initial surgery for lagophthalmos one-third required a further surgery as the outcome of surgery did not reduce the gap to less than 5 mm. The longitudinal study of ocular leprosy found that lagophthalmos already present at diagnosis has little chance (less than 20%) of full recovery with conventional steroid treatment while incident lagophthalmos has a 60% cure rate. The early diagnosis of lagophthalmos and treatment with steroids cannot be overemphasized but the large number of cured leprosy patients with lagophthalmos either with a need for surgery or resurgery present a serious surgical therapeutic option that need to be resolved.[33]

The need for lagophthalmos surgery is quite obvious in eyes with severe dry eye symptoms, exposure keratitis, corneal abrasions, corneal ulcers and useful vision only in the eye with lagophthalmos. In patients with a large gap of the palpebral fissure on gentle closure but having clear corneas, good corneal sensation, ability to take care of the eyes and with regular follow-up visits with an ophthalmologist, the decision to operate however, remains an unresolved issue. There is a need to educate patients and ophthalmologists on the importance of TMT surgery that is an effective surgery in the hands of an experienced surgeon. Patients needing surgical correction are usually reluctant to undergo the procedure, the reasons mainly are attributed to lack of full awareness of the availability of good surgical care.[34-36]

Ectropion (Fig. 27.21)

Since ectropion leaves the cornea irritated and exposed, the cornea is more susceptible to drying. This can lead to corneal abrasions and ulcers, which in turn can cause permanent loss of vision. As in lagophthalmos, lubricating eyedrops and ointments can help to protect the cornea and prevent damage until the ectropion is corrected surgically by lid shortening and/or tightening surgeries.

Entropion

Entropion may require surgery and there are a variety of surgical procedures described to correct this anomaly.

Trichiasis

Misdirection of the lashes can cause irritation of the hypoesthetic cornea and induce excessive rubbing of the eye that can result in an abrasion or a corneal ulcer. If the misdirected lashes are less than five, they can be plucked out or epilated. Epilation with forceps is an easy procedure but the eye lashes can grow back in a few weeks. Laser ablation of the hair follicle prevents recurrence. It must be remembered that trachoma that causes lid deformities including trichiasis can coexist with leprosy in endemic areas.[37]

CORNEAL INVOLVEMENT

Dry Eye

The tear film in leprosy can be deficient in several ways but usually develops due to lid deformities such as lagophthalmos, ectropion and entropion. Tear breakup time was found to be lower in lepromatous patients and in those having these eyelid deformities. Tear production observed by doing a Schirmer's test appeared not to be affected.[38-40] Elevated lactoferrin levels in tears were associated with type 2 reactions.[41] Surgical correction is required for dry eyes associated with eyelid deformities. All forms of dry eyes require tear substitutes in keeping the cornea moist and healthy (see treatment under lagophthalmos).

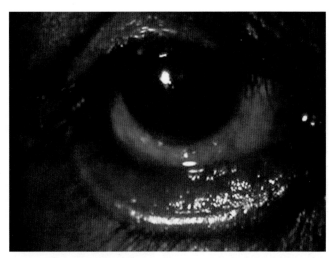

Fig. 27.21: A large ectropion of the lower lid with the palpebral conjunctiva exposed

Corneal Sensation

Loss of sensation is the hallmark of leprosy. Injuries in the hand and legs are predominantly the result of decreased sensation in the extremities. Reduced corneal sensation (corneal hypoesthesia) or rarely complete corneal sensory impairment (corneal anesthesia) is likely to be present in long-standing LL. During a routine ocular examination, these patients sometimes present with small foreign bodies embedded in their corneas with no accompanying painful symptoms, with an increased risk of developing a secondarily infected corneal ulcer.[42,43] Corneal sensory impairment and anterior segment pathology are strongly correlated. Ocular leprosy complications such as lagophthalmos, chronic uveitis, iris atrophy, and blindness are five-fold more frequent in eyes that have impaired corneal sensation.[44,45]

The traditional method of estimating corneal sensation is to use a sterile cotton wisp. The wisp is brought from the side of the face to touch the cornea gently in the 6 o'clock position, 2 mm inner to the limbus and the reaction of the patient is noted. If there is a blink or a reaction to the touch then corneal sensation is recorded as being intact. The longitudinal study of ocular leprosy showed that the cotton wisp method for testing corneal sensation was extremely subjective and inconsistent in reproducibility. Using cotton wisp for testing corneal sensation in the field should be discouraged because of the danger of producing iatrogenic abrasions on the corneal epithelium during testing. Unfortunately, many manuals on preventing disability in leprosy still persist in describing this method as an important component of ocular examination in leprosy even though WHO had discouraged its use. The method is mentioned here only because of its widespread use and must be avoided unless it is done by an experienced ophthalmologist with recourse to follow-ups and good equipment to conclude that after the testing there has been no epithelial damage.[46,47]

A standardized method of measuring corneal sensation is performed by using the Cochet and Bonnet esthesiometer. Using this methodology it has been shown that loss of corneal sensation can occur while there is no clinically detectable eye pathology in MB patients.[45] Cost of the equipment and its maintenance preclude its use in field situations.

There is a need to evaluate and establish a better tool than the cotton wisp for estimating corneal sensation in the field.[46] A substitute for decreased corneal sensation could be the presence of hypopigmented or hypoesthetic patches over the face. Investigations with adequately powered studies are required to test these correlations, which show promise as an alternative to direct corneal sensory testing with a cotton wisp.[48-50]

Corneal Ulcer (Infectious Keratitis)

Leprosy patient's corneas are extremely vulnerable to injury and secondary infection but there is very little data from published studies to understand the prevalence, incidence, risk factors, etiopathogenesis, and treatment of corneal ulcers. In the longitudinal study of ocular leprosy, none of the patients presented with corneal ulcers and none developed corneal ulcers while under MDT, but three patients developed an ulcer after completion of MDT during the follow-up period, reporting with eye symptoms and so made unscheduled visits.[3] Data from a tertiary care leprosy hospital in India show that corneal ulcers tends to occur more commonly in males presumably related to the outdoor work and inpatients belonging to the lepromatous spectrum of the disease and in those who had Grade 2 hand deformities. Lagophthalmos and reduced corneal sensation increase the risk of developing corneal ulcers. Nearly half of the eyes having surgically treated lagophthalmos developed corneal ulcers demonstrating that eyelid surgery does not provide complete protection against development of corneal ulcers. Only one-fifth of patients who presented with a corneal ulcer gained visual acuity after treatment, enhancing the importance of aggressive and early treatment of these ulcers.[42]

In leprosy, corneal ulcers usually occur when abrasions of the cornea become secondarily infected by bacteria or fungus. These ulcers are not caused by *M. leprae*. Patients, especially lepromatous with longstanding disease, may be unaware of injuries to the cornea when there is reduced corneal sensation and are likely to present at a healthcare center for treatment when their corneal ulcers are in an advanced stage. Patients with agricultural jobs can present with a fungal corneal ulcer following a vegetable/stick injury. Patients with ulcers on hands and insensitive corneas can transmit bacteria from the hand ulcer to the cornea after abrading the corneal surface with inadvertent vigorous rubbing (Fig. 27.22). Abrasions of the cornea involving only the epithelium usually heal without

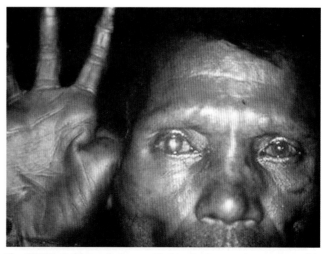

Fig. 27.22: Rubbing the eye with impaired corneal sensation with an ulcerated hand produced a corneal ulcer. The same organism, *Pneumococcus*, present in the hand ulcer was cultured from the corneal ulcer. Healed opacity can be seen in the right eye

an opacity but involvement of the underlying stroma usually leaves behind a corneal opacity.

Corneal ulcers should be considered medical emergencies and appropriate aggressive treatment should commence immediately. Taking a good history is important to document injury and coexisting systemic diseases such as diabetes mellitus that can hamper the healing process. Examination of the eyes must be done carefully to document the extent and depth of the ulcer, presence of inflammatory cells in the anterior chamber and hypopyon, patency of the nasolacrimal duct and the presence of other risk factors such as reduced corneal sensation (Fig. 27.23) and lagophthalmos. If laboratory facilities are available, a specimen must be taken from the base and edge of the ulcer and sent for culture and sensitivity before commencing treatment.

A broad-spectrum antibiotic must be started immediately (never waiting for the culture and sensitivity results), instilling the drops as frequently as every 5 minutes initially and then reducing it to every waking hour as the corneal ulcer heals. The drops are usually continued until the ulcer heals. Antibiotic drops may need to be changed according to the results of the culture and sensitivity or if there is no improvement with the drops or if the ulcer worsens despite treatment or the causative organism is a fungus. The resident bacteria in the ulcer may be gram-positive or gram-negative and common isolates include *Staphylococcus aureus, Eschericha coli, Pseudomonas, Streptococcus viridans, Enterocoli* and *Nocardia*. Fluoroquinolone antibiotics such as gatifloxacin, moxifloxacin, ofloxacin are excellent broad-spectrum antibiotics. Other antibiotic drops include *Tobramycin, Gentamicin* and *Vancomycin*. Depending on the severity of the corneal ulcer a combination of two broad-spectrum antibiotics can be used, instilling them

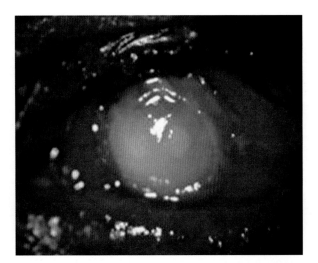

Fig. 27.23: Lepromatous leprosy patient with endophthalmitis. The patient presented late from a corneal ulcer because of impaired corneal sensation and good vision in the other eye

alternatively. Sometimes fortified antibiotic drops as in the case of Vancomycin may be used. Fortification increases the strength of the antibiotic drops by adding an antibiotic injection into the eyedrop bottle. Antibiotic drops should be tapered only after improvement is confirmed by decreasing pain, redness and infiltrates and continued for a few days after healing has taken place as evidenced by cessation of symptoms and complete epithelial resurfacing. Superficial small ulcers usually heal within a week but larger and deeper ulcers may take several weeks to heal.

Supportive therapy such as pain medication (Acetaminophen or Ibuprofen) may be given. If the corneal ulcer is not mild and there is inflammatory reaction evidenced by flare and cells in the anterior chamber, cycloplegics such as homatropine or atropine drops may be given (three drops daily) to dilate the pupil and relieve any ciliary spasm. Deep ulcers or descemetoceles (bulge caused by an ulcer that has eroded the stroma completely to reach the decemets membrane) may require conjunctival grafts or even corneal transplantation. Slow healing or nonhealing ulcers may be the result of local ocular factors such as lagophthalmos for which either a temporary or permanent tarsorrhaphy must be performed. Healing may be delayed due to blockage of the nasolacrimal duct for which a dacryocystorhinostomy or dacryocystectomy must be done. Healing may take longer in leprosy patients with diabetes mellitus, which must be treated adequately.

Topical steroids are contraindicated. They must be stopped if they were being used to treat uveitis in a patient who develops a corneal ulcer. The corneal ulcer must be taken care of and healed before continuing treatment with topical steroids for uveitis. Even though in recent times, there are ongoing large trials investigating if topical steroids hasten recovery and decrease scarring in corneal ulcers, steroid drops should remain a contraindication in treating corneal ulcers in leprosy patients until such time there is compelling proof to advocate its usage.

A corneal ulcer that does not respond to vigorous topical antibiotic therapy may be due to bacterial resistance or have a fungal etiology. Fungal ulcers are not uncommon in leprosy patients.[51-53] If the patient comes with a history of trauma, especially with plant or stick injury then a fungal corneal ulcer must be suspected. Corneal ulcers that received prior treatment with plant-based native medicines (still a common practice in some rural areas) should also be suspected of fungal etiology. Fungal ulcers usually are more severe and deeper with intense inflammatory reaction and may present with a plaque and have satellite lesions. They will not get better on antibiotic therapy. Broad-spectrum antifungal eye drops like Natamycin, Amphotericin B, Clotrimazole, and Econazole can be instilled every waking hour. They can be supplemented by Ketaconazole orally 200–400 mg/day. Adequate liver function tests must be done while on oral ketaconazole. Fungal eye drops are sometimes not available and in such circumstances a tablet of Ketaconazole or Natamycin may be powdered and mixed with methylcellulose and applied as drops. If the ulcer continues to deteriorate in spite of good compliance with antibiotic or antifungal eyedrops, the patient needs to be referred to a cornea specialist who will investigate the etiology further and use remedies that are appropriate.

Corneal Opacity

The cornea is a transparent organ but any injury or ulcer that is deep enough to involve the stroma will leave behind an opacity that is not amenable to medical treatment. Depending on the location and severity of the ulcer, the remnant opacity can be faint (nebulous) or dense (leucomatous). If the corneal ulcer had perforated and the scar or opacity has the iris incarcerated, then it is called an adherent leucoma. The treatment of dense corneal opacities in the visual axis is surgical. In cases where penetrating keratoplasty is not feasible an optical iridectomy sometimes provides improved visual acuity. There are not many reports on the outcome of penetrating keratoplasty in leprosy patients. A case report in the 1960s showed a good outcome to keratoplasty.[54] Local ocular problems, if any, such as dry eye, lid deformities and uveitis need to be taken care of before surgery can be undertaken. The risks of the surgery such as graft rejection and infection must be clearly understood by the patient before giving consent for surgery.

OCULAR INFLAMMATIONS

Episcleritis

Episcleritis is an inflammation affecting the episcleral tissue between the conjunctiva (the clear mucous membrane lining, the inner eyelids and sclera) and the sclera (the white part of the eye). It can be nodular or localized, patchy redness with mild soreness but not associated with mucous discharge or reduction in visual acuity. It usually manifests in LL patients and can occur long after bacteriological cure has been achieved.[55] It can present as part of a type 2 reaction but usually presents independent of any reaction. Episcleritis occurring in a leprosy patient could be due to other systemic diseases such as rheumatoid arthritis and systemic lupus erythematosus.

A study done in Japan, suggests that HLA-Cw3 antigen confers susceptibility to development of episcleritis among Japanese leprosy patients and conversely the DRB1 and/ or DQB1 alleles might provide protection against leprous episcleritis.[56] Episcleritis generally is innocuous and clears without any treatment. Topical steroids or oral anti-inflammatory drugs sometimes are used to relieve pain and in chronic or recurrent cases. Topical steroids such as prednisone 1% eye drops are typically prescribed one to three times/day.

Scleritis

Inflammation of the sclera is more serious than episcleritis. It is also a manifestation of LL. It can present as nodular scleritis, deep red and tender patchy scleritis or as necrotizing scleritis. Repeated episodes of scleritis can lead to thinning of the sclera and anterior staphyloma, not an uncommon feature in old LL patients. Similar to episcleritis, scleritis can occur long after bacteriological cure.[57]

It can also occur in a leprosy patient due to other causes such as rheumatoid arthritis. Unlike episcleritis, scleritis must be treated immediately and rigorously and the inflammation must be taken care of before permanent damage is produced. For the treatment of mild nodular anterior scleritis, topical steroid drops such as prednisone 1% and nonsteroidal anti-inflammatory drugs are sufficient. Oral steroids are given in more severe cases of scleritis. Subconjunctival steroid injections have been used in refractory cases. Although its use in leprosy scleritis is not known, immunosuppressive drugs have been used in scleritis caused by a noninfectious diseases and may be useful in treating refractory recurrent scleritis that occurs in patients after bacteriological cure.

Iridocyclitis (Iritis, Uveitis, Anterior Uveitis)

Iridocyclitis is inflammation of the iris and ciliary body and a few decades ago was considered the most common cause of blindness in leprosy. Leprosy remains one of the important causes of infectious iridocyclitis. Although traditionally thought to occur in LL patients as part of a type 2 reaction, iridocyclitis most often occurs without ENL reactions.[58] In rare instances, it has been seen in patients presenting with a type 1 reaction.[59] During the dapsone monotherapy era from the 1940s to the 1980s almost all studies on ocular leprosy reported iridocyclitis as a significant ocular complication of leprosy patients. It was probably perceived as such due to selection bias as most subjects included in ocular leprosy studies were derived from leprosy rehabilitation villages and from patients treated in hospitals or clinics. Some studies however, continue to report iridocyclitis and its complications as the predominant causes of visual disability among leprosy patients.[60] Although cataract is now considered the most common cause of decreased vision in leprosy, iridocyclitis remains a more dangerous complication of leposy.

Iridocyclitis can appear as an acute inflammation with sterile pus in the anterior chamber called hypopyon. This type of acute manifestation has rarely been reported in recent times.[61,62] Acute iridocyclitis should be treated aggressively by dilating the pupil and by instilling topical steroid drops frequently. Before dilating the pupil with strong mydriatics such as atropine, the angle of the anterior chamber should be examined for potential angle closure and also for signs of any anterior synechia. Anterior synechia is the attachment of the iris to the inner surface of the cornea. Before starting topical steroid drops, usually prednisone acetate 1%, instilled every waking hour at the commencement of therapy, the corneal epithelium's integrity should be checked with a slit lamp. Occasionally, acute iridocyclitis can become recalcitrant and aggressive and will progress despite intensive treatment with topical steroids. In such instances, oral steroids should be given, starting with 60–80 mg Prednisolone daily, tapering only after the inflammation begins to settle down. If oral corticosteroids also do not produce the desired anti-inflammatory effect or if they are harmful to the patient, immunosuppressive drugs may be considered with adequate precautions in bacteriologically cured leprosy patients, after carefully weighing the risk benefits of the drug. Methotrexate, and mycophenolate mofetil have been used in several forms of severe noninfectious iridocyclitis with good results but their efficacy and side effects in patients with intractable iridocyclitis in leprosy have not been evaluated.

An imprecisely defined but nevertheless an important form of iridocyclitis is the subclinical iridocyclitis. There is histopathological evidence that leprosy bacilli can be sequestered within the uveal tissue long after MDT had been successfully completed.[63] The persistence of the organism within the uveal tissue may be a stimulus for continuing subclinical inflammation in bacteriologically cured leprosy patients. The histopathology of enucleated lepromatous eyes have shown that even in florid lepromatous infections the bacteria do not get beyond the anterior segment of the eye and are restricted to an area in front of the equator of the eye.[64] The inflammation is therefore confined to the anterior uveal tissue (iris and ciliary body) and does not usually cause choroidopathy or retinopathy. Rare instances of severe ENL causing perforation of the sclera and bacillary involvement of the choroid has been reported.[65]

Iridocyclitis can become chronic with development of posterior synechia (posterior surface of the iris attached to the anterior surface of the lens). Effort to release such synechia by treating the eye with the application of strong mydriatic drops such as atropine may be undertaken but usually are unsuccessful in old synechia. Chronic iridocyclitis may sometimes exacerbate into acute episodes and must be treated with topical steroid drops. Such acute episodes can be prevented by maintaining the patient on long-term Clofazimine. The two most common ocular complications secondary to iridocyclitis are glaucoma and cataract.

When iridocyclitis occurs in leprosy patients the most probable cause is the host response to *M. leprae*. But it is possible that, especially in MDT treated and bacteriologically cured leprosy patients, other common causes of iridocyclitis may exist and it is important to rule out these diseases. Common infectious diseases that can coexist with leprosy and cause iridocyclitis are HIV, herpes simplex and zoster, syphilis, onchocerciasis, leptospirosis and tuberculosis.[66-69] Other noninfectious causes of iridocyclitis include HLA-B27

associated iridocyclitis. The occurrence of HLA-DR2 has been found to be significantly higher in leprosy patients with iridocyclitis than patients without iridocyclitis.[70] The basic workup for an anterior uveitis in leprosy cured patients must include an HLA-B27, fluorescent treponemal antibody-absorption (FTA-Abs) and a chest X-ray. Iridocyclitis in leprosy has been observed to occur more in patients who have severe hand and foot deformities. This could be a reflection of the increased amounts of reactions that occur in leprosy patients who develop these deformities.

Iris Atrophy

It is a well-known ocular complication in longstanding lepromatous patients. Patients initially develop small patches of atrophy in the iris that are pale depigmented areas on the anterior surface of the iris. They can remain as a small localized area or spread circumferentially. Iris atrophy is associated with chronic low degree or subclinical inflammation of the iris. It can progress with repeated episodes of acute iridocyclitis. The destruction of the intraocular musculature and the preferential atrophic changes in the dilator muscle of the iris have been demonstrated histopathologically and correlate well with the clinical finding of chronic iridocylitis.[71,72] Progressive atrophy can lead to deeper excavations and eventually to polycoria where apertures other than the pupil would distort vision (Fig. 27.24).

The longitudinal study of ocular leprosy showed that one-third of the MB patients who were followed up developed at least one sign of intraocular inflammation that included iris atrophy. This extensive but subtle iris involvement is different from the overt acute iridocyclitis that is observed in some patients. Two histopathological studies support these results; a histopathological study on 33 iris specimens collected during cataract surgery from LL patients from

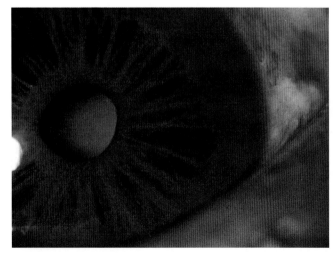

Fig. 27.24: Iris atrophy showing the atrophied musculature of the iris

north India showed features of chronic iridocyclitis. A significant aspect of the study was that 60% of these patients never had any clinically detectable uveal involvement. Those patients who had completed a 2-year fixed MDT had similar amounts of uveal involvement as those who had received Dapsone monotherapy only.[73] A similar study on iris tissue from patients in south India showed chronic inflammatory reactions in the iris of 11 patients, seven of whom did not have any clinically demonstrable evidence of iridocyclitis, proving that histopathology disclosed far more silent chronic iridocyclitis in leprosy patients than that are diagnosed clinically.[63]

Iris atrophy occurring after completion of MDT and the mycobacterial load at the time of leprosy diagnosis show a direct relationship. Higher load of *M. leprae* appears to be an important risk factor in the development of late iris atrophy (Fig. 27.25).[74] Tuberculoid granulomas have been observed in the iris tissue of polar lepromatous patients proving that upgrading reactions can occur in lepromatous patients within the iris tissue.[75,76] These upgrading reactions may account for some cases of iridocyclitis seen in leprosy and the reactions could occur locally without any association with the upgrading reactions seen in the skin or peripheral nerves.

There is uncertainty on how best to treat an inflammation that is largely silent and hidden and whether such inflammation can eventually culminate in more serious ocular problems such as glaucoma and cataract. Because detection and management of minimal iridocyclitis requires a slit lamp, it seems reasonable that MB patients should be examined by an ophthalmologist at least once a year. Ophthalmologists may prefer to use corticosteroid treatment only when there is clinical evidence of active iridocyclitis

(cells in the anterior chamber). Flare (protein in the anterior chamber) alone without cells may need careful supervision and/or treatment with low-dose oral Clofazimine. Evidence of past inflammation such as old keratic precipitates and iris atrophy do not require treatment with steroids.

CATARACT

Cataract is clouding or loss of transparency of the lens and most commonly denoted as opacity in the lens. It is currently the leading cause of blindness in leprosy and can manifest in several ways, the most common being advancing age (age-related cataract), intraocular inflammation (secondary to iridocyclitis) and corticosteroid therapy (steroid induced).

Age-related Cataract

Although this form of cataract is a significant global problem the magnitude and severity of its occurrence is not uniform throughout the world.[77] India has the largest number of treated and untreated leprosy patients and the largest number of cataract patients in the world. As the preventable risk factors attributed to age-related cataract such as exposure to ultraviolet light, smoking, diabetes and protein calorie malnutrition are common among leprosy patients, it is obvious that age-related cataracts will continue to be a significant ocular problem among leprosy patients in the coming decades.[78,79]

Complicated/Secondary Cataract

Iridocyclitis can locally impede the nutrition of the lens with subsequent development of cataract. Overt and severe iridocyclitis has been historically recognized as a potent risk factor for cataract. Recent research has revealed that insignificant amount of inflammation that often go unnoticed is an important risk factor as well in producing cataract in leprosy patients. In MB patients with the high bacterial index subclinical iridocyclitis is not uncommon and has more than a three-fold risk for developing cataract.[80]

Steroid-induced Cataract

Oral and topical corticosteroids are known risk factors for developing cataract. Typically they appear as posterior subcapsular cataracts. Leprosy patients who develop iridocyclitis are treated with steroid drops and those with neuritis are often treated for long periods with oral corticosteroids. Treatment with corticosteroids may add to the development of cataracts among leprosy patients although, not to the extent of age-related or iridocyclitis-induced cataract.

Diagnosis of cataract can be done in the field by using an oblique flash light illumination in a dark room when a

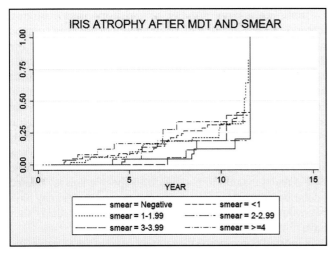

Fig. 27.25: Graph of iris atrophy developing after completion of MDT and the smear bacterial index at enrollment. A proportional direct correlation can be seen between iris atrophy and increasing loads of Mycobacterium

yellowish or white coloration of the lens is noticed. Cataract associated with decrease in vision is more important than cataract without a decrease in vision. In a clinic, the ophthalmologist would diagnose cataract by using slit-lamp examination or retroillumination.

Treatment of Cataract

The only treatment currently available for cataract is surgical removal of the opaque lens and implantation of a synthetic lens. Prevention or more accurately prolonging the cataract-free period in a patient's life can possibly be achieved by good nutrition, less exposure to ultraviolet light, avoiding obesity and cessation of smoking. The mere presence of a cataract does not require surgery. If there is good vision that allows the patient to do all of the things that needs to be done in daily activity then there is most likely no need for surgery. On the other hand, if any amount of decreased vision due to cataract, however small, interferes with the patient's lifestyle, surgery may be beneficial.

Older leprosy affected persons who lived through the pre-MDT era, especially ones with obvious hand and foot deformities face stigma in accessing good ophthalmic care including surgery for the blinding cataract. Cataract surgery in a leprosy patient presents with some unique features that are unlike those found in other patients and these must be taken into consideration by caregivers such as surgeons, nurses as well as policy makers. Stigma and poverty are important social factors and can lead to unnecessary and prolonged blindness and it is not uncommon for leprosy patients to present with mature, over-ripe cataracts called Morgagnian cataracts. These cataracts have fragile capsules surrounding a liquefied and milky lens content and can pose problems during conventional surgery.

Just a few decades ago, when eye camps were in vogue, it was not unusual to stall cataract surgery for leprosy patients until the very end of the eye camp and then to have them operated by fresh postgraduate students. Patients who had desperate need for the best expertise available, ended up having been operated on by the least experienced and the visual outcome results were predictably poor. It must be recognized that stigma of these deformed patients still exists and while they were accepted for surgery at these free eye camps, regular ophthalmology clinics might not be easily accessible for leprosy patients. Education about the disease among ophthalmologists and other personnel associated with the surgery may be necessary.

Deformity, Ocular Comorbidity and Cataract Surgery

It must be recognized that although the overall deformity rate in leprosy may be declining, the number of deformed patients who need surgery will only increase in the coming decade. Apart from stigma, this significant proportion of patients

present with some unique challenges. It is known that patients with severe deformity are likely to have potentially blinding ocular complication that are five to six times more than those who do not have similar deformities. The ocular comorbidities that coexist with the cataract can prevent a successful surgical outcome. During the postoperative healing period, patients with reduced corneal sensation must be taught not to rub the eye. Patients with callosities on hands may have partial corneal hypoesthesia giving rise to irritation and inducing the patient to rub the eyes, which can be disastrous. Deformed patients are often unable to perform tasks such as instilling eyedrops by themselves.[81]

Cataract Surgery

Even after the advent of safe and effective cataract surgery with intraocular lens implantation worldwide was established, there was an extended period of time where resistance to having an intraocular lens implanted in the eye of a leprosy patient was the norm because of the long held belief that introducing a foreign body into the eye would precipitate a catastrophic inflammation ending in not only complete failure of the surgery but with a dismal visual acuity outcome that left a patient with minimal vision before surgery completely blind after surgery. Other than in extremely rare cases where the patient has only one eye with some useful vision and that eye had experienced a long history of ocular inflammation and there is a high possibility of a bad outcome, it is safe to perform cataract surgery with intraocular implantation in all leprosy patients. Caution must however, be observed to undertake surgery when the eye has been made quiescent from any intraocular inflammation and there is coverage with oral steroids during the perisurgical period to prevent any increased inflammatory response to surgery.

There are a large number of variations to the surgical techniques and the kind of intraocular lens that the surgeon might implant and the options are only limited by the decisions that the patient and surgeon collectively make taking into consideration the cost, the expertise and the nature of the cataract. Local ocular manifestations such as impaired corneal sensation, lagophthalmos and iridocyclitis also can modify the timing and type of cataract surgery. Although it is safe to have the operation done in patients who are highly positive for *M. leprae* in skin smears, very little evidence is available on the surgical outcomes of patients with type 1 and type 2 reactions and in patients with specific leprosy related ocular complications. Although, cataract surgeries may have been done on patients with reactions and foot ulcers they have not been reported widely.

Reported outcomes from cataract surgery are variable and depend upon the period in which they had been performed. Studies that were done when phasing out intracapsular surgery for extracapsular surgeries report comparable outcomes for extracapsular cataract surgery with intraocular lens implantation for patients with and without leprosy. The type of patients that undergo cataract surgery also would dictate overall visual outcomes. One study reported a 3% prevalence of blindness in patients who had undergone cataract surgery. Another reported that 35% of patients had vigorous (3+ anterior chamber cellular reaction) inflammatory response in the immediate postoperative period, but noted that the inflammation responded well to treatment with topical corticosteroids.[81-86] In general, despite having leprosy related ocular complications, visual acuity outcomes for cataract surgery in leprosy patients should not be different from those that do not have the disease. This would be true if adequate precautions were taken before, during and after surgery.

INTRAOCULAR PRESSURE

Glaucoma

Elevated intraocular pressure can be a serious ocular complication in leprosy. In the pre-MDT era most ocular clinical examinations did not include a fundus examination and intraocular pressures were measured with a Shiotz tonometer.[87] Glaucoma is now recognized to be a complex disease with raised or normal intraocular pressure, optic disc and visual field abnormalities. In a field setting all that would be possible by a health worker would be to estimate crudely large increases in intraocular pressure by gentle finger palpation over the upper lid. In an ophthalmologist's clinic intraocular pressure estimation is usually done using the Goldman applanation tonometer and pressures of more than 20 mm Hg are considered as ocular hypertension and require further investigation for glaucoma by visual field and retinal fundus examinations. Treatment is usually instituted to keep the pressure under 21 mm Hg.

Two broad categories of glaucoma are recognized in the general population; primary open angle glaucoma and the primary closed angle glaucoma. Both types can occur in leprosy patients but glaucoma in leprosy is most commonly associated with secondary open angle or closed angle glaucoma.

Secondary open angle glaucoma is usually the result of either uveitis or steroid therapy. In secondary open angle glaucoma, the angle can be mechanically obstructed by uveitic debris, protein, inflammatory cells or the endothelium of the trabecular meshwork which can be swollen and damaged. Treating either the uveitis itself with topical and/or oral corticosteroids or using oral corticosteroids over a long period of time in treating neuritis can produce corticosteroid-induced open angle glaucoma. The glaucoma is dependent on the dose, chemical structure of the corticosteroid compound, frequency and route of delivery, duration of treatment, and the patient's susceptibility to steroid response. Clinically, a corticosteroid response usually develops 2–6 weeks after initiating corticosteroid therapy, but may occur at any time. It is often difficult to distinguish between the raised IOP effects of the corticosteroids and the underlying uveitic inflammation. Secondary open angle glaucoma can produce irreversible damage to the optic nerve causing visual field defects without the patient being aware of the harmful process. Because it can lead to blindness, patients with uveitis and those receiving steroid therapy should have their eyes examined at regular intervals for any rise in intraocular pressure or changes in the optic nerve head.

Secondary open angle glaucoma once diagnosed requires treatment and follow-up by an ophthalmologist in a clinic setting. If uveitis is the primary cause of the glaucoma, both the ocular inflammation and the glaucoma will be treated by various combinations of anti-inflammatory and antiglaucoma drugs. Actively controlling the inflammation should be the first priority and this will often take care of the glaucoma as patients aggressively treated with anti-inflammatory therapy have a better clinical course of uveitic glaucoma. In some patients, surgery for glaucoma may be necessary and may include trabeculectomy and drainage implants.

Secondary angle-closure glaucoma is usually the result of uveal inflammation. Angle closure may occur because of a pupillary block which is produced when there is 360 degrees of posterior synechia (attachment of the posterior iris to the anterior surface of the lens) blocking the flow of aqueous from the posterior chamber into the anterior chamber or because of peripheral anterior synechia (attachment of the anterior iris to the posterior surface of the cornea close to the angle of the anterior chamber; peripheral anterior synechia). Patients usually present with severe pain. The ophthalmologist will treat the angle closure glaucoma with a laser iridotomy that opens up the passage for the aqueous to flow from the posterior chamber to the anterior.

Multibacillary patients with chronic low-grade or subclinical inflammation should be followed up carefully with fundus examination, visual field and intraocular pressure estimation at every visit. Of particular concern is the large number of cured lepromatous patients who have subclinical inflammation and/or iris atrophy and whose clinical course on a long-term basis is unclear.[74] Although the 5-year follow-up of MB patients in the longitudinal study of ocular leprosy both in India and the Philippines did not reveal any patients with severe glaucoma,[88] cross-sectional studies examining MB patients have found the prevalence of glaucoma to vary from around 3.6% (population-based) to 10% (leprosy institution based).[89,90] The population-based study found 1.3% had primary open-angle glaucoma, 1.8% had primary angle-closure glaucoma, and 0.5% had secondary angle closure glaucoma.[89] The institution-based study found that more than half of the glaucoma occurred as a result of uveitis.[90]

Reduced Intraocular Pressure

Low intraocular pressures have been observed among leprosy patients especially in those who have had a long duration of the disease with untreated chronic iridocyclitis.[91,92] Although hypotony (defined as < 5 mm Hg IOP) seems to be rare among leprosy patients, the mean IOP appears to be significantly less among leprosy patients with signs of uveitis.[93] Several earlier reports suggested that postural changes in intraocular pressure and lower intraocular pressures were associated with autonomic nerve dysfunction and instead of being considered only as a feature of the late stage of the disease could actually be an early change in leprosy and thereby would have the potential for being markers of an early infection.[94] However, a later study found that although patients had ocular autonomic dysfunction it was not the primary cause for low intraocular pressure in leprosy.[95] Leprosy patients with no clinical anterior segment pathology had similar intraocular pressures to an age-matched control group of normal individuals suggesting that intraocular pressures may not be the best indicators of early leprosy in the eye.[96]

OCULAR DEFORMITY CLASSIFICATION IN LEPROSY

The objective of having a deformity grading system in leprosy is to facilitate monitoring and evaluation of the progress of deformity in individuals and cohorts of patients with the disease, so that interventions and programs can be planned. Any increase in the severity of an ocular deformity should alert the healthcare worker for referral to a specialist. A good grading system needs to be quantitative, easy to document by any trained personnel examining patients in a field setting or screening camps and must confirm to standards used worldwide.

In 1987, the WHO Expert Committee on Leprosy substantially simplified the eye deformity grading into a three-grade system which in 1988 was endorsed with an amendment that lagophthalmos, iridocyclitis and corneal opacities should be considered as grade 2 deformities.[97] While the limb deformity classification had found wide use, the deformity grading recommended for eyes did not seem to have received such wide acceptance and usage.

The current WHO eye deformity grading assumes that the examiner can distinguish between leprosy related and nonleprosy related eye problems while documenting grade 1 and 2 eye deformities. Even for an experienced ophthalmologist this poses difficulties; ocular problems commonly perceived to be associated with leprosy could result from other causes; lagophthalmos due to Bell's palsy, trichiasis due to trachoma, age-related ectropion are some examples. Ocular complications such as corneal opacities, iridocyclitis and cataract can be due to multiple other causes. The healthcare worker, operating in the field without an in-depth ophthalmic knowledge or adequate equipment cannot be expected to make distinctions that would differentiate leprosy related

causes, especially if these occur after bacteriological cure. In patients having other comorbidities such as diabetes mellitus or hypertension, there could be reduced vision without apparent reason because the health worker is not adequately experienced in diagnosing retinal problems.

A new simpler more user-friendly classification that can be used by a general healthcare worker in the field is proposed. The fundamental unit of measurement in this ocular grading system is the visual acuity of each eye measured using a Snellen's chart. The Snellen's chart should be an essential part of the field workers kit as much as a Semmes Weinstein's filament is for testing sensation in the skin. With adequate training and experience, anyone should be able to record vision using a Snellen's chart and grade the deformity of the eye (Table 27.2). Visual acuity in this grading supplants anesthesia in the grading of deformities of the hands and feet. It also removes the distinction between leprosy related and nonleprosy related pathology that can reduce visual acuity. A study has shown that over two-thirds of ocular complications seen among leprosy patients were not related to the disease.[98]

Integration of leprosy services into the general health care has resulted in healthcare workers coming across a variety of ocular problems, some related to the disease itself, but many having other local or systemic causes. The proposed new grading for eye deformities in leprosy patients aims to take away from the healthcare worker the responsibility for determining the differential diagnosis, and to provide clear guidelines on referral. Movement of a patient from grade 0 to grade 1 suggests that a local or systemic treatment for the eye needs to be considered. Movement from grade 1 to grade 2 indicates a significant complication requiring rapid referral for ophthalmic intervention to a specialized eye center, whereas movement from grade 0 to grade 2 implies that a nonleprosy cause is responsible for the visual deterioration, also necessitating referral to a specialist eye clinic. The new classification proposed for ocular deformity is broad based but still does not adequately cover important vision measurements such as near vision. The near vision of the patient should also be recorded separately whenever possible.

Table 27.2: Proposed eye deformity grading in leprosy	
Grade	**Description of grade**
0	No leprosy related visible eye abnormality present;* visual acuity 6/6[†]
1	Visible leprosy related eye abnormality present or absent; visual acuity ≥6/60
2	Visible leprosy related eye abnormality present or absent; visual acuity <6/60

*Leprosy related visible eye abnormality includes, face patches involving zygomatic area or lids, orbicularis oculi weakness, lagophthalmos, conjunctival or scleral redness particularly if patchy or around the cornea, signs of iridocyclitis and cataract.
[†] Visual acuity as measured by a Snellen's chart in each eye.

CONCLUSION

All healthcare providers in leprosy must understand that systematic ocular examination at regular intervals, especially in patients with known risk factors for developing ocular complications, will help reduce ocular morbidity by enabling early diagnosis and treatment of potentially blinding ocular complications. Preliminary screening can be performed by trained leprosy workers who are not ophthalmologists, but clear guidelines should exist for referral. Ocular leprosy complications continue to occur long after bacteriological cure. The risks of developing serious ocular complications are higher in elderly, heavily infected and deformed patients. An aging leprosy population will develop significant amounts of nonleprosy related ocular pathology that will contribute to the total visual disability among them. It is increasingly difficult to differentiate ocular complications that are directly related to leprosy from those that are not directly related to the disease, but in the integrated primary care setting this differentiation may not be of much importance.

It is regrettable that there are not more evidence-based outcomes that can help in establishing best clinical practice guidelines in ocular leprosy related care. There have been some excellent studies and descriptions on various ocular complications in leprosy but we are often forced to rely on old anecdotal material that predates the MDT era. Literature on ocular leprosy has not kept pace with the wonderful advances that have been taking place in ophthalmology. Many ophthalmologists, optometrists, nurses, physiotherapists, occupational therapists and field workers in leprosy perform wonderful service in several areas of ocular leprosy and undertake training but do not realize that their work would be more meaningful and have a longer lasting effect if they would organize and execute important ocular leprosy research. Examples of some research would include finding consensus for the indications of lagophthalmos surgery, collecting prospective long-term outcomes of various cataract surgeries, finding an effective substitute for cotton wisp corneal sensation testing and discovering best methods of treatment for chronic mild iridocyclitis. It is my hope that these and many other obvious gaps in our knowledge on the myriad clinical issues of ocular leprosy would find answers in the coming years. It will help equip the 21st generation leprosy worker to be competent and confident than their peers in administering the best possible ocular care for leprosy patients.

Finally, it is the right of every leprosy patient to expect the best eye care available and our responsibility to see that they can access such care in the primary, secondary and tertiary hospitals. Impediments to accessing such care which unfortunately still exist in many places on account of stigma should be rigorously eradicated using aggressive advocacy and education. Information on ocular manifestations in the pre-MDT era and incident ocular abnormalities developing in a cohort of MB patients on MDT, may be useful to field workers, clinicians, ophthalmologists, epidemiologists, programmers and other caregivers in the field of leprosy, helping them to provide good eye care for these patients.[99-102]

ACKNOWLEDGMENT

I am grateful to Dr Margaret Brand and Mr Eli Smith for their inputs in the form of photographs and diagram in improving the chapter. I also acknowledge the support of the managers of International Journal of Leprosy and Other Mycobacterial Diseases for the use of some of the material from my old publications.

REFERENCES

1. Courtright P, Daniel E, Sundarrao, et al. Eye disease in multibacillary leprosy patients at the time of their leprosy diagnosis: findings from the Longitudinal Study of Ocular Leprosy (LOSOL) in India, the Philippines and Ethiopia. Lepr Rev. 2002;73:225-38.
2. Daniel E, Ffytche TJ, Sundar Rao PS, et al. Incidence of ocular morbidity among multibacillary leprosy patients during a 2 year course of multidrug therapy. Br J Ophthalmol. 2006;90:568-73.
3. Daniel E, Ffytche TJ, Kempen JH, et al. Incidence of ocular complications in patients with multibacillary leprosy after completion of a 2-year course of multidrug therapy. Br J Ophthalmol. 2006;90:949-54.
4. Parikh R, Thomas S, Muliyil J, et al. Ocular manifestation in treated multibacillary Hansen's disease. Ophthalmology. 2009;116:2051-7.
5. Daniel S, Arunthathi S, Rao PS. Impact of integration on the profile of newly diagnosed leprosy patients attending a referral hospital in South India. Indian J Lepr. 2009;81:69-74.
6. Pandey A, Rathod H. Integration of leprosy into GHS in India: a follow-up study (2006-2007). Lepr Rev. 2010;81:306-17.
7. Daniel S, Arunthathi S, Rao PS. Impact of integration on the profile of newly diagnosed leprosy patients attending a referral hospital in South India. Indian J Lepr. 2009;81:69-74.
8. Pandey A, Uddin MJ, Patel R. Epidemiological shift in leprosy in a rural district of central India following introduction of multidrug therapy (April 1986 to March 1992 and April 1992 to March 2002). Lepr Rev. 2005;76:112-8.
9. Nepal BP, Shrestha UD. Ocular findings in leprosy patients in Nepal in the era of multidrug therapy. Am J Ophthalmol. 2004;137:888-92.
10. Dana MR, Hochman MA, Viana MA, et al. Ocular manifestations of leprosy in a noninstitutionalized community in the United States. Arch Ophthalmol. 1994;112:626-9.
11. Malaty R, Togni B. Corneal changes in nine-banded armadillos with leprosy. Invest Ophthalmol Vis Sci. 1988;29:140-5.
12. Malaty R, Beuerman RW, Pedroza L. Ocular leprosy in nine-banded armadillos following intrastromal inoculation. Int J Lepr Other Mycobact Dis. 1990;58:554-9.
13. Ebenezer GJ, Daniel E. Expression of protein gene product 9.5 in lepromatous eyes showing ciliary body nerve damage and a "dying back" phenomenon in the posterior ciliary nerves. Br J Ophthalmol. 2004;88:178-81.
14. In: Basic and clinical science course (BCSC) Section 2: Fundamentals and Principles of Ophthalmology. San Francisco, CA: American Academy at Ophthalmology, 2010.

15. Peitersen E. The natural history of Bell's palsy. Am J Otol. 1982;4:107-11.

16. Daniel E, Rao PS, Courtright P. Facial sensory loss in multibacillary leprosy patients. Lepr Rev. 2013;84:194-8.

17. Hogeweg M, Kiran KU, Suneetha S. The significance of facial patches and type I reaction for the development of facial nerve damage in leprosy. A retrospective study among 1226 paucibacillary leprosy patients. Lepr Rev. 1991;62:143-9.

18. Daniel E, Chacko S, Arunthathi S. Lid retraction as an indicator of lagophthalmos in leprosy; a preliminary report. Int J Lepr Other Mycobact Dis. 1994;62:436-7.

19. Daniel E, Thompson K, Ebenezer GJ, et al. Pterygium in lepromatous leprosy. Int J Lepr Other Mycobact Dis. 1996;64:428-32.

20. Daniel E, Arunthathi S. Climatic droplet keratopathy in leprosy. Int J Lepr Other Mycobact Dis. 1996;64:66-8.

21. Shorey P, Krishnan MM, Dhawan S, et al. Ocular changes in reactions in leprosy. Lepr Rev. 1989;60:102-8.

22. Citirik M, Batman C, Aslan O, et al. Lepromatous iridocyclitis. Ocul Immunol Inflamm. 2005;13:95-9.

23. Kiran KU, Hogeweg M, Suneetha S. Treatment of recent facial nerve damage with lagophthalmos, using a semistandardized steroid regimen. Lepr Rev. 1991;62:150-4.

24. Turkof E, Richard B, Assadian O, et al. Leprosy affects facial nerves in a scattered distribution from the main trunk to all peripheral branches and neurolysis improves muscle function of the face. Am J Trop Med Hyg. 2003;68:81-8.

25. Ranney DA, Furness MA. Results of temporalis transfer in lagophthalmos due to leprosy. Plastic Reconstructive Surg. 1973;51:301-11.

26. Chang Y, Cantelmi D, Wisco JJ, et al. Evidence for the functional compartmentalization of the temporalis muscle: a 3-dimensional study of innervation. J Oral Maxillofac Surg. 2013;71:1170-7.

27. Das P, Kumar J, Karthikeyan G, et al. Efficacy of temporalis muscle transfer for correction of lagophthalmos in leprosy. Lepr Rev. 2011;82:279-85.

28. Anderson JG. Surgical treatment of lagophthalmos in leprosy by the Gillies temporalis transfer. Br J Plast Surg. 1961;14:339-45.

29. Soares D, Chew M. Temporalis muscle transfer in the correction of lagophthalmos due to leprosy. Lepr Rev. 1997;68:38-42.

30. El Toukhy E. Gold weight implants in the management of lagophthalmos in leprosy patients. Lepr Rev. 2010;81:79-8

31. Kuntheseth S. Reanimation of the lagophthalmos using stainless steel weight implantation; a new approach and prospective evaluation. Int J Lepr Other Mycobact Dis. 1999;67:129-32.

32. Courtright P, Kim SH, Tungpakorn N, et al. Lagophthalmos surgery in leprosy: findings from a population-based survey in Korea. Lepr Rev. 2001;72:285-91.

33. Lewallen S, Tungpakorn NC, Kim SH, et al. Progression of eye disease in "cured" leprosy patients: implications for understanding the pathophysiology of ocular disease and for addressing eyecare needs. Br J Ophthalmol. 2000;84:817-21.

34. Mpyet C, Hogeweg M. Lid surgery in patients affected with leprosy in North-Eastern Nigeria: are their needs being met? Trop Doct. 2006;36:11-3.

35. Thompson K. Lid surgery to reduce discomfort produces an unexpected improvement in visual acuity-a case presentation. Indian J Lepr. 1998;70:123-5.

36. Courtright P, Lewallen S. Current concepts in the surgical management of lagophthalmos in leprosy. Lepr Rev. 1995;66:220-3.

37. Khanduja S, Jhanji V, Sharma N, et al. Trachoma prevalence in women living in rural northern India: rapid assessment findings. Ophthalmic Epidemiol. 2012;19:216-20.

38. Koshy S, Daniel E, Kurian N, et al. Pathogenesis of dry eye in leprosy and tear functions. Int J Lepr Other Mycobact Dis. 2001;69:215-8.

39. Lamba PA, Rohatgi J, Bose S. Evaluation of precorneal tear film in leprosy. Indian J Ophthalmol. 1987;35:125-9.

40. Lamba PA, Rohatgi J, Bose S. Evaluation of precorneal tear film in leprosy. Indian J Ophthalmol. 1987;35:125-9.

41. Daniel E, Duriasamy M, Ebenezer GJ, et al. Elevated free tear lactoferrin levels in leprosy are associated with Type 2 reactions. Indian J Ophthalmol. 2004;52:51-6.

42. John D, Daniel E. Infectious keratitis in leprosy. British J Ophthalmol. 1999;83:173-6.

43. Daniel E, Brand ME. An unusual presentation of recurrent corneal abrasion in a lepromatous patient with impaired corneal sensation. Int J Lepr Other Mycobact Dis. 1995;63:450-2.

44. Karacorlu MA, Cakiner T, Saylan T. Corneal sensitivity and correlations between decreased sensitivity and anterior segment pathology in ocular leprosy. Br J Ophthalmol. 1991;75:117-9.

45. Hieselaar LC, Hogeweg M, de Vries CL. Corneal sensitivity in patients with leprosy and in controls. Br J Ophthalmol. 1995;79:993-5.

46. Daniel E, Thompson K. Corneal sensation in leprosy. Int J Lepr Other Mycobact Dis. 1999;67:298-301.

47. WHO Expert Committee on Leprosy. Seventh Report. Geneva. World Health Organization. 1998, Tech Rep Series 847. pp. 25.

48. Daniel E, Premkumar R, Koshy S, et al. Hypopigmented face patches; their distribution and relevance to ocular complications in leprosy. Int J Lepr Other Mycobact Dis. 1999;67:388-91.

49. Premkumar R, Daniel E, Suneetha S, et al. Quantitative assessment of facial sensation in leprosy. Int J Lepr Other Mycobact Dis. 1998;66:348-55.

50. Daniel E, Rao PS, Courtright P. Facial sensory loss in multibacillary leprosy patients. Lepr Rev. 2013;84:194-8.

51. Daniel E, Mathews MS, Chacko S. Alternaria keratomycosis in a lepromatous leprosy patient. Int J Lepr Other Mycobact Dis. 1997;65:492-4.

52. Anandi V, Suryawanshi NB, Koshi G, et al. Corneal ulcer caused by Bipolaris hawaiiensis. J Med Vet Mycol. 1988;26:301-6.

53. Gopalakrishnan K, Daniel E, Jacob R. Bilateral Bipolaris keratomycosis in a borderline lepromatous patient. Int J Lepr Other Mycobact Dis. 2003;71:14-7.

54. Jones RF. Keratoplasty in the keratitis of leprosy. Br J Ophthalmol. 1963;47:248-9.

55. Díaz-Valle D, Miguélez Sánchez R, Toledano-Fernández N, et al. [Immunomediate scleritis in a patient with lepromatous leprosy]. Arch Soc Esp Oftalmol. 2002;77:155-8. (Spanish).

56. Joko S, Numaga J, Fujino Y, et al. Immunogenetics of episcleritis in leprosy. Jpn J Ophthalmol. 1998;42:431-6.

57. Poon A, MacLean H, McKelvie P. Recurrent scleritis in lepromatous leprosy. Aust N Z J Ophthalmol. 1998;26:51-5.

58. Sharma N, Koranne RV, Mendiratta V, et al. A study of leprosy reactions in a tertiary hospital in Delhi. J Dermatol. 2004;31:898-903.

59. Spindler E, Deplus S, Flageul B. Acute uveitis in reversal reactions. Acta Leprol. 1991;7:331-4.

60. Nepal BP, Shrestha UD. Ocular findings in leprosy patients in Nepal in the era of multidrug therapy. Am J Ophthalmol. 2004;137:888-92.

61. Rathinam S, Prajna L. Hypopyon in leprosy uveitis. J Postgrad Med. 2007;53:46-7.

62. Citirik M, Batman C, Aslan O, et al. Lepromatous iridocyclitis. OculImmunol Inflamm. 2005;13:95-9.

63. Daniel E, Ebenezer GJ, Job CK. Pathology of iris in leprosy. Br J Ophthalmol. 1997;81:490-2.

64. Ebenezer GJ, Daniel E. Pathology of a lepromatous eye. Int J Lepr Other Mycobact Dis. 2000;68:23-6.

65. Rathinam SR, Khazaei HM, Job CK. Histopathological study of ocular erythema nodosum leprosum and post-therapeutic scleral perforation: a case report. Indian J Ophthalmol. 2008;56:417-9.

66. Murray KA. Syphilis in patients with Hansen's disease. Int J Lepr Other Mycobact Dis. 1982;50:152-8.

67. Trindade MA, Manini MI, Masetti JH, et al. Leprosy and HIV co-infection in five patients. Lepr Rev. 2005;76:162-6.

68. Agarwal DK, Mehta AR, Sharma AP, et al. Coinfection with leprosy and tuberculosis in a renal transplant recipient. Nephrol Dial Transplant. 2000;15:1720-1.

69. Rafi A, Feval F. PCR to detect *Mycobacterium tuberculosis* DNA in sputum samples from treated leprosy patients with putative tuberculosis. Southeast Asian J Trop Med Public Health. 1995;26:253-7.

70. Joko S, Numaga J, Maeda H. Immunogenetics of uveitis in leprosy. Jpn J Ophthalmol. 1999;43:97-102.

71. Job CK, Ebenezer GJ, Thompson K, et al. Pathology of eye in leprosy. Indian J Lepr. 1998;70:79-91.

72. Ffytche TJ. Role of iris changes as a cause of blindness in lepromatous leprosy. Br J Ophthalmol. 1981;65:231-9.

73. Thompson K, Job CK. Silent iritis in treated bacillary negative leprosy. Int J Lepr Other Mycobact Dis. 1996;64:306-10.

74. Daniel E, Sundar Rao PS, Ffytche TJ, et al. Iris atrophy in patients with newly diagnosed multibacillary leprosy: at diagnosis, during and after completion of multidrug treatment. Br J Ophthalmol. 2007;91:1019-22.

75. Daniel E, Ebenezer GJ, Ffytche TJ, et al. Epithelioid granuloma in the iris of a lepromatous leprosy patient: an unusual finding. Int J Lepr Other Mycobact Dis. 2000;68:152-4.

76. Brandt F, Shi ZR, Zhou HM, et al. A histological study of the eye lesions in 12 leprosy patients with tuberculoid lesion in 4 eyes. Lepr Rev. 1993;64:44-52.

77. Rao GN, Khanna R, Payal A. The global burden of cataract. Curr Opin Ophthalmol. 2011;22:4-9.

78. Chaterjee A, Milton RC, Thyle S. Cataract prevalence and aetiology in Punjab. Brit J Ophthalmol. 1982;66:35-42.

79. West SK, Valmadrid CT. Epidemiology of risk factors for age related cataract. Survey Ophthalmol. 1995, 39:323-34.

80. Daniel E, Sundar Rao PS. Evolution of vision reducing cataract in skin smear positive lepromatous patients: does it have an inflammatory basis? Br J Ophthalmol. 2007;91:1011-3.

81. Mpyet C, Dineen BP, Solomon AW. Cataract surgical coverage and barriers to uptake of cataract surgery in leprosy villages of north eastern Nigeria. Br J Ophthalmol. 2005;89:936-8.

82. Frucht-Pery J, Feldman ST. Cataract surgery in a leprosy population in Liberia. Int J Lepr Other Mycobact Dis. 1993;61:20-4.

83. Suryawanshi N, Richard J. Cataract surgery on leprosy patients. Int J Lepr Other Mycobact Dis. 1988;56:238-42.

84. Daniel E, Koshy S. Intraocular lens implantation in leprosy. Int J Lepr Other Mycobact Dis. 2002;70:9-15.

85. Daniel E, Ebenezer GJ, Abraham S, et al. Posterior chamber intraocular lens implantation in smear-positive leprosy patients; a preliminary report. Int J Lepr Other Mycobact Dis. 1997;65:502-4.

86. Girma T, Mengistu F, Hogeweg M. The pattern of cataract and the postoperative outcome of cataract extraction in Ethiopian leprosy patients as compared to nonleprosy patients. Lepr Rev. 1996;67:318-24.

87. Malla OK, Brandt F, Anten JG. Ocular findings in leprosy patients in an institution in Nepal (Khokana). Br J Ophthalmol. 1981;65:226-30.

88. Ravanes JM, Cellona RV, Balagon M, et al. Longitudinal ocular survey of 202 Filipino patients with multi-bacillary (MB) leprosy treated with 2 year WHO-multiple drug therapy. Southeast Asian J Trop Med Public Health. 2011;42:323-30.

89. Thomas R, Thomas S, Muliyil J. Prevalence of glaucoma in treated multibacillary Hansen disease. J Glaucoma. 2003;12:16-22.

90. Walton RC, Ball SF, Joffrion VC. Glaucoma in Hansen's disease. Br J Ophthalmol. 1991;75:270-2.

91. Brandt F, Malla OK, Anten JG. Influence of untreated chronic plastic iridocyclitis on intraocular pressure in leprous patients. Br J Ophthalmol. 1981;65:240-2.

92. Karaçorlu MA, Cakiner T, Saylan T. Influence of untreated chronic plastic iridocyclitis on intraocular pressure in leprosy patients. Br J Ophthalmol. 1991;75:120-2.

93. Daniel E, Rao PS, Ffytche TJ, et al. Ocular hypotension and hypotony in multibacillary leprosy patients; at diagnosis, during and after completion of multidrug therapy. Indian J Lepr. 2010;82:181-8.

94. Hussein N, Courtright P, Ostler HB, et al. Low intraocular pressure and postural changes in intraocular pressure in patients with Hansen's disease. Am J Ophthalmol. 1989;108:80-3.

95. Lewallen S, Courtright P, Lee HS. Ocular autonomic dysfunction and intraocular pressure in leprosy. Br J Ophthalmol. 1989;73:946-9.

96. Daniel AE, Arunthathi S, Bhat L, et al. Intraocular pressure in leprosy patients without clinically apparent anterior segment pathology. Indian J Lepr. 1994;66:165-72.

97. World Health Organization. WHO Expert Committee on Leprosy: Seventh Report. WHO Technical Report Series 874, Geneva; 1998.

99. Mpyet C, Solomon AW. Prevalence and causes of blindness and low vision in leprosy villages of north eastern Nigeria. Br J Ophthalmol. 2005;89:417-9.

100. Daniel E. Factors associated with ocular complications in multi-bacillary leprosy patients [PhD dissertation]. Schieffelin Leprosy Research and Training Centre; 2007. The Tamilnadu Dr MGR Medical University Library, Chennai, India.

101. Brand MB. Care of the Eye in Hansen's Disease (Leprosy). TAMILEP 2nd Edt. 1987.

102. Brand MB, Ffytche T. The eye in leprosy. In Leprosy. Hastings R (Ed). Edinburgh: Churchill Livingstone; 1985.

103. Courtright P, Lewallen S. A guide to ocular leprosy for health workers. A training manual for eye care in leprosy. Singapore: World Scientific Publishing Co Pte Ltd; 1993.

SECTION 5

Disease Complications (Nerve Involvement, Neuritis and Reactions)

CHAPTERS

28
CHAPTER

Neuritis: Definition, Clinicopathological Manifestations and Proforma to Record Nerve Impairment in Leprosy

P Narasimha Rao, Sujai K Suneetha, Gigi J Ebenezer

INTRODUCTION

Most important consequences of leprosy are due to the direct result of the involvement of peripheral nerves. But for the involvement of peripheral nerves and consequent deformities, leprosy would have been a simple disease and definitely a disease without stigma. In this chapter we have described the definition of neuritis, neuropathology of leprosy neuritis, clinical manifestations and proformas to record nerve impairment.

DEFINITIONS

Neuritis/Neuropathy

Neuritis is defined as the inflammation of nerves. Although "neuritis" is a pathological term, in parlance of leprosy it also denotes the clinical involvement of peripheral nerves. The terms neuropathy and neuritis are used interchangeably in leprosy literature and denote the same process. Neuritis in leprosy is usually a subacute, demyelinating and nonremitting event involving cutaneous nerves and larger peripheral nerve trunks. Invasion of Schwann cells and axons by *Mycobacterium leprae* leads to demyelination and axonal degeneration.[1,2]

Nerve Damage/Nerve Function Impairment

Nerve function impairment (NFI) and nerve damage are often used interchangeably to denote the sensory, motor and autonomic nerve deficits or combination of these that occur as a consequence of the pathological processes resulting from *M. leprae* infection of the nerve(s).

Silent Neuritis/Quiet Nerve Paralysis

Silent neuritis or quiet nerve paralysis is defined as progressive sensory or motor impairment in the absence of symptoms such as pain, paresthesia or tenderness of the nerve and no obvious signs of reaction.

Neuritis Associated with Reactions

Reactions are acute inflammatory episodes which occur during the course of leprosy and are of two types; type 1 or reversal reaction and type 2 or erythema nodosum leprosum (ENL) reaction. Although neuritis can occur at any time during the course of leprosy; it is more common and severe during these phases of leprosy reactions and more so during type 1 reaction. Overall neuritis, and that occurs as a consequence of type 1 and type 2 reactions, together account for a significant proportion of nerve damage occurring in leprosy.

Neuropathic Pain

Neuropathic pain (NP) or nerve pain is defined as pain "initiated" or "caused" by a primary disease, lesion or dysfunction in the peripheral or central nervous system (CNS).[3] Excessive firing of pain mediating nerve cells that are insufficiently controlled by segmental and nonsegmental inhibitory circuits causes it. It includes a wide spectrum of symptoms, including paresthesia, dysesthesia, hyperesthesia (increased sensitivity to normally painful stimuli) and allodynia (pain in response to a stimulus that is not normally painful) along the nerve and in its area of distribution which can be quite debilitating. The importance of NP in leprosy is being increasingly recognized recently.

PATHOLOGICAL BASIS OF NEURITIS

Localization of *M. leprae*

Leprosy neuropathy is a slowly progressive sensorimotor polyneuropathy. *M. leprae* has the unique ability to invade peripheral nerves and its presence within a nerve fiber is a pathognomonic sign of leprosy. Various theories have been proposed for the entry of *M. leprae* into the peripheral nerves. *M. leprae* prefers to localize in the distal cooler regions of the body and inflammatory collections are predominantly observed in segments of nerve trunk that are in close contact with the skin.[4] Studies have shown that *M. leprae* first binds to the exposed *Remak* Schwann cells in the dermis probably through skin abrasion, directly ascend from cutaneous nerves to the nerve trunks that carry mixed sensory and motor nerve fibers. However, studies in experimentally infected armadillos have suggested that the entry and further multiplication of *M. leprae* could occur through endoneurial blood vessels.[5,6]

After decades of laboratory research, several pathological mechanisms have been proposed for nerve damage in leprosy: interference of *M. leprae* cell wall proteins with host cell (macrophage) metabolism, immune mediated inflammation triggered by T-cell/Schwann cell interactions, and a "bystander" type of nerve injury due to the large influx of cells and edema during the course of immune and inflammatory responses to *M. leprae*.[7,8]

Analysis of Sensory Nerve Fibers

Skin Lesions

Nerves innervating the skin arise within the dorsal root and sympathetic ganglia. These heterogeneous peripherally directed populations of axons run in distal peripheral nerves, branch and form small dermal nerve bundles, course through the dermis and end as free nerve endings in the epidermis. Thus, the skin is densely innervated by sensory and autonomic fibers. Sensory nerves are classified as unmyelinated (C) and myelinated fibers (A) and these afferent fibers transmit the sensations of pain, pressure, temperature, vibration, and itch.[9] Thermal sensitivity is mediated by thin myelinated Aδ fibers. Nociceptive (pain and itch) and non-nociceptive (warmth, pleasant touch) sensations are mediated by unmyelinated C fibers. In the dermis, the unmyelinated fibers lose their Schwann cell sheathing and end as free nerve endings in the epidermis and are "not visible" for nerve conduction tests.[10] *M. leprae* targets sensory (unmyelinated and myelinated), autonomic and motor nerve fibers of the peripheral and cutaneous nerves. Sensory nerve involvement occurs early in the course of the disease, as evidenced by the fact that the earliest reliable clinical sign is loss of sensation in a skin lesion, commonly accompanied by a peripheral nerve enlargement. Skin lesions across the spectrum of leprosy exhibit significant destruction of cutaneous nerves. Although leprosy neuritis has been well-described clinically and histologically, study of various components of the nociceptive fibers as diagnostic biological markers in early leprosy lesions is limited.

Recent studies suggest that sensory nerve conduction particularly sensory nerve action potentials (SNAP) and warm perception testing are sensitive tools for early detection of leprosy.[11,12]

Role of Schwann Cells

Mycobacterium leprae has a special affinity for Schwann cells. Intact acid-fast bacilli are found within swollen Schwann cells of unmyelinated nerve fibers of lepromatous leprosy (LL) patients.[13] A recent advance in the understanding of the pathogenesis of leprosy has been the identification of host Schwann cell proteins that bind to *M. leprae*. These binding proteins mediate the entry of the organism into the nerve as the first step in the pathogenesis of the disease. It has been shown that the organism binds to the G domain of the laminin alpha-2 chain which is expressed on the surface of the Schwann cell-axon unit through a receptor on *M. leprae* which was shown to be a 21 kDa histone-like protein.[14,15] This protein, laminin-binding protein 21, coded by the *ML1683* gene, is a major surface exposed antigen on *M. leprae*, and probably serves as an adhesin for its interaction with peripheral nerves. In addition, a 25 kDa phosphorylated glycoprotein of human peripheral nerve has been identified to bind to *M. leprae*.[2] Similarly, the terminal trisaccharide of phenolic glycolipid 1 (PGL-1) which is a surface exposed *M. leprae*-specific antigen, was shown to bind to laminin-2, indicating that PGL-1 also plays a part in the invasion of *M. leprae* into Schwann cells.[16,17] Furthermore, there is evidence that *M. leprae* induced demyelination is a result of direct bacterial ligation and activation of ErbB2 receptor of neuregulin-1 that regulates normal myelination.[18-20]

Schwann cells are also found to be actively phagocytic and able to engulf *M. leprae*. Intact acid fast bacilli are found within swollen Schwann cells of unmyelinated nerve fibers of LL patients.[13] It is not clear, however, whether Schwann

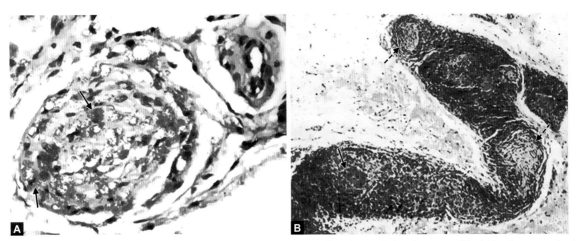

Figs 28.1A and B: (A) Neurovascular bundle in dermis showing clumps of *M. leprae* (arrows), on modified Fite-Faraco stain; (B) Large granulomatous inflammatory cell collection consisting of epithelioid cell clusters (arrow) and dense aggregates of lymphocytes infiltrating small dermal nerve bundles (broken arrows)

cells are involved in presenting *M. leprae* antigens to T-cells *in vivo*, although there are suggestions that they might be able to do so *in vitro*.

In all forms of leprosy neuropathy, bacilli are first seen lying in Schwann cells without producing any cellular response. Subsequently, they alter the interior milieu of the cell producing metabolic and functional changes (Figs 28.1A and B). The events that follow in nerves that progress to develop severe form of disease are; Schwann cell proliferation, segmental demyelination of the nerve and ultimately axonal degeneration. The sequence of pathomechanism of nerve damage in leprosy is as follows:

- *M. leprae* infection of the Schwann cells triggers the immune system resulting in recruitment of lymphocytes and macrophages to the nerve.
- Release of cytokines and other mediators of inflammation and accompanying inflammatory edema produce segmental demyelination of the nerves.
- The inflammatory cells make an attempt to form granuloma. The volume of the granuloma as well as intra- and perineural edema plays a crucial part in causing the pressure on the axons and producing axonal damage.
- The initial axonal damage is predominantly due to the formation of granuloma within the nerve and subsequently due to the release of pharmacological mediators produced by the inflammatory cells. Recruitment of inflammatory cells to this site of *M. leprae* infection, granuloma formation and accompanying edema contribute to the process and severity of nerve damage.

The precise mechanisms of axonal damage at the tuberculoid end may differ from that at the lepromatous end

of leprosy.[21] Furthermore, these changes are accentuated by leprosy reactions when they occur.

MECHANISMS OF NEURITIS ACROSS THE SPECTRUM OF LEPROSY

It should be noted that involvement of nerves by formation of granuloma within them is observed across the leprosy spectrum. At the lepromatous end (LL), the granuloma is of the typical macrophage type, whereas at the tuberculoid end the granuloma is like that of delayed hypersensitivity type with predominance of epithelioid cells. The granulomas consisting of epithelioid cells, Langhans giant cells and lymphocytes infiltrate the nerve followed by destruction of nerve tissue and in some instances there is caseous necrosis.[22] In between, in one-third to one-half of the borderline leprosy cases there may be discordance as to the type of granuloma seen in nerves.[23] In other words, when some patients with a histological diagnosis of borderline tuberculoid (BT) leprosy in the skin were studied, the granuloma in the nerve biopsies showed histopathology of LL with presence of acid-fast bacilli. In general nonetheless, the cellular infiltrate of granuloma within peripheral nerves usually mirrors the type of cellular infiltrate seen in the granulomas of the skin. When the lesion is paucibacillary, there is typical epithelioid cell granuloma in the nerve with presence of high proportion of CD4 lymphocytes. Where the lesions are of multibacillary (MB) type, T lymphocytes are less evident with lowered CD4/CD8 ratio.

The size of granuloma also varies with the type of leprosy. In the nerve, the sizes of cellular infiltrates in tuberculoid and BT leprosy are greater than in LL. The infiltrate and the accompanying edema causes compression of the nerves at "sites of predilection" and in fibro-osseous canals causing severe nerve injury, equivalent to crush injury, resulting in Wallerian degeneration of the nerve. This explains the more severe nerve damage observed in tuberculoid leprosy as compared to LL. Nonetheless, even in LL extensive segmental demyelination, Wallerian degeneration and axonal degeneration can take place insidiously. However, concurrently, there is some regeneration of Schwann cells and small nerve fibers within areas of fibrosis. With passage of time, the severe endoneural fibrosis leads to permanent damage to nerve function. Vascular changes in the nerves are found early in LL patients and these changes include development of fenestrations (gaps) between endothelial cells of capillaries, thickening of basement membrane and rarely can progress to endarteritis with partial or total occlusion of capillaries.[24]

The nerve damage in leprosy is substantiated by evidence of some reduction of myelin sheath and loss of unmyelinated axons in nerves of BT and borderline lepromatous (BL) leprosy patients compared to controls. Also, on the basis of immunohistochemistry studies it was observed that there is almost a total absence of sensory and autonomic neuropeptide immunoreactivity in nerve fibers across the leprosy spectrum. Although nerve damage as a result of neuritis can occur at any time throughout the course of the disease; it is more severe during the phases of leprosy reactions, especially during type 1 reactions.[25]

The effects of neuritis occur very early during leprosy; they continue during the phase of active disease and can cause secondary effects long after the disease has been arrested. Based on the type of pathology, neuritis in leprosy was described by Ridley as intrafascicular, mainly as a result of Schwann cell involvement; extrafascicular mainly due to reactional episodes, and extra neural as a result of compression in the fibro-osseous canals due to swelling and edema of the nerve.[24] Essentially, peripheral nerve trunks carry sensory, motor and autonomic nerve fibers within them and when they are involved, the effects of nerve damage observed clinically are either motor, sensory or autonomic impairments or combination of these, depending on the severity of involvement. NFI is the term used to denote the outcome of such involvement.

MECHANISM OF NEURITIS DURING REACTIONS

During type 1 reaction, the inflammatory response in the nerve is due to the increased immunological activity secondary to the increased delayed type hypersensitivity or cell-mediated immunity (CMI) response to mycobacterial antigens. During type 2 reaction the inflammatory response is secondary to circulating immune complexes.[26]

As already stated, type 1 reactions occur due to an enhanced CMI response to the organism or its antigens. The benefit is

the containment and localization of infection. However, there are also deleterious effects in the form of immune-mediated damage to the tissues and nerves. During a reaction there is exacerbation of the inflammatory granuloma in the nerve with marked increase in inflammatory cells infiltrating the nerve and accompanying edema. Damage to smaller cutaneous nerves is mainly due to compression of the nerve fibers due to edema although more complex damage due to inflammatory mediator release is also implicated in case of larger nerves. The edema which occurs during reactions increases the pressure inside the larger nerves, and the nerve cannot expand much due to the encircling fibrous sheath of perineurium. This leads to the compression of the axons in the endoneural fascicles, leading to demyelination, damage to the axons and consequent loss of nerve conduction. If the edema persists, it causes pressure effects on the vasa nervorum traversing obliquely through the perineurium, compressing the venules which leads to the dilatation of capillaries within the endoneurium causing further edema.[24] In effect, the endoneurial blood flow is compromised leading to relative anoxemia and more damage.

Type 2 or ENL reaction, is an immune complex reaction wherein, antigen-antibody complexes are deposited in various tissues of the body including the nerves. The immune complexes could be formed in the nerve directly with the mycobacterial antigen released locally or may be from the immune complexes in the circulation. The inflammation is initiated by the direct activation of alternate complement pathway by the breakdown products of *M. leprae* and the deposited immune complexes.[27] Such activation leads to migration of polymorphonuclear neutrophils (PMN) to these sites resulting in increase in edema and inflammation, and further nerve damage. In addition, in areas where the nerves are damaged, the metabolites, free radicals and cytokines released due to continued antigen-antibody deposition and activated PMN leukocytes play a significant part in keeping the inflammation smoldering, leading to the chronicity and recurrence of neuritis. However, during type 2 reactions, the nerve damage is usually patchy, limited to sites where PMN leukocytes infiltrate is in significant numbers.

CLINICAL PRESENTATIONS OF NEURITIS

Neuritis or neuropathy in leprosy can broadly be classified into four clinical types based on their period of occurrence and type of presentation. However, it should be noted that they are not mutually exclusive and can overlap one another:
1. Neuritis associated with the disease, which is usually chronic and low-grade
2. Neuritis associated with reactions, which is usually acute and severe
3. Silent neuropathy or quiet nerve paralysis, and
4. Neuropathic pain in leprosy.

NEURITIS ASSOCIATED WITH THE DISEASE

Neuritis in leprosy begins very early in the disease process with subperineurial edema and some loss of unmyelinated axons.[13] Clinically, neuritis associated with the disease is usually chronic and low-grade and is due to the presence of granuloma and the resulting inflammatory response in the nerve. It is clear from available pathological data that extensive neuropathy is already present before the patient notices any signs and symptoms of neural impairment.[28]

The peripheral neuropathy of leprosy has been neurologically classified by many workers as "mononeuritis multiplex" as it is widespread, but not homogeneous or systemic in nature.[29] One part of the nerve may show extensive destruction, while a nearby section of the same nerve may have an almost normal appearance. Similarly, among adjacent fascicles some may be affected, while others appear normal. Since nerves progressively give off branches in their proximal to the distal course, the more proximal the nerve damage, greater is the likelihood of a more extensive nerve deficit and sensory loss.[30] Apart from "mononeuritis multiplex", mononeuritis affecting single nerve trunk without skin lesions is characteristic of "pure neuritic leprosy" which is not an uncommon clinical type of leprosy in India.[31]

In many patients, significant nerve involvement and its effects are observed at the time of first diagnosis of the leprosy itself, so the proportion of disability may be quite high among the new leprosy patients. In a study based at West Bengal, India, it was observed that in adult new leprosy patients, 11.5% had grade 1 and 8.6% had grade 2 deformity at the time of diagnosis, more so in patients with pure neuritic type of leprosy.[32] In a study of 374 leprosy patients who were reporting for the first time to different leprosy referral centers in Northern India, the reason for visiting the hospital was for impairment of sensations in 22% and reaction in 16% of patients. At the time of reporting 9% and 14% patients had WHO grade I and II disability respectively, and 34% were prescribed steroids along with multidrug therapy (MDT) at the first visit.[33] In another study on children with leprosy, it was observed that 16% had already developed WHO grade 2 deformity. Multiple nerve involvement was seen in a quarter of these children.[34]

NEURITIS ASSOCIATED WITH REACTIONS

Neuritis associated with reactions can occur during both type 1 and type 2 reactions. It is usually more frequent and severe in type 1 reactions and NFI more pronounced than in type 2 reactions. Type 1 reactions can have changes both in cutaneous lesions and nerves as its feature or can only be limited to the cutaneous component, or the nerves. In a follow-up study of leprosy patients in Nepal, type 1 reaction was cutaneous in 43% of patients, neural in 24% patients and mixed (both cutaneous and neural) in 33% of patients.[32,35]

In a study based at Bangladesh, it was observed that 7.9% of MB patients developed NFI while on MDT, 4.0% with NFI at diagnosis showed complete recovery at completion of MDT,[36] indicating that NFI can develop even while on treatment and that at the same time it is reversible if attended to early.

Although majority of the patients have single episode of neuritis, recurrent episodes of neuritis are known to occur and can cause severe nerve damage. Nerve damage occurs during reactions at various levels; one, at the level of cutaneous nerve endings, second, at the level of subcutaneous nerves and third at the level of nerve trunks. Damage to cutaneous and subcutaneous nerves lead to an increase in the area of loss of sensations and autonomic nerve function such as sweating. Damage to nerve trunks is seen as enhanced autonomic effects such as increased xerosis and fissuring of an extremity, apart from new motor deficits. Such damage when it occurs in a major nerve trunk carrying all three types of nerve fibers: (1) sensory, (2) motor, and (3) autonomic, such as in posterior tibial, ulnar, median, lateral popliteal and facial nerves, results in considerable NFI.

The type 1 reactions occurring as erythematous skin patches at certain sites such as face need special attention as these are associated with higher frequency of ocular NFI (Fig. 28.2). The significance of facial patches in type 1 reaction for the development of facial nerve damage in leprosy has been demonstrated in a study on a large group of PB patients.[37] Other risk factors for neuritis include large skin patches on the limbs, patches overlying trunk nerves, skin and nerve involvement of more than one body area, previous history of type 1 reaction or neuritis.[38] In general, the NFI effects are more extensive and pronounced during type 1 reaction than in type 2 reaction. Nonetheless, chronic and recurrent type 2 reactions in BL and LL patients can lead to

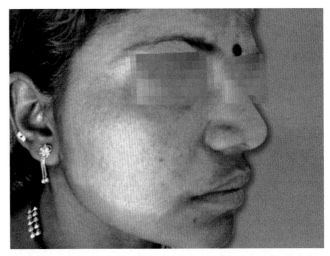

Fig. 28.2: Borderline tuberculoid (BT) patch on face in type 1 reaction. These patients should be followed for possible NFI of facial nerve

considerable NFI in the long run, as more number of nerve trunks are involved bilaterally in these forms of leprosy.

SILENT NEURITIS OR QUIET NERVE PARALYSIS

Silent neuritis/neuropathy is quiet in the sense that the patient does not complain or give history of pain or tenderness of the nerve associated with the recent event of motor and/or sensory deficit. Some workers have also referred it to as "quiet nerve paralysis." It does not refer to the chronic insidious destructive neuropathy of LL, but rather to the episodes of neuropathy that cause clinical nerve damage within a relatively short period of weeks to months.[39] It has also been defined as sensory or motor impairment without skin signs of reversal reaction or ENL, without nerve tenderness or complaints of nerve pain or paresthesia.[40] Although it has been observed across the spectrum of leprosy, it is probably more common in the borderline group.

Silent neuritis has been observed in three clinical settings:
1. First, the patient who comes to the leprosy clinic with only skin lesions without reference to nerve pain or deficit but is found to have sensory and/or motor deficit.
2. Second, the patient who during or after MDT, develops new sensory or motor deficit insidiously without clinical features of type 1 or type 2 reaction.
3. Third, the patient who presents with an obvious motor paralysis and/or sensory deficit (usually presenting as neuropathic ulcers) of recent onset, but without apparent skin lesions of leprosy or history of reactions.[29] The third pattern is consistent with pure neuritic type of leprosy.

The exact process of silent neuritis is not known. Some workers consider it as a mild reversal reaction limited to the affected nerve. Others disagree, as they point out that the patients with silent neuritis can have episodes of obvious reversal reactions, hence argue that it cannot be a manifestation of a mild reaction. It has also been suggested that fibrosis following inflammation of nerve tissue can insidiously produce silent nerve impairment.[41] Such a silent fibrosis of a nerve is possible as it has been shown that in a nerve involved in tuberculoid leprosy, a fairly normal appearing nerve fascicle can be seen alongside the fascicle infiltrated by granuloma.

Neuropathic Pain (NP)

The importance of neuropathic or nerve pain in leprosy was recognized only in the last two decades. NP is defined as "pain initiated or caused by a primary lesion or dysfunction in the peripheral nerves or CNS."[42] Since leprosy is known to cause severe sensory loss leading to hypo/anesthesia, it is generally assumed that pain is uncommon in leprosy. However, peripheral nerve pain or NP can complicate leprosy both during and after treatment. During active disease, patients who usually complain of NP are patients of pure neuritic leprosy and patients at the tuberculoid end of the leprosy spectrum with type 1 reactions, although LL patients with recurrent and severe type 2 reactions can have bouts of intense nerve pain involving multiple nerve trunks associated with other symptoms.

Neuropathic pain which is often debilitating is being increasingly recognized not only in patients with active disease and reactions, but also in patients who have completed their MDT. It could be the chief complaint in some patients who have been "released from treatment" and it could last for months to years. It includes a wide spectrum of symptoms, including paresthesia, dysesthesia, hyperesthesia and allodynia along the nerve and in its area of distribution. The occurrence of paresthesia could be in as high as 24% of the patients as observed in an Indian study.[43] Although NP can be present at rest, it is appreciated more during or after a strenuous and repetitive physical activity of the limb involved, such as along the ulnar nerve in a weaver, or along the sural nerve or lateral popliteal nerve in a tailor. It is usually described as "shooting" "dragging" "pulling" or "electric shock like," and also as "Jhum Jhum" in nature and can force the patient to keep the limb in a position of rest.[44] NP can be moderate or severe and either continuous or intermittent. When it is severe, it could disturb sleep.

In patients who have completed their treatment, NP can occur due to continued damage to the peripheral nerves, probably due to the persistent low-grade inflammation and its sequel. It was observed that a majority of patients of NP have nerve tenderness and their nerve biopsies showed evidence of ongoing inflammation. Excessive firing of pain mediating nerve cells that are insufficiently controlled by segmental and nonsegmental inhibitory circuits causes NP. Some workers have found severely impaired perception of tactile stimuli and mechanical and thermal pain, indicating damage of Aβ, Aδ and C fibers at the painful site. Others have suggested that it could be a small fiber sensory neuropathy which predominantly affects small nerve fibers and its functions with painful paresthesia as the most common effect of its occurrence.[45]

There are no controlled trials to assess the efficacy of simple analgesics in this condition. Tricyclic antidepressants and several antiepileptic drugs have a good efficacy in various neuropathic states.[46] However, no evidence-based study is available to study the efficacy of these described drugs in patients with NP due to leprosy.

CLINICAL MANIFESTATIONS OF NEURITIS

Nerve thickening is the main presenting feature of peripheral nerve involvement in leprosy, which can be clinically appreciated in most leprosy patients. In a study investigating the pathogenesis of neuropathy in North India, 94% of patients had nerve enlargement as the most common sign of leprosy.[43] This is often accompanied by mild to moderate nerve tenderness. Although nerve swelling could rarely occur in other conditions, the nerve enlargement due to leprosy is fusiform and less circumscribed, compared to the swelling observed in chronically traumatized nerve due to other causes.[47] Associated skin lesions corroborate to confirm leprosy as the cause of nerve thickening in most cases (*See* Chapter no. 22 on Differential Diagnosis of Neurological and other disorders in relation to Leprosy).

Major peripheral nerves most frequently affected in leprosy are the posterior tibial nerve, followed by the ulnar, median, lateral popliteal and facial nerves.[48] These nerves are involved at the most superficial locations of their course, at their specific sites of predilection. The sites of predilection of major nerve trunks in leprosy are at their most superficial and cooler sites where they are also prone to trauma: ulnar nerve in the upper arm just above the elbow; median nerve at wrist behind the flexor retinaculum; radial nerve in the upper arm in the radial groove; lateral popliteal nerve behind the knee as it winds round the neck of the fibula and posterior tibial nerve at the ankle below and behind the medial malleolus are such sites. Of these, the ulnar nerve is most accessible and easily palpable for a longer part of its course in the arm. Others nerves are accessible for palpation for a shorter part of their course and hence need more clinical expertise to appreciate the changes in their thickness. Although these are the common sites of early involvement clinically and pathologically, nonetheless, the whole length of the other nerves could be involved in severe forms of the disease as observed in LL (*See* Chapter no. 17 on Methods of Nerve Examination).

Apart from these main peripheral nerves, any cutaneous nerve near or supplying an area of a skin lesion of leprosy (e.g. great auricular nerve, ulnar and radial cutaneous nerves, digital nerves and for that matter any other cutaneous nerve) could be involved and thickened (Fig. 28.3). These cutaneous nerves could be palpated and occasionally seen along their course against a taut muscle.

The main risk factor for nerve involvement is the presence of skin lesions overlying nerve trunks. Such a presence increases the risk of NFI by three to four times compared to those nerves without overlying skin lesions.[43] Type 1 reaction in these skin lesions further increases this risk six to eight times. Hence, patients with skin lesions overlying peripheral nerve trunks should be carefully monitored periodically for the development of NFI, especially during reactions.

Nerve function impairment as a result of damage to nerves includes autonomic, sensory and motor nerve functions, depending on the type and severity of the nerve involved (Box 28.1). In a developing skin lesion of leprosy, loss of sweating precedes the loss of temperature sensation, which is followed by impairment of pain and then touch sensation.

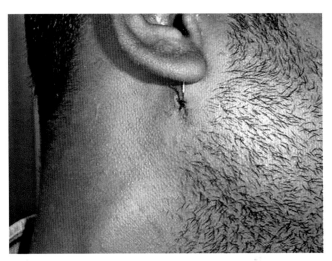

Fig. 28.3: Thickened right great auricular nerve

Box 28.1: Manifestations of neuritis
Nerve thickening
Nerve tenderness
Nerve pain
Sensory NFI
Altered heat and cold sensitivity
Hypoesthesia and anesthesia
Motor NFI: motor weakness
Motor paralysis
Autonomic NFI
Loss of sweating
Xerosis of skin and fissuring
Secondary sequelae of NFI
Deformities and ulcers

Abbreviation: NFI, nerve function impairment.

Motor paralysis never occurs independent of sensory impairment in leprosy.[30] Early manifestations of neuritis are xerosis of skin secondary to reduced sweating, mild hypoesthesia and muscle weakness. Late manifestations include severe xerosis, anesthesia of the skin, motor paralysis, wasting of the muscles supplied by the involved nerve and deformities. It is to be noted that the wasting of muscles encountered in leprosy patients with neuropathy is secondary to neurogenic atrophy and not due to direct muscle involvement. In leprosy, deep tendon reflexes are normal as the CNS is not involved as a rule. However, in severe neuritis a small proportion of patients can show abnormal tendon reflexes and joint position sense.[43]

In a study of childhood leprosy in India, it was observed that about 24% of them had associated type 1 reaction at the time of initial examination and neuritis was the presenting symptom in 65% of these reactions, emphasizing the importance of careful neurological examination at the time of diagnosis and appropriate use of steroids in children to prevent deformities.[49] Trials in prevention of disability using corticosteroid therapy indicate that nerve function recovers spontaneously and that prednisolone is safe, but there are limits to its usefulness.[50] The best way to prevent disabilities occurring as a result of nerve damage is early diagnosis and treatment of leprosy and leprosy reactions.

The methodology and proforma for testing of peripheral nerves in a patient is given later in the section. In this context, it is important to be familiar with the sensory and motor supply and distribution of major peripheral nerves to accurately diagnose their involvement by appropriate testing.

METHODOLOGY TO RECORD NERVE INVOLVEMENT (BOX 28.2)

Examination of Peripheral Nerves

Examination of peripheral nerves in leprosy patients is an integral part of a clinical examination. Confirmation of nerve thickening by palpation is important as it is one of the clinical criteria for the diagnosis of leprosy in a patient. Proper technique of clinical examination of peripheral nervous system is mandatory to assess with reasonable accuracy the extent of its involvement based on the symptoms and signs elicited. While palpating a peripheral nerve, thickening should be assessed by palpating the affected nerve and comparing it to the corresponding contralateral nerve. However, when thickening of nerves occur bilaterally, which occurs rather infrequently, it would be difficult to correctly assess the

Box 28.2: Clinical assessment of neuritis
• Palpation of peripheral nerves
• Grading of nerve thickening, tenderness and pain
• Assess NFI
– Tools to assess sensory NFI
- Semmes-Weinstein monofilaments
- Sensory ENMG
– Tools to assess motor NFI
- Modified MRC scales for VMT
- EMG
– Tools to assess autonomic NFI
- Sweat test

Abbreviations: NFI, Nerve function impairment; ENMG, Electroneuromyography; VMT, Voluntary muscle testing.

grade of nerve thickening. The peripheral nerves commonly palpated in a leprosy patient are greater auricular, ulnar, radial, radial cutaneous, lateral popliteal, posterior tibial, sural and superficial peroneal nerve. Median nerve at wrist is behind the flexor retinaculum and hence, is very difficult to palpate normally. Apart from these, any visibly thickened nerve can be palpated and assessed, such as supraclavicular nerves, ulnar cutaneous nerve, cutaneous nerves of fore arm and thigh and digital nerves of fingers. These can be felt, more readily when they are involved, under the surface of skin along their anatomical course against a taut muscle or bone.

Proper examination for nerve thickening by physical palpation cannot be over emphasized. Although nerve conduction studies proved to be sensitive in detecting NFI, the combination of physical palpation for nerve thickening, voluntary muscle testing (VMT) and use of graded nylon for sensory testing was closely comparable to the nerve conduction studies in detecting neuritis.[51] Nerve tenderness is elicited by applying mild to firm pressure on the nerve during palpation.

Good amount of expertise in clinical examination is necessary for making these assessments as these are comparative in nature.

CLINICAL GRADING OF NERVE THICKENING, TENDERNESS AND PAIN

There is no objective clinical grading available to assess thickening and tenderness of the nerves as they are subjective in nature. High resolution ultrasonography has recently been used objectively to measure the thickness of nerves.[52] A clinical grading of thickness and tenderness of nerves based on subjective assessment would help in recording the extent and severity of nerve involvement by the disease process. Such a clinical grading of thickening and tenderness is useful not only in the initial assessment, but also during the follow-up of such patients for clinical improvement. Moreover, a standardized clinical grading of clinical parameters of neuritis could be a means of communication between leprosy workers, form a basis for its recording and provide a parameter for institution of appropriate therapy and evaluation. Although such a clinical grading of nerve thickening was practiced in a few research studies,[49] it is not widely practiced in leprosy clinics. Recently, however, one such grading of nerve thickness, tenderness and pain was detailed in a leprosy website.[53] Given further is the clinical grading of nerve thickening, nerve tenderness and nerve pain as practiced at Blue Peter Research Centre, in Hyderabad, India.[54,55]

Grading of Nerve Thickening

A four-grade scale (0–3) is used to grade nerve thickening (Table 28.1). The nerves are palpated at their most superficial locations and sites based on the methodology and technique

Table 28.1: Grading of nerve thickness

Grade	Degree	Description
0	Not thickened	Nerve not thickened and feels normal*
1	Mild thickening	Thickened compared to contralateral nerve
2	Moderate thickening	Thickening is rope like
3	Severe thickening	Nerve thickened and also nodular or beaded

*Normal nerve feels soft to firm, flattish and slightly compressible.

Table 28.2: Grading of nerve tenderness

Grade	Degree	Description
0	None	Palpation is not painful even when asked about it
1	Mild	Palpation is painful only when asked about it
2	Moderate	Indicates palpation is painful by wincing during palpation or says so
3	Severe	On palpation, tries to withdraw the limb or is clearly distressed by any pressure on the nerve

Table 28.3: Grading of neuropathic pain

Grade	Degree	Description
0	None	Does not complain of nerve pain; says "no nerve pain" even when asked about it
1	Mild	Complains of nerve pain even when not asked about it
2	Moderate	Complains of severe nerve pain and points to the areas of its radiation. The pain does not interfere with sleep. It is aggravated by repeated use of the limb such as manual labor, tailoring, etc.
3	Severe	Says "pain is severe, and that it interferes with sleep;" the patient keeps the limb in a position of rest and avoids/restricts its movement

Table 28.4: Assessment of NFI associated with neuritis

Early manifestations of NFI	Late manifestations of NFI
Sensory: Altered heat and cold sensitivity Hypoesthesia	Sensory: Hypoesthesia and anesthesia leading to neuropathic ulcers
Motor: Mild motor weakness VMT score equal or less than 4	Motor: Severe motor weakness progressing to paralysis. VMT score 0–3
Autonomic: Decreased sweating	Autonomic: Severe dryness with fissuring

described under nerve palpation. Palpate each nerve for at least 5–10 cm of its length to detect pattern of thickening including rope like, beaded or nodular.

Grading of Nerve Tenderness

This is a highly subjective assessment, but an experienced examiner can make reasonable grading. A four-grade scale (0–3) is used to grade tenderness (Table 28.2). Only apply mild to moderate but firm pressure on the nerve while palpating it. While palpating the nerve, look for the patient's response, such as wincing, expression of distress on face or pulling away of limb, to evaluate the grade of tenderness. Repeated palpation of tender nerves should be avoided.

Grading of Neuropathic Pain

Neuropathic pain, also called "nerve pain" is increasingly recognized as a symptom associated with the severe involvement of peripheral nerves in leprosy. It is observed not only in patients with active disease and reactions, but also in patients who have completed MDT. Such pain is complained more often after strenuous physical activity. Patients describe the pain usually as "shooting," "dragging," "pulling," or "electric shock like" in nature. The grading of nerve pain is based on the symptoms of the patients and does not need palpation of the nerve. A four-degree scale (0–3) is used (Table 28.3).

Application of Clinical Grading

When nerve tenderness is more than or equal to grade 2; it requires immediate institution of corticosteroid therapy along with other measures to prevent further NFI. NFI associated with neuritis should be assessed periodically in these patients with the help of specific tests mentioned in the later part of this chapter (Table 28.4).

TOOLS TO ASSESS SENSORY AND MOTOR NFI AND INTEGRITY OF PERIPHERAL NERVES

In leprosy as in other diseases of the peripheral nervous system, identification of neuropathy in a patient is dependent upon the results of the tests employed and the criteria for abnormality used. It is very important that the tests performed should be relevant to the population group being examined. Keeping note of this is very relevant because, the touch sensibility thresholds when tested with Semmes-Weinstein (SW) filaments and recorded in a large group of healthy normal Indians were not only higher than those reported in populations of developed nations, but also showed an increased deterioration with ageing.[43,56] It was also observed that women compared to men had higher sensibility in palms. Many a times in a given patient, the worsening of test score may reflect the onset of neuropathy, but the test score may still be within the range of normal value. These factors should be kept in mind while performing tests for evaluation of neuropathy in a leprosy patient. Some of the tests mentioned below are such that they can be performed very easily in all leprosy and general clinics with minimal facilities and are reproducible.

Sensory Testing by Monofilaments

Semmes-Weinstein monofilaments are used to measure both diminishing and returning cutaneous sensations. These are nylon monofilaments made from polyhexamethylene dodecandiamide, better known as nylon 612, which absorbs very little water (less than 3% in 100% humidity) and can be cleaned by alcohol. They have indefinite shelf life.[57] SW monofilaments provide a repeatable instrument stimulus with a small standard deviation in contrast to other hand-held test instruments, making them an optimum choice for objective sensory testing of NFI in leprosy patients.

Sensory NFI is usually tested using a standard set of SW monofilaments. These nylon monofilaments are precisely calibrated and are of equal length. The monofilaments are calibrated so as to produce a force of 0.05 gm (green), 0.2 gm (blue), 2 gm (purple), 4 gm (red), 10 gm (orange) and 300 gm (light red) of pressure on the surface of the skin on application. A color coded six-monofilament set is used to test normal, diminished light touch, diminished protective sensation, loss of protective sensation for hands, loss of protective sensation for feet and for deep pressure sensation, in that order (Fig. 28.4). Each filament is mounted on holders (such as needle bottoms or small plastic bases) and they should be applied perpendicularly to each specified site with mild pressure until the filament forms a "C" curve (Fig. 28.5). The standard sites tested are; on the hands, three sites each for the ulnar and median nerves, and one for radial nerve; on feet, seven sites on the sole for the posterior tibial nerve, and one site on the dorsum of the foot for deep peroneal nerve (Figs 28.6A and B). Application should be started with the finest (the green) filament and built up to the orange one. The details of the score should be recorded on a hand and foot examination card-form of the patient. Testing should be done once a month for the first 6 months and subsequently once in 3 months.[58]

Criteria for Sensory Impairment

The reference value for normal sensation level/threshold for population of Indian subcontinent for all sites on the hand is 0.2 gm pressure and for the foot is 2 gm pressure, as felt by the graded SW filaments.[59,60] 0.05 gm pressure is the threshold for facial skin sensation. Sensory impairment is diagnosed in

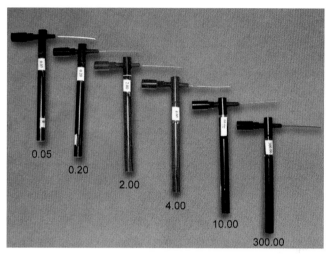

Fig. 28.4: Standard set of SW filaments of various calibers

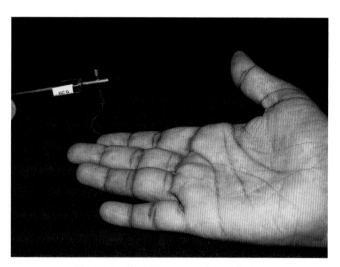

Fig. 28.5: The "C" curve produced during examination with SW filaments

the following situations: when the monofilament threshold sensation is increased by 3 or more levels at any one site or when threshold is increased by 2 levels in one site and 1 level in another site or when it is increased by 1 level in all three sites for a nerve tested.

Indentation of the skin quantifiable by Semmes-Weinstein monofilaments is an accepted method of measuring perception of touch. Silent neuropathy is a well-defined entity that can be accurately detected with the help of SW monofilaments.[58] Periodic examination for nerve function assessment, at least during their first year of treatment, with the help of SW fibers and VMT, which could easily be performed in an outpatient leprosy clinic, would enable us to detect early occurrence of such a silent impairment. Regular assessment of nerve function is essential as early detection

Table 28.5: Sites for testing with SW filaments on hands and feet (Figs 28.6A and B)

Sites for testing on hand	Sites for testing on feet
Sites in the distribution of ulnar nerve	**Sites in distribution of deep peroneal nerve**
Distal phalanx of little finger	Dorsum of the big toe
Head of fifth metacarpal	**Sites in the distribution of posterior tibial nerve**
Hypothenar eminence	Plantar surface of the distal phalanx of the little toe
Sites in the distribution of median nerve	Head of fifth metatarsal
Distal phalanx of index finger	Lateral border of foot
Head of second metacarpal	Plantar surface of the heel
Distal phalanx of thumb	Medial border of foot
Sites in the distribution of radial nerve	Head of first metatarsal
Dorsum of the thumb	Plantar surface of the distal phalanx of the big toe

and treatment with steroids limits impairment and eventual disabilities associated with it.

(Reference values for normal individuals: 0.2 gm for the hand and 2 gm for the foot).

Sites for Testing

The sensory testing with SW filaments is being practiced widely to diagnose various types of peripheral neuropathies, including those secondary to diabetes mellitus and leprosy. The pertinent sites of testing for sensation on hands and feet of importance are given in Table 28.5 and depicted in Figures 28.6 A and B. While testing for sensation with SW filaments, subjects should be placed in a chair in a quiet room, made comfortable and explained about the methodology of testing. During testing, they should keep their eyes closed to avoid a visual influence. The SW filaments are tested on hands at seven sites and on the feet at eight sites starting from right to left, using the staircase method.

A series of monofilaments in decreasing order are applied starting with the highest (usually 300 gm) target force until the approximate threshold is determined. A minimum of five monofilaments should be selected and used sequentially in three cycles of ascending and descending order. The lowest target force consistently detected in three threshold crossings should be considered as the threshold force. Rapid and repeated testing at or nearby sites should not be done to avoid spatial and temporal summation of stimuli. To prevent false positives, subjects are also given mock exercises, without the probe touching the skin.

Testing for Hot and Cold Sensibilities

Hot and cold sensibilities are tested using instruments that can test both sensations one after the other. The WHO has designed one such small pen-shaped battery operated instrument for thermal testing in the field. Some workers prefer test tubes with hot and cold water for testing the same. However, in most clinical settings, testing for hot and cold sensibilities is seldom practiced.

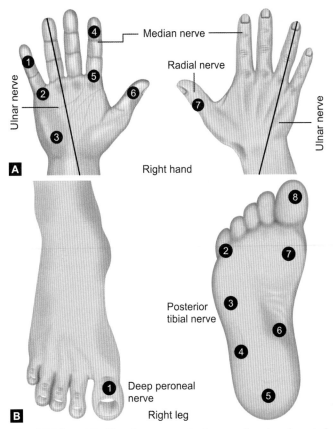

Figs 28.6A and B: Sites for sensory testing on dorsal and ventral aspects of hand and foot representing areas supplied by ulnar, median and radial nerves on hand and posterior tibial and deep peroneal nerves on foot

Laboratory Tools to Test for Sensory Impairment

Nerve Conduction Studies

Formerly electromyography (EMG) and nerve conduction studies required large and sophisticated instrumentation which required high levels of expertise. More recently, however, these are becoming bedside procedures with much smaller "laptop" kind of instruments to assess motor and sensory nerve conduction. However, these instruments are still not in routine use and such tests are performed mostly in neuroscience laboratories.

Abnormalities in nerve conduction studies include the following:
- Segmental slowing of conduction at common sites of entrapment
- Prolonged distal latencies and reduced sensory or motor nerve conduction velocities
- Absent or low-amplitude SNAP, reduced amplitude of compound muscle action potentials, and abnormalities in nerve conduction studies suggesting mononeuropathy, entrapment neuropathy, or generalized polyneuropathy may also be observed.

The ulnar, common peroneal, median and tibial nerves are most commonly involved and studied in leprosy. Changes in nerve conduction are more severe if the nerves are clinically affected than if they are not. In detecting early nerve damage in clinically asymptomatic nerves, prolongation of the refractory period and decreased nerve-conduction velocity are considered more sensitive parameters than conventional motor or sensory conduction.[61,62] In LL, nerve thickening is not correlated with impaired nerve conduction. Palpably enlarged nerves may be functional, though they may eventually fail. Abnormalities in visual and brainstem auditory evoked potentials have been reported in LL, suggesting CNS involvement.[63]

Neurophysiological studies of ulnar nerves in patients with type 1 and type 2 reactions indicate axonal and demyelinating processes across the elbow. In type 2 reactions, changes of demyelination, seen as conduction block, is a primary event, occurring as an acute phenomenon, while in type 1 reactions, temporal dispersion, a subacute phenomenon, is seen.[64]

Electrophysiological Study by Needle Electromyography[65]

Electromyography helps in detection and recording of the electrical activity from a portion of a muscle by recording of motor unit potentials. The muscles usually examined in leprosy include abductor pollicis brevis for testing the function of the median nerve, abductor digiti minimi for testing the ulnar nerve and extensor digitorum brevis for testing the lateral popliteal nerve. For each muscle EMG is to be recorded in three phases: (1) during insertion of needle, (2) at rest, and (3) at full volition.

In the normal EMG, complete electric silence is observed at rest and with minimal voluntary contraction; individual motor unit potentials represent the summation of membrane action potentials of many muscle fibers. With increasing contraction, firing rate increases indicating increased motor fibers recruitment, referred to as a complete interference pattern. In an abnormal EMG indicating neuropathy, findings

include fibrillation, fasciculation, giant motor unit potentials and reduced interference or recruitment pattern. Motor nerve conduction variables and sensory nerve conduction variables can also be measured and recorded by EMG. In cases of myopathy, EMG demonstrates a motor unit potential that is lower in amplitude and shorter in duration than normal, and there is reduced interference pattern.

Imaging of the Nerves

Recent advances in imaging of peripheral nerves by magnetic resonance imaging (MRI) and ultrasonography (USG) have helped to observe and record structural changes in the nerves, objectively. Many studies have reported the efficacy of USG and MRI in identifying of peripheral nerves over last two decades. In leprosy, as important peripheral nerves are involved at their most superficial locations along their course and imaging of these nerves in patients of leprosy provides useful information on their state and extent of involvement.

Although MRI has been shown to depict soft tissues with excellent resolution, it is expensive compared with USG. Moreover, it is difficult to follow the peripheral nerves along its superficial course for identification of pathology with MRI as can be done easily with USG. Because of new technical developments, the resolution of USG has improved considerably and is sometimes even better than standard MRI.[66]

Imaging by USG reveals structure of normal peripheral nerves and gross changes in its structure due to pathology. Peripheral nerves have a typical USG pattern that correlates with histologic structure[67] and can be done with reasonable precision with broadband frequency of 10-14 MHz; CD frequency of 6-13 MHz and linear array transducer. Normal peripheral nerves of extremities have been described as markedly echogenic tubular structures with parallel linear internal echoes on longitudinal sonograms with round to oval cross-section on transverse scans with occasional internal punctuate echoes.[68,69] Healthy nerves show in transverse section a honeycomb like appearance made of hypoechoic fascicles surrounded by hyperechoic epineurium. Nerve thickness may be quantified on longitudinal scan by measuring the anterior-posterior diameter or on transverse scan by measuring the diameters and calculating the cross-sectional area, accurate to the tenth of a millimeter.

Results of high resolution USG imaging on ulnar, radial, median, femoral, common peroneal, posterior tibial, sciatic nerves and on brachial plexus in healthy subjects and various disease states have been reported.[66,70] Sonographic imaging of affected nerves in leprosy patients allows complete analysis of median, ulnar, lateral popliteal and posterior tibial nerves. Studies have shown that the site of maximum involvement was limited to 6-10 cm above the flexor retinaculum for median nerves, 8-12 cm proximal to the cubital groove for ulnar nerves, and 4–10 cm proximal to the medial malleolus for posterior tibial nerve.[71] Not only the above mentioned nerves, but also any peripheral nerve of reasonable thickness can be imaged by USG. Color Doppler (CD) imaging of each nerve can be performed to look for absence or presence of blood flow signals in the perineural plexus and interfascicular vessels of nerve trunks. In health, neither the fascicles nor the epineurium show CD signals indicating normal (hypo) vascularity of nerve trunks. The increased blood flow signals seen in CD in thickened and tender peripheral nerves of leprosy indicate the hyperemic changes secondary to the inflammation leading to alteration of an effective blood-nerve barrier during reversal reactions[55] while being independent of the extent of destruction of nerve fascicles. As neuritis in leprosy reactions varies in intensity, the detection of blood flow signals in those nerves with greater nerve cross-sectional area and tenderness, points to its usefulness as a tool in assessing the severity of the neuritis. Significant correlation was observed between clinical parameters of grade of thickening, sensory loss and muscle weakness and USG abnormalities of nerve echotexture, endoneural flow and cross-sectional area (CSA) of nerves.[54]

On the whole, use of imaging of nerves with the help of high-resolution USG has significant advantage over clinical assessment of peripheral nerve involvement. Imaging assesses enlargement objectively apart from providing information about the integrity of fascicular structure, type of enlargement, edema and state of neural vascularity of nerves in leprosy patients. In addition, imaging can support clinical and electrophysiologic testing for detection of a variety of nerve abnormalities, including entrapment neuropathies, trauma, infectious disorders and tumors.[72]

TOOLS TO ASSESS MOTOR NFI

Voluntary Muscle Testing

Motor NFI is assessed by VMT using the modified Medical Research Council (MRC) scale of 0–5.[73] VMT score is recorded using a modified version of the scale that was first introduced by MRC of UK in 1940s and is known as MRC scale. It has six levels that are easily assessed during clinical examination. The modified MRC grading score used for VMT is given in Table 28.6.

Different muscles are tested for each of the motor nerves commonly affected by leprosy.

The movements tested for the muscles for each of the nerves are:
- *Ulnar nerve*: Abductor digiti minimi—little finger abduction
- *Median nerve*: Abductor pollicis brevis—abduction of thumb
- *Radial nerve*: Extensor muscles of the wrist (wrist extension), Extensor pollicis brevis and longus causing extension of thumb.

Table 28.6: Description of grades of voluntary muscle testing (VMT) for voluntary muscles

VMT score	Description of motor power
Grade 5	Normal power. Full strength in all movements against normal degree of resistance
Grade 4	Full range of movements but less than the normal strength. Movement against gravity present, but not of normal degree
Grade 3	There is full range of movements sufficient to overcome gravity, but not against added resistance
Grade 2	There is some contraction of the muscle, the range of active movement is incomplete, effective neither against gravity nor resistance
Grade 1	Perceptible contraction of muscles(s) not allowing joint movement
Grade 0	No movement or power representing total paralysis

- *Lateral popliteal nerve*: Tibialis anterior, peroneus longus and brevis-dorsiflexion of foot and big toe
- *Facial nerve*: Orbicularis occuli—forced closure of eyes.

Criteria for Motor Impairment

If the VMT score for any muscle or group of muscles is equal or less than 4 on the MRC scale, it is considered as motor impairment.

TOOLS TO ASSESS AUTONOMIC NFI

Damage to autonomic nerve supply of the sweat glands in the dermis leads to reduced or absent sweating. However, in tuberculoid leprosy, sweating could also be reduced due to the direct infiltration and destruction of sweat glands by granulomatous infiltration.

Sweat Test

A simple method is to observe the suspected area of skin lesion for presence of moisture and/or sweating after mild exercise. The typical tuberculoid patch looks very dry and wrinkled due to xerosis secondary to diminished sweating. However, to confirm the absence of sweating, starch iodine test can be performed on the suspected area of skin.

Starch Iodine Test

Absence of sweating can be established by injecting 0.2 mL of 1 in 1,000 solution of pilocarpine nitrate into the lesion to be tested and paint the test site with tincture iodine and then dust with starch powder. Sweating causes bluish discoloration of the starch powder due to its reaction with iodine in the presence of moisture, absence of which indicates anhidrosis.[74]

Bromophenol Blue Test

Presence or absence of sweating can also be established with the help of bromophenol blue test paper. Pilocarpine nitrate 0.2 mL of 1 in 1,000 solution is injected into the lesion to be tested (as described before). Before applying the test paper, the skin is carefully dried with cotton wool. The paper is than placed in position and held firmly in contact with the skin for 30 seconds to 1 minute by the help of a plastic/metal plate. The prepared paper is yellow in color, turning dark blue in the presence of sweat.

The test paper is prepared by soaking filter paper (Whatman No. 2) in a 10% solution of bromophenol blue in anhydrous ether. The paper is stored in sealed metal boxes.

EXAMINATION OF EYES IN LEPROSY

Pathological Basis of Eye Involvement in Leprosy

Many of the clinically observed ocular manifestations in leprosy have been attributed to the presence of the bacilli and its fragments within the eye or of neuritis in the zygomatic branch of the facial nerve or the ophthalmic branch of the trigeminal nerve.[37,75] Quantitative assessment of the visibility of unmyelinated corneal nerves in a large cohort of leprosy patients have revealed a significant reduction in the visibility of these nerves as the spectrum of the disease moved from the tuberculoid to the lepromatous pole.[76,77] Corneal nerves exhibiting morphological changes such as beading and thickening have been observed in LL patients. The changes could probably be due to bacillary and inflammatory cell collections in and around the nerves in the stroma of lepromatous eyes resulting in impaired corneal sensation.[78,79] Some of the ocular manifestations of autonomic dysfunctions described in LL patients are denervation of iris and miotic pupil.[80]

Examination of Eye for NFI

Assessment of NFI is never complete without examination of the eye, as the eye is an important organ affected by neuritis in leprosy. Involvement of the eye could occur either directly as a result of invasion of *M. leprae* into ocular structures as happens in LL or more commonly as an indirect result of neuritis of the zygomatic branch of the facial nerve or the ophthalmic branch of the trigeminal nerve. The strong association between the frequency of eye involvement in leprosy and the presence of type 1 reaction on facial patches has been demonstrated.[37] Existing eye involvement in leprosy could be further exacerbated during both type 1 and type 2 reactions; while reduction in the corneal sensation and its sequelae are observed more often due to type 2 reactions; decrease in the motor function of orbicularis oculi leading to lagophthalmos and its effects are observed more often

in type 1 reaction. While grading VMT for orbicularis oculi muscle (Table 28.7), please note that lid gap when present, is indicative of advanced motor deficit and is not an early sign.

DISABILITY IN LEPROSY AND ITS GRADING

Unattended, neuritis in leprosy can result in a wide range of NFI especially of hands, feet and eyes, ultimately leading to anesthesia, muscle weakness, deformities, neuropathic ulcers and resultant disabilities. The WHO proposed deformity grading of these impairments in 1988.[81] Periodic grading of such deformities in a leprosy patient (Table 28.8) would assist in providing appropriate care and attention required for them.

Each limb and eye should be assessed and classified separately. If any deformity is found in the patient due to causes other than leprosy, that fact should be noted. To record overall deformity grading for the patient, the highest leprosy deformity grade for any part of the body should be taken.

The best ways to prevent disabilities, which are the result of nerve damage, is early diagnosis and prompt treatment of leprosy and leprosy reactions. Simple ways to care for insensitive hands and feet, and the need for eye care and protection should be explained and taught to the patient. Daily self-care by the patient to minimize the effects of NFI is very important in preventing the progression of the existing deformity.

Table 28.7: Description of grading of VMT for orbicularis oculi

VMT score	Description of motor power for eye
Grade 5	Normal forced eye closure
Grade 4	Full closure against reduced resistance
Grade 3	Full closure without resistance
Grade 2	Partial closure (lid gap present)
Grade 1	Muscle flicker with no closure
Grade 0	Complete paralysis

Table 28.8: WHO disability grading with its modifications[82]

Hands and feet	
Grade 0	No anesthesia, no visible deformity or damage
Grade 1	Anesthesia present but no visible deformity or damage
Grade 2	Visible deformity or damage present
Eyes	
Grade 0	No eye problem due to leprosy, no evidence of visual loss
Grade 1	Eye problem due to leprosy present, but vision not severely affected (vision 6/60, can count fingers at 6 meters)
Grade 2	Severe visual impairment (vision worse than 6/60, inability to count fingers at 6 meters. Also include lagophthalmos, iridocyclitis and corneal opacities)

PROFORMA TO RECORD NERVE FUNCTION IMPAIRMENT

Form for Sensory Testing of Hands and Feet

Area of testing	Site	SW filament* Score/grade	
		Right	Left
Hand			
Ulnar nerve	1		
	2		
	3		
Median nerve	4		
	5		
	6		
Radial nerve	7		
Foot			
Deep peroneal nerve	1		
Posterior tibial nerve	2		
	3		
	4		
	5		
	6		
	7		
	8		

*The SW monofilaments are calibrated so as to produce a force of 0.05 gm (green), 0.2 gm (blue), 2 gm (purple), 4 gm (red), 10 gm (orange) and 300 gm (light red) of pressure on the surface of the skin on application. The SW filaments could be numbered/graded from 1 to 6 or as A to F.

Reference values of threshold pressure by the graded SW filaments
The reference value for normal sensation threshold for all sites on the hand is 0.2 gm pressure and for the foot is 2 gm pressure.

Sensory impairment is diagnosed in the following situations:
- The monofilament threshold is increased by three or more levels in any one site or
- By two levels in one site and one level in another site, or
- By one level in all three sites for a nerve tested.

MOTOR FUNCTION ASSESSMENT OF IMPORTANT NERVES BY VOLUNTARY MUSCLE TESTING

Nerve	Muscles to be tested	VMT score	
		Right	Left
Ulnar nerve	Abductor digiti minimi		
Median nerve	Abductor pollicis		
Radial nerve	Wrist extensors and extensors of thumb		
Lateral popliteal nerve	Tibialis anterior/Peroneus longus—dorsiflexion of foot		
	Extensor hallucis longus—dorsiflexion of big toe		
Facial nerve	Orbicularis oculi (VMT)		
	Lid gap on light closure (in mm)		
	Lid gap on strong closure (in mm)		

PROFORMA AS FOR RECORDING NFI IN THE EYE

		Right	Left
Eyelid	Power in orbicularis oculi muscles [try to open on forceful closure (VMT grade)]		
	Blink		
	Lid gap on light closure (in mm)		
	Lid gap on strong closure (in mm)		
	Obvious Lagophthalmos		
Conjunctiva	Redness		
	Conjunctival congestion		
	Ciliary congestion		
	Watering of eyes		
Cornea	Corneal sensation		
	Corneal ulcer		
	Corneal opacity/leucoma		

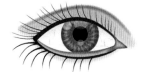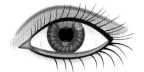

VMT score	# Description of motor power for eye
Grade 5	Normal forced eye closure
Grade 4	Full closure against reduced resistance
Grade 3	Full closure without resistance
Grade 2	Partial closure (lid gap present)
Grade 1	Muscle flicker with no closure
Grade 0	Complete paralysis

PROFORMA TO RECORD CLINICAL GRADING OF NERVE INVOLVEMENT IN LEPROSY

Nerves		Grade of thickening	Grade of tenderness	Grade of nerve pain
Ulnar nerve	Right			
	Left			
Radial cutaneous nerve	Right			
	Left			
Lateral popliteal nerve	Right			
	Left			
Posterior tibial nerve	Right			
	Left			
Sural nerve	Right			
	Left			
Greater auricular nerve	Right			
	Left			
Median nerve	Right	Not applicable		
	Left	Not applicable		
Other nerve				
Other nerve				

PROFORMA TO RECORD DISABILITY, DEFORMITIES AND ULCERS

	WHO grade of disability (0/1/2)	Type of deformity	Ulcer(s)
Right hand			
Left hand			
Right foot			
Left foot			
Right eye			
Left eye			

Highest disability for any part should be taken as its disability grade. Mention the type of deformity when present. Mention the number, location and type of ulcers when present.

REFERENCES

1. Job CK. Nerve damage in leprosy. Int J Lepr Other Mycobact Dis. 1989;57:532-9.
2. Suneetha LM, Satish PR, Korula RJ, et al. *Mycobacterium leprae* binds to a 25-kDa phosphorylated glycoprotein of human peripheral nerve. Neurochem Res. 1998;23:907-11.
3. Treede RD, Jensen TS, Campbell JN, et al. Neuropathic pain: redefinition and a grading system for clinical and research purposes. Neurology. 2008;70:1630-5.
4. Ebenezer GJ, Arumugam S, Job CK. Dosage and site of entry influence growth and dissemination of *Mycobacterium leprae* in T900r mice. Int J Lepr Other Mycobact Dis. 2002;70:245-9.
5. Dastur DK. Cutaneous nerves in leprosy; the relationship between histopathology and cutaneous sensibility. Brain. 1955;78:615-33.
6. Scollard DM. *M. leprae* infection of vascular and lymphatic endothelial cells of the epineurium and perineurium in experimental lepromatous neuritis. Nihon Hansenbyo Gakkai Zasshi. 1999;68:147-55.

7. Spierings E, De Boer T, Zulianello L, et al. Novel mechanisms in the immunopathogenesis of leprosy nerve damage: the role of Schwann cells, T-cells and *Mycobacterium leprae*. Immunol Cell Biol. 2000;78:349-55.

8. Scollard DM, Adams LB, Gillis TP, et al. The continuing challenges of leprosy. Clin Microbiol Rev. 2006;19:338-81.

9. Peng YB, Ringkamp M, Campbell JN, et al. Electrophysiological assessment of the cutaneous arborization of Adelta-fiber nociceptors. J Neurophysiol. 1999;82:1164-77.

10. Ebenezer GJ, Hauer P, Gibbons C, et al. Assessment of epidermal nerve fibers: a new diagnostic and predictive tool for peripheral neuropathies. J Neuropathol Exp Neurol. 2007;66:1059-73.

11. van Brakel WH, Nicholls PG, Wilder-Smith EP, et al. Early diagnosis of neuropathy in leprosy—comparing diagnostic tests in a large prospective study (the INFIR cohort study). PLoS Negl Trop Dis. 2008;2:e212.

12. Capadia GD, Shetty VP, Khambati FA, et al. Effect of corticosteroid usage combined with multidrug therapy on nerve damage assessed using nerve conduction studies: a prospective cohort study of 365 untreated multibacillary leprosy patients. J Clin Neurophysiol. 2010;27:38-47.

13. Shetty VP, Antia NH, Jacobs JM. The pathology of early leprous neuropathy. J Neurol Sci. 1988;88:115-31.

14. Rambukkana A, Yamada H, Zanazzi G, et al. Role of alpha-dystroglycan as a Schwann cell receptor for *Mycobacterium leprae*. Science. 1998;282:2076-9.

15. Shimoji Y, Ng V, Matsumura K, et al. A 21-kDa surface protein of *Mycobacterium leprae* binds peripheral nerve laminin-2 and mediates Schwann cell invasion. Proc Natl Acad Sci USA. 1999;96:9857-62.

16. Rambukkana A, Zanazzi G, Tapinos N, et al. Contact-dependent demyelination by *Mycobacterium leprae* in the absence of immune cells. Science. 2002;296:927.

17. Harboe M, Aseffa A, Leekassa R. Challenges presented by nerve damage in leprosy. Lepr Rev. 2005;76:5-13.

18. Michailov GV, Sereda MW, Brinkmann BG, et al. Axonal neuregulin-1 regulates myelin sheath thickness. Science. 2004;304:700-3.

19. Tapinos N, Ohnishi M, Rambukkana A. ErbB2 receptor tyrosine kinase signaling mediates early demyelination induced by leprosy bacilli. Nat Med. 2006;12:961-6.

20. Chen S, Velardez MO, Warot X, et al. Neuregulin 1-erbB signaling is necessary for normal myelination and sensory function. J Neurosci. 2006;26:3079-86.

21. Turk JL, Curtis J, De Blaquiers G. Immunopathology of nerve involvement in leprosy. Lepr Rev. 1993;64:1-6.

22. Chandi SM, Chacko CJ, Fritchi FP, et al. Segmental necrotising granulomatous neuritis of leprosy. Int J Lepr. 1980;48:41-7.

23. Ridley DS, Ridley MJ. Classification of nerves is modified by the delayed recognition of *Mycobacterium leprae*. Int J Lepr. 1986;54:596-606.

24. Ridley DS. Pathogenesis of leprosy and related diseases. London: Butterworth & Co. Publishers; 1988.

25. Lienhardt C, Fine PE. Type 1 reaction, neuritis and disability in leprosy. What is the current epidemiological situation? Lepr Rev. 1994;65:9-33.

26. Ramu G, Desikan KV. Reaction in borderline leprosy. Indian J Lepr. 2002;74:115-28.

27. Ramanathan VD, Curtis J, Turk JL. Activation of the alternate pathway of complement by Mycobacteria and cord factor. Infect Immun. 1980;29:30-5.

28. Pearson JM, Ross WF. Nerve involvement in leprosy -pathology, differential diagnosis and principles of management. Lepr Rev. 1975;46:199-212.

29. van Brakel WH. Peripheral neuropathy in leprosy-the continuous challenge [Thesis]. Utrecht: University Utrecht; 1994.

30. Job CK, Chandi SM. Differential diagnosis of leprosy—a guide to histopathologists. Karigiri Leprosy Education Programme. SLRTC, Vellore Chummy Printer; 2001.

31. Suneetha S, Arunthathi S, Kurian N, et al. Histological changes in the nerve, skin and nasal mucosa of patients with primary neuritic leprosy. Acta Leprol. 2000-2001;12:11-8.

32. Sarkar J, Dasgupta A, Dutt D. Disability among new leprosy patients, an issue of concern: an institution based study in an endemic district for leprosy in the state of West Bengal, India. Indian J Dermatol Venereol Leprol. 2012;78:328-34.

33. John AS, Pitchaimani G, Rao PS. Early nerve function impairment in leprosy and its correlates in the post elimination era. Book of abstracts, 18th International leprosy congress; 2013 Sep 16-Sep 19; Brussels. p. 237.

34. Horo I, Rao PS, Nanda NK, et al. Childhood leprosy: profiles from a leprosy referral hospital in West Bengal, India. Indian J Lepr. 2010;82:33-7.

35. Roche PW, Theuvenet WJ, Le master JW, et al. Contribution of type 1 reaction to sensory and motor function loss in borderline leprosy patients and the efficacy of treatment with prednisolone. Int J lepr. 1998;66:340-7.

36 Richardus JH, Finlay KM, Croft RO, et al. Nerve function impairment in leprosy at diagnosis and at completion of MDT: a retrospective cohort study of 786 patients in Bangladesh. Lepr Rev. 1996;67:297-305.

37. Hogeweg M, Kiran KU, Suneetha S. The significance of facial patches and type 1 reaction for the development of facial nerve damage in leprosy. A retrospective study among 1226 paucibacillary leprosy patients. Lepr Rev. 1991;62:143-9.

38. Suneetha S. Key issues in the management of reactions and relapse in leprosy. Proceedings of round table conference-Ranbaxy science foundation; 2002; Agra. pp. 103-117.

39. Srinivasan H, Rao KS. Steroid therapy in quiet nerve paralysis in leprosy. Indian J Lepr. 1982;54:412-9.

40. van Brakel WH, Khawas IB. Silent neuropathy: an epidemiological description. Lepr Rev. 1994;65:350-60.

41. Cheroskey CB, Gatti JC, Cardama JE. Neuropathies in Hansen's disease. Int J Lepr. 1983;51:576-86.

42. Hietaharju A, Croft R, Alam R, et al. The existence of chronic neuropathic pain in treated leprosy. Lancet. 2000;356:1080-1.

43. van Brakel WH, Nicholls PG, Das L, et al. The INFIR Cohort Study: investigating prediction, detection and pathogenesis of neuropathy and reactions in leprosy. Methods and baseline results of a cohort of multibacillary patients in North India. Lepr Rev. 2005;76:14-34.

44. Lemaster JW, John O, Roche PW, et al. Jhum-Jhum–a common paraesthesia in leprosy. Lepr Rev. 2001;72:100-01.

45. Haanpaa M, Lockwood DN, Hietaharju A, et al. Neuropathic pain in leprosy. Lepr Rev. 2004;75:7-18.

46. Lund C, Koskinen M, Suneetha S, et al. Histopathological and clinical findings in leprosy patients with chronic neuropathic pain: a study form Hyderabad, India. Lepr Rev. 2007;78:380.

47. Martinoli C, Derchi LE, Bertolotto M, et al. US and MR imaging of peripheral nerves in leprosy. Skeletol Radiol. 2000;29:142-50.

48. Croft RP, Richardus JH, Nicholls PG, et al. Nerve function impairment in leprosy: design, methodology, and intake status of a prospective cohort study of 2664 new leprosy cases in Bangladesh (The Bangladesh Acute Nerve Damage Study). Lepr Rev. 1999;70:140-59.

49. Jain S, Reddy RG, Osmani SN, et al. Childhood leprosy in an urban clinic, Hyderabad, India: clinical presentation and the role of household contacts. Lepr Rev. 2002;73:248-53.

50. Croft R. Editorial. Lepr Rev. 2003;74:297-9.

51. Samant G, Shetty VP, Uplekar MW, et al. Clinical and electrophysiological evaluation of nerve function impairment following cessation of multidrug therapy in leprosy. Lepr Rev. 1999;70:10-20.

52. Beekman R, Visser LH. High-resolution sonography of the peripheral nervous system—a review of the literature. Euro J Neuro. 2004;11:305-14.

53. Srinivasan H. Nerve thickening standards. AIFO leprosy mailing list archives. [online]. Available from http://www.aifo.it/english/resources/online/lml-archives/2008/210908-3.htm. [Accessed Feb, 2009].

54. Jain S, Visser LH, Praveen TL, et al. High-resolution sonography: A new technique to detect nerve damage in leprosy. 2009. PLoS Negl Trop Dis. 3(8):e498.

55. Rao PN, Jain S. Newer management options in leprosy. Indian J Dermatol. 2013;58:6-11.

56. Jain S, Muzzafarullah S, Peri S, et al. Lower touch sensibility in extremities of healthy Indians: further deterioration with age. J Peripheral Nervous Sys. 2008;13:47-53.

57. Bell Krotoski JA. Pocket filaments and specifications for Semmes-Weinstein monofilaments. J Hand Ther. 1993;3:26-9.

58. Santhanam A. Silent neuropathy: Detection and monitoring using Semmes-Weinstein monofilaments. Indian J Dermatol Venereol Leprol. 2003;69:350-2.

59. Malaviya GN, Hussain S, Girdhar A, et al. Sensory functions in the normal persons and leprosy patients with peripheral trunk damage. Indian J Lepr. 1994;66:157-64.

60. Kets CM, van Leerdam ME, van Brakel WH, et al. Reference values for touch sensibility thresholds in healthy Nepalese volunteers. Lepr Rev. 1996;67:28-38.

61. Chopra JS, Kaur S, Murthy JM, et al. Clinical, electrophysiological and teased fibre study of peripheral nerves in leprosy. Indian J Med Res. 1983;77:713-21.

62. Gourie-Devi M. Molecular mechanisms underlying nerve damage: some aspects of leprous neuropathy. In: Rao BS, Bondy SC. Molecular Mechanisms Underlying Neuronal Response to Damage: National Institute of Mental Health and Neurological Sciences; Bangalore, India. 1990:267-76.

63. Kochar DK, Gupta DV, Sandeep C, et al. Study of brainstem auditory-evoked potentials (BAEPs) and visual-evoked potentials (VEPs) in leprosy. Int J Lepr Other Mycobact Dis. 1997;65:157-65.

64. Garbino JA, Naafs B, Ura S, et al. Neurophysiological patterns of ulnar nerve neuropathy in leprosy reactions. Lepr Rev. 2010;81:206-15.

65. Ramdan W, Mourad B, Fadel W, et al. Clinical, electrophysiological, and immunopathological study of peripheral nerves in Hansen's disease. Lepr Rev. 2001;72:35-49.

66. Beekman R, Visser LH. High-resolution sonography of the peripheral nervous system: A review of the literature. Eur J Neurol. 2004;11:305-14.

67. Silvestri E, Martinoli C, Derchi LE, et al. Echotexture of peripheral nerves: Correlation between USG and histologic findings and criteria to differentiate tendons. Radiology. 1995;197:291-6.

68. Fornage BD. Peripheral nerves of the extremities: Imaging with USG. Radiology. 1988;167:179-82.

69. Graif M, Seton A, Nerubai J, et al. Sciatic nerve: sonographic evaluation and anatomic-pathologic considerations. Radiology. 1991;181:405-8.

70. Visser LH. High resolution sonography of the common peroneal nerve: Detection of intraneural ganglia. Neurology. 2006;67:1473-5.

71. Martinoli C, Derchi LE, Bertolotto M, et al. USG and MR imaging of peripheral nerves in leprosy. Skeletol Radiol. 2000;29:142-50.

72. Martinoli C, Bianchi S, Cohen M, et al. Ultrasound of peripheral nerves. J Radiol. 2004;86:1869-78.

73. Brandsma JW. Basic nerve function assessment in leprosy patients. Lepr Rev. 1981;52:161-70.

74. Jopling WH, McDougall AC. Hand book of leprosy, 5th edition. New Delhi: CBS Publishers and Distributors; 1996.

75. Parikh R, Thomas S, Muliyil J, et al. Ocular manifestation in treated multibacillary Hansen's disease. Ophthalmol. 2009;116:2051-7.e1.

76. Daniel E, Thompson K. Corneal sensation in leprosy. Int J Lepr Other Mycobact Dis. 1999;67:298-301.

77. Daniel E, David A, Rao PS. Quantitative assessment of the visibility of unmyelinated corneal nerves in leprosy. Int J Lepr Other Mycobact Dis. 1994;62:374-9.

78. Ebenezer GJ, Daniel E. Expression of protein gene product 9.5 in lepromatous eyes showing ciliary body nerve damage and a "dying back" phenomenon in the posterior ciliary nerves. Br J Ophthalmol. 2004;88:178-81.

79. Zhao C, Lu S, Tajouri N, et al. In vivo confocal laser scanning microscopy of corneal nerves in leprosy. Arch Ophthalmol. 2008;126:282-4.

80. Daniel E, Sundar Rao PS, Ffytche TJ, et al. Iris atrophy in patients with newly diagnosed multibacillary leprosy: at diagnosis, during and after completion of multidrug treatment. Br J Ophthalmol. 2007;91:1019-22.

81. WHO expert committee on leprosy. Sixth report. Technical report series 768. Geneva: WHO; 1988.

82. Rao PN. Recent advances in the control programme and therapy of leprosy. Indian J Dermatol Venereol Leprol. 2004;70:269-76.

Leprosy Reactions: Pathogenesis and Clinical Features

Hemanta Kumar Kar, Amrita Chauhan

INTRODUCTION

Leprosy reactions are immunologically mediated episodes of acute or subacute inflammation which interrupt, the relatively uneventful usual chronic course of disease affecting the skin, nerves, mucous membrane and/or other sites. Reactions may occur in any type of leprosy except the indeterminate type. Unless promptly and adequately treated, they can result in deformity and disability.

To the patients, the appearance of reactions not only indicates worsening of the disease, but also raises doubts about curability of the disease. Repeated attack of reactions also affects drug compliance.

TYPES OF LEPROSY REACTIONS

Three types of reactions recognized are classified as follows:

Type 1 Reaction

The type 1 reaction (T1R) is a delayed hypersensitivity reaction associated with sudden alteration of cell-mediated immunity associated with a shift in the patient's position in the leprosy spectrum. The T1R is usually observed in borderline spectrum of the diseases except very rare reports in lepromatous leprosy (LL).[1] The skin or nerves or both may be affected. Even when only skin is affected not all lesions may show acute increase in swelling and redness. In some patients, however, there may be sudden appearance of inflamed, new lesions and/or new nerve affection; with or without impairment of nerve function.

Upgrading or Reversal Reaction

If there is increase in the immunity, the shift is from borderline spectrum toward the tuberculoid pole and is called upgrading or reversal reaction (RR). The term, 'reversal reaction' is used because of the natural tendency for subpolar tuberculoid and borderline leprosy to downgrade slowly toward the lepromatous pole, without treatment, which is reversed with treatment.

Downgrading Reaction?

On the other hand, if there is sudden shift toward the lepromatous pole with reduction of immunity, it is called as downgrading reaction. However, there are conflicting opinions regarding the existence of this form of T1R. There were two explanations proposed in the past to explain the concept of downgrading reactions. One is that, during an upgrading reaction, the immunity is directed against antigenic determinants that are essential for the bacterium to survive and during a downgrading reaction, the reaction is directed against the antigenic determinants of secreted antigens, remnants of dead or dying bacteria or against antigenic determinants of the host that are in common with *M. leprae*. The other concept that in both upgrading and downgrading reactions, the same antigenic components may be involved is the one most likely and it is the orchestration of the cytokines resulting from immunological events that are responsible for the final effect, up- or downgrading. Different antigenic determinants induce different cytokine profiles in different individuals depending on their genetic make-up and immunological history, including their contact with environmental microorganisms.

In clinical practice, this distinction is clearly evident. However, the laboratory tests to confirm the upgrading or downgrading of immunity may not be helpful. Moreover, as the management is same, no distinction is recommended to be made and all T1Rs are labeled as RRs. Henceforth, in this text, the term RRs will be used for all types of T1Rs.

Type 2 Reaction or Erythema Nodosum Leprosum

This type is an immune complex syndrome which is observed in LL and rarely in borderline lepromatous (BL) leprosy. Occasionally, both T1R and type 2 reactions (T2R) are observed in BL spectrum of the disease, very rarely they may occur simultaneously in the same person.

The Lucio Phenomenon

This is a type of reaction observed in untreated, uniformly diffuse shiny infiltrative, non-nodular form of LL which is chiefly encountered in Mexicans, called as Lucio leprosy. This is associated with necrosis of arterioles whose endothelium is massively invaded by *M. leprae*.[2]

EPIDEMIOLOGY

Published reports indicate that the frequency of RRs at the time of diagnosis varies between 2.6% and 6.4%.[3] However, higher figures were reported from different countries; 28% in a hospital-based study from Nepal,[4] 16.5% from Ethiopia,[5] and 24.1% in one center from India.[6] Probably it reflects a variable proportion of paucibacillary (PB)/multibacillary (MB) cases and the mixed case definitions used.[6] Figures for the percentage of patients manifesting RRs at any time vary from 3.5% among PB cases in Malawi[7] to 47.5% among MB cases in Zaire.[3]

An attempt was made by the Indian Association of Leprologists (IAL) in 2003 to find out the incidence of reactions in leprosy collecting, both hospital (9 centers) and field (4 centers) based data of previous 10 years from different zones of India.[8] The cumulative crude incidence rates from hospital and field samples for both types of reactions were found to be 24.4 and 3.7 per 100 patients respectively and the corresponding crude annual incidence rates were 2.4 and 0.37 per 100 patients respectively (Table 29.1).

The Table 29.1 also shows that in both field and hospital situations, T1R rates are significantly higher than T2R. Late T1R and T2Rs after completion of multidrug treatment (MDT) have been observed among 1.5% and 0.6% of patients with fixed duration treatment of 6, 12 months and MDT till inactivity, respectively. Neuritis without skin manifestations of reactions is observed in quite appreciable number. Combining both T1R and T2Rs, 30% of the cases suffered more than one episode of reaction. About 34% had two to three episodes and few (5%) even had four or more episodes or recurrent reactions which points to the need for longer duration of follow-up.[8]

At a fully monitored field control unit [Koraput Leprosy Eradication Project (KORALEP)], the data showed that T1R occurred in 3.9% of borderline cases and T2R in 23.7% of LL and BL cases. Majority of these were of mild or moderate degree and could be treated as outpatients. Of the borderline cases, borderline borderline (BB) type showed maximum rate of reactions. The BL type can present with both T1R and T2R with a total incidence of 12.8%. While borderline tuberculoid (BT) type constituted 74% of the total cases, T1R occurred in only 3.1% of cases. Reactions also occurred in 0.8% of release from treatment (RFT) cases.[9] At Post Graduate Institute of Medical Education and Research (PGIMER), Chandigarh, India, 30.9% of cases presented with reaction at the time of first visit, late RR occurred in 9.5% of all cases and was noted up to 7 years after treatment.[6] Overall 33% of all patients in the above study developed RR at some time during treatment and follow-up, including those with a reaction at presentation.

Reversal reactions usually occur during the first 6 months of therapy in BT and BB patients, but longer intervals have been seen in BL patients. Data on time of onset of the reactions collected by IAL in 2003, both from the field and hospital combined, shows that 42% of all T1R cases present at the time of registration and initiation of therapy, 33% develop within first 6 months after starting MDT, 16% developed in

Sample	Number of cases registered	Type 1 reaction number (%)	Type 2 reaction number (%)	Combined type 1 and 2 reactions number (%)	Only neuritis number (%)	Total number (%)*
Hospital	6,017	1,132 (18.8)	287 (4.8)	12 (0.2)	38 (0.6)	1,469 (24.4)*
Field	26,403	708 (2.7)	196 (0.7)	0 (0.0)	75 (0.3)	979 (3.7)*
Total	32,420	1,840 (5.7)	483 (1.5)	12 (0.03)	113 (0.4)	2,448 (7.6)*

Table 29. 1: Incidence of reactions, according to type of reaction

* Cumulative crude incidence rate calculated for approximately 10 years is 7.6 and the annual incidence rate is 0.76/100 patients (hospital: 2.4/100 patients and field: 0.37/100 patients)

between 7 months and 12 months after starting therapy and 10% after RFT called late RR.[8]

Erythema nodosum leprosum (ENL) reactions were reported to occur in more than 50% of LL cases and in about 25% of BL cases in the pre-MDT era.[10] Since the introduction of WHO-recommended MDT which includes clofazimine, the prevalence of ENL seems to have decreased.[11] Of the two hospital-based studies, the one from Nepal reported high incidence of ENL reactions (28.6%) in LL, but only 7.5% in BL cases,[12] whereas the other study from north India reported 47.4% in LL cases and 10.5% in BL cases.[6] The result of field studies from Bangladesh and Ethiopia reported comparatively lower incidence of ENL, such as 12% in LL and 3.6% in BL from Ethiopia,[13] and 2.1% of all MB patients from Bangladesh.[14]

The higher institutional figures may be related to the referral of cases particularly with severe, chronic or recurrent episodes of reaction from peripheral health care facilities.

TYPE 1 REACTION (REVERSAL REACTION)

Type 1 reactions (Figs 29.1 to 29.5) usually occur in borderline leprosy (BT, BB and BL), and very rarely in LL.[15]

The Risk Factors for Type 1 Reactions

- Borderline group of patients (BT, BB and BL) are the most vulnerable group with the highest risk of developing T1R.[16] BL and BB patients have a higher risk than BT patients.[17] However, reactions occur earlier in BT patients.[5]

- Patients who have one episode of reaction are more likely to develop a second episode of reaction.
- Female gender carries a higher risk than men.[6] This could be due to hormonal fluctuations.[18] Pregnancy and delivery carry an increased risk which is found to be the highest in the first 6 months after delivery (postpartum).
- Older age group is at a higher risk than the younger age group.
- Patients with multiple and disseminated patches involving larger body areas and multiple nerve involvement are at increased risk of developing RR.[4,6,19]
- Patients with large facial patches and lesions near the eyes are at risk of developing lagophthalmos due to a reaction.[20]
- Nerve enlargement, paresthesia and tenderness on palpation are associated with an increased risk of a reaction.[21]

The ILEP Nerve Function Impairment and Reaction (INFIR) was done with an aim to find predictors of neuropathy and reactions. Three hundred and three subjects were enrolled in the study. Altogether, 115 subjects had a reaction or NFI event at registration. The main finding in this cross-sectional analysis is that skin lesions overlying major nerve trunks increase the risk of nerve damage in these nerves significantly, irrespective of whether these lesions show signs of a skin reaction. Absent joint position sense or tendon reflexes appear to indicate more advanced neuropathy. Nerve enlargement and tenderness on palpation were associated with an increased risk of a reaction or a NFI event at diagnosis:[21]

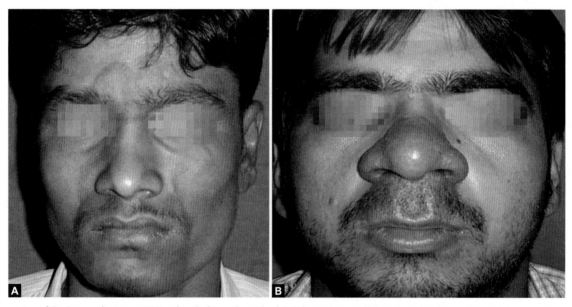

Figs 29.1A and B: Reversal reaction (RR) in borderline tuberculoid (BT) leprosy. Note the existing lesions on face become erythematous, shiny and swollen in both patients. Also note a new lesion on the right cheek of the patient (R)

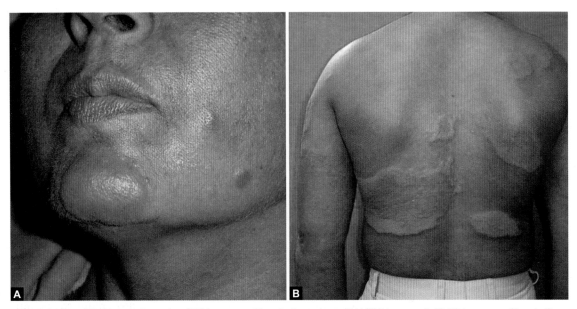

Figs 29.2A and B: Reversal reaction (RR) in a case of borderline tuberculoid (BT) leprosy, (left), RR in a case of borderline borderline (BB) leprosy (right), note the shiny erythematous and edematous plaques

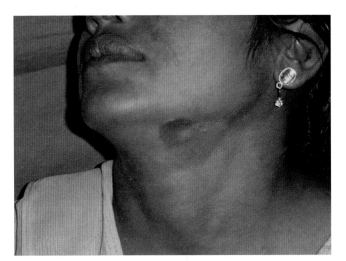

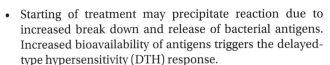

Fig. 29.3: Development of a single erythematous plaque of borderline tuberculoid (BT) leprosy with type 1 reaction in a HIV positive patient, 7 weeks after start of HAART (IRIS). The CD4+ counts rose from 125 cells (pre-HAART level) to 333 cells/mm³ during this period

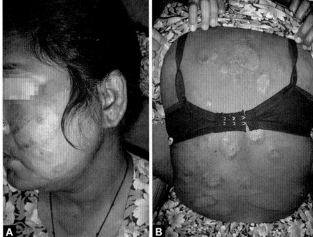

Figs 29.4A and B: Borderline borderline (BB) leprosy with reversal reaction. The plaques are prominent with erythema and edema

- Starting of treatment may precipitate reaction due to increased break down and release of bacterial antigens. Increased bioavailability of antigens triggers the delayed-type hypersensitivity (DTH) response.
- Reaction may be present at the time of presentation or develop during treatment and even after RFT[6]
- Incidence of RRs is observed to be relatively higher when MDT is administered combined with immunotherapy *Mycobacterium indicus pranii (MIP)* as compared to those under MDT alone.[22,23]

- Hepatitis B or C may be risk factors for developing RRs.[24]

Immunopathomechanisms (Box 29.1)

Reversal reactions are caused by increased cellular immune responses (DTH reaction) to *M. leprae* antigens in the skin and nerves that are presented by macrophages in the skin; and Schwann cells in the nerves. This is marked by infiltration of activated CD4 T lymphocytes, especially of Th1 class, with

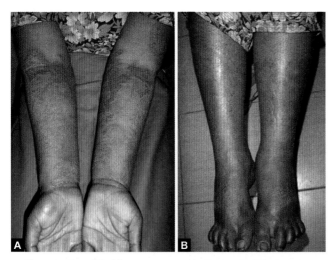

Figs 29.5A and B: The same case as in Figure 29.4. The reaction may be associated with edema of hands and/or feet

---

Box 29.1: Salient features of reversal reactions (RRs):
Immunology and histopathology

- Increased cell-mediated (Type IV) immune response to *Mycobacterium leprae* antigens
- Activation of CD4+ lymphocytes (Th1 type) and increased expression of adhesion molecules on endothelium, increased IL-2 and IFN-γ leading to increased lymphocytic infiltration in skin and nerves (clinically manifesting as inflamed skin lesions, neuritis, nerve damage)
- Histopathological features show lymphocytic infiltration, extracellular edema in and around epithelioid cell granuloma. It also manifests in nerves showing Schwann cell destruction, ischemia of nerve fibers (clinically manifesting as neural pain and loss of function).

Abbreviations: RR, reversal reaction; IL, interleukin; IFN, interferon.

---

increased expression of adhesion molecules on endothelium of blood vessels resulting in local DTH. Associated with it are the raised IL-2 receptor and INF-γ with resultant increased cellularity (lymphocytes) in the skin and nerves. Clinically, it manifests as localized inflammatory lesions of the skin and nerve; producing neuritis and nerve damage. It is not known as to which antigen(s) or antigenic determinant(s) of *M. leprae* are involved in the causation of RR. Again, the role of autoimmunity is not clear, though it has been shown that human nerve and skin have a number of antigenic determinants in common with *M. leprae*. Thus, there could be alternate immune mediated pathways for inflammation, triggered by host-derived antigens or by the process of molecular mimicry.[25,26]

Histopathological Features

The lesions show all characteristics of a DTH reaction. At initial stage only mild extracellular edema with some proliferation of fibroblasts may be seen with increased

number of lymphocytes in the leprosy granuloma. Later, there is further increase in the edema and a change in the cellular composition in and around the epithelioid cell granuloma, due to influx of lymphocytes that are mainly of CD4 subtype, especially of the Th1 class.[27-30]

Inflammatory edema and infiltration within the nerves results in the destruction of Schwann cells by CD4 lymphocytes, as well as ischemia resulting in pain and functional loss.

Immunological Studies

In last few years various studies have demonstrated the increased expression of proinflammatory cytokines, tumor necrosis factor alpha (TNF-α), interleukin 1b (IL-1b), IL-6, interferon gamma (IFN-γ) and IL-12, and immunoregulatory cytokines, transforming growth factor beta (TGF-β) and IL-10 in reactional skin lesions, along with evidence of macrophage activation. Using messenger ribonucleic acid (mRNA)-based polymerase chain reaction and *in situ* hybridization, it was observed that a higher percentage of cells expressed IFN-γ (Th1 type of response) in RRs than in ENL lesions.[31] In addition to the above, higher signals for human serine esterase (a cytotoxic T-cell marker) were noted in the lesions of RR than in those of ENL. In general, in RRs, the cytokine responses are of Th1 type and in ENL the responses are of Th2 type. The increased production of interleukins like IL-2 and TNF-α confirms a shift to the Th1 subtype during a RR.[32-34] Possibly, due to this shift the humoral immunity during RR seems to be diminished.[34] However, there also may occur a shift to Th2 activity in the course of a reaction since there is a mRNA for IL-4 in some of the lesions.[28-30] In a recent study from Brazil for identification of potential markers for reactions, the plasma levels of CXC-Chemokine-10 (CXCL10/IP10) and IL-6 were found to be elevated in T1R, which may serve as potential laboratory marker tools.[35]

The finding of high levels of antibodies against stress proteins in patients with RRs, especially to 18 kDa antigen, along with a heightened lymphoproliferative response to *M. leprae* soluble extract (MLSE), is suggestive of a coexistence of cell-mediated and humoral immunity in leprosy patients during T1R.[36] During the reaction and when it subsides, the relative number of CD8+ (suppressor/cytotoxic) cells increases.[37] The regulatory interleukin, IL-12 was noted in higher percentage of patients of RRs as compared with those having ENL.[38] Further, Th1 type of response may persist in patients for 6–7 months after the onset of reactions.[39] In summary, in RR there is an influx of CD4 T-cells into the granuloma and a mantle of CD8, with increase in Th1 type cytokine pattern with increased expression of IFN-γ, IL-2 and TNF-α.

Changes in plasma cytokine levels are not consistently associated with RRs, however, IFN-γ and TNF-α response of peripheral blood lymphocytes to *M. leprae* antigens are increased in RRs, which fall with therapy, but rise again as corticosteroids are withdrawn. It has been shown that during RR the peripheral blood lymphocytes show an increased immune response to *M. leprae* antigens as demonstrated *in vitro* using lymphocyte migration inhibition tests. These immune responses decrease with subsidence of reaction.

However, it is still not known which antigens or antigenic determinants are responsible for RRs.[34,37] Since *M. leprae* are very difficult to find in PB patients especially in those with RR, the autoimmune phenomena have been incriminated by some to play a role in the reactional process. It has been shown that human nerve and skin have a number of antigenic determinants in common with *M. leprae*.[40-42] Many of these epitopes are heat-shock proteins. In animal models, it has been shown that *M. leprae*-primed macrophages attack the Schwann cells, not only in the presence, but also in the absence of detectable *M. leprae*.[43] It was also observed *in vitro* that T-cells that reacted with *M. leprae* also reacted with components of Schwann cells.

A recent study shows that toll-like receptor 2 polymorphisms are associated with RRs in leprosy and provide new insights into the immunogenetics of the disease.[44] The microsatellite and the 597T polymorphism both, influenced susceptibility of the host to RRs. Although the 597T allele had a protective effect, homozygosity for the 280 bp allelic length of the microsatellite strongly increases the risk of RRs. These associations are consistently observed in the different ethnic groups.[44]

Clinical Features

Clinical Terms

The various clinical terms used to describe the course of the reaction, under different clinical situations are as follows:

- *Acute*: Symptoms persisting up to or less than 1 month
- *Subacute*: Symptoms persisting for more than 1 month up to 6 months
- *Chronic*: Symptoms persisting for more than 6 months
- *Recent*: Covers both acute and subacute types
- *Recurrent/Repeated reactions*: Episodes recurring after 3 months of stopping antireaction treatment
- *Late reversal reaction (LRR)*: (RR occurring any time after completion of MDT)
- Sometimes, RR develops after the full course of antileprosy treatment, any time with in first 2 years after release from treatment. This happens particularly in those individuals who used to develop repeated reactions during the course of treatment or even before starting therapy. It is usually seen over the patches and plaques present over the face and other exposed areas like forearms. It is frequently confused with relapse clinically. The differentiating points are outlined in the Table 29.2.

At times the differentiation between the two conditions is so difficult; one may have to prescribe a course of oral steroids (1 mg/kg/day) for a period of 4–6 weeks. During this period the lesions of LRR would show some subsidence or may clear to a large extent. If the lesions do not show any regression, the patient should be considered as a case of relapse and be treated with a fresh course of MDT for PB or MB leprosy, depending on the number of fresh skin and nerve lesions.

Type 1 reactions as a part of immune reconstitution inflammatory syndrome (IRIS) in human immunodeficiency virus (HIV) positive patients:

In coexisting conditions of leprosy and HIV, a phenomenon akin to T1R is observed after the patient is put on highly active antiretroviral therapy (HAART). The patient may be having active leprosy patches which become inflamed and show

Table 29.2: Criteria helping in distinguishing a relapse from a reversal reaction

Criteria	Reversal reaction	Relapse
Type of leprosy	Observed in BT, BB, BL and subpolar leprosy	Can occur in all types of leprosy after it becomes inactive with treatment
Onset	Sudden	Insidious
Time	Any time during treatment and within 3 years after release from treatment (RFT)	More than 3 years after RFT
Progression of signs and symptoms	Fast	Slow
Site of skin lesions	Over old patches	In new places
Pain, tenderness or swelling	Present over skin lesions and nerves	Not usually present, however, rarely relapse may present with clinical manifestation of RRs
Nerve damage	Sudden onset	Occurs slowly
Constitutional symptoms	May be encountered (mild symptoms like body-aches and fever)	Not present
Response to steroids	Good	Not effective, disease may progress

(Source: Adapted from "Global strategy for further reducing the leprosy burden and sustaining leprosy control activities", 2006–2010, Operational Guidelines, WHO, 2006)

features of T1R. Alternatively, the leprosy patches may appear for the first time after starting HAART, in a situation when the patient may not be having any patch (subclinical infection). Usually this phenomenon occurs anytime within 3 months (usually 3–6 weeks) after start of HAART and is frequently associated with a two- to three-fold rise in the CD4+ counts (as compared to the pre-HAART level) (Fig. 29.3). A detailed account of IRIS in leprosy is given in Chapter 24 'Leprosy and Human Immunodeficiency Virus Coinfection'.

The possible underlying mechanisms for this phenomenon could be that HAART may provide the immunological 'trigger' to the antigens present leading to development of subpolar tuberculoid form of disease. Secondly, there could be a sudden unexplained switching-on of Th1 type responses to *M. leprae*, induced by HAART, even though HIV may not impair immune responses to *M. leprae*. Thirdly, HIV coinfection could result in a degree of suppression of host responses to *M. leprae* infection which is reversed after commencing HAART.[45]

Clinical Manifestations

Symptoms

Patients may complain of burning, stinging sensations in the skin lesions. They may have aches and pains in the extremities and of loss of strength and/or sensory perception. They may suddenly start dropping things from their hands and/or stumble when walking.

Signs

- Increased inflammation of some or all of the pre-existing skin patches or plaques which become erythematous, swollen and may be tender looking like erysipelas. Necrosis and ulceration can occur in severe cases. Lesions desquamate as they subside.
- Crops of fresh inflamed skin lesions in the form of plaques may appear in previously clinically uninvolved skin. The pattern of these skin lesions are of upgrading nature clinically as compared to the existing skin lesions.
- Edema of extremities or face, frequently accompanied by nerve involvement.
- *Neuritis*: Rapid swelling with severe pain\tenderness of one or more peripheral nerves is common. The peripheral nerve affected is usually close to the inflamed skin lesion or situated over the area innervated by the corresponding nerve. In the severe form of T1R nerve abscess may be formed.
- Tinel sign may be positive, i.e. pressure exerted on the nerve gives distally a tingling pain.
- Sometimes loss of nerve function occurs suddenly without other signs of inflammation, making it much less obvious— the so called 'silent neuritis', i.e. without apparent neuritis, producing claw hand, foot drop and facial palsy.

Rare or Uncharacteristic Presentations

- Tenosynovitis due to synovial inflammation manifested with a moderately painful swelling over the dorsum of one or both hands and very rarely over the dorsum of the feet (Fig. 29.5). It is commonly associated in BT and BL leprosy.[46]
- Very severe reaction may be characterized by necrosis and deep ulceration. This is presumably the result of exaggerated hypersensitivity in T1R.
- Systemic manifestations like fever, malaise, vomiting, epistaxis and joint pain are unusual.[46]

Grading of Reversal Reactions

Reversal reactions (RRs) can be graded as mild or severe in form. This is essential for management and for the purpose of referral from primary health care level to middle or tertiary care level, for admission and management by the specialists.

Mild

Few skin lesions with features of reaction clinically; without any nerve pain or loss of function.

Severe

- Nerve pain or paresthesia
- Increasing loss of nerve function
- Fever or discomfort
- Edema of hands, feet
- Mild reaction persisting for more than 6 weeks
- Reaction of skin lesion on the face
- Ulcerative skin lesion.

Diagnosis

Clinical

Usually RR is diagnosed clinically when a patient has erythema, tenderness and edema over all or some of the existing skin lesions; with or without appearance of fresh similar reacting skin lesions and/or neuritis. There may be accompanying edema of the hands, feet and face with or without peripheral nerve involvement.

Criteria

A criteria system for clinical diagnosis of T1R has been proposed by Naafs and his team, which can be used for research purposes or for operation under field conditions. It includes presence of one major criterion or, at least two minor criteria (without signs of ENL) for the diagnosis of T1R, as shown in Table 29.3.[47]

Table 29.3: Criteria for diagnosis of type 1 reaction (T1R)

Major	Pre-existing and/or new skin lesions become inflamed, red and swollen
Minor	• One or more nerves become tender and may be swollen • Crops of new (painless) lesions appear • Sudden edema of face and extremities • Recent loss of sensation in hands and feet or signs of recent nerve damage (loss of sweating, sensation, muscle strength) in an area supplied by a particular nerve

Histopathological Examination[48]

Before the reaction is clinically apparent, there may be some diffuse extracellular edema in and around the granuloma and in the superficial dermis and a diffuse proliferation of fibrocytes in the dermis. However, when the reaction is clinically apparent, the histological response is not altogether predictable, it varies greatly in degree. Edema and proliferation of fibroblasts may be profuse or barely significant. If the DTH reaction upgrades further, the granuloma becomes completely composed of the epithelioid cells and giant cells. Foreign body giant cells may appear at this stage and if edema is profuse they acquire vacuoles due to intracellular edema. These could be confused with lepromatous vacuoles but they contain no acid-fast bacilli (AFB), and are not present unless there is much extracellular edema. An important feature of a severe reaction with ulceration is the breakdown and dispersal of the granuloma or even liquefaction necrosis. Small accumulations of polymorphs are sometimes present, but unlike ENL they are associated with the presence of epithelioid cells. Heavy granuloma formation or even caseation may be seen in the small nerve bundles of the skin. Fibrinoid necrosis, if present, signifies strong upgrading to TTs (subpolar tuberculoid leprosy), and it is followed by fibrosis. More details are given in Chapter 9 'Pathology'.

Lepromin Reaction

Due to strong DTH response in RR, the positivity of lepromin will be stronger in BT and TTs and may become positive from earlier negativity in BB and BL.

Other Laboratory Tests

No laboratory criterion is available for the assessment of reaction. Further research is needed for new markers, e.g. neuropeptides, specific antigens and recently reported potential markers like CXCL10 and IL-8 for early diagnosis of RRs.[35] Recently, Scollard et al. have shown that increased CXCL10 in lesions and serum is characteristic of T1R.[49] A recent study has specified that serum circulatory levels of IL-17F are elevated during T1Rs in the borderline spectrum

of the disease and thus may play a role in the regulation of inflammatory responses associated with reactions in leprosy.[50]

Differential Diagnosis

Reversal reaction, particularly late RR, must be differentiated from relapse (Table 29.2) and the other skin conditions like acute urticaria, erysipelas, cellulitis and insect bite.

The problem in the diagnosis of late RR in leprosy is how to differentiate relapse from reactions. This is emphasized in a study by Shetty et al.[51] who investigated biopsies of 25 BT leprosy cases presenting with recurrent lesions, 1–13 years after RFT. Although none of these cases showed overt signs of reaction, 13 out of 25 cases were histologically characterized as T1R, whereas the others showed features of BT leprosy only. However, mouse foot pad (MFP) inoculations detected live bacteria in five and seven cases respectively. Therefore, cases with recurrent lesions with clinical/histopathological features of RRs having live bacilli (5 out of 13) probably indicates relapse presenting as RR. Since differentiation of RR and relapse is necessary, in doubtful cases a few weeks of steroids course may help to differentiate between two. Possibility of multiplication of *M. leprae* with steroid administration should be kept in mind, at least theoritically.[51]

Recently a new diagnostic criterion for MB relapses in leprosy has been proposed by Linder et al. taking into account the time factor, risk factors and clinical presentation at relapse using a scoring system (Table 29.4). This scoring system

Table 29.4: Diagnostic scoring system for multibacillary (MB) relapse in leprosy[52]

	Factor	Parameter	Score*
I	Time factor (time after RFT) in month	≤12	0
		13–24	1
		25–60	2
		>60	3
II	Risk factor	Initial BI ≥ 3+	1
III	Clinical factor (presentation at relapse)	BI in a single lesion ≤ 2+ higher than the expected BI**	1
		Average BI is ≥ 2+ higher than the expected BI**	1
		No signs of reaction***	1

*Relapses are diagnosed with a score of ≥3; the maximal score = 7; the maximal score for the time factor = 3, the maximal score for the additional factors = 4, these scores are added to give the final score.

**Expected BI = calculated BI with an assumed fall of 1 log-unit/year. If the initial BI was negative, a positive BI at relapse is sufficient to score.

***Clinical signs of inflammation of the nerve or the skin or erythema nodosum leprosum.

needs further validation in a prospective study to confirm its superior sensitivity and to evaluate the specificity of these criteria by using MFP in patients presenting with signs of activity after treatment including late RR.[52]

Course

The T1R, if properly and adequately treated, seldom persists for more than a few months. Recurrences usually indicate inadequate therapy.

TYPE 2 REACTIONS

Type 2 reaction, popularly known as ENL is an immune complex syndrome (antigen-antibody reaction involving complement), causing inflammation of skin, nerves and other organs, and generally malaise. It is an example of type III hypersensitivity reaction (Coombs and Gell classification) or Arthus phenomenon. IgG, IgM, complement (C_3) and mycobacterial antigens are all identified at the site of ENL. Therefore, immune complex formation is implicated in the pathogenesis of T2R. The major clinical lesions on the skin are of erythema nodosum type; hence the term "ENL" is used as an alternative term for T2R.

Type 2 reaction occurs mostly in LL and sometimes in BL leprosy. Those patients with high bacillary index are more prone to get ENL.[53]

The Risk Factors for Type 2 Reactions

- Lepromatous leprosy with skin infiltration[54]
- Antileprosy drugs except clofazimine
- Bacterial index (BI) of >4+[54]
- Patients with < 40 years of age[54]
- *Intercurrent infections*: Streptococcal, viral, intestinal parasites, filariasis, malaria
- Trauma
- Surgical intervention
- Physical and mental stress
- Protective immunizations
- A strongly positive Mantoux test
- Pregnancy and parturition
- Ingestion of potassium iodide.

Immunopathomechanisms (Box 29.2)

Initially, there is minimal increase in the number of lymphocytes, especially perivascularly. Majority of these cells are CD4+ Th2 cells.[55] With the progression of reaction, the number of these cells increases further and surpasses the number of CD8 cells (suppressor cells) that normally form the majority in a LL lesion.[37] This goes in parallel with an increase in mRNA for IL-4, IL-5, IL-13 and perhaps IL-10 cytokines, which are indicative of a Th2 type of reaction.[28,56]

The reflections of both immune-complex and enhanced T-cell reactivity are observed, both in the blood and tissues.

During early phase of ENL in the lepromatous granuloma, in between the foamy cells, smaller cells like monocytes, become active macrophages and probably destroy the inert foamy macrophages. Antigens released from these foamy macrophages are presented by fresh macrophages to the immune system that further stimulate CMI. Those antigens which could not be engulfed by macrophages; form immune complexes with the locally present antibodies.[57]

Immunology (Box 29.2)

The involvement of CMI is proved by observation that the number of IL-2 receptors on the immune competent cells increases, as does the HLA-DR expression, not only within the infiltrate; but also on the keratinocytes of the overlying epidermis.[37,55] Within the lesions the plasma cells, which can be stimulated by the IL-4 producing cells, are able to produce antibodies. These antibodies combine with the ubiquitous antigens and form immune complexes.[55,58]

Mycobacterium leprae antigens, IgG, IgM antibodies, complement (C3d) and IL-4 mRNA are all identified in ENL skin lesions. IL-4, known to be a B-cell stimulator, increases the HLA-DR expression and is a growth factor for mast cells. In a full-blown ENL lesion, polymorphonuclear granulocytes dominate the picture; a few leu7-positive (natural killer) cells can be seen along with increased number of mast cells.[37,59]

Evidence of involvement of both, immune complexes and CMI, in ENL has been shown in the peripheral blood also. During ENL there is an *in vitro* increase in the response of peripheral blood leukocytes to mitogens, indicating a generalized increase in the CMI. The complement factor C3d is increased in the peripheral blood which indicates complement activation and is probably a spill-over from the tissues and not a sign of a classic Arthus phenomenon.

The most prominent cytokines present during ENL reaction are IL-4, IL-5, TNF-α, and INF-γ. TNF-α is known to be a

---

Box 29.2: Salient features of type 2 reactions (immunology and histopathology)

- Initial histopathological features are of LL or BL leprosy.
- Dense infiltration of dermal and subcutaneous tissue by neutrophils (sometimes forming microabcesses), superimposed on existing lepromatous diffuse granuloma.
- Vasculitis, damage to collagen and elastic fibers are common features clinically manifesting as skin necrosis and ulcerations.
- Increased expression of IL-4, IL-5, IL-13 and IL-10 cytokines (Th2 type response) and TNF-α and INF-γ.
- Local reduction of bacterial load, presence of *M. leprae* debris and replacement of neutrophils by lymphocytes are other histopathological features of type 2 reaction.
- Evidence of presence of both immune complex mediated (type III) and cell-mediated (type IV) immune response in ENL.

pyrogen which may be responsible for the rise of temperature and further tissue damage during ENL reaction.[60] A recent study from Brazil for identification of potential markers of reactions has reported the elevated levels of IL-7, platelet derived growth factor BB (PDGF BB) and IL-6 could serve as the laboratory markers of T2R.[35]

Similar to T1R, during ENL, autoimmunity might also play a role in the tissue damage. Histopathological examination of ENL tissue shows an increase in neural cell adhesion molecules (NCAM) and NCAM-positive CD8+ cells are isolated from the nerve tissue. During active ENL reaction, when peripheral blood monocytes are exposed to *M. leprae,* there is an increase in cytolysis of NCAM expressing Schwann cells by CD8+ NCAM-positive cells. IL-15 which is capable of inducing NCAM expression has been found in excess in leprosy tissue.[61]

Since many sign and symptoms described above can occur without classical ENL lesions, the term T2R is used to describe this type of leprosy reaction rather than ENL. However, ENL term is often used by the physicians or dermatologists or leprologists for those patients who have clinical evidence of ENL with or without other signs and symptoms of T2R.

Histopathology (Box 29.2)

The ENL lesion shows features of either LL or BL histopathology depending on the clinical spectrum the patient belongs to and there is dense infiltration of the superficial and/or deep dermis and/or subcutaneous tissue by neutrophils. Thus neutrophilic infiltration is superimposed on an already existing lepromatous granuloma. Often the influx of neutrophils is so intense as to form microabscesses. Vasculitis is a predominant feature in some cases. Damage to collagen and elastic fibers is common. In some variants known as necrotizing ENL, there is also necrosis and ulceration of skin. There is a local reduction in the bacterial load. Most of the bacilli are fragmented and granular. During healing phase, the neutrophils are gradually replaced by lymphocytes.

In neuritis associated with T2R, there is inflammatory edema, and cellular exudates in the perineurium.

Clinical Manifestations

Time of Onset

Type 2 reaction occurs mostly during the course of antileprosy treatment. A few cases present for the first time with features of reaction before leprosy is diagnosed and treatment started. Data on time of onset of the reactions collected by IAL in 2003 both from the field and hospital shows that 21% of all cases present as ENL lesions at the beginning, 17.6% present within 6 months after starting MDT, 16.6% during second half of the year of MDT, and 44.5% have the episodes even beyond 1 year of therapy.[8] A Chandigarh study also showed similar figures, 19.4% (in BL) and 20.1% (in LL) at registration, 10.5% (in BL),

12.9% (in LL) within 6 months, 17.2% (in BL) and 17.4% (in LL) in second half of first year, 32.8% (in BL) and 27.2% (in LL) in second year, 20% (in BL) and 21.8% (in LL) in third year and beyond.[6] A recent report from Nepal showed similar figures (30% of patients presented with ENL at the time of diagnosis, 41% developed during the first year of MDT).[62]

Mode of Onset

Cutaneous Onset

There may be appearance of crops of skin lesions in the form of painful/tender evanescent maculopapular, papular, nodular or plaque type of lesions before the appearance of constitutional signs and symptoms.

Rheumatic Onset

In one-third of the cases, pain and swelling in the joints precede or are a component of other constitutional symptoms. The patient may sometime get admitted in the internal medicine department with suspicion of rheumatic or rheumatoid fever. There are case reports of T2Rs with manifestations mimicking systemic lupus erythesmatous (SLE), polyarteritis nodosa, and Behçet's syndrome.[63]

Mixed Onset

Fever, joint pain and other constitutional signs and symptoms; and skin lesions develop together, and fever immediately follows the appearance of skin lesions.

Skin Lesions

Erythema Nodosum Leprosum

In classical T2R, usually no clinical change is noticed in the original clinical skin lesions of leprosy in contrast to the T1R, where the lesions become more prominent, erythematous, edematous and sometimes tender. ENL lesions may appear anywhere, deep in the dermis and subcutaneous tissue and these may not be clinically apparent on the surface of the skin.

There is sudden appearance of crops of evanescent (lasting for few days) pink (rose) colored tender papules, nodules or plaques variable in size. They are painful and tender to touch (Figs 29.6 and 29. 7). These lesions may be present inside the dermis and visible clearly or may be deep enough involving subcutaneous tissue forming subcutaneous nodule (SCN) where they are palpable rather than visible. The nodules are dome-shaped and ill-defined. These skin lesions are known as ENL. The common sites of appearance of ENL are outer aspects of thighs, legs and face. However, they may appear anywhere on the skin except the hairy scalp, axillae, groin and perineum, the warmer areas of the body. These may be few or multiple, if multiple they tend to be distributed bilaterally

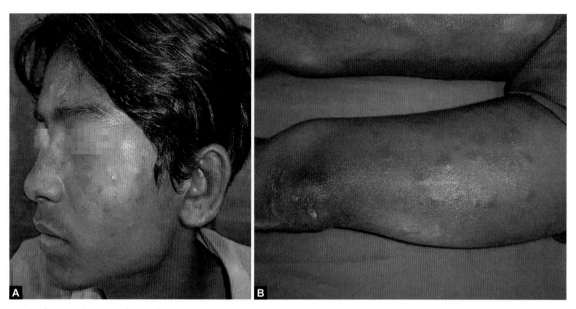

Figs 29.6A and B: Erythema nodosum leprosum (ENL) in a case of LL. Note the shiny erythematous papules and nodules (usually tender) over face and thighs. The lesions are evanescent and usually associated with systemic features like fever, malaise, joint pain, etc.

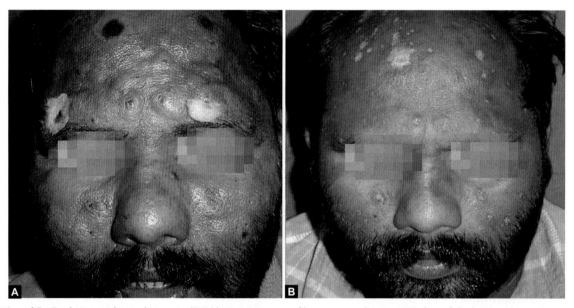

Figs 29.7A and B: Erythema nodosum leprosum (ENL) lesions in a case of lepromatous leprosy (LL), few of the lesions show necrotic changes and break down (erythema nodosum necroticans) (left). The lesions healed leaving behind depigmentation and scarring, following 4 weeks course of thalidomide along with MDT (right)

and symmetrically. They are tender, warmer, and blanch with light finger pressure. The fresh crops of ENL lesions usually appear in the evening when endogenous cortisol production is at its lowest.[12] New ENL lesions appear, as old lesions subside. An individual ENL lesion after a period of 24–48 hours shows a change of color from pink/red to bluish and brownish and finally dark, in a week or 10 days. ENL lesions may not uncommonly become vesicular, pustular, bullous

and necrotic and break down to produce ulceration called as erythema nodosum necroticans.[64,65] In certain cases the lesions may be hemorrhagic resembling Lucio phenomenon. The ENL lesions subside with desquamation or there may be peeling of the superficial skin (Figs 29.8A and B). Pustular lesions scab or leave shallow ulceration followed by scarring of the involved skin. Erythema multiforme type of skin lesions are also described.[66]

There may be edema of the hands, feet or face. When the inflammatory edema on the dorsum of the hand is associated with SCN and arthritis of the interphalangeal (IP) joints; it constitutes the clinical condition known as the 'reaction hand'.

Skin lesions sometimes tend to recur at the same sites. If they do not subside completely; a chronic painful panniculitis develops which may persist for months or years. Large areas of inflamed skin and subcutaneous tissues get fixed to underlying fascia, muscle, bone and may thus immobilize a hand or foot or even the face. This fixed fibrous tissue is poorly vascularized and may ulcerate with slightest trauma, and heals with difficulty.

Another peculiar form of ENL described by some authors is 'lazarine leprosy', the term which itself is a subject of nonconsensus. Cochrane described it as a chronic progressive form of ENL in which individual SCNs tend to break down and ulcerate, and the patient's condition is very distressing.[67] However, according to Ramu and Dharmendra, lazarine leprosy is a rare form of leprosy that occurs near tuberculoid end of borderline spectrum of leprosy in debilitated patients, it is characterized by extensive ulceration of the lesions, which commonly involve the trunk and the extremities.[66] The features of lazarine leprosy are further discussed in the section on lucio phenomenon.

Lepromatous Exacerbation

The term lepromatous exacerbation has been used in older literature for certain type of reaction in LL. This type of reaction is characterized by exacerbation of the LL skin lesions; they are swollen, red, painful and tender. There may be constitutional symptoms. Lesions may ulcerate and involve cartilage of pinna giving a rat bitten appearance. Exacerbation may involve the mucosa, leading to nasal stuffiness and hoarseness of voice. Rarely, laryngeal edema may require emergency tracheostomy.

Acute exacerbation of the disease is mainly seen in very advanced lepromatous patients with nodular and plaque-like lesions. The author has recently noticed a similar clinical form, where some of the shiny papulonodular histoid-looking LL lesions suddenly underwent central necrosis and ulceration (Figs 29.9A and B). Histologically there are small localized areas of necrosis in the middle of a large sheet of macrophages eliciting a localized infiltration of neutrophils. Vasculitis is rarely seen. The macrophages contain a relatively large load of AFB with many solid staining organisms which differentiate acute exacerbation from ENL. This may be due to sudden burst of bacterial multiplication which overgrows the macrophage population, resulting in localized cell necrosis and acute inflammation. Recently, a case report of histoid leprosy with ENL has been described with complains of fever and bilateral pitting edema of feet and softening in the center of existing skin lesions with no ENL, but histopathologically suggestive of ENL in the altered existing skin lesions.[68] However, Ridley and Job (1985) described ulceration in histoid lesions and in other large hyperactive lesions, nodular or otherwise, mimicking ENL histologically.[69]

Unusual Pattern of Vesiculobullous Type 2 Reactions:[70]

Atypical bullous lesions in T2Rs arranged in an annular fashion on the extensor aspects of arms and lower legs have been described in a pregnant lady after ingestion of ofloxacin

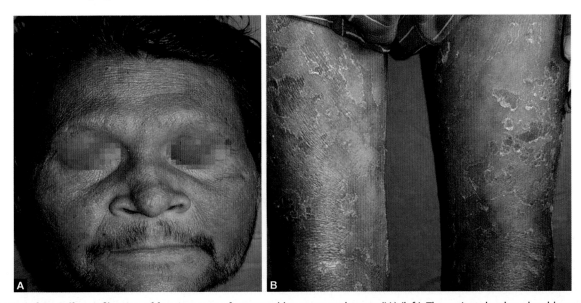

Figs 29.8A and B: Diffuse infiltration of face in a case of untreated lepromatous leprosy (LL) (left). The patient developed sudden red-bluish ill-defined painful slightly indurated diffuse lesions and plaques over the limbs which underwent exfoliation after a period of 1 week without blistering. Such type of reactional phenomenon can be observed in Lucio leprosy called Lucio phenomenon. This patient improved with starting MDT. However, later on, developed classical pattern of ENL

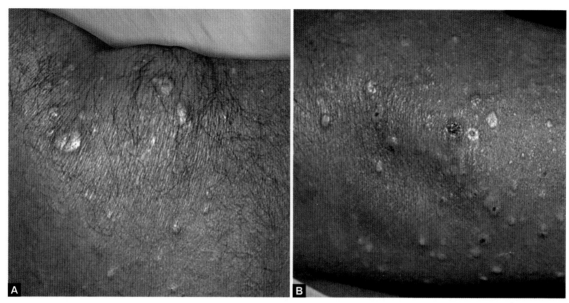

Figs 29.9A and B: The shiny papules and nodules over the back of upper trunk in a case of lepromatous leprosy (LL), resembling the lesions of histoid leprosy (left). Similar type of lesions over shoulder region showing central necrosis and ulceration. This unusual presentation with acute exacerbation of leprous lesions is rare in type 2 reaction (right)

for urinary tract infection.[70] The authors also observed similar type of lesions in a young unmarried female, an untreated case of BL leprosy who suddenly developed T2R with the appearance of papulovesicular lesions in an annular form over the inner margin of the BL plaques after taking a course of ofloxacin (a bactericidal drug for *M. leprae*) for treatment of acute urinary tract infection (Figs 29.10A and B).

Systemic Manifestations

In T2R, the systemic manifestations like fever, malaise, prostration, headache, muscle, joint and bone pain, usually confining to tibia are common, may precede the appearance of ENL. The rise of temperature is usually of intermittent type in the acute stage with the fastigium in the evening. As the reaction subsides, the temperature comes down. In very severe types, the fever may be remittent in nature with diurnal variations.

Nerve Involvement

Nerve damage may occur in T2R, but not as quickly as it occurs in T1R. Due to inflammatory edema and cellular exudates in the perineurium; the nerve is unable to accommodate the increase in its bulk contents. Compression of the vasa nervorum and of the nerve fibers, results in precipitation of acute symptoms. Added compression is provided by points of entrapment of certain sites, e.g. the ulnar groove, the

median nerve in the carpal tunnel, the lateral popliteal in the fibroosseous canal at the neck of fibula, and the posterior tibial nerve in the tarsal tunnel. In addition, the facial, radial and cutaneous nerves may also be involved.

In severe T2R there may be swollen, painful, and tender nerve trunks with loss of function. Careful nerve examination is essential to detect recent nerve function impairment (sensory, motor and autonomic functions) of the respective affected nerves during and after each episode of T2R. However, skin involvement may not be always associated with manifest nerve lesions.

Other Associated Features

The associated features of T2R are myositis, arthritis, synovitis, rhinitis, epistaxis, laryngitis, iridocyclitis, glaucoma and painful dactylitis. There may be periosteal pain (particularly in tibia), tender and swollen lymph nodes (especially inguinal and femoral groups), acute epididymo-orchitis, nephritis and proteinuria, renal failure, hepatosplenomegaly, anemia and amyloidosis.

Acute Myositis

Muscle involvement in T2R is not uncommon which may be invaded by an extension of the process of SCN formation, from the subcutis to deep into the muscle through deep fascia. The entire involved region feels woody hard. In some cases painful,

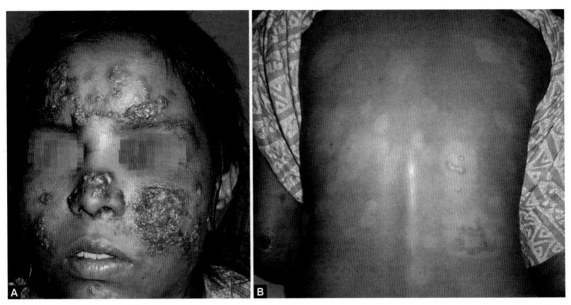

Figs 29.10A and B: Type 2 reaction with presence of vesico-bullous and crusted lesions (erythema nodosum necroticans), some of these lesions are arranged in annular fashion, over the existing lesions of BL, a rare form of ENL[70]

tender, firm nodular lesions occur in the muscle fibers *per se*. The movement of the muscles is painful. In both instances the histopathological features of myositis are observed.

Arthritis

In one-third of the cases, T2R is heralded by the rheumatic type of onset. The presenting features consist of joint swelling, pain, tenderness, with limitation of movements. Synovial effusions and bursitis are found and in certain cases joint effusions appear very rapidly. The joints commonly affected are knee, metacarpophalangeal, IP, wrist and ankle joints; in order of frequency. In recurrent T2R, nonparalytic deformities and limitation of movement at the joint and radiological changes may develop without or with inadequate treatment.

Involvement of Nose

The infiltration and nodules present in the nasal septum and inferior turbinate may be swollen with blocking of the nose leading to difficulty in breathing. It may be associated with pain and epistaxis. In severe cases the nodules may ulcerate, the cartilage may be involved resulting in perforation of the septum.

Soft Palate Involvement

The soft palate, fauces, base of the uvula may be hyperemic and may ulcerate. Repeated ulceration may lead to complete destruction.

Hard Palate Involvement

Hard palate may similarly be hyperemic and swollen during reactive states. Erosion of these reacting lesions involves the bone with destruction and eventually a perforation of the palate may result.

Involvement of Larynx

In presulfone era the inflammatory reaction involving the larynx was a life threatening complication. The edema of the epiglottis or of the false vocal cords led to respiratory embarrassment which sometimes necessitated tracheostomy as a life-saving procedure.

Bone Changes

- *Osteoperiostitis*: Osteoperiostitis particularly over the anterior aspect of the tibia is very common. There are severe bone pains and soft tender swelling of the anterior aspect of tibia. X-ray picture reveals elevation of the periosteum at the site of swelling with soft shadow underneath. Repeated attacks may lead to laying down of new bone with thickening of the cortex and increased anterior curvature of the bone looking like 'sabre tibia' of syphilis. Besides tibial involvement it may also involve the phalanges (dactylitis) producing spindle-shaped swellings with tenderness. This can occur at the upper end of ulna, the lower end of fibula, and the calcaneum.
- *Osteoporosis*: Osteoporosis may occur without accompanying arthritis. The phalanges and metacarpals

are common sites of predilection. It has been observed in long bones and ribs. It may occur in the form of demineralization or as punched out areas of rarefaction seen in the skiagrams. The rarefaction may result in pathological fractures. The pull of the contracting muscles over the rarefied phalanges may lead to subarticular collapse of the bones. Demineralization is an acute process as evidenced by increased excretion of calcium in the urine during reaction phase.

Lymph Node Enlargement

During ENL episodes, there is often acute and painful enlargement of inguinal, axillary, cervical and epitrochlear lymph nodes along with constitutional signs and symptoms. Occasionally, large abscesses are formed which break open through lymph node capsule and skin producing sinuses with discharge of pus. On acid-fast stain the pus shows numerous *M. leprae* inside the neutrophils and macrophages.

Involvement of Liver

Hepatic enlargement below the costal margin is sometimes observed. The liver is soft and tender.

Involvement of Kidneys

Acute glomerulonephritis in leprosy may be associated with ENL, due to the immune complex deposition involving antigens of *M. leprae*. However, in majority of cases the blood pressure is not elevated. Routine examination of urine reveals albuminuria many times in T2R, from a trace to 1+. Microscopic examination of the sediments after centrifuging the urine sample reveals plenty of red blood cells (RBCs), pus cells, epithelial cells, casts (from RBC, pus cells) and granular casts. In few instances frank hematuria, and rarely oliguria is observed. Kidney involvement is observed with repeated attacks of T2R, rarely ending fatally. In others, repeated reaction favors the onset and progress of the amyloidal process of which renal amyloidosis forms a part.

Suprarenal Involvement

The blood pressure remains low due to hypofunction of the suprarenal gland during reactive phases. The treatment with corticosteroid should be prompt and in adequate doses to compensate for the decrease of the hormone.

Acute Epididymo-orchitis

There may be acute pain, tenderness and swelling in the scrotum during T2R due to acute inflammation of the testes and epididymis. There may be concomitant swelling and tenderness of the breast. Repeated attacks of reaction result in testicular atrophy and gynecomastia.

Hematological Changes

Occasionally, a hemolytic crisis may be encountered with a dangerous fall in the RBC count and hemoglobin. There is sudden pallor; the patient develops breathlessness on the slightest exertion. The condition calls for prompt treatment with steroids and blood transfusion. Megaloblastic anemia has been documented possibly because of toxic or depressive effect on bone marrow. Therefore, there may be dimorphic anemia.

Type 2 Reactions without ENL

It is possible that the manifestations of the reaction may not be confined to the skin, and the patient may develop neuritis or systemic involvement or both, depending upon the target organs where immune complexes deposition occurs.

Severity of Type 2 Reaction

Presence of one or more of the features mentioned under severe reaction (Table 29.5) is considered as severe T2R which needs treatment with steroids; albeit in older times it was graded as mild, moderate and severe. In milder grade, the temperature does not go above 100°F; and the reacting skin lesions (ENLs) are few, confined to one or two extremities. In moderate degree, the temperature goes up to 102°F the skin lesions are more numerous, affecting all the four limbs, with few on the trunk, face and perhaps occasionally vesiculation. Extracutaneous signs may also be present. In the severe grade, the temperature rises above 102°F, tends to be remittent. Vesiculation and postulation are frequent. Visceral involvement is not uncommon.

Reaction Severity Assessment System (Table 29.6)

A reaction severity score may play an important role in making clinical decisions about reactions, the choice of treatment and monitoring progress. Reaction severity assessment for both types of reaction (type 1 and type 2) can be calculated more accurately using reaction severity scale formulated and tested by van Brakel and his team.[71] This group assessed 21 items as the basis for a reaction severity scale. These included assessment of skin signs, fever, edema and forms of neuritis plus changes in sensory and motor function assessed using monofilaments (200 mg, 2 g, 4 g, 10 g and 300 g) and voluntary muscle testing (VMT) respectively. Monofilament assessment at each test point is scored 0 where the 200 mg monofilament is felt through to 5 where the 300 g is not felt. Muscle testing is scored using the standard Medical Research Council grading, normal (5), full range of movement but reduced resistance (4), full range of movement but no resistance (3), movement but reduced range (2), muscle flicker (1) and paralyzed (0). For the eye, any gap on strong closure was substituted for movement but reduced range.

Table 29.5: Differentiation between mild and severe form of type 2 reaction

S. No.	Clinical feature	Mild	Severe
1	Skin lesions and extent of involvement	Few lesions	Multiple red, painful nodules in skin, with or without ulceration
2	Ulceration/necrosis of skin lesion	Absent	Present
3	Constitutional symptoms like fever, arthralgia or fever	Absent	Present
4	Neuritis	Absent	Pain and tenderness in one or more nerves
5	Edema of limbs	Mild	Marked edema of the hands, feet or face
6	Eye involvement (pain/tenderness of eye, with or without loss of visual acuity)	Absent	May be present
7	Recurrent ENL	Nil	Four or more episodes in a year
8	Response to oral steroids	Usually responds in 6 weeks	Persists for long
9	Tender lymphadenopathy	Absent	Frequently present
10	Systemic involvement (like epididymo-orchitis)	Absent	May be present

Table 29.6 summarizes test points for hands and feet and the method of calculation of a severity score ranging from 0 to 70, higher score being associated with more severe reactions. However, this scoring system requires formal testing for validation and reliability.

Originally, the scoring of the items in the 'A section' of the severity scale was weighted in such a way that a score of '3' or more on any individual item would trigger the diagnosis that the outcome event (reaction or nerve function impairment) was severe and required steroid treatment. In section 'B' a score of '2' or more triggered the diagnosis 'severe'.

Diagnosis

Clinical

Classical ENL and other rarer types of T2R with different morphological patterns with or without other constitutional features and associated manifestations are diagnostic (Table 29.7). Criteria for diagnosis of T2R (ENL) may be used for research or in the field proposed by B Naafs and his team includes the major criterion or at least three minor criteria.[47]

Clinical Tests

Certain clinical tests are used as a clue for diagnosis of T2R.

Ryrie Test

Stroking the sole of the foot with the back of a reflex hammer elicits a burning pain which also may be noticed when watching the patient walk, which seems as if he is walking on hot coals.

Ellis Test

Squeezing the wrist during ENL elicits a painful reaction; this does not occur in RRs unless the radial cutaneous nerve is tender.

Histopathological Features of the Skin from the ENL Lesions

Classical histopathological features of active ENL lesions of the skin are increased vascularity with dilated capillaries in the upper dermis, and in the lower dermis, an intense infiltration with neutrophils which have predilection for surrounding blood vessels and invading the walls. There is edema of the endothelium of veins, arterioles and small arteries. In case of erythema necroticans there is obliterative angiitis and endarteritis. Bacilli are few and are mostly fragmented and granular. The acid-fast bacilli are usually scanty. However, it is possible to demonstrate mycobacterial antigen by the immunoperoxidase technique.

In bullous ENL, immunofluorescence studies have revealed IgG deposits at the basement membrane zone in occasional cases; only fibrinogen deposits in one case,[64] while negative immunofluorescence in others.[65]

Laboratory Tests

There is need for development of laboratory tests to assist in the assessment of severity and resolution of ENL. Further research is needed on the evaluation of recently reported laboratory markers IL-7, PDGF-BB and IL-6, as the indicators of T2R.

There is no definitive criterion for histopathological diagnosis.

Section A: Signs and symptoms of reactions: Score in the right hand column

	Scoring	0	1	2	3	4	Score
					Table 29.6: Reaction severity assessment[71]		
A1	Number of raised and inflamed lesions	None	1–3	4–10	>10		
A2	Degree of inflammation of skin lesions or nodules	None	Erythema or nodules	Erythema, raised plaques or nodules	Ulceration		
A3	Peripheral edema due to reaction	None	Minimal	Visible, but not affecting function	Edema affecting function		
A4	Fever due to reaction	<37.5	37.6–38.9		≥39		
A5	Involvement of other organs (eye, testes, etc.)	None			Mild	Definite	
A6	Nerve pain and/or paresthesia	None	Intermittent, not limiting activity		Sleep disturbed and/or activity diminished		
A7	Nerve tenderness on gentle palpation	None	Absent if attention is distracted		Present if attention is distracted	Withdraws limb forcibly	

Section B: Sensory assessment: Score in the right hand column

	Scoring	0	1	2	3	Score
B1	Ulnar-left	No recent worsening	1–2 points worse	3–8 points worse	9–16 points worse	
B2	Ulnar-right	No recent worsening	1–2 points worse	3–8 points worse	9–16 points worse	
B3	Median-left	No recent worsening	1–2 points worse	3–8 points worse	9–16 points worse	
B4	Median-right	No recent worsening	1–2 points worse	3–8 points worse	9–16 points worse	
B5	Lat. Pop.-left	No recent worsening	1–2 points worse	3–8 points worse	9–16 points worse	
B6	Lat. Pop. right	No recent worsening	1–2 points worse	3–8 points worse	9–16 points worse	

Section C: Motor assessment : Score in right hand column

	Scoring	0	1	2	3	Score
C1	Facial left	No recent worsening	1 point worse	2 points worse	3–5 points worse	
C2	Facial right	No recent worsening	1 point worse	2 points worse	3–5 points worse	
C3	Ulnar left	No recent worsening	1 point worse	2 points worse	3–5 points worse	
C4	Ulnar right	No recent worsening	1 point worse	2 points worse	3–5 points worse	
C5	Median-left	No recent worsening	1 point worse	2 points worse	3–5 points worse	
C6	Median-right	No recent worsening	1 point worse	2 points worse	3–5 points worse	
C7	Lat. Pop. left	No recent worsening	1 point worse	2 points worse	3–5 points worse	
C8	Lat. Pop. right	No recent worsening	1 point worse	2 points worse	3–5 points worse	

Total score, sections A + B + C

Table 29.7: Criteria for diagnosis of T2R

Major	A sudden eruption of tender (red) papules, nodules or plaques, which may ulcerate
Minor	Mild fever, the patient is unwell Tender enlarged nerves Increased loss of sensation or muscle power Arthritis Lymphadenitis Epididymo-orchitis Iridocyclitis or episcleritis Edema of extremities or face Positive Ryrie or Ellis test

Hematological changes: There is always a leukocytosis during reaction; the count varies from 20,000/mm³ to 50,000/mm³. The ESR is markedly elevated. C-reactive proteins appear in the blood. Megaloblastic anemia has been observed due to bone marrow depression. Occasionally, hemolytic crisis may be observed with dangerous fall in the RBC count and hemoglobin.

Routine and microscopic urine examination is must for detection of albuminuria, RBC, pus cells, epithelial cells and casts to exclude kidney involvement.

Liver function tests: In certain number of cases there is mild rise of serum bilirubin of 1–2 mg/100 mL. Rise in serum transaminases [serum glutamic oxaloacetic transaminase (SGOT) and serum glutamic-pyruvic transaminase (SGPT)] indicates hepatic and muscular damage.

Differential Diagnosis

Type 1 reaction must be differentiated clinically from T2R (Table 29.8). However, acute EN can occur due to other common causes like sarcoidosis, tuberculosis, streptococcal infections, intestinal infections and drugs. They are usually up to 10 lesions, but in severe cases many more may be found, more common in young adult women, bilaterally symmetrical, usually located on the pretibial area and lateral shins.

Erythema nodosum leprosum is frequently associated with malaise, leg edema, and arthritis or arthralgia.

Rheumatic fever, rheumatoid arthritis, collagen disorders like SLE; and drug reactions are to be kept in mind and need to be excluded.

It is not unusual to notice both types of reactions (type 1 and type 2) observed in same individual with BL or subpolar type of leprosy while under MDT.

LUCIO PHENOMENON (BOX 29.3)

This is a special type of reaction observed in uniformly diffuse shiny infiltrative non-nodular form of LL leprosy, called as Lucio leprosy which is chiefly encountered in Mexicans. Its unique feature is that it is seen only in untreated cases. This form of leprosy and its unique form of reaction were described by Lucio and Alvardo in Mexico in 1852 and later, by Latapi and Zamora in 1948. It has also been reported from other countries such as Costa Rica, the USA, Hawaii, and Brazil. Few cases of lucio leprosy have also been reported in the

Table 29.8: Differences between type 1 and type 2 reactions

Features	Type 1	Type 2
Type of immunological reaction	Delayed type hypersensitivity reaction	Antigen antibody immune complex reaction (Arthus reaction)
Type of patients affected	Borderline types (BT, BB, BL, rarely subpolar LL)	LL, rarely BL
Constitutional signs and symptoms like fever, malaise, arthralgia, myalgia	None or rare	Common
Type of the skin lesions	Existing skin lesions (few or many or all) suddenly becomes reddish, swollen, warm, painful, tender	Fresh red, painful, tender, cutaneous nodules, plaques. The existing skin lesions remain unchanged
Nerve involvement	Nerves close to skin lesions may be enlarged, painful and tender due to acute neuritis with loss of nerve functions (loss of sensation and muscle weakness). Neuritis may also appear suddenly	Nerves may be affected but not as common or as severe; as in type 1 reaction
Eye involvement	Corneal anesthesia and lagophthalmos (weakness of eyelid closure) may occur due to nerve involvement (5th and 7th cranial nerves)	Internal eye diseases like iritis, iridocyclitis, glaucoma, cataract, are common
Other organs	Not affected	May be affected: (lymphadenitis, epididymo-orchitis, painful dactylitis, periosteal pain, myositis, arthritis, and glomerulonephritis, are common

Abbreviations: BT, borderline tuberculoid; BB, borderline borderline; BL, borderline lepromatous; LL, lepromatous leprosy.

recent past from India.[72,73] The authors also diagnosed a case of Lucio leprosy with initial attack of Lucio's phenomenon; subsequently after starting MDT he developed classical ENL lesions (Fig. 29.10).

The etiopathogenesis of this phenomenon is less well-understood. *M. leprae* are found unusually in large numbers in the endothelial cells of superficial blood vessels, and this finding may be responsible for the serious vascular complications seen during the reactive phase. There is marked vasculitis and thrombosis of the superficial and deep vessels resulting in hemorrhage and infarction of the skin. Lucio phenomenon might be another unusual variant of ENL, like necrotizing ENL.

Clinical Manifestations

- The reaction begins with slightly indurated red-bluish plaques on the skin with an erythematous halo, usually on one of the limbs, but may also develop on other areas of the body. The lesions are ill-defined, but painful and rarely palpable. The shape of lesions is irregular or triangular (Fig. 29.11). After a few days they become purplish at the center, a central hemorrhagic infarct may develop with or without blister formation. Later, this becomes a necrotic eschar, which detaches easily, leaving an ulcer of irregular shape. The ulcer heals leaving a superficial scar (Fig. 29.12).
- Sometimes larger inflamed bullous lesions also develop, which burst leaving a deep ulcer with jagged edges. It heals slowly and secondary cellulites may complicate (Figs 29.11 and 29.12).
- Usually, the patients have lesions that are at different stages of evolution. It takes about 3 weeks for a lesion to develop an ulcer from the initial lesion. It may take many months to heal.
- Patients remain afebrile.

Box 29.3: Salient features of Lucio phenomenon

- Unique form of leprosy reaction, observed in Lucio leprosy, mainly reported from Mexico, Costa Rica, USA, Hawaii, Brazil and recently from India.
- Lucio leprosy characterized by diffuse skin infiltration, loss of facial skin creases (leading to youthful appearance-beautiful leprosy) and absence of papules and nodular lesions *M. leprae* are found in.
- *Classical clinical picture of Lucio phenomenon:* Usually afebrile, appearance of erythematous diffuse or plaque type lesions which becomes purpuric, becomes necrotic followed by black eschar formation. The eschar falls off in a few days leaving behind big ulcers of irregular shape.
- *Specific histopathological features:* Ischemic epidermal necrosis, necrotizing vasculitis of small blood vessels in the upper dermis, severe focal endothelial proliferation of mid-dermal vessels, and by presence of large number of AFB in endothelial cells.
- The condition improves after starting MDT.

- However, later on few of them may develop typical ENL after starting antileprosy treatment (MDT). In one report, 4 out of 10 patients... developed typical ENL in 3 months to 3 years after starting dapsone therapy.[73]

Histopathological Features

Rea and Ridley have compared the histology of ENL and lesions of Lucio phenomenon. They distinguish Lucio phenomenon from ENL by ischemic epidermal necrosis,

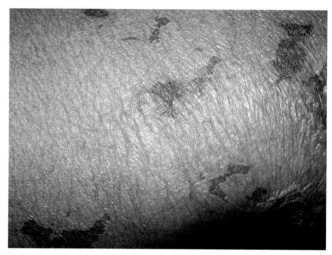

Fig. 29.11: Slightly indurated red-bluish plaques of irregular and triangular shaped lesions in a case of lucio leprosy, reported from India (Reproduced with permission from Dr DM Thappa, JIPMER, Puducherry, India)

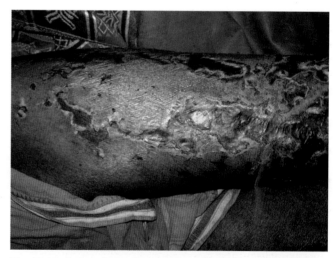

Fig. 29.12: Bullous lesions leading to deep ulceration and necrosis, resulting into formation of eschar, which on falling leaves a deep ulcer with jagged margins, as observed in a fatal case of lucio phenomenon (Reproduced with permission from Dr DM Thappa, JIPMER, Puducherry, India)

Table 29.9: Differentiating features between Lucio's phenomenon and type 2 leprosy reaction with vasculonecrotic phenomenon[74]

Lucio phenomenon	Type 2 leprosy reaction with vasculonecrotic phenomenon
Occurs only in the diffuse form of leprosy when no nodules appear. Erythematous spots appear without localized infiltrations (diffuse leprosy that never presents papules, plaques or lepromas in the course of disease) and evolves into small superficial ulcerations, generally triangular or angular, that heal leaving atrophic and hypochromic scars	Occurs in leprosy with plaques and nodules, vasculonecrotic lesions with eschars are formed.
Occurs in untreated individuals, a few years after onset of disease and, disappears with treatment being sometimes replaced by erythema nodosum	More frequent in the first months of treatment
Reddish 0.5–1.0 cm spots that ulcerate	Extensive and deep necrotic lesions, regular and round or oval ulcerations overlying a nodule
Burning sensation	Ischemic pain
Usually afebrile, never appear to be acutely ill, except in severe cases of extensive necrosis	Presents with fever and constitutional symptoms
Does not affect nerves	It may be accompanied by neuritis
No general symptoms or visceral damage	Arthralgia, iridocyclitis, orchitis, lymphadenopathy, nephritis, hepatitis
Positive Medina test*	Negative Medina test
Histopathology shows colonization of the endothelial cell by acid fast bacilli, ischemic epidermal necrosis, necrotizing vasculitis of the small vessels of the superficial dermis, endothelial proliferation of the medium-sized vessels of the mid-dermis with passive venous congestion, and neutrophilic infiltration	Histopathology shows panvasculitis. It starts in the hypodermis, where the affected vessels are of variable caliber, with larger necrosis resulting in fibrotic scars
Does not respond to thalidomide	Responds to thalidomide
Resolution in 15 days	Slow resolution
Small hypochromic scars with hyperchromic border	Large deep ulcers result in fibrotic, hypertrophic and radiating scars

*Medina test: This test is similar to lepromin test except that the antigen is prepared from the lesions of Lucio leprosy.

necrotizing vasculitis of small blood vessels in the upper dermis, severe focal endothelial proliferation of mid-dermal vessel, and by presence of large numbers of bacilli in endothelial cells.[2] A comparative account of clinical features of lucio phenomenon and vasculonectrotic ENL has been presented by Leticia et al. (Table 29.9).[74]

Diagnosis

- *Geographical distribution*: Chiefly encountered in Mexicans. It is rarely reported from India.[73,75]
- Observed in untreated long standing Lucio leprosy (diffuse non-nodular form of LL)
- *Classical clinical picture*: Appearance of erythematous diffuse or plaque type lesions which become purpuric, then necrotic followed by black eschar formation. The eschar falls off in a few days leaving behind big ulcers of irregular shape.
- Absence of constitutional symptoms
- *Specific histopathological features*: The clinical diagnosis is confirmed by microscopic pathology marked by ischemic epidermal necrosis, necrotizing vasculitis of small blood

vessels in the upper dermis, severe focal endothelial proliferation of mid-dermal vessels, and by presence of large number of AFB in endothelial cells[76]
- The condition improves after starting MDT.

REFERENCES

1. Kar BR and Job CK. Very rare reversal reaction and Mitsuda conversion in secondary lepromatous leprosy, a case report. Lepr Rev. 2005;76:258-62.
2. Rea TH, Ridley DS. Lucio phenomenon: a comparative histopathological study. Int J Lepr. 1979;47:161-6.
3. Lienhardt C, Fine PE. Type 1 reaction, neuritis and disability in leprosy. What is the current epidemiological situation? Lepr Rev. 1994;65:9-33.
4. Van Brakel WH, Khawas IB, Lucas S. Reactions in leprosy: an epidemiological study of 386 patients in West Nepal. Lepr Rev. 1994;65:190-203.
5. Saunderson P, Gebre S, Byass P. Reversal reactions in the skin lesions of AMFES patients: incidence and reaction factors. Lepr Rev. 2000;71:309-17.
6. Kumar B, Dogra S, Kaur I. Epidemiological characteristics of leprosy reactions: 15 years experience from North India. Int J Lepr Other Mycobact Dis. 2004;72:125-33.

7. Becx-Bleumink M, Berhe D. Occurrence of reactions, and their diagnosis and management in leprosy patients treated with multidrug therapy: experience in the leprosy control programme of the All Africa leprosy and Rehabilitation Training Centre (ALERT) in Ethiopia. Int J Lepr Other Mycobact Dis. 1992;60:173-84.

8. IAL workshop on reactions in leprosy, Jamnagar, Gujarat, 11-12 January 2003. Indian J Lepr. 2003;75:295-303.

9. Desikan KV, Sudhakar KS, Tulsidas I, et al. Observations on reactions of leprosy in the field. Indian J Lepr. 2007;79:1-7.

10. Lockwood DN. The management of erythema nodosum leprosum: current and future options (editorial). Lepr Rev. 1996;67:253-9.

11. Post E, chin-A-Lein RA, Bouman C, et al. Lepra in Nederland in de periode 1970-1991. Ned Tijdschr Geneesk. 1994;138:1960-3.

12. Jopling WH, McDougall AC. In: Handbook of Leprosy, 5th edition. New Delhi: CBS Publishers; 1996.pp.10-47.

13. Lockwood DN, Vinayakumar S, Stanley JN, et al. Clinical features and outcome of reversal (type 1) reactions in Hyderabad, India. Int J Lep Other Mycobact Dis. 1993;61:8-15.

14. Naafs B. Treatment of reactions and nerve damage. Int J Lepr Other Mycobact Dis. 1996;64:S21-8.

15. Ridley DS. Reaction in leprosy. Lepr Rev. 1969;40:77-81.

16. Roche PW, Theuvenet WJ, Britton WJ. Risk factors for type-1 reactions in borderline leprosy patients. Lancet. 1991; 338:654-7.

17. De Rijk AJ, Gabre S, Byass P, et al. Field evaluation of WHO-MDT of fixed duration at ALERT, Ethiopia. The AMFES Project-II: Reaction and neuritis during and after MDT in PB and MB leprosy patients. Lepr Rev. 1994;65:320-32.

18. Lockwood DN, Sinha HH. Pregnancy and leprosy: a comprehensive literature review. Int J Lepr Other Mycobact Dis. 1999;67:6-12.

19. Ramu G, Desikan KV. Reactions in borderline leprosy. Indian J Lepr. 2002;74:115-28.

20. Hogeweg M, Kiran KU, Suneetha S. The significance of facial patches in type1 reaction for the development of facial nerve damage in leprosy: a retrospective study among 126 paucibacillary patients. Lepr Rev. 1991;62:143-6.

21. van Brakel WH, Nicholls PG, Das L, et al. The INFIR Cohort Study: investigating prediction, detection and pathogenesis of neuropathy and reactions in leprosy. Methods and baseline results of a cohort of multibacillary leprosy patients in north India. Lepr Rev. 2005;76(1):14-34.

22. Kar HK, Sharma AK, Misra RS, et al. Reversal reaction in multibacillary leprosy patients following MDT with and without immunotherapy with a candidate for an antileprosy vaccine, *Mycobacterium w.* Lepr Rev. 1993;64:219-26.

23. Wilkinson RJ, Lockwood DN. Antigenic trigger for type 1 reaction in leprosy. J Infect. 2005;50:242-3.

24. Rego VP, Machado PR, Martins I, et al. Type 1 reaction in leprosy: characteristics and association with hepatitis B and C viruses. Rev Soc Bras Med Trop. 2007;40:546-9.

25. Shetty VP, Antia NH. Pathology of nerve damage in leprosy. In: Shetty V, Antia NH (Eds). The peripheral nerve in leprosy and other neuropathies. Calcutta: Oxford University Press; 1997. pp. 79-137.

26. Fiallo P, Cardo PP, Nunzi E. Identification of sequence similarities between *Mycobacterium leprae* and the myelin proteolipid protein by computational analysis. Indian J Lepr. 1999;71:1-10.

27. Yamamura M, Uyemura K, Deans RJ, et al. Defining protective responses to pathogens: cytokine profiles in leprosy lesions. Science. 1991;254:277-9.

28. Yamamura M, Wang XH, Ohmen JD, et al. Cytokine patterns of immunologically mediated tissue damage. J Immunol. 1992;149:1470-81.

29. Modlin RL, Yamamura M, Salgame P, et al. Lymphokine patterns in leprosy skin lesion. In: Burgdorff WH, Katz SI (Eds). Dermatology; Progress and Prospectives. London: Parthenon Publishing Group; 1993. pp. 893-6.

30. Verhagen CE, Wieringa EE, Buffing AA, et al. Reversal reaction in borderline leprosy is associated with a polarized shift to Type 1 like Mycobacterium leprae T-cell reactivity in lesional skin: A follow-up study. J Immunol. 1997;159:4474-83.

31. Cooper CL, Mueller C, Sinchaisri TA, et al. Analysis of naturally occurring delayed type hypersensitive reactions in leprosy by in situ hybridization. J Exp Med. 1989;169:1565-81.

32. Khanolkar-Young S, Rayment N, Brickell PM, et al. Tumour necrosis factor alpha synthesis is associated with skin and peripheral nerve pathology of leprosy reversal reaction. Clin Exp Immunol. 1995;99:196-202.

33. Verhagen CE, van der Pauw Kraan TC, Buffing AA, et al. Type 1- and type 2- like lesional skin derived M. leprae-responsive T- cell clones are characterized by co-expression of IFN-gamma/TNF-alpha and IL-4/IL-5/IL-13 respectively. J Immunol. 1998;160:2380-87.

34. Verhagen CE, Faber WR, Klatser PR, et al. Immunohistological analysis of in situ expression of mycobacterial antigens in the skin lesions of leprosy patents across the histopathological spectrum. Am J Path. 1999;154:1793-1804.

35. Stefani MM, Guerra GK, Sousa AL, et al. Potential plasma markers Type 1 and Type 2 leprosy reactions: a preliminary report. BMC Infect Dis. 2009;9:75.

36. Mohanty KK, Joshi B, Katoch K, et al. Leprosy reactions: humoral and cellular immune responses to *M. leprae*, 65 kDa, and 18 kDa antigens. Int J Lepr Other Mycobact Dis. 2004;72:149-58.

37. Naafs B. Reactions in leprosy. In: Ratledge G, Stanford JL, Grange JM (Eds). Biology of Mycobacteria. London: Academic Press Ltd; 1989.pp.359-403.

38. Sengupta U. Immunopathology of leprosy (Symposium paper). Indian J Lepr. 2000;72:381-91.

39. Sreenivasan P, Misra RS, Wilfred D, et al. Lepromatous leprosy patients show T- helper 1- like cytokine profile with differential expression of interleukin-10 during type 1 and type 2 reactions. 1998;95:529-36.

40. Naafs B, Kolk AH, Chin A lien RA, et al. Anti-*Mycobacterium leprae* monoclonal antibodies cross-reactive with human skin. An alternative explanation for the immune responses in leprosy. J Invest Dermatol. 1990;94:685-8.

41. Van den Akker TW, Naafs B, Kolk AH, et al. Similarity between mycobacteria and human epidermal antigens. Brit J Dermatol. 1992;127:352-8.

42. Rambukkana A, Burggraaf JD, Faber WR, et al. The mycobacterial secreted antigen 85 complex possesses epitopes that are differently expressed in human leprosy lesions and *Mycobacterium leprae* infected armadillo tissues. Infect Immunol. 1993;61:1835-45.

43. Stanley JN. Pathological changes in the sciatic nerves of mice with leprosy neuropathy—an electromicroscopic study. 1988 [PhD thesis]. Oxford, UK quoted by Naafs B in symposium

paper "Current views on reactions in leprosy". Indian J Lepr. 2000;72:97-122.

44. Bochud PY, Hawn TR, Siddiqui MR, et al. Toll-like receptor 2 (TLC2) polymorphisms are associated with reversal reaction in leprosy. J Infect Dis. 2008;197:253-61.

45. Ustianowski AP, Lawn SD, Lockwood DN. Interactions between HIV infection and leprosy. Lancet Infect Dis. 2006;6:350-60.

46. Kar HK, Saxena AK, Jain RK, et al. Type 1 (reversal) lepra reaction in borderline leprosy with unusual clinical presentations—a case report. Indian J leprosy. 1987;59:219-22.

47. Naafs B. Treatment and duration of reversal reaction: a reappraisal. Back to the past. Lepr Rev. 2003;74:328-36.

48. Ridley DS. Reactions. In: Ridley DS (Ed). Skin Biopsy in Leprosy, 3rd edition. Basle: CIBA-GEIGY Limited; 1990.pp. 53-8.

49. Scollard DM, Chaduvula MV, Martinez A, et al. Increased CXC Ligand 10 levels and gene expression in type I leprosy reactions. Clinic Vaccine Immunol. 2011;18:947-53.

50. Chaitanya S, Lavania M, Turankar RP, et al. Increased serum circulatory levels of interleukin 17F in type I reactions in leprosy. J Clin Immunol. 2012;32:1415-20.

51. Shetty VP, Wakade A, Antia NH. A high incidence of viable Mycobacterium leprae in post-MDT recurrent lesions in tuberculoid leprosy patients. Lepr Rev. 2001;72:337-44.

52. Linder K, Zia M, Kern WV, et al. Relapses vs. Reactions in multibacillary leprosy: proposal of new relapse criteria. Trop Med Int Health. 2008;13:295-309.

53. Saunderson P, Gebre S, Byass P. ENL reactions in the multibacillary cases of AMFES cohorts in central Ethiopia: Incidence and risk factors. Lepr Rev. 2000;71:318-24.

54. Manandhar R, LeMaster JW, Roche PW. Risk factors for erythema nodosum leprosum. Int J Lepr. 1999;67:270-8.

55. Naafs B. Leprosy reactions: New knowledge. Trop Geogr Med. 1994;46:80-4.

56. Modlin RL, Mehra R, Bloom BR, et al. *In situ* and *in vitro* characterization of the cellular immune-response in erythema nodosum leprosum. J Immunol. 1986;123:1813-7.

57. Naafs B. Symposium paper "Current views on reactions in leprosy". Indian J Lepr. 2000;72:97-122.

58. Variham G, Douglas JT, Moad J. Immune complexes and antibody levels in blisters over human leprosy skin lesions with or without erythema nodosum leprosum. Clin Immunol Immunopathol. 1992;63:230-6.

59. Shetty VP, Antia NH. Pathology of nerve damage in leprosy. In: Antia NH, Shetty VP. The peripheral nerve in leprosy and other neuropathies. Mumbai: Oxford University Press; 1997.pp. 79-137.

60. Sarno EN, Sampaio EP. The role of inflammatory cytokines in the tissue injury of leprosy. Int J Lepr. 1996;64:S69-S74.

61. Julien D, Sieling PA, Uyemura K, et al. IL-15, an immunomodulator of T cell responses in intracellular infection. J Immunol. 1997;158:800-06.

62. Feuth M, Brandsma JW, Faber WR, et al. Erythema nodosum leprosum in Nepal: a retrospective study of clinical features and response to treatment with prednisolone or thalidomide. Lepr Rev. 2008;79:254-69.

63. Danda D, Cherian AM. Rheumatological manifestations of leprosy and lepra reaction. Indian J Lepr. 2001;73:58-62.

64. Sethuraman G, Jeevan D, Srinivas CR, et al. Bullous erythema nodosum leprosum (bullous type 2 reaction). Int J Dermatol. 2002;41:362-4.

65. Rai VM, Balachandran C. Necrotic erythema nodosum leprosum. Dermatol Online J. 2006;12:12.

66. Ramu G, Dharmendra. Acute exacerbations (reactions) in leprosy. In: Dharmendra (Ed). Leprosy. Mumbai: Kothari Medical Publishing House; 1978.pp.108-39.

67. Cochrane RG. Complicating conditions due to leprosy. In: Cochrane RG, Davey TF (Eds). Leprosy in Theory and Practice, 2nd edition. Bristol: John Wright & Sons Ltd; 1964. pp.152-82.

68. Vassavi S, Reddy BS. Histoid leprosy with erythema nodosum leprosum—a case report. Indian J Lepr. 2012;84:27-9.

69. Ridley DS, Job CK. The pathology of leprosy. In: Hastings RC (Ed). Leprosy, 1st edition. Edinburgh: Churchill, Livingstone. pp. 100-33.

70. Kar HK, Raina A, Sharma PK, et al. Annular vesiculobullous leprosy: a case report. Indian J Lepr. 2009;81:205-8.

71. van Brakel WH, Nicholls PG, Lockwood DN, et al. A scale to assess the severity of leprosy reactions. Lepr Rev. 2007;78:161-4.

72. Saoji V, Salodkar. Lucio leprosy with Lucio phenomenon. Indian J Lepr. 2001;73:267-72.

73. Kumari R, Thappa DM, Basu D. A fatal case of lucio phenomenon from India. Dermatology Online J. 2008;14(2):10.

74. Leticia F, Elemir MS, Maria LC, et al. Vasculonecrotic reactions in leprosy. Brazilian J Infect Dis. 2007;11:378-82.

75. Rea TH, Levan NE. Lucio's phenomenon and diffuse non-nodular lepromatous leprosy. Archi Dermatol. 1978;114:1023-8.

76. Jopling WH, McDougall AC. Leprosy reactions (reactional states). Handbook of Leprosy, 5th edition. New Delhi: CBS Publishers; 1996.pp.82-91.

SECTION 6

Therapeutics (Medical and Surgical), Prophylaxis and Vaccines

30
CHAPTER

Chemotherapy of Leprosy

Paul R Saunderson

INTRODUCTION

The chemotherapy of leprosy has been remarkably successful in recent years in the management of individual cases. The pivotal point in the treatment of leprosy came in 1981 when the World Health Organization (WHO) called together a Study Group on the Chemotherapy of Leprosy for Control Programmes.[1] The group recommended two so-called multidrug regimens [multidrug therapy (MDT)], containing the powerfully bactericidal drug rifampicin and either one or two additional drugs to replace dapsone monotherapy, which was becoming increasingly ineffective because of drug resistance. The drugs in routine use since then (rifampicin, dapsone and clofazimine) have been well-tolerated and highly effective (*See* Chapter 31 on the WHO-MDT Regimens).

However, chemotheraphy has been surprisingly ineffective in preventing the spread of disease. When the bactericidal multidrug regimens were launched in 1981, a major goal was to reduce the transmission of the disease to contacts, but epidemiological surveillance in subsequent years has shown very little effect on the incidence of disease, which has exhibited a constant, but very gradual decline for several decades, preceding the introduction of MDT.[2,3] Recent evidence from Cebu,[4] for example, suggests that the decline in case detection in recent years is no faster than the decline in Norway in the late nineteenth century, despite good coverage with *Bacillus Calmette-Guérin* (BCG) in infants, and chemotherapy for all new cases detected—interventions which were not available a 100 years ago, of course.

The reason for this surprising result is not known, but it is likely that the disease is spread to contacts of new cases during the incubation period, before clinical signs and symptoms of disease have developed, and before treatment can be started. For this reason, more effective treatment regimens are not the answer to interrupting the transmission of leprosy—people who are incubating leprosy need to be started on treatment much earlier, a task that is not possible at present, while subclinical disease remains undetectable. The only practical way to tackle this issue is to consider postexposure prophylaxis—giving some sort of prophylactic treatment to people who have been in contact with a case of leprosy. Chemoprophylaxis for household contacts of new cases using single-dose rifampicin is being studied in this context.[5] The possibility of immunoprophylaxis for this group is also being examined.[6] The two approaches may be complimentary in that chemoprophylaxis has a rather short-term effect, while immunoprophylaxis may provide lower level protection for a longer period.

The discovery of new bactericidal drugs for leprosy, since the 1982 report, allows the possibility of new drug regimens, which could be fully supervised (i.e. monthly administration, without any unsupervised treatment), and perhaps of shorter duration than the standard MDT regimens. These drugs include the fluoroquinolones, minocycline and clarithromycin, although the latter drug is less well-tolerated. Because of cost and the fact that the MDT regimens continue to be donated free-of-charge by Novartis, these newer regimens have not yet been widely taken up within routine leprosy control programs.

This chapter will look in more detail at the drugs that have been, or could be, used to treat leprosy. New antileprosy drugs are most likely to be found among drugs being developed for tuberculosis (TB) and in most cases knowledge of the genomes of the two organisms will permit an estimation of the likely activity of a new antituberculosis (anti-TB) drug against leprosy. Thus, two new drugs (PA824, or delamanid; and linezolid) being tested against drug-resistant TB have less activity against *Mycobacterium leprae*, and will not be discussed further.[7]

After a brief discussion of so-called persisters, and reviewing the issue of relapse after treatment, regimens that may be considered for future use will be discussed. Drug resistance is an important topic of great relevance here, but it will be fully discussed in a separate chapter (See Chapter 40).

DAPSONE

History

Dapsone monotherapy was the mainstay of treatment for leprosy for 30 years, from the early 1950s until MDT was introduced in 1981. The drug was first synthesized in 1908, but only much later were such chemical compounds tested for possible antibacterial activity. Sulfonamide drugs proved to be useful in various bacterial infections in the 1930s and 1940s, so they and related drugs, such as the sulfones were tested in leprosy by GH Faget at Carville, in Louisiana. Dapsone, the parent sulfone, was initially thought to be too toxic as it was tested in the high doses required for the sulfonamides, but it was eventually realized that it was effective in much lower doses and it became the drug of choice from the 1950s onwards.

Dapsone is extremely cheap to produce and has a long shelf-life, making it suitable for widespread distribution in leprosy endemic areas. Because of these characteristics and its extremely high therapeutic ratio (the lethal dose of the drug, divided by the minimum effective dose), it was retained in the multidrug regimens developed in 1981.[1]

Activity

Dapsone, like all the active sulfonamide and sulfone drugs, inhibits the synthesis of dihydrofolic acid by blocking the enzyme dihydropteroate synthetase. It is weakly bactericidal for *M. leprae*.

Dapsone is also used as an immune-modulatory drug in certain skin conditions, such as dermatitis herpetiformis and pemphigoid, although the mechanism of action is not well understood.

Uses and Dosage

Dapsone can be given orally once a day (half-life just over 24 hours), being rapidly absorbed from the gastrointestinal tract; the adult dose is 100 mg daily.

Adverse Effects

A wide range of adverse effects have been associated with dapsone, the most important being anemia (through a variety of mechanisms) and the dapsone hypersensitivity syndrome.

Hemolytic anemia is frequently seen, especially in patients with G6PD deficiency. In communities where borderline anemia is common, dapsone therapy may often precipitate clinically significant anemia, especially in women.[8] Methemoglobinemia is less common and rarely of any significance. Agranulocytosis is rare but serious, usually resulting in the death of the patient.

The dapsone hypersensitivity syndrome is a rare but sometimes fatal complication of dapsone therapy, characterized by fever, skin rashes (sometimes progressing to exfoliative dermatitis and Stevens-Johnson syndrome), generalized lymphadenopathy, hepatitis and hepatospenomegaly.[9,10]

Less serious adverse effects, including gastrointestinal complaints, mild skin rashes, headaches and psychosis are managed by stopping the drug and using an alternative.

Because of the serious nature of some adverse effects of dapsone, and the fact that the drug is only weakly bactericidal, many clinicians would like to see it replaced by a safer and more potent drug for routine use in the treatment of leprosy.

RIFAMPICIN

History

Rifampicin is one of the ansamycins, first synthesized in 1959 and was introduced for the treatment of TB in 1967. It has a powerful bactericidal effect and is well-tolerated. While known to be active against *M. leprae*, it was at that time too expensive for widespread use in leprosy programs.

As with dapsone in leprosy and streptomycin in TB, monotherapy with rifampicin quickly led to the development of drug resistance. As dapsone resistance in leprosy became more widespread during the 1970s, it was clear that a combination of several active drugs (MDT) would be needed to preserve the efficacy of any drug regimen. Following the WHO Study Group report of 1982,[1] rifampicin replaced dapsone as the cornerstone of antileprosy chemotherapy, where it has remained ever since.

Resistance to rifampicin is a major issue in the control of TB, and is a potential problem for the treatment of leprosy, which could lead to treatment failure or relapse. Up to now, there is little evidence of drug resistance, but it has not been systematically searched for. A surveillance program has been established by WHO to monitor drug resistance (described in more detail in Chapter 40).

Activity

Rifampicin inhibits deoxyribonucleic acid dependent (DNA-dependent) ribonucleic acid (RNA) synthesis, by blocking RNA polymerase. A single dose of 1,500 mg in human patients reduces the number of viable bacilli to such a low level as to be undetectable in the mouse foot pad system.[11] Rifapentine was synthesized in 1965 as a derivative of rifampicin; it has a longer half-life in the body, so is theoretically more suited to being given intermittently than rifampicin.

Uses and Dosage

Because of the slow rate of growth of *M. leprae,* doubling in number every 14 days or so, rifampicin can be administered orally on a monthly basis, at an adult dose of 600 mg. For TB, rifampicin is given daily in a dose of 600 mg for adults (or 10 mg/kg).

An interesting development in the use of rifampicin is the possibility of using significantly higher doses than in the past and tolerance for higher doses is now being tested. Initially, using the lowest effective dose of rifampicin was regarded as an important cost-saving strategy. The rationale for exploring higher doses is that, because of fibrosis and other pathological processes, some bacilli may not be exposed to the same concentration of the drug as is present in the circulation and may be able to survive standard doses of rifampicin: regimens that use a higher dose may turn out to be more effective, or allow a shorter duration of treatment.[12] The relative cost of rifampicin is now greatly reduced.

Adverse Effects

A common but insignificant effect of rifampicin is to color bodily secretions (tears, urine, etc.) red or orange—this can be alarming for some patients who should be warned of the effect.

The most important adverse effect is hepatitis, which is usually not serious, unless compounded by another drug which also affects the liver. For this reason, it is unwise to give rifampicin with another hepatotoxic drug, such as ethionamide. Rifampicin also induces liver enzymes so that some other drugs may be rendered less effective, because they are metabolized more quickly—this applies in particular to oral contraceptives.

Several other reported adverse effects of rifampicin are more common when it is given 2 or 3 times per week. These include a flu-like syndrome, renal failure and thrombocytopenia. The monthly dosage used in leprosy greatly reduces the risk of these adverse effects and makes rifampicin a very safe component of MDT.

CLOFAZIMINE

History

Clofazimine, often referred to in its early days as B663, is an orange-colored iminophenazine dye, which was first synthesized in 1954 and tested with poor results as an anti-TB drug. After being found to have activity against *M. leprae* during the 1960s, it was marketed in 1969 as lamprene. At the WHO Study Group in 1981, mentioned above, clofazimine was the third drug to join dapsone and rifampicin in the multidrug regimens, which have been used throughout the world since that time.

The MDT regimens were designed by the WHO Study Group to be effective in the presence of dapsone resistance, which was known to be quite widespread at the time. In paucibacillary disease, it is calculated that the maximum bacillary load is about 10^6 organisms, which means that the problem of drug resistant mutants is insignificant; in this case rifampicin can be given alone with dapsone, even if the dapsone is ineffective.[1] In multibacillary (MB) disease, however, the large bacillary load means that an additional drug is essential to prevent the development of drug resistance, as resistant mutants can be expected to be present. Clofazimine was chosen as the additional drug because of the low risk of adverse effects, the fact that it is weakly bactericidal and the lack of any proven resistance developing to it. An additional feature that was attractive to the study group was the fact that while clofazimine is normally given either daily or three times per week, because it persists for weeks in the tissues, a monthly supervised dose could also be given to help maintain a therapeutic effect.[1]

Activity

The mode of action of clofazimine is unknown and it has minimal activity against other mycobacterial pathogens.

It has been known for some time that clofazimine has a mild immunosuppressive effect which may help in the management of erythema nodosum leprosum (ENL) reactions, although it seems not to have a useful effect in reversal reactions. It was noted, for example, that when the standard MDT regimen for MB leprosy was reduced from 24 months to 12 months, ENL appeared to be more of a problem.[13] A controlled trial of the prevention of ENL, using additional clofazimine in those at risk, is now under way.

Uses and Dosage

Clofazimine is an essential component of MB-MDT. It is given orally in a dose of 50 mg daily, with a supervised dose of 300 mg on a monthly basis.

In the treatment of ENL, higher doses may be used, but the adverse effects of high doses must be borne in mind. A suitable regime would be 300 mg daily for 1 month, 200 mg daily for the next 3–6 months and 100 mg daily thereafter, while symptoms remain.

Adverse Effects

Clofazimine causes discoloration and darkening of the skin, which is generally reversible when the drug is stopped.

In some cultures, this is regarded as major problem by some patients, but usually this can be overcome by good health education concerning the value of the drug in treating the disease.

At high doses, clofazimine builds up in the tissues and can precipitate out to form crystals, especially in the intestinal mucosa, lymph nodes and in fatty tissue. The formation of crystals in the gastrointestinal tract may lead to abdominal pain, nausea and diarrhea, which may be fatal in severe cases.

ETHIONAMIDE/PROTHIONAMIDE

History

Ethionamide and prothionamide have very similar profiles, so will be considered together. Discovered in the 1950s, the drugs are bactericidal for *M. leprae*, but less powerful than rifampicin. They have been used to treat leprosy and were considered as candidates for the new MDT regimens in 1981. The higher risk of adverse effects relegated them to a role in patients who did not wish to take clofazimine.

Before the development of MDT, prothionamide was included in a combined tablet known as isoprodian, which also contained isoniazid and dapsone. The goal was to have one tablet for the treatment of both leprosy and TB, but better and safer regimens for both diseases were soon available and its use quickly declined.

Activity

Ethionamide is similar in action to isoniazid, which inhibits the synthesis of mycobacterial cell wall components. It is bactericidal for both *M. leprae* and *M. tuberculosis*. At the present time, its only use is in the treatment of multidrug resistant TB.

Uses and Dosage

The drug may be given orally in a dose of either 250 mg or 500 mg daily. Adverse effects are more common with the higher dose.

Adverse Effects

Hepatotoxicity is the most important side effect, particularly when the drug is given with rifampicin. Gastrointestinal symptoms are also common.

FLUOROQUINOLONES

History

The quinolones include a range of broad-spectrum antibiotics, related to nalidixic acid, which was discovered in 1962. The newer fluoroquinolones have been developed since the 1980s and two in particular have a potential role in the treatment of leprosy, namely ofloxacin and, more recently, moxifloxacin. In the 1990s, ciprofloxacin, which was becoming widely used for many infections, was shown to be inactive against *M. leprae* while ofloxacin was the most active of the commercially available fluoroquinolones at that time, with a strongly bactericidal effect in mice.[14]

In the 1990s, there were a number of trials involving a combination of rifampicin, ofloxacin and minocycline (known as ROM). The seventh WHO Expert Committee on Leprosy reviewed the evidence and indicated that a single dose of ROM would be a cost-effective and suitable treatment for leprosy cases with only a single lesion.[15]

Moxifloxacin is a newer fluoroquinolone with a bactericidal activity close to that of rifampicin.[16,17]

Activity

The fluoroquinolones are broad-spectrum antibiotics through DNA-gyrase inhibition, blocking cell replication.

Uses and Dosage

Ofloxacin and moxifloxacin are both given orally in an adult dose of 400 mg monthly for leprosy, although a daily dose is used for other indications, as well as for the treatment of proven rifampicin-resistant leprosy.

Adverse Effects

Adverse effects are generally mild and include nausea, diarrhea and various effects on the nervous system, such as headaches, insomnia and dizziness. Because of an effect on the growth cartilage in young animals, the fluoroquinolones are not recommended for use in children. There is a risk of tendonitis and even tendon rupture with both ofloxacin and moxifloxacin. The monthly dosage used in leprosy reduces the likelihood of serious adverse effects with these drugs.

MINOCYCLINE

History

Minocycline is one of the tetracycline antibiotics and was synthesized in 1972. It is strongly bactericidal for *M. leprae*,[18] although bacteriostatic for other bacteria. Used in combination with rifampicin and ofloxacin (ROM) or with rifapentine and moxifloxacin (PMM),[16] minocycline could form part of a fully supervised and potent antileprosy regimen.

Activity

Minocycline has a broader spectrum of activity than the tetracyclines to which it is related. Like its relatives, the drug becomes dangerous when past its expiry date as the degradation products can cause renal damage.

Uses and Dosage

Minocycline is given orally in a dose of 100 mg monthly, as part of a supervised regimen including other bactericidal drugs, such as rifampicin and ofloxacin. Otherwise it may be given daily.

Adverse Effects

Minocycline can cause a variety of adverse effects, including nausea, diarrhea, dizziness, drowsiness, mouth sores and headache. It causes discoloration of the teeth, if given to infants or young children. As with other drugs used in leprosy, however, monthly administration greatly reduces the problem of side effects.

CLARITHROMYCIN

History

Clarithromycin is a macrolide antibiotic, related to erythromycin. Its spectrum of activity is broader than that of erythromycin, extending to a number of mycobacteria, including *M. leprae* and *M. ulcerans*. It is bactericidal for *M. leprae*, although less potent than minocycline.[18]

Activity

Clarithromycin inhibits bacterial protein synthesis.

Uses and Dosage

The normal dose of clarithromycin is 500 mg daily. Monthly use in leprosy has not been tested in a clinical trial, but it would most likely be as effective as other bactericidal drugs used in this way.

Adverse Effects

Clarithromycin can cause gastrointestinal upset and effects on the central nervous system, such as dizziness, irritability, hallucinations, a metallic taste in the mouth and confusion. There may be interactions with other drugs, especially those used in the treatment of human immunodeficiency virus (HIV) infection.

BEDAQUILINE

History

Bedaquiline is a diarylquinolone that has been heralded as the first major new drug for TB control to be developed for several decades. It was launched in 2004 after years of preclinical development and efficacy trials began to appear in the literature after 2010. Previously known as R207910, it was shown to have an activity against *M. leprae* in mice similar to that of rifampicin and moxifloxacin.[7]

Activity

Bedaquiline affects the proton pump for adenosine 5′-triphosphate (ATP) synthetase, thus disrupting bacterial energy metabolism.

Uses

Bedaquiline is being used for TB, especially for drug-resistant cases. While it is potentially useful in leprosy, its current high cost and the availability of other alternatives for leprosy, make it less likely to be used routinely in the near future.

Adverse Effects

Bedaquiline, like clofazimine, persists for long periods in the tissues, and can cause arrhythmias and a prolongation of the QT interval.

PERSISTERS

Bacilli are termed persisters when they show tolerance to antibacterial agents, without having developed genetic mutations associated with drug resistance. It is assumed that such bacilli are present in a dormant and nondividing state, as they can later be shown to be sensitive to the antibiotics being used.

The underlying mechanisms for this phenomenon are obscure, but it has been known for many years that viable, drug-sensitive leprosy bacilli can sometimes be grown from patient material, after an adequate course of treatment.[19,20]

RELAPSE

Relapse denotes the reappearance of clinical leprosy after the successful completion of a course of recommended antileprosy treatment. The reappearance of leprosy may be indicated by new skin lesions and/or an increase in the bacteriological index of two or more units. There are a number of situations, which can mimic a true relapse and also a number of possible causes of a true relapse, and it may be difficult to know what has, in fact, happened in any particular case. The important question for the clinician, however, is whether the patient needs further antibiotic treatment and, if so, which regimen should be prescribed.

Situations that mimic a relapse include:
- It may be that the first course of treatment was inadequate, either because the drugs were not taken as prescribed, or

because of a misclassification—cases may be classified and treated as paucibacillary, when they are in fact MB, a situation that may be more common when skin smears are not routinely done. A few cases with less than six lesions do have MB disease, indicated by a positive smear. In these cases, a new course of MDT is required.

- The reappearance of leprosy lesions may be a manifestation of a reversal reaction, rather than a relapse; this is often difficult to resolve, although the timing of the supposed relapse may give an indication in that most reversal reactions occur within 5 years after the end of treatment, whereas most true relapses occur more than 5 years after the end of treatment.[21] Histopathology may be helpful in deciding the appropriate management of the case.

A true relapse may be caused by a number of underlying problems:

- Relapse due to 'persisters' in which the bacilli remain sensitive to the standard antibiotics.
- Reinfection from an outside source, which cannot be distinguished from a true relapse, unless strain-typing has been done at the time of the original diagnosis and again at the time of the new episode.
- Relapse may be due to drug resistance, which has prevented the complete clearance of the disease with the first course of treatment.[22]

In general, relapse after MDT is rare, although published studies give rates anywhere between 0% and 20%, probably reflecting differences in previous treatment history, treatment adherence, definition of relapse, length of follow-up, and pretreatment bacillary index.[23]

The vast majority of relapse cases can be treated with a full course of standard MDT, although every effort should be made to test for drug resistance. A regimen for rifampicin resistant cases is available, but because it is an onerous regimen for the patient, it should not be prescribed unless rifampicin resistance has been proven in the laboratory—clinical suspicion alone is not acceptable as sufficient grounds for using this regimen. The WHO has recommended a drug regimen for the rare cases of proven rifampicin resistance—this involves daily treatment for 6 months, comprising clofazimine 50 mg and any two of the following: ofloxacin 400 mg, minocycline 100 mg or clarithromycin 500 mg—followed by daily treatment for 18 months, with clofazimine 50 mg and either ofloxacin 400 mg or minocycline 100 mg.

FUTURE REGIMENS

The goals for future regimes include the following essentials:

- Well-tolerated with a minimal risk of adverse effects.
- Highly bactericidal effect in order to minimize the duration of treatment.
- Fully supervised regimen in order to minimize noncompliance.
- Suppressive effect on leprosy reactions in order to minimize complications.
- Acceptable cost.

A most likely new regimen for leprosy would include rifampicin (or rifapentine as a longer acting alternative), a fluoroquinolone, such as ofloxacin or moxifloxacin, and minocycline due to their potent bactericidal effects

Table 30.1: Characteristics of antileprosy drugs (Adapted from WHO[1] and Ji and Grosset[16])

Drug	MIC (μg/mL)	Daily adult dosage (mg)[a]	Ratio of peak serum concentration to MIC[b]	Bactericidal activity	Killing power of a single dose: % M. leprae killed[c]
Rifampicin	0.3	600	30	High	92.1
Dapsone	0.003	100	500	Low	
Clofazimine[d]		50		Low	
Ethionamide	0.05	375	60	Intermediate	
Clarithromycin		500		High	74.9
Moxifloxacin		400		High	92.1
Ofloxacin		400		High	60.2
Rifapentine		600		High	99.6
Minocycline		100		High	

MIC is the Minimal Inhibitory Concentration.

[a] Antibiotics are typically given daily for most infections, but because of the very slow growth of *M. leprae,* monthly administration of bactericidal drugs (using the same dose as is normally given daily) has proved effective in leprosy, which reduces both the cost and the incidence of adverse effects.

[b] Ratio of peak serum concentration in man, after a single dose, to MIC determined in the mouse.

[c] The calculation is based on the proportions of viable organisms in the mouse foot-pad system, between untreated controls and treated groups.

[d] Because of uneven distribution, estimate of the MIC was not possible.

(Table 30.1).[16] This could be given as a monthly regimen under full supervision, but it is not clear yet whether the duration could be less than 12 months for all cases. Further research would be needed to indicate the length of time required for treatment in order to minimize relapses. It is also too early to say whether a higher dose of rifampicin or rifapentine would permit a much shorter regimen to be used, and if so, how much shorter than 12 months it could be. Bedaquiline could be part of a future regimen, although it remains to be seen whether adverse effects will limit how widely it can be used.

CONCLUSION

Chemotherapy for leprosy is highly successful in curing the bacterial infection and there are a number of potent antibiotics which have not yet been used routinely for leprosy, but are still in reserve.

There are two aspects of treatment for leprosy in which the current regimens have failed. Firstly, as mentioned in the introduction to this chapter, transmission has not been interrupted and it appears that we need new tools to be able to break the chain of transmission in leprosy.

Secondly, a considerable proportion of people who develop leprosy go on to develop signs and symptoms of nerve damage, and much of this damage remains as permanent impairment causing disability and severe social consequences. Chemotherapy does not reduce nerve damage once it is present, although if treatment is started early enough, much of the potential risk for future nerve damage is removed. Many people affected by leprosy do not consider themselves 'cured', if they still have signs of nerve damage and other stigmata of the disease, while from a bacteriological standpoint they are labeled as cured once they have completed a course of MDT.

REFERENCES

1. World Health Organization. Chemotherapy of leprosy for control programmes. Technical Report Series No.675, Geneva. 1982.
2. Meima A, Gupte MD, van Oortmarssen GJ, et al. Trends in leprosy case detection rates. Int J Lepr Other Mycobact Dis. 1997;65(3):305-19.
3. Meima A, Richardus JH, Habbema JD. Trends in leprosy case detection worldwide since 1985. Lepr Rev. 2004;75(1):19-33.
4. Scheelbeek PF, Balagon MV, Orcullo FM, et al. A retrospective study of the epidemiology of leprosy in Cebu: an eleven-year profile. PLoS Negl Trop Dis. 2013;7(9):e2444.
5. Moet FJ, Pahan D, Oskam L, et al. Effectiveness of single dose rifampicin in preventing leprosy in close contacts of patients with newly diagnosed leprosy: cluster randomised controlled trial. BMJ. 2008;336:761-4.
6. Duthie MS, Saunderson P, Reed SG. The potential for vaccination in leprosy elimination: new tools for targeted interventions. Mem Inst Oswaldo Cruz. 2012;107:190-6.
7. Ji B, Chauffour A, Andries K, et al. Bactericidal activities of R207910 and other newer antimicrobial agents against *Mycobacterium leprae* in mice. Antimicrob Agents Chemother. 2006;50:1558-60.
8. Deps P, Guerra P, Nasser S, et al. Hemolytic anemia in patients receiving daily dapsone for the treatment of leprosy. Lepr Rev. 2012;83(3):305-7.
9. Agrawal S, Agarwalla A. Dapsone hypersensitivity syndrome: a clinico-epidemiological review. J Dermatol. 2005;32:883-9.
10. Pandey B, Shrestha K, Lewis J, et al. Mortality due to dapsone hypersensitivity syndrome complicating multi-drug therapy for leprosy in Nepal. Trop Doct. 2007;37:162-3.
11. Levy L, Shepard CC, Fasal P. The bactericidal effect of rifampicin on *M. leprae* in man: a) single doses of 600, 900 and 1200 mg; and b) daily doses of 300 mg. Int J Lepr Other Mycobact Dis. 1976;44(1-2):183-7.
12. Steingart KR, Jotblad S, Robsky K, et al. Higher-dose rifampin for the treatment of pulmonary tuberculosis: a systematic review. Int J Tuberc Lung Dis. 2011;15(3):305-16.
13. Balagon M, Saunderson PR, Gelber RH. Does clofazimine prevent erythema nodosum leprosum (ENL) in leprosy? A retrospective study, comparing the experience of multibacillary patients receiving either 12 or 24 months WHO-MDT. Lepr Rev. 2011;82(3):213-21.
14. Ji B, Grosset J. Ofloxacin for the treatment of leprosy. Acta Leprol. 1991;7(4):321-6.
15. World Health Organization Expert Committee on Leprosy. Seventh report. Technical Report Series No. 874, Geneva. 1998.
16. Ji B, Grosset J. Combination of rifapentine-moxifloxacin-minocycline (PMM) for the treatment of leprosy. Lepr Rev. 2000;71:S81-7.
17. Pardillo FE, Burgos J, Fajardo TT, et al. Powerful bactericidal activity of moxifloxacin in human leprosy. Antimicrob Agents Chemother. 2008;52:3113-7.
18. Ji B, Perani EG, Grosset JH. Effectiveness of clarithromycin and minocycline alone and in combination against experimental *Mycobacterium leprae* infection in mice. Antimicrob Agents Chemother. 1991;35(3):579-81.
19. Waters MF, Rees RJ, Pearson JM, et al. Rifampicin for lepromatous leprosy: nine years' experience. Br Med J. 1978;1(6106):133-6.
20. Shetty VP, Mistry NF, Wakade AV, et al. BCG immunotherapy as an adjunct to chemotherapy in BL-LLpatients - its effect on clinical regression, reaction severity, nerve function, lepromin conversion, bacterial/antigen clearance and 'persister' *M. leprae*. Lepr Rev 2013;84(1):23-40.
21. Balagon MF, Cellona RV, Cruz ED, et al. Long-term relapse risk of multibacillary leprosy after completion of 2 years of multiple drug therapy (WHO-MDT) in Cebu, Philippines. Am J Trop Med Hyg. 2009;81(5):895-9.
22. Williams DL, Hagino T, Sharma R, et al. Primary multidrug-resistant leprosy, United States. Emerg Infect Dis. 2013;19(1):179-81.
23. Maghanoy A, Mallari I, Balagon M, et al. Relapse study in smear positive multibacillary (MB) leprosy after 1 year who-multi-drug therapy (MDT) in Cebu, Philippines. Lepr Rev. 2011;82(1):65-9.

Chemotherapy: Development and Evolution of WHO-MDT and Newer Treatment Regimens

VV Pai, RR Rao, V Halwai

INTRODUCTION

Leprosy, one of the major diseases of mankind, has been declared eliminated in many endemic countries (despite seemingly unsurmountable odds), primarily due to the WHO multidrug therapy (MDT), political will, donor agencies, non-governmental organizations (NGOs) and committed health workers. Development and implementation of MDT has transformed leprosy into a curable disease. As per WHO documents, since the introduction of MDT in 1981, an estimated 16 million patients have been cured globally and disabilities have been prevented in some 4 million individuals.[1,2] The seemingly great success of MDT had prompted the World Health Assembly in 1991 to call for elimination of leprosy as a public health problem by the year 2000.[3]

However, a recent review of the public health aspects of scenario of leprosy by Rao observed that though most countries have succeeded in achieving the target of elimination, the incidence rates have continued to remain high in several countries.[4] Despite free MDT being available through integrated health facilities, owing to stigma and other factors, many patients especially of multibacillary (MB) type, delay treatment resulting in irreversible disabilities and continued transmission of the disease. Inadequate surveillance, poor research and lack of dissemination of accurate information have added to the problem of not developing more effective strategies to eradicate leprosy.

SOME SIGNIFICANT LANDMARKS IN THE TREATMENT OF LEPROSY AND THE EVOLUTION OF MDT

Until 1941, there was no truly effective antileprosy drug, apart from hydnocarpus (*Chaulmoogra*) oil which was in use since centuries in India and China. The only remedy for leprosy patients was isolation/segregation.

Dapsone

In 1941, Guy Faget first used a disubstituted derivative of dapsone (Promin) intravenously in treating leprosy at the National Leprosarium, Carville, USA. It was first used for the treatment of leprosy by Cochrane in India in 1946.[5] Later, Lowe and Smith in 1949 reported on the successful use of oral diaminodiphenylsulfone (DDS).[5] Dapsone is administered orally in a daily dose of 1–2 mg/kg body weight and it shows clinical improvement within 3–6 months. It is remarkably well-tolerated and side effects are uncommon.

Rifampicin

The first results of treatment of leprosy patients with rifampicin were reported in 1970.[6-8] In the 1970s, there were wide differences of opinion about rifampicin dosage (150–900 mg daily), dose intervals (daily, twice weekly, weekly or on 2 consecutive days every 4 weeks) and duration (from a single dose to up to 7 years) of treatment. Later the recommended dosage of rifampicin was 450–600 mg daily.

Languillon et al. were the first to report on the high efficacy, good tolerability and practicability of the supervised once monthly (1,200 mg oral dose) schedule as a component of the combination therapy in lepromatous leprosy (LL).[9]

Later, Yawalkar et al. confirmed these findings on the basis of Ciba-Geigy's International, multicentric, single-blind, comparative trial carried out in Brazil, India and Senegal.[10] In this trial the clinical, bacteriological and histopathological effects of adding rifampicin (450 mg daily or 1,200 mg once monthly) in a supervised single dose to dapsone 50 mg daily, in 93 previously untreated with lepromatous leprosy patients were practically identical.

Clofazimine

In 1962, Brown and Hogerzeil first reported on the efficacy of clofazimine in leprosy patients in Nigeria.[11] The drug has a mild bactericidal action on *Mycobacterium leprae* and its accumulation within the macrophages is advantageous and results in inhibition of intracellular multiplication of *M. leprae*. Clofazimine is effective when given daily or on alternate days. The clinical response to a 50–100 mg daily dose of clofazimine is almost similar to that seen with 100 mg of dapsone although the effect is slightly slow to come.

Sequence of Significant Events in Treatment of Leprosy[12]

In 1941, Guy Faget first used a disubstituted derivative of dapsone in the treatment of leprosy. In 1962, clofazimine was confirmed to be effective in treatment of leprosy based on evidence in mouse foot pad responses. In 1964, the first confirmed case of dapsone resistance was reported by Petit and Rees.[13] In 1970, Rees et al. demonstrated rifampicin as the most potent bactericidal drug against leprosy.[7] In 1972, Shepard suggested use of combined rifampicin and acedapsone therapy to reduce drug resistance.[14] In 1974, Waters et al. demonstrated the existence of persistence of viable *M. leprae* in lepromatous patients treated with dapsone for 10–12 years.[15]

In 1982, WHO Study Group recommended multidrug regimens for the treatment of both MB and PB leprosy patients.

Reasons for Shift from Monotherapy to MDT

Until 1982, the chemotherapy of patients with leprosy relied almost entirely on dapsone monotherapy. It is interesting to note that the first multidrug combination project to treat MB leprosy patients was started in 1972, in Malta, by Professor E Freerkson of Borstel, Germany. All the registered patients with leprosy were treated with a combined regimen,

comprising initially a daily oral administration of dapsone, prothionamide and isoniazid called isoprodian. Later dapsone, rifampicin, prothionamide and isoniazid were given in a combined tablet named Isoprodian-R.[16] The duration of treatment was dependent on initial clinical, bacteriological and histopathological status. Minimum treatment was for 5 months and the longest was for 89 months.[16]

A recent report on the follow-up investigation of the first MDT Malta project indicates that the overall response to the therapy was excellent with an extremely low relapse rate. During the 30 years of the project the incidence of leprosy steadily decreased, continuing a decline that had started at least two decades earlier and Freerkson declared the disease eradicated from Malta in 2001.[17]

Three main factors have been responsible for the development of MDT: (1) drug resistance, (2) bacterial persistence, and (3) defaulting. In addition, some of the other reasons in favor of introducing MDT were:

- To eliminate persisters and reduce the incidence of post-treatment relapse as compared with monotherapy.
- To reduce side effects due to prolonged use of a drug.
- Increase cost-effectiveness by a shorter duration of treatment leading to an earlier release of patients from control.

Persisters

Persisters are viable, drug susceptible, bacilli that can be recovered from lepromatous patients after many years of apparently successful treatment with antileprosy drugs.

Approximately 37% of the 131 patients with lepromatous leprosy (LL) admitted into the THELEP controlled clinical trials in Bamako and Chingleput were found to have dapsone resistant organisms indicating primary dapsone resistance demonstrating the need for MDT regimens. However, the primary objective of the THELEP controlled clinical trials in Bamako and Chingleput was to compare several combination drug regimens among previously untreated lepromatous leprosy patients to detect persisting *M. leprae*. The results demonstrated that persisting *M. leprae* were detected in approximately 9% of all patients without relation to regimen and duration of treatment. This study established the strong support to the multidrug regimen recommended for treatment of MB leprosy.[18] The significance of surviving drug sensitive persisters has remained debatable until recently. It has been suggested that they die a natural death during and subsequent to treatment and thereafter are of not much consequence. In the past, it had been thought that relapses were due to emergence of resistance. However, recent findings based on long-term follow-up suggest drug-sensitive bacilli to be a cause of relapse, as the relapsed patients treated with same regimens showed good response indicating persisters as the probable cause.

Rifampicin-Based Combined Therapy for MB Patients

In a study, rifampicin was given in a single dose of 1,500 mg in 12 untreated lepromatous leprosy patients followed by dapsone 10 mg daily for 4 weeks and later dapsone given in a dose of 50 mg daily. Mouse foot pad results indicated no multiplication of *M. leprae*.[19] In another study of 17 untreated lepromatous leprosy patients, rifampicin was administered in a dose of 600 mg daily for a short period (duration not specified). Mouse foot pad studies indicated no evidence of multiplication of *M. leprae*.[20] The studies strongly indicated the powerful bactericidal effect of rifampicin against *M. leprae* paving the way for future investigations.

In fact, during the decade between the mid-1970s and the mid-1980s, 12 rifampicin containing combined regimens were tested among lepromatous leprosy patients in the Institute Marchoux.[21] In another study, 384 cases were followed up for more than 1 year, the mean duration of follow-up being 63 ± 30.3 months after completion of treatment. Relapse was confirmed by the presence of viable *M. leprae* in skin biopsy specimens. Relapses occurred late, about 5 ± 2 years after stopping treatment, the shorter the duration of rifampicin administration the earlier the appearance of relapse. The total relapse rates ranged from 2.9% to 27.8% and the relapse rates per 100 patient—years of observation ranged from 0.8 to 6.9. Among the 12 regimens, only the WHO-MDT yielded an acceptable relapse rate.[22]

WHO STUDY GROUP ON CHEMOTHERAPY OF LEPROSY[23]

When WHO Study Group on Chemotherapy of leprosy met in 1981, leprosy control programs faced a variety of serious constraints. Widespread secondary dapsone resistance was reported in 19% of patients when treated with dapsone monotherapy. Primary dapsone resistance mostly of low-grade was detected in 50% of newly diagnosed cases. Further cases of resistance of *M. leprae* to rifampicin and thioamides had been reported among these patients receiving these drugs as monotherapy.

After reviewing the situation related to dapsone resistance, persisters, early development of resistance to monotherapy even with potent drugs and no consensus on duration of therapy, WHO Study Group on Chemotherapy of Leprosy for control programs, in 1981 recommended treatment with more than one drug for 24 months or till smear negativity in MB leprosy and for 6 months in paucibacillary leprosy.[24] Because subsequently most data on the effects of limiting therapy to a 24 month course (rather than continuing until skin smear results are negative) were favorable, the WHO Study Group on Chemotherapy of Leprosy recommended at its meeting in 1994 that all MB patients be given the standard WHO MDT regimen for a fixed period of 24 months.[25]

Multibacillary leprosy—for adults, the recommended regimen is:

Rifampicin: 600 mg once a month—supervised

Dapsone: 100 mg daily—self-administered

Clofazimine: 300 mg once a month—supervised and 50 mg daily—self-administered

Duration: 24 months

Paucibacillary leprosy— for adults the recommended standard regimen is:

Rifampicin: 600 mg once a month—supervised

Dapsone: 100 mg daily—self-administered

Duration: 6 months

Children should receive appropriately reduced doses of the above drugs. MB patients should complete 24 monthly doses within 36 months period and paucibacillary patients 6 monthly doses within 9 months period. It was recommended that patients receive their drugs in monthly calendar blister packs.

In 1981, WHO also recommended that patients be classified as PB leprosy with bacteriological index (BI) of up to 2+ and as MB leprosy with BI more than 2+ at any site in the initial skin smear. It was introduced to simplify disease recognition and to ensure that patients were apparently treated with MDT.[23] In 1988, it was recommended that a positive smear at any site was sufficient for inclusion of the patient in MB category. Later the need for skin smear was dropped altogether so that the current classification includes any patient with 6 or more lesions under MB.·

HISTORY OF MDT

Bombay Leprosy Project (BLP) as an NGO engaged in research in leprosy, initiated rifampicin and clofazimine along with dapsone for the treatment of smear-positive leprosy cases (BL, LL types) for the first time in the slums of Bombay in 1977–1978, during which time WHO coordinated THELEP trials were on in Chingleput in Tamil Nadu state of India and in Bamako, Mali.

Rifampicin was administered as a single dose of 1,200 mg to 1,500 mg once a month along with daily dapsone till bacteriological negativity was achieved. Since then, several studies on rationalization of treatment have been taken up from time to time but at a slower pace.

Controversy over Intensive Treatment with Rifampicin

Soon after WHO recommended MDT in 1981, BLP was one of the first to start WHO-MDT to treat leprosy patients in

Bombay. The drugs were supplied by the Government of India in a small quantity. Initially all the skin smear positive MB leprosy patients were administered rifampicin daily for 21 days. This was followed by monthly pulse doses. The patients were treated till smear negativity was reached.

The Indian Association of Leprologists (IAL) organized a workshop in Karigiri in 1983 and recommended the use of rifampicin 600 mg daily for 21 days followed by the monthly pulse dose as recommended by WHO. National Leprosy Eradication Program (NLEP) accepted this recommendation initially and later changed over to 14 days intensive therapy for their district MDT programs.

The multidrug combination project on a mass scale was implemented in Wardha, in 1981. Intensive therapy for 14 days with rifampicin was practiced.

In a study conducted in seven leprosy colonies in and around Bombay city, it was observed that after 21 days of initial intensive therapy and continued MDT till bacteriological smear negativity and follow-up after 13 years of 100 smear-positive cases, no relapses were encountered. This study of highly smear-positive cases showed that there was no bacteriological relapse or reaction over a period of 10 years of post-MDT follow-up.[26]

Switching over to Monthly Dose of Rifampicin

Bombay Leprosy Project reported its findings in 1986 on the comparable outcome of conversion of smear positive to negative, with and without initial intensive therapy with rifampicin.[27]

This study indicated the efficacy of WHO regimen over daily rifampicin therapy. Pharmacologists and dermatologists were initially hesitant to accept the efficiency of rifampicin given as monthly pulse dose.

Fixed Duration Treatment for 24 Months

A key question for the study group was whether the WHO-MDT regimen for MB disease could now be fixed at 24 months. Most control programs started practicing WHO MDT for 24 months.[28] Becx-Bleumink reviewed the literature and recommended that treatment for MB patients should be limited to 24 months for operational reasons.[29]

Analysis of BI of 584 MB leprosy patients who had completed MDT as per recommendations of the WHO and IAL, showed a smear conversion rate of 56% at 24 doses and 66% at 36 doses. This study also indicated that daily initial administration of rifampicin for 21 days did not show any distinct advantage over WHO regimen. Taking BI as a parameter of evidence, the results indicated distinct improvement over the performance achieved through dapsone monotherapy during earlier period.[27.]This contribution assisted the policy makers to shorten the duration of treatment from "till smear negative" to a fixed duration of 24 months. In spite of the WHO recommendations, leprologists were hesitant to stop

treatment after 24 months. At the first meeting on this issue called by NLEP, in Delhi, selected leprologists were asked to stop treatment after 24 months on a trial basis especially in cases with low BI.

It was only in 1990 that the NLEP introduced 24 months fixed MDT (FDT-24) in modified MDT district programs for the convenience of the PHC doctors who were supposed to look after treatment of leprosy patients. Later, since 1992, the rest of the country started practicing FDT-24 irrespective of BI grading.[30] Some leprologists and pathologists did have reservations earlier, in following the FDT-24 regimen especially in patients with high BI.

Fixed Duration Treatment for 12 Months

In 1991, BLP reported its observations on stopping treatment after 12 months of MDT in skin smear-positive MB leprosy patients and provided follow-up data on 190 patients which influenced policy makers to further reduce the duration of MDT from 24 months to 12 months. WHO meanwhile started double-blind field trial of MDT 12 months and other regimens in 1992. In 1997, the WHO Expert Committee on Leprosy and NLEP recommended FDT, MDT-12 months for MB leprosy and MDT-6 months for PB leprosy in the program.[24] This was not accepted by all clinicians and they continued to treat MB patients with 24 doses. Even today, selected NGOs still practice FDT-24 especially in cases with high BI as their organizational policy. Their fear is based on the report from Bamako, Mali and JALMA, Agra, who reported high relapses in patients with BI more than 4.0+. This fear is still haunting many clinicians and even policy makers. NLEP of India "In training manual for medical officers, 2009" put a foot note stating "Rarely, specialists may consider treating a person with high BI for more than 12 months; decision is based on clinical and bacteriological evidence."

Bombay Leprosy Project reported its findings as early as 1984, on smear conversion in smear-positive drop out patients after receiving treatment for less than 12 months. The findings of this investigation were considered (along with those collected by WHO worldwide on treatment of drop out patients), by the "WHO Expert Committee on Leprosy" in 1997 as an important authentic data to reduce the duration of treatment from 24 months to 12 months. Earlier BLP had reported their observations on very low number of relapses in patients given FDT for 24 or even 12 months. BLP observed 11 relapses in patients with initial BI of 3+ and above over a period of 5–25 years of follow-up among patients treated with FDT-24 (six relapses) as well as FDT-12 (five relapses) regimen.[31]

In a retrospective analysis of 730 MB (545 males, 185 females) patients included since 1999–2010 and treated with 12 months MDT-MB with a follow-up period ranging from 9 months to 10 years, it was observed that nearly all patients had clearance of skin lesions including histopathological/bacteriological improvement. Only 13 (1.7%) patients relapsed and it was concluded that the recommendation for 12 months MDT-MB for all MB leprosy patients is robust and operationally practical, a decision which seems logical.[32]

Rationale for Shortening the Duration of MDT to 12 Months

In 1997, the 7th WHO Expert Committee on Leprosy explored the possibility of shortening the duration of MDT (MB) to 12 months as it would facilitate better treatment compliance if the duration of MDT could be further shortened without significantly compromising the efficacy.[24]

The rationale being that rifampicin kills more than 99.999% of the viable organisms with 3 monthly doses and rifampicin resistant mutants are likely to be eliminated by 3–6 months with coadministration of dapsone and clofazimine. It was therefore, considered that the elimination of drug susceptible organisms is almost entirely due to the bactericidal effect of the initial few doses of rifampicin. The major role of the dapsone-clofazimine component in MDT is to ensure the elimination of rifampicin resistant mutants from the bacterial population.

The efficacy of standard and shorter MDT regimens for MB leprosy has also been compared in Malawi in which 305 MB patients were treated with 18 or 30 monthly doses of MDT. No relapses were observed in either group after treatment was completed. It was concluded that 18 monthly doses of MDT taken within 24 months may be sufficient for the treatment of MB leprosy.[24,33]

Information on the clinical and bacteriological progress of patients who fail to complete treatment may shed some light on the efficacy of MDT regimens of shorter duration than the standard WHO regimen. In a separate retrospective study, 234 defaulters with MB leprosy were examined at the time of retrieval after a mean period of 7.5 years. 139 patients had taken treatment for 12 months or less and 95 were treated with 13–23 month doses and the results were comparable to the group treated for 24 months. In 1998, skin smear was done away with as the reports from several field laboratories were not found to be dependable in the sense that they would not match with the clinical diagnosis. There could be many causes for such problems pertaining to several operational factors and skills of the field staff, e.g. (poor staining, poor quality of smears taken, etc.).

In a recent review, Malathi and Thappa commenting on FDT and its limitations and opportunities, observed that a fine balance needs to be maintained between achieving a cure for the patients and at the same time protecting the society from a public health point of view.[34]

Multidrug Therapy Adherence[35]

Adherence is defined as the extent to which the patient's behavior matches recommendations from the prescriber. In general, adherence can be categorized into factors related to the patient, social environment, the health system including health facility and workers, the disease and its causative agent and treatment factors.

Adherence with MDT or for that matter any form of chemotherapy in the treatment of leprosy is important to complete the duration of treatment and to minimize the risk of relapse and also avoid the emergence of drug resistance. Poor adherence with MDT has also been associated with the risk of reactions and disability. Leprosy program routinely use treatment completion and defaulter rates as indirect measures of treatment adherence. Patients with PB and MB leprosy must complete their courses of six doses and 12 doses of MDT within a time frame of 9 months and 18 months respectively. The supervised monthly dose, use of patient friendly blister calendar packs and shortened regimens are all health system factors that can improve adherence. Few studies assessing adherence have been published in the past 15 years and therefore the issue demands further investigations in the context of current integrated scenario.

A recent epidemiological study from Brazil by Chichava et al. which included 1,076 individuals diagnosed with leprosy identified 351 (32.6%) participants who had interrupted MDT.[36] The median time of interruption was 15 days and a maximum of 3 years. In this open questionnaire based study, the most common reason given by the respondents was nonavailability of medicines at the health care center, forgetfulness to take medicines, and drug related adverse events. The less common findings reported were acknowledging not having leprosy, difficult to access health care center, pregnancy and stigma related issues.

In another literature search study by Weiand et al. observed that a number of methods have been used to assess adherence including questionnaires, pill counts, testing urine for presence of dapsone besides treatment completion rates as proxy measures of adherence.[35] Adherence is therefore very important in leprosy and regular assessment of medication adherence with constructive feedback and counseling of patients is likely to be beneficial.

POST-TREATMENT SURVEILLANCE

The responsibility of health system toward the patients does not cease with the completion of chemotherapy. Surveillance has two main objectives, detection of a relapse and the recognition of reactive phenomenon occurring after completion of MDT. Patients should continue to have access to health facilities for detection and treatment of relapse and management of reactions.[37]

Since many relapses occur late, 5-year post-treatment follow-up period may not be adequate. Surveillance period of 8–10 years or even more will be ideal.

Stating reaction as a sign of activity have led to the interpretation that reaction warrants chemotherapy even after completion of MDT in certain number of patients who do not respond to oral steroid therapy for few weeks. In our experience, even macular lesions reappearing during surveillance respond to steroid therapy, which is generally recommended for classical reversal reaction. Experience is to be gained with respect to the further follow-up of such patients.[38]

Relapses after MDT

Relapse after MDT remains low even after almost 30 years of its widespread use. Some reports suggest that the risk of relapse is higher in a subset of patients with a pre-MDT average BI of 4+ or more. Recently published WHO Operational Guidelines recommend that it may be advisable to treat an MB patient with high BI for more than 12 months, taking careful consideration of the clinical and bacteriological evidence. A number of studies have reported that retreatment of relapses following dapsone monotherapy or MDT with another course of standard MDT regimens is highly successful.

Although demonstration of organisms resistant to dapsone is relatively common probably because of pre-existing dapsone-resistant strains, there are reports on organisms resistant to rifampicin, clofazimine or quinolones after completion of treatment with MDT. Most investigators consider that a relapse after MDT is most likely to be due to persisters and only rarely due to resistance. This is borne out by the results of molecular tests on biopsies from a small number of relapsed cases[2] and also due to the fact that patients with true relapse respond well to the WHO-MDT on same duration.

Several risk factors for relapses in leprosy have been suggested, including persisters, reinfection, drug resistance, inadequate/irregular therapy, use of monotherapy, high initial BI, number and even size of skin lesions and lepromin negativity. The risk of relapse in patients coinfected with HIV

is a possibility and needs further investigation. Currently, diagnosis of relapse is based mainly on clinical features such as appearance of a new lesion and a significantly increased BI. Some studies have demonstrated the utility of histopathological changes and simple serological tests in confirming the diagnosis of relapse. There is a possibility of developing molecular tests based on PCR for early identification of relapses. There are several PCR methods to amplify different gene stretches of *M. leprae.* The RNA targeting probes are 10–100 fold more sensitive than deoxyribonucleic acid (DNA) targeting probes and can be used to monitor responses to therapy and also for diagnosing true relapses while differentiating them from reactions.[39]

The current recommendations for leprosy control program include stopping active surveillance in view of the very low relapse rates and a phased integration of leprosy services with the general health services.[40] However, it is necessary to identify the relapses early before they transmit the infection to a large segment of the densely populated urban population. Though relapses are few in relation to the number of leprosy cases who completed treatment, it has not been adequately documented at the community level. Relapses have been detected in MB patients treated with MDT and various other short course chemotherapy (SCC) regimens of variable period at BLP (Mumbai) after a mean period of 8–10 years of RFT (Fig. 31.1).[41]

Biological factors influencing relapse following any duration of MDT may be quite different from those influencing decline of BI and attainment of negativity. Long-term observation to assess relapse after FDT for 12 months is required.[38]

The issue of relapses following WHO MDT is obviously of great significance and several studies have been initiated to provide estimates of the risk involved. The ultimate test of chemotherapeutic effectiveness of any regimen is the relapse rate among patients who have completed the prescribed

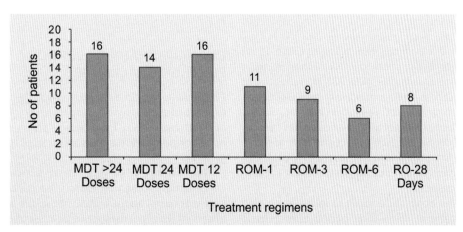

Fig. 31.1: Relapse (BI +ve) after various treatment regimens
Abbreviations: MDT, multidrug therapy; ROM, rifampicin, ofloxacin and minocycline; RO, rifampicin and ofloxacin.

course of treatment. In leprosy, relapse occurs long after completion of treatment with any regimen, so a prolonged follow-up of treated patients is required.

Relapse rates after MDT for 24 months have been negligible. Thus in the two THELEP supported field trials carried out in Karigiri and Polambakkam in Tamil Nadu, India, not a single relapse was reported for at least 4 years among the 2,000 MB patients whose treatment was stopped after achieving smear negativity.[22]

In a study conducted in Malawi, relapses were reported after 4 years at the rate of 0.65 per 100 person-years and from Indonesia 0.12 per 100 person-years after 5 years.

In a survey organized by WHO, the cumulative risk of relapse was 0.77% for MB leprosy treated for 24 months or till skin smear negativity and 1.07% for PB leprosy, 9 years after completion of MDT. Similar results have been reported in several leprosy elimination programs and research projects indicating that the overall relapse rate was less than 1.0%.[24] In a pilot survey in which 92,194 MB patients were covered, 467 relapses were reported, giving an overall relapse rate of 0.23 per 100 person-years. In the second extended questionnaire survey, information was obtained from 28 selected centers on patients treated with MDT for 24 months or till smear negativity between 1982 and 1990. A total of 20,141 MB patients were observed of whom 1,414 were followed for 9 years. Sixty seven patients were reported as relapse during a follow up period of 80,000 person-years giving a cumulative relapse rate of 0.77%.[42] It was reported at the IAL workshop on Cure of Leprosy held at Konark, Orissa, India, that till March 2003, only 2,563 cases have been diagnosed as relapse out of 743,224 cases treated with MDT.[43] In a study by Jamet et al. the overall relapse rate was reported to be as high as 20% in a group of 35 MB patients treated with 2 years of MDT, after a mean period of 27–84 months of follow-up.[44]

In our experience, a total of 51 cases of true relapses in MB leprosy with bacterial positivity were observed as late as 10–15 years after stopping the treatment irrespective of the treatment regimens.[45] All relapses were diagnosed in the clinic and in the referral center and as they were not from a defined and specific population, relapse rate cannot be worked out. However, it indicates that relapses occur in all types of regimens irrespective of any combination of drugs.

In patients who relapsed after WHO-MDT, retreatment with the same regimen showed a good response indicating persisters or drug sensitive bacilli to be the cause of relapse. In line with such relapses, Shetty and coworkers have found persisters (viable *M. leprae*) in 20% of skin and 30% of nerve biopsies of MB patients treated with 24 months of MB-MDT.[46] The same workers have also reported persistence of viable bacilli in treated PB patients.

A study by Desikan et al. undertaken to follow-up highly bacillated leprosy patients for a long period after release from treatment (RFT) reported a low relapse rate.[47] About

660 patients with an initial bacterial positivity of 4+, 5+ or 6+ who had undergone WHO MB MDT-24 were followed up. They were reviewed twice, once 4–9 years after RFT and again 7–12 years after RFT, 516 patients were available in the second review. Five patients were found to have relapsed giving a relapse rate of 0.103 per 100 person-years. With well-supervised and regular MDT, relapse rate is very low.

Human Immunodeficiency Virus and Leprosy Relapse

In the 1980s, it was feared that the HIV pandemic might have the same effect on leprosy as it has on tuberculosis. It was predicted that patients with leprosy and human immunodeficiency virus (HIV) co-infection would be at increased risk of lepromatous disease and faster clinical evolution and that leprosy would be more difficult to treat. None of these fears has materialized and the interaction between HIV and *M. leprae* is known to be far more subtle than that between HIV and *Mycobacterium tuberculosis*. There have been many studies performed and documented that the course of leprosy is not influenced by HIV infection. The conclusive studies of the association between HIV and leprosy are lacking.

On the other hand, there is some evidence that immune-mediated reactions (particularly type 1) occur more often in coinfected patients.

There are several reports of leprosy presenting as an immune reconstitution disease among patients starting highly active antiretroviral treatment (HAART), probably as a result of the unmasking of an existing subclinical infection or incubating disease.[2]

In a recent investigation by Pai et al. undertaken to study the coassociation of leprosy and HIV.[48] It was observed that out of 11 patients with leprosy and HIV, four (36.4%) were found to have relapsed with the disease after an average period of 2 years and 2 months after smear negativity, indicating that relapses might occur earlier, as compared to the relapses seen in HIV seronegative patients.

CHEMOTHERAPY OF LEPROSY: FURTHER CHALLENGES[49]

Paucibacillary leprosy in our view is the most ill-understood aspect of the disease with respect to the rational management of such cases. WHO advocated regimen (1992) based on bacillary population seems to be improperly understood in general.

The validity of several trials drawing conclusion that continuation of chemotherapy is necessary to achieve clinical cure was based on the conclusion of the few authors who had observed that "persistence of patches after 6 months of MDT warrant continuation of treatment".

In our own experience only 17% of the patients with PB leprosy showed clinical activity after 3 years of surveillance, whereas 98.8% of patients with single lesion healed at the end of 2 years of surveillance.[50] In a study from Malawi, Boerrighteret et al. reported 4.3% patients with active skin lesions in 483 PB patients after WHO-MDT, while Katoch et al. reported 29.6% cases with activity (personal communication) after completion of therapy.[51]

The occurrence of type 1 reaction or appearance of new lesions during treatment or surveillance seems to be yet another grey area. Experience is to be gained with respect to further follow-up of such patients. It is not clear whether determination of the duration of treatment for PB leprosy should be influenced by episodes of reaction or appearance of new lesions. However, follow-up of these cases is necessary to ascertain the long-term efficacy of such an approach. This is precisely the area where research on FDT for PB leprosy is inadequate.

In an investigation reported by Kar et al. to study clinical events of development of new skin and/or nerve lesions during or after fixed duration of MDT, both in MB and PB leprosy observed that the new lesions could be due to reaction, relapse due to multiplication of persisting or drug resistant bacilli or reinfection due to reentry of lepra bacilli from outside.[52] It is relatively easier to recognize the lesions due to classical reaction, both clinically and histopathologically. However, the differentiation could be difficult in other situations, especially when many of the cases may present with features of reaction at the onset. Similarly, sometimes in late reversal reaction in addition to development of classical acute inflammation of old lesions, many of the patients developed multiple fresh new lesions without any sign of inflammation. It was observed in this study comprising a group of 28 relapsed leprosy cases, who developed new skin and/or nerve lesions at greatly varying time intervals (3 months to 22 years) after stopping MDT that 11 were MB (1 LL, 6 BL and 4 BB) and 17 were PB (12 BT, 4 TT and 1 Neuritic) at their first registration. The likely cause of new lesions in group A (< 6 months interval) could be either (1) mild type 1 reaction or (2) early relapse due to inadequate MDT. Similarly, the new lesions appearing in group B (0.5–3 years) could also represent mild type 1 reaction following improvement of CMI or a true early relapse. The possible causes of early relapse may be because of original misclassification or inadequate chemotherapy/irregular treatment or insufficient duration of therapy. In group C (3–10 years), the cause would most probably be late relapse, the possible causes of late relapse is either due to drug resistance and *M. leprae* persisters. When the time interval goes beyond 10 years (Group D), as in six of the cases, the possibility of reinfection cannot be excluded besides causes of late relapse, since this period is usually considered equivalent to the maximum incubation period of lepra bacilli. All doubtful cases with new lesions, with clinical presentation of type 1 reaction were diagnosed as relapse,

through the therapeutic trial with oral prednisolone for 4–6 weeks. All other cases with new lesions were treated with a second course of MDT (MB or PB) as per classification of new lesions.

A number of reports on relapses in PB patients were published which used different definitions and were based on number of criteria. In spite of wide variety of definitions the relapse rates in these reports, after revision and standardization by WHO are minimal, ranging from 6.5 to 30 per 1,000 person-years.[50] In the two PB trials, the relapse rate on follow-up were, 0.65 per 100 person-years after 4 years in Malawi and 0.12 per 100 person-years after 5 years in Indonesia. Results from the program providing annual information on cohorts of patients on treatment from 1982 and 1990 revealed that the risk of relapse indeed was very low 1.07%, 9 years after stopping MDT. The risk was thus 10 times lower than for dapsone monotherapy.[53] Scollard et al. observed that successful treatment of leprosy has had a profound effect on the management of the disease not only at individual patient level but also at levels of public policy and medical training.[54] In fact chemotherapy has made leprosy hospitals obsolete as outpatient treatment is the norm. As MDT can be taken at home it maintains patient's family and social connections, employment, etc., and therefore permits the patients to keep their jobs and contribute to the economy.

CHEMOTHERAPY AND RELATED CLINICAL ISSUES

Multibacillary Leprosy

Though the success of MDT is well-known, some of the deficiencies and difficulties reported are slow fall of BI especially in those with high BI of more than or equal to 3+. After the introduction of FDT, leprosy program were doing away with slit-skin smear and even clinical status at the end of the treatment which is of fixed duration. Persistence of lesions occurs in MB disease also.

Paucibacillary Leprosy

A study by Boerrigter et al. reported new or worsening of disabilities in 2.5% patients in a total of 499 PB leprosy patients followed up over 4 years in Malawi.[55] Another study from Thailand also reported worsening of nerve function impairment in MB patients from 8% to 13% and in PB patients from 4% to 7%.[56] The development of new or worsening of disabilities is not due to MDT but because of inflammatory process possibly triggered by antigen related nerve damage.

Though MDT has been largely successful, delayed response in some patients as observed in the same study reported 29% of patients being clinically active even after 3 years of follow-up.[56] In a clinical study by Shetty et al. in Mumbai undertaken to investigate effects of therapeutic usage of corticosteroids on *M. leprae* killing and clearance, granuloma clearance and nerve damage in MB leprosy patients (100 patients receiving MDT + steroids) compared with (100 patients receiving MDT alone), it was concluded that treatment with MDT + corticosteroids does not adversely affect the *M. leprae* killing, clearance of the granuloma, and of *M. leprae* and/or their antigens.[57] However, the continued presence of viable bacteria in greater than 14% of BL-LLs patients indicated that 12 months MDT may be insufficient for complete bacterial killing. In both groups nerve conduction studies indicated that deterioration of nerves was high, suggesting that MDT with corticosteroids was not very efficacious in the prevention of nerve damage.

Drug Safety with MDT

Drug safety has not been a major problem with MDT. In one large study involving 10,426 patients with MB disease and 35,013 with PB disease, only 17 patients had hepatitis, three had renal failure and four had cutaneous hypersensitivity reactions.[58]

Toxic reactions to rifampicin such as renal failure or thrombocytopenia are rare. It has been reported that delayed-type hypersensitivity reactions to dapsone are more common among patients receiving MDT, but there are few data to support this.[59,60] In one program report with 98,000 patients (PB and MB), there were 24 cases of adverse effects like hepatitis, renal failures and hypersensitivity reactions observed over a period of 5 years. There have been isolated case reports of hypersensitivity reactions to dapsone.

The most common adverse effects reported were:
- Pigmentation with clofazimine
- Gastrointestinal side effects in (8.5%) with daily dose of rifampicin and hepatitis in (0.8%) and allergic reaction in (0.2%) patients with monthly dose therapy[60]

In practice, toxicity and side effects due to MDT are not a major problem and one needs to ensure the early detection of any difficulties for better patient compliance.[61]

It has been recently reported that dapsone hypersensitivity syndrome (DHS) occurs in approximately 2% of the patients in Nepal.[62] A retrospective study from Vitoria, Espiritu Sanctu, Brazil using good case definitions found that 45% of patients had adverse effects attributable to MDT with 43.85% having effects attributable to dapsone, 12.3% to rifampicin and 9.25% to clofazimine.[63]

In a Genomewide association analysis, Zhang et al. observed that SNP rs2844573, located between the HLA-B and MICA loci, was significantly associated with dapsone hypersensitivity syndrome among patients with leprosy.[64] In fact HLA-B*13:01 was confirmed to be a risk factor for the dapsone hypersensitivity syndrome. The presence of HLA-B*13:01 had a sensitivity of 85.5% and a specificity of 85.7% as a predictor of the dapsone hypersensitivity syndrome and its absence was associated with a reduction in risk by a factor of 7 (from 1.4% to 0.2%). HLA-B*13:01 is present in about 2–20% of Chinese persons, 1.5% of Japanese persons, 1–12% of Indians, and 2–4% of Southeast Asians but is largely absent in Europeans and Africans.

Though MDT has been largely successful some of the issues that need to be kept in mind are the frequent changes in the definitions of classification of leprosy, operational guidelines, change in schedules, rationale for microbiological cure only, nerve involvement not considered in classification of leprosy, delayed response and healing of lesions in some patients.

Newer Chemotherapeutic Agents in Leprosy[65]

The most crucial effective usage of new drugs is to develop an ideal combination and ascertain the optimal duration of treatment. The reasons for development of new drugs and regimens are:
- From the operational point of view the recommended duration of treatment, particularly for MB leprosy is still too long.
- Two of the components of currently administered drugs for MB leprosy, i.e. dapsone and clofazimine are weakly bactericidal against *M. leprae*. Hence, further shortening the duration of treatment by this regimen might result in higher relapse rate.
- Administration of the daily components dapsone and clofazimine cannot be supervised.
- Patients who cannot tolerate any of the drugs in standard WHO-MDT-MB need safer and effective alternative.

How concepts on duration of treatment for MB and PB leprosy have changed over the years is portrayed below (Table 31.1). It will be interesting to know that keeping antibacterial activity alone in mind, it is possible to reduce the period of treatment in a drastic manner. How rational it is to form impressions by attributing clinical improvement or deterioration to the duration of administration of any antileprosy drug is likely to be clear, when long-term results of the suggested regimens are available. Chemotherapy coupled with immunotherapy, the research on which is still very scanty may alone be the answer for those who are eager to achieve maximum clinical results.

To further improve the efficacy of treatment and shorten the duration of treatment, several newer drugs are being studied in combination with rifampicin to achieve a better cure in PB and MB leprosy.

A combination consisting of newer drugs is the regimen which was recommended at the Pre-Congress Workshop (Proceedings of 17th International Leprosy Congress, Hyderabad, 2008) on Chemotherapy. The regimen consists of combination of rifapentine (900 mg) or rifampicin (600 mg)—moxifloxacin (400 mg)—clarithromycin (1,000 mg) (or minocycline 200 mg) (PMM_x), all drugs administered once monthly under supervision (the doses are for adults).[66]

Table 31.1: Evolution of treatment regimens in leprosy

Sr. No.	Regimen	Classification	Duration
1	DDS monotherapy	MB PB	Lifelong (continuous) 10 years
2	WHO-MDT (21 days intensive therapy)	MB	24 months or till skin smear negativity
3	WHO-MDT (modified)	MB	24 months or till skin smear negativity
4	WHO-MDT (FDT-24)	MB	24 months
5	WHO-MDT (FDT-12)	MB	12 months
6	WHO-MDT (FDT-6)	PB	6 months
7	ROM-12	MB	12 months (monthly)
8	ROM-6	PB	6 months (monthly)
9	RO	PB/MB	28 days (daily)
10	ROM-1	SSL	1 day (single dose)
11	PMMx-1	MB	1 day (single dose)
12	MxRM – 12	MB	Intermittent (monthly)
13	MxRM – 6	PB	Intermittent (monthly)

Abbreviations: R, rifampicin; O, ofloxacin; M, minocycline; P, rifapentine; Mx, moxifloxacin.
No. 1–4: Not in vogue; No. 5 and 6: Universally recommended by WHO; No. 7, 8, 9, 11–13: Trials in progress; No. 10: In vogue for some time, now given up

The following are the various group of drugs:

- *Fluoroquinolones:*[67] Ofloxacin, pefloxacin, sparfloxacin, temafloxacin, moxifloxacin and sitafloxacin. Fluoroquinolones the nalidixic acid derivatives are effective against both gram-positive and gram-negative bacteria. This group of drugs acts by blocking DNA gyrase, thereby inhibiting the coiling and supercoiling of DNA. Studies in lepromatous leprosy patients have demonstrated remarkable efficiency of ofloxacin, as over 99.99% killing of viable *M. leprae* was observed with less than 1 month of therapy. This degree of *M. leprae* killing suggests that with their use any naturally occurring mutants would be killed in a month time.

- *Tetracyclines:* Minocycline is bactericidal: It inhibits protein synthesis by binding to the 30s ribosomal subunits of bacteria. Minocycline being tremendously lipophilic easily enters the bacteria and results in inhibition of protein synthesis. A good clinical and bacteriological response has been observed with its use in lepromatous patients. Minocycline is a time tested drug as far as its safety record is concerned.

- *Macrolides:* Clarithromycin bactericidal: It inhibits protein synthesis by binding to the 50s ribosomal subunits of bacteria. Clarithromycin at 0.125 µg/mL concentration was found to have potent anti *M. leprae* activity. Mouse foot studies have confirmed the bactericidal action of clarithromycin. These newer macrolides formulated as enteric coated tablets have the advantage of being acid stable resulting in more reliable absorption and fewer abdominal side effects. Using clarithromycin in leprosy patients, a rapid clinical improvement has been observed together with significant decline in MI and loss of viable bacilli. On account of the sequential action of minocycline and clarithromycin in inhibiting protein synthesis, a marked synergism of action has been found in leprosy.

- *Ansamycins:* Rifabutin, rifapentine, R-76-1 (bactericidal —Its effect is based on blocking the DNA-dependent RNA-polymerase of the bacteria).

- *Dihydrofolate reductase inhibitors:* Brodimoprim and K-130 (Bacteriostatic—It inhibits the multiplication of several bacteria by acting sequentially in blocking folate synthesis).

- Fusidic acid (bacteriostatic: It inhibits protein synthesis by preventing the translocation of elongation factor G from the ribosome).

- *Beta-lactam antibiotics:* Cephaloridine, cefuroxime and amoxicillin plus clavulanic acid (bactericidal: act by inhibiting the synthesis of the peptidoglycan layer of bacterial cell wall).

- Diarylquinoline R207910[68] (bactericidal: It targets the subunit c of mycobacterial ATP synthase).

RECOMMENDATIONS FOR RESEARCH TRIALS

Rifampicin with Ofloxacin Trials (Continuous Treatment for 28 Days)

Trials were undertaken to reduce the duration of treatment to 28 days in MB and PB leprosy with combination of rifampicin (R) and ofloxacin (O). Double-blind multicenter trial co-coordinated by WHO was undertaken in which 1,651 MB smear positive patients (BI $\geq$ 2+) were recruited and equally divided into four different groups, viz. (I) MDT-12 doses, (II) MDT-12 doses + ofloxacin for 28 days, (III) Rifampicin + ofloxacin, (RO) for 28 days, and (IV) MDT—24 doses. Review of the results after 5 years showed that the BI fall in all the groups was comparable and no relapses were encountered in group I, group II and group IV.[69]

As regards Group III, a recent report by WHO shows that in Brazil there were 19 relapses after 5 years of follow-up in the group treated with RO for 1 month indicating a high relapse rate of 38.8%.[70] This group was one of the comparative arms with 12 months, 24 months MDT regimen and 12 months plus ofloxacin regimen which was a double-blind control study as referred to above.

In an "open trial" conducted by BLP, 56 MB smear positive patients were administered 28 days RO on the basis of WHO protocol. During the follow-up period lasting for 6 years, BI fall in RO group was compared with BI fall in 24 doses (214 patients) and 12 doses (190 patients) WHO-MB-MDT groups. In all the groups, the fall in BI was comparable.[71] The first case of relapse following short course (RO28) chemotherapy which occurred after 7 years was reported by Ganapati et al.[72] On follow-up of all patients, it was observed that RO group was associated with far more risk of relapse than expected.[73]

In a WHO study comprising of 1,815 PB leprosy patients, the efficacy of 4 weeks ofloxacin-containing regimen and the standard WHO-MDT regimen for PB leprosy was compared to study the rate and timing of relapse after treatment completion, the results of which so far are not available.[69] Balagon et al. conducted a trial to study the rate and timing of relapse after treatment completion 66 patients received the standard 6 month WHO-MDT regimen and 58 patients received 28 daily doses of rifampicin 600 mg with ofloxacin 400 mg, plus 5 months of placebo.[74] They reported one early relapse at 3 years after treatment completion and two late relapses at 8 and 12 years. Both were classified as PB relapses, concluding that both regimens appeared generally efficacious with few relapses.

Rifampicin, Ofloxacin and Minocycline Trial (Single Dose Therapy)

Based on laboratory and clinical studies, WHO 7th Expert Committee (1997) recommended the use of single dose of rifampicin, ofloxacin and minocycline (ROM) rifampicin (600 mg) + ofloxacin (400 mg) + minocycline (100 mg) for single skin lesion PB leprosy.

A multicentric randomized double-blind controlled clinical trial by WHO to compare the efficacy of ROM with that of the WHO PB-MDT in 1,483 patients with one skin lesion and no peripheral nerve trunk involvement was conducted in India.[75] At 18 months follow-up of 1,381 patients who completed the study, marked improvement was observed in 51.8% in ROM as against 57.3% in the WHO group, while complete cure was observed in 46.9% in the ROM group as against 54.7% in WHO PB-MDT group. Twelve out of 1,381 (0.9%) treatment failures were observed as they either did not improve or showed deterioration at the 18 months examination. This study showed that ROM is almost as effective as the standard WHO PB-MDT in the treatment of single lesion PB leprosy. No further observations were reported as ROM for single skin lesion leprosy was withdrawn from the program for operational reasons.

In another study from Bangladesh, long-term follow-up of ROM treatment was done for 310 SSL PB cases treated from 1998 to 2000. 87% were retrieved having an average follow-up of 6.3 years. Of these, in 76% of patients, complete clearance of lesion was observed and in 10 cases (3.6%) evidence of relapse (PB) was seen. None of them had nerve function impairment. Possibility of increased relapse in patients who receive ROM for single lesion leprosy should be kept in mind.[76]

A study by Girdhar et al. undertaken to assess whether the addition of another effective drug like clarithromycin increases the efficacy of ROM treatment in single lesion patients observed that addition of clarithromycin does not seem to improve on the efficacy of ROM in the short term.[77] It was also observed that healing of the lesions was seen in 73% and 78% patients in the ROM and C-ROM groups respectively at the end of 6 months. Over 90% of patients in both the groups were observed to have healed lesions within 24 months of single-dose treatment.

Rifampicin, Ofloxacin and Minocycline Trial (Intermittent Therapy)

World Health Organization later initiated further clinical trials with ROM given intermittently in both MB and PB leprosy. The supervised dose was given once a month without any treatment in between. Short-term objective of such intermittent therapy for both MB and PB leprosy was to study, besides clinical response any side effects and reactions (ENL and reversal) which might occur during and after the end of treatment. The other objective was to make chemotherapy of leprosy simpler and operationally feasible for mass programs particularly in all difficult situations and ensure better treatment compliance.

1,500 MB patients and 1,800 PB patients were enrolled in the study in three countries, viz. Guinea, Myanmar and Senegal. MB patients were given as intermittent therapy of

12 or 24 doses of ROM once a month. PB patients were given intermittent therapy of three or six doses of ROM once a month.[69,78] Follow-up data on this study is not yet available. However, only two other studies have been reported using multiple doses of ROM in lepromatous leprosy (LL). One in the Phillipinnes by Villahermosa et al.[79] comprising 21 patients with BL and LL given either monthly ROM or the standard MDT for 24 months. These patients had a mean BI of 4+ at entry to the study and it fell to 1.18 at the end of therapy. Those on WHO MB-MDT had similar fall in their BI. Skin lesions improved as did the histological changes in their skin biopsies during treatment. Another study done in Brazil with a similar design mostly had LL patients and both groups had a similar fall in BI (3.5+ to 2.5+) and similar clinical and histological improvements after 24 months of treatment.[80] In the Philippines study, the BI continued to fall after the completion of treatment and no relapses were recorded during the subsequent 64 months (>5 years) after treatment. No toxicities were recorded in patients receiving ROM whereas all patients on WHO-MDT developed clofazimine-induced pigmentation. These are important and encouraging studies which should be repeated on a larger scale with a randomized design.[81]

In 1995, a field trial was implemented in Senegal in order to evaluate the efficacy of ROM intermittent therapy in 102 PB and 118 MB patients.[82] During the first year of trial, patients tolerated the drugs well, none of the patients showed any side effects. 11 PB and 10 MB patients developed reaction (type 1 and 2) during the first 6 months of treatment. Short-term observations showed BI decline and clinical regression in a similar manner as seen with WHO MDT (PB and MB).

Rifampicin, Ofloxacin and Minocycline Trial (Single Dose) and WHO PB-MDT (Two to Three Lesions)[83]

In a multicentric double-blind controlled clinical trial to compare efficacy of ROM administered as a single dose with that of standard WHO-PB-MDT in a total of 236 smear-negative untreated cases with two or three skin lesions without nerve trunk involvement, comparable clinical improvement was seen in most patients with both the regimens. Marked improvement at 18 months of follow-up seen in 46.2% and 53.4% of patients in ROM and standard WHO regimens. But significant difference was noticed in favor of WHO-MDT-PB regimen in patients with three lesions and in patients with more than one body part affected. Reversal reactions and adverse drug reactions were minimal in both the groups.

In another longitudinal study[84] of 51 PB patients with two to three lesions to compare efficacy of ROM administered as a single dose with that of standard WHO-PB-MDT and followed up for 2 years showed good clinical and histopathological improvement which was similar in both the groups.

In another study, 93 PB leprosy patients with two to three skin lesions, treated with a single dose of ROM showed good clinical regression. Five (5.3%) patients developed reaction.[85]

A long-term follow-up study of 634 patients treated with single-dose ROM in single skin lesion and in those with two to five lesions showed lack of any correlation between the problems encountered and the chemotherapy interventions adopted.[86] In the same study, it was reported that most of the clinical events including reaction were manageable.[87] It was also concluded that the delayed clinical problems in the form of relapses/treatment failures observed in single skin lesion leprosy and those with two to five lesions leprosy cases were not encountered in alarming proportion and were within limits manageable by field workers.[88]

Similar trials were undertaken in Bombay by BLP. 230 PB patients having two to three skin lesions and 43 patients having more than 10 lesions (smear negative) were treated with three and six doses of ROM respectively. All the patients showed clinical improvement. 6.5% of patients developed leprosy reactions in both the groups.[89]

A recent randomized double-blind trial by Manickam et al. was conducted to investigate the efficacy of single-dose-ROM in PB leprosy patients with two to five skin lesions compared to WHO-PB-MDT in 1,526 patients from five centers (ROM-762; WHO-PB-MDT-764) followed for 36 months post-treatment during 1998–2003.[90] It was observed that complete clearance of skin lesions was similar in both the arms. Clinical scores declined steadily and equally. Difference in relapse rates was statistically highly significant (ROM=1.13 and WHO-PB-MDT=0.35 per 100 person-year). Twenty eight of the 38 total relapses were reported within 18 months. The study was extended to follow-up for 48 months for 1,082 of the 1,526 patients from two program-based centers, wherein no further relapses were reported. They concluded that single-dose ROM, though less effective than the standard WHO-PB-MDT regimen, conceptually offers an alternative treatment regimen for PB leprosy patients with two to five lesions only when careful follow-up for relapse is possible.

However, ROM therapy as single dose for single skin lesion, and two to three lesions was withdrawn by WHO and NLEP from the program for operational reasons.

Uniform MDT[91]

The objective of the investigation was to provide 6 months MDT for all types of leprosy patients and assess the treatment response in terms of relapse rates. Seven centers participated (five in India and two in China), treating a total of 3,396 patients. An interim analysis available for 2,930 patients out of 3,396 at the end of 3 years, showed that uniform multidrug therapy (U-MDT) appears to be promising with respect to clinical status of skin lesions (Table 31.2).[92]

In another study U-MDT of 6 months duration in PB and MB patients was compared with the existing WHO PB and

Table 31.2: Showing status of patients after Uniform MDT (U-MDT)

Sr. No.	Particulars	WHO/TDR[91,92] (India and China) 2008	Rao PN[93] (India) 2008						Penna LM et al.[94] (Brazil) 2012			
1	Number of patients	3,396	127						U-MDT = 323 WHO-MDT = 290			
2	Duration of Follow-up	3 Years	2 Years						1 Year			
3	Outcome	New Lesions = 53 patients 6 Relapses PB patients responded better than MB patients	Response						BI <3+		BI >3	
			PB		MB				WHO-MDT	U-MDT	WHO-MDT	U-MDT
			WHO MDT	U-MDT	Good		Poor		39.10%	52.91%	53.72%	57.8%
			82%	100%	WHO MDT	U-MDT	WHO MDT	U-MDT				
					77%	25%	23%	75%	Observations on reactions only			
4	Conclusion	U-MDT appears promising with respect to clinical status of skin lesions.	MDT of 6 months duration was well-tolerated and effective in patients with PB leprosy but was too short a regimen to adequately treat patients with MB leprosy						High BI had a higher frequency of first reaction than those with BI <3+ Incidence of recurrent reaction was directly associated with high BI and with U-MDT			

Abbreviations: MDT, multidrug therapy; U-MDT, uniform multidrug therapy.

MB regimen based on clinical and histological parameters: 64 patients were followed up over a period of 24 months. It was concluded that U-MDT of 6 months duration was well-tolerated and effective in patients with PB leprosy but was too short a regimen to adequately treat patients with MB leprosy (Table 31.2).[93]

In an open label randomized comparative clinical study by Penna et al. reporting on preliminary findings on U-MDT (323 patients) and WHO standard MDT (290 patients) and reaction frequency in MB patients observed that those on U-MDT have more reactions than those on WHO-MDT.[94] After 1 year in the subgroup with initial BI of less than 3+, 39.10% presented with at least one reaction episode in the WHO-MDT subgroup and 52.91% in the U-MDT subgroup. Those with BI greater than 3+, presented with reaction 53.72% in WHO-MDT and 57.8% in U-MDT subgroup in the same time interval. Those with high BI had a higher frequency of first reaction than those with BI less than 3+ throughout the observation time. The incidence of recurrent reaction presented a positive association with BI greater than 3+ and with the U-MDT group (Table 31.2).

Accompanied MDT[95]

Accompanied MDT (A-MDT) was recommended by WHO to address frequent problems in the field program by providing certain patients with a full course of treatment on their first visit to the leprosy clinics after diagnosis. WHO recommends that A-MDT is user friendly. It is suitable for mobile population and for patients living in remote areas and in areas of civil strife. Though MDT coverage is reported as 100% by all countries there are still some underserved populations such as those living in hard to reach border areas or in urban slums or the migrant laborers. As an innovative approach to ensure that such underserved groups have access to MDT and other services, WHO strongly recommended that A-MDT would give better access to MDT for patients in general and in particular for those unable to visit the health center regularly for a variety of reasons. In an operational study conducted by Damien Foundation of India Trust in Bihar a total of 462 PB patients (168 given A-MDT and 294 given routine MDT) and 125 MB patients (58 A-MDT and 67 routine MDT) were recruited. The results of this study showed that in PB leprosy patients treatment adherence for monthly pulse doses was 80% for the A-MDT group but only 54% for the routine MDT group, whereas in MB leprosy, treatment adherence for monthly pulse doses was 79% for the A-MDT group, but only 42% for the routine MDT group. In the routine MDT group the main reasons for missing treatment were distance from the health facility, MDT drugs out of stock and closed health facility. For A-MDT the main reasons were loss of drugs and damaged drugs.[53]

Moxifloxacin-based Regimens

The flouroquinolone moxifloxacin, has been shown to be the most powerful bactericidal agent against *M. leprae*. It is a synthetic broad spectrum 8-methoxyfluoroquinolone. The bactericidal action of moxifloxacin and other flouroquinolones results from inhibition of the DNA gyrase required for the bacterial DNA replication and is reported to have strong bactericidal activity. Comparative bactericidal activity of various drugs used for leprosy is given in Table 31.3.

A combination regimen of moxifloxacin with rifapentine and minocycline was recommended for human trials by Ji and Grosset in 2000.[33] However, no reports of clinical trials using this combination are still available. In a clinical trial in eight MB patients, Eleanor et al. in 2008 reported moxifloxacin alone to be highly effective.[95]

Similar preliminary observations in an open trial on 54 patients have recently been reported from Bombay in a moxifloxacin containing regimen (rifampicin 600 mg + moxifloxacin 400 mg + minocycline 200 mg) given once monthly for 12 months in smear positive MB patients and for 6 months in smear-negative patients.[96]

- Remarkable clinical regression observed within 2–3 months in all cases
- No side effects of the drugs were seen.

In a recent investigation, Halwai et al.[97] reported occurrence of leprosy reactions in 22 skin smear-positive patients following monthly supervised administration of MRM [Moxifloxacin (400 mg) + Rifampicin (600 mg) + Minocycline (200 mg)] compared with another group of 25 patients that received MRM plus clofazimine (300 mg) given monthly under supervision along with 50 mg daily self-administered.[97] It was observed that most of the reactions (13 out of 15) were encountered in the first 6 months after starting the therapy. Addition of clofazimine had no influence on the occurrence of reactions. A small sample of 28 patients in both groups with BI greater than 3 showed a steady decline over 12 months. Follow-up is in progress to study observations from a long-term point of view.

Table 31.3: Shows comparative bactericidal activity of drugs

Drug	Class	Bactericidal activity in mice	Bactericidal activity in human
Pefloxacin	Fluoroquinolone	++	++
Ofloxacin		++	++
Moxifloxacin		+++	+++
Clarithromycin	Macrolide	++	++
Minocycline	Tetracycline	++	++
Rifapentine	Rifamycin	+++	Not done

Other Regimens for Special Situations[24]

Special regimens are required for individual patients who cannot benefit from rifampicin because of allergy or intercurrent diseases such as chronic hepatitis, or who have been shown to be infected with rifampicin-resistant *M. leprae*. Patients who refuse to accept clofazimine because of the coloration it causes also require a safe and effective alternative.

For patients who do not accept clofazimine, the 1993 Study Group recommended using ofloxacin 400 mg daily, or minocycline 100 mg daily as substitutes for clofazimine, the committee suggested that they could also be treated by monthly administration of ROM for 24 months. Patients harboring rifampicin-resistant *M. leprae* are very often also resistant to dapsone and their treatment depends almost entirely on clofazimine. Daily treatment with the combination of ofloxacin plus minocycline shows promising bactericidal activity against *M. leprae* in mice and in patients. MB patients who cannot tolerate rifampicin may be treated with the following WHO recommended regimen for adults.

Daily administration of 50 mg clofazimine together with 400 mg of ofloxacin and 100 mg of minocycline or 500 mg of clarithromycin for 6 months followed by daily administration of 50 mg clofazimine together with 100 mg of minocycline or 400 mg of ofloxacin for at least an additional 18 months.

Severe Dapsone Toxicity[29]

If dapsone has any severe toxic effects the drug should be stopped immediately. No further modification is required for patients with MB leprosy. However clofazimine may be substituted for dapsone for a period of 6 months in the dose employed in WHO-MDT regimen for PB leprosy.

CONCLUSION

It is remarkable that chemotherapy of leprosy has come a long way and has shown great promise and hope in the management of leprosy. The evolution of WHO-MDT treatment regimens has undergone a sea change due to consistent research and painstaking follow-up which is necessary in a chronic disease like leprosy to draw practical conclusions to understand the efficacy of several drugs and their different combination regimens. WHO-MDT is still the main tool and the strategy for the control of the disease.

The benefits of chemotherapy have therefore, come at the expense of education and maintenance of expertise regarding leprosy. As thousands of new patients are detected every year and many more are missed and remain untreated, this poses a major public health challenge as regards maintaining good quality treatment and training new physicians and several health workers to recognize and treat this disease.[54.]

In an exhaustive review on chemotherapy of leprosy from a historical perspective, Gelber et al. observed that leprosy can generally be cured by MDT and is less often an incurable disease that needs lifelong chemotherapy.[98] However, after MDT, completion, there is a substantial subset of MB patients with a high bacterial burden at risk for relapse. Thus, leprosy chemotherapy development remains a considerable concern, while leprosy now may well be more neglected than previously. The substantial extent of what the "elimination" campaign has accomplished also remains controversial. What is clear is that though in the 1960s both tuberculosis and malaria were declared controlled, currently both are acknowledged to be major causes of mortality in the developing world. What is also clear is that worldwide the number of leprosy clinicians and researchers has diminished greatly, and fundamental tools used to properly evaluate leprosy patients, such as skin smears, skin histopathology and mouse footpad facilities, and leprosy control such as case finding, supervised drug administration and follow-up are almost nonexistent and therefore probably the stage for leprosy to reemerge is surely set.

Meanwhile newer drugs and the regimens hold a great promise for future but have to be observed carefully for long term to study their efficacy. Further, research is also required into an important area to find a new drug or combination of drugs and immunotherapy capable of eradicating persisting organisms as well as *M. leprae* derived antigens causing adverse reactions and nerve damage.

ACKNOWLEDGMENTS

The authors gratefully acknowledge the assistance provided by Mr Rahul Gupta and Mr Sanjay Kulkarni of Bombay Leprosy Project in preparing the manuscript. The authors are also thankful for all the clinical and secretarial assistance by the staff of BLP and the patients who have cooperated in helping us to understand the disease better.

REFERENCES

1. WHO regional strategy for sustaining leprosy services and further reducing the burden of leprosy, 2006-2010. Indian J Lepr. 2006;78:33-47.
2. WHO Expert Committee on Leprosy, 8th Report, WHO Technical Report Series, 968; 2012.
3. WHO weekly epidemiological record 30 August 2013;88(35): 365-80.
4. Rao PS. Worldwide elimination of leprosy. Expert Rev Dermatol. 2012;7:513-20.
5. Dharmendra. Sulphone therapy general considerations. In: Dharmendra (Ed). Leprosy. Samant DR, Bombay, 1985. pp.359-412.
6. Lowe J, Smith M. The chemotherapy of leprosy in Nigeria. Int J Lepr. 1949;17;181-95.
7. Rees RJ, Pearson JM, Waters MF. Experimental and clinical studies on rifampicin in treatment of leprosy. Br Med J. 1970;1:89-92.
8. Leiker DL, Kamp H. First results of treatment of leprosy with rifadin. Lepr Rev. 1970;41:25-30.
9. Languillon J, Yawalkar SJ, McDougall AC. Therapeutic effects of adding rimactane (rifampicin) 450 milligrams daily or 1200 milligrams once monthly in a single dose to dapsone 50 milligrams daily in patients with lepromatous leprosy. Int J Lepr Other Mycobact Dis. 1979;47:37-43.
10. Yawalkar SJ, McDougall AC, Languillon J, et al. Once monthly rifampicin plus daily dapsone in initial treatment of lepromatous leprosy. Lancet. 1982;1:1199-202.
11. Brown SG, Hogerzeil LM. "B 663" in the treatment of leprosy, Preliminary report of a pilot trial. Lepr Rev. 1962;33:6-10.
12. Ellard GA. The chemotherapy of leprosy. Part 1. Int J Lepr Other Mycobact Dis. 1990;58:704-16.
13. Petit JH, Rees RJ. Sulphone resistance in leprosy. An experimental and clinical study. Lancet. 1964.pp.673-4.
14. Shepard CC. Combinations of drugs against *Mycobacterium leprae* studied in Mice. Int J Lepr. 1972;40:33-9.
15. Waters MF, Rees RJ, McDougall AC, et al. Ten years of Dapsone in Lepromatous Leprosy: Clinical, Bacteriological and Histological assessment and the finding of viable leprosy bacilli. Lepr Rev. 1974;45:288-98.
16. Freerksen E, Rosenfeld M, Bonnici E, et al. Combined therapy in Leprosy, background and findings. Chemotherapy. 1978;24:187-201.
17. Jacobson RR, Gatt P. Can leprosy be eradicated with chemotherapy? An evaluation of the Malta Leprosy Eradication Project. Lepr Rev. 2008;79:410-15.
18. Subcommittee on clinical trials of the chemotherapy of leprosy (THELEP) scientific working group of the UNDP/World Bank/ WHO special programme for research and training in tropical diseases, persisting *M. leprae* among THELEP trial patients in Bamako and Chingleput. Lepr Rev. 1987;58:325-37.
19. Levy L, Shepherd CC, Faisal P. Death of *M. leprae* following treatment of leprosy patients with 1500 mg rifampicin in a single dose. Int J Lepr. 1973;41:489-90.
20. Faisal P, Shepherd CC, Levy L. Death of *M. leprae* during treatment of leprosy patients with 600 mg rifampicin daily. Int J Lepr. 1973;41:489-90.
21. Marchoux Chemotherapy Study Group. Int J Lepr. 1992;60:4; 525-35.
22. Ellard G. The Chemotherapy of Leprosy. Part 2; Editorial; Int J Lepr. 1991;59:82-94.
23. WHO Study Group. Chemotherapy of Leprosy for control programmes, Geneva: World Health Organisation; Technical Report Series; 675;1982.
24. WHO Expert Committee of Leprosy, Seventh Report; WHO Technical Report Series; 874;1998.
25. Ganapati R, Revankar CR, Pai VV. History of MDT in India—Role of Bombay Leprosy Project. NLO Bulletin; April–June 2002.
26. Naik SS, Shere SS, Ganapati R. Thirteen years of follow up of 100 smear positive leprosy cases after completion of multidrug therapy. Indian J Lepr. 1995;67:483-4.
27. Ganapati R, Revankar CR, Pai RR. Three year assessment of multidrug therapy in multibacillary leprosy cases. Indian J Lepr. 1987;59:44-9.
28. WHO Study Group. Chemotherapy of Leprosy, Report of a WHO Study Group, WHO Geneva; 1994.
29. BecxBleumink M. Experience with WHO recommended multidrug therapy for multibacillary leprosy patients in

the leprosy control program of the All Africa Leprosy and Rehabilitation Training Centre (ALERT) in Ethiopia, appraisal of the recommended duration of MDT for MB patients. Int J Lepr. 1991;59:558-68.

30. Proceedings of Annual Meeting of State Leprosy Officers, Delhi, Leprosy Division, DGHS, Ministry of Health and Family Welfare, Nirman Bhavan, New Delhi, 29–30th Dec;1995,32.

31. Ganapati R, Pai VV, Rao R. Leprosy: control and rehabilitation. In: Valia RG, Valia A (Eds). IADVL Textbook of Dermatology, 3rd edition. Mumbai: Bhalani Publishing House; 2008. pp. 2139-54.

32. Dogra S, Kumaran MS, Narang T, et al. Clinical characteristics and outcome in multibacillary (MB) leprosypatientstreated with 12 months WHOMDT-MBR: a retrospective analysis of 730 patients from a leprosy clinic at a tertiary care hospital of Northern India. Lepr Rev. 2013;84:65-75.

33. Baohong Ji, Grosset J. Combination of Rifapentine—Moxifloxacin, Minocycline for the treatment of leprosy, Asian Leprosy Congress, 2000, Agra.

34. Malathi M, Thappa DM. Fixed-Duration Therapy in Leprosy: Limitations and Opportunities. Indian J Dermatol. 2013;58:93-100.

35. Weiand D, Thoulass J, Smith CW. Assessing and improving adherence with multidrug therapy. Lepr Rev. 2012;83:282-91.

36. Chichava AO, Ariza L, Oliveira RA, et al. Reasons for Interrupting Multidrug therapy against Leprosy: The Patients Point of View. Lepr Rev. 2011;82:78-9.

37. WHO Expert Committee on Leprosy, Sixth Report, Technical Report Series, 768; 1988.

38. Ganapati R, Pai VV. Field experience with multidrug therapy in leprosy. VNS Prescribers Monthly Guide; 1994.

39. Katoch VM. New investigative techniques in leprosy. In: Valia RG, Valia AR (Eds). Dermatology Update. Mumbai: Bhalani Publishing House; 1998. pp. 165-74.

40. Ganapati R, Halwai V, Pai VV, et al. Relapses after Chemotherapy in Leprosy. Fontilles Rev Leprol. 2011;28:89-94.

41. Annual Report, Bombay Leprosy Project 2011.

42. Isaac S, Christian M, Jesudasan K, et al. Effectiveness of Multidrug therapy in multibacillary leprosy: A long-term follow-up of 34 multibacillary leprosy patients treated with multidrug regimens till skin smear negativity. Lepr Rev. 2003;74:141-7.

43. Patnaik PK. Recommendations of the seminar on "cure of leprosy". 14th Feb 2009, Konark, Orissa.

44. Jamet P, Ji B. Relapse after long-term follow-up of multibacillary patients treated by WHO Multidrug regimen. Int J Lepr Other Mycobact Dis. 1994;62:195-201.

45. Annual Report: Bombay Leprosy Project; 2008, Mumbai.

46. Shetty VP, Suchitra K, Uplekar MW, et al. Persistence of *M. leprae* in the peripheral nerve as compared to the skin of multi drug treated leprosy patients. Lepr Rev. 1992;63:329-36.

47. Desikan KV, Peri S, Tulsidas I, et al. An 8-12 year follow-up of highly Bacillated Indian leprosy patients treated with WHO Multi-Drug therapy. Lepr Rev. 2008;79:303-10.

48. Pai VV, Tayshete PU, Ganapati R. Observations in 11 patients with leprosy and human immunodeficiency virus co-association. Indian J Dermatol Venereol Leprol. 2011;77:714-6.

49. Pai VV. Chemotherapy of leprosy–Further challenges. Health Administrator, 2006; Vol XVII; Number 2:72-76.

50. Revankar CR, Karjivkar VG, Gurav VJ, et al. Clinical assessment of paucibacillary leprosy under multidrug therapy—three years followup study. Indian J Lepr. 1989;61:355-9.

51. Boerrigter G, Ponnighaus J, et al. Preliminary appraisal of a WHO-recommended multidrug regimen in paucibacillary leprosy patients in Malawi. Int J Lepr. 1988;56:408-17.

52. Kar HK, Sharma P. New lesions after MDT in PB and MB leprosy: a report of 28 cases. Indian J Lepr. 2008;80:247-55.

53. WHO Study Group. Multidrug therapy against leprosy. Development and implementation over the past 25 years, Geneva: World Health Organisation; Technical Report Series; 2004. pp. 60-2.

54. Scollard MD. Chemotherapy of leprosy has changed (almost) everything. Lepr Rev. 2012;83:245-6.

55. Boerrigter G, Ponnighaus J, et al. Four-year follow-up results of a WHO-recommended multiple-drug regimen in paucibacillary leprosy patients in Malawi. Int J Lepr. 1991;59:255-61.

56. Dasanjali K, Schreuder P, Pirayavaraporn C. A Study on the effectiveness and safety of the WHO/MDT regimen in the northeast of Thailand; a prospective study, 1984–1996. Int J Lepr. 1997;65:28-36.

57. Shetty VP, Khambati FA, Ghate SD, et al, The effect of corticosteroids usage on bacterial killing, clearance and nerve damage in leprosy; part 3—Study of two comparative groups of 100 multibacillary (MB) patients each, treated with MDT + steroids vs. MDT alone, assessed at 6 months post-release from 12 months MDT. Lepr Rev. 2010;81:41-58.

58. Ekambaram V, Rao MK. Changing picture of leprosy in North Arcot district, Tamil Nadu after MDT. Indian J Lepr. 1989; 61:31-43.

59. Richardus JH, Smith TC. Increased incidence in leprosy of hypersensitivity reactions to dapsone after introduction of multidrug therapy. Lepr Rev. 1989;60:267-73.

60. Reeve PA, Ala J, Hall JJ. Modification of multidrug treatment of leprosy in Vanuatu. Int J Lepr. 1992;60:655-6.

61. Gilbody JS. Impact of Multidrug therapy on the treatment and control of leprosy. Int J Lepr Other Mycobact Dis. 1991;59: 458-78.

62. Sapkota BR, Kancha S, Pandey B, et al. A retrospective study of the effect of modified multi-drug therapy in Nepali leprosy patients following the development of adverse effects due to dapsone. Lepr Rev. 2008;79:425-8.

63. Deps PD, Nasser S, Guerra P, et al. Adverse effects from multi-drug therapy in leprosy: a Brazilian study. Lepr Rev. 2007;78:216-22.

64. Zhang FR, Liu H, Irwanto A, et al. HLA-B*13:01 and the dapsone hypersensitivity syndrome. N Engl J Med. 2013;369:1620-8.

65. Ganapati R, Pai VV. Newer chemotherapeutic agents in leprosy. Indian J Dermatol. 1996;41:1-4.

66. Proceedings of Pre Congress Workshop at 17th International Leprosy Congress, 2008, Hyderabad, India.

67. Girdhar BK. Flouroquinolones and their adverse effects. Indian J Lepr. 1993;65:69-9.

68. Gelber R, et al. The diarylquinoline R207910 is bactericidal against *M. leprae* in mice at low dose and administered intermittently. Department of antimicrobial Research, Tibotec BVBA, Johnson & Johnson, Beerse, 2009 Belgium.

69. WHO meeting on chemotherapy research in leprosy, Madras. Lepr Rev. 1997;68:285-7.

70. World Health Organization. (2008). WHO report of the ninth meeting of the technical advisory group on leprosy control, Cairo, Egypt, 6-7th March 2008. [online]. Available from http://

www.searo.who.int/entity/global_leprosy_programme/publications/9th_tag_meeting_2008.pdf. [Accessed June, 2014].

71. Ganapati R, Pai VV, Shroff HJ, et al. Rate of decline in bacterial index in leprosy; observations after three different chemotherapeutic interventions. Int J Lepr. 1997;65:264-6.

72. Ganapati R, Pai VV, Revankar CR, et al. Relapse of multibacillary leprosy after rifampicin and ofloxacin for 28 days; a case report. Int J Lepr. 1998;66:56-8.

73. Ganapati R, Pai VV, Revankar CR, et al. A Decade of experience with ofloxacin in leprosy—An update. Dermacon 2003, 31st National Conference of IADVL; 2003; Kolkata. p. 145.

74. BalagonMarivic F, Cellona RV, Abalos RM, et al. The efficacy of a four-week, ofloxacin containing regimen compared with standard WHO-MDT in PB leprosy. Lepr Rev. 2010; 81:27-33.

75. WHO single lesion multicentre trial group. Efficacy of Single dose multidrug therapy for the treatment of single-lesion paucibacillary leprosy. Indian J Lepr. 1997;69:121-9.

76. Alam K, Butlin RC, Pahan D, et al. Long-term follow-up of ROM treated cases. Lepr Rev. 2007;78:160.

77. Manickam P, Nagaraju B, Selvaraj V, et al. Efficacy of single-dose chemotherapy (rifampicin, ofoxacin and minocycline-ROM) in PB leprosy patients with 2 to 5 skin lesions, India: randomized double-blind trial. Indian J Lepr. 2012;84:195-207.

78. Pannikar VK. Milestones towards the elimination of leprosy. Int J Lepr. 1996;64:S11-S12.

79. Villahermosa LG, Fajardo TT, Abalos RM, et al. Parallel assessment of 24 monthly doses of rifampicin, ofloxacin and minocycline versus two years of World Health Organization multi-drug therapy for multi-bacillary leprosy. Am J Trop Med Hyg. 2004;70:197-200.

80. Ura S, Diaro SM, Carreira BG, et al. Estudio Terapeitico comparando a associao derifampicina, of loxacina Emino cyclinacom a assocacaorifampicina, clofazimiaedaps on eempacientes com hanseniasemultibacilar. Hansenologia Internationalis. 2007;32:57-65.

81. Lockwood DN, Cunha Mda G. Developing new MDT regimens for MB patients; time to test ROM 12 months regimens globally. Lepr Rev. 2012;83: 241-4.

82. Mane I, Cartel JL, Grosset JH. Field trial on efficacy of supervised monthly dose of 600 mg rifampicin, 400 mg ofloxacin and 100 mg minocycline for the treatment of leprosy, first result. Int J Lepr. 1997;62:224-9.

83. WHO Single Lesion Multicentre Trial Group. A comparative trial of single dose chemotherapy in paucibacillary leprosy patients with two to three skin lesions. Indian J Lepr. 2001;73:131-43.

84. Emmanuel M, Gupte MD. Lesional characteristics and histopathology in paucibacillary leprosy patients with 2 or 3 skin lesions, Comparison between ROM and PB-MDT regimens. Indian J Lepr. 2005;77:19-25.

85. Pai VV, Revankar CR, Chavan RG, et al. Single dose of rifampicin, ofloxacin and minocycline for PB leprosy patients with 1-3 lesions. 20th Biennial Conference of Indian Association of Leprologists; 1997; Bhopal.

86. Ganapati R, Revankar CR, Pai VV, et al. Single-dose treatment for paucibacillary leprosy; feasibility of long-term follow-up. Int J Lepr Other Mycobact Dis. 1999;67:308-9.

87. Pai VV, Bulchand HO, Revankar CR, et al. Single-dose treatment for paucibacillary leprosy; clinical problems and management. Int J Lepr. 1999;67:310-2.

88. Revankar CR, Pai VV, Samy A, et al. Single-dose treatment for paucibacillary leprosy; field implications. Int J Lepr Other Mycobact Dis. 1999;67:312-4.

89. Ganapati R, Pai VV, Chavan RG, et al. Reactions after intermittent therapy with ROM in PB leprosy—Preliminary observations. 20th Biennial Conference of Indian Association of Leprologists; 1997, Bhopal.

90. Girdhar A, Kumar A, Girdhar BK. A randomised controlled trial assessing the effect of adding clarithromycin to Rifampicin, Ofloxacin and Minocycline in the treatment of single lesion paucibacillary leprosy in Agra District, India. Lepr Rev. 2011;82;46-54.

91. World Health Organization (2009). WHO Report of the Tenth Meeting of the WHO Technical Advisory Group on Leprosy Control. [online] Available from http://www.searo.who.int/entity/global_leprosy_programme/publications/10th_tag_meeting_2009.pdf. [Accessed June, 2014].

92. WHO/TDR multicentric trial on 'Uniform MDT regimen for all types of leprosy patients. (2007-08). [online] Available from http://www.icmr.nic.in/annual/2007-08/nie/leprosy.pdf. [Accessed June, 2014].

93. Rao PN, Suneetha S, Pratap DV. Comparative study of uniform MDT in pauci- and multibacillary leprosy patients over 24 months on observation. Lepr Rev. 2009;80:143-55.

94. Penna LM, Sekula SB, Pontes AM, et al, Primary results of clinical trial for uniform multidrug therapy for leprosy patients in brazil (U-MDT/CT-BR): reactions frequency in multibacillary patients. Lepr Rev. 2012;83:308-19.

95. Pardillo F, Burgos J, Fajardo TT, et al. Powerful bactericidal activity of moxifloxacin in human leprosy. Antimicrob Agents Chemother. 2008;52:3113-7.

96. Ganapati R, Pai VV, Khanolkar SA, et al. Clinical trials with moxifloxacin based regimen in leprosy—a preliminary communication. Rev De Fontilles Leprol. 2009;27:49-55.

97. Halwai V, Ganapati R, Pai VV, et al. Leprosy reactions in smear positive patients receiving moxifloxacin based regimens. Fontilles Rev Leprol. 2011;28:159-63.

98. Gelber R and Grosset J. The chemotherapy of leprosy: An interpretive history. Lepr Rev. 2012;83:221-40.

Management of Leprosy Reactions

Hemanta Kumar Kar, Ruchi Gupta

CHAPTER OUTLINE

- Early diagnosis of reaction
- Management of type 1 reaction or Reversal Reaction
- Treatment of late Reversal Reaction
- Management of Type 2 Reaction
- Management of Lucio Phenomenon

INTRODUCTION

Leprosy reactions are immunologically mediated episodes of acute or subacute inflammation affecting the skin, nerves, mucous membrane and/or other sites which interrupt the chronic and placid course of leprosy. Unless promptly and adequately treated, these reactions can result in deformity and disability. Two types of reaction occur in leprosy: type 1 reaction (T1R) or reversal reaction (RR), a type IV hypersensitivity, occurring mostly in borderline tuberculoid (BT), borderline borderline (BB) and borderline lepromatous (BL) patients and rarely in lepromatous leprosy (LL) (subpolar). Type 2 reaction (T2R) or erythema nodosum leprosum (ENL) is a type III hypersensitivity reaction, occurring commonly in LL and sometimes in BL patients. Recently, ENL has been described in patients with histoid leprosy also.[1] Lucio phenomenon is another rare form of reaction observed only in Lucio leprosy.

EARLY DIAGNOSIS OF REACTION

Timely initiation of treatment for reaction can reduce morbidity and prevent deformities. With the current level of understanding about leprosy reactions it is neither possible to predict their occurrence nor is it always possible to prevent them altogether. However, the following steps can be taken for early diagnosis and prompt treatment of reactions:

- Build capacity of the peripheral or primary level healthcare staff to enable them to suspect reaction from its early signs and symptoms, and refer them to the next higher healthcare center for confirmation of diagnosis and prompt treatment.

> **Box 32.1:** Early signs and symptoms suggestive of reaction
>
> - Inflammation of existing skin lesions, redness, pain, tenderness, swelling
> - Sudden appearance of painful nodular swellings on the skin
> - Numbness, tingling and loss of sensation in limbs
> - Weakness and paralysis of the muscles of limbs
> - Infrequent blinking of the eye
> - Incomplete closure of eyelids
> - Red painful eye(s)
> - Diminution of vision.

- The patients must be counseled, so also their family members regarding importance of continuing multidrug therapy (MDT) along with treatment of leprosy reactions.
- Patients and the family members must be educated to identify early signs and symptoms of reactions and neuritis, and asked to report immediately on their appearance. The early features which can give some clue to the reactions are given in Box 32.1.
- Persons at higher risk should be examined frequently, at least once a month.
- Defaulters should be retrieved.

MANAGEMENT OF TYPE 1 REACTION OR REVERSAL REACTION

Type 1 reaction is characterized by exacerbation of existing skin lesions (EEL), seen clinically as erythema, edema and tenderness of lesions and/or appearance of new inflamed skin lesions with/without neuritis, i.e. pain and tenderness of enlarged nerve trunk with sensory ± motor weakness. The management should be on the following lines:

Antileprosy Treatment

Multidrug therapy has to be started or continued, if already started, since this is required for continuous killing of *M. leprae* to reduce the bacterial/antigenic load in the skin and nerves. Antileprosy drug, clofazimine is known for its anti-inflammatory action and in higher doses has been observed to have a role in the prevention of neuritis.

Specific Treatment of Reaction

Specific treatment has to be initiated depending on the severity of the reaction (mild or severe type).

Mild Reaction[2]

Characterized by inflammation (moderate to marked erythema, swelling, pain, tenderness) in few of the existing skin lesions.

Nonsteroidal anti-inflammatory drug (NSAIDs, e.g. aspirin or paracetamol) in adequate doses is given for few weeks. Reassurance is very important to the patient as well as to family members. They should be educated that the development of reaction is an indicator of bacterial killing, which in patients on treatment is a sign of immunological upgradation.

Severe Reaction[2]

Characterized by the presence of one or more of the following features:

- Involvement of more number of existing skin lesions (EEL) as well as appearance of new inflamed skin lesions
- Nerve pain, tenderness or paresthesia or increasing nerve function impairment (NFI) in the form of loss of sensation or muscle weakness
- Red, swollen skin plaque on the face, or overlying another major nerve trunk
- Fever, discomfort, arthralgia
- Edema of hands and/or feet
- Ulcerative skin lesions
- Reaction persisting for more than 6 weeks with the usual dose of analgesics. It is noteworthy that facial involvement is considered as an emergency due to risk of facial nerve palsy and its associated ocular complications. It needs prompt treatment with corticosteroids.[3]

Corticosteroids (Prednisolone)

Corticosteroids are the cornerstone of therapy and considered to be the drug of choice.

Mechanisms of Action

- *Genomic*: via modulation of gene and thence protein synthesis, which results in slow and delayed action.
- *Nongenomic*: via interaction with cell surface receptors and via alteration of physiochemical properties of cell membrane. It is responsible for early effects of steroids.

The recent work on the relative genomic and nongenomic potencies of glucocorticoids suggests that methylprednisolone has a high ratio of nongenomic to genomic activity, and may be needed for early, high level of immunosuppression.[4] This compound acts by the dual mechanism of reducing the inflammatory edema, and inducing immunosuppression, thus forming the basis of pulse therapy in management of severe T1R.[5] However, in any patient, the response to corticosteroid therapy is modulated by expression of toll-like receptors (TLRs), 2 and 4.[6]

Dose and Duration of Prednisolone

Standard dose schedule for field purpose (World Health Organization, 1998): World Health Organization recommends a standard field regimen of 12 weeks therapy with prednisolone (Table 32.1).[7] However, with the standard steroid dose schedule of WHO, the recovery does not seem to be sustained.[8]

Standard dose schedule at referral center[9]: Steroids need to be given at the earliest and in sufficient doses, not only to regain the sensory and motor functions of the affected nerves, but also to prevent irreversible nerve damage. Starting dose 1 mg/kg body weight, given once in the morning after breakfast, to be continued till improvement of skin lesions is visible/nerve tenderness and pain subsides. Then the dose should be cut by 5 mg every 1—2 weeks. The crucial maintenance dose should be around 15–20 mg for several weeks/months. In the follow-up period, the dose should be cut by 5 mg every 2-4 months. Graded sensory testing with monofilaments and voluntary muscle testing can guide the tapering of prednisolone. The duration should be long enough to cover the period during which the antigen (Ag) load is able to trigger the CMI response (BT: 4–9 months, BB: 6–12 months, BL: 6–24 months).

The ideal duration and dose of steroids to be administered is still a matter of debate. The WHO regimen lasting for 3 months (mentioned above) has been criticized in view of high recurrences. Longer regimens have been warranted not only for effective treatment of reactions and to prevent NFI after stopping treatment but also to control the recurrence of reactions. The efficacy of a longer duration of steroid therapy has been described by Rao et al.[8] wherein they

Table 32.1: Standard treatment schedule of oral prednisolone for management of type 1 reaction (under field conditions)

Dose	Weeks of treatment
40 mg daily	1st and 2nd week
30 mg daily	3rd and 4th week
20 mg daily	5th and 6th week
15 mg daily	7th and 8th week
10 mg daily	9th and 10th week
05 mg daily	11th and 12th week

demonstrated better response rates and lesser additional steroid requirements in regimens of longer duration (5 months) than the shorter ones (3 months). They have advocated that as RRs in multibacillary (MB) leprosy persist over many months, duration of the steroid treatment matters more than the dose. They have emphasized that initial dose of steroids does not affect the efficacy of the antileprosy regimen. In a recent clinical trial comparing high dose (60 mg) with low dose (40 mg) steroid in the management of T1R, recurrence was noted in 16% and 48.3% patients in high and low dose groups, respectively. Both regimens were equally efficacious and no major adverse effects were observed in either groups.[10] Similarly, Walker et al. lend further support to the use of more prolonged courses of corticosteroids to treat T1R.[11] Further, another interesting observation concluded that in the low dose regimen majority of recurrence occurred within a period of 6 months after completion of the regimen, whereas only 25% patients had recurrence within 6 months in the high dose regimen indicating that recurrences may occur earlier in low dose regimen.[10]

To conclude, longer duration of treatment depending on the spectrum of the leprosy (longer duration of treatment in MB cases) with higher starting dose (1 mg/kg body weight) of steroid is the most ideal regimen for appropriate management as well as to prevent recurrence of T1R.

Outcome of Timely and Adequate Corticosteroid Administration[12]

- Improvement in inflammation over the skin lesions, both old and new.
- Improvement in NFI in 30–70% of the patients. Response is better in those with recent nerve damage and more in BT group than in others, especially when nerves are rested. Median nerve shows better response than the ulnar nerve.

Adverse Effects

It is surprising that the adverse effects with corticosteroids during treatment of T1R are not many in contrast to those observed while treating ENL with prednisolone. This is particularly relevant in view of steroid dependency and the associated metabolic problems. The adverse effects seen most commonly are:

- Skin changes include striae, steroid acne, purpura, ecchymosis, xerosis, persistent erythema of the skin in sun exposed areas and erythromelanoses. Last three skin complications, viz., xeroris, persistent erythema in the exposed areas and erythromelanoses which can also be observed due to clofazimine which is a component of MDT in MB leprosy. The most common change is development of cushingoid features due to the alteration in fat distribution, like buffalo hump, facial fullness (moon face), increased supraclavicular and suprasternal fat,

protuberant or pendulous abdomen, and flattening of buttocks and gynecomastia (it can also occur *per se* in LL, as a result of orchitis and liver involvement). In addition, there is hair loss, thinning of hair and the hair becoming brittle and fracturing along the shaft. There may be hair growth on the beard area, on the arms and back, and coarsening of fine vellus hair, especially in women.

- Gastrointestinal (GIT) side effects, like hematemesis, peptic ulcer or perforation.
- Metabolic complications include diabetes mellitus, hypertension, edema due to sodium retention, hypokalemia due to increased potassium excretion, hyperlipidemias, secondary amenorrhea, decreased efficacy of anticoagulants and oral contraceptives. These side effects call for alternate or second line drugs, such as other immunosuppressive drugs referred to earlier.[13]
- Ocular side effects like cataracts and glaucoma.
- *Bone changes*: Osteoporosis, pathological fractures and aseptic necrosis of the bone.
- The prolonged use of steroids may also result in central nervous system (CNS) complications, like psychosis and pseudotumor cerebri.
- Opportunistic infections, including tuberculosis, mucormycosis and chromoblastomycosis, have been reported in MB leprosy patients under prolonged corticosteroid and thalidomide therapy to control T2R.[14]

The patient should carry a steroid card giving details of the steroid dosing, with durations. The reason for carrying such a card is that injury, intercurrent infection and surgical operation demand extra supplies of endogenous cortisol, and these cannot be produced by an already atrophic adrenal cortex due to prolonged steroid therapy. Rarely, the patient may die of adrenal shock unless adequate doses of steroid are administered during the crisis period. As a precautionary measure, it is essential to check the patient for hypertension, diabetes mellitus, infections, particularly tuberculosis, worm infestations, before the start, and during course of steroid treatment, as these may get worse with prolonged corticosteroid therapy.

Other Immunosuppressant Drugs for Treatment of T1R

The side effects associated with prolonged use of corticosteroids sometimes warrant discontinuation of their usage for flaring up of conditions like diabetes mellitus or hypertension. Many a times it becomes necessary to reduce the corticosteroid doses to a minimal functioning level because of their side effects. A number of other compounds have been tried, some not so successfully.

- *Methotrexate*: Methotrexate is known to reduce the production of Th1 cytokines, and increase the expression of anti-inflammatory Th2 cytokines. Recently, low-dose methotrexate (5–7.5 mg/week) was reported to be successful in reducing the steroid dose in BL patient with steroid intolerance.[15]

- *Cyclosporine A (CyA)*: It inhibits transcription of interleukin-2 (IL-2) mRNA, thereby blocking proliferation of T-cells. It is found to be associated with decrease in antinerve growth factor antibodies.[16] This drug is useful in chronic neuritis and can be tried in those cases who do not respond well to prednisolone. It improves sensory impairment, muscular force and pain. CyA has been administered for up to 12 months without significant side effects with a starting dose of 5 mg/kg/day followed by gradual reduction of the dose.[17] However, close monitoring of blood pressure and kidney function test are warranted.
- *Azathioprine*: It inhibits T- and B-cell proliferation, antibody (Ab) synthesis and tumor necrosis factor-α (TNF-α). It acts much more slowly, but has been reported to reduce the requirement of steroids when given in combination with them.[18]
- *Mycophenolate mofetil*: This is a reversible inhibitor of inosine monophosphate dehydrogenase, an enzyme essential for *de novo* purine synthesis that is needed for lymphocyte proliferation. As this compound affects both T and B lymphocyte activity resulting in immunosuppression, it should theoretically work both for T1Rs and T2Rs. However, it was not found to be useful in any type of the reactions in reducing and withdrawing the steroid dose after several months of its addition.[19]
- *Miscellaneous*: Recently, topical tacrolimus 0.1% ointment was favorably used to treat a case of BL leprosy with severe reversal reaction without nerve involvement, which was resistant to oral prednisolone (1 mg/kg daily).[20]

Although treatment of T1R is primarily based on inducing immunosuppression, report of its occurrence in patients of liver transplantation on triple immunosuppressive therapy consisting of low-dose prednisolone (10 mg/day), tacrolimus (6 mg/day) and mycophenolate mofetil (MMF) (2 g/day) has appeared recently in the literature. The reaction was successfully treated with 0.5 mg/kg prednisolone.[21] The occurrence of reaction in patients on optimal doses of immunosuppressive drugs suggest that probably the action of various immunosuppressive drugs is selective, whereas corticosteroids have a broader immunosuppressive effect, especially with respect to the range of target cells which include monocytes, macrophages, and CD4+ T-cells. They also reduce the production of inflammatory mediators, including cytokines, prostaglandins (PGE) and nitric oxide.

Additional Measures for Neuritis/Nerve Function Impairment

In acute phase the inflamed nerves must be kept in resting position. Appropriate splinting and padding gives relief. When the acute phase is over, passive and active exercises should be initiated. Oil massage and other modalities like short wave diathermy (SWD) or ultrasonic therapy (UST) help in restoring the motor function and preventing disability. Additional nonsteroidal anti-inflammatory drugs (NSAIDs) may be required for relieving pain.

Surgical Decompression[22]

In spite of the best efforts with medications and other supportive measures, a few cases continue to have nerve pain and tenderness and/or functional impairment in one or few nerves. This is because of the persistence of increased intraneural pressure due to formation of an abscess, as a result of acute inflammation, leading to ischemia in the nerve. In such patients there is need for surgical nerve decompression, which adds to the benefit of steroids in relieving pain, and stops further deterioration of sensory and motor functions. Surgical decompression involves exposing the affected nerve trunk at the point of maximal thickness, and giving longitudinal incisions into the nerve up to epineurium layers of nerve bundles. Continuation of steroids during and after surgery prevents postoperative edema and decreases postoperative scarring.

TREATMENT OF LATE REVERSAL REACTION

Prednisolone (1 mg/kg body weight per day) for 4–6 weeks, makes the lesions disappear completely or show early signs of subsidence as evidenced by decrease in infiltration/erythema. Steroids may be continued till complete subsidence of the lesions. If reactive skin and nerve lesions do not show improvement within 3 months of steroid therapy, the case should be considered as relapse presenting in the form of T1R, and MDT should be restarted for another course and oral steroids gradually tapered off with complete subsidence of reactional features.[23]

MANAGEMENT OF TYPE 2 REACTION

This reaction is characterized by crops of tender, evanescent, erythematous, subcutaneous nodules associated with fever and malaise. There may be accompanying neuritis, iritis, arthritis, orchitis, dactylitis and/or lymphadenopathy. The reactions may continue to occur even after completion of MDT. The very first dose of MDT can lead to precipitation of a reaction of mild to severe nature. To prevent the occurrence of a reaction, some leprologists suggest that in cases with high initial bacterial load, MDT should preferably be started under the cover of oral steroids, which may be withdrawn after a period of 2–4 weeks.[11]

Grade Severity of Type 2 Reaction

It may be of mild or severe type. Mild type is defined when the patient has only a few ENL skin lesions and no signs of involvement of other organs. Patients with any one or more of the following signs and symptoms should be treated as severe: (1) high fever, severe bodyaches and pains, myalgia and other constitutional symptoms, (2) extensive ENL with or without pustular/necrotic lesions, (3) pain or tenderness (neuritis) in one or more nerves, with or without loss of nerve function, (4) recent NFI, (5) pain and/or tenderness of the eye (iridocyclitis) with or without loss of visual acuity, (6) painful swelling of the testes (orchitis), (7) marked arthritis and/or lymphadenitis. They should preferably be admitted in the hospital for bed rest and daily monitoring.

Severity of T2R can be assessed and efficacy of anti-reactional drugs can be monitored using RSS (reaction severity scale) designed and modified by van Brakel et al.[24] (*See* Chapter 29 on Leprosy Reactions).

Treat Precipitating Factors (Figs 32.1A and B)

It is important (and sometimes rewarding also) to look for any precipitating factor which could be providing a trigger for reaction. It may be any intercurrent infection like sore throat (streptococcal), viral (especially common is herpes simplex), intestinal parasites and protozoa, filaria, or malaria, which all need appropriate treatment. Psychological stress should not be overlooked and must be dealt with by counseling by the doctor, nurses, or a trained counselor. Sedation with tranquilizers helps in reducing stress.

Continue or Start Multidrug Therapy

Multidrug therapy has to be continued uninterrupted and, if not started earlier, should be started along with specific treatment for T2R.

Specific Treatment of Type 2 Reaction

Mild Type 2 Reaction

Mild T2R can be managed with analgesics and anti-inflammatory drugs such as aspirin and other NSAIDs. Aspirin is given in the dose of 600 mg 6 hourly with meals. The dosage is reduced slowly as signs and symptoms are controlled. NSAIDs decrease prostaglandin synthesis, and help in mild suppression of Ag-Ab reaction and Ab production, and thus help to alleviate the reaction.[25]

Colchicine inhibits vascular injury by inhibiting neutrophil chemotaxis and may be helpful in mild to moderate type of ENL.[25] It is given orally in the dose of 0.5 mg, three times daily with a tapering course. The adverse reactions in decreasing order of severity are bone marrow depression, peripheral neuritis, purpura, myopathy, loss of hair, reversible azoospermia and diarrhea.

Severe Type 2 Reaction

1. *Oral corticosteroids*: Oral corticosteroids constitute the first line armamentarium in the management of severe T2R. They act by inhibiting both the early and late phases of inflammation. Corticosteriods decrease chemotaxis of neutrophils and inhibit the enzyme prostaglandin synthetase. Steroid administration is also associated with suppression of cell-mediated immunity (CMI) by depletion of T-cells, particularly helper T-cells, with consequent restoration of altered helper/suppressor T-cells ratio and resultant decrease in the liberation of proinflammatory lymphokines.

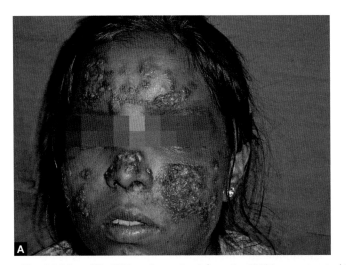 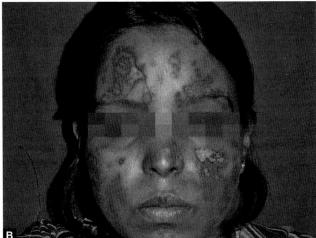

Figs 32.1A and B: (A) Type 2 reaction (ulcerative ENL) in an untreated BL patient after a course of ofloxacin given for urinary tract infection; (B) Clinical improvement after 5 weeks oral prednisolone along with MDT

World Health Organization (1998) recommends prednisolone for severe ENL reaction in doses similar to those prescribed for RR (Table 32.1). Prednisolone should be started in a dose of 1 mg/kg/day till clinical improvement, then tapered every week by 5–10 mg over 6–8 weeks. A maintenance dose of 20–30 mg may be needed for several weeks to prevent recurrence of ENL. No doubt, quick response to prednisolone is observed in most of the cases in the first attack of T2R.

However, in addition to usual side effects observed with steroid administration (described earlier), steroid dependence is a very important problem to handle. Tapering the dose of steroid is often associated with recurrence of reaction.

2. *Clofazimine*: The biochemical basis for the antimicrobial action of clofazimine remains to be elucidated. The drug possibly acts by blocking the template function of DNA, by increasing lysosomal enzyme synthesis and by increasing phagocytic capacity of macrophages.[26] It binds preferentially to GC-rich region of mycobacterial (not mammalian) DNA. Stimulation of PGE2 synthesis, inhibition of neutrophil motility, together with selective suppression of Th-1 subtype of T-helper cells contribute to its role in T2R.[27] Clofazimine selectively block the Kv1.3 potassium channel activity, perturbing the oscillation frequency of the calcium-release activated calcium channel, which in turn led to the inhibition of the calcineurin-nuclear factor of activated T-cells (NFAT) signaling pathway.[28] Thus, it has immunomodulatory effect also.

It is administered in the dose of 300 mg daily, orally in an adult for a period of 1–3 months, followed by 200 mg daily for 3 months and 100 mg daily for as long as the symptoms remain. Clofazimine is slow to act and does not relieve acute manifestations of reaction. However, with the use of higher initial dose of clofazimine (300 mg) given over several weeks, it is possible to reduce the dose or even withdraw the steroids under its cover. This also prevents requirement of frequent increment of the steroid dose to control T2R. A recent study comparing the efficacy of clofazimine in control of ENL in MB leprosy patients receiving either 12 months or 24 months WHO-MDT suggested that an extended period of coverage with clofazimine may reduce the severity of ENL in relatively small number of high-risk patients (LL, or average initial BI of 4 or more).[29] Further research is required to identify the best way of using clofazimine to minimize the occurrence of ENL.

3. *Thalidomide*: Although thalidomide is the treatment of choice for the management of severe T2R, this is kept as second option because of its teratogenic effects, difficulty in monitoring at all healthcare levels, cost and nonavailability at all places.

Thalidomide was developed in 1954 and subsequently marketed in Europe, Australia and Canada as a sedative and antiemetic; useful in morning sickness. The drug was not approved by United States Food and Drug Administration (US-FDA). It was banned in 1962 in view of worldwide criticism following serious teratogenic effects (discussed below). In 1965, Sheskin reported the effectiveness of thalidomide in the management of ENL. It was licensed in the Unites States of America (USA) for use in leprosy on July 16, 1998.

Structure and metabolism: Thalidomide is a racemic glutamic acid analogue composed of two enantiomers R- and S- thalidomide which interconvert under physiological conditions. Two enantiomers have different properties; one is a more potent suppressor of TNF-α release by stimulated peripheral blood mononuclear cells, whilst the other is sedative. Thalidomide undergoes hydrolysis at pH 7 in aqueous solution and this degradation leads to the formation of more than 20 products, which are responsible for the activity.

Mechanism of action: The exact mechanisms of action are not clear, but TNF, interferon-γ, IL-10 and IL-12, cycloxygenase-2, and possibly the proinflammatory transcription factor κB [nuclear factor-kappa B (NF-κB)], p38 and ERK1/2 are all affected. Elucidation of the activation mechanisms in cells stimulated with *M. leprae* can lead to the development of new therapeutic applications to modulate NF-κB activation and to control the inflammatory manifestations due to enhanced TNF-α response as observed in leprosy and in leprosy reactions.[30] The various modes of anti-inflammatory actions are summarized in Box 32.2.

Indications: WHO expert committee and The International Federation of Anti-leprosy Associations' (ILEP) Technical Bulletin acknowledges the effectiveness of thalidomide and states that it has fewer adverse effects than corticosteroids. Therefore, thalidomide is a good choice for men and postmenopausal women with difficulty to manage ENL, particularly for the patients with recurrent ENL and for steroid dependent cases. However, women of childbearing age should also not be denied an effective and sometimes life-saving drug, provided that they and their physicians understand the risk associated with it, and all precautionary measures are taken for administration of this drug prior to therapy as described under System for Thalidomide Education and Prescribing Safety (STEPS) program (Box 32.3).

Clinical effects: Thalidomide is able to suppress all clinical manifestations of T2R within 48–72 hours. Its action is faster and more effective than aspirin, clofazimine and pentoxyphylline. Although response is faster to both thalidomide and prednisolone, improvement is better and recurrence is less frequent with thalidomide.[31] It quickly reduces the fever and number of skin lesions. Effect on nerve and eye involvement is less pronounced. This drug is essentially nontoxic and well-tolerated even during

Box 32.2: Mechanism of action of thalidomide
• It reduces chemotactic factors and IgM synthesis which is important in ENL
• Thalidomide causes significant reduction in CD4+ lymphocytes and thus normalizes CD4/CD8 ratio. It also decreases dermal infiltration of polymorphonuclear leukocytes and T-cells
• It inhibits inflammatory cytokines TNF-α, IFN-γ, VEGF, and bFGF. It reduces plasma soluble IL-2 receptor, a marker of inflammation
• It causes significant reduction of TNF-α, the most important mechanisms of action in suppressing ENL. *In vitro* study has demonstrated that *M. leprae* induce activation of NF-κB in a Schwann cell line mediated by TNF-α. Thalidomide causes repression of transcription of TNF-α and thereby inhibit NF-κB. Recurrence of the ENL after cessation of thalidomide is associated with an elevation in serum TNF levels
• Thalidomide has effects on angiogenesis in addition to those over immune function and inflammation
• It causes down regulation of ICAM-1 and MHC class-I Ags expression on keratinocytes
• Induction of NF-κB activation and DNA binding activity is inhibited by thalidomide. The drug also reduces *M. leprae* induced TNF-α production and inhibits p38 and ERK1/2 activation.

Abbreviations: IgM, immunoglobulin M; ENL, erythema nodosum leprosum; TNF, tumor necrosis factor; IFN-γ, interferon gamma; VEGF, vascular endothelial-derived growth factor; bFGF, basic fibroblast growth factor; IL, interleukin; NF, nuclear factor; ICAM, intercellular adhesion molecule; MHC, major histocompatibility complex; ERK, extracellular signal-regulated kinases; Ag, antigen.

Box 32.3: Thalidomide monitoring guidelines [As under System for Thalidomide Education and Prescribing Safety (STEPS)]
Baseline
Determine the patient's ability to comprehend the drug risks and willingness to sign the consent form, and to participate in ongoing monitoring programs
Laboratory testing   • *Pregnancy test*: Serum (or urine) test of adequate sensitivity in women of child bearing potential   • CBC with platelet count
Neurological evaluation   • Clinical neurological examination   • *Nerve conduction studies for amplitude of SNAP*: If suggested by history and physical examination
Follow-up
Laboratory testing   • *Pregnancy test*: In women with regular menses, Weekly for 4 weeks, then monthly.
In women with irregular menses: Every 2 weeks   • CBC with platelet count   • *Clinical neurological examination*: Monthly for 3 months, thereafter at 1–6 months as indicated   • *Nerve conduction studies for amplitude of SNAP*: If decrease by 30%—decrease the dose, if by 40%—stop thalidomide.

Abbreviations: CBC, complete blood count; SNAP, sensory nerve action potential.

long-term administration and can be tried as a complimentary medication for tapering the steroid dose. However, the side effects of this drug must be kept in mind (see below).

Dosage: In severe ENL, it is suggested to start thalidomide at a dose of 400 mg at bedtime or 100 mg, four times daily. This dose easily controls the reaction within 48 hours in most of the cases. The dose is then reduced more slowly by 100 mg each month.[31] During this period, the patient should be assessed regularly and should be stabilized on the lowest dose that controls the symptoms and continue at this dose for a period of 2–3 months. This is essential since several studies have recorded high relapse rates and flare-ups of ENL including precipitation of necrotic ENL in patients upon sudden withdrawal of thalidomide.[32,33] Welsh et al.[34] also reported a patient of ENL who had relapsed when thalidomide dose was decreased to 50 mg/day, which was managed with pentoxifylline 400 mg TDS and clofazimine 100 mg TDS within 8 days. Although the exact mechanism of these relapses remains unelucidated, Mahajan et al.[34] have suggested that thalidomide has only a suppressive effect. Premature withdrawal of thalidomide without tapering doses perhaps causes a sudden spurt of various inflammatory cytokines [TNF-α, IFN-γ, vascular endothelial-derived growth factor (VEGF) and basic fibroblast growth factor (bFGF)], reversal in CD4/CD8 ratio which was normalized by thalidomide and neutrophil-lymphocytes chemotaxis as a rebound phenomenon.

In such cases prolonged maintenance therapy is required. Instead of discontinuing the drug, a maintenance dose of 100 mg daily (with a range of 100 mg on alternate days; to 100 mg two or more times, daily) should be given for a sufficient period. Every 6 months, attempts should be made to discontinue the drug after gradual tapering of the dose. If again there is recurrence of reaction, this drug can be restarted for another period of 6 months. This process is repeated until reaction no longer recurs when the drug is discontinued. Recently, Japan has proposed their local guidelines on use and application of thalidomide. They suggest starting thalidomide from 50–100 mg/day and then adjusting the dose according to the symptoms of each patient, not to exceed the maximum recommended dose of 300 mg/ day, for the treatment of ENL.[35] If a patient is already receiving prednisolone for T2R, but difficult to control and needs to be switched over to thalidomide, first prednisolone should be tapered to a level until the reaction recurs. Then at that level of corticosteroid, thalidomide should be introduced and tapered. In few patients, the drug may have to be continued till skin-smear negativity is achieved.[36] However; controlling ENL by replacing steroids with thalidomide is more difficult than using thalidomide from the beginning.

Adverse effects of thalidomide:

- *Teratogenicity*[37]: Intrauterine exposure to thalidomide during pregnancy between days 20 and 36 after conception leads to development of a condition known as phocomelia (Gk. *Phok*; seal, *melos*; limb) due to resemblance of the limbs with that of seal (Fig. 32.2). The other associated abnormalities with phocomelia are deficient or absent ears, hearing loss, absent or extra digits, visual disturbances, cardiac, renal and GIT anomalies, cleft palate, saddle nose, etc.

An *in vitro* study in myeloma cells has shown that thalidomide intercalate into guanine rich promoter sequences of insulin growth factor-1 (IGF-1) and fibroblast growth factor (FGF) genes which act in combination to stimulate limb initiation and thereby suppress guanine rich promoter sequences resulting in limb defects.[38] The drug is also distributed into human semen after oral dosing.[39] But there is no report of teratogenicity so far caused through semen exposure.

During the use of thalidomide in women of childbearing age, it is absolutely mandatory to invoke contraception as mentioned under STEPS Program (Box 32.3). Reliable contraception is indicated even where there has been a history of infertility, unless due to hysterectomy or because the patient has been postmenopausal for at least 24 months. Although there is a strict legislation for the prescription and use of thalidomide,

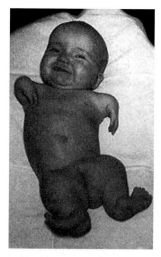

Fig. 32.2: Phocomelia baby
Source: www.documentingreality.com

two new cases of thalidomide embryopathy (TEP) were identified in Brazil.[40] A recent study suggests that TEP has probably increased in recent years, which coincides with the period of greater thalidomide availability. The high frequency of leprosy and the large use of thalidomide reinforce the need for a continuous monitoring of TEP across Brazil.[41]

- *Neuropathy*: Peripheral neuropathy occurs in 20% of individuals during first year of treatment.[42] It is characterized by painful paresthesia and numbness in a glove and stocking distribution. It affects the lower limbs initially, followed by the involvement of upper limbs. It may be associated with weakness. Neuropathy correlates with the daily dose administered, but continues to progress for some time, even after cessation of therapy, then gradually shows improvement. However, it remains permanent in 50% of the cases. Nerve conduction studies reveal a sensory, predominantly axonal, length-dependent neuropathy (small fiber axonopathy). Nerves show loss of large myelinated fibers and little inflammation when examined histopathologically.[43]

- *Thromboembolism:* In thalidomide treated cases of multiple myeloma, thromboembolism has been reported in 3% of cases.[44] This rate increases to 14% when it is combined with dexamethasone. There is sudden emergence of multiple reports of deep venous thrombosis (DVT) when corticosteroid and thalidomide are coadministrated for the treatment of ENL.[45] There have been two case reports from India describing occurrence of iliac vein thrombosis in a woman with ENL treated with a combination of thalidomide, prednisolone and cyclophosphamide.[46] Another case of deep vein thrombosis in a 43-year-old man with lepromatous leprosy who was being treated with thalidomide and prednisolone for a type 2 leprosy reaction has been reported recently.[47] The patient also had transiently positive antiphospholipid Ab results. Hence, antiphospholipid Ab levels should be measured in high-risk patients before starting thalidomide.

- *Somnolence*: Drowsiness, a common side effect, can be avoided by giving the drug at bed time. It may be of severe nature in up to 11% of patients.[48]

- *Cutaneous adverse reactions:* These have been reported in 3% of cases.[48] Rare, but severe, cutaneous adverse effects are erythema multiforme (EM), erythroderma and toxic epidermal necrolysis (TEN).

- *Other side effects:*[48] Conditions like constipation, nausea, dizziness, peripheral edema, and hypothyroidism have also been reported.

- Recently, a case of left thigh phlegmon caused by *Nocardia farcinica* in a 54-year-old Italian man affected by MB leprosy with ENL reaction being treated with MDT plus thalidomide and steroid has been described.[49]

Treatment of Chronic and Recurrent Type 2 Reaction

Drug regimens: A combination of prednisolone plus thalidomide or clofazimine is preferable for management of chronic and recurrent T2R. The ideal duration and dose of steroid and other drug combinations is still a matter of debate.

An open prospective single center study at New Delhi was conducted to assess the comparative efficacy of combination of prednisolone plus thalidomide in one group versus prednisolone with clofazimine in another group in chronic and recurrent T2R.[31]

Prednisolone was given in the dose of 1 mg/kg/day to start with, then gradually tapered as (10 mg every 2 weeks upto 30 mg, than 5 mg every 2 weeks up to 5 mg, then 2.5 mg for 2 weeks-for a total of 20 weeks) *plus either thalidomide* (200 mg BD × 7 days and then tapered by 100 mg every month to a dose of 100 mg daily, then every alternate day for 20 weeks) or *clofazamine* (300 mg/day to start for 12 weeks, and then 200 mg/day × 4 weeks, then 100 mg/day × 4 weeks given over 20 weeks).

Patients were followed-up for 6 months after 20 weeks course of treatment to note any further recurrence of T2R. The response rate based on the clinical outcome was 82.35% in thalidomide plus prednisolone group, and 60% in clofazimine and prednisolone group. In the follow-up period of 6 months, 2 of 16 patients in prednisolone plus clofazimine group developed fresh episode of T2R whereas none (0/17) in the prednisolone plus thalidomide group had recurrence. It was concluded that thalidomide has good efficacy when administered in combination with prednisolone for chronic and recurrent T2R. Clofazamine has a definite role when thalidomide cannot be administered (women in child bearing age). The duration of combination treatment should be judged depending on the frequency of recurrence and chronicity of lesions even beyond 20 weeks, which may vary from individual patient to patient.

A recent study from Bangladesh showed that nine cases of recurrent/chronic ENL not controlled by a combination of prednisone with clofazimine could be managed with a combination of prednisolone with methotrexate (prednisolone dose: 40 mg/day × 3 months, reduced to 20 mg/day × 3 months, then reduced by 5 mg/week × 3 months, reduced by 5 mg a/d, then weekly twice, then weekly once: 30–36 months (total) and methotrexate dose: 7.5 mg/week: 24–30 months).[50]

Algorithm for managing severe ENL reaction is summarized in Box 32.4 and Flow chart 32.1.

Immunotherapy: Several immunomodulators, including Mw (MIP) vaccine along with MDT, have been tried in the past in patients with MB leprosy for faster clearance of dead bacilli from the body. Theoretically, it is expected that they would help to prevent T2R and may even be helpful in the treatment of reaction through their effectiveness for quick bacterial clearance.[51]

Alternate therapies for type 2 reaction:

- *Betamethasone pulse therapy*: Slow infusion of 40 mg betamethasone daily in 5% dextrose for three consecutive days and every 4 weeks has been recommended for recurrent ENL. Though well-tolerated, it does not offer significant advantage over conventional way of managing ENL—chronic and recurrent ENL. However, side effects of

---

Box 32.4: Summary of treatment for severe type 2 reaction

- *For first attack of severe ENL*

  – *Option 1: Prednisolone*

  Initial high dose (1 mg/kg body weight till clinical improvement, then taper every week by 5–10 mg over 6–8 weeks. A maintenance dose of 20–40 mg may be needed for several weeks to prevent recurrence of ENL

  or

  Combination of prednisolone and clofazimine: Prednisolone as above in first option + clofazimine as below.
  Clofazimine 100 mg tds for first 4 weeks followed by 100 mg bd for next 4–12 weeks followed by 100 mg od for 4–12 weeks or till the symptoms/signs persist
  Clofazimine is useful in reducing or withdrawing prednisolone. Total duration of clofazimine therapy should not exceed 12 months

  – *Option 2: Thalidomide*

  200 mg BD, for 3–7 days or till reaction is under control, followed by tapering within 3–4 weeks or taper more slowly if recurrence occurs quickly:
  100 mg morning + 200 mg evening for 4 weeks
  200 mg evening for 4 weeks
  100 mg evening for 4 weeks
  50 mg daily evening or 100 mg every alternate day evening for 8–12 weeks

- *For recurrent or chronic ENL: Combination treatment is always preferred*

  – *Option 1: Clofazimine + Prednisolone*

  Prednisolone: 1 mg/kg body weight OD till clinical improvement followed by 5–10 mg reduction every 2 weeks
  Clofazimine 100 mg tds for 3 months
  100 mg bd for 3 months
  100 mg od as long as symptoms persist

  – *Option 2: Thalidomide + Prednisolone*

  Prednisolone in the same dose as above
  Thalidomide 200 mg bd for 3–7 days
  100 mg morning + 200 mg evening for 4 weeks
  200 mg evening for 4 weeks
  100 mg evening for 4 weeks
  50 mg daily evening or 100 mg every alternate day evening for 8–12 weeks
  For any relapse of reaction or deterioration raise the dose immediately by 200 mg, and then slowly reduce to 100 mg on alternate day or 50 mg daily for several months, to manage chronic ENL

Abbreviations: tds, thrice a day; bd, twice a day; od, once a day.

Flow chart 32.1: Algorithm for management of severe erythema nodosum leprosum

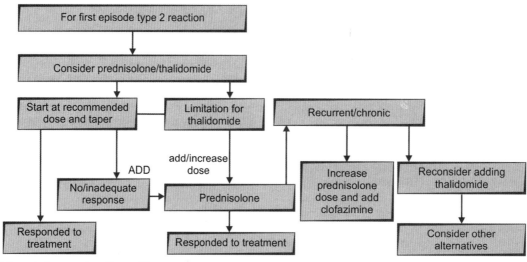

Source: Kar HK, Gupta L. Comparative efficacy of four treatment regimens in type 2 leprosy reactions (prednisolone alone, thalidomide alone, prednisolone plus thalidomide and prednisolone plus clofazimine). Presented at 18th International Leprosy Congress; 2013 Sept 16 – Sept 19; Brussels, Belgium. Abstract No: O-070.

monthly infused steroids were not progressive in contrast to the side effects observed in daily steroid regimen.[52]

- *Dexamethasone pulse therapy with azathioprine*: This regimen may be considered as a daily steroid sparing regimen for steroid dependent chronic ENL reaction. It is given in a dose of 100 mg dexamethasone in 500 mL glucose IV infusion on three consecutive days, every month, along with 50 mg daily azathioprine.[53] This combination pulse therapy may help in reducing the steroid requirement.

- *Azathioprine*: Literature contains few experiences in the use of glucocorticosteroids sparing agents, such as azathioprine in leprosy reactions.[54] It has been tried in preventing recurrence of reaction in patients with recurrent ENL and was reportedly effective in the dose of 2 mg/kg/day given for 6–8 months in weaning a female patient of thalidomide.

- Recent reports of its use in severe ENL reactions have concluded that patients who began treatment with azathioprine at the first reaction episode required a much shorter treatment with high doses of glucocorticoids than those who began azathioprine after initial ENL reaction. It was also noted that control of leprosy reactions with azathioprine prevented the progression of neural damage, but there was no recovery of lost neural functions.[53]

The drug is usually well-tolerated but there is a large interindividual variability related to genetic polymorphisms in metabolic enzymes, thiopurine s-methyltransferase (TPMT) and xanthine oxidase (XO). Decreased TPMT or XO activity results in increased production of toxic metabolites. A TPMT check value is recommended before introducing azathioprine to avoid potentially fatal myelotoxicity.

- *Pentoxifylline*: This is a methyl xanthine derivative used in the management of peripheral vascular diseases. It has been shown to inhibit the production of TNF-α both *in vivo and in vitro*. A double-blind study from Brazil showed that pentoxifylline 1,200 mg daily is not as effective as thalidomide given in a dose of 300 mg daily. It could be a good option for patients with human immunodeficiency virus (HIV) coinfection where long-term steroids are contraindicated.[55] However, all leprologists do not enjoy the same amount of good response with pentoxyphylline.

- *Cyclosporine A*: Cyclosporine A has been used because of its immunosuppressant action. It inhibits T-helper (Th) cells and restores the Th:Ts (T-suppressor) cells balance. However, in short series of clinical trials, it has provided ambiguous results with controversial outcome.

- *Plasma exchange*: Plasma exchange removes Ag, Ab and immune complexes. It may be helpful in difficult cases when this facility is available and cost factor is not a hindrance.

- *Methotrexate*: Methotrexate acts by increasing the adenosine levels, reducing proinflammatory cytokines and increasing the levels of anti-inflammatory cytokines. It was found to be effective as a steroid sparing agent in a case of steroid resistant ENL.[50]

- *Mycophenolate mofetil*: It is an inhibitor of *de novo* purine synthesis in T and B lymphocytes. But the results so far have not been promising, as discussed in the section on T1Rs.

Newer Drugs in the Management of Erythema Nodosum Leprosum

Leukotriene Inhibitors (Zafirlukast, Montelukast)

Zafirlukast has been tried in an open phase II cohort using an initial dose of 40 mg twice, daily. It was found to be effective in six patients of ENL, but end points are not defined.[56]

Thalidomide Derivatives-IMiDs-[Lenalidomide (Revimid), Pomalidomide (Actimid)]

Immunomodulatory analogs of thalidomide's (lenalidomide, CC-5013; pomalidomide, CC-4047) represent a novel class of compounds with numerous effects on the immune system. IMiDs inhibit TNF-α, IL-1β, IL-12, and granulocyte macrophage-colony stimulating factor (GM-CSF). They also had an inhibitory effect on the production of IL-6, IFN-γ, CXCL9 and CXCL10, but stimulate IL-10. A recent study found reduced levels of mRNA for TNF-α after treatment with lenalidomide and pomalidomide, suggesting post-transcriptional effects.[57] The compounds had no effect on cell viability. These IMiDs drugs appear to be even more potent than thalidomide and do not appear to have any adverse effects. However, these molecules require human clinical trials.

Anti-TNF-α Agents (Infliximab, Etanercept, Adalimumab)

Infliximab has been reported to be effective in a case of recurrent ENL without any complications.[58] Recently, the effectiveness of etanercept has been shown in a 33-year-old woman with ENL who failed to respond adequately to conventional therapy over a 6-year period.[59] Hence, use of anti-TNF-α agents appears to be a promising approach for chronic/resistant ENL reactions. However, these drugs should be used with caution in leprosy patients, since the occurrence of type 1 leprosy reaction manifesting after discontinuation of adalimumab therapy have been reported.[60,61] Also, TNF-α blockade carries an increased risk of fungal infection and also with *M. tuberculosis*.

Treatment of Other Manifestations

Discussed in detail in separate chapters and summarized in Table 32.2.

MANAGEMENT OF LUCIO PHENOMENON

It is a rare variant of T2R occurring primarily in the evolution of Lucio leprosy and rarely in other forms of LL, which is encountered in certain parts of the world, like Mexico and the Caribbean. This form of reaction typically occurs in untreated patients and the patients remain afebrile throughout.

Table 32.2: Treatment of other complications

Motor deficits	Physiotherapy Splints Surgical correction
Acute iridocyclitis	Oral/local steroids (1% hydrocortisone, hourly; eye drops and eye ointment at night) Atropine eye drops bd
Acute epididymo-orchitis	Bed rest Oral corticosteroids Scrotal suspensory bandage

Patients respond excellently well when MDT is started. They also respond to oral steroids but thalidomide is of no value. However, after initial good response to MDT, many of these patients may develop the classical ENL. Recently, Montero et al. reported a case of lepromatous leprosy on irregular treatment that developed Lucio phenomenon, which was diagnosed by classical histopathological findings, and was treated with MDT, antibiotics, steroids and thalidomide with favorable outcome.[62]

Although presentation as angular purpuric ulcers is the most common presentation, involvement of bone marrow and lymph nodes has also been described in Lucio phenomenon.[63]

CONCLUSION

Borderline leprosy patients have to be monitored very closely for RR and neuritis, both during antileprosy treatment and thereafter. Adequate initial dose of steroids is the key to control reactions and even reverse the nerve damage. Adequate duration of steroid therapy is also important to prevent recurrence and nerve recovery.

As per the severity of ENL, the choice of suitable drugs has to be made. Recurrent and chronic ENL pose a difficult problem for the physician to manage. Recurrent and chronic ENL reactors need combination of steroids and thalidomide/clofazimine in adequate doses and duration. For steroid dependent cases, better treatments need to be available.

The reactions are the basis for neuritis; and neuritis is the basis for deformities, disabilities and the stigmatizing figure of a leprosy patient. So the identification of predictors of neuropathy and reactions, as well as treatment at an early stage is important. The presently ongoing cohort INFIR study[64] may throw some light on better management of reactions in future. At the current juncture, there is a need to enhance the research for newer drugs in the management of reactions. There should be a good patient monitoring scheme. Quality of life studies in patients with ENL would help to determine the social and financial impact of these conditions.

REFERENCES

1. Vasavi S, Reddy BS. Histoid leprosy with erythema nodosum leprosum—a case report. Indian J Lepr. 2012;84(1):27-9.
2. Naafs B. Current views on reactions in leprosy. Indian J Lepr. 2000;72(1):97-122.
3. Marzano AV, Tosi D, Cusini M, et al. Facial reversal reaction: a dermatological emergency. J Dermatol. 2012;39(2):203-5.
4. Lipworth BJ. Therapeutic implications of non-genomic glucocorticoid activity. Lancet. 2000;356(9224):87-9.
5. Lu PH, Lin JY, Tsai YL, et al. Corticosteroid pulse therapy for leprosy complicated by a severe type 1 reaction. Chang Gung Med J. 2008;31(2):201-6.
6. Walker SL, Roberts CH, Atkinson SE, et al. The effect of systemic corticosteroid therapy on the expression of toll-like receptor 2 and toll-like receptor 4 in the cutaneous lesions of leprosy type 1 reactions. Br J Dermatol. 2012;167(1):29-35.
7. WHO Expert Committee on leprosy. Technical Report Series No. 874.1998.pp.1-48.
8. Rao PS, Sugamaran DS, Richard J, et al. Multi-centre, double blind, randomized trial of three steroid regimens in the treatment of type-1 reactions in leprosy. Lepr Rev. 2006;77(1):25-33.
9. Girdhar A, Chakma JK, Ravinderan A, et al. A comparative study of high vs. low dose corticosteroid therapy in reversal reactions in leprosy. Indian J Lepr. 2005;77:350-1.
10. Pai VV, Tayshetye PU, Ganapati R. A study of standardized regimens of steroid treatment in reactions in leprosy at a referral centre. Indian J Lepr. 2012;84(1):9-15.
11. Walker SL, Nicholls PG, Dhakal S, et al. A phase two randomised controlled double blind trial of high dose intravenous methylprednisolone and oral prednisolone versus intravenous normal saline and oral prednisolone in individuals with leprosy type 1 reactions and/or nerve function impairment. PLoS Negl Trop Dis. 2011;5(4):e1041.
12. Girdhar BK, Girdhar A, Chakma JK. Advances in the treatment of reactions in leprosy. Indian J Lepr. 2007;79(2-3):121-34.
13. Papang R, John AS, Abraham S, et al. A study of steroid-induced diabetes mellitus in leprosy. Indian J Lepr. 2009;81(3):125-9.
14. Basílio FM, Hammerschmidt M, Mukai MM, et al. Mucormycosis and chromoblastomycosis occurring in a patient with leprosy type 2 reaction under prolonged corticosteroid and thalidomide therapy. An Bras Dermatol. 2012;87(5):767-71.
15. Biosca G, Casallo S, Lupez-Velez R. Methotrexate treatment for type 1 (reversal) reactions. Clin Infect Dis. 2007;45(1):e7-9.
16. Sena CB, Salgado CG, Tavares CM, et al. Cyclosporine A treatment of leprosy patients with chronic neuritis is associated with pain control and reduction in antibodies against nerve growth factor. Lepr Rev. 2006;77(2):121-9.
17. Chin-A-Lien RA, Faber WR, Naafs B. Cyclosporine A treatment in reversal reaction. Trop Geogr Med. 1994;46(2):123-4.
18. Marlowe SN, Hawksworth RA, Butlin CR, et al. Clinical outcomes in a randomized controlled study comparing azathioprine and prednisolone and prednisolone alone in the treatment of severe leprosy type 1 reaction in Nepal. Trans R Soc Trop Med Hyg. 2004;98(10):602-9.
19. Burdick AE, Ramirez CC. The role of mycophenolate mofetil in the treatment of leprosy reactions. Int J Lepr Other Mycobact Dis. 2005;73(2):127-8.
20. Safa G, Darrieux L, Coic A, et al. Type 1 leprosy reversal reaction treated with topical tacrolimus along with systemic corticosteroids. Indian J Med Sci. 2009;63(8):359-62.
21. Trindade MA, Palermo ML, Pagliari C, et al. Leprosy in transplant recipients: report of a case after liver transplantation and review of the literature. Transpl Infect Dis. 2011;13(1):63-9.
22. Pre-congress workshop on reactions and neuritis. Lepr Rev. 2008;79:216-20.
23. Kar HK, Sharma P. New lesions after MDT in PB and MB leprosy: a report of 28 cases. Indian J Lepr. 2008;80(3):247-55.
24. vanBrakel WH, Nicholls PG, Lockwood DN, et al. A scale to assess the severity of leprosy reactions. Lepr Rev. 2007;78:161-4.
25. Lucas SB, Naafs B, Waters MF, et al. Reactions in leprosy. In: Ratledge C, Stanford JL, Grange JM (Eds). Biology of Mycobacteria, Clinical Aspects of Mycobacterial Disease. London: Academic Press Ltd. 1989. pp. 359-403.
26. Morrison ME, Morley GE. Clofazimine binding with deoxyribonucleic acid. Int J Lepr. 1976;44(4):475-81.
27. Anderson R. Enhancement by clofazimine and inhibition by dapsone of production of prostaglandin E2 by human polymorphonuclear leucocytes in vitro. Antimicrob Agents Chemother. 1985;27:257-62.
28. Ren YR, Pan F, Parvez S, et al. Clofazimine inhibits human kv1.3 potassium channel by perturbing calcium oscillation in T lymphocytes. PLoS One. 2008;3(12):e4009.
29. Balagon M, Saunderson PR, Gelber RH. Does clofazimine prevent erythema nodosum leprosum (ENL) in leprosy? A retrospective study, comparing the experience of multibacillary patients receiving either 12 or 24 months WHO-MDT. Lepr Rev. 2011;82(3):213-21.
30. Hernandez Mde O, Fulco Tde O, Pinheiro RO, et al. Thalidomide modulates Mycobacterium leprae-induced NF-kB pathway and lower cytokine response. Eur J Pharmacol. 2011;670(1):272-9.
31. Kar HK, Gupta L. Comparative efficacy of four treatment regimens in type 2 leprosy reactions (prednisolone alone, thalidomide alone, prednisolone plus thalidomide and prednisolone plus clofazimine). Presented at:18th International Leprosy Congress; 2013 Sept 16 – Sept 19; Brussels, Belgium. Abstract. No: O-070.
32. Rattan R, Shanker V, Tegta GR, et al. Severe form of type 2 reaction in patients of Hansen's disease after withdrawal of thalidomide: case reports. Indian J Lepr. 2009;81(4):199-203.
33. Mahajan VK, Chauhan PS, Sharma NL, et al. Severe vasculonecrotic erythema nodosum leprosum following thalidomide withdrawal without tapering doses: do we have something unusual? Braz J Infect Dis. 2011;15(1):90-1.
34. Welsh O, Gómez M, Mancias C, et al. A new therapeutic approach to type II leprosy reaction. Int J Dermatol. 1999;38(12):931-3.
35. Ishii N, Ishida Y, Okano Y, et al. Japanese guideline on thalidomide usage in the management of erythema nodosum leprosum. Nihon Hansenbyo Gakkai Zasshi. 2011;80(3):275-85.
36. Walker SL, Waters MF, Lockwood DN. The role of thalidomide in the management of erythema nodosum leprosum. Lepr Rev. 2007;78(3):197-215.
37. Stephens TD, Blunde CJ, Fillmore BJ. Mechanism of action in thalidomide teratogenesis. Biochem Pharmacol. 2000;59(12):1489-99.
38. Drucker L, Uziel O, Tohami T, et al. Thalidomide down regulates transcript levels of GC- rich promoter genes in multiple myeloma. Mol Pharmacol. 2003;64(2):415-20.

39. Teo SK, Harden JL, Burke AB, et al. Thalidomide is distributed into human semen after oral dosing. Drug Metab Dispos. 2001;29(10):1355-7.
40. Vianna FS, Schüler-Faccini L, Leite JC, et al. Recognition of the phenotype of thalidomide embryopathy in countries endemic for leprosy: new cases and review of the main dysmorphological findings. Clin Dysmorphol. 2013;22(2):59-63.
41. Vianna FS, Lopez-Camelo JS, Leite JC, et al. Epidemiological surveillance of birth defects compatible with thalidomide embryopathy in Brazil. PLoS One. 2011;6(7):e21735.
42. Bastuji-Garin S, Ochonisky S, Bouche P, et al. Incidence and risk factors for thalidomide neuropathy: a prospective study of 135 dermatologic patients. J Invest Dermatol. 2002;119(5):1020-6.
43. Chaudhry V, Cornblath DR, Corse A, et al. Thalidomide-induced neuropathy. Neurology. 2002;59:1872-5.
44. Sharma NL, Sharma V, Shanker V, et al. Deep vein thrombosis: a rare complication of thalidomide therapy in recurrent erythema nodosum leprosum. Int J Lepr Other Mycobact Dis. 2004;72(4):483-5.
45. Yamaguchi S, Yamamoto Y, Hosokawa A, et al. Deep venous thrombosis and pulmonary embolism secondary to co-administration of thalidomide and oral corticosteroid in a patient with leprosy. J Dermatol. 2012;39(8):711-4.
46. Glasmacher A, Hahn C, Hoffmann F, et al. A systematic review of phase-II trials of thalidomide monotherapy in patients with relapsed or refractory multiple myeloma. Br J Haematol. 2006;132(5):584-93.
47. Hebe Petiti-Martin G, Villar-Buill M, de la Hera I, et al. Deep vein thrombosis in a patient with lepromatous leprosy receiving thalidomide to treat leprosy reaction. Actas Dermosifiliogr. 2013;104(1):67-70.
48. Knable AL, Davis LS. Miscellaneous systemic drugs. In: Comprehensive Dermatologic Drug Therapy, ed Stephen E. Wolverton, 3rd edition, Saunders, USA, pp. 439-40.
49. De Nardo P, Giancola ML, Noto S, et al. Left thigh phlegmon caused by Nocardia farcinica identified by 16S rRNA sequencing in a patient with Leprosy: a case report. BMC Infect Dis. 2013;13:162.
50. Hossain D. Using Methotrexate to treat patients with ENL unresponsive to steroids and clofazimine: A Report on 9 patients. Lepr Rev. 2013;84:105-12.
51. Sharma P, Kar HK, Misra RS. Reactional states and neuritis in multibacillary leprosy patients following MDT with/without immunotherapy with Mw antileprosy vaccine. Lepr Rev. 2000;71:193-205.
52. Girdhar A, Chakma JK, Girdhar BK. Pulsed corticosteroid therapy in patients with chronic recurrent ENL: a pilot study. Indian J Lepr. 2002;74:233-6.
53. Mahajan VK, Sharma NL, Sharma RC, et al. Dexamethasone pulse therapy with azathioprine in ENL. Lep Rev. 2003;74:171-4.
54. Verma KK, Srivastava P, Minz A. et al. Azathioprine and recurrent ENL. Lep Rev. 2006;77:225-9.
55. De Carsalade GY, Achirafi A, Flageul B. Pentoxifylline in the treatment of erythema nodosum leprosum. J Dermatol. 2003;30:64-8.
56. Vides EA, Cabrera A, Ahem KP, et al. Effect of zafirlukast in leprosy reactions. Int J Lepr Other Mycobact Dis. 1999;67:71-5.
57. Mazzoccoli L, Cadoso SH, Amarante GW, et al. Novel thalidomide analogues from diamines inhibit pro-inflammatory cytokine production and CD80 expression while enhancing IL-10. Biomed Pharmacother. 2012;66:323-9.
58. Faber WR, Jensema AJ, Goldschmidt WF. Treatment of recurrent erythema nodosum leprosum with infliximab. N Eng J Med. 2006;355:739.
59. Ramien ML, Wong A, Keystone JS. Severe refractory erythema nodosum leprosum successfully treated with the tumor necrosis factor inhibitor etanercept. Clin Infect Dis. 2011;52:e133-5.
60. Camacho ID, Valencia I, Rivas MP, Burdick AE. Type 1 leprosy reaction manifesting after discontinuation of adalimumab therapy. Arch Dermatol. 2009;145:349-51.
61. Oberstein EM, Kromo O, Tozman EC. Type I reaction of Hansen's disease with exposure to adalimumab: a case report. Arthritis Rheum. 2008;59:1040-3.
62. Monteiro R, Abreu MA, Tiezzi MG, et al. Lucio's phenomenon: another case reported in Brazil. Ann Bras Dermatol. 2012;87:296-300.
63. Huits RM, Oskam L, van Raalte JA. Lucio's phenomenon in a patient with leprosy on Aruba. Ned Tijdschr Geneeskd. 2012;156:A4285.
64. van Brakel WH, Nicholls PG, Das L, et al. The INFIR Cohort Study: investigating prediction, detection and pathogenesis of neuropathy and reactions in leprosy. Methods and baseline results of a cohort of multibacillary leprosy patients in north India. Lepr Rev. 2005;76(1):14-34.

Management of Neuritis and Neuropathic Pain

Bhushan Kumar, Sunil Dogra

CHAPTER OUTLINE

INTRODUCTION

Neuritis, literally translated, means inflammation of the nerve. *Mycobacterium leprae* is the only bacillus which is able to invade the peripheral nerves, produces inflammation in the nerve (neuritis) and consequent nerve function impairment (NFI) with attendant deformity and increased risk of stigma. A patient with leprous neuritis can have any of the following symptoms—spontaneous nerve pain, paresthesia, sensory, motor or autonomic impairment. Different clinical types of leprosy produce different patterns of nerve involvement. Nerve inflammation can be acute, chronic, acute on chronic or smoldering type. Neuritis is not always symptomatic, and can have minimal symptoms and even the damage can go on silently (silent neuropathy).

A neuron is the building block of a nerve. Neuron has cell body and multiple cytoplasmic projections including axons and dendrites. Each axon has an insulating lining of myelin formed of a fatty material inside the Schwann cells. The interstitial layer outside neurilemma around each individual nerve fiber is called endoneurium. Nerve fascicle is made up of a group of axons encased by perineurium bathing together in endoneurial fluid. Between the fascicles is a fatty material called the interfascicular epineurium. The nerve is then wrapped in the main epineurium. Even if the sensitive living axons are damaged, the conduit made up of epineurium and perineurium will often survive and provide a pathway for regrowing of the nerve fibers.

Nerve damage in leprosy occurs by three distinct mechanisms:

1. *M. leprae* directly damages neurons via mechanisms involving Schwann cells[1] and by contact demyelination as described by Rambukkana.[2]
2. Damage mediated by inflammatory and immune mediated processes.
3. Damage due to edema and mechanical processes.

Neuritis and NFI can occur in the setting of immunological reactions but occur more commonly independent of them because of the disease *per se*. Some patients develop neuropathy after completion of multidrug therapy (MDT) in the absence of reaction or visible leprous activity.[3] A study has suggested an experimental evidence for the autoimmune mechanism of nerve damage in leprosy.[4] All leprosy patients do not develop neuritis and NFI. The Bangladesh Acute Nerve Damage Study (BANDS) study identified the bacillary status and nerve function loss (NFL) at presentation as the significant risk factors for further development of the NFI.[5] Leprosy patients were divided into three risk groups based on the presence of these risk factors. Paucibacillary (PB) leprosy patients with no NFL at presentation had 1.3% risk (low-risk) of developing NFI within 2 years of follow-up; PB leprosy patients with NFL and multibacillary (MB) leprosy patients without NFL had 16% risk; and MB patient with NFL at the time of presentation had a 65% risk of development of new NFI within 2 years of registration. Another prospective 5-year follow-up study concluded that new episodes of NFI are common, particularly in MB patients with long standing NFI at registration. This emphasizes that a clinician should keep a vigil on early signs and symptoms of NFI, particularly up to 2 years of registration.[6]

A recent study has described adjusted NFI prediction rule that replaces longstanding NFI at diagnosis with antiphenolic glycolipid 1 (PGL-1) antibodies. This would help in predicting NFI even before it occurs for the first time. Though the adjusted prediction rule could identify a substantially higher number of new NFI cases than either routine or BANDS rule-based surveillance, it needs to be validated to find place in routine screening to predict NFI.[7]

The INFIR (ILEP Nerve Function Impairment and Reactions) cohort study from North India has described presence of skin lesions overlying nerve trunks as the main risk factor for neuropathy, increasing the risk by 3–4 times and further by 6–8 times, if reactional signs are present in the lesions.[8]

According to a recent study, early diagnosis and treatment of neuritis on ambulatory basis is more cost-effective and avoids the negative effect of hospitalization on patients' view of the disease.[9]

A clinician should be aware of the varied presentations of leprous neuritis, so as to individualize therapy and prognosticate the patient. The different clinical presentations are:

Acute neuritis: Patient presents with acute neuritic pain or nerve tenderness and/or swelling due to nerve abscess and/or recent onset neurological deficit of usually less than 6 months duration. This mostly occurs in the setting of type 1 or type 2 leprosy reactions and should be treated vigorously as the clinical deterioration is fast. It shows good response to treatment.

Chronic neuritis: Patient presents with long-standing (> 6 months duration), gradually progressive neurological deficit with nerve tenderness or pain. It shows poor response to treatment.

Recurrent neuritis: An episode of neuritis recurring after a symptom free interval of at least 3 months and it indicates poor prognosis and the NFI deteriorates further.

Silent neuropathy: Patient has only neurological deficit, which is mostly progressive in the absence of nerve pain and tenderness with no evidence of reaction.

Subclinical neuropathy: Patients have normal values for voluntary muscle testing (VMT) and monofilament testing, but have impaired nerve conduction studies (NCS) and/or warm detection threshold (WDT).[10] In a study, 16% of such patients subsequently developed clinical NFI.[11]

Catastrophic paralysis: Patient develops sudden paralysis. It is an emergency which needs urgent attention.

Completely destroyed nerves: When patient has no residual nerve function and electrophysiological studies show no conduction.

DIAGNOSIS AND MONITORING

When patient presents in the clinic, detailed examination should be done to make note of the extent of NFI, if any, at the time of presentation. Patients at high risk of development of NFI or having it at presentation should be put on close follow-up. Risk factors for development of new NFI are MB leprosy,[5] NFI at diagnosis[5] and those with detectable PGL-1 antibodies.[12] This would help in detecting the fresh NFL at the earliest and also help in gauging the efficacy of the treatment.

An international workshop on neuropathology in leprosy, held at Soesterberg, Netherland, in June 2007, concluded that the nerve function assessment (NFA) should be performed at different times and frequencies according to the type of leprosy, presence of NFI and the context of the case:[13]
- At the start and end of treatment with MDT in all types of disease.
- If NFI present at diagnosis then NFA at every visit—3 monthly approximately.
- In MB patients, assessment should continue after MDT, every 3 months, for 2 years.

Assessment of patient includes clinical examination and the specialized investigations.

Clinical Examination

Nerve examination includes nerve palpation and NFA:
- Nerve palpation is done to look for tenderness, thickening, consistency and abscess formation.
- NFA
  - Sensory function evaluation in the distribution of nerves for touch, pain and temperature.
    John et al. demonstrated that using 0.2 g and 4 g Semmes Weinstein filaments for sensory testing in the field would be a cost-effective method to enhance the prevention of disability by detecting NFI at an earlier stage.[14]
  - VMT and grading the power.
  - Autonomic function evaluated from skin dryness, hair loss, skin color and temperature.

Investigations

Specialized investigations include fine needle aspiration (FNA), nerve biopsy, electrophysiological studies and laser Doppler fluxometry. These investigations are done only in selected cases.
- *Fine needle aspiration*: It is a simple, quick, less invasive procedure which does not affect the nerve adversely and, therefore, can be done from any accessible nerve which

seems to be affected clinically. It provided diagnostic aspirate in 67–92% patients in different studies.[15,16] It is mainly useful in establishing the diagnosis of pure neuritic leprosy.

- *Nerve biopsy*: It is an invasive procedure done on superficial cutaneous sensory nerves. Tissue can be used for histopathological examination and PCR for *M. leprae*. It is useful in establishing the diagnosis of pure neuritic leprosy when it is a diagnostic problem.

  A study has demonstrated nerve biopsy as a useful tool for the differential diagnosis of post-MDT peripheral neuropathy, given that detection of acid-fast bacilli in the samples may favor the decision regarding relapse; however, this decision should be strongly supported by clinical and neuro-electrophysiological data.[17]

- *Electrophysiological studies*: Electrodiagnostic findings early in the disease reveal demyelinating features, such as slowing of conduction velocity and prolongation of latencies, but as the disease progresses, secondary axonal damage ensues. These studies are the most sensitive. They help in early detection of NFI, and provide a baseline and an objective measure for gauging the response to therapy.

  A study correlating the detection of immunoglobulin M (IgM) antibodies to gangliosides in sera of leprosy patients with presence or absence of demyelinating pattern in electroneurographical (ENG) examination found 45.4% of those showing demyelination on ENG to be positive for at least one antibody (GA1, GM1, GM2, GD1a, GD1b, GQ1b), while 37.5% of patients without demyelination were immunoreactive for antiganglioside antibodies. This suggested that serological studies may be a useful tool for diagnosis and follow-up of demyelination in leprosy neuropathy.[18]

- *Laser Doppler Fluxometry*: It measures the cutaneous blood flow in fingertips and toes using laser light. This technique is utilized to measure vasomotor reflex in leprosy patients with prominent autonomic nerve lesion.

- *Nerve imaging*: High resolution sonography [ultrasonography (US)] and color Doppler imaging provide objective measure of nerve dimensions and structural changes resulting from nerve damage and inflammation in leprosy. They have several advantages such as being noninvasive, ability to assess nerves at sites that cannot be biopsied and more cost-effective than magnetic resonance imaging (MRI). The nerve can be probed for a longer length with US than MRI examination which is limited to defined segments. These tools have important role in following up patients and deciding when to stop treatment in neuritis, rather than just relying on clinical signs and symptoms.[19]

A study comparing different methods to detect peripheral neuropathy in leprosy concluded NCS and WDT measurements to be the most promising tests for early detection of nerve involvement in leprosy.[20]

A randomized controlled trial (RCT) has found these tests to be beneficial in detecting subclinical neuropathy. However, such tools are expensive and need to be carried out in an air conditioned room (20–25°C).[10]

- *Thermography*: It is a noninvasive tool that provides consistent images with reproducible thermal patterns in sites affected by leprosy bacilli. The results correlate well with abnormal functioning of sensory and sympathetic nervous system, even before the occurrence of clinical signs, and hence may play an important role in early diagnosis of nerve injury. In a recent study that measured palm and sole temperature using infrared video camera, 70% (14/20) of the patients showed temperature variations between hemispheres of the body. Temperature variations in grade-0 disability patients were not significant while 83.4% with grade 1 disability presented an average difference of 2.5°C between right and left limbs and 77% with grade-2 disability had average temperature variation of 10°C between limbs.[21]

Newer objective measures, like grip or pinch dynamometer, pressure specified sensory device, or electronic esthesiometer, electrodiagnostic recording, etc. can be standardized to improve the accuracy and reproducibility of sensory and motor evaluation in research protocols.[22]

Portable glove embedded tactile sensors can predict pressure thresholds and ulcer prone areas on hands and feet in leprosy patients while involved in daily activities. According to a recent study in 100 patients, it was found that the pressure is maximal in the middle of an activity, and minimal at the onset and end of the activity. The buzzer set in the glove alerts the patient on the activity which causes prolonged high pressures to the hand.[23]

In a study evaluating Schwann cell and epidermal nerve fiber density (ENFD) in the distal leg of nine-banded armadillos with experimental leprosy neuropathy, progressively decreasing epidermal densities in naïve armadillos and increasing proliferation of Schwann cells in infected armadillos were found. They proposed quantification of ENFD and Schwann cells to be an important tool for investigating early sensory neuropathy in leprosy.[24]

MANAGEMENT

Early detection and appropriate treatment of neuritis and lepra reactions is the key issue in leprosy management. The principles of management of neuritis are:

- Continuing the treatment of leprosy (MDT)
- Treating complicating reactional states, i.e. type 1 and type 2 reactions
- Effective and prolonged anti-inflammatory therapy
- Physical therapy and rest during the phase of active neuritis
- Surgery when indicated
- Physiotherapy during recovery phase

Recovery of NFI depends on several factors, like degree of damage, severity of reaction, duration of NFI, age of the patient, general health condition, type of leprosy and adequacy of treatment.

Multidrug therapy should be continued or started if the patient has not received it before. Though MDT does not improve neuritis but is still an important part of treatment as it would kill the bacilli and reduce the bacterial antigenic load responsible for the reactions and neuritis. In a study involving 46 leprosy patients with progressive or new nerve impairment that showed no improvement after steroid therapy, nerve biopsy was carried out to define the cause of the insidious nerve impairment. AFB were found in 67% samples suggesting patients may not respond to corticosteroid treatment due to the persistence of infection which requires specific antileprosy MDT.[25] Those patients at greater risk of developing neuritis should be educated regarding their occurrence at the start of MDT as patients tend to panic and default when they develop new NFI while on MDT.

Anti-Inflammatory Therapy

Corticosteroids are the most commonly used anti-inflammatory agents for the management of leprosy neuritis. Other agents include clofazimine, azathioprine, thalidomide and cyclosporine.

CORTICOSTEROIDS

Corticosteroids with dual anti-inflammatory and immunosuppressive actions form the mainstay in the treatment of leprous neuritis. Steroids produce rapid improvement in most, but not all the patients, by quickly reducing the edema and number of inflammatory cells, and bringing down the intraneural pressure considerably. Their action is via genomic[26] and nongenomic[27] effects. Genomic effects are produced by binding to steroid nuclear receptors which in turn alter the production of various cytokines. These effects take time while the nongenomic effects are responsible for the immediate action and are mediated via steroids cytoplasmic receptors and via nonspecific physiochemical activity. Steroids with relatively high nongenomic potencies like methylprednisolone would be needed for early and greater immunosuppression.[28] Steroids also reduce the postinflammatory scar formation during the prolonged healing phase, which is very important for the improvement of nerve function after the reaction is controlled.[29]

The World Health Organization recommended corticosteroid regimen for treating nerve damage starts with 40 mg prednisolone daily and tapered over the next 12 weeks (Table 33.1).[30]

Earlier the treatment is started, higher is the chance of reversal of NFI.[31,32] Recovery of NFL is more likely when the

Table 33.1: Corticosteroid regimen for treating nerve damage recommended by World Health Organization

Dose once a day (mg)	Weeks of treatment
40	1, 2
30	3, 4
20	5, 6
15	7, 8
10	9, 10
5	11, 12

duration of NFI has been less than 6 months.[29,31] But doubts have been expressed about the need for treatment of very early nerve damage with steroids.[33]

The optimal dose and duration of therapy for neuritis has not been established. Rao et al.[34] in an optimal steroid dose finding study compared three steroid regimens in leprosy patients with type 1 reaction and they concluded that prolonged duration of therapy was more effective than high dose therapy. In another RCT by Garbino et al.,[35] it was found that the higher dose (2 mg/kg/day) of steroids produced better results than the lower dose (1 mg/kg/day) during the first month of treatment for ulnar neuropathy.

Various studies have found that prolonged prednisolone treatment may be more effective in the treatment of severe reactions and in reversing the nerve damage, and that the WHO recommended 12 weeks therapy is inadequate.[31,36,37]

In support of this, a RCT comparing prednisolone therapy (1 mg/kg/day) for 32 weeks versus 20 weeks is ongoing to determine the effective treatment duration. The results of this trial will help in establishing new guidelines for management of acute neuritis.[10] However, at present the best is to tailor therapy to individual patient.

High doses of intravenous methylprednisolone were found to be safe and effective in preventing neuropathy, and subsequent disabilities due to nerve damage.[38] Another RCT involving 60 MB leprosy patients suggested that use of low dose prophylactic prednisolone (20 mg/day from the beginning of treatment for 6 months and tapering in 7th and 8th month) during the first 8 months of multidrug treatment reduces the incidence of new reactions and the benefit is sustained at one year.[39]

In a recent study[40] investigating the efficacy of corticosteroids in MB leprosy patients, treatment with MDT and corticosteroids did not affect the killing of *M. leprae*, clearance of its antigens and granuloma. Percentage cases showing viable bacilli in mouse foot pad inoculation 6 months post-release from MDT were not significantly different between MDT and steroids versus MDT only group. NCS found an overall nerve function deterioration in 22% compared to improvement in 9% cases. Deterioration of sensory nerves was significantly higher in the group that received steroids and MDT-MB compared to MDT-MB alone, while motor nerve worsening was comparable in both groups, thereby concluding that MDT and adjunct corticosteroid therapy is not very efficacious in the prevention or reversal of nerve damage and a better immunomodulatory drug may be required.

Efficacy of Steroids in Acute Neuritis

Many studies report spontaneous improvement in nerve function in leprosy patients over a period of time and this is a big confounding factor for steroid dose and duration efficacy studies.[41,42]

In a RCT, mild sensory impairment of less than 6 month duration was treated with tapering doses of steroids for 16 weeks starting at 40 mg/day. Sensory improvement at the end of 1 year was seen in 80% of cases in prednisolone group and 79% in placebo group.[33]

In another retrospective cohort study, 35% of patients having complete anesthesia and 67% with moderate sensory impairment improved to good function in 3 months after the start of corticosteroid treatment.[43] For patients with complete motor paralysis or moderate motor impairment, 11% and 55% of the patients, respectively, recovered to good function.

Data from Ethiopia ALERT MDT Field Evaluation Study (AMFES) showed that the patients with acute neuropathy, when treated with steroids, had full recovery in 88% cases, while patients with recurrent or chronic NFI had poor prognosis with only 51% of involved nerves showing full recovery in the long term.[41]

Data from nonrandomized studies show that the steroids are effective in acute neuritis though the recent RCT does not support it.[33]

Efficacy of Steroids in Chronic and Recurrent Neuritis

TRIPOD 3 study investigated the role of steroids in patients with long standing neuritis.[44] In a multicenter, randomized, double-blind placebo-controlled trial conducted in Nepal and Bangladesh, patients with untreated NFI between 6 months and 24 months duration were randomized to either tapering doses of prednisolone starting at 40 mg/day for 16 weeks, or to placebo. Assessment was done at 4, 6, 9, and 12 months from the start of treatment. There was no demonstrable additional improvement in nerve function, or in the prevention of further leprosy reaction events in the prednisolone group. Overall, improvement of nerve function at 12 months was seen in about 50% of patients in both groups. The trial concluded that it is not advisable to treat long-standing NFI with prednisolone.

Saunderson[45] found steroids to be disappointing in recurrent neuritis. All nerve fibers are not destroyed even in

badly damaged nerves and axon sprouting, and regeneration of nerves have been demonstrated in long standing cases of leprosy.[46] However, some clinicians still believe in giving a trial of treatment with corticosteroids, even in long standing cases of neuritis.

Acute neuritis shows better response while the patients with recurrent and chronic neuritis respond poorly to the steroids. So earlier the treatment is started; higher are the chances of reversal of NFI.

Though steroids are the most efficacious drugs among all anti-inflammatory agents for the treatment of leprous neuritis but there are few drawbacks and limitations. Steroids are not uniformly effective in all patients and a significant number of patients do not respond to steroids.[41,47,48] Variability of response to steroids is due to different processes of nerve damage working in different combinations in different patients.

It is not known if steroids interfere with the killing of bacilli and clearance of antigen from the body. So there is a concern regarding potential of growing of lepra bacilli in patients on long-term steroids, and increasing the chances of relapse and late reactions. Therefore, patients of neuritis or chronic reactions who have completed MDT but are on steroids should be given some antileprosy treatment. Clofazimine alone is considered better because of its additional anti-inflammatory properties.

Steroids have minor and major side effects and these side effects become all the more significant in patients with leprous neuritis who receive steroids for long periods. Data from three TRIPOD trials, in which standardized regimens of corticosteroids for prophylaxis and treatment of NFI were given, was evaluated for incidence of adverse events with prednisolone.[49] It revealed minor adverse events in 20% and major adverse events in 2% of the test group which received prednisolone. Minor adverse events included acne, fungal infections and gastric pain. Major adverse events were peptic ulcer, diabetes and infections like sepsis.

To minimize side effects steroids should be given in combination therapy, which will complement other anti-inflammatory agents like clofazimine.

Efficacy of Steroids in Subclinical Neuropathy

A RCT is going on in which patients with subclinical neuropathy will be receiving prednisolone (1 mg/kg/day) tapered down over 20 weeks. If this intervention prevents development of clinical NFI, it would significantly reduce the burden of patients presenting with clinical NFI. However, this would be feasible only where such sophisticated tools and controlled conditions to detect the subclinical neuropathy are available.[10]

However, according to a recent prospective cohort study of 365 untreated MB patients, addition of corticosteroid to

MDT for neuritis/reaction failed to prevent deterioration in nerve function when compared to MDT alone as assessed by NCS. This encourages the search for alternative drugs or appropriate treatment regimens.[50]

OTHER ANTI-INFLAMMATORY AGENTS

Treatment of leprosy reactions and neuritis is largely dependent on steroids. Clofazimine and thalidomide are other anti-inflammatory agents with well-established role in the management of leprosy reactions. All of these drugs have significant adverse effects when given for long duration and, also, all patients do not show good response. So there is an ongoing hunt for new agents. This has led to clinical trials of azathioprine and cyclosporine under the INFIR research program to identify second-line treatments for severe leprosy type 1 reactions (T1R).

CLOFAZIMINE

Clofazimine is a phenazine derivative with both antileprosy and anti-inflammatory properties. It acts by reducing the granulocyte chemotaxis and stabilizing the lysosomal membrane. It has limited role in the management of acute stage of lepra T1R but has been found to reduce its incidence[51,52] and that of neuritis[53] as well. It is a steroid sparing drug in the treatment of recurrent and chronic erythema nodosum leprosum (ENL) reactions.[54,55]

As clofazimine acts slowly, it should be used in combination therapy with steroids. Later steroids can be gradually withdrawn while patient continues on clofazimine alone. There is an added advantage with clofazimine that its addition to therapy takes off any fear of growing bacilli when patients with lepra reaction or neuritis are on prolonged immunosuppression with steroids.

It is given in doses of 300 mg daily in three divided doses for a maximum period of 12 weeks. Dose is then reduced to 200 mg daily and after few months to 100 mg daily, which may be continued for more months.

The drug accumulates in the body especially in the skin, mucous membrane, reticuloendothelial system and tissues with large number of macrophages. The side effects are related to the dose and are more common and severe at higher cumulative dose. Most important side effects are gastrointestinal disturbances and cutaneous pigmentation.

A recent double-blind randomized trial including 30 patients who received 6 months of standard WHO MDT-PB along with clofazimine (50 mg daily and 300 mg once a month) and 30 patients who received WHO MDT-PB only, found no significant difference in improvement or deterioration of NFI with or without clofazimine.[56]

THALIDOMIDE

Thalidomide is a nonpolar glutamic acid derivative. It is an anti tumor necrosis factor-alpha (anti-TNF-α) agent with immunomodulatory, anti-inflammatory and hypnosedative effects. It is the drug of choice for lepra type 2 reactions and there are reports of satisfactory response of neuritis in these patients.[57]

But the problem with thalidomide is that it itself produces peripheral neuropathy. Peripheral neuropathy most commonly presents with symmetrical painful paresthesias of the hands and feet frequently associated with a lower limb sensory loss. Mild proximal muscle weakness can occur but severe motor impairment and proprioceptive failure occurs only occasionally. The cardinal sign of drug related neuropathy is a 50% decrease in the sensory nerve action potential (SNAP) amplitude, with relative conservation of nerve conduction velocities on nerve electrophysiological studies (NES).

Reaction patients with neuritis when treated with thalidomide should be monitored closely, both clinically and with NES.

AZATHIOPRINE

Azathioprine has immunosuppressive and anti-inflammatory effects. Its active metabolite 6-thioguanine is structurally similar to endogenous purines adenine and guanine. It gets incorporated into the DNA and RNA, subsequently inhibiting cell division. It affects the function of both the T as well as the B-cells.

Azathioprine is used as steroid sparing agent in various immune mediated cutaneous disorders. This has led to clinical trial of azathioprine under the ILEP coordinated INFIR research program to find its efficacy as a second-line treatment for severe T1R.[58] The trial concluded that a 12-week course of azathioprine at 3 mg/kg/day plus an 8 week reducing course of prednisolone starting at 40 mg/day is as effective as a 12 week reducing course of prednisolone starting at 40 mg/day and that the combination therapy is well-tolerated in leprosy patients with severe T1R.

The significant adverse effects of azathioprine are pancytopenia, liver toxicity and gastrointestinal intolerance.

In a recent double-blind RCT comparing placebo, or 24, 36 and 48 weeks of azathioprine (50 mg/day) added to a 20 week course of prednisolone in patients with T1R and new neuritis, there was a significant benefit for all treatments for the skin component of the severity score and addition of azathioprine increased the benefit. Azathioprine also led to improvement in motor scores, but this was not clinically significant and no improvement was seen in sensory scores. Azathioprine did not reduce recurrences and 72 patients who had recurrences of T1R and neuritis required a further course of prednisolone.[59]

Further studies are needed to establish its role in the management of neuritis.

CYCLOSPORINE

Cyclosporine is a potent immunosuppressant which acts directly on CD4+ T-cells. The drug inhibits calcineurin and this leads to decreased activity of transcription factor NFAT-1, inhibiting the IL-2 production. Reduced IL-2 levels result in decreased activation of T-cells and thereby the B-cells and antibody production.

Cyclosporine has been used in the management of chronic ENL[60] and reversal reactions.[61] Cyclosporine has been found to produce pain relief in chronic neuritis patients along with the recovery of the neural functions.[62] Cyclosporine was given in a 12 months reducing course starting at 5 mg/kg/day. The author proposed that the mechanism of action of cyclosporine was through reduction of antinerve growth factor (anti-NGF) autoantibodies titers. NGF is trophic to the neurons and anti-NGF autoantibodies deplete the NGF in leprosy patients.

Marlowe et al.[63] in an open prospective trial treated 41 patients of severe T1R with cyclosporine (5–7.5 mg/kg/day) for 12 weeks with good response of skin lesions as well as the nerve function.

The significant adverse effects, like renal dysfunction, hypertension, electrolyte imbalance, neurological side effects, gum hyperplasia and high cost, are an important limiting factor with cyclosporine.

Analgesics

Aspirin, ibuprofen, paracetamol and other nonsteroidal anti-inflammatory drugs (NSAIDs) can be used in full doses for the pain control in patients with acute neuritis.

INTRANEURAL ADMINISTRATION OF DRUGS

Some workers have tried giving drugs via intra- or perineural injections in patients whose acute severe neuritic pain was not controlled with medical therapy alone. Various drugs given via this route include the vasodilator drugs, like duvadilan or priscol, spreading factor hyalase and the corticosteroids. As the intraneural injections are very painful, the drug was combined with local anesthetics. Garrett[64] was first to use this technique.

Results of this technique are inconsistent. While Sepaha et al.[65] recommended the use of this technique, Ramanujam[66] reported results to be unsatisfactory. Recently Nashed et al.[67] reported successful treatment of right claw hand deformity in a 60 year old male with monthly intraneural injection of corticosteroids over a 6 month period.

This mode of drug administration has not been very popular because of two reasons. First, the pain during and for few minutes immediately following the injection is extremely severe and second, there is a potential danger of damaging the nerve fibers.

CHRONIC NEUROPATHIC PAIN

Nerves carry the pain sensation, but when some primary lesion or dysfunction of the nerve itself produces pain, it is termed as neuropathic pain. Leprosy related chronic neuropathic pain has received scant attention in literature. It is a common late complication of leprosy. Its diagnosis is made when patient after completion of MDT presents with pain in the absence of leprosy reaction and new NFI. It is predominantly of continuous burning type with glove and stocking distribution.[68,69]

Different pathophysiological mechanisms possibly leading to leprosy related neuropathic pain are small fiber neuropathy and persistent intraneural inflammation.[68]

In a recent cross-sectional prevalence study from India, out of 101 recruited patients who had completed MDT, 22 (21.8%) had neuropathic pain. The main sensory symptoms were numbness (86.4%), hypoesthesia to touch (81.2%) and pinprick (72.7%) and tingling (68.2%). Pain was significantly associated with nerve enlargement and tenderness suggesting that ongoing inflammation may be important in its causation. Psychological morbidity was present in 41% of patients with neuropathic pain, thereby further increasing the magnitude of problem.[70]

Simple analgesics like NSAIDs are usually ineffective. Though there are no RCTs, but in corollary with the management of neuropathic pain of other etiologies like post herpetic neuralgia and diabetic neuropathy, tricyclic antidepressants, anticonvulsants and opioids can be/have been tried.

Tricyclic Antidepressants (TCAs)

There is no major difference between different drugs of this group. Amitriptyline and nortriptyline are most commonly used. The drug is started at doses of 10–25 mg and dose escalation is done every 3–7 days till adequate pain relief is attained. The common side effects of TCA are sedation, tiredness, dry mouth, constipation, disturbances of micturition and orthostatic hypotension. Less common side effects are disturbances of sexual functions and arrhythmias.

Anticonvulsants

Carbamazepine is effective in neuropathic pain of varied etiologies. Dosage regimen is similar to that in epilepsy. Drug is started at a dose of 100 mg daily and escalation of drug dose is by 100 mg after every 3–5 days. Adequate pain relief is usually attained at doses of 400–600 mg daily. The common side effects are tiredness, vertigo, hyponatremia. Total blood cell counts and liver enzyme assay should be done at start of therapy.

Gabapentine is another anticonvulsant found to be effective in management of neuropathic pain. It is started at dosage of 300 mg daily at bed time. The dose is escalated by 300 mg every 1–3 days till a maximum dose of 3,600 mg. The most common adverse effects are vertigo, tiredness and edema.

Pregabalin

Pregabalin received FDA approval for treating epilepsy and neuropathic pain in 2004, and for post herpetic neuralgia in 2005. Pregabalin increases neuronal gamma amino butyric acid (GABA) levels by producing a dose-dependent increase in glutamic acid decarboxylase activity. Enzyme glutamic acid decarboxylase converts the excitatory neurotransmitter glutamate into inhibitory GABA which produces pain relief. It is given in a dose of 150 mg daily at bed time and the dose can be up to 450 mg/day. Dizziness, drowsiness, ataxia and peripheral edema are uncommon side effects. Rarely neutropenia has been reported.

A study from Japan involving 21 leprosy patients with chronic neuralgia showed marked improvement in pain in 90% cases with a mean daily dose of 60 mg of pregabalin. It suggested that pregabalin can be effective in leprosy patients who complain of intractable pain of nerves that are fibrosed.[71]

Opioids

Tramadol is a weak opioid with proven efficacy in neuropathic pain. It produces little dependence and tolerance.

A recent study has shown efficacy of long-term corticosteroids in relieving pain in late onset neuropathy in leprosy patients released from treatment suggesting that pain may be the result of chronic immune mediated process in response to antigens of *M. leprae,* and relapse or reaction should be ruled out clinically and histologically in such a clinical scenario.[72]

SURGERY

Surgery of the nerve is done primarily to improve its function. There is a consensus regarding the validity of nerve surgeries but there is no uniformity of opinion on its indications, achieved benefits and timing of surgery. Surgery should be done under corticosteroid coverage as the two modalities are complimentary and not competitive. While steroids would overcome the inflammation, surgery would help steroids to reach in adequate concentration. Indications for surgery are not well-defined but are based on common practice. The important indications are:[22]

- No improvement or deterioration while on steroids for several weeks, particularly in cases presenting with symptoms of more than 3 months duration.

- Nerve abscess.
- Intractable pain despite adequate dose of anti-inflammatory drugs and vigorous immunosuppressive therapy.
- Increasing pain while receiving MDT and corticosteroid treatment for NFI.

It is believed that axonal damage is due to the inflammatory response of the body against *M. leprae* and ischemia. Ischemia is the result of increased intraneural pressure compromising the blood flow in vasa nervorum. The affected nerve is swollen and is unable to accommodate edema in the rigid fibro-osseous channels with limited space, resulting in increased external pressure and obstructing the axoplasmic flow. Also, the perineurium does not give way to the swollen inflamed nerve, again compromising the function of nerve axonal cylinders. Basis of nerve surgeries is to relieve the mechanical compression, restoring the blood flow and functioning of nerve axonal cylinders.

As with steroids, early intervention with surgery results in complete recovery or arrest of progression of damage.[73] Different surgeries are:

- *Extraneural neurolysis*: This is a decompression surgery in which constricting fibrous bands and ligaments are excised and rigid fibro-osseous channels opened. This procedure relieves the external pressure only. Fibro-osseous channels in relation to the important nerve trunks are:
  - *Ulnar nerve*: Cubital tunnel at elbow, medial intermuscular septum, aponeurosis of flexor carpi ulnaris muscle, Guyon's canal (wrist).
    - *Median nerve*: Carpal tunnel at wrist
    - *Radial nerve*: Spiral grove of humerus
    - *Common peroneal nerve*: Retrofibular tunnel at neck of fibula
  - *Tibial nerve*: Tarsal tunnel (behind medial malleolus)

  All the vessels supplying nerve should be carefully saved and the nerve should not be subjected to undue trauma or tension or traction or displacement from its bed.
- *Intraneural neurolysis or longitudinal epineurotomy*: Longitudinal incisions are given in the sheath of the nerve trunk, i.e. epineurium taking care not to injure the vasa nervorum. This procedure has to be preceded by extraneural neurolysis.
- *Interfascicular neurolysis*: It is a meticulous and delicate procedure in which individual nerve bundles are dissected and separated. This procedure is now almost abandoned as it damages the nerve tissue and its vascularity producing fibrosis, which is far more crippling than the advantage it offers. It can be combined with intraoperative electrodiagnostics to identify skip areas with abnormal impulse transmission.[22]
- *Nerve abscess drainage*: Nerve abscess should always be drained. Longitudinal incision is given over abscess and then all the caseous liquid material is drained. If there

is subcutaneous collection of the material then a collar stud extension into the nerve must be anticipated. Whole procedure should be done meticulously to avoid trauma to the surviving nerve fibers. After complete drainage skin is closed by sutures of suitable material.

Nerve transposition by means of medial epicondylectomy: This procedure is done for the ulnar nerve at elbow. The objective is to avoid stretching of the nerve with movement of the elbow joint to increase the blood supply and protecting it from injury by burying it into the muscles.

Nerves with multiple sites of entrapment should be decompressed at multiple sites to minimize "double crush effects".[74]

Which surgery to be done is the decision of operating surgeon based upon the gross appearance of the nerve at dissection and extent of its damage.

Evidence from RCTs for the effectiveness of decompressive surgery is scarce. The most consistently reported benefit is the relief of nerve pain and tenderness while nerve function improvement is also frequently reported. Response to surgery depends on several factors and surgery results will be better in cases of:
- Partially damaged nerve.
- Duration of neuritis before surgery less than 6 months.

Trial by Pannikar et al.[75] and Ebenezer et al.[76] compared the added benefits of medial epicondylectomy and external decompression over corticosteroids for participants with ulnar neuritis of less than 6 months duration. They did not find any added benefit with surgical intervention as compared to steroid therapy alone in the treatment of early ulnar neuritis.

Boucher et al.[77] carried out a RCT of medical versus medico-surgical treatment of leprous neuritis. They performed longitudinal epineurotomy for ulnar, median, common peroneal and posterior tibial nerve involvement of less than 6 months duration. There was no significant statistical difference between the two groups according to the nerve involved, duration of the deficit, type of leprosy and the type of antileprosy treatment. However, the medico-surgical treatment had a significant better result on pain and on major but incomplete nerve involvement. Malaviya[78] suggested that surgery should be considered as add on therapy to the steroids as they remove the external compression, and improve the circulation so that steroids can reach faster and lead to rapid improvement of nerve function.

It has recently been proposed that timing of surgical intervention should be earliest, preferably within 3 months of onset as fibrosis and axonal death accumulate with passage of time. However, more RCTs are needed to establish the effectiveness of medical and surgical treatment versus medical treatment alone.[22]

A RCT is in progress to determine the value of surgical nerve decompression in leprosy neuropathy in association with corticosteroid treatment.[79]

Complications of decompressive surgery are painful scars, wound problems, hematoma, infection and damage to nerves, arteries or tendons.

GENERAL MEASURES

Acutely inflamed nerve should be put to strict rest as any kind of trauma would further aggravate the inflammation. In addition rest also reduces the reactive fibrosis. This is done by immobilizing the limb in semi-relaxed functional position using padded splints. Graduated exercises are to be done as the clinical improvement occurs.

Heat therapy in the form of short wave diathermy, ultrasonic therapy and transcutaneous nerve stimulation are different physical modalities which can be used for pain control not fully responding to immunosuppressants.

Hand and foot care advice is given to the patient to prevent the development of nerve deficit related deformities and complications. Patient should be explained that the anesthetic area will gradually contract with time as the other nerve fibers supplying in neighboring areas will take over the function.

Correct counseling of the patient is important. It should be emphasized that the reversal of NFI is highly unpredictable and the duration of therapy is going to be long. Many patients tend to default from MDT when their long-standing NFI does not improve or when they develop new NFI while on MDT. The importance of continuation of MDT should be explained to ensure compliance.

PREVENTION

Only the early diagnosis of leprosy and regular treatment can prevent the nerve damage by killing all *M. leprae* before they infect the nerves. The goal could be partially achieved by increasing awareness about the early signs and symptoms of leprosy among the general public and removing the barriers (like social stigma), which prevent people from reporting for treatment. Much of the nerve damage occurs during reactions. Therefore, patients at higher risk of reactions should be educated about these reactional episodes in detail and emphasized to present early for treatment.

Patients who are at increased risk of reaction and neuritis can be identified and put on prophylactic treatment. TRIPOD 1 trial[80] investigated the role of low dose steroid in the prevention of T1Rs in MB patients. One group of patients received 20 mg of prednisolone during initial 4 months of MDT while the other group received placebo. Incidence of T1R was lower in the trial group during the 4 months but the difference was not significant at the end of 1 year.

Arunthathi et al.[81] tested the usefulness of clofazimine as a prophylactic agent against neuritis and nerve damage. Sixty five patients received high doses (300 mg daily) of clofazamine for initial 3 months of MB-MDT and the control group received only MB-MDT. Patients were followed for 2 years and the incidence of neuritis was significantly low in the test group (5.66%) as compared to control group (26.1%).

NEWER APPROACHES OF TREATMENT

Till now we largely rely on anti-inflammatory agents for the treatment of leprosy related neuritis. With the advancement in the knowledge of pathophysiology of leprosy and leprosy related neuritis, newer approaches of treatment are designed which are in experimental stages.

- *Drugs and vaccines blocking the attachment of mycobacteria to the Schwann cell-axon unit:* With the identification of neural targets on Schwann cells and the specific bacterial component responsible for neural tropism, agents blocking the attachment of the two can be designed.[82] These agents would prevent the entry of bacilli into the nerve.
- *Neruotropic factors:* Schwann cells play significant role in the maintenance and regeneration of axons of the neurons in the peripheral nervous system. These cells are regulated by neurotropic factors (NTFs). NTF have been found to increase the transmission of impulses between fibers of collateral axons blocked by mycobacterial antigens in the axoplasm.[83] These NTFs could be the drug molecules of future promoting the nerve regeneration and conduction in existing fibers.

HUMAN IMMUNODEFICIENCY VIRUS AND LEPROUS NEURITIS

Presently, coinfection with HIV-1 and *M. leprae* is a rare event. With increasing HIV prevalence, in future we are likely to get more number of cases suffering from both ailments. HIV, per se, produces neuropathy and so would aggravate it in leprosy patients. Steroids have to be given cautiously in these patients with strict monitoring for adverse effects.

Neuritis and T1Rs were found to be more common in HIV seropositive MB cases as compared to HIV seronegative MB cases, while the same did not hold true for PB cases.[63] HIV seronegative and seropositive patients showed a similar response to steroid therapy for the management of acute neuritis.

CONCLUSION

Early and appropriate management of leprous neuritis is the key to prevention of disabilities in leprosy patients. Our understanding of pathogenetic mechanisms involved in nerve damage is incomplete and more research is needed for development of new principles in therapy and prophylaxis.

REFERENCES

1. Spierings E, de Boer T, Wieles B, et al. *Mycobacterium leprae*-specific, HLA class II-restricted killing of human Schwann cells by CD4+ Th1 cells: a novel immunopathogenic mechanism of nerve damage in leprosy. J Immunol. 2001;166(10):5883-8.
2. Rambukkana A, Zanazzi G, Tapinos N, et al. Contact-dependent demyelination by *Mycobacterium leprae* in the absence of immune cells. Science. 2002;296(5569):927-31.
3. Rosenberg NR, Faber WR, Vermeulen M. Unexplained delayed nerve impairment in leprosy after treatment. Lepr Rev. 2003;74(4):357-65.
4. Umerov Z. Leprosy neuropathy: a study both cross-reacting epitope on the *Mycobacterium leprae* and human peripheral nerve. A novel autoimmune mechanism of nerve damage and appropriate therapeutic strategy. International Leprosy Congress; 2013 September 16 - September 19; Brussels, Belgium. Abstract No. P-364.
5. Croft RP, Nicholls PG, Steyerberg EW, et al. A clinical prediction rule for nerve-function impairment in leprosy patients. Lancet. 2000;355(9215):1603-6.
6. Richardus JH, Nicholls PG, Croft RP, et al. Incidence of acute nerve function impairment and reactions in leprosy: a prospective cohort analysis after 5 years of follow-up. Int J Epidemiol. 2004;33(2):337-43.
7. Schuring RP, Richardus JH, Steyerberg EW, et al. Preventing nerve function impairment in leprosy: validation and updating of a prediction rule. PLoS Negl Trop Dis. 2008;2(8):e283.
8. Van Brakel WH, Nicholls PG, Das L, et al. The INFIR Cohort Study: investigating prediction, detection and pathogenesis of neuropathy and reactions in leprosy. Methods and baseline results of a cohort of multibacillary leprosy patients in north India. Lepr Rev. 2005;76(1):14-34.
9. HN Ravi, George R, Eapen EP, et al. A comparison of economic aspects of hospitalization versus ambulatory care in the management of neuritis occurring in lepra reaction. Int J Lepr Other Mycobact Dis. 2004;72(4):448-56.
10. Wagenaar I, Brandsma W, Post E, et al. Two randomized controlled clinical trials to study the effectiveness of prednisolone treatment in preventing and restoring clinical nerve function loss in leprosy: the TENLEP study protocols. BMC Neurol. 2012;12:159.
11. Van Brakel WH, Nicholls PG, Wilder-Smith EP, et al. Early diagnosis of neuropathy in leprosy—comparing diagnostic tests in a large prospective study (the INFIR cohort study). PLoS Negl Trop Dis. 2008;2(4):e212.
12. Roche PW, Theuvenet WJ, Britton WJ. Risk factors for type-1 reactions in borderline leprosy patients. Lancet. 1991;338(8768):654-7.
13. Van Brakel WH, Saunderson P, Shetty V, et al. International workshop on neuropathology in leprosy--consensus report. Lepr Rev. 2007;78(4):416-33.
14. John AS, Rao PS, Pitchaimani G. Early detection of sensory nerve function impairments in the field. International Leprosy Congress: Hidden challenges; 2013 September 16 - September 19; Brussels, Belgium. Abstract No. P-239.
15. Vijaikumar M, D'Souza M, Kumar S, et al. Fine needle aspiration cytology (FNAC) of nerves in leprosy. Lepr Rev. 2001;72(2):171-8.

16. Jayaseelan E, Shariff S, Rout P. Cytodiagnosis of primary neuritic leprosy. Int J Lepr Other Mycobact Dis. 1999;67(4):429-34.

17. Antunes SL, Jardim MR, Vital RT, et al. Post-MDT leprosy neuropathy: differentially diagnosing reactional neuritis and relapses. International Leprosy Congress; 2013; Brussels, Belgium. Abstract No. O-200.

18. Vital RT, Jardim MR, Sales AM, et al. Demyelination in leprosy neuropathy: correlation between electroneurographical alterations and detection of serum antiganglioside antibodies International Leprosy Congress; 2013 September 16 - September 19, 2013; Brussels, Belgium. Abstract No. P-365.

19. Jain S, Visser LH, Praveen TL, et al. High-resolution sonography: a new technique to detect nerve damage in leprosy. PLoS Negl Trop Dis. 2009;3(8):e498.

20. Van Brakel WH, Nicholls PG, Das L, et al. The INFIR Cohort Study: assessment of sensory and motor neuropathy in leprosy at baseline. Lepr Rev. 2005;76(4):277-95.

21. Cunha AC, Araújo S, Goulart IM, et al. Thermography as an early indicator of nerve injury in leprosy patients. International Leprosy Congress; Brussels, Belgium. Abstract No. P-065.

22. Nickerson DS, Nickerson DE. A review of therapeutic nerve decompression for neuropathy in Hansen's disease with research suggestions. J Reconstr Microsurg. 2010; 26(4):277-84.

23. Paul SK, RV, Sivarasu S. Effect of tactile sensors in detecting pressure threshold of anesthetic hand. International Leprosy Congress; 2013; Brussels, Belgium. Abstract O-027.

24. Ebenezer GJ, Truman R, Scollard D, et al. Epidermal nerve fibre and Schwann cell densities in the distal leg of nine banded armadillos with experimental neuropathy. International Leprosy Congress; 2013; Brussels, Belgium. Abstract No. O-153.

25. Jardim MM, Vital RT, Antunez SL, et al. Revisiting the worsening of nerve impairment after MDT. International Leprosy Congress; 2013. Brussels, Belgium. Abstract No. O-093.

26. Barnes PJ. Anti-inflammatory actions of glucocorticoids: molecular mechanisms. Clin Sci (Lond). 1998;94(6):557-72.

27. Buttgereit F, Wehling M, Burmester GR. A new hypothesis of modular glucocorticoid actions: steroid treatment of rheumatic diseases revisited. Arthritis Rheum. 1998;41(5):761-7.

28. Lipworth BJ. Therapeutic implications of non-genomic glucocorticoid activity. Lancet. 2000;356(9224):87-9.

29. Britton WJ. The management of leprosy reversal reactions. Lepr Rev. 1998;69(3):225-34.

30. World Health Organization, Action Programme for the Elimination of Leprosy. A guide to eliminate leprosy as a public health problem, 1st edition; 1995.

31. Becx-Bleumink M, Berhe D, Mannetje W. The management of nerve damage in the leprosy control services. Lepr Rev. 1990;61(1):1-11.

32. Naafs B. Bangkok Workshop on Leprosy Research. Treatment of reactions and nerve damage. Int J Lepr Other Mycobact Dis. 1996;64(4 Suppl):S21-8.

33. Van Brakel WH, Anderson AM, Withington SG, et al. The prognostic importance of detecting mild sensory impairment in leprosy: a randomized controlled trial (TRIPOD 2). Lepr Rev. 2003;74(4):300-10.

34. Rao PS, Sugamaran DS, Richard J, et al. Multi-centre, double blind, randomized trial of three steroid regimens in the treatment of type-1 reactions in leprosy. Lepr Rev. 2006;77(1):25-33.

35. Garbino JA, Virmond Mda C, Ura S, et al. A randomized clinical trial of oral steroids for ulnar neuropathy in type 1 and type 2 leprosy reactions. Arq Neuropsiquiatr. 2008;66(4):861-7.

36. Naafs B, Pearson JM, Wheate HW. Reversal reaction: the prevention of permanent nerve damage. Comparison of short and long-term steroid treatment. Int J Lepr Other Mycobact Dis. 1979;47(1):7-12.

37. Naafs B. Treatment duration of reversal reaction: a reappraisal. Back to the past. Lepr Rev. 2003;74(4):328-36.

38. Frade MA, Tomaselli P, Marques VD, et al. High doses of intra venous methylprednisolone re-establishes the nerve function in leprosy neuritis: A pilot study. International Leprosy Congress; 2013; Brussels, Belgium. Abstract No. P-381.

39. Sahay G, Kar HK. Evaluation of nerve function impairment (NFI) in multibacillary (MB) leprosy patients on multidrug therapy (MDT-MB) along with or without prednisolone. International Leprosy congress; 2013; Brussels, Belgium. ABstract No. P-458.

40. Shetty VP, Khambati FA, Ghate SD, et al. The effect of corticosteroids usage on bacterial killing, clearance and nerve damage in leprosy; part 3—Study of two comparable groups of 100 multibacillary (MB) patients each, treated with MDT + steroids vs. MDT alone, assessed at 6 months post-release from 12 months MDT. Lepr Rev. 2010;81(1):41-58.

41. Saunderson P, Gebre S, Desta K, et al. The pattern of leprosy-related neuropathy in the AMFES patients in Ethiopia: definitions, incidence, risk factors and outcome. Lepr Rev. 2000;71(3):285-308.

42. Schreuder PA. The occurrence of reactions and impairments in leprosy: experience in the leprosy control program of three provinces in northeastern Thailand, 1987-1995 [correction of 1978-1995]. III. Neural and other impairments. Int J Lepr Other Mycobact Dis. 1998;66(2):170-81.

43. Van Brakel WH, Khawas IB. Nerve function impairment in leprosy: an epidemiological and clinical study-part 2: Results of steroid treatment. Lepr Rev 1996;67(2):104-18.

44. Richardus JH, Withington SG, Anderson AM, et al. Treatment with corticosteroids of long-standing nerve function impairment in leprosy: a randomized controlled trial (TRIPOD 3). Lepr Rev. 2003;74(4):311-8.

45. Saunderson P. The epidemiology of reactions and nerve damage. Lepr Rev. 2000;71 Suppl:S106-10.

46. Miko TL, Le Maitre C, Kinfu Y. Damage and regeneration of peripheral nerves in advanced treated leprosy. Lancet. 1993;342(8870):521-5.

47. Croft RP, Nicholls PG, Richardus JH, et al. The treatment of acute nerve function impairment in leprosy: results from a prospective cohort study in Bangladesh. Lepr Rev. 2000;71(2):154-68.

48. Lockwood DN, Vinayakumar S, Stanley JN, et al. Clinical features and outcome of reversal (type 1) reactions in Hyderabad, India. Int J Lepr Other Mycobact Dis. 1993;61(1):8-15.

49. Richardus JH, Withington SG, Anderson AM, et al. Adverse events of standardized regimens of corticosteroids for prophylaxis and treatment of nerve function impairment in leprosy: results from the 'TRIPOD' trials. Lepr Rev. 2003;74(4):319-27.

50. Capadia GD, Shetty VP, Khambati FA, et al. Effect of corticosteroid usage combined with multidrug therapy on nerve damage assessed using nerve conduction studies: a prospective cohort study of 365 untreated multibacillary leprosy patients. J Clin Neurophysiol. 2010;27(1):38-47.

51. Ross WF. Does clofazimine have any value in the management of reversal reaction? Lepr Rev. 1980;51(1):92-3.

52. Imkamp FM. Clofazimine (lamprene or B663) in lepra reactions. Lepr Rev. 1981;52(2):135-40.

53. Pfaltzgraff RE. The control of neuritis in leprosy with clofazimine. Int J Lepr Other Mycobact Dis. 1972;40(4):392-8.

54. Ramu G, Girdhar A. Treatment of steroid dependant cases of recurrent lepra reaction with a combination of thalidomide and clofazimine. Lepr India. 1979;51(4):497-504.

55. Schreuder PA, Naafs B. Chronic recurrent ENL, steroid dependent: long-term treatment with high dose clofazimine. Lepr Rev. 2003;74(4):386-9.

56. Poulkar CB, Kar HK, Gupta L. Evaluation of nerve function impairment (NFI) in paucibacillary leprosy (PB) on WHO paucibacillary multidrug therapy (PB-MDT) along with or without clofazimine. International Leprosy Congress: Hidden challenges; Brussels, Belgium. Abstract No. P-063.

57. Theophilus S. Treatment with thalidomide in steroid dependency and neuritis. Lepr India. 1980;52(3):423-8.

58. Marlowe SN, Hawksworth RA, Butlin CR, et al. Clinical outcomes in a randomized controlled study comparing azathioprine and prednisolone versus prednisolone alone in the treatment of severe leprosy type 1 reactions in Nepal. Trans R Soc Trop Med Hyg. 2004;98(10):602-9.

59. Lockwood DN, John AS, Joydeepa D, et al. RCT of azathioprine versus prednisolone in the treatment of type 1 reaction and neuritis. International Leprosy Congress; 2013; Brussels, Belgium. Abstract No. O-024.

60. Miller RA, Shen JY, Rea TH, et al. Treatment of chronic erythema nodosum leprosum with cyclosporine A produces clinical and immunohistologic remission. Int J Lepr Other Mycobact Dis. 1987;55(3):441-9.

61. Chin-A-Lien RA, Faber WR, Naafs B. Cyclosporin A treatment in reversal reaction. Trop Geogr Med. 1994;46(2):123-4.

62. Sena CB, Salgado CG, Tavares CM, et al. Cyclosporine A treatment of leprosy patients with chronic neuritis is associated with pain control and reduction in antibodies against nerve growth factor. Lepr Rev. 2006;77(2):121-9.

63. Marlowe SN, Leekassa R, Bizuneh E, et al. Response to ciclosporin treatment in Ethiopian and Nepali patients with severe leprosy type 1 reactions. Trans R Soc Trop Med Hyg. 2007;101(10):1004-12.

64. Garrett AS. Hyalase (hyaluronidase) injections for lepromatous nerve reactions. Lepr Rev. 1956;27(2):61-3.

65. Sepaha GC, Sharma DR. Intraneural cortisone and priscol in treatment of leprosy. Lepr India. 1964;36:264-8.

66. Ramanujam K. A note of the use of intra-neural corticoids in acute leprous neuritis. Lepr India. 1964;36:261-3.

67. Nashed SG, Rageh TA, Attallah-Wasif ES, et al. Intraneural injection of corticosteroids to treat nerve damage in leprosy: a case report and review of literature. J Med Case Rep. 2008;2:381.

68. Lund C, Koskinen M, Suneetha S, et al. Histopathological and clinical findings in leprosy patients with chronic neuropathic pain: a study from Hyderabad, India. Lepr Rev. 2007;78(4):369-80.

69. Hietaharju A, Croft R, Alam R, et al. Chronic neuropathic pain in treated leprosy. Lancet. 2000;356:(9235)1080-1.

70. Lasry-Levy E, Hietaharju A, Pai V, et al. Neuropathic pain and psychological morbidity in patients with treated leprosy: a cross-sectional prevalence study in Mumbai. PLoS Negl Trop Dis. 2011;5(3):e981.

71. Goto M, Sugio Y, Sawada S, et al. Effect of pregabalin on the chronic neuropathic pain of leprosy. International Leprosy Congress; 2013 September 16 - September 19; Brussels, Belgium. Abstract No. O-156.

72. Cardoso Fde M, De Freitas MR, Escada TM, et al. Late onset neuropathy in leprosy patients released from treatment: not all due to reactions? Lepr Rev. 2013;84(2):128-35.

73. Husain S, Mishra B, Prakash V, et al. Results of surgical decompression of ulnar nerve in leprosy. Acta Leprol. 1998;11(1):17-20.

74. Williams EH, Williams CG, Rosson GD, et al. Combined peroneal and proximal tibial nerve palsies. Microsurgery. 2009;29(4):259-264.

75. Pannikar VK, Ramprasad S, Reddy NR, et al. Effect of epicondylectomy in early ulnar neuritis treated with steroids. Int J Lepr Other Mycobact Dis. 1984;52(4):501-5.

76. Ebenezer M, Andrews P, Solomon S. Comparative trial of steroids and surgical intervention in the management of ulnar neuritis. Int J Lepr Other Mycobact Dis. 1996;64(3):282-6.

77. Boucher P, Millan J, Parent M, et al. Randomized controlled trial of medical and medico-surgical treatment of Hansen's neuritis. Acta Leprol. 1999;11(4):171-7.

78. Malaviya GN. Shall we continue with nerve trunk decompression in leprosy? Indian J Lepr. 2004;76(4):331-42.

79. Virmond M, Garbino JA, Cury Filho M, et al. Proposal for a prospective, randomized trial to determine the role of nerve decompression in leprosy neuropathy. International Leprosy Congress; 2013; Brussels, Belgium. Abstract No. P-304.

80. Smith WC, Anderson AM, Withington SG, et al. Steroid prophylaxis for prevention of nerve function impairment in leprosy: randomised placebo controlled trial (TRIPOD 1). BMJ. 2004;328(7454):1459.

81. Arunthathi S, Satheesh KK. Does clofazimine have a prophylactic role against neuritis? Lepr Rev. 1997;68(3):233-41.

82. Rambukkana A. Molecular basis of the interaction of *Mycobacterium leprae* with peripheral nerve: implications for therapeutic strategies. Lepr Rev 2000;71(Suppl):S168-9.

83. Anand P. Neurotrophic factors and their receptors in human sensory neuropathies. Prog Brain Res. 2004;146:477-92.

Chemoprophylaxis in Leprosy

BK Girdhar

INTRODUCTION AND THE NEED

All efforts at elimination of leprosy during the last 50 years or so have been directed at early detection and treatment of patients with the aim of reducing the pool of infection in the community and thus preventing spread of infection to the uninfected members of the society. Most people with leprosy are noninfectious as the *Mycobacterium* remains intracellular. Patients with lepromatous leprosy, however, shed *Mycobacterium leprae* from their nasal mucosa and skin, and are infectious before starting treatment with multidrug therapy. Such an approach of early detection and institution of therapy, though likely to be effective, is sure to take long to result in perceptible reduction in the incidence rate. For an effective outcome, in other words for disease elimination and zero incidence in the near future, the efforts based only on chemotherapy of known patients alone, may not be sufficient. Raising the herd immunity of the community is considered important so that the individuals are no longer susceptible to the infection, even if the causative organism is present in the surrounding environment. However, for this as of now, we do not have the really effective tool—the vaccine. The next best is aborting the infection so that the disease manifestation does not occur.

Consequent to the spread of any infection in the community, on active case detection or voluntary reporting, manifest disease is detected only in a small proportion of population. In contrast, many individuals with subclinical infection remain unidentified and, if left alone, some of them may later develop disease. It has long been considered that prophylactic treatment of the individuals, who are exposed to infection and might be incubating the disease, may be helpful in killing the infecting organism and preventing the disease. Such an approach has been remarkably effective in containing yaws. Similar reduction in occurrence of tuberculosis in the families, by giving isoniazid to the healthy familial contacts of 'open' cases, had led to the thinking in leprosy that chemoprophylaxis could be useful in reducing the incidence rates in leprosy.

The mechanism by which chemoprophylaxis works, possibly involves killing of the causative organisms before the onset of pathology or when given later, killing of the pathogen and allowing the microscopic pathology to reverse/subclinical disease to heal or both. In leprosy, as the incubation period is very long, both the mechanisms may be involved, though the later appears to be more relevant.

WHO NEEDS CHEMOPROPHYLAXIS?

An issue of importance appears to be who needs protection—entire community or a select group? In theory, everyone who lives in an endemic area should get protection. In leprosy, providing protection to the entire community, apart from reducing the pool of infection, does not seem cost effective and/or feasible—as the disease affects only a small fraction of the society, prevalence and incidence rates being very low even in endemic areas. If it is not possible to cover all the individuals in an endemic area, can the efforts be limited to any particular or select group in whom the disease is likely to occur more frequently?

In tuberculosis transmission, 'stone-in-the-pond' concept has been suggested,[1] meaning that the risk of infection gradually decreases as one moves away from the open case. Familial contacts are at greater risk than neighbors, who in turn are at increased danger than their neighbors and so on. This implies that as one moves away from the pool of infection—the index case, the risk of infection decreases. Indeed, the available data does indicate that the risk of contracting leprosy, too, decreases with increasing physical distance from the patient or the duration and intimacy of contact. This increased risk of infection determines the need for prophylaxis.

It is a common observation that only 30% patients have an index case in the family and the rest neither have any known case of leprosy in the family or neighborhood or at place of work. The former group, on account of closeness of contact, is at higher risk than the noncontacts. Thus, among the small number of familial or close contacts, a third of the total patients occur. So, for leprosy, chemoprophylaxis focus had long been on the contact population, i.e. on siblings within the family who stand a higher chance of infection and disease.

In the endemic areas the remaining population, with no known contact with any leprosy patient, accounts for rest of the cases. Even though the leprosy prevalence rate in this population, extrafamilial or noncontacts, is very small, the total number of patients who appear in this population is not insignificant as nearly 70% of the patients come from this category. In view of this, work has also been undertaken to find ways to prevent disease in the general population.

The High-risk Group

In both tuberculosis and leprosy, contact examination has received a lot of importance. Based on the above mentioned 'stone-in-the pond' concept, familial contacts of the index case have been considered to be the most important group. Household contacts, in particular, have been the focus of attention. Workers have defined household contacts in very varied fashion taking the social structure of the society into consideration. However, all seem to agree that a person with prolonged, frequent or intimate contact with an infectious case is at a greater risk.

It has also been observed that the risk of disease among the contacts not only depends upon the closeness of contact but also the type of disease in the index case, risk being 6–8 times greater in contacts of multibacillary (MB) cases than paucibacillary (PB) patients, but still are at twice the risk than noncontacts. Likewise, contacts of smear positive cases are at a much higher risk of getting infected as compared to the contacts of skin and nasal smear negative cases.[2,3] A follow-up study of household contacts of patients in Indonesia,[3] has shown that household contacts of index patients with *M. leprae* DNA in the nose, skin smear positive MB patients and seropositive patients, were significantly at a higher risk of disease. Males were observed to be at twice the risk than females. The authors further report that the risk of disease transmission was three times higher among household contacts when the family size was more than seven, as compared to smaller families (members less than 4).

Apart from the increased exposure, the susceptibility of the individuals also seems to play some role.[4] Higher prevalence among the familial contacts has been suggested to be due

to similar genetic makeup. In this regard, observations of more than twice the risk of leprosy in monozygotic twins, as compared to dizygotic twins, are relevant. Human leukocyte antigen (HLA) (DR2) and non HLA genes appear to contribute to genetic susceptibility to either leprosy, *per se*, or the type of disease a person acquires. Locus on chromosome 6q25 appears to control part of susceptibility. Studies from India have shown that a locus on chromosome 10p13 is linked to the increased risk with PB leprosy.[5]

Younger children have been observed to be more susceptible to leprosy[6]—there being a strong relationship between the risk of developing clinical leprosy and the age at exposure. Bimodal distribution of the disease has been observed in several studies. This could also be on account of long incubation period of the disease, or due to infection later in life. Disease attack rates are higher in the males possibly on account of increased exposure. If there are any biological factors to account for this increased risk in the males, is not clear. Less occurrence of the disease in the educated class, as also those with better housing conditions and less household crowding, indicates that individuals with poor socioeconomic conditions are at a greater risk of infection and disease.[7] This could possibly be on account of several factors, such as poor personal hygiene, closeness of contact, poor nutrition, poor sanitation, etc.

Delayed detection or diagnosis and consequent delayed start of treatment of leprosy patients, especially the smear positive ones, exposes the community to prolonged contact and, thus, increases chances of infection. Many individuals in endemic areas may already be infected before the index case, in the family or neighborhood, is detected or diagnosed and put on treatment. Therefore, even when only a few patients are detected and diagnosed in the field, there may be several members in the community who have already been infected but have not yet developed disease manifestations, because of the long incubation period of the disease.

Based on the above understanding, studies were initiated in the sixties to see if chemoprophylaxis could reduce the risk of developing the disease among both the contacts and the general population.

DAPSONE CHEMOPROPHYLAXIS

During the last 50 years, workers were involved in testing the efficacy of various drugs that could be used for chemoprophylaxis. Expectedly, initially dapsone was tested for its utility in preventing the disease.

Studies in Contacts

Early work in this regard was carried out in India and Africa. In the trial undertaken at Bombay (Mumbai),[8] none of the 51 contacts who received dapsone chemoprophylaxis developed leprosy in contrast to leprosy manifesting in 9.35% of 524 contacts who had not been administered dapsone. Working with children of leprosy parents, Lew and Kim[9] reported that only two of the 325 DDS administered familial contacts developed disease. This is in contrast to 31 of the 425 contacts not given DDS, developing the disease during the same 2-year period. Similar protective effect was observed on long-term (3–10 years) follow-up in larger familial contact population.[9] Work undertaken in Philippines showed a reduction of 44% in occurrence of leprosy over a period of 3 years in child contacts of leprosy patients, who had been given DDS, as compared to those without the drug.[10] Observations made in Vietnam[11] also indicated marked efficacy of dapsone in children. Contacts staying with their lepromatous parents, who received dapsone, had less cases of leprosy as compared to those not given the drug.

Two systematic investigations had been made on the utility of DDS prophylaxis in the familial contacts. One study was undertaken in South India.[12,13] In this placebo-controlled, randomized and double-blind investigation, half of the familial contacts had been given DDS for a minimum of 3 years and the remaining received a placebo. Comparison made over 5 years revealed that there was an overall reduction of 52% in the treatment group as compared to the control group—the difference being statistically significant. In both the groups, most of the patients were of tuberculoid type—an effect of early detection possibly on account of periodic check-up. Though no contact developed lepromatous disease in either of the groups, three patients in the control group had skin-smear positive leprosy. In contrast, only one patient had bacteriologically positive disease in the dapsone treated group. None of the children, staying with their lepromatous parents and receiving DDS, for a mean period of 30 months, was observed to have developed leprosy. *In all the above studies, the source or the index case had been treated side by side.*

With these observations of disease protection with dapsone and the knowledge that the number of contacts, who develop disease, form a small percentage of the total incident cases, it was considered that, if chemoprophylaxis was limited to contacts alone, this might not help much in the control of leprosy. With this in mind, workers have continued to assess, if chemoprophylaxis given to the entire population would be useful in this regard.[14]

Dapsone Chemoprophylaxis Given to the Entire Endemic Population

Initial work, in this direction, was undertaken in Srikakulam district of Andhra Pardesh.[15,16] The study was carried out in 54 villages divided randomly into two groups. In one group, all the healthy individuals below 25 years of age received DDS twice a week for four and a half years, whereas persons in the other 27 villages were given placebo tablets for the entire duration of observation. Yearly assessment carried over four and a half years showed reduction in the incidence in the prophylaxis group to the tune of 49% more than in the control group—wherein a decrease of 41% had been observed, possibly consequent to reducing load of infection in the community due to simultaneous treatment of all diagnosed cases. Continued DDS administration beyond this period was found to have lesser protective role. Like in other contact studies, benefit of disease protection was more among the younger age group.

Whereas mass chemoprophylaxis, as above, appears effective in reducing new leprosy cases, its application to very large populations in the endemic countries does pose challenges. Not only because large numbers of individuals have to be given the drug, but also because of the long duration for which the drug administration has to be continued, especially to children. Since self-administration of any drug, even for symptomatic diseases over long periods of time, is fraught with the dangers of irregularity and the consequences of resistance and adverse effects, self-intake of drugs for long duration for prophylaxis, is even more likely to be erratic.

Acedapsone (Diacetyl Diamino Diphenyl Sulfone or DADDS) for Chemoprophylaxis

With the understanding that minimum inhibitory concentration (MIC) of dapsone against *M. leprae* was very low and that even a small daily dose of 1–2 mg resulted in drug levels that were almost ten times higher than the MIC for *M. leprae*, an injectable depot preparation of dapsone, diacetyl diamino diphenyl sulfone, in short called acedapsone, had been developed. Injections of acedapsone (225 mg) given deep intramuscularly every two and a half months (11 weeks) were advocated for leprosy. One shot of acedapsone gave serum levels above MIC for almost 3 months. As the drug had to be injected, this supervised and ensured form of dapsone administration was tested for its prophylactic value against leprosy, in Micronesia and later in Chinglepet.

In the work undertaken in three villages of Ponape district of Micronesia,[17,18] which had high prevalence of active disease, all the under treatment leprosy patients were switched on to acedapsone from oral treatment and the entire leprosy-free population, more than 6 months in age, was given acedapsone injections every 75 days for 3 years. Yearly examination of the population revealed less than half the expected cases during the first year and no new case in the next 2 years. Continued follow-up showed emergence of five cases in the subsequent 2 years, four among those who had not taken full course of acedapsone prophylaxis. In the two nearby villages, where acedapsone administration had been better supervised, the results were better as compared to the third village which was far away and thus had lesser supervision. This indicated considerable role of preventive treatment, when given to the entire population. The important issue here was the essentiality of continuing therapy of all known cases. A double-blind placebo-controlled study, undertaken in *contacts* of lepromatous patients in south India, confirmed a significant protection with acedapsone administration over 2-year-period.[19]

In short, all the studies on the subject, controlled (*vide supra*) and uncontrolled, indicated that chemoprophylaxis with dapsone or acedapsone, afforded protection to the extent of 55–60% during the period of administration, with gradual loss of protection after stoppage of the drug both in contacts and the entire population. Further, to prevent occurrence of a case of leprosy, the numbers of individuals that had to be treated was relatively small among the contacts and fairly large in the general population. The main problem with this mode of prophylaxis was that dapsone/acedapsone had to be given for long periods and, hence, the possibility of being irregular, especially in case of dapsone, on account of self-administration. Another cause of concern had been the risk of increasing dapsone resistance on account of irregularities and low drug concentrations, as with acedapsone, which had already been observed to be a worldwide phenomenon.

RIFAMPICIN FOR PROTECTION AGAINST LEPROSY

Following the demonstration of its potent bactericidal action against *M. leprae,* and thus the efficacy of rifampicin in treatment of leprosy, its utility in prophylaxis of the disease was considered. As the drug had been shown to kill over 99% *M. leprae* following a single dose, it had been considered that a limited administration of rifampicin may be useful for prophylaxis of the disease. In the initial work, undertaken in Southern Marquesas,[20,21] wherein the entire population was given one dose of rifampicin, 25 mg/kg body weight, a protection of 40–50% was observed. As the superiority of giving bolus dose of 1,500 mg rifampicin over efficacy of 600 mg, given only once or on two days, had not been proved, this dose has not been used in any further trials.

Bakker and his coworkers[22] have undertaken controlled studies in five Indonesian islands. Comparing the outcome of two doses of rifampicin given 3 months apart, to all residents of the three islands (the blanket group), with the drug administered the same way to only the child and neighborhood contacts in one island—the contact group and no chemoprophylaxis in the fifth island, the authors have reported that the cumulative incidence after 3 years was significantly lower in the blanket group, as compared with control group. The protection afforded was to the tune of 75%. On long-term follow-up of 6 years, the effectiveness of the rifampicin protection was reduced and was not significantly more than in the control group. To prevent occurrence of one case of leprosy, the number which needs to be treated at 3 years was 127 and it increased to 244 at 6 years. The protection, in the spatially defined contacts, with rifampicin was not significantly different than in the control group.

Placebo-controlled, randomized double-blind study giving single dose of rifampicin to the contacts of leprosy patients (household and compound members, immediate neighbors and neighbors of neighbors, and close social and business contacts) has been conducted in Bangladesh.[23,24] First follow-up made after 2 years showed a significant reduction of 56% in the incidence of leprosy in the rifampicin protected contacts as compared to the controls. However, the protection was no longer significant in the third and fourth year. The protective efficacy was observed to be more in the comparatively less high-risk group, i.e. in neighbors of neighbors and social, and business contacts than among the family (close) contacts. A possible reason suggested is that the load of *M. leprae* and, hence, intensity of infection in the household contacts could be much higher in the immediate contacts than among the noncontacts and thus relative inability of one dose of rifampicin to kill the bacilli. Like in the earlier study, the numbers needed to be given chemoprophylaxis to prevent a case of leprosy was 272.

A similar multicentric, double-blind, randomized and placebo-controlled trial in over 7,500 household contacts in India has shown protection against leprosy.[25] A significant decrease in new case occurrence in the ensuing 4–5 years was observed in contacts who received a single dose of rifampicin (10 mg/kg body weight). However, the numbers needed to be treated to prevent the occurrence of one case of the disease was 1,556—a large population!

Utility of a combination of three drugs—rifampicin, ofloxacin and minocycline (ROM) has also been looked into. Work undertaken in Micronesia[26] with ROM has shown protective efficacy similar to that observed in studies using rifampicin alone. This is in line with the findings in mice, that ROM is no more bactericidal than single dose of rifampicin alone.[27] Further, in view of the small bacterial load that may be present in the exposed individuals and thus very little possibility of *de novo* rifampicin resistance, addition of accompanying drugs is sure to make it less cost-effective and possibly more toxic and, hence, has not found favor with the leprosy workers. In contrast to the above, a study conducted in Myanmar, among the contacts followed up for 6 years, has shown no protective efficacy of single dose ROM when compared to placebo (vitamins).[28]

In short, the studies indicate that chemoprophylaxis, particularly when given to the entire community, has a significant protective effect in reducing the incidence of leprosy but the protective effect lasts for a limited period and then wanes. In contrast to the prolonged intake of dapsone required, single or two doses of rifampicin are better options. However, the important need is simultaneous and still better, earlier start of treatment of all the patients in the family and the community.

Concerns have been expressed regarding the applicability and feasibility of rifampicin chemotherapy application in the field, i.e. to very large populations in the endemic countries.

This is because, as has been observed, that to prevent a case of leprosy, large numbers of healthy persons have to be given chemoprophylaxis. Fear of selection of resistant bacteria of varied types, including *M. leprae* and *M. tuberculosis,* has been another concern. It is considered that this may pose problems in the treatment of leprosy and/or tuberculosis. Therefore, it is essential that the contacts/healthy population be screened for both leprosy and tuberculosis prior to consideration of chemoprophylaxis, which should only be given under supervision.

APPLICATION OF CHEMOPROPHYLAXIS

Contacts of leprosy patients are at increased risk of infection, chemoprophylaxis reduces this risk but the logistics, ethics and cost-effectiveness of providing chemoprophylaxis are not simple. How should chemoprophylaxis be made use of, has been the subject of discussion. Whether this would be cost-effective at national level in reducing the incidence rates of the disease in a community, depends upon the number of individuals who need to be treated to prevent a case of leprosy and thus on the endemicity of leprosy in the region. For blocking the transmission at the community level, large number of apparently healthy individuals in the endemic areas needs to be given the drug in a supervised fashion. All the studies indicate that to prevent one case of leprosy, hundreds and may be thousands of subjects need to be treated.[29] With the decreasing case load and, hence, reduced pool of infection and subsequent transmission, the number of individuals who need to be given prophylaxis will be still more. These numbers are bound to increase making chemoprophylaxis for control less and less cost-effective in future as the incidence of the disease goes down. So, it would require very high direct and indirect cost in implementing chemoprophylaxis. In a study conducted in Bangladesh[30] between 2002 and 2007, approximately $6,000 was spent to prevent 38 patients (incremental cost-effectiveness ratio of $158—cost of preventing occurrence of one case). The authors reported that prevention was most cost-effective in neighbors of neighbors, social contacts and household contacts in that order.

Chemoprophylaxis of whole population or close contacts is not only difficult, time and manpower intensive, but may not be well-accepted by several healthy individuals in the community. For chemoprophylaxis to high-risk groups, it may often be required to let the contacts know the likely source of possible spread of infection. Newly diagnosed, concerned and understanding patients may indeed want to protect their household contacts but may not like their diagnosis/disease to be known to their contacts and/or neighbors on account of stigma that continues with the disease.[31] A recent study has shown that whereas index cases do not object to disclosure of their diagnosis to household members, they are unwilling to let the neighbors know about their disease. This indicates that even though chemoprophylaxis may be more effective in close contacts, mass therapy without disclosing the source may not be easily acceptable and thus may be less feasible.[32] Further, many individuals, even educated ones, continue to believe that leprosy is a disease of the poor or deprived, or of a particular group and thus may not accept prophylaxis.

Despite above reservations rifampicin chemoprophylaxis for leprosy could be useful and acceptable in high endemic pockets where clustering of cases is found, provided thorough screening for leprosy and tuberculosis is made before hand, and the community is well educated in health issues and understands that prophylaxis afforded by rifampicin is significant, though not complete.

Chemoprophylaxis has shown a good protection among the high-risk groups. Therefore, its application in protection of household contacts, in particular those of skin-smear positive patients, is more likely to be useful. Here, only a small numbers of individuals, more often child contacts of index cases are to be protected. *As protection is more often asked by the family,* not only the contacts are brought for examination to rule out pre-existing leprosy but also can be thoroughly examined to rule out tuberculosis. It has been suggested that that chemoprophylaxis would be more useful, and feasible in contacts of patients in low endemic and high resource countries.[25] As stated earlier, for any protection using chemoprophylaxis to be effective, the essential thing is the treatment of the index cases side by side, if not earlier.

Multidrug therapy has enabled us to contain the disease and has resulted in reduction of prevalence of disease globally with almost all countries having achieved elimination of leprosy. However, it is being observed that new cases continue to appear in not insignificant numbers in all earlier endemic areas despite continued application of MDT. It is now being argued that simultaneous chemoprophylaxis of the high-risk group may help in reducing the number of incident cases.[33] In view of the perceived increase in *M. leprae* resistance against rifampicin, a suggestion has been made that one or two doses of ROM chemoprophylaxis be given to household of leprosy patients to achieve better results in disease elimination.[34] Should this become a routine is yet not clear.

Giving one or two doses of rifampicin has been another issue. A second dose given the very next day is not likely to add to the efficacy. Whether repeating the dose 3 months or 6 months later, and/or repeating the prophylactic dose to the contacts after the index case has become skin-smear negative, would be of any benefit is not clear. Is there a subgroup among the close contacts who in turn is more prone to disease is not clear, as we still lack tools, serological and others, to identify them. Whether combination of chemoprophylaxis and immunoprophylaxis would be more useful, needs to be seen.

REFERENCES

1. Veen J. Micro-epidemics of tuberculosis: the stone-in–the-pond principle. Tuber Lung Dis. 1992;73(2):73-6.
2. Moet FJ, Meima A, Oskam L, et al. Risk factors for development of clinical leprosy among contacts, and their relevance for targeted intervention. Lepr Rev. 2004;75:310-26.
3. Bakker MI, Hatta M, Kwenang A, et al. Risk factors for developing leprosy—a population based cohort study in Indonesia. Lepr Rev. 2006;77:48-61.
4. Fitness J, Tosh K, Hill AV. Genetic susceptibility to leprosy. Genes Immun. 2002;3(8);441-53.
5. Siddiqui MR, Meisner S, Tosh K, et al. A major susceptibility locus for leprosy in India maps to chromosome10p13. Nat Genet. 2001;27(4):439-41.
6. Fine PE, Sterene JA, Ponnighaus JM, et al. Household and dwelling contact as risk factor for leprosy in northern Malawi. Am J Epidemiol. 1997;146(1):91-102.
7. Kumar A, Girdhar A, Yadav VS, et al. Some epidemiological observations on leprosy in India. Int J Lepr Other Mycobact Dis. 2001;69(3):234-41.
8. Figueredo N, Balakrishnan V. Risk of infection in leprosy. Part 2. Chemoprophylaxis. Lepr Rev. 1967;38:87-92.
9. Lew J, Kim YS. Chemoprophylaxis of leprosy contacts with DDS. Int J Lepr. 1968;36(7):47-51.
10. WHO Expert Committee on Leprosy. WHO Tech Report Series # 459: 1970.
11. Nhu TQ, Mong Don TK. Chemotherapy in children living in leprosy institutions. Presented at: 10th Leprosy Congress; 1973; Bergen, Norway. Abstract pp. 136. Int J Lepr. 1973;41:618.
12. Dharmendra, Noordeen SK, Ramanujam K. Prophylactic value of DDS against leprosy—a further report. Lepr India. 1967;39:100-6.
13. Noordeen SK. Chemoprophylaxis in leprosy. Lepr India. 1969;41:247-54.
14. Louvey M, Saint-Andre P, Giraudeu P. Role of chemoprophylaxis in prevention of leprosy. Med Trop. 1976;36:153-7.
15. Wardekar RV. DDS prophylaxis against leprosy. Lepr India. 1967;39:155-9.
16. Wardekar RV. Chemoprophylaxis in leprosy. Lepr India. 1969;41:240-6.
17. Sloan NR, Worth RM, Jano B, et al. Acedapsone in leprosy chemoprophylaxis; Field trial in three high prevalence villages in Micronesia. Int J Lepr Other Mycobact Dis. 1972;40(1):40-7.
18. Russell DA, Worth RM, Scott GC, et al. Experience with acedapsone (DADDS) in the therapeutic trial in New Guinea and the chemoprophylaxis trial in Micronesia. Int J Lepr Other Mycobact Dis. 1976;44(1-2):170-6.
19. Noordeen SK, Neelan PN, Manaf A. Chemoprophylaxis against leprosy with acedapsone—an interim report. Lepr India. 1980;52(1):97-103.
20. Cartel JL, Chanteau S, Moulia-Pelat JP, et al. Chemoprophylaxis of leprosy with a single dose of 25 mg per kg rifampin in the south Marquesas; results after four years. Int J Lepr Other Mycobact Dis. 1992;60(3):416-20.
21. Ngyur LN, Cartel JL, Grosset JH. Chemoprophylaxis of leprosy in the south Marquesas with a single dose of 25 mg/kg rifampicin. Results after 10 years. Lepr Rev. 2000;71 Suppl;S33-6.
22. Bakker MI, Hatta M, Kwenang A, et al. Prevention of leprosy using rifampicin as chemoprophylaxis. Am J Trop Med Hyg. 2005;72(4); 443-8.
23. Moet FJ, Oskam L, Faber R, et al. A study on transmission and trial of chemoprophylaxis in contacts of leprosy patients: design, methodology and recruitment findings of COLEP. Lepr Rev. 2004;75(4):376-88.
24. Moet FJ, Pahan D, Oskam L, et al. Effectiveness of single dose rifampicin in preventing leprosy in close contacts of patients with newly diagnosed leprosy: cluster randomized controlled trial. BMJ. 2008;336(7647):761-4.
25. Oskam L, Mi B. Report of the workshop on use of chemoprophylaxis in the control of leprosy held in Amsterdam, the Netherlands on 14 December 2006. Lepr Rev. 2007;78(2):173-85.
26. Diletto C, Blank L, Levy L. Leprosy chemoprophylaxis in Micronesia. Lepr Rev. 2000;71(Suppl):S21-5.
27. Ji B, Sow S, Perani E, et al. Bactericidal activity of single-dose combination of ofloxacin plus minocycline, with or without rifampicin, against *M. leprae* in mice and in lepromatous patients. Antimicrobial Agents Chemother. 1998;42(5): 1115-20.
28. Oo KN, Wai KT, Myint K, et al. Effectiveness of single dose of rifampicin,ofloxacin and minocycline (ROM) chemoprophylaxis in preventing leprosy. Mynamar Hlth Sci Res J. 2010;22:62-4.
29. Noordeen SK. Prophylaxis—scope and limitations. Lepr Rev. 2000;71(Suppl):S16-9.
30. Idema WJ, Majer IM, Pahan D, et al. Cost effectiveness of chemoprophylactic intervention with single dose rifampicin in contacts of new leprosy patients. PLoS Negl Trop Dis. 2010;e874.
31. Smith WC. Chemoprophylaxis in prevention of leprosy. BMJ. 2008;336(7647):730-1.
32. Feenstra SG, Nahar Q, Pahan D, et al. Acceptability of chemoprophylaxis for household contacts of leprosy patients in Bangladesh: a qualitative study. Lepr Rev. 2011;82(2): 178-87.
33. Shen J, Zhou M, Yang R, et al. Features of leprosy transmission in pocket villages at low endemic situation in China. Indian J Lepr. 2010;82(2);73-8.
34. Senior K. Stigma, chemoprophylaxis and leprosy control. Lancet Infec Dis. 2009;9(1):10.

Leprosy Vaccines: Immunoprophylaxis and Immunotherapy

Kiran Katoch

CHAPTER OUTLINE

- Immunoprophylaxis
- Chemoprophylaxis

- Immunotherapy

INTRODUCTION

Leprosy is a chronic granulomatous disease caused by *Mycobacterium leprae* and has a long and variable incubation period. The manifestation of the disease depends to a large extent on the immune response of the host. Majority of the individuals exposed to the disease organism, do not manifest the disease, and/or in a few cases self-heal. A small proportion of the exposed individuals, however, manifest the disease in the skin, and/or peripheral nerves, and in a vast majority of patients, in both. In some patients, as a result of immunological alterations evoked by the organism they suffer from acute inflammatory episodes also known as leprosy reactions [type 1 or reversal reactions (RRs) and type 2 or erythema nodosum leproticum (ENL) reactions], which may lead to deformities and are the main cause of morbidity due to the disease. It is also believed that besides, the live pathogen which triggers the immunological response, the dead bacilli or its products also can induce immune responses associated with leprosy reactions and nerve damage. Leprosy reactions have also been observed to be precipitated and triggered by endocrinal changes occurring in the host (physiological changes like puberty, pregnancy and lactation) as well as by intercurrent illnesses like acute viral infections, human immunodeficiency (HIV) coinfection, malaria and other parasitic diseases.

Large scale and successful implementation of present day multidrug therapy (MDT) has brought down the prevalence of disease substantially. However, new cases are still being reported globally, and need to be addressed for ultimate eradication of the disease and achieving the goal of "World without leprosy and its deformities". Chemotherapy/MDT kills most of the susceptible live organisms but "persisters"/metabolically dormant bacilli and dead organisms remain in the body for long and variable duration, and many a times precipitate a leprosy reaction, nerve damage and resultant deformities. Therefore, besides MDT/chemotherapy, which primarily targets the infecting live organism, immune modulators are required to modulate the immune response which damages the nerves in the host and are a cause of continued morbidity in some leprosy patients.

Vaccines are biological substances that improve the immunity to a particular disease (Wikipedia). These vaccines/immunomodulators are substances which help to regulate the immune system and optimize the immune response. This immune response is essential not only for recovery from the infection, but also for prevention and the development of disease on exposure to the pathogen (immunoprophylaxis). Over the last few decades, a large number of immuno-modulators have been investigated for their potential as immunoprophylactic as well as immunotherapeutic agents to optimize the immune response in the host. This has been used in general population for prevention of the disease, and in leprosy patients for rapid clinical and bacteriological improvement, granuloma clearance, and for treatment, and decreasing the incidence and severity of reactions, and preventing nerve damage (immunotherapy). These are being reviewed and discussed.

IMMUNOPROPHYLAXIS

Generally, immunoprophylactic agents or vaccines (as more commonly called) have the capacity to provoke an immune response which enables the host to effectively deal with the infecting organism and confer protection from disease. The word "vaccine" is derived from the French word *"la vacche"* meaning the cow. This is in reference to the first "vaccine", cowpox extract used by Jenner, in 1812, for prevention of smallpox in human beings. The global eradication of smallpox could be achieved mainly because of widespread use and availability of a cheap and effective vaccine, and is a very good and successful example of use of vaccine to prevent disease. The same is being tried in prevention of other diseases also.

The issue of a need for a vaccine to prevent leprosy has been, and is still being, debated. With the changing profile of the disease, curability of the disease with effective and widely available MDT coupled with the low prevalence of the disease, vaccine development has taken a backseat by most research groups and funding agencies. Moreover, with a limited knowledge of the transmission dynamics and spread of the disease, a vaccine for use in the general population is probably not urgently required. However, it may still be important to consider its administration in specific areas/groups, like pockets of high endemicity, close family contacts and other high-risk groups. With the increased survival of acquired immunodeficiency syndrome (AIDS) patients and manifestation of the immune reconstitution inflammatory syndrome (IRIS) associated with the wide spread use of antiretroviral therapy, leprosy has been reported to clinically manifest in some patients, while "leprosy reactions" are being reported in some other patients with AIDS. Considering these developments, the debate on immunoprophylaxis is still alive and needs attention.

Vaccines are generally antigenically similar to the pathogen and are capable of evoking an immune response in the host. They are broadly prepared/classified as:
a. Using killed organisms that have lost its infectivity but has retained its "protective" antigens and can provoke an immune response
b. Using live attenuated organisms that provoke a protective response in the host against the pathogen, but do not cause disease *per se*
c. Using a related nonpathogenic organism that antigenically cross-reacts with the pathogen and evokes a immune response in the host
d. More recent is the use of only the immunogenic "subunit(s)" of the organism prepared by recombinant deoxyribonucleic acid (DNA) technology, amplified by polymerase chain reaction (PCR) which evokes a protective host response
e. Drugs.

Vaccines have been developed from all the above (a–d) categories and have elicited a variable degree of immune response in the recipient host. Besides, the inherent different responses evoked by the use of these various vaccines, some other factors may also influence the protective effect. These include:
• Route of administration
• Age of the recipient at the time of vaccination
• Coverage of vaccination in the population
• Duration of follow-up

• Nutritional status of the vaccinated persons
• Endemic diseases in the population
• Environmental bacteria prevailing in the environment and geographical location.

All these factors singularly, or in combination, may influence the outcome of the immunoprophylactic agent and needs to be kept in mind while evaluating the outcome of the vaccination. Vaccines which have been tried in general population for prevention of leprosy are detailed below.

Bacillus Calmette-Guerin: Bacillus Calmette-Guerin (BCG), the live attenuated strain of *M. bovis* has been used worldwide as a live attenuated vaccine for prevention of mycobacterial diseases: tuberculosis and leprosy. It was first described by Calmette during the early 20th century for its use in the cattle. Animal studies demonstrated that BCG has a protective effect against *M. leprae* in mice.[1] It was later found to be useful in humans also.[2,3] BCG as an antileprosy vaccine was tried in Karinaul, Papua, New Guinea and was reported to be efficacious.[3,4] The results were however varied in different population groups.[5,6] Other case control studies showed that it could be of value in preventing borderline disease.[7] In a large scale study in South India, where BCG was given in one of the four limbs to the general population, it was observed that the overall prophylactic effect of BCG was 34.1% [confidence interval (CI) 13.5–49.8] in the second resurvey (5 years after vaccination).[8] In the meta-analysis of use of BCG for prevention of leprosy, Sethia et al.[9] have analyzed and included seven experimental and 19 observational studies from the reported literature. They report that the experimental studies demonstrated an overall protective effect of 26% (95% CI 14–37%). However, the observational studies overestimated the protective effect which has been reported as 61% (95% CI 51–70%). The age at vaccination did not predict the protective effect of BCG. An additional dose of BCG was more protective in the prevention of leprosy compared with a single dose. The authors opine that an additional dose of BCG may be warranted for contacts of leprosy patients in areas where leprosy continues to be a public health problem.[9]

Bacillus Calmette-Guerin + killed M. leprae: Convit et al.[10] showed the immunogenicity of *M. leprae* was enhanced by the addition of BCG and a mixed vaccine containing a mixture of heat-killed armadillo-derived *M. leprae* + BCG could evoke a better immunological response and could be used for vaccination purposes. He reported his findings with both BCG and BCG + killed *M. leprae* in immunoprophylactic trials undertaken by him and observed that both BCG as well as the combination provided protection, but the combination did not provide significant additive effect as compared to BCG alone.[11]

In the comparative leprosy vaccine trial, four vaccines, namely BCG, BCG + killed *M. leprae*, *Mw* [now named as *Mycobacterium indicus pranii*, (MIP)], Indian Cancer Research Centre *(ICRC)* vaccine and normal saline as placebo was administered to about 1,71,000 population. The protective efficacy after 5 years follow-up was observed to be 64% for BCG + killed *M. leprae*.[8] However, with a longer follow-up, this protection to BCG + killed *M. leprae* decreased considerably. Results for vaccine efficacy in the above study are based on examination of more than 70% of the original vaccinated cohort population, in both the first and the second resurveys. The author's opine that the incidence rates were not sufficiently high to ascertain the protective efficacy of the candidate vaccines against progressive and serious forms of leprosy.

Mycobacterium indicus pranii (MIP): This was initially isolated from a lepromatous patient, is a saprophytic cultivable mycobacteria. It is administered as a killed vaccine. This vaccine was administered in one of the arms of the study as a single dose in the South India comparative vaccine study[8] (also referred to with BCG and BCG + killed *M. leprae* and ICRC section). As indicated above, the results of vaccine efficacy in this study is based on examination of more than 70% of the original vaccinated cohort population. The study group noted that the placebo group showed a significant decline in leprosy incidence during the three resurveys from 23.6/10,000 during the first, to 12.8/10,000 during the second and 6.1/10,000 during the third resurvey, and reported that the incidence rates of leprosy were not sufficiently high to ascertain the protective efficacy of the candidate vaccines against progressive and serious forms of leprosy. It was observed that the protective efficacy of MIP was 34.1% at the end of second resurvey. On further analysis, to observe its effect on household contacts of index cases, protection was observed to be 60% in household contacts who received a single dose of killed MIP (Gupte et al. unpublished reports).

Another large field-based, double-blind placebo-controlled clinical study was undertaken in family contacts of index leprosy cases, in Ghatampur tehsil of Kanpur district, India, using two doses of killed MIP administered at an interval of 6 months.[11] On follow-up of the household contacts, a protective efficacy of 68% and 60% was observed after a follow-up of 3–4 years and 7–8 years, respectively. However, the efficacy decreased to 39.3%, 10 years after vaccination. This waning of protection probably indicates a need for a second booster around 8–10 years.[11]

Indian Cancer Research Centre: ICRC is a cultivable mycobacteria belonging to the *M. avium intracellulare* (MAI) complex which shares several antigens with *M. leprae*. It has been used as a killed vaccine and has been administered to both lepromin positive and negative healthy household contacts (HHC) of multibacillary (MB) leprosy patients in Maharashtra, India.[5] However, the results of the same have not been reported. In the comparative South Indian vaccine study,[8] ICRC was also administered in one of arms of the study. The protective effect observed was 65% during the second follow-up after 5 years of vaccination.

Mycobacterium vaccae: M. vaccae is a rapidly growing, nontuberculous mycobacterium species that is generally not considered a human pathogen. This mycobacteria also shares some antigens with *M. leprae* and has been shown to induce *in vitro* and *in vivo* immune reactivity in leprosy patients[12-14]It is administered as a killed vaccine intradermally in the dose of 10[8] organisms/mL and it produces a similar scar as BCG. It has also shown immunomodulatory useful properties, like leprosin conversion in previously negative patients, as well as children of leprosy patients who were previously leprosin negative. Its immunomodulatory effects were enhanced when combined with BCG.[14] Long-term effects on protection in leprosy have not been reported.

Long-term studies of immunoprophylaxis with BCG and MIP have been undertaken, and are well documented. They are both safe and well tolerated, have some effect on both leprosy and tuberculosis, and are available commercially.

CHEMOPROPHYLAXIS

More recently, studies have been undertaken on the use of chemoprophylaxis for the prevention of leprosy.[15-17] In these studies, a single dose of rifampicin is administered to contacts of patients of leprosy in a cohort cluster. Bakker et al.[15] tried it in endemic five islands of Indonesia, wherein contacts of index cases were given a single dose of rifampicin/placebo administered orally in a randomized blind manner. These contacts were followed up for 3 years. A reduced incidence of leprosy was reported in the rifampicin group as compared to the placebo group. However, due to the very short follow-up it could not be ascertained if this was just a postponement of the occurrence of symptoms or was truly the prevention of disease. Leprosy has a long and variable incubation period, ranging from few months to several years. Moreover, in some patients the lesions self-heal (which person and in what proportion is not known), and what proportion of exposed individuals will manifest the disease and when, is not predictable and uncertain. Such short follow-up for assessing the effect of an immunoprophylactic agent is not justifiable. Furthermore, the causative organism cannot be cultured in any known artificial culture medium and a much longer follow-up is required to reach any conclusion on the role of the agent in providing protection from infection. Thus, a much longer follow-up is required to reach any conclusion.

Similar double-blind studies have also been undertaken in Bangladesh by Oskam et al.[16] as well as Moet et al.[17] Due to the very small follow-up of 2 years, it is difficult to conclude the role of single dose of rifampicin in such trials. Theoretically speaking, with the available knowledge, a single dose of rifampicin *per se* cannot induce prophylaxis and long-term follow-up studies are required to establish the role of chemoprophylaxis due to it. Rifampicin is a highly bactericidal drug and acts by killing rapidly multiplying organisms with no established immunomodulatory effects. It may be argued that rifampicin merely causes a postponement of the manifestation of the disease rather than true protection.

IMMUNOTHERAPY

Although the present day chemotherapy has helped in reducing the prevalence, incidence of the disease and achieving the elimination goal at the national level, some problems do remain. These include:

- Relatively long duration of treatment
- Strict adherence to the treatment regimen
- Persistence of disease activity after stoppage of therapy
- Occurrence of reactions and nerve damage before, during, as well as after stoppage of therapy
- Relapses and recurrences after stoppage of fixed duration treatment (FDT).

These call for better and efficient management of the disease.[18] The addition of immunotherapy to chemotherapy has been considered by several investigators to overcome the above deficiencies, optimize the treatment and aims at the following:

- Achieving more efficient killing of viable bacilli, including the persister organisms
- Faster clearing of dead bacilli and their components from the body
- Reducing the incidence and severity of reactions
- Restoration of effective immunity so that relapses/reinfection can be prevented.

The immunomodulators being used can be broadly classified into:

- Related mycobacteria which share antigens with *M. leprae*
- Drugs
- Other miscellaneous agents and/or components of *M. leprae* which mount an immunogenic response.

Antigenically Related Mycobacteria

Mycobacteria, which share some antigens/or show cross reactivity with *M. leprae,* have been studied and evaluated for their immunomodulatory potential in animals as well as in humans. Mycobacteria which have been tried in humans include BCG, BCG + killed *M. leprae*, MIP, ICRC bacillus, *M. vaccae* alone and in combination with BCG and *M. habana.*

M. bovis BCG: This was one of the first mycobacteria to be tried in humans as an immunomodulator, is used as a live vaccine and has shown both nonspecific, as well as specific immunomodulatory effect in leprosy. Fernandez, in 1939, demonstrated lepromin conversion in 30–100% individuals vaccinated with BCG.[3] Immunotherapy with BCG showed enhanced bacterial killing and clearance in borderline lepromatous (BL)/lepromatous leprosy (LL) smear positive patients treated for 2 years with standard MB-MDT and BCG administered at the end of treatment.[19] In another study, BCG was given with MDT from the start of MDT and every 6 months till the end of treatment.[20] The vaccine was well

tolerated and there was a blister/nodule formation at the local site of vaccination which healed of its own, leaving a small scar. There was faster bacteriological attainment of smear negativity, faster fall in bacterial index (BI), more rapid killing of viable bacilli [as observed by mouse foot pad inoculation and estimation of adenosine triphosphate (ATP) from tissue biopsies]. The severity and incidence of reactions was decreased in comparison with patients receiving MDT alone. It was observed that in the MDT + placebo group, the reactions persisted for a longer period[20] and the degree of severity was more. Natrajan et al. reported faster granuloma clearance and histological upgrading in these patients.[21] Similar results were observed by Narang et al.[22] in their study where BCG was given every 3 months till 12 months in MB patients undergoing World Health Organization (WHO) recommended MB-MDT for 1 year. They reported statistically significant difference in the time to achieve smear negativity, granuloma clearance, and reduction in the incidence of type 2 reactions in the BCG + MDT group as compared to controls who received MDT + placebo.

BCG + killed M. leprae: Shepard et al., in 1980, studied the protective effect of BCG + killed *M. leprae* in mice.[23] Convit et al., in 1974[10] and in 1982,[24] in combination with killed *M. leprae* reported lepromin conversion and enhanced bacterial clearance in treated LL patients. He also reported beneficial immunological changes in indeterminate leprosy patients, Mitsuda negative contacts and LL patients. Meyers et al., in 1988, reported histological upgrading in patients receiving this therapy[25] while Samuel et al., in 1985,[26] studied the lepromin conversion in contacts of leprosy patients receiving the vaccine. Both of them reported beneficial effects in the form of lepromin conversion in their respective studies.

Mycobacterium indicus pranii: MIP is a rapid growing, nonpathogenic, cultivable mycobacteria belonging to Runyon Group IV classification of mycobacteria. It shares several antigens with *M. leprae* and *M. tuberculosis.*[27,28] It is administered as a killed vaccine. Its immunomodulatory effect has been tested *in vitro* and experimental animals.[29] It has recently been characterized molecularly and whole genome sequenced.[30] It has also been tried in humans.[18,20,22,31-37] It is well tolerated and safe with only a blister/nodule formation at the local site of inoculation. The blister/nodule appears in 3–4 weeks and heals by its own in another 6–8 weeks. The results in MB cases have shown an earlier achievement of smear negativity, a more rapid bacterial clearance and rapid killing of viable bacilli[37] in patients receiving MIP + MDT as compared to MDT alone. Natrajan et al. observed a more rapid granuloma clearance and histological upgrading in MIP + MDT group as compared to MDT + placebo.[21] Mukherjee et al.[38] also reported a significantly higher percentage of patients showing upgrading and/or enhanced clearance of dermal granuloma in MIP + MDT group as compared to the MDT alone group in a independent study.

In the studies undertaken at JALMA, Agra, MIP was given along with MDT every 6 months in highly bacillated BL/LL patients till 24 months.[18,20,37] To summarize, the results observed at the center, MIP was well tolerated and there were no side effects except for blister/nodule formation at the local site of injection, which appeared in 2–4 weeks and regressed within the next 1–2 months with a small scar. The fall in BI in the MIP + MDT and MDT + placebo group is shown in Figure 35.1. It can be seen that there was a rapid fall in the BI in the MIP + MDT group as compared to MDT + placebo.

The fall in BI was as a result of killing of viable bacilli as measured by mouse foot pad inoculation and measuring the ATP in the tissue biopsies of these patients, as well as clearing of dead bacilli from the tissues.[18,20,21,37] The patients in MIP + MDT group became smear negative in 32 months while patients in the MDT + placebo group took 52 months to attain smear negativity. Besides, the granuloma fraction also decreased more rapidly and there was more lymphocytic infiltration in the MIP group as compared to MDT+ placebo group.[20,21,37] In the studies undertaken at Postgraduate Institute (PGI), Chandigarh,[22,34,35] the vaccine was given with MDT every 3 months for four doses. A similar, more rapid fall in BI was noted in the MDT + immunotherapy group as compared to MDT + placebo group. In these studies only bacterial clearance was noted, but killing of viable bacilli was not assessed. Similar results were also observed by Sharma et al.[36] in a hospital based study at New Delhi, where MIP was given along with MDT every 3 months for four doses with MDT.

There was no increase in the incidence of reactions (both reversal and ENL), rather the reactions stopped earlier in the MIP + MDT group as compared to MDT + placebo group.[37]

Kar et al.[32] observed a slightly increased incidence of RR in BL/LL patients given MIP + MDT (MIP was given at 3 monthly interval along with MDT). The RR was of mild nature, short lasting and not leading to any significant morbidity. Similar results were also observed by Narang et al.[22] and Kaur et al.[35] The investigators have opined that this is due to protective defense immunity mounted by the host to the antigenic challenge.

More recently, placebo-controlled double-blind study using MIP + MDT and MDT + placebo in borderline leprosy patients [borderline tuberculoid (BT), borderline borderline (BB) and BL cases] has also been published[39] from JALMA, Agra. The authors reported a marked clinical improvement, rapid fall in BI, faster granuloma clearance and lesser RRs in MIP + MDT group as compared to the MDT + placebo group. *ICRC bacillus:* This is a cultivable leprosy derived mycobacteria probably belonging to MAI complex. This organism was isolated from leprosy patients and showed cross-reactive antigens to *M. leprae* in *in vitro* and *in vivo* experiments.[27,28,40] It has also been used in humans with reported beneficial effects.[5,40-44] The authors observed that when killed ICRC vaccine was given to lepromatous patients along with chemotherapy, a significant and rapid fall in BI was observed in addition to RRs and lepromin convertibility.[5,41,44]

Mycobacterium vaccae: It is a rapidly growing, nonpathogenic mycobacteria which also shares some antigens with *M. leprae* and *M. tuberculosis.* It has been shown to induce *in*

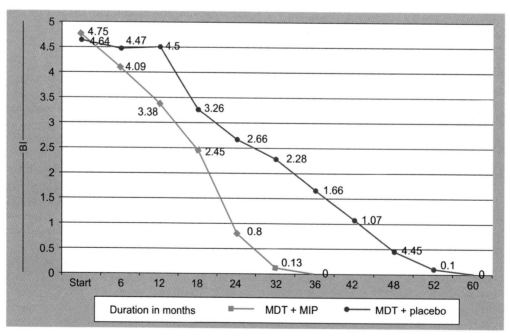

Fig. 35.1: Graph shows the fall of BI-MIP + MDT and MDT + placebo group in highly bacillated leprosy cases

vitro and *in vivo* immune reactivity in leprosy patients.[12,45] It is administered as a killed vaccine intradermally in the dose of 10^8 organisms/mL and it produces a similar scar as *BCG and is well tolerated.* Stanford et al.,[45] observed that intradermal injection of a suspension of killed *M. vaccae* promotes cell-mediated responses to antigens common to all mycobacteria and switches off the tissue-necrotizing aspects of the Koch phenomenon. There is a more rapid faster fall in bacteriological indices when administered along with chemotherapy in leprosy patients. These immunomodulatory effects were enhanced when combined with BCG and the authors opine that BCG with killed *M. vaccae* is likely to be a better vaccine for leprosy than BCG alone.[46]

Besides the related mycobacteria discussed above, there are a few more mycobacteria which have been investigated and possess some antigenic similarity with *M. leprae* and show some degree of cross-sensitization. These include *M. habana,*[47,48] *M. phlei* and *M. gordonnae.*[26] *M. habana* has also been tested in animals and was observed to have a protective effect in mice and monkeys which was observed after the animals were challenged with *M. leprae* after vaccination with the organism.

M. phlei and *M. gordonnae*[26] also have cross-reactive antigens with *M. leprae* as observed by *in vitro* tests. However, these mycobacteria have not been adequately investigated/ promoted as immunotherapeutic agents for use in leprosy (Table 35.1).

Immunomodulatory Drugs

Levamisole: This is a broad spectrum antihelminthic, which acts by influencing the host defenses and modulating the cell-mediated human response as seen by *in vitro* and *in vivo* experiments.[49,50] It is believed to have an immunomodulatory effect on defective T lymphocyte function and has been tried in LL patients. Sher et al. administered levamisole daily for two consecutive days each week for 6 weeks in a group of lepromatous patients.[49] Although there was no significant clinical improvement at the end of 6 weeks, there was a significant change histologically in the biopsies and in the erythrocyte (E) and erythrocytes coated with antibody and complement (EAC) rosettes formation in patients who took levamisole.[49] Martinez and Zaiasin, in 1976, used levamisole as an adjunct to dapsone therapy and reported improvement in the clinical lesions and decrease in the incidence of reactions as compared to placebo.[51] In another study, 150 mg of levamisole was given twice a week for 6 weeks in persistently skin-smear positive LL patients who had received continuous dapsone treatment for 5 years. Most of the patients became skin-smear negative within 1 year of treatment.[52] Beneficial effects have also been reported by Sharma et al.[53] The use of levamisole as an adjunct to MDT has been reported by Kar et al.[54] Although there was no conversion of Mitsuda reactivity and no change in leukocyte migration inhibition in both control (only MDT) and the experimental group (levamisole + MDT), in the experimental group statistically significant clinical and bacteriological improvement and increase in the EAC rosette counts were observed at the end of 1 year. No adverse effect due to levamisole was observed.[54] With the changed profile and prevalence of the disease, further reports of its use are not available.

Zinc: Zinc has also been tried as an immunomodulator in treatment of LL. When given in therapeutic dosages, it inhibits the complement dependent immune complex formation and polymorphonuclear leukocyte chemotaxsis.[55] It has also been tried in recurrent ENL reaction and it was observed that after giving zinc therapy steroids could be withdrawn completely, and the duration and severity of reaction could be reduced.[56] Cases treated with zinc showed faster clinical improvement, regrowth of the eyebrows and rapid fall in BI of the skin and in the granuloma as seen histologically. Histological upgrading was observed in six of the 15 cases (40%) treated

Table 35.1: Shows the *in vitro* and *in vivo* effects of the various mycobacteria

Agent	LMIT	LTT	Lepromin convertibility	Tuberculin response	Protection in mice/animals
BCG	+	+	+	+	+
BCG + killed Mycobacterium leprae	Not done	+	+	+	+
MIP	+	+	+	+	+
ICRC	+	+	+	+	+
M. habana	+	+	+	+	+
M. vaccae	+	+	+	+	+
M. phlei	+	+	+	Not done	+
M. gordonnae	+	+	+	Not done	Not done

Abbreviations: LMIT, leukocyte migration inhibition test; LTT, leukocyte transformation test; BCG, Bacillus Calmette-Guerin; MIP, Mycobacterium indicus pranii; ICRC, Indian Cancer Research Centre.

with zinc + dapsone as compared to one of ten (10%) treated with dapsone alone. Five of the six patients, who showed upgrading in the trial study group, became epromin positive while one of the six in the control group (BL case) showed lepromin conversion.[56] However, the effect of zinc with MDT is not well documented. Subsequently, studies investigating the beneficial effect of zinc have not been reported, although it is being used as supportive supplementation with MDT by several medical practitioners.

Other drugs: Various other drugs, like corticosteroids, thalidomide, high doses of clofazimine (300–400 mg daily), colchicine, cyclosporine, have been used for treatment of reactions, neuritis and ENL reactions. These also act by immunomodulation of host response in addition to other effects.

Other Miscellaneous Immunomodulators

Other miscellaneous agents used as immunomodulators in leprosy include:

Transfer factor: This was used by Hastings and Job and has been shown to induce lepromin conversion, granuloma formation and increased influx of lymphocytes at the local site of injection, However, these effects were short-lived, could be demonstrated at the local site of inoculation, and not observed systemically.[57]

Cytokines/Interleukins: The use of gamma interferon (IFN-γ) has been shown to activate macrophages and cause intracellular killing of *M. leprae.*[58] However, it had to be injected and the results were confined locally and remained for a short period. Intralesional injections of recombinant IFN-γ have demonstrated a distinct fall in the BI at the local site, formation of epithelioid granuloma and occurrence of RR in some cases.[58-61] Enhanced bacterial clearance at the local site of injection has also been observed by Sivasai et al.[62] The administration of recombinant interleukin-2 (IL-2) has also been reported to produce similar effects by Kaplan et al.[63]

Acetoacetylated M. leprae: This is a carrier modified *M. leprae* and a single injection produced a positive lepromin response in seven out of the 13 patients who were repeatedly lepromin negative.[64] Further, investigations on its use have not been reported.

Delipified cell components of M. leprae: Mahadevan and Robinson observed that defective macrophages of leprosy patients were able to recognize delipified cell components (DCC) as antigen, which led to production of desired lymphokines.[65] Mice vaccinated with DCC could mount good cell-mediated immunity (CMI) response and control the growth of *M. leprae.*[66] Further use and investigations in this direction have not been documented.

Soluble protein component obtained from cell wall of M. leprae: The soluble cell wall component acts as antigen, causes stimulation of T-cell and show protection in mice.[65-68]

Table 35.2 Summarizes the observations on the effect of various immunomodulators as used in leprosy and various systemic effects of immunotherapy.

Immunotherapy leads to systemic changes in the host in the form of improved CMI responses, better killing of mycobacteria, clearance of organisms, granuloma clearance and related pathology, and ultimately the clinical recovery. However, the major limitations of IL-2 and IFN-γ are that the effects are seen locally at the site of injection and last for a limited period, whereas the effect of the related mycobacteria is longer lasting, systemic, i.e. is observed throughout the body, besides the local area of inoculation.

CONCLUSION

Most of the studies cited above were undertaken when the profile of the disease was different than that seen presently, and several highly bacillated patients were reporting and were also being detected in field conditions. The treatment was for longer duration and several patients were reporting with reactions. The disease profile has since changed, more smear negative cases are detected and FDT is now used for treating patients. However, leprosy reactions continue to occur, before, during and after stoppage of therapy and are a cause of concern for the resulting continued morbidity. Understanding the beneficial effects of use of immunotherapy with chemotherapy will help in reducing reactions, faster granuloma clearance and may help in further reducing the duration of treatment by helping in both killing of viable bacilli and clearing of dead bacilli from the host. Despite available effective MDT, persisting viable organisms as well as persisting clinical activity are significant problems in a section of leprosy patients.[72] Immunotherapy is a good option to overcome this problem.[18,37]

The use of single dose of rifampicin for chemoprophylaxis in leprosy should not be recommended at present as most of the studies are with a short follow-up considering the long incubation period of the disease and also does not have a sound theoretical basis. Single dose chemotherapy even for treatment of single lesion leprosy was abandoned after observing high relapse rates with longer follow-up although the initial response to therapy was considered encouraging. Similarly, in cluster, randomized trials in close household contacts of newly diagnosed leprosy, no difference was seen between the placebo and rifampicin groups beyond 2 years.[16] However, as pointed out above, this is too short a period for analyzing the results, and even without a single dose of antileprosy drugs, patients do self-heal and do not manifest the disease throughout the life. The effect of immunoprophylaxis has been studied and observed with long follow-up, are safe

Table 35.2: Systemic effects of immunotherapy as used in leprosy

Agent used	Lepromin conversion			Histological response		Clinical regression of skin lesions	Bacterial killing	Clearance of bacilli	Reduction in reactions	
	Contacts	Indeterminate leprosy	BL leprosy	Upgrading	Granuloma clearance				RR	ENL
BCG[2,10,14, 18.21,27,30,45-46,69]	+	+	+	+	+	Good	+	+	Not reported	Decreased duration and severity
BCG + *killed M. leprae*[10,14, 24,25,27,28]	+	+	+	+	−	Good	Not tested	+	Not reported	±
MIP[11,18,21,22,26, 27,30-34,36-38,70,71]	+	+	+	+	+	Good	+	+	Mild increase, less severity, lesser duration	Decreased duration and severity
ICRC[5,27,30, 41-44]	+	+	+	±	±	Good	Not tested	+	+	−
BCG + *M. vaccae*[12,14, 28,45-46,69]		+	+	+	-	Good	Not tested	+	+	−
IL-2[58,59,63]		+	+	+ (local)	+ (local)	Local only		−		+
IFN-γ[61,62]			+	+ (local)	+ (local)	Local only		−		+

Abbreviations: BL, borderline lepromatous; RR, reversal reaction; ENL, erythema nodosum leprosum; IL-2, interleukin-2; IFN-γ; gamma interferon.

and well-tolerated and are more promising. In addition, they have a protective effect on both leprosy and tuberculosis.

The use of MIP as immunomodulator has been documented by several workers and also importantly in all types of leprosy patients. It is approved for human use and marketed in India. The whole genome of MIP has been mapped and sequenced.[30] Further studies can be planned to identify parts of the genome which impart the immunomodulatory properties to the organism. Immunotherapy combined with chemotherapy is a good and viable option to overcome problems with present day MDT.[37] Agents like BCG and MIP (Immuvac) can be used as they are safe, well tolerated and available commercially.

Although leprosy elimination has been achieved in most countries, eradication probably cannot be achieved by MDT alone.[73,74] The issue of using mass immunization in selected endemic pockets and other situations is also worth considering.[73] Both BCG and MIP have a potential immunoprophylactic role against leprosy and tuberculosis.[3,6,7,18,19,71] Both these agents are safe, well-tolerated and beneficial *in vitro*, *in vivo*, experimental animals, as well as large scale hospital-based and field based studies, with a long follow-up of 10–15 years.[11,37,71] The role of BCG against adult pulmonary tuberculosis was not considered significant in India,[3] although there is some amount of protection imparted against leprosy.[3] MIP has the advantage of being potentially useful against both tuberculosis[71] and leprosy[11,70]

and may be a better option. It merits consideration and in depth investigations, especially with co-occurrence of leprosy with the HIV infection and IRIS manifestations associated with its treatment.

ACKNOWLEDGMENT

The author gratefully acknowledges the contributions of patients of the institutes as well as its field unit for their co-operation, members of the SAC, and scientific and technical staff of the institutes, as well the editors in writing and editing the chapter.

REFERENCES

1. Shepard CC. Vaccination against human leprosy bacillus infections of mice: Protection by BCG given during the incubation period. J Immunol. 1966;96(2):279-83.
2. Fernandez JM. Use of BCG in immunoprophylaxis of leprosy. Rev Arg Dermatol. 1939;23:435.
4. Bagashawe A, Scot GC, Russel DA, et al. BCG vaccination in leprosy: final results of the trial in Karinaul, Pappua New Guinea, 1963-79. Bull World Health Organ. 1989;67(4):389-99.
5. Kartikeyan S, Chaturvedi RM, Deo MG. Anti-leprosy vaccines: current status and future prospects. J Post Grad Med. 1991;37(4):198-204.
6. Mulyil JP, Nelson KE, Diamond EL. Effect of BCG on the effect of leprosy in endemic area: a case control study. Int J Lepr. 1991;59(2):229-36.

7. Convit J, Smith PG, Zuniga M, et al. BCG vaccination protects against leprosy in Venezuela: a case control study. Int J Lepr Other Mycobact Dis. 1993;61(2):185-91.

8. Gupte MD, Vallishayee RS, Ananathramanan DS, et al. Comparative leprosy vaccine trial in south India. Indian J Lepr. 1998;70(4):369-87.

9. Setia MS, Steinmaus C, Ho CS, et al. The role of BCG in prevention of leprosy: a meta-analysis. Lancet Infect Dis. 2006;6(3):162-70.

10. Convit J, Pinnardi ME, Rodriguez OC, et al. Elimination of Mycobacterium leprae by other mycobacteria. Clin Exp Immunol. 1974;17(2):821-6.

11. Sharma P, Mukherjee R, Talwar P, et al. Immunoprophylactic effects of anti-leprosy vaccine in household contacts of leprosy patients: clinical field trials with a follow-up of 8-10 years. Lepr Rev. 2005;76(2):127-43.

12. Stanford JL, Stanford CA, Ghazi Saudi K, et al. Vaccination and skin test studies on children of leprosy patients. Int J Lepr Other Mycobact Dis. 1989;57(1):38-44.

13. Ghazi Saudi K, Stanford JL, Stanford CA, et al. Vaccination and skin test studies in children living in villages of different endemicity of leprosy and tuberculosis. Int J Lepr. 1989;57(1):45-53.

14. Ganapati R, Revankar CR, Lockwood DN, et al. A study of three potential vaccines of leprosy in Bombay. Int J Lepr. 1989;57:33-7.

15. Bakker MI, Hatta M, Kwenang A, et al. Prevention of leprosy using rifampicin as chemoprophylaxis. Am J Trop Med Hyg. 2005;72(4);443-8.

16. Oskam L, Bakker MI. Report of the workshop on use of chemoprophlaxis in the control of leprosy held in Amsterdam, The Netherlands on December 14 2006. Lepr Rev. 2007;78(2):173-85.

17. Moet FJ, Pahan D, Oskam L, et al. Effectiveness of single dose of rifampicin in preventing leprosy in close contacts of patients with newly diagnosed leprosy, cluster randomized controlled trial. BMJ. 2008;336(7647):761-4.

18. Katoch K. Immunotherapy of leprosy. Indian J Lepr. 1996;68(4):349-61.

19. Katoch K, Natrajan M, Narayan RB, et al. Immunotherapy of treated BL/LL cases with BCG: histological, immunohistological and bacteriological assessment Acta Leprol. 1989;7(Suppl 1): 153-5.

20. Katoch K, Katoch VM, Natrajan M, et al Treatment of bacilliferous BL/LL cases with combined chemotherapy and immunotherapy. Int J Lepr Other Mycobact Dis. 1995;63(2):202–12.

21. Natrajan M, Katoch K, Bagga AK, et al. Histological changes with combined chemotherapy and immunotherapy in highly bacillated lepromatous leprosy. Acta Leprol. 1992;8(2):79-86.

22. Narang T, Kaur I, Kumar B, et al. Comparative evaluation of immunotherapeutic efficacy of BCG and Mw vaccines in patients of borderline lepromatous and lepromatous leprosy. Int J lepr Other Mycobact Dis. 2005;73(2):105-14.

23. Shepard CC, Van Landinghaun R, Walker LL. Searches among mycobacterial cultures for antileprosy vaccines. Infect Immun. 1980;29(3):1034-9.

24. Convit J, Aranzau N, Ulrich M, et al. Immunotherapy with a mixture of Mycobacterium leprae and BCG in different forms of leprosy and Mitsuda negative contacts. Int J Lepr Other Mycobact Dis. 1982;50(4):415-24.

25. Meyers W, McDougall AC, Fleury RN, et al. Histological responses in sixty multibacillary patients inoculated with autoclaved Mycobacterium leprae and live BCG. Int J Lepr Other Mycobact Dis. 1988;56(2):302-9.

26. Samuel NM, Neopani K, Louden J, et al. Vaccination of leprosy patients and healthy contacts. Indian J Lepr. 1985;57(2):288-96.

27. Mustafa AS, Talwar GP. Five cultivable mycobacterial strains giving blast formation and leukocyte migration inhibition of leukocyte analogous to Mycobacterium leprae. Lepr India. 1978;50(4):498-508.

28. Govil DC, Bhutani LK. Delayed hypersensitive skin reaction to leprosin and antigens prepared from other mycobacteria. Lepr India. 1978:50(4):550-4.

29. Talwar GP, Zaheer SA, Mukherjee R, et al. Immunotherapeutic effect of vaccine based on saprophytic cultivable Mycobacterium w in multibacillary patients. Vaccine. 1990;8(2):121-39.

30. Ahmed N, Saini V, Raghuvanshi S, et al. Molecular analysis of a leprosy immunotherapeutic bacillus provides insights into Mycobacterium evolution. PLoS One. 2007;2(10):e968.

31. Chaudhari S, Fotedar A, Talwar GP. Lepromin conversion in repeatedly lepromin negative BL/LL patients after immunization with autoclaved Mycobacterium w. Int J Lepr Other Mycobact Dis. 1983;51(2):159-68.

32. Kar HK, Sharma AK, Mishra RS, et al. Reversal reaction in multibacillary leprosy patients following MDT with and without immunotherapy with candidate anti leprosy vaccine, Mycobacterium w. Lepr Rev. 1993;64(3):219-26.

33. Zaheer SA, Mukherjee R, Beena HR, et al. Combined multidrug and Mycobacterium w in patients with multibacillary leprosy. J Infect Dis. 1993;167(2):401-10.

34. De Sarkar A, Kaur I, Radotra BD, et al. Impact of combined Mycobacterium w vaccine and 1 year MDT on multibacillary leprosy patients. Int J Lepr Other Mycobact Dis. 2001;69(3):187-94.

35. Kaur I, Dogra S, Kumar B, et al. Combined 12 month WHO/MDT MB regimen and Mycobacterium w vaccine in multibacillary patients: a follow-up of 136 patients. Int J Lepr Other Mycobact Dis. 2002;70(3):174-81.

36. Sharma P, Misra RS, Kar HK, et al. Mycobacterium w vaccine —a useful adjuvant to multidrug therapy in multi bacillary patients; a report in hospital based immunotherapeutic trial with a follow-up of 7-10 years after treatment. Lepr Rev. 2000;71(2):179-92.

37. Katoch K, Katoch VM, Natrajan M, et al. 10-12 years follow-up of highly bacillated BL/LL leprosy patients on combined chemotherapy and immunotherapy. Vaccine. 2004;22:3049-57.

38. Mukherjee A, Zaheer SA, Sharma P, et al. Histological monitoring of a immunotherapeutic trial with Mycobacterium w. Int J Lepr. 1992;60:28-34.

39. Kamal R, Natrajan M, Katoch K, et al. Clinical and histopathological evaluation of the effect of addition of immunotherapy with Mw vaccine to standard chemotherapy in borderline leprosy. Indian J Lepr. 2012;84(4):287-306.

40. Bapat CV, Modak MS, DeSouza NG, et al. Reversal reaction in lepromatous leprosy patients to M. leprae lepromin and to ICRC in antigen from cultivable acid fast bacilli isolated from lepromatous nodules Lepr India. 1977;49(4):472-84.

41. Deo MG, Bapat CV, Chullawalla RG, et al. Potential anti-leprosy vaccine from killed ICRC bacilli—a clinicopathological study. Indian J Med Res. 1981;74:164-77.

42. Deo MG, Bapat CV, Bhalerao V, et al. Anti-leprosy potential of ICRC vaccine: A study in patients and healthy volunteers. Int J Lepr Other Mycobact Dis. 1983;51(4):540-9.

43. Bhakti WS, Chulawala RG, Bapat CV, et al. Reversal reaction in lepromatous leprosy patients induced by a vaccine containing killed ICRC bacilli—a report of 5 cases. Int J Lepr Other Mycobact Dis. 1983;51(4):466-72.

44. Bhakti WS, Chulawala RG. Immunotherapeutic potential of of ICRC vaccine—A case control study. Lepr Rev. 1992;63 (4):358-64.

45. Stanford JL, Rook GA, Bahr GM, et al. Mycobacterium vaccae in the immunoprophylaxis and immunotherapy of leprosy and tuberculosis. Vaccine. 1990;8(6):525-30.

46. Ganapati R, Revankar CR, Lockwood DN, et al. A study of three potential vaccines of leprosy in Bombay. Int J Lepr Other Mycobact Dis. 1989;57(1):33-7.

47. Singh NB, Lowe C, Rees RJ, et al. Vaccination of mice against *M. leprae* infection. Infect Immun. 1989;57:633-655.

48. Singh NB, Srivastava A, Gupta HP, et al. Induction of lepromin positivity in monkeys by a candidate antileprosy vaccine: Mycobacterium habana. Int J Lepr. 1991;59(2):317-20.

49. Sher R, Wade AA, Jaffer M, et al. The in vitro and in vivo effect of levamisole in patients of lepromatous leprosy. Int J Lepr. 1981;59:317-20.

50. Shepard CC, Van Landinghan R, Walker LL. Effect of levamisole in *Mycobacterium leprae* in mice. Infect Immun. 1977;16(2):564-7.

51. Martinez D, Zaias N. Levamisole as an adjunct to dapsone in lepromatous leprosy. Lancet. 1976;2:209.

52. Ramu G, Sengupta U. Preliminary trial of intervention levamisole in persistently bacteriologically positive lepromatous leprosy. Lepr India. 1983;55:64-7.

53. Sharma L, Thalliath GH, Girgia HS, et al. A comparative evaluation of Levimasole in leprosy. Indian J Lepr. 1985;57;11-6.

54. Kar HK, Bhatia VN, Kumar V, et al. Evaluation of levamisole, an immunomodulator, in the treatment of lepromatous leprosy. Indian J Lepr. 1986;58:592-600.

55. Mathur NK, Bumb RK, Mangal HN. Zinc in recurrent erythema nodosum leprosum reaction. Lepr India. 1983;55(3):547-52.

56. Mathur NK, Bumb RK, Mangal HN, et al. Oral zinc as an adjuvant to dapsone in lepromatous leprosy. Int J Lepr. 1984;52 (3):331-8.

57. Hastings RC, Job CK. Reversal reaction in lepromatous leprosy following transfer factor therapy. Am J Trop Med Hyg. 1978;27(5):995-1094.

58. Nathan CF, Kaplan G, Lewis WR, et al. Local and systemic effects of intradermal recombinant interferon gamma in patients with lepromatous leprosy. New Engl J Med. 1986;315(1):6-15.

59. Samuel NM, Grange LM, Samuel S, et al. A study of effect of intradermal administration of gamma interferon in lepromatous leprosy patients. Lepr Rev. 1987;58:389-96.

60. Kaplan G, Mathur NK, Job CK, et al. Effect of multiple interferon gamma injection in the disposal of *Myobacterium leprae*. Proc Natl Acad Sci USA. 1989;86(20):8073-7.

61. Mathur NK, Mittal A, Mathur D, et al. Long term follow-up of lepromatous leprosy patients receiving intralesional gamma interferon. Int J Lepr. 1992;60:98-100.

62. Sivasai KS, Prasad HK, Mishra RS, et al. Effect of recombinant interferon gamma administration on lesional monocytes/macrophages in lepromatous leprosy patients. Int J Lepr. 1993;61:259-69.

63. Kaplan G, Britton WJ, Hancock GE, et al. The systemic influence of recombinant interleukin 2 on the manifestation of lepromatous leprosy. J Exp Med. 1991;173(4):993-1006.

64. Talwar GP. Vaccines against leprosy. Lepr India. 1983;55:525-30.

65. Mahadevan PR, Robinson P. An antigen complex that restores ability of leprosy patients to kill *Mycobacterium leprae*—the probable molecular events identified by in vitro experiments. Trop Med Parasitol. 1990;41(3):310-3.

66. Mahadevan PR, Robinson P, Varmani M, et al. Delipified cell wall component of *M. leprae* and its application. Indian J Lepr. 1991;63:371-87.

67. Gelber RH, Breenar DJ, Hunter SW, et al. Effective vaccination of mice against leprosy disease with sub-unit of *Mycobacterium leprae*. Infect Immun. 1990;58(3):711-8.

68. Gelber RH, Murray L, Sui P, et al. Vaccination of mice with a soluble protein fraction of *M. leprae* provides consistent and long term protection against *M. leprae* infection. Infect Immun. 1992;60(5);1840-4.

69. Ghazi Saudi K, Stanford JL, Stanford CA, et al. Vaccination and skin test studies in children living in villages of different endemicity of leprosy and tuberculosis. Int J Lepr. 1989;57:45-53.

70. Gillis T. Is there a role of vaccine in leprosy control? Lepr Rev. 2007;78:238-42.

71. Jacobson RR, Gati P. Can leprosy be eradicated with chemotherapy? An evaluation of Malta Leprosy Eradication Project. Lepr Rev. 2008;79;410-5.

72. Tuberculosis prevention trial of BCG vaccines in South India for tuberculosis prevention. Indian J Med Res. 1979;70:349-63.

73. Katoch VM, Gupta UD. Vaccines against leprosy. In: SK Sharma, (Ed). Adult Immunization. API Publication; 2009. pp. 116-20.

74. Katoch K, Singh P, Adhikari T, et al. Potential of Mw as a prophylactic vaccine against pulmonary tuberculosis. Vaccine. 2008;26(9):1228-34.

Nursing Care in Leprosy Patients

Vineet Kaur, Gurmohan Singh

CHAPTER OUTLINE

INTRODUCTION

Leprosy is a chronic disease with significant potential for disability from nerve damage and reactional states. The National Leprosy Eradication Programme has undoubtedly achieved success through the use of multidrug therapy (MDT) but with its incorporation into the general health services, some aspects, such as early detection of new cases, identification of lepromatous cases and care of deformities, have perhaps become a greater challenge and put additional strain on the healthcare resources. Healthcare providers at all levels must now strive to continue to be vigilant and look for new cases, help detecting early signs of impending nerve damage and educate patients about prevention and self-care.

Institutional care of leprosy patients is becoming increasingly less common. The care and support should be community based. Poverty, poor hygiene and lack of clean drinking water are some of the challenges that need to be addressed.

There is ample evidence that the emphasis has to now shift from mostly medical management to promoting culturally acceptable health education about leprosy and the stigma surrounding it. The World Health Organization states that India's healthcare system, although among one of the less privatized in the world, leaves lot to be desired in terms of a stronger public health sector to ensure provision of healthcare to the common man. This lack of governmental healthcare provision makes it hard to provide good nursing care which is increasingly becoming an invaluable resource in our battle against leprosy.

Health education is one of the most effective tools against leprosy as a public health problem. Early detection, prompt and regular treatment, prevention of disability and care of deformities/ulcers through self-care are the cornerstones of leprosy management. A qualified nurse with good communication skills, who has the sensitivity to select the most appropriate method of health education, keeping in mind the gender and cultural characteristics of the patient, will be one of the key players. In India, verbal information is more important than written due to high rates of illiteracy. Also, in cases of women, there is a greater need to promote early reporting and treatment without disturbing their domestic roles for any intervention to be sustainable. Quality nursing care not only includes effective health education and patient empowerment, but also teaching patients and their families on improved hygiene at low cost.

NURSING ASSESSMENT OF A LEPROSY PATIENT

Through Interview

Understanding of Diagnosis

The nurse must reiterate that leprosy is a completely treatable disease that is acquired through air borne route and to a smaller extent, by skin to skin contact. It is neither hereditary nor the result of wrath of gods. The disease, however, has the potential to cause deformity in a small percentage of patients.

Understanding of Multidrug Therapy

Once MDT has been instituted, the nurse must emphasize that it is absolutely essential that it should be continued without interruption for the prescribed period. The patient must be instructed to report any perceived side effects immediately. The nurse must also ensure that the patient has understood how the drugs have to be taken.

Understanding of the Course of Disease Including Reactions

After the diagnosis is understood, the nurse must take the opportunity to assess if the patient understands that the disease might go through reactional phases which might seem like worsening of the disease to the patient.

Understanding of Prognosis

The nurse must assess if the patient understands what to expect from treatment. The patient must accept that all of the sensory loss will not be reversed and in some cases deformity will remain.

Communicability Status of Disease

Because of the stigma attached to leprosy, the patient must be assessed for his understanding of the noncommunicability to those in close contact with him, if regular treatment is taken.

Effect on Employment

Once a diagnosis of leprosy is made, the patient might have concerns about whether it will affect his employment for which the nurse must assure him/her that according to the present laws, a diagnosis of leprosy should not jeopardize his/her job.

Lifestyle Changes

On initial assessment, the nurse must ascertain if the patient is aware that a diagnosis of leprosy may warrant some day to day lifestyle changes both at home and at the work place. These may include cycling and not walking to work, using modified utensils in the kitchen, wearing special footwear, etc. The patient should be able to understand that the aim is to prevent disability from setting in and from its worsening.

Family Support

The success of treatment in leprosy depends to a very large extent on the support extended to the patient at home, at the work place and by society at large. The nurse should pick up clues that point towards this while interviewing the patient and not try to elicit answers from direct questioning. This information will help the nurse to involve family members in care of the patient.

Social Rehabilitation

Once a diagnosis of leprosy is made, in some cases, especially in the villages, there might be problems with acceptance of the patient in the community. This can be a major hurdle for some patients in their rehabilitation.[1] The nurse should ascertain if there are any such issues.

Post-assessment Nursing Intervention

- The nurse must explain that MDT is the global standard treatment for leprosy. She must reiterate that the patient must not miss taking medication at any time and that the duration of treatment as prescribed by the doctor is based on type of leprosy [paucibacillary (PB) or multibacillary (MB)].
- The patient must be explained that intake of clofazimine may turn the skin coppery and in lactating mothers can also darken the color of breast milk. Rifampicin causes the urine to be tinged orange is an important fact that must be explained to the patient, since it can cause unnecessary alarm. Rare side effects, like flu like syndrome with rifampicin, jaundice with dapsone/rifampicin and acute renal failure with rifampicin, should all be flagged up.
- The nurse must explain that even after completing the prescribed course of MDT, some anesthesia will remain. MB cases, in particular, must be explained about the possibility of occurrence of reactions while on treatment and the fact that these do not indicate a worsening of the disease. They should be explained how to recognize the signs of reactions and ask the patient to report at the earliest.
- Those with existing deformity must be prognosticated with regard to the extent of likely recovery.
- Pregnant mothers on MDT should be reassured about the safety and the usefulness of continuing MDT. They should be encouraged to breastfeed their newborns as usual.
- Lifestyle changes (e.g. use of special utensils to avoid thermal injury, not being able to sit in front of the community fire in winters, etc.) must be impressed upon by the nurse and their significance explained. This is specially so because patients without paralytic or anesthetic disabilities are unlikely to realize their long-term impact.
- It is important that the patient and the nurse form a close bond of confidence and the patient is able to discuss his or her family problems related to the disease or its management. It is also important for the nurse to involve at least one other family member in the ongoing care of the patient, and to try and solicit the family's support in general.

Through Examination

General Examination of Skin

The nurse should expose the patient's skin in good light and look for the clinical signs of leprosy [hypopigmented macules, infiltrated lesions, lesions of erythema nodosum leprosum (ENL), etc.] for record keeping and follow-up, and also the general condition of the skin, especially dryness.

Examination for Sensory Loss

The areas of sensory loss should be mapped out by the nurse and these should be subsequently used during follow-up visits.

Examination for Motor Functions of the Six Commonly Affected Nerves

Although there are many methods detailed on testing methods for motor functions,[2] the nurse must adopt a quick check approach. The relevance being to be able to identify impending deformity at the earliest:

The motor function of the following nerves which are most commonly affected in leprosy is to be assessed:

- Ulnar nerve
- Radial nerve
- Median nerve
- Common peroneal nerve
- Posterior tibial nerve
- Facial nerve.

To test the first three together, ask the patient to bring all the fingers tips together with the thumb, and then to flex and extend this hand at the wrist. In case of ulnar nerve paralysis, the little and ring finger will lag (Fig. 36.1), in case of median nerve paralysis, there will be inability to join the index finger (Fig. 36.2) and in case of radial nerve paralysis, there will be difficulty in dorsiflexion at the wrist.

To examine the common peroneal nerve, ask the patient to dorsiflex the foot at the ankle. Inability to do this shows nerve paralysis.

For the posterior tibial nerve, a quick test is to ask the patient to fan out his toes (Fig. 36.3), paralysis of this nerve will not allow the patient to do this.

To test the facial nerve, ask the patient to close his eyes, a lid lag (inability to completely close the eye) will be observed.

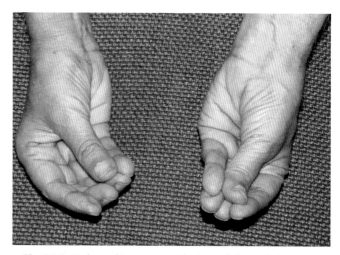

Fig. 36.2: Early median nerve paralysis—inability to bring index finger together with the others in the right hand

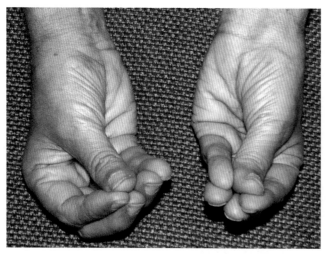

Fig 36.1: Early ulnar nerve paralysis—inability to bring little finger together with the others in the right hand

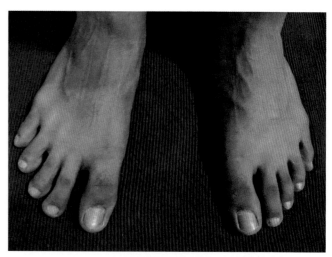

Fig. 36.3: Inability to fan out toes of left foot—early paralysis of posterior tibial nerve

All these quick tests can be carried out by the nurse in a very short time and are a useful tool even during follow-up.

Examination for Deformity

The nurse should document any claw hand, wrist drop, foot drop or lagophthalmos in the patient. Anesthetic deformities resulting in resorption of digits must also be noted.

Impending deformity from a swollen and tender major nerve must be picked up as early as possible.

Examination for Ulcers

The hands and feet are most likely to get ulcerated due to anesthesia. The nurse should examine any ulcer for:
- Location—this will give an idea of the possible cause, e.g. is it at a pressure point? Is it at a point of friction?
- Appearance of the ulcer—this will give an idea of the duration for which it has been present. Longstanding ulcers will be deeper with more hyperkeratotic tissue around it. Infection of the ulcer will indicate the level of care of an ulcer.

ASSESSMENT DURING REPEAT VISITS

Checking Regularity of Multidrug Therapy

The nurse must ask the patient to describe how he is taking medication. Indirect questioning will reveal if rifampicin is being taken (patient will report high colored urine).[3]

Checking for Side Effects

The nurse must ask for any fever, discoloration of urine on days other than when rifampicin is taken (indicating jaundice), loss of appetite, and dryness/cracking of skin from the patient.

Re-examination of Skin, Nerves, Ulcers and Deformity

To be quickly repeated as described in "Examination for Sensory Loss", "Examination for Motor Functions of the Six Commonly Affected Nerves" and "Examination for Deformity".

Checking for Exercises being Performed

As described in "Intervention in Deformity due to Leprosy".

Checking Splints, Footwear and Assistance Aids

As described in "Intervention in Deformity due to Leprosy".

ASSESSMENT OF "RISK" STATUS

The nurse working in leprosy should be able to broadly classify leprosy patients into 'high-risk' and 'low-risk' after initial assessment. This classification is important to be able to prognosticate the patient, as well as flag up issues that might warrant an immediate consultation by a specialist. Also, 'low-risk' patients can be reviewed less frequently as compared to 'high-risk' ones who need to be seen more frequently.

This stratification is broadly based on:
- Age of the patient
- Type of disease (MB vs. PB)
- Nerve/organ involvement
- Past or present reactional status
- Presence/absence of disability and deformity.

Low-Risk

Young patients with PB leprosy having no significant damage to nerves and no reaction/disability can be included in this group. There is a less likelihood of them going into a reactional state in future or developing deformity.

High-Risk

Patients with MB leprosy, having past or present reactions and nerve trunk involvement, are included in this group. Patients with sensory loss on the limbs and eye involvement, as also pregnant women, belong to this high-risk group. They are more likely to develop fresh deformity or worsening of the existing one and so must be followed up closely.

Note: The nurse must reassess the risk status of the patient at every repeat visit because it is not unusual for the risk status of the patient to change.

ASSESSMENT OF ACTIVITIES OF DAILY LIVING

Since nerve involvement, reactional states and disability, all directly or indirectly affect the daily activities of a leprosy patient, it is important that the nurse be able to assess the patient's ability to carry these out on a routine basis.

Nurses can easily be trained to use the Green Pastures Activity Scale (GPAS),[4] which consists of grading, namely:
- Daily activities
- Interpersonal relationship
- Use of assistive devices
  - The daily activities are assessed as:
    - 4-Not difficult
    - 3-A bit difficult
    - 2-Very difficult
    - 1-Impossible

- The interpersonal relationship can be scored as:
  - 4-No problem
  - 3-Some problem
  - 2-More problem
  - 1-No relation
- For the use of assistive devices:
  - 4-Not necessary
  - 3-Not difficult
  - 2-Difficult
  - 1-Very difficult

The scores allotted to each of the three dimensions are then added and used for assessment of activities of daily living.

Nursing Intervention

Such a scoring system done at initial visit, and then at follow-up, can help the nurse pick-up early deformity and steps can be taken to prevent further deterioration. Also, such information is required to optimize the assistive devices being used by the patient. Family support too can be tailored to the daily needs of the patient.

ROLE IN THE CARE OF ANESTHETIC LIMBS

The nurse has a major role to play in helping to care for anesthetic upper and lower limbs.

Anesthetic Upper Limb

Assessing the extent of anesthesia is described in section "Examination for Sensory Loss". This assessment is a prerequisite for advising on the care of such a limb. Once the nurse has established this, she can then proceed to advice on the following:

Nursing Intervention

The success of a nursing intervention is that eventually the patient learns self-care. Various models around the world emphasize transferring this skill to the patient.[5]

Teaching Daily Self-examination

Since insensitive hands do not experience pain and temperature, trauma goes unnoticed. Therefore, the patient has to be taught that in order to identify injury early, he should inspect his hands daily in good light. They must wash their hands with clean water at room temperature and then look for:

- Areas of redness
- Blisters
- Swelling
- Ulcers

Once an injury has been identified, the nurse must reiterate the need to identify how it might have occurred. This is necessary to prevent further injury from the same cause.

Avoidance of Injury

The nurse should train the patient to think about possible injury even before beginning the activity. One of the most common injuries to the anesthetic hands is thermal—in women while cooking and in men in rural areas who sit around fire in cold winter months. The women patients must be demonstrated the use of cotton oven gloves (Fig. 36.4) or, simpler still, a piece of cloth wrapped around utensil handles. The ideal solution is to have long wooden handles for all utensils (Fig. 36.5) and molded handles for deformed hands. They must also be told not to cook chapattis directly on the fire but to use tongs because burns can be caused in this situation.

Men should be instructed to cover up with extra layers of woolens instead of sitting around a fire. Likewise, cigarette smoking is not only harmful to the lungs but can also burn the digits of an unsuspecting hand in leprosy. Those working as manual laborers in many different fields need to protect their hands from trauma by the use of protective bandaging or gloves. Patients must be advised to drink hot tea, etc., in cups with handles or hold the cups with a cloth piece.

Those patients with involvement of the eye must be instructed to always wear protective glasses and use artificial tears.

Teaching Self-care

For those patients who do develop blisters or ulcers, the nurse can teach them basic steps of skin care as below:
- *Cleansing*: The patient should wash their hands with soapy water at room temperature to remove all the dirt

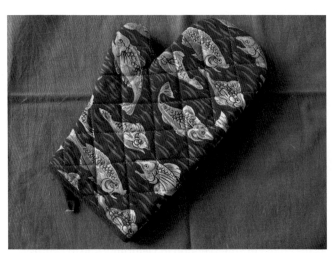

Fig. 36.4: Oven gloves

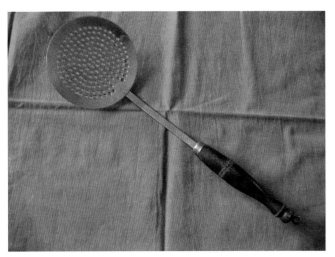

Fig. 36.5: Kitchen implement with wooden handle

and mop them dry. Later, oil/petroleum jelly/any other moisturizer must be applied.

• *Dressing*: Any raw area should be covered with sterile gauze and a clean bandage or cloth. If the wound looks infected (explain signs of infection, i.e. redness, pain, pus discharge, foul smell), an antiseptic ointment should be applied and he should be seen by the treating physician.

• *Care of the bandage*: The patient should be instructed to keep the bandage dry and clean. While engaging in any chores, the hand can be put in a polythene disposable bag. In case the dressing gets wet, it must be changed. Now-a-days self-care kits are available. Use of this kit can be taught by the nurse (described in detail in Ulcer Care Chapter no. 37).

• *Elevation*: In case the hand is swollen, the nurse can show the patient how to elevate it by putting it in a sling.

• *Splinting*: The nurse must emphasize that only rest may not help the ulcer heal. Often splinting is required for this. The patient can be shown how to use materials, such as cardboard, plastic, wood, etc., wrapped in cotton and then a bandage or cloth to be used to support the hand. While explaining the use of a splint, the nurse must ensure that the patient understands that:
  – The edges of the splint must be smooth
  – The bandage used to secure the splint must not be too tight
  – A part of the fingertip and nail must be kept exposed so that any color changes in the digits can be noticed easily.

Nursing Advice on Follow-up Visits

She should check for any raw areas, blisters, ulcers, etc., and whether they are infected. Dressings must be assessed for their correctness. The patient should be asked to bring along any mittens they might be using so that the nurse can see if they are not worn out and are thick enough to protect the hand from heat. Splints should be checked for any sharp edges.

Anesthetic Lower Limb

As in the upper limb, the nurse has a crucial role in helping leprosy patients protecting their feet from development of ulcers, disability and deformity. As compared to the upper limb, the lower limb is more difficult to protect and preserve because of its weight bearing role. In fact, injury occurs most commonly on the plantar aspect of the feet due to walking on bare anesthetic feet. Other causes like injury from heat, walking on rough and uneven surfaces, and friction from ill-fitting footwear are not uncommon.

Nursing Intervention

The nurse has an important role in explaining to the patient, through demonstration, that his feet are anesthetic. The fact that walking on such feet, for what might be normal distances for others, causes blistering and ulceration, must be emphasized. These ulcers heal with scarring, which is a weak point in the foot and can break down again. Repeated ulceration finally causes deformity.

Teaching Daily Self-examination

The nurse must demonstrate soaking the feet in water (soapy, if possible) for 10–15 minutes. The areas between the toes must be cleaned and any foreign bodies like splinters, dust, sand, etc., removed. After this, the patient must examine his feet and look for:
• Cracks/fissures
• New areas of redness or blistering
• Ulcers

Also, the nurse must show the patient how to examine the footwear and look for worn out areas that might be causing friction. Very often the patient does not notice a nail sticking out of the footwear, which may be the cause of repeated trauma and a subsequent ulcer.

Care of Fissures and Callosities

The nurse must explain to the patient that because of anesthesia and decreased sweating the sole becomes thickened at places where there is repeated pressure. This localized area of thickening (callosity) is more prone to cracking and secondary infection. The patient must be shown the five most common sites of callosities:
• Tips of toes (especially if clawed)
• Creases between toes and ball of the foot

- Area under the fifth metatarsal
- Center of the heel
- Margins of the heel.

The aim of treating callosities is to prevent cracks and further infection. To achieve this aim, it is important that the feet are kept supple and soft by:
- Soaking feet in water for 15–20 minutes.
- Using a pumice stone/any rough surface to remove dead friable skin.
- Applying petroleum jelly/urea cream to moist skin.

The nurse should flag up the following points for callosities in special situations:
- Callosities on the lateral malleolus are mainly due to pressure while squatting. This can be avoided by advising the patient to either change his posture or put a thick padding on it while squatting.
- When callosities are present on the top of the feet on the outer margin, they are most often a result of friction with ill-fitting footwear. This can be avoided by using footwear specially designed for that individual's foot deformity.

Care of Ulcers on the Feet

The first requirement for treating ulcers on the feet is to teach the patient to recognize an early ulcer. The patient must be made to understand that the more superficial the ulcer, the faster it will heal. Deeper and infected ulcers may take up to several weeks to months to re-epithelize and are the commonest cause of deformity. The nurse must judge if there is a need for referral to a specialist in a higher center.

The basic principles of care are the same as for the upper limb except that, since the lower limb is weight bearing, a much greater emphasis on rest has to be given. If the ulcer is uncomplicated, the patient may be allowed to carry out daily activities using crutches, but if it is deep, rest in bed, perhaps with limb elevation must be suggested.

Teaching Self-care

Since deformity depends on repeated injury to the limb, it is prudent to explain to the patient that his efforts to look after his lower limb will go a long way in preventing deformity. The patient must carry out the following on a daily basis:
- Soaking feet in water before retiring to bed and then examining them for any blisters or ulcers.
- Applying petroleum jelly to moist feet to prevent cracks and fissures.
- Changing any dirty or wet bandage.
- Regular use of soft footwear.
- Examining footwear for any rough areas that might have developed from constant usage and might be causing friction.

Care on Revisits

A review visit is an opportunity for the nurse to reiterate what she had discussed and taught the patient in the past. These visits must never be hurried, and it should not be presumed that the patient has understood and is carrying out all the instructions given so far.

The following could be a handy check list for the nurse:
- Has the area of sensory loss increased?
- Is there any increase in motor deficit (has the patient developed a foot drop/has the foot drop worsened)?
- Is the patient able to carry out his daily checking routine at bed time?
- Has he developed any new raw areas (blisters/ulcers), if yes, how do they look?
- Does the patient need special footwear?
- Is the footwear fitting correctly?
- Are any assistive aids like crutches required?

INTERVENTION IN DEFORMITY DUE TO LEPROSY

The nurse has to help prevent deformity as well as preventing deformity from worsening.

Deformity in leprosy primarily involves the hands, feet and eyes. They could be a result of the disease itself (saddle nose), result from nerve damage or a consequence of repeated trauma to any anesthetic body part.

The nurse should first briefly explain the cause of the deformity. This initiation will go a long way in the patient understanding how to avoid injury and subsequent damage. For the sake of simplicity, deformities can be divided into paralytic and anesthetic.

Paralytic Deformity

Patients must be explained that because leprosy primarily involves nerves, damage to these nerve trunks causes weakness and sometimes paralysis of the muscles supplied by them. In the upper limb, this results in partial claw hand, complete claw hand and wrist drop. In the lower limb, the most common deformity is foot drop. Lagophthalmos (inability to completely close the eye on blinking) and subsequent exposure keratitis (dry eye) are common deformities encountered in the eye.

Anesthetic Deformity

Loss of sensation of touch, pain and temperature compounded by the loss of sweating can cause the affected area to get damaged. It is important for the nurse to make the patient understand the relevance of this so that he is able to take measures at all times to protect such body parts.

At the same time, the nurse must reiterate that leprosy does not necessarily mean deformity, and that with proper care and prevention these are avoidable.

Deformity of Upper Limb

Since the hand is our connection with the world, being used all the time for picking, touching, feeling, etc., it is the part most likely to be damaged by thermal and other injuries. The need for care is perhaps most important here because the mind has to be retrained to do things differently, that are a reflex.

Nursing Intervention

The nurse must teach the patient to:
- Recognize early signs of paralysis (As described in "Examination for Motor Functions of the Six Commonly Affected Nerves").
- Recognize early areas of impending ulceration.

The patient must remember at all times that the aim is to:
- Prevent ulceration.
- Prevent deformity from getting worse.
- Avoid stiffness of deformed hand.

Once a deformity has been identified, the nurse should take the patient through the care routines that he will then have to follow henceforth.

Massage and Exercises for Hands with Paralytic Deformity

Massage and exercises for the fingers: The nurse must demonstrate to the patient the correct technique for massage. First take some oil and smear it on the fingers (both palmar and dorsal surfaces). The patient should rest the hand on the thigh and gently stroke them with the flat of the opposite hand trying to straighten the fingers without applying too much pressure. This should be repeated twice daily for at least 20 times each.

To exercise the fingers, the patient should keep the hand bent at the knuckles and press the back of the hand against the thigh or a table top (Figs 36.6 and 36.7). Then using the other hand he should attempt to straighten his fingers till the back of the fingers touch the thigh or table top.

Massage and exercises for the thumb: Ask the patient to rest the palm on the edge of the table. Then he should gently but firmly try to pull the thumb to straighten it. Too much force should not be applied while stretching for fear of producing cracks. The nurse must instruct the patient that no massage is to be done if the hand has blisters, raw areas, or is swollen.

The patient should steady the thumb with the opposite hand. Then he should try to lift up the tip of the thumb in order to straighten it.

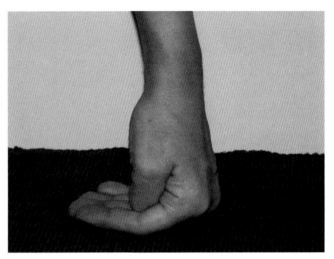

Fig. 36.6: Exercise for fingers

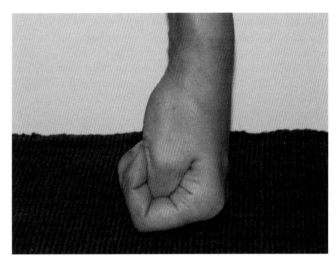

Fig. 36.7: Another exercise for the hand

Taking a soft rubber ball and making a small hole in it to squeeze out the air can be a useful aid for exercising the hand muscles. In addition, there are devices such as foam balls (Fig. 36.8) and hand grips that are available locally at very low costs to help exercise the hand.

Use of Splints for the Hand

In case where paralytic deformity is of recent onset, the nurse must explain to the patient that it can be prevented from getting worse. If it is not yet stiff, splints play a useful role. The nurse must demonstrate the use of splints for passive stretching after taking the patient through the full range of movements of a normal hand. The principle in paralytic deformities is that one set of muscles is not working. So the

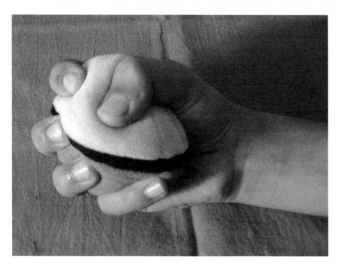

Fig. 36.8: Hand exercise using soft ball

muscles with opposite action overact to create an imbalance, e.g. in a claw hand, the extensors are paralyzed, so the over action of the flexors causes the hand to claw. Other than active stretching through exercises, the nurse must demonstrate the use of splints for passive stretching, especially at night. These have been described in some detail in section under "Teaching Self-care" for upper limb.

Deformity of Lower Limb

Since the feet are weight bearing and used all day for walking, there are more chances of injury than perhaps on other body parts.

Nursing Intervention

As in the upper limb, the nurse must teach the patient for early paralytic deformity or anesthetic injury. A simple check list can be discussed with the patient to be used both by the patient and the nurse, as given below:
- Check if the toes are bent rather than straight.
- Check if the tips of the toes rather than the pads are making contact with the ground.
- Whether the heel and the ball of the big toe are in contact with the ground.
- Check if fanning of the toes is possible.
- The patient has a "foot drop" gait rather than a normal heel-to-toe gait. Here the patient has to lift the leg high in order to clear the ground.
- To look for any breaks in the skin, blisters or ulcers on the sole or dorsum.
- Ask the patient to lift his toes and then his heels. Inability to do so or to sustain it for more than 30 seconds signifies muscle weakness.

The nurse must emphasize that deformities like foot drop and weakness of any muscle cause an uneven transmission of load in the foot leading to further friction and ulceration. This information will help elicit cooperation from the patient in caring for the foot, recognizing early paralysis and helping to prevent further deformity.

Care of Anesthetic Foot

This has been dealt with in detail in section "Anesthetic Lower Limb".

Care of Foot Drop

Once early weakness is picked up, the nurse must refer the patient to the doctor for institution of therapy in addition to MDT. The nurse must explain to the patient in detail the side effects to watch for while on corticosteroids and also detail the precautions to be taken. She must monitor if the patient is taking the prescribed additional drugs, doing exercises and using splints, etc., as advised. The nurse will have to teach the patient the following:

Splinting of knee: When there is acute neuritis of the common peroneal nerve and foot drop, the knee and ankle must be splinted to prevent repeated bending. This will allow rest to the inflamed nerve and result in quicker healing. A splint can easily be made at home by taking a stiff board. This should be well padded with a lump of extra padding in the middle and at the lower end (these parts will sit behind the knee and the ankle). Bandage this splint to the leg at the knee (Fig. 36.9). Even at night when the patient is in bed, the dropped foot should be supported. Again a simple homemade splint, as shown, can be used (Fig. 36.10).

Stretching the calf muscles: Whenever there is a foot drop, normal stretching of the calf muscles as it occurs during

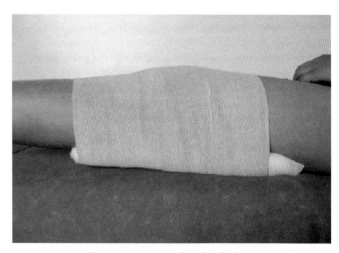

Fig. 36.9: Homemade splint for knee

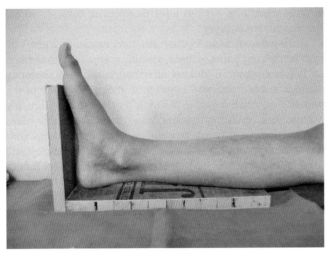

Fig. 36.10: Night time splint for foot drop

walking on heel-toes does not occur. This leads to development of contracture and the patient lands up permanently walking on the toes, which get damaged from over use. In order to prevent this, the nurse must demonstrate to the patient simple calf stretching exercises.

Ask the patient to stand straight in front of a wall, keeping the feet about one foot away. Without lifting the toes or bending the knees, he should lean forward supporting his body with his palms against the wall. He should stay like this for 10 seconds and repeat this about ten times.

Foot supporting devices: These devices help to support the dropped foot and prevent it from falling when the patient walks. In addition, equal weight distribution to the sole can be ensured. Most of these devices work on a simple principle—an above ankle strap has a spring or an elastic band, the other end of which is attached to the sandal or the shoes at the point of the third/fourth toe. Each time a step is taken, it pulls the front of the foot up and on setting the foot down does not allow it to fall. Thus the high stepping gait can be abolished. The nurse can show the patient the use of such a device and also suggest a place where one can be obtained or ordered.

Use of Protective Footwear

Once there is a deformity, whether anesthetic or paralytic, the nurse needs to reiterate the need for protection of such a foot at every follow-up visit. There is now sufficient evidence that regular use of protective footwear and foot orthoses can help plantar ulcers heal faster.[4]

The nurse has to make the patient understand the vulnerability of his feet. This alone will ensure that he complies with the special footwear that will be needed.

There is a wide variety of specialized footwear options available for the patient; however, the nurse must ascertain the most suitable option for each individual case.[6]

Wearing shoes with soft upper and insoles but a hard sole are necessary. Although a variety of such specialized shoes made from microcellular rubber are available in some set-ups, there are simpler versions that are readily available at ordinary shoe stores. The simplest thing to suggest is a soft sports shoe. However, if there is significant scarring and deformity, especially molded shoes are essential. Once the patient understands the function of such shoes, he is more likely to comply with their constant use. The nurse must ensure that the patient understands that the protective footwear is to be worn both inside and outside the house.

The challenge is far greater in getting women to comply because of the social taboo in rural areas regarding women wearing shoes. It is better to suggest a protective sandal, since it is more likely to be used. They too must be told to wear footwear at all times, both inside and outside the house. The patient must also be taught to take care of footwear and examine it from time to time for worn out or rough areas.

INTERVENTION FOR CARE OF THE EYES IN LEPROSY

The eyes can get affected in leprosy. Estimates reveal that at first presentation 3.2% of patients have leprosy related blindness.[7] The two most common complications resulting from leprosy are lagophthalmos and exposure keratitis. The nurse can play a crucial part in preventing ocular complications and in preventing the damaged eye from worsening. Her role includes:

- Informing patients considered 'at risk' on the first visit itself to recognize early signs of lagophthalmos (explain to the patient in simple terms that it manifests as inability to close the eye completely on voluntary closure or during sleep).
- Checking for signs of early facial paralysis (inability to screw up eyes tight on affected side and asymmetry on showing teeth) and identifying lagophthalmos through examination at every repeat visit.
- If the patient has already developed lid lag, he should be explained that this can lead to repeated infections and a dry eye.
- Educate the patient regarding an 'acute red eye' (uveitis) that must be reported immediately.
- Educating the patient about the need to use protective glasses at all times and checking for the same at repeat visits.
- Stressing on the need to use of artificial tears at least twice daily.
- Early referral to a specialist in case of need.

ROLE IN THE CARE OF WOMEN WITH LEPROSY

Gender inequalities in health have a significant impact on women's health.[8] Being a woman puts a leprosy patient in double jeopardy. Her status in the family, in society and in special situations, like pregnancy, puts her at higher risk for developing disability, deformity and social stigma. It is important for the nurse to take these aspects into consideration while following up and caring for a woman leprosy patient.

Status in the Family

For most unmarried girls this might not be a big issue, but once the woman is married, her treatment and care depends to a very large extent on her place in the family. Using indirect clues, e.g. the delay in bringing the patient for treatment, the regularity with which she is taking MDT, the state of her hands and feet, if anesthetic, her footwear, etc., the nurse can assess her status. Then using this information the nurse can foresee difficulties she will encounter and be able to find solutions sensitively.

Status in Society

A woman leprosy patient's status in her family directly influences her place in society. Those who have no support at home are ostracized by society and ill-treated by all. Such examples are still common in spite of leprosy having been said to be 'eliminated'. The role of the nurse is to support the patient, educate the family and bring about a change in attitude, and finally influencing the acceptance of such patients by society.

Leprosy and Pregnancy/Lactation

Hormonal changes during pregnancy can cause a variation in the host immunity. The first appearance of disease, its reactivation and relapse in 'cured' patients is most likely to occur in the third trimester. It is well known that both type 1 and type 2 reactions extend into the postpartum and lactation period. If the nurse is aware of these special circumstances, she can look out for any signs of worsening of disease or development of reactions and similarly educate the patient. The fact that MDT has to be continued throughout pregnancy must be reiterated at every follow-up visit. Clofazimine can sometimes be excreted through breast milk and this may alarm the patient. The nurse can allay any fears the mother might have about the effect of leprosy and its treatment on the unborn child or on the breastfed baby.

ROLE IN THE CARE OF INDOOR PATIENTS

Leprosy patients sometimes need hospital admission due to a variety of reasons. These most commonly include reactions, severe neuritis, trophic ulcers and for reconstructive surgery.

During reactions in leprosy, the patient can be quite sick with fever, joint pains, nausea, vomiting, etc. The nurse plays an important role in looking after hydration, cold sponging for high grade fever, and helping to alleviate anxiety of the patient and relatives by explaining that these reactions are not unusual. Splinting to immobilize the affected limb helps to prevent deformity due to neuritis. For those patients with nonhealing ulcers, the nurse helps in the daily cleansing and dressing of the wound, as well as in teaching the patient how to care for a trophic ulcer. Patients who undergo reconstructive surgery need the input of a nurse not just for daily dressings but also for limb elevation and helping the patient to carry out daily bodily functions while a limb is immobilized after surgery. While in the hospital, the nurse has the opportunity to show the patient how important it is to protect limbs from thermal injury even while carrying out daily activities like feeding and drinking tea.

CONCLUSION

In this chapter, an attempt has been made to highlight the invaluable role nurses can play in the eventual outcome of the management of a leprosy patient. In some settings they might be the only healthcare professionals available for advice to a leprosy patient and so their role must not be underestimated. The combined efforts of all the members of the team can ensure that some day we will live in a leprosy free world.

REFERENCES

1. Scott J. The psychological needs of leprosy patients. Lepr Rev. 2000;71(4):486-91.
2. Brandsma JW, Schreuders TA. Sensible manual muscle strength testing to evaluate and monitor strength of intrinsic muscles of the hand: a commentary. J Hand Ther. 2001;14(4):273-8.
3. Harries AD, Chilemba PE, Greya D, et al. Monitoring rifampicin compliance by visual inspection of urine color. Trop Doct. 1999;29(4):243-4.
4. Chitra W. Impairment of activities of daily living among leprosy patients. Indian J Comm Med. 2006;31:4-6.
5. Benbow C, Tamiru T. The experience of self-care groups with people affected by leprosy. Lepr Rev. 2001;72(3):311-21.
6. Saunderson PR, Seboka G. Protective footwear for leprosy patients with sole sensory loss or ulceration of foot. Lepr Rev. 1995;66(3):257.
7. Ffytche TJ. The prevalence of disabling ocular complications of leprosy: a global study. Indian J Lepr. 1998;70:49-59.
8. Le Grand A. Women and leprosy: a review. Lepr Rev. 1997;68(3):203-11.

37

CHAPTER

Deformities of Face, Hands, Feet and Ulcers and their Management

Atul Shah, Neela Shah

INTRODUCTION

The word leprosy is derived from the Greek word "lepros" which means "scaly". The Indian word "kushtha" is derived from Sanskrit word "kushnati" which means eating away. The abhorrent images often seen in the pictures and depictions about leprosy-affected individuals with eaten away fingers and toes are no longer a trend of the disease. The incurability, transmission to other individuals because of nonavailability of the effective treatment, is also a chapter bygone. However, we cannot ignore the fact that amongst us, we have more than a million individuals with leprosy related deformities and disabilities living in homes and colonies surrounding us.

Leprosy bacilli, discovered by GA Hansen in 1873, are pleomorphic, slightly curved, rod shaped, Gram-positive organisms seen in the slit-skin smear, lying singly or in clumps, in cases of borderline to lepromatous leprosy, often called multibacillary (MB) leprosy. It is this spectrum of the disease, which over a period tends to exhibit greater disabilities. The other part of the spectrum, borderline to tuberculoid leprosy, called (PB) leprosy, has up to five patches on the body including peripheral nerve involvement, and may show evidence of deformity associated with the affected nerve trunk. The development of different clinical types from the indeterminate leprosy to the whole spectrum depends on susceptibility and resistance of the individual. Greater the immunity, better are the chances of the disease tending towards tuberculoid type manifestations. Pure neuritic (without any identifiable skin lesions) type of leprosy is mostly seen in the Indian subcontinent. Any type of leprosy which shows bacilli on laboratory examination is considered as MB disease.

CLINICAL MANIFESTATIONS

Leprosy affects skin as well as nerves. Deformities due to skin infiltration are more obvious on the face with resultant sagging of skin, wrinkled skin appearance, enlarged ear lobules, loss of eyebrows, etc. Mucosa of the nose is also affected in some cases leading to depressed or saddle nose.

The effect on nerves may be limited to cutaneous nerve thickening in line with a cutaneous patch or may extend to peripheral nerve trunk with or without palpable thickening in its course. In majority of the cases, presenting with disabilities like claw hand, the enlarged (thickened) nerve with corresponding loss of sensation in the skin clinches the diagnosis of leprosy. Sometimes, skin smears are required for making a diagnosis or judging the improvement in the status while on MDT. The demonstration of *Mycobacterium leprae* in skin smears is one of the cardinal signs for the diagnosis of the disease.

Episodes of Reactions

An acute episode of sudden inflammation during the chronic course of disease is defined as 'reaction'. There are two types of reactions: the "reversal reaction (RR)" and "erythema nodosum leprosum (ENL)". The former occurs on account of enhanced cell-mediated immunity whereby a skin patch becomes pinkish and inflamed while the affected nerves become painful and tender causing onset of loss of sensation or weakness in motor power. In the ENL reaction (considered as immune complex mediated), the typical inflammatory nodular eruptions, which may even ulcerate, and constitutional symptoms like fever, joint pain, malaise,

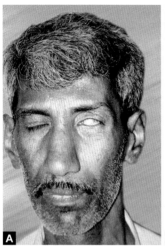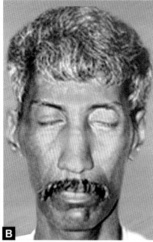

Figs 37.1A and B: Recovery in lagophthalmos
with steroid therapy

etc. may be seen. When any of these reactions involve nerves, they are classified as "severe" on account of their propensity to cause functional impairment in nerves and deformities.

Next to inflamed skin lesions, acute neuritis is the most common manifestation of a reaction in leprosy. Early identification of reactional episodes, particularly in the field areas, and early recognition of nerve damage help tremendously to prevent the development of deformities or to bring about the sensorimotor recovery with prednisolone therapy. World Health Organization (WHO) recommended prednisolone therapy for management of reactions is considered safe for use in the field. Figures 37.1A and B show recovery in a case of lagophthalmos following this regimen. It is well accepted that effective management of the reactions can bring down the occurrence of disabilities to a great extent. Not all cases tend to exhibit signs of reactions. There is also an entity called as "silent neuritis" or "quiet nerve palsy" wherein some cases develop deformity gradually without pain or sign of tenderness, despite the fact that nerve damage continues to occur.

DISABILITIES AND DEFORMITIES IN LEPROSY: TERMINOLOGY

Development of a hypopigmented patch, associated with loss of sensations, is considered essential for making a diagnosis of leprosy. Often the terms anesthetic patches or anesthetic extremities are used to describe decreased sensations in the affected areas. The term *anesthesia* denotes the complete loss of sensations while the term *hypoesthesia* denotes impairment of sensations like touch, temperature and pain. Clinically, it is established that at first, the temperature sensation is affected followed by touch and pain. Thus, early recognition often depends on testing with hot and cold test

tubes. However, since this technique is not feasible in the field, loss of sensations to touch is tested by a ballpoint pen and/or cotton wool and pinprick as a routine.

The term *impairment* is a term denoting the loss or abnormality of the anatomical/physiological structure or function. Van Brakel and associates have popularized nerve function impairment (NFI) assessment to draw attention towards disability prevention.

It is classified as:
- *Primary impairment:* Changes in the structures and functions of the body tissues directly due to disease process like damage to the nerve, e.g.:
  - Anesthesia of area supplied by the affected nerve
  - Impairment of motor function
  - Impairment of autonomic function
- *Secondary impairment:* Changes in the structures and function of the body parts due to neglect, excessive use, careless and improper care of parts with primary impairment, e.g.:
  - *Insensitive hand or foot:* Development of cracks, ulcer, septic hand/foot, shortening of fingers/toes, even mutilation of hands or feet and disorganization of foot or wrist.
  - *Weak/paralyzed parts:* Joint stiffness or formation of contractures.

The most common term *deformity* is defined as the visible alteration in the form, shape or appearance of body due to impairment produced by the disease. It occurs due to infiltration of the tissue by the bacteria or damage to the peripheral nerve trunk by invasion of bacteria. Anesthesia of the sole is not deformity, but presence of ulcer/loss of eyebrows/claw hand or foot are deformities.

Disability, on the other hand, is the lack of ability to perform an activity considered normal for a human being of the same age, gender and culture. This includes any impairment, activity limitation or participation restriction that affects a person. Thus, in leprosy, slipping of pen or objects from the hands constitutes a disability even without an apparent deformity. It is due to the deformity and precisely the disability that a person is not able to play the role of a normal individual and becomes handicapped. For example, he cannot earn his living or cannot perform activities of daily living as a result of the handicap caused due to leprosy.

People working in the field of leprosy often use the term "POD" which means "prevention of disabilities". Any activity, which is directed at the prevention of either primary or secondary disabilities, is included under this term. Some people suggest more specific terms like *POWD*, which means "prevention of worsening of disabilities". Technically, in certain cases, it refers to activities at the field level, more accurately in cases that may deteriorate unless cared for. The health services often use the term "deformity care program" or "disability care program", whereby patients are examined to provide disability care services. These are colloquial terms

Table 37.1: World Health Organization's grading of disabilities in leprosy

Grade	Hands and feet	Eyes
Grade 0	No disability found	No disability found
Grade 1	Nonvisible damage (Loss of sensation)	No grade 1 for eye
Grade 2	Visible damage (Disability, wounds (ulcers), deformity due to muscle weakness, (such as foot drop, claw hand, loss or partial resorption of fingers/toes, etc.)	Inability to close, obvious redness, visual impairment, blindness

often used as synonyms and, in general, include activities related to caring of the leprosy disabled persons. These programs are aimed at prevention, correction and care of various disabilities witnessed in a leprosy-affected person with various aids and appliances, as well as selection for referral for reconstructive surgery (RCS). In the holistic approach, is also included socioeconomic rehabilitation of the leprosy-disabled person.

Recently, the Government of India has rechristened the prevention of disability (POD) as "DPMR", which means "Disability Prevention and Medical Rehabilitation". It includes all activities aimed at prevention and care for disabilities, RCS for leprosy related deformities and other rehabilitation measures.

In their sixth report, WHO Expert Committee on Leprosy recommended that "prevention and management of impairments and disabilities", which have long been recognized as essential components of leprosy control programs, should be implemented effectively. The best way to prevent disabilities (Table 37.1) is through early detection of patients and their treatment with multidrug therapy (MDT), which is provided free of charge to patients throughout the world. Hence, it should not be difficult to bring down the disability rate in the population if this effort continues. Van Brakel has worked extensively on grading of impairment in leprosy and the eye, hand and foot (EHF) score. He advocates its use to assess the patient's condition after any service, which can be reported as stable, improved or worse.

NERVE INVOLVEMENT

Involvement of nerves produces loss of sweating, loss of sensations and loss of motor power in its territory just distal to the site of affection. Palpation reveals the enlargement of the nerve and that clinical examination of sensory and motor loss is charted in order to judge its recovery or downgrading.

Clinical examination of nerves starts from the greater auricular nerve in the neck, which shows thickening in cases of facial patches. One must remember that the greater auricular nerve is visibly enlarged in some normal individuals: laborers, sports persons, etc. but in such cases, the enlargement is usually bilateral. Unilateral thickening invariably points towards diagnosis of leprosy. It is followed by examination of radial cutaneous nerve at wrist. The ulnar nerve is affected just proximal to the elbow and is easily palpable behind the medial epicondyle. Enlargement is just above the medial epicondyle and often continues as a fusiform segment higher up in tuberculoid leprosy cases, and as general thickening in lepromatous type. Median nerve is affected just above the wrist but is difficult to palpate unless grossly enlarged. In some cases, tenderness on pressing firmly at the proximal wrist crease can be elicited. In case of the radial nerve, the main trunk is affected in very few cases and when affected it can be rolled as thickened cord in the humeral groove, in the arm. In the legs and feet, the thickening of any superficial nerve is generally diagnostic and confirmatory for leprosy. Sural nerve can be palpated on the back of the leg, running along the lower portion of tendo-Achilles. Its thickening almost confirms the diagnosis. The lateral popliteal nerve at the neck of the fibula when affected can be palpated extending proximally towards popliteal fossa in its course. The posterior tibial nerve is palpated just behind the medial malleolus and is occasionally found painful even in normal individuals on exertion of deep pressure. Unless the enlargement of any affected nerve is unilateral and associated with anesthesia or deformity, it should not be considered as the sole criteria for diagnosis. The electromyography and nerve conduction velocity when available can serve as a tool in aiding the diagnosis of the disease in difficult cases.

Surgery on Nerves

The common indications for surgery on nerves are obtaining a biopsy of a funicle for establishing diagnosis in certain cases, e.g., pure neuritic leprosy, or to evacuate a nerve abscess to get back the sensory and motor recovery through tunnel decompression. External entrapment is relieved by deroofing of the nerve tunnel while the internal entrapment can be released by hemicircumferential epineurotomy.

Ideally, as a base for the diagnosis, especially in pure neuritic leprosy, biopsy of an affected nerve is required to be done. However, one cannot take the biopsy from the proximal nerve trunk due to fear of causing damage where none may exist. Therefore, superficial nerves are considered for biopsy, among which radial cutaneous or its index branches and sural nerves are preferred. Electron microscopy can reveal the neural affection even in clinically uninvolved nerves.

TESTING FOR NERVE DAMAGE

Frequent signs and symptoms of gradually progressive nerve damage are tingling and numbness, altered sensibility towards touch, temperature and pain sensations, and muscular weaknesses which are noticed ultimately in the form of deformities.

Sensory Testing

There are many different techniques to test the loss of sensations in the hands and feet, however, a quick method is to test the area supplied by the nerve with a ballpoint pen or pinprick. Figures 37.2A and B show the points on the hand and foot for quick testing. In the detailed testing technique utilized by physiotherapists, many points in the palm have to be tested and results are to be noted down for future comparisons. For the ulnar nerve, the little finger and for the median nerve the index finger is tested respectively as they generally do not have any overlapping sensory supply by the adjacent nerve. Lateral popliteal nerve supplies a minor area of the first web space and hence, generally does not require testing. For the posterior tibial nerve, loss of sensations occurs in the sole of the foot. The areas to be tested include first and fifth toe until metatarsal head and heel in the center. It is necessary to remember that instep area and lateral side of the foot have sensory overlap, hence, one need to be careful in deriving inferences.

Motor Testing

Deformities arise due to loss of power in certain muscles supplied by the affected nerve. Unopposed action of the normal muscles of the opposite group (extensors in case of flexor paresis) produces instability at the joints giving rise to characteristic deformities like claw hand.

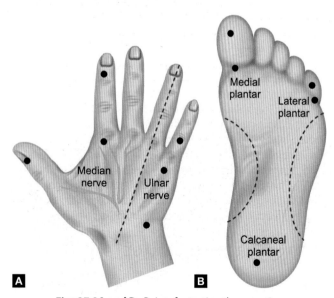

Figs 37.2A and B: Points for testing the sensation in hand and foot

A Quick Test to Assess Motor Damage in Hands

The person should be asked to make a five finger pinch in the wrist-extended position with metacarpophalangeal (MP) joints in flexion and interphalangeal joints in extension, as shown in Figure 37.3A (called as "Beak Test"; after the shape attained by hand, looking similar to that of beak and the extended neck of a bird). If he is able to maintain this position for about 30 seconds, there is no motor damage to the hand (after Fritschi).

For the ulnar nerve, a simple test is to teach a patient to spread the fingers and apply pressure with one little finger to the other little finger. The weak one will give way and turn towards the ring finger (Fig. 37.3B). For the median nerve, the affection of the thumb is tested by asking the patient to raise the thumb. The weakness will be evident when compared with the normal thumb (Fig. 37.4A) and show the method of testing and the weakness of little finger and the thumb (Fig. 37.4B). In radial nerve affection there is a weakness in raising the wrist.

In the lower extremity, if lateral popliteal nerve affection is present, the foot cannot be raised from the ankle (foot drop). If a patient is explained properly, he can test the weakness himself by keeping both feet on the table (or ground) and the foot which is weak, will be seen to be lagging behind while actively taking the ankle upwards. Figure 37.5A shows the weakness on the right side, which is lagging behind in dorsiflexion. Patient will also notice a slight limp while walking.

In facial nerve affection resulting in lagophthalmos, the weakness in closure of the eye is evident and the globe of the eye remains visible while attempting to close the eye. However, the patient is unlikely to realize the same, as he cannot see when his eyes are closed. What he generally feels is heaviness and somebody else points out to him that his eyelids do not seem to close. Figure 37.5B shows early weakness in eye closure on left side with sclera visible on the medial aspect. The weakness can be tested with the examiner's hands trying to lift the eyelid and comparing it with the opposite side. One may also observe the uneven blinks. In the lower facial palsy, which is quite uncommon nowadays and affects the mouth, the patient will notice that there is a change in his facial appearance, and it can be confirmed by asking him to show his teeth and observing that the affected side does not move properly. For all cases, a proper disability record of nerve function assessment is mandatory and Jean Watson gives a detailed format, while Brandsma offers an excellent review on monitoring the nerve function. As he mentions, not all muscles innervated by the nerve at risk need to be tested and that many muscles cannot be tested in isolation.

Deformities in Leprosy

Deformities in leprosy arise due to tissue infiltration and nerve damage. Loss of eyebrows, depressed nose and wrinkled skin

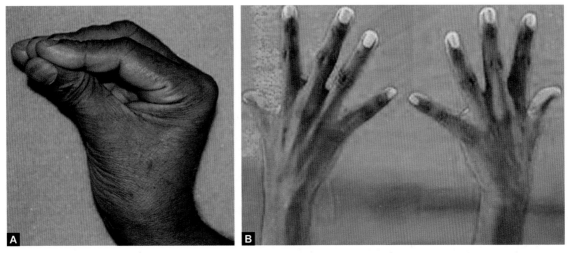

Figs 37.3A and B: (A) The Beak Test; (B) Testing for weakness in little finger and thumb

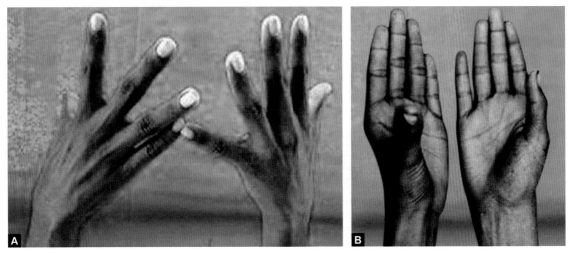

Figs 37.4A and B: Testing for weakness in little finger and thumb can be taught to patient

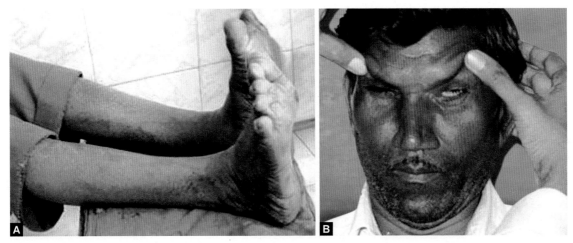

Figs 37.5A and B: (A) In lateral popliteal nerve palsy weakness does not allow foot to be lifted upwards at the level of the ankle, which can be compared with the other side; (B) In facial palsy affecting eyelids, the eye does not close completely and eyelid can be lifted with ease as orbicularis oculi is paralyzed

of the face are deformities due to tissue infiltration. These are commonly seen in lepromatous leprosy. The nerve damage is due to leprous neuritis and reactions which affects peripheral nerves at a particular site, resulting in paralysis, of which the most common example being the claw hand, which is usually chronic and not sudden like in a case who has injury to the nerve.

Primary and Secondary Deformities

A deformity is the visible consequence of impairment. Loss of sensation due to nerve damage is primary impairment (as already described above) and is classified as a grade 1 disability. Claw hand is also a primary impairment and is called as claw hand deformity due to it being a visible consequence, and hence, it is classified as a grade 2 disability. Secondary impairment/deformities are joint stiffness and volar skin contractures in the hands, and ulcers due to anesthesia, injury and neglect of self-care. Absorption and shortening are the examples of secondary impairment/deformities in the hands and feet. In the eyes, corneal ulcers and loss of vision can occur secondary to lagophthalmos. Figures 37.6A to D show various deformities that occur in leprosy.

DEFORMITIES OF HANDS

Claw Hand

Affected ulnar nerve paralyses small muscles of the hands, i.e. intrinsic muscles like interossei and lumbricals. Extensors exert the force and pull MP joints in extension bringing about compensatory flexion at the proximal interphalengeal (PIP) joints. When it affects only ulnar nerve, both the ring and the little finger are involved, and it is called ulnar claw. When both ulnar and median nerves are affected, often the median nerve is involved partially, i.e. thumb is not involved, it is called

ulnar and partial median claw hand or subtotal claw. When all fingers and the thumb are involved causing ape-thumb deformity along with claw of all fingers, it is called ulnar and median claw hand or "total" claw hand.

The fitness of the hand for RCS can be assessed by Bouvier's maneuver. When holding the MP joint in flexion and asking the patient to extend the PIP joints, if he is able to extend completely, the hand is fit for surgery. If PIP joints cannot be extended, it is likely that there is damage to extensor expansion at the PIP level. It may be associated with contracture of volar skin. In such cases, it is necessary to make such hands fit with preoperative exercises and splinting. Other deformities of hands include swan-neck deformity, which is very rare and occurs generally in reactions. Similarly, wrist drop is rare but may occur and needs RCS.

Management of Hand Deformities

A clear understanding of the duration of the disease, neuritis and the deformity is necessary. The best treatment would be to operate on the nerve within 6 months of onset of symptoms of neuritis in order to get better sensory and motor recovery. One must remember that RCS cannot get the sensations back. However, if a patient presents with a mobile claw hand, immediate reconstruction is advisable. This will also prevent the occurrence of secondary deformities.

Dryness of hands due to the involvement of autonomic fibers sometimes exhibits cracks in the palmar skin. The use of oil at home generally takes care of the dryness. Only when the cracks are infected and deep crevices are noticed, that it requires dressings. Other secondary deformities following unprotected use of anesthetic hands are burns and cuts or wounds, which need medical care with dressings. Untreated wounds become deeper with development of osteomyelitis and eventually lead to resorption and/or amputations.

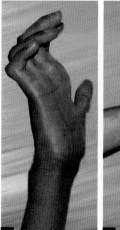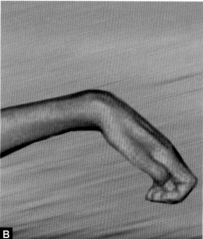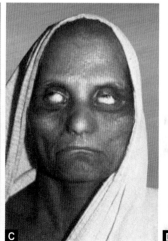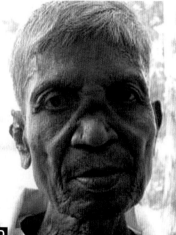

Figs 37.6A to D: Deformities in leprosy: Total clawhand (including thumb paralysis), a case of wrist drop, lagophthalmos and face of a patient showing wrinkling, collapse of nose and loss of eyebrows

Physical Measures

A mobile claw hand is one where there is no stiffness and range of movements is not affected. This type represents a hand that needs RCS at the earliest. However, if such a facility is not available or surgery is deferred to a later date, then exercises are advocated to prevent stiffness. The best exercise is to put all joints through their range of movement several times a day with the help of the normal hand. Specific exercise for clawed fingers is aimed at movement of PIP joint to prevent its stiffness. Patient is taught to hold his clawed fingers with his thumb and index finger in total flexion at MP joint and move PIP joints up and down (flex and extend). Mostly, the patients do not continue the exercise for long. Therefore, it would be advisable to give finger loop splint to carry out exercises. The aim is to prevent secondary complications like stiffness, skin contracture and extensor hood damage (Figs 37.7A to C).

Physiotherapy is very useful in the management of deformities and is essential in both preoperative as well as postoperative care of patients with deformity. RCS requires the patient to use a different muscle in place of the paralyzed muscle. Therefore, the intelligent cooperation of the patient and the active involvement of the physiotherapist trained in leprosy are essential before the surgery is performed.

Splints

Four main types of splints have been used by the authors in the field areas. The health workers deliver these on their routine rounds. These prefabricated lightweight splints have been the mainstay in the management of deformities in leprosy. These are adductor band splint, finger loop splint, opponens loop splint and gutter splint (Figs 37.8A to D).

Splints prevent deterioration and render the hands fit for reconstruction. In early cases of abduction deformity or in splayed fingers before or after reconstruction, an adductor band splint helps to keep fingers together and in case of ulnar claw hand indirectly allows common extensors to act on the paralyzed fingers. In late cases with stiffness, dynamic gutter splints made of elastic materials are very helpful in stretching out the skin contractures and relieve the joint stiffness. Gutter splints are of two types: (i) static splints, those made of rigid materials and (ii) dynamic splints made up of flexible materials. Authors prefer to use elastic materials, like a hosepipe split into half, to make the dynamic gutter splint. On account of its elasticity, it tends to exert antagonistic pressure on the contracture or stiff joint and gradually stretches it out. Another method is to give plaster cylinder to each individual finger. Wax bath may be offered to loosen out the stiff joints wherever available. Finger loop splint not only maintains the lumbrical position but also helps strengthen the small muscles of the hand. Figures 37.9A to C show a patient who recovered from the deformity with corticosteroid therapy and splintage.

Grip-aids

In the advanced deformities of hands, like absorption and amputations, grip-aids may be required for activities of daily living, which minimizes the dependency on others for day-to-day tasks. Epoxy-resin grip-aids (Modulan®) applied on articles of work help patients to hold objects and increase his/her efficiency in the working environment. However, it takes time to make an epoxy resin grip-aid and is not easy to use it in the field area. Recently, Neela Shah demonstrated the quick solution with an instant grip-aid kit for immediate

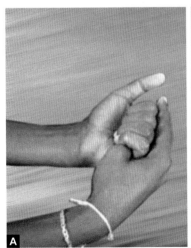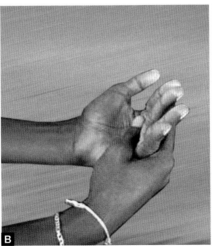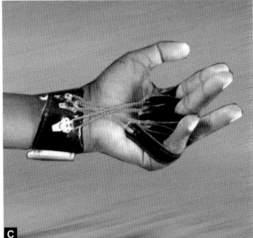

Figs 37.7A to C: A single most important exercise for a clawhand is to hold MP joint and move the PIP joints of the fingers several times in a day. Finger loop splint helps to carry it out with better efficiency

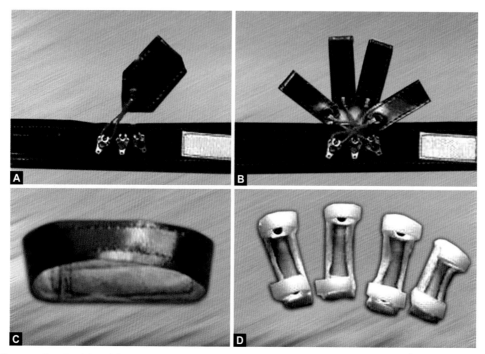

Figs 37.8A to D: (A) Prefabricated opponens loop; (B) Finger loop; (C) Adductor band and (D) Gutter splints
These have been incorporated in the disability care program in the field areas

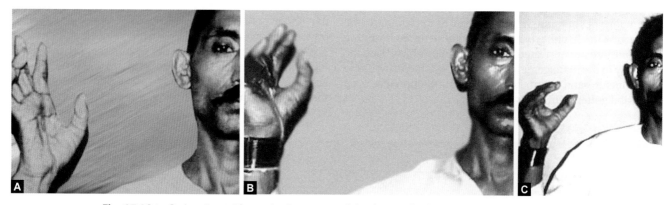

Figs 37.9A to C: A patient with reaction in nerves and developing clawhand was put on corticosteroid
and splints with exercises which resulted in total recovery from deformity

benefit in eating, drinking, combing and other activities of daily living. It has caught the attention of many rehabilitation specialists and has been provided free of cost across India and Africa by Novartis Foundation. Figures 37.10A to C show how it facilitates eating, drinking water and brushing the teeth almost as soon as it is applied.

Reconstructive Surgery

Reconstructive Surgery of the claw hand is a complex subject, and the very fact that there are many procedures described show that there is no uniformity and that no single technique is the best. However, following extensive work on the Zancolli's lasso procedure, lasso as done by many surgeons, is considered simple and effective with minimal rehabilitation requirements. Shah described lasso in 1984–1985. Currently, Shah advises 1:4 lasso for subtotal or total claw (Figs 37.11A to C) and transverse arch correction (TRAC) operation for ulnar claw hand. Malaviya used flexor digitorum superficialis (FDS) of middle or index finger and found good results in nearly 60% cases with FDS middle finger while Shah uses FDS ring finger after checking that flexor digitorum profundus (FDP) is not

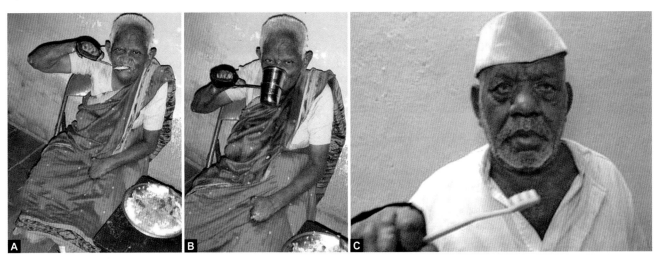

Figs 37.10A to C: Instant grip-aid kit contains rubber Velcro strap to tie it on shortened or amputated stump of the hand, a spoon, a glass, a toothbrush and a comb holder. Patients can do activity of daily living like eating, drinking water or tea, brushing teeth, etc. almost immediately

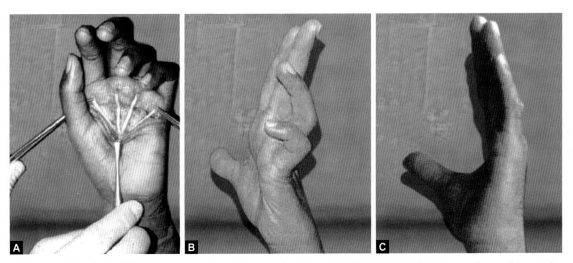

Figs 37.11A to C: Atul Shah's Lasso procedure is done under vision with FDS slip divided into two or four and inserted to itself after forming a loop (Lasso) around A1 pulley. Photographs show clawhand before and after reconstruction

weak. When one does not want to sacrifice the sublimis of any finger, indirect lasso can be done using palmaris longus as a motor muscle. Contraindication for lasso would be PIP joint stiffness. In such cases, it is better to insert the transferred slip into the extensor expansion like original Stiles-Bunnel or Antia's palmaris longus four-finger many tail operation. Palande, however, prefers insertion into the intrinsic muscles, which though slightly difficult, gives good results including correction of transverse arch. In some instances, Brand's *extensor carpi radialis longus* (ECRL) transfer and Fowler's operation are also useful. Ape thumb deformity, i.e. thumb paralysis is corrected by transfer of FDS of the ring finger to the thumb, split into two and inserted at the adductor tendon

by routing over the neck of metacarpal and the other slip into the *extensor pollicis longus* at the distal interphalangeal joint level. Long-term results of opponens plasty have been extensively studied at Schiffelin Institute and correction within 3 years of origin of deformity has been found superior than that performed at a later stage. Swan neck deformity is a rare occurrence. For the wrist drop correction, generally, *pronator teres* is transferred to ECRL and brevis at the forearm, *palmaris longus* is transferred to thumb extensors and FDS of ring finger is transferred for the *extensor digitorum communis*. All reconstructive procedures are followed by proper re-education exercises for maximization of the result and the improvement. In the long-term results studied at

Schiffelin again, long flexor contracture was one of the factors affecting outcome.

For flexion deformities due to forearm pathology in the form of long flexor contracture—shortened musculotendinous units' fascia release in the upper forearm or along with aponeurosis release of long flexors (author's personal technique) could help reduce the deformity and extend the fingers.

Once functional correction of the hand deformities is done, surgery for correction of the esthetic deformity of sunken webspaces can take the form of lipofilling or dermofat graft placement in the sunken webspaces.

DEFORMITIES OF FEET

The common deformities seen in the feet are foot drop and claw toes, besides plantar ulcers. If neglected, these deformities can worsen with time and make a person dehabilitated. Therefore, empowering a person with proper knowledge and supplementing the care with required materials is the only solution for deformity prevention and better foot care.

Foot Drop and Claw Toes

Foot drop occurs when the lateral popliteal nerve, near the knee joint is affected. Patients cannot lift the foot from the ankle in the upward direction and it affects the normal gait. In addition, paralysis of the muscles causes uneven distribution of loads and stresses in the foot. Unsupported or uncorrected foot drop in the long run cripples the patient by contracture of tendo-Achilles and equinus deformity.

Strengthening of weak dorsiflexion is carried out by tying gradually increasing load on the foot and asking the patient to dorsiflex the foot. The tightening effect of strong tendo-Achilles is counteracted by stretching exercises in which a bandage cloth is tied in such a way that the patient himself can dorsiflex the foot by pulling it. Standing on a slope by which the foot is everted outward will nullify the inversion effect of the posterior compartment muscles.

A foot drop splint is provided at the earliest sign of weakness in the leg to support the foot. So far, the common splint used was a spring splint attached to the microcellular rubber (MCR) footwear. The spring action can be offered at ankle or by a splint tied at the knee with an elastic strap. A simple solution has evolved recently with the use of polymers in the form of prefabricated foot ankle arthrosis. The advantage is that it is prefabricated and modified at the time of application and will be useful for a lifetime. If the patient does not want to get operated, the foot drop splint serves as the next best solution. No major complications have been reported in long-term follow-up of 10–30 years conducted at Schieffelin Institute, Vellore, Tamil Nadu, India.

Claw toes generally do not cause any problem to the patient, except sometimes rubbing against the footwear and/or development of ulcers on the tips. They are correctable by RCS with long flexor to extensor transfer. Often following foot-drop surgery, claw toes deformity develops or gets accentuated, therefore, tenotomy of flexors at the time of foot drop correction has been advised.

Plantar Ulcers

Ulcers on the insensitive feet occur due to injuries from outside or burns , neglected and infected cracks and fissures in dry and hard skin (due to loss of sweating). It may be due to body weight itself. While walking, pressure on insensitive feet is normally countered by contraction of intrinsic muscles which elevate the metatarsophalangeal (MTP) joint region upwards and forwards. When posterior tibial nerve is affected this mechanism is not available due to paralysis of small muscles. Moreover, there is sagging at MTP joint resulting in increased pressure at localized areas causing local ischemia, traumatic inflammation and breakdown of subcutaneous fat underneath the MTP joints. If sensation in the foot is normal it is recognized as fatigue and person tends to rest the part providing time to heal; but persons with insensitive skin cannot realize the situation and continue to use the foot causing further damage to the tissue. Area of traumatic inflammation undergoes necrosis and liquefaction resulting in formation of blister. If neglected, covering skin of the blister may break down resulting in formation of ulcer. Therefore, all persons with anesthetic feet are advised regular use of padded or MCR footwear.

The common sites of ulcerations on the sole of the foot are the weight bearing areas like metatarsal heads in the forefoot, followed by heel and lateral border. On examination, the ulcer may be found to have purulent discharge or be dry with unhealthy granulations in the base. The former needs to be treated with systemic and/or local antibiotics, and the latter needs more of the local antiseptic measures to promote healing. On movement of the toes or on pressing the ulcer site, if serosanguineous discharge is seen coming out, it can be said to be a deeper ulcer affecting probably the joint space. True plantar ulcer is also called trophic ulcer as it is devoid of proper nutrition. It has a typical punched out margin, which is thickened as a result of the body's protective response to further weight bearing and continued walking on the painless foot.

Management

If ulcer is present, rest is essential. All simple ulcers will heal, if given sufficient rest. The decision on what advice and reference is to be given depends on some simple criteria. The first and foremost is the depth of the involvement. Deep ulcers are less likely to respond to conservative treatment and will need scraping (pairing) or scooping surgically, followed by dressing and in a case of nonhealing ulcer, skin replacement with graft or flaps will be required. However, majority of cases need only self-care at home.

Author's work over a decade in obtaining healing with self-care kit has been well recognized and adopted by the government and nongovernment organizations making their own self-care kits. A typical self-care kit contains scraper to scrape gently the thick margin of the ulcer, an antiseptic cream, an antiseptic solution to pour into water at the time of soaking the feet, sterile gauze pieces to cover the ulcer after ointment application, a bottle of Vaseline, or any oil or cream, which is used to hydrate the skin or retain hydration in the skin, and bandage with scissors and sticking plaster.

A typical session of empowerment of patients in the rural area is carried out as group therapy with instructions and demonstrations on every step. Self-care groups have been started in some communities. A number of people with self-care needs meet together to discuss the practicalities of self-care. These groups are often surprisingly supportive and can be very motivating for the members. In addition, these groups also advice on how to care for feet even without a kit, replacing with the home made materials when materials in self-care kit are over. On the other hand, Hugh Cross advises reliance more on the self-care with available materials at home and teaching patients what to do on a daily basis. The most important instructions in use of the kit are:

- Do not use the scraper on the dorsal surface.
- Do not scrape as to cause bleeding.
- Do not use too many gauze pieces for dressing.
- Do not tie the bandage too tight to cause swelling distally.
- Not to use more than four rounds of the bandage, so as to keep the ulcer area in good aeration.

The plastic tub and MCR footwear forms an integral part of the materials to be given in these camps.

As per the author's experience, nearly 40% of cases are able to heal their ulcers with the use of the self-care kit.

Figure 37.12A shows the sample of the self-care kit designed by authors and Figures 37.12B and C show the healing of ulcer with its use. Empowerment happens when individuals or group of people recognize that they themselves can change their situation and then begin to do so. Although 85% feet improve considerably well, it is the cardinal rule that those cases in which ulcers do not heal in about 4 months' time, are referred for RCS. The cases with grade 1 disability with anesthetic feet, dryness and cracks, who were given only the moisturizing cream or oil and taught to keep their feet hydrated, were able to prevent worsening of disability. In some cases with ichthyosis on legs, improvement was noticed with the application of moisturizing cream. Furthermore, all these cases are also supplied MCR footwear at the disability care program.

Surgery for Plantar Ulcers

About 10–15% cases of plantar ulcers need RCS. If there is deeper tissue infection or bone involvement, one of the three procedures is performed. These are: (1) sesamoidectomy, (2) subtotal metatarsectomy, and (3) transmetatarsal amputation. Besides split skin graft in cases with large raw areas, a flap cover is required for the chronic heel ulcers and metatarsal head ulcers as these are weight-bearing areas. The author has described an advanced myocutaneous flap for chronic heel ulcers. However, often local transposition flap suffices. His original technique of Neurovascular Island flap to first and second metatarsal region offers sensory skin and often prevents or delays the recurrence. However, it can only be performed by a specialist plastic surgeon. Alternately, the author advocates a distally based flap for 1st metatarsal head ulcers (Figs 37.13A and B) which is simple and effective to provide skin cover over the region and can be easily carried out by a general surgeon.

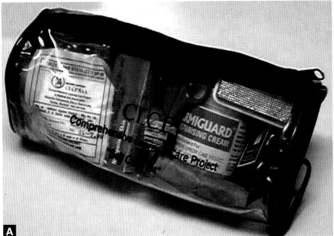
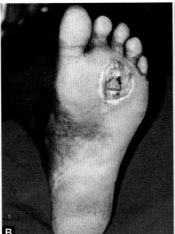
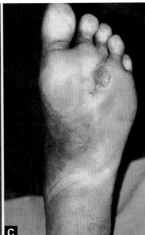

Figs 37.12A to C: Self-care kit and result in healing of ulcer in about 3 months. Patient is empowered to carry out self-care at home in a training session at DPMR camp

Footwear

Microcellular rubber footwear is considered the best for evenly spreading out the body weight as well as preventing external injuries with a hard sole. Considering the paucity of its availability, a criterion for its distribution was standardized by the authors as a first priority to those with ulcers and healed ulcers for next 3 years, secondly to those with cracks and history of infection and swelling in the feet off and on; followed by all other cases. If specialized footwear is not available, the insole of MCR also can be used in patients own footwear, as an alternative. Finally, it is necessary to explain to the patient that any footwear, which will prevent injury, has to be used by them and they need to learn to diagnose the initial symptoms of impending ulcerations by looking at their feet, palpating for increase in temperature in certain areas and any unusual swelling, on regular day-to-day basis. To overcome the stigma associated with conventional MCR footwear, some designer (and fancy!) MCR footwear has also been made available for use. The pictures of some designer footwear, prosthesis and splints made commercially available at subsidized cost by ALERT, a nongovernmental organization (NGO) are given in the end of this chapter.

DEFORMITIES OF FACE

The common deformities of face are wrinkling of face giving an aged appearance, saddle nose changing the personality of the person, loss of eyebrows making him an obvious notable person with an unusual face in the crowd. These are generally due to tissue infiltration and can be corrected once the chemotherapy treatment is completely satisfactory.

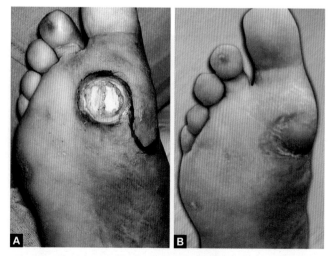

Figs 37.13A and B: Distally based flap to provide skin cover for 1st metatarsal head ulcer with exposed tendon

Depressed Nose (Collapsed Nose)

It occurs due to destruction of anterior nasal spine and loss of cartilaginous support to the nose following mucosal infiltration, secondary infection and destruction of cartilage. The lining of the nose shrinks inwards, pulling the end of the nose upward. The upper lip then seems unusually long. Destruction of anterior maxillary spine and later lack of support to upper central incisors may also be noted in advanced cases. Replacement of mucosa is invariably required with either skin graft or nasolabial flaps. Replacement of mucosa, described by Antia as inlay graft, is one of the standard procedures when there is a snarl present on the nose. The author has modified Antia and Buch's approach and prefers to insert the nasolabial flaps as lining, wherever possible, with a U-shaped incision. The nasolabial flaps are inserted horizontally, giving bulk to the nose and it generally does not require any prosthesis to be held for prevention of contracture, as for inlay. In both procedures, a cantilever bone graft can be performed after 6 months to give a better dorsal line. In the inlay, at that time, the oral incision is closed and prosthesis discontinued. In cases where one finds adequate lining, either a silicone implant or a bone graft may be put to correct the dorsum of the depressed nose. Behavior of silicone implant is unpredictable and it may come out after a period varying from few days to few years. But it is an easy procedure and bone graft can always be done later on, if required. Figures 37.14A and B show a patient in whom silicone implant was put offering quick correction without any associated morbidity. It remained for few months and was extruded due to infection. However, he did not need any further surgery.

Wrinkled Face

Nasolabial facelift has been the standard as generally there is greater laxity in these areas making it an obvious choice. However, the disadvantage is the visible incisions, at least for some time. The author has also performed the typical plastic surgery facelift procedure when the patient is relatively younger and when one wants to avoid the scars on the face (Figs 37.15A and B). Sometimes, enlarged ear lobules also need to be tackled with triangular excision.

Loss of Eyebrows

Reconstruction is undertaken with superficial temporal artery flap (either pedicle or island). In the former case, the flap is divided after 15 days and the extra portion is discarded. When island flap is done occasionally, necrosis in medial portion may occur and need secondary reconstruction with free full thickness hair graft from the occipital area. Some surgeons prefer directly the full thickness hair graft, which initially looks as if it has necrozed but the thin line of hair eventually remains and grows. The flap cover also needs a secondary

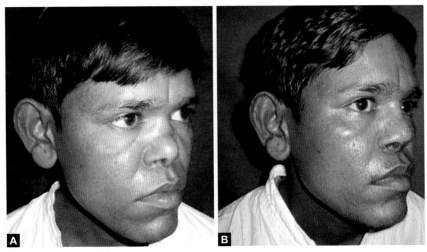

Figs 37.14A and B: Depressed nose in which silicone implant was inserted to shape the dorsum of the nose

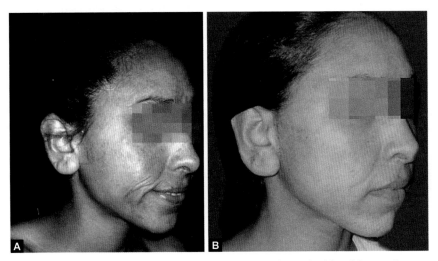

Figs 37.15A and B: Wrinkles on the face corrected with standard face-lift procedure

procedure for trimming the bushy growth, which is not liked by the patients.

Lagophthalmos

Lagophthalmos generally occurs due to involvement of the zygomatic branch of the facial nerve. It is important to recognize this complication early and if possible treat it with prednisolone therapy to get motor recovery. In the established cases, reconstruction may be in the form of the temporalis musculofascial sling (Figs 37.16A and B) or gold implant in the upper lid (Figs 37.16 C to E). Lateral tarsorrhaphy, though a simple procedure, often shows an unsatisfactory outcome in terms of the eye closure.

Ectropion

In the old age, and in patients from colonies with long standing disease, one also comes across the ectropion of the lower eyelid, which may need correction with full thickness skin graft and/or by triangular excision of the everted eyelid margin.

RECONSTRUCTIVE SURGERY (IN DISABILITY PREVENTION AND MEDICAL REHABILITATION)— A GOVERNMENT OF INDIA INITIATIVE

It is estimated that around one million leprosy patients with disabilities exist in the country. There is a greater need to introduce RCS at all medical colleges and district hospitals. Authors have been closely associated with RCS megacamp experiment in Gujarat where nearly 7,500 operations have been performed. The Government of India (GOI) labeled it as the Gujarat Model and asked other states to follow it, to reach the benefits to a majority of disabled cases. Disability prevention and medical rehabilitation (DPMR), initiated by GOI and enthusiastically implemented by the National Leprosy Program Manager, has RCS built in for all DPMR Institutes, Government Medical Colleges and District Hospitals. All patients undergoing RCS and centers performing RCS, either at their center or in the camps, are being supported with cash incentives per operation as per PIP guidelines of GOI. In the year 2012–2013 itself, this has resulted in about 2,400 RCSs being performed, of which nearly 865 were performed in the government institutions indicating good progress being made to integrate leprosy RCS in the medical services. However, load of RCS is so extensive that it will take many years to reach these services to all those in need.

ECONOMIC REHABILITATION

Leprosy handicapped persons form a very distinct entity, even for the rehabilitation strategy. Often leprosy sufferers, especially those with stigmatizing signs and deformities, are not accepted well even within their own families. Fortunately, instances of dehabilitation leading to social ostracism are now on decrease following extensive education about leprosy and the availability of a cure in the form of MDT. Nevertheless, some of the patients lose their self-esteem and find it difficult to earn money, causing a strain on the family income. Often they do not have the means and resources to get back to work. As mentioned in the ILEP Social and Economic Rehabilitation (SER) Guidelines, "although many people are resilient enough to cope with the effects of leprosy, others need help if they are to resume their previous way of life. These individuals are the focus of SER programs".

The leprosy workers identify such people who are in need of economic rehabilitation, try to understand what they can do and in consultation with them and their family, identify what could best serve them and for their betterment, as an appropriate economic rehabilitation, e.g. sewing machines, handcarts, kits for bicycle repair, carpentry, masonry work, agricultural tools, etc. After their assessment, the project personnel provide the required aids (Figs 37.17A to C). In the account on leprosy sufferers, i.e. "Don't Fence Me In", Tony Gould writes from the expedition of Dr Tonkins that "despite the repulsive appearance, the public have no active objection to it. I have frequently seen them tailoring, selling second hand clothes, and presiding at provision stores". Yo Yuasa claims that the final goal is not only the healing of leprosy as a disease; but total restoration of leprosy patient as a whole person in community.

The publicity provided at public functions is of great help in increasing awareness about leprosy as a disease, and the plight of the sufferers, which sensitizes the community regarding their restoration in the community. One can also

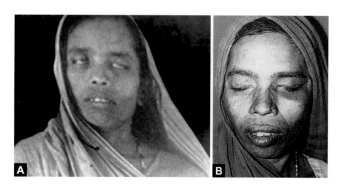

Figs 37.16A and B: Temporalis sling was performed on both sides in this patient for correction of lagophthalmos

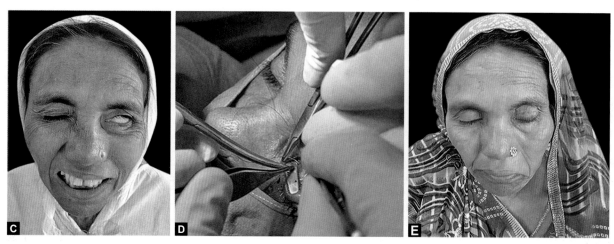

Figs 37.16C to E: (C) Preoperative lagophthalmos; (D) Intraop gold; (E) Postoperative result after 3 months

equate this activity as community based rehabilitation (CBR). CBR is a strategy, which targets social inclusion, and aims to overcome activity limitations and participation restrictions, and thus improve the quality of life for persons with disabilities. The impact of the economic rehabilitation with articles of income generation for the disabled individual and their families is dramatic and it has transformed the quality of lives of hundreds of people.

On account of integrated approach of disability prevention, correction and care including rehabilitation, this approach by authors Atul Shah and Neela Shah for Novartis Foundation has been hailed as a successful "model" of the holistic approach. The enhanced strategy for 2010–2015, by WHO, has endorsed the goal of reducing grade 2 disabilities by 35% from the baseline level of 2010. Improving the quality of services for prevention of disabilities and rehabilitation are also the objectives of the enhanced strategy.

In the end, authors have to reiterate the fact that "leprosy is curable, do not fear it or its consequences but face them and fight back to emerge happy and victorious in life".

HEALTH EDUCATION TO A PERSON AFFECTED WITH LEPROSY

Advice to Patients on Completion of Multidrug Therapy

- Skin patches will take much longer time to disappear or get back the original color and texture.
- Skin color will return to normal within few months of MB MDT when dark coloration of the skin is due to clofazimine.
- Reactions in the skin or nerves may occur in a few instances even after completion of the treatment (after being cured). If the skin patches become reddish, if there is a sudden loss of sensation in the hands or feet or weakness in the muscles, report back immediately for a check-up.

- Tingling, numbness or heavy feeling is the initial sign of neural damage. Do not neglect it and report for a check-up.

Advice to Patients with Loss of Sensations in Hands and Feet (Fig. 37.18)

- Daily inspection of hands and feet for signs of injury.
- Keep the hands and feet moist—use water to wet hands and feet often; rub a few drops of oil or use moisturizing creams.
- Do not exert undue pressure while working, for this can cause friction on the skin.
- Do not touch any hot objects without wrapping a cloth on your hands.
- Use wooden handles while cooking food at home and never lift the cooking vessels with bare hands; use thick cotton cloth for the same or use cotton gloves.
- Do not walk barefoot, particularly on tar roads. Walk a small distance at a time, walk slowly and take rest frequently. If possible, use of cycle is much safer than walking on anesthetic feet.
- Use comfortable footwear without nails and check your feet daily for injuries or burns.

Advice to Patients who have Deformities

- Follow advice meant for patients with loss of sensations.
- Carry out simple physiotherapy exercises at home to keep the joints mobile.
- Deformity is a consequence of the disease and is often reversible or mostly correctable.
- Deformity is not contagious and cannot transmit the disease.
- Do not allow deformities to worsen; get the specialist's advice as soon as possible.

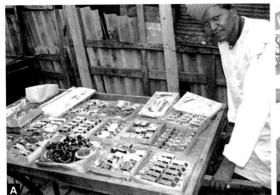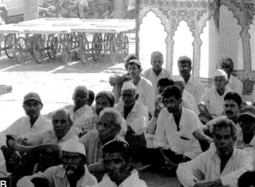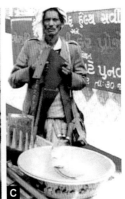

Figs 37.17A to C: (A) Economic rehabilitation program, a person followed up was selling toys and earning good amount; (B) Leprosy affected persons at the regular community gathering to discuss their health and social problems; (C) While another was using farming equipment to earn more

NUMBNESS? NO SENSATION IN YOUR HANDS OR FEET?

Don't ignore it. Consult a doctor immediately. Take the following precautions:

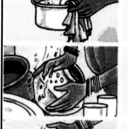

- Never touch a hot vessel with bare hands. Always use a cloth/napkin.

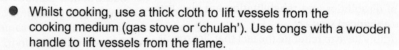

- Treat your hands with gentle care. Whilst washing clothes or vessels, don't exert pressure on them.

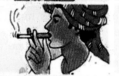

- Whilst cooking, use a thick cloth to lift vessels from the cooking medium (gas stove or 'chulah'). Use tongs with a wooden handle to lift vessels from the flame.

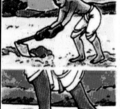

- Avoid smoking. If you must smoke occasionally, make sure the cigarette is fixed on a holder, so that the burning end does not touch your fingers/lips.

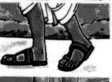

- Whilst working in th fields, use cloth gloves/ wrap a cloth on the axe and other field equipment.

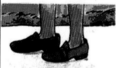

- Always use footwear.

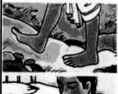

- Wear comfortable shoes which are stitched and do not have nails.

- Walking barefoot is dangerous. More so on tarred/rough surfaces, it can hurt your feet badly.

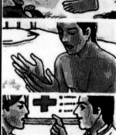

- Every morning and every night inspect your hands and feet. Wash them in hot water, massaging them gently. Rub oil or moisturizing cream.

- Do not ignore any injury to your hands or feet. Consult a doctor immediately.

Fig. 37.18: Health education pamphlet shown above has been translated in various languages and used in many countries to educate patients who have loss of sensations
Courtesy: Novartis CLC Association

Other Aids and Appliances Available from NGO Alert India

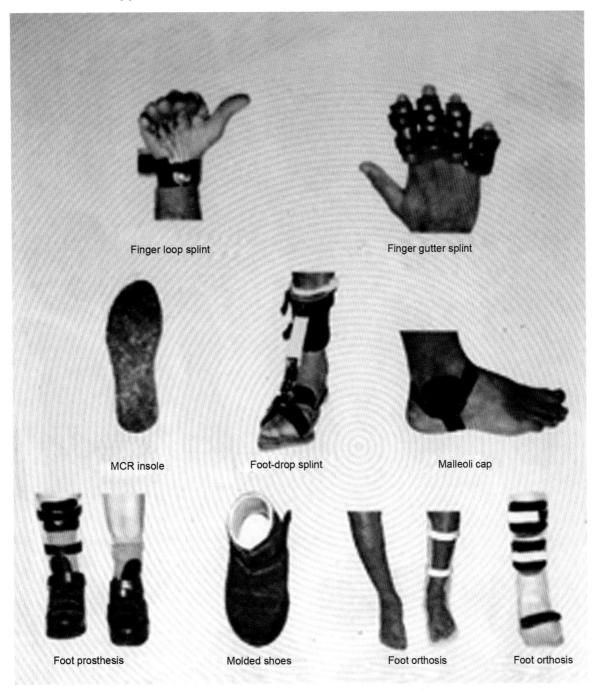

Finger loop splint

Finger gutter splint

MCR insole

Foot-drop splint

Malleoli cap

Foot prosthesis

Molded shoes

Foot orthosis

Foot orthosis

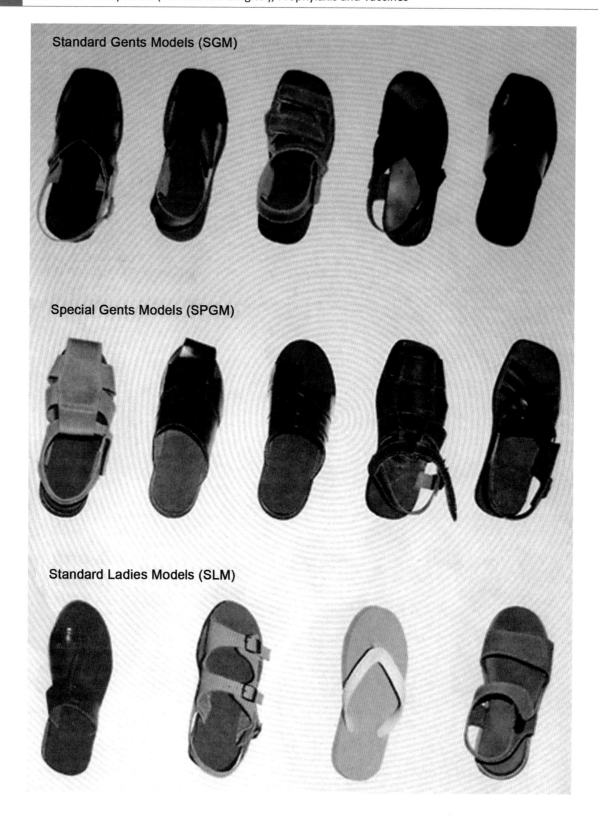

Special Ladies Models (SPLM)

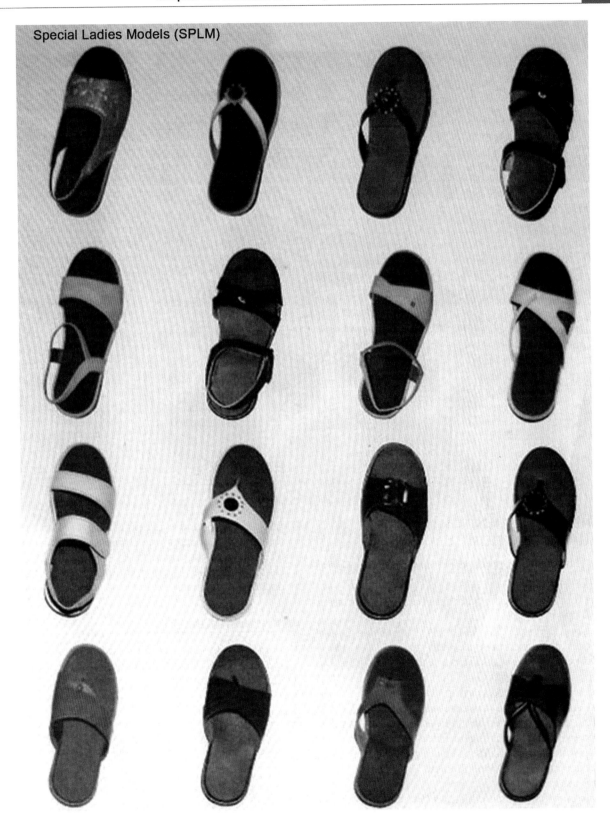

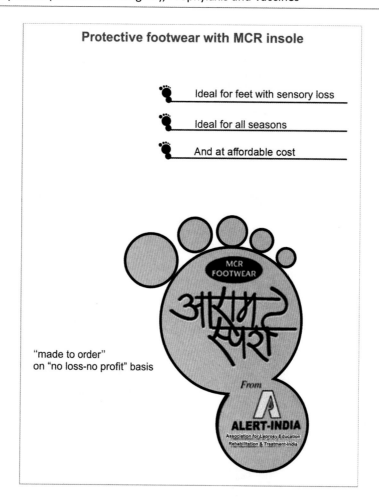

NUMBNESS? NO SENSATION IN YOUR HANDS OR FEET?

Do not ignore it. Consult a doctor immediately. Take the following precautions.

- Never touch a hot vessel with bare hands. Always use a cloth/napkin.
- Treat your hands with gentle care. Whilst washing clothes or vessels, don't exert pressure on them.
- Whilst cooking, use a thick cloth to lift vessels from the cooking medium (gas stove or "chullah"). Use tongs with a wooden handle to lift vessels from the flame.
- Avoid smoking. If you must smoke occasionally, make sure the cigarette is fixed on a holder, so that the burning end does not touch your fingers/lips.
- Whilst working in the fields, use cloth gloves/wrap a cloth on the axe and other field equipment.
- Always use footwear.
- Wear comfortable shoes which are stitched and do not have nails.
- Walking barefoot is dangerous. More so on tarred/rough surfaces, it can hurt your feet badly.
- Every morning and every night inspect your hands and feet. Wash them in hot water, massaging them gently. Rub oil or moisturizing cream.
- Do not ignore any injury to your hands or feet. Consult a doctor immediately.

ACKNOWLEDGMENT

Authors thank Dr Vinita Puri, Professor of Plastic Surgery, KEM Hospital, Mumbai, Maharashtra, India for her contribution in revision of the manuscript.

BIBLIOGRAPHY

1. Antia NH, Buch VI. Correction of nasal deformity with nasolabial flaps. Indian J Plast Surg. 1972;5:23-5.
2. Antia NH. Reconstructive surgery of the face. In: Cochrane RG, Davey TF (Eds) Leprosy in Theory and Practice, 2nd edition. Bristol: Wright; 1964. pp. 497-508.
3. Antia NH. The "temporalis musculofascial sling" for the correction of lagophthalmos. Indian J Surg. 1966;28:389-96.
4. Antia NH. The palmaris longus motor for lumbrical replacement. The Hand. 1969;1(2):139-45.

5. Bakhtha Reddy NB, Doris P. Schieffelin Leprosy Research and Training Centre, Karigiri, 2000:12.
6. Brand PW. Neuropathic ulceration, quademi di cooperazione sanitaria, Browne SG, Nunzi E, pub; Associazione Italiana Amici di Raoul Follereau. 1981;93-107.
7. Brand PW. Paralytic claw hand, with special reference to paralysis in leprosy and treatment by sublimis transfer of the Stiles and Bunnell. J Bone Joint Surg Am. 1958;40-B(4):618-32.
8. Brandsma JW. Monitoring motor nerve function in leprosy patients. Lepr Rev. 2000;71(3):258-67.
9. Central Leprosy Division. Disability prevention and medical rehabilitation. Guidelines for primary, secondary and tertiary level care. New Delhi: Ministry of Health and Family Affairs, Government of India; 2007. pp. 11-92.
10. Dingle A. Guidelines for the social and economic rehabilitation of people affected by leprosy. London: The International Federation of Anti-Leprosy Association; 1999.
11. Dutch Coalition on Disability and Development. (2007). Brochure on community-based rehabilitation, towards an inclusive policy. [online]. Available from www.dcdd.nl/. [Accessed June, 2014].
12. Ebenezer M, Kumar S, Partheebarajan S. Factors affecting functional outcome of opponens replacement in median nerve palsy in leprosy. Indian J Lepr. 2012;84(2):131-6.
13. Ebenezer M, Rao K, Partheebarajan S. Factors affecting functional outcome of surgical correction of claw hand in leprosy. Indian J Lepr. 2012;84(4):259-64.
14. El Toukhy E. Gold weight implants in the management of lagophthalmos in leprosy patients. Lepr Rev. 2010;81(1):79-81.
15. Fritschi EP. Etiological considerations in leprous neuritis and their implication in treatment. Proceedings of the workshop on reactions in leprosy. Pub: Indian Association of Leprologists, Sponsored by World Health Organisation and Government of India, New Delhi; 1986.pp.133-5.
16. Ganapati R. Studies on leprosy, Bombay Leprosy Project, 1988:6.
17. Gokhale SG, Sohoni N. Human Face of Leprosy. International Leprosy Union; 2001.pp.168-9.
18. I can do it myself. Tips for people affected by leprosy who want to prevent disability. [online]. Available from www.searo.who.int/entity/global_leprosy_programme/publications/prevention_disability.pdf. [Accessed June, 2014].
19. Job CK, Selvapandian AJ, Rao CK. Aetiology, pathogenesis and pathology, In: Job CK (Ed). Leprosy diagnosis and management, 4th edition. New Delhi: Hind Kusht Nivaran Sangh; 1991. pp. 9-13.
20. Malaviya GN. Lasso procedure to correct finger clawing in leprosy using index or middle finger flexor digitorumsuperficialis split into four tails - a long term follow up study. Indian J Lepr. 2004;76(3):207-14.
21. Mendis M. Physiotherapy in leprosy, 2nd edition. Bristol: John Wright and Sons; 1965.
22. Nilsson T, Sparell G. Skin smears for leprosy, 1st edition, ALERT, Addis Ababa, Ethiopia, printed by GLRA, Wurzburg, Germany, produced under TALMILEP with financial support of CIBA-Geigy, Basle, 1989:3.
23. Novartis. (2005). Improving access to leprosy treatment. [online]. Available from www.novartisfoundation.org/platform/apps/Publication/getfmfile.asp?id=614&el=824&se=9668314&doc=45&dse=4. [Accessed June, 2014].
24. Orsi AT, Santos M, Miranda AE, et al. Hand atrophy in a leprosy patient—treatment with polymethyl methacrylate. Lepr Rev. 2010;81(3):216-20.
25. Partheebarajan S, Soloman S, Ebenezer M. Long term results of tibialis posterior tendon transfer for foot drop in leprosy. Indian J Lepr. 2012;84(2):145-9.
26. Pfaltzgraf RE. How to diagnose and classify leprosy: a study guide. New Jersey: American Leprosy Mission; 1988.
27. Prevention of disability in leprosy. ILEP Tech Bull. 1995; December(8):1-3.
28. Renital L, Pulimood SA, Eapen EP, et al. Health care utilization in Indian leprosy patients. Lepr Rev. 2010;81(4):299-305.
29. Salafia A, Chauhan G. Claw toes correction: personal technique. Indian J Lepr. 2011;83(2):71-4.
30. Shah A, Bhagat N. Rehabilitation Surgery for leprosy handicapped at a rural leprosy colony. Int J Rehabil Res. 1985;8(3):345-7.
31. Shah A, Pandit S. Reconstruction of the heel with chronic ulceration with flexor digitorum brevis myocutaneous flap. Lepr Rev. 1985;56(1):41-8.
32. Shah A, Saluja K. Rehabilitation in Hansen's Disease. India Disabil Stud. 1991;13(4):125-33.
33. Shah A, Shah N. Prevention and Care of Disability in Leprosy, Pub; Novartis Comprehensive Leprosy Care Association, Mumbai, 2006;20-4.
34. Shah A, Yawalkar SJ, Ganapati R. Modulan Grip-Aids for Rehabilitation in Leprosy, Ciba Geigy Leprosy Fund, Novartis Foundation for Sustainable Development, Basle, Switzerland.1993.
35. Shah A. A new technique for correction of reversal of transverse metacarpal arch and ulnar claw hand. In: Maneksha RJ (Ed). Transactions of 9th International Congress of Plastic and Reconstructive Surgery: New Delhi, India, March 1-6, 1987. New Delhi: Tata McGraw Hill; 1987. pp. 533.
36. Shah A. Correction of ulnar claw hand by a loop of FD superficialis motor for lumbrical replacement. J Hand Surg Br. 1984;9(2):131-3.
37. Shah A. Multiple Superficialis Motor for Opponens and Lumbrical replacement: One stage correction of leprous claw hand. J Hand Surg Br. 1984;9(3):285-8.
38. Shah A. One in four flexor superficialis lasso for correction of clawhand. J Hand Surg Br. 1986;11(3):404-6.
39. Shah A. Physiotherapy and surgery. In: Koticha KK (Ed). Leprosy A concise text. DK Koticha; 1990. pp. 189-214.
40. Shah A. Prevention and Correction of Claw Hand by Splintage. A New Approach to Deformity Care. Ciba-Geigy Leprosy Fund – Comprehensive Leprosy Care Project, 1992.
41. Shah N, Shah A. Grip-aid kit—a simple method for instant benefit in activity of daily living in advanced hand deformities. Presented at 17th International Leprosy Congress; 2008; Hyderabad, India.
42. Srinivasan H, Palande DD, World Health Organization. Action Programme for the Elimination of leprosy. Essential surgery in leprosy: techniques for district hospitals. Geneva: World health organization; 1996.
43. Tony G. Don't Fence Me In. Bloomsbury, 2005:229.
44. Van Brakel WH, Reed NK, Reed DS. Grading impairment in leprosy. Lepr Rev. 1999;70(2):180-8.

45. Vieira R, Felicíssimo P. Surgical treatment of three cases of plantar foot ulceration in leprosy. Lepr Rev. 2008; 79(3):325-30.
46. Watson JM. Essential action to minimise disability in leprosy patients, 2nd edition. Leprosy Mission; 1994. pp. 4-5.
47. Wheate HW, Pearson JM. How to examine for enlargement of nerves, In: Wheate HW, Pearson JM (Eds). A practical guide to the diagnosis and treatment of leprosy in the basic health unit, 3rd edition. Wurzburg: German Leprosy Relief Association; 1985.pp.13-7.
48. WHO/ILO/UNESCO CBR Guidelines, pub; WHO, 2007:5.
49. Workshop for Health service Managers in Charge of Leprosy Control Programs, World Health Organisation, 2007, printed in India Feb. 2008.pp.90-91.
50. World Health Organization. Report of the Global Program Managers Meeting on Leprosy Control Strategy. New Delhi: World Health Organization; 2009.
51. Yawalkar SJ. Historical Background. In: Leprosy: For medical practitioners and paramedical workers, 7th edition. Basle: Novartis Foundation for Sustainable Development; 2002.p.2.
52. Yuasa Y. International Seminar on leprosy control, Seoul, Korea, 1991, quoted in Annotated Bibliography on Leprosy. Pub: CASPPLAN, Pune, 2001:395.

SECTION 7

Miscellaneous

CHAPTERS

Deformity and Disability Prevention

GN Malaviya

INTRODUCTION

Leprosy deforms and disables but seldom kills. These deformities evoke varied responses in the individual, his/her family and the community as a whole like aversion, hatred, fear, stigma, discrimination and ultimately socioeconomic dehabilitation. A considerable portion of disability load is the result of failure to incorporate activities relating to prevention of disabilities using simple technologies and patient motivation into leprosy management. Where leprosy is common, it is identified with deformity and disability by the public. The failure of control programs to master the problem of deformity is seen by public as failure to cure the disease. With the availability of newerdrugs and new treatment regimens leprosy patients can be completely cured in 6–12 months without any disabilities. Most serious consequences of cured leprosy patients are caused by permanent peripheral nerve function impairments. So, it is important to minimize nerve damage during its course.

Prevention of impairments and disability (POID) is integral part of the successful management of leprosy affected persons as well as national leprosy eradication program. The objectives of managing disabilities in leprosy, therefore, are to prevent: (1) onset of new disabilities, and (2) worsening of existing disabilities. In addition to any direct benefit to the patient, attention to disabilities has a favorable influence on attendance at clinics and thus on the control of leprosy. Prevention of deformities increases the confidence of the patient and his peers in therapy.

Disability and deformity words have been used interchangeably while referring to the physical problems in leprosy patients. Deformity is an alteration in the appearance and is usually associated with some incapability especially if the limbs are involved. Disability is actually an incapability of the patient and it may exist even without any obvious disfigurement.

TYPES OF DEFORMITIES

The deformities due to the direct result of disease process and infiltration with *M. leprae* are called specific. The deformities in this group are due to the bacterial load of the patient and its local damaging effect on tissues, for example, leonine facies, sagging of ear lobules, loss of eyebrows, etc. Deformities which are produced due to indirect effects of disease, e.g. motor paralysis and recurrent ulcers due to anesthesia of extremities are grouped separately as paralytic and anesthetic deformities respectively. Table 38.1 summarizes various deformities seen in leprosy patients. Fortunately, the deformities which are difficult to treat can be easily prevented if little attention is paid, e.g. anesthetic deformities. The deformities, which are difficult to prevent, are amenable to treatment at least partially if not totally, e.g. motor paralysis.

Table 38.1: Disabilities and deformities which can develop in leprosy patients

S. No.	Organ	Specific deformities	Motor paralytic deformities	Anesthetic deformities	Miscellaneous deformities
1.	Face	Nodulation; loss of facial hair in males; nasal defects-full thickness loss of nasal wall, depressed dorsal crest, alar deformities and distortion, facial wrinkles	Lagophthalmos; facial palsy	Anosmia	Paresthesia; loss of taste; crocodile tear syndrome; nasal crusting and blockage
2.	Eyes	Loss of eye brows		Blurring due to corneal abrasions	Complicated cataracts; ectropion and entropion; loss of vision
3.	Ears	Sagging of ear lobules; Rat bitten appearance of helix			
4.	Larynx	Hoarseness of voice			
5.	Hard and soft palate	Palatal perforation			Nasal speech
6.	Hands	Reaction hand, Frozen hands, Twisted fingers, Intrinsic plus fingers	Ulnar claw hand; ulnar median claw hand; wristdrop; 'z' thumb and weak pinch; reversal of distal transverse metacarpal arch; interphalangeal joint contracture of the thumb	Anesthesia	Paresthesia, pain loss of grip power
7.	Legs and feet	Frozen foot, twisted toes	Clawing of toes, drop foot partial or complete	Ulcers, absorption, disorganization of foot	Warty out growths on the dorsum of foot; chronic lymphedema
8.	Skin	Scarring due to recurrent reactions			
9.	Testes	Testicular atrophy			Gynecomastia; gynecothelia, impotence, sterility

GRADING OF DISABILITIES AND DEFORMITIES

Some form of grouping or grading of deformities is necessary to assess the patients in field surveys, leprosy control programs and rehabilitation work. Different methods of grading do offer some convenience to the field workers but in a clinical setup it is always better to record the actual disability/deformity.

World Health Organization in 1970[1] suggested one such grouping of disabilities (Table 38.2). The main drawback of this classification is the failure to recognize the significance of individual defects which seem to have a lot of bearing on the overall function of the part. In the hand, for example, wrist drop is grouped with stiff joints and severe resorption of bones. Wrist drop can be easily corrected with surgery. Similarly, drop foot deformity has been grouped with ulcers. Drop foot is a severe disability but that responds fairly well to surgical correction. The altered gait mechanics of the drop foot predisposes to ulceration because weight distribution

patterns are altered. In 1988, WHO grading was revised (Table 38.3).[2] It considered only three grades and appears to be meant for grading the disabilities for statistical purposes and not for recording the progress of individual patients from the point of rehabilitation.

The need is being felt for a simple disability record for field use from which the problems can be immediately identified and appropriate action taken on a priority basis. A modified scheme for grading is shown in Table 38.4. Here grade I and grade II which include anesthesia and ulcers problems can be taken care of by physio-technician and other personnel participating in the leprosy control program. Grade III disabilities are paralytic deformities and can be corrected by surgery and therefore should be referred to the centers offering surgical services at the earliest. Grade IV disabilities are gross mutilations needing the attention of rehabilitation team and social workers who then can organize the institutional or community care for them.

Table 38.2: World Health Organization (1970) grading of disabilities

S. No.	Grade	Hands and feet	Eyes
1.	Grade 0	No anesthesia, no visible deformity or damage*	No eye problems due to leprosy† No evidence of visual loss
2.	Grade I	Anesthesia present but no visible deformity or damage	Eye problems due to leprosy present but vision not severely affected as a result of these (vision 6/60 or better; can count fingers at 6 meters)
3.	Grade II	Visible deformity or damage present	Severe visual impairment; (vision 6/60 or less inability to count fingers at 6 meters

* Damage in extremities means ulcer, shortening, stiffness, disorganization, and loss of part or all of the hand or foot.
† Eye problems due to leprosy include corneal anesthesia, lagophthalmos and iridocyclitis.
  Each hand, foot and eye is to be assessed and classified separately.
  If any disability found in the patient, is due to causes other than leprosy the fact should be recorded.

Table 38.3: World Health Organization (1988) grading of disabilities

S. No.	Grade	Hands	Feet	Eyes
1.	Grade I	Insensitive hand	Insensitive feet	Redness of conjunctiva
2.	Grade II	Ulcers and injuries and/or mobile claw hand, and/or slight absorption	With trophic ulcer and /or claw toes or foot drop and/or slight resorption	Lagophthalmos and/or blurring of vision and/or inflammation of globe
3.	Grade III	Wrist drop and/or clawing of fingers with stiff joints and/or severe absorption of fingers	Contracture and/or severe resorption of foot (1/5 of the sole area is lost)	Severe loss of vision

Table 38.4: Grading of disabilities according to their management

S. No.	Grade	Hands	Feet	Eyes
1.	Grade I	Insensitive hand	Insensitive foot	Redness of conjunctiva
2.	Grade II	Ulcer and injuries and/or and/or slight resorption	Trophic ulcers and/or claw toes	Blurring of vision and/or inflammation of the globe
3.	Grade III	Mobile claw fingers and/or paralyzed thumb and/or wrist drop	Foot drop	Lagophthalmos
4.	Grade IV	Stiff finger joints and/or resorption of fingers	Contracture and/or severe resorption of the foot	Severe loss of vision or blindness

FACTORS AFFECTING THE ONSET AND PROGRESSION OF DISABILITIES

Existence of an effective leprosy control/eradication program influences the deformity rate and all leprosy patients do not suffer from disability. The available reports quote that 4–10% of patients suffer from some form of disability.[3]

Age

The deformities are more commonly seen in 20–40 years age group probably because of the fact that self-limiting forms of disease occur in younger age groups and the duration of disease is also shorter in them. The 20–40 years age group is comparatively more active and thus forms a vulnerable group.

Sex

The deformities are less common in females because of lower incidence of disease, occurrence of milder forms of disease and also lesser involvement of nerve trunks in them and also due to reduced trauma due to their less exposure to outdoor occupations.

Duration of the Disease

It has been observed that shorter the duration of active disease lesser the number of deformities that develop later, because of better control of the disease under treatment and lesser degree of involvement of nerves and other body tissues.

Type of Disease and Immune Status

The immunity to disease varies with the type of leprosy, being maximum in tuberculoid variety and almost absent in lepromatous leprosy. Tissue damage, when it occurs, is severe in patients with higher cell-mediated immunity. The nerve damage occurs fairly early in tuberculoid form of the disease. Excessive cell-mediated immune response in the nerves in tuberculoid leprosy results in rapid destruction of the nerve progressing even to caseation, and is often irreversible.

In lepromatous patients, multiple nerve trunks are involved but damage occurs quite late. However, the disease takes longer to be controlled. Due to wide spread nerve involvement, deformities are observed in larger proportion of lepromatous patients. In lepromatous forms of the disease, there is slow fibrosis in the nerve with the result that over a period of several years multiple nerves are affected. Since the nerve fibers are damaged even by intraneural fibrosis, deformities might appear even in cases where the disease appears to be clinically subsided. A sudden onset of leprosy reactions (type 1 or 2) may also damage the nerves.

Borderline forms of leprosy are notorious because the immunity is unstable and fluctuating. In these patients, reactional states produce acute nerve damage which, at times, may recover fully under appropriate treatment.

Occupation

Injuries, single or repeated, often cause damage to the anesthetic limb. Heavy manual labor and specific occupations causing repeated trauma to an anesthetic part are likely to cause ulcerations which may progress to mutilation if not attended to. Females suffer damage to the fingers due to burns because of their role as homemakers.

Attitude of the Patient

Living with anesthetic extremities is difficult. Patients, who do not have clear concepts about the value of sensations and its protective function preventing tissue damage, suffer more and develop serious deformities due to minor trauma occurring in routine activities of life. Due to extreme emotional upset, sometimes the patients develop apathy toward their disease and ignore their injuries. Such cases also suffer severe mutilations.

Treatment

Effectiveness of the antileprosy treatment in preventing the occurrence of deformities is still debated. An attempt has been made to establish an association between dapsone treatment and development of deformities.[4] A possible neurotoxic effect of dapsone was suggested because it was observed that deformities were more common in patients who had regular dapsone therapy.[4] A report on military personnel where treatment was supervised, said that only 1.5% of patients developed deformities after they were put on therapy.[5] In another report, where workers have emphasized the need for anti-inflammatory drugs together with dapsone during reactional states, none of the patients developed deformity after starting the therapy.[6]

Srinivasan and Noordeen reported higher deformity rates in patients taking regular treatment as compared to the group who has not taken any treatment.[7] They suggested that under field conditions the treatment is carried out on a mass scale and on a routine basis where facilities for individualizing treatment for management of complications and for satisfactory follow-up are not adequate as in an institution. This probably could explain to some extent the contradictory reports from various centers.

It is likely that patients who developed deformities under treatment visited more regularly because they were deeply concerned about their deformities and disease. Regularity of treatment indicated the clinical symptomatic state of the patients.[8] Furthermore, dapsone given in doses for treatment of leprosy is not neurotoxic at least in experimental situations.

Availability of Medical Care

Areas where adequate medical attention is available, the deformities tend to be lesser in number and milder in form.

Quiet Nerve Paralysis

Clinically evident acute or subacute neuritis of nerve trunks is a sign of impending paralysis. However, thickened nerve trunks quite frequently become paralyzed without manifesting any nerve pain and the damage is recognized only after it is physically manifest. The use of corticosteroids in substantial doses over a period of 3–6 months is reported to facilitate the recovery in high proportion of such cases when the disease in them is identified and treated before the nerve is completely paralyzed.[9]

CAUSATION OF DEFORMITIES

The deformities can develop due to:
- Direct result of infiltration of tissues by *M. leprae*
- Muscle imbalance secondary to motor paralysis and
- Secondary effects of impaired sensations and anesthesia
- These factors operate singly or in combination in various patients but to emphasize the individual contributions of each, these are discussed separately.

EFFECTS OF INFILTRATION OF TISSUES BY *M. LEPRAE*

Nerve Damage

Involvement of major nerve trunks of extremities results in sensory–motor deficits. Sensory loss almost always precedes motor paralysis. The sites and sequence of nerve trunk involvement in leprosy follows a definite pattern, but the causes for such specificity of nerve involvement have not been fully established. It has been suggested that the tissues in a more superficial position where core temperature is less, favor the growth of *M. leprae*.[10] The nerves which commonly get involved pass through a narrow osseo-fascial tunnel across the joints. During movements of these joints nerve trunks suffer minor damage due to stretching. The inflammatory process starts at these sites and is perpetuated in the presence of infection. The reactionary edema and infiltration add to the swelling of the nerve which is further aggravated by the preexisting external compressive forces. The unyielding fibrous epineurium adds to the compression. The end result is ischemic, inflammatory nerve damage.

Brand suggested three chief factors which determine whether an infected nerve will be paralyzed or not.[11] These factors are: (1) number of nerve fibers in the nerve trunk, (2) the depth of location of the nerve from the body surface, and (3) immunological status of the patient. Higher the immunity severe is the nerve damage. More the number of nerve fibers in a nerve trunk more is the susceptibility of nerve to damage because intervening areolar tissue is less and compression can occur more easily. More superficially located nerves are involved than the deeper ones.

Most commonly involved nerve is ulnar at the level of elbow just above the medial epicondyle. Posterior tibial and common peroneal nerves are involved at the ankle and just behind the neck of the fibula respectively. Median nerve is involved at the level of wrist. The radial nerve is involved in the upper arm, but is usually not damaged enough to manifest clinically in most of the patients.

The sequence of paralysis is also characteristic. The usual paralysis is high ulnar (at the elbow) followed by combined high ulnar-low median type. The least common combination is high ulnar-low median and radial paralysis. Isolated paralyses of these nerves have been reported but are rather uncommon. Lateral plantar component of posterior tibial nerve is more commonly affected and so is the deep peroneal component of common peroneal nerve which innervates tibialis anterior and extensor muscles of the toes. The zygomatic branch of the facial nerve is more commonly involved producing lagophthalmos, complete facial paralysis being uncommon.

Accompanying sensory loss is a major handicap. Since anesthesia is generally irreversible, continued trauma can result in ulceration, infection, osteomyelitis and absorption of digits even after the disease is cured. In addition to the sensory-motor damage, the autonomic fibers innervating the sweat glands and cutaneous vessels are also damaged. The capability of vessels to respond to inflammatory process therefore decreases. In the beginning, there occurs only partial ischemia of the nerves which causes a reversible paralysis due to loss of conduction in the nerve. Later Wallerian degeneration sets in which, if mild, the nerve recovers.

This reversible stage of damage lasts up to 1 year in majority of the patients. After that paralysis is considered as established, and the corrective measures should be undertaken.

Table 38.5 depicts the effects of nerve damage and associated deformities. Deformities of the hands being more common are seen in all types of leprosy followed by those of the feet and face.

Skin Damage

Most of the obvious lesions in leprosy occur in skin and a lower temperature than the body core has been put to blame. Some of the most marked infiltration occurs in these regions but the sparing of axilla and groin is far from clear. The axilla has a much lower temperature than the oral cavity.

When the skin and subcutaneous tissues are infiltrated, the collagen and elastic fibers, which maintain the shape and form of skin, are largely replaced by granulation tissue. The skin, first of all, looks swollen and shiny but later when disease subsides it becomes wrinkled and loose. The skin appendages are also destroyed leading to the loss of hairs, sweat and sebaceous glands. Recurrent reactional episodes in lepromatous patients with pustulation produce scarring on the body surface.

Oronasal Defects

The nose is affected because of its lower temperature. The cooler epithelium of nasopharynx favors growth of *M. leprae*. Granuloma has been shown to be present in nose even before the disease manifests clinically.[12] Nasal stuffiness develops first followed by superficial ulcers in nasal mucosa due to trauma while picking the nose. These get secondarily infected and repeated inflammatory episodes lead to the destruction of nasal cartilage and scarring. The nasal tip is pulled posteriorly presenting as typical nasal deformity with depressed dorsal crest and anteriorly facing nostrils. The alar cartilage can also be damaged and its margins show various forms of irregular outline. Excessive nasal discharges putrefy and dry up forming crusts attracting flies. The larvae of these flies hatch out and burrow deeper tunnels into local tissues producing intense cellulitis of the face. Sometimes, destruction is so extensive that full thickness of the nasal wall is lost producing severe facial disfigurement.

The lepromatous nodules occurring over palate may ulcerate and an oronasal fistula can form making eating and drinking difficult. The scarring around soft palate may restrict its movements resulting in nasal speech.

Lesions of leprosy may develop on lips—both upper and lower, inside the mouth and also on gums and inside of cheek, especially in borderline leprosy. These lesions may be small independent lesions or a part of larger lesion affecting the face. Diffuse infiltration and plaques have been noted in these areas in lepromatous leprosy. In cases that have

S. No.	Nerve trunk	Site	Muscles paralyzed	Deformity	Sensory loss
			Table 38.5: Physical manifestations of nerve damage in leprosy		
1.	Ulnar nerve	Wrist	All interossei; lumbrical for ring and little fingers; hypothenar muscles; adductor pollicis and sometimes flexor pollicis brevis	Clawing of ring and little fingers 'Z' pinch	Ulnar side of ring finger and complete palmar aspect of little finger and hypothenar area
		Elbow	All the above plus flexor carpi ulnaris and flexor digitorum profundus of little and ring fingers	As above	As above plus anesthesia on the dorsum of ring and little fingers
2.	Median nerve	Wrist	Thenar muscles	Loss of abduction-opposition of thumb; thumb lies in the plane of palm	Palmar aspect of thenar eminence, index and middle fingers
		Forearm	Long flexors of fingers and thumb	Loss of active flexion of fingers; deformity becomes obvious while gripping an object	As above
3.	Radial nerve	Upper arm	Paralysis of wrist and finger extensors and abductor pollicis longus	Wrist drop; finger clawing if present becomes less obvious	Over dorsum of thumb web
4.	Common peroneal nerve	Just behind the neck of fibula	Evertors and dorsiflexors of the foot	Drop foot	Over dorsum of foot
5.	Posterior tibial nerve	Just above and behind medial malleolus	Intrinsic muscles of the foot	Clawing of toes	Over sole of the foot
6.	Facial nerve	Over zygomatic bone;	Orbicularis occuli	Lagophthalmos	Nil
		In facial canal	All the muscles of the facial expression	Complete facial paralysis of the affected side	Nil

extensive nasal involvement, the nasal spine of the maxilla may get absorbed.

Gynecomastia and Associated Changes

Atrophy of testes can occur due to its complete destruction by granulomatous infiltration, in lepromatous patients. The resulting hormonal imbalance leads to gynecomastia and impotence. Such patients may also develop sterility.

Damage to Other Tissues

Leprosy by itself does not cause gross bone destruction, but it does cause bone to become fragile by trabacular absorption and decalcification so that it is no longer able to withstand normal strains. These changes are reversible and recalcification takes place leaving functionally normal bones if adequate protection is given during acute reactional episodes. The granuloma has been found to occur in the subarticular regions of small bones of the hands and feet in lepromatous patients which may gradually increase in size. During reactional episodes, these granulomata swell up. Accompanying osteoporosis and misuse of hands precipitate pathological fractures at these sites. These fractures heal spontaneously, in bizarre positions if not splinted properly producing deformities of the hands and feet. There are number of other abnormalities in bones associated with trophic changes and accompanying sepsis.

Damage to tendon sheath and joint capsules does occur in leprosy. The synovial inflammation due to infiltration might present clinically as cystic swellings over dorsum of the hands.[13] Damage to joint capsules during reactional episodes may produce contractures. Invasion of cartilage can also occur during reactional states. There may be painful arthritis as the joint capsules are infiltrated and swollen.[14] The patients keep their fingers in extended position relaxing the ligaments. In due course, these ligaments contract producing stiffness of the joints and contractures. If the fingers are kept partially flexed throughout the acute phase, the healing and scarring will be in a functional position and the hand remains functionally useful.

EFFECTS OF MOTOR PARALYSIS

Motor paralysis results in loss of function performed by the paralyzed muscle(s). When some muscles around a particular joint are paralyzed the normal balance of forces acting on that joint is disturbed, and a new equilibrium is achieved in conformity with the new system of forces. Achieving the new equilibrium involves adopting new postures by the concerned joints and this postural alteration is seen as deformity. The disturbed muscle balance across the joints produce a deformity of the part, for example, the clawing of the finger results due to paralysis of small muscles of the hand—the lumbricals and the interossei.

Motor paralysis may also contribute to the resorption of fingers by altering the gripping patterns. When a patient tries to hold an object with his clawed hands, the fingertips come in contact with the object, not the pulp of the fingers (Figs 38.1A and B). Thus, the actual strain of bearing the weight of the object is confined to the tip of the fingers. The pressure exerted by the object/mm^2 of contact area will be much more as compared to the situation where whole hand grasps the object. Furthermore, due to anesthesia of hands and fingers, the amount of force exerted by the patient in order to hold an object is excessive. This adds to the traumatic forces and is one of the causes of finger resorption in leprosy patients.

EFFECTS OF ANESTHESIA AND ANALGESIA

Inability to appreciate the temperature and pain sensations causes damage to the hands and feet. The protective reflexes are lost. Without pain sensation many occupations become hazardous, especially those requiring heavy manual work and working with hot objects.

The loss of pain allows the patient to use his burnt or injured fingers as actively as if it were unwounded or uninfected. The reflex splinting action due to pain is absent in these patients and they need a conscious effort to avoid further injuries to the already injured hand. If neglected, these minor injuries have a cumulative effect leading to tenosynovitis and osteomyelitis.

Much of the deformities and mutilations that occur in the anesthetic hands and feet in leprosy are mostly due to the excessive and unreasonable strains which they have to bear. The denervated tissues are somewhat less able to bear even normal physiological strains. Healing response of the tissues to inflammation and trauma is also not effective.

PREVENTION OF DISABILITIES

Early case detection followed by full treatment is the most important step to prevent and or to minimize nerve function impairment (NFI). Early signs and symptoms of leprosy should be known well to the community to promote self-reporting in its early stages so that cure is evident without the development of NFI. The disease may leave residual effects of nerve damage, in the form of sensory, motor and autonomic nerve paralysis, in the eyes, hands and feet. If a recent onset nerve damage remains untreated for 3–6 months it may become permanent. The sensory and autonomic nerve fiber damage occurs almost simultaneously because cross-sectional damage to the nerve trunk occurs at certain levels in leprosy affected nerve trunks. If unattended, it may progress further and motor fibers are also damaged leading to muscle paralysis, wasting, postural changes and contractures.

To prevent further progression of disabilities in a fresh case efforts should be made to recognize early signs of damage to

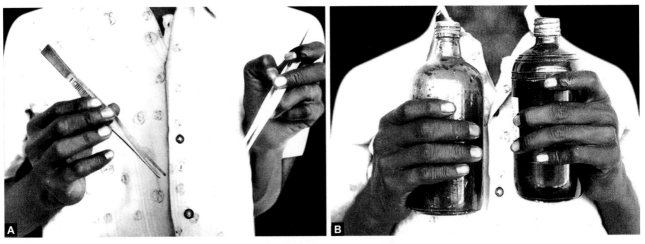

Figs 38.1A and B: Gripping by normal and intrinsic palsied fingers. (A) Pinching; (B) Gripping

the nerves and eyes, so that supportive/preventive measures and treatment could be given at the earliest. The deformities are surgically corrected if needed. Attempts need to be made to provide a life with dignity and fellowship for the severely disabled regardless of their physical condition.

ANTICIPATING NERVE FUNCTION IMPAIRMENT

We need to anticipate the impending neural damage and thereby identify high-risk patients. These patients can then be given extra attention and some form of prophylactic treatment to bring down the numbers of those developing deformities. Risk factors have been identified, which can help in pointing out cases that are more likely to develop reactive episodes and NFI.[15] Previous nerve damage, multibacillary (MB) disease especially borderline leprosy, multiple nerve trunk involvement, pregnancy, inter-current illness like tuberculosis—all can precipitate a reactive episode. Predicting the onset of a reactive episode based on serological changes have not been successful so far,[16] and diagnosis of reaction is a clinical exercise based on the changes appearing in the skin lesions, neural swelling, nerve pain and tenderness along with nerve function changes.

ROLE OF STEROIDS

Steroids have been used to treat NFI, reactive episodes and also as prophylactic agents against reactions.[17-22] In a report, it was concluded that 60% of patients who were treated with steroids for NFI had useful recovery of sensory-motor functions. It might be possible that if detected in early stages of NFI, patients can have full recovery. However, defining early has its own problems—early in terms of duration of clinical manifestations or early in terms of severity of clinical manifestations. Some studies have suggested that steroids if given along with multidrug therapy (MDT) can prevent NFI and reactions.[20,22] Optimal steroid regimens and duration still need to be worked out.

ROLE OF NERVE TRUNK DECOMPRESSION

The timing of nerve trunk decompression is not very clear.[23-26] It has been reported that nerve damage of 3 months or lesser duration and with muscle strength of Medical Research Council grade 3 or more has a favorable prognosis.[24]

CARE OF THE EYES

The impairment of vision is a devastating disability in leprosy since it is often associated with sensory loss in hands and feet. The eyes need special care, because in the absence of sensory feedback from palms and soles, they take-up the additional responsibility of warning the patient about imminent dangers

from noxious stimuli. Basic screening of the eye functions is easy and quick. The eyes should be examined initially in every patient and all MB patients should be reexamined at regular intervals.

In leprosy, eyes can be damaged either as a direct result of disease process or following nerve damage which affect the blinking and closure of the eyes. It is through tears and blink that the surface of the eye is kept moist and clean. The blinking is an involuntary (reflex) process initiated by a feeling of dryness or irritation in the eye. Damage to the corneal sensory nerve endings results in impaired sensory perception which affects reflex blinking. Damage to facial nerve branches may result in paralysis of orbicularis oculi muscle so that the eyes cannot be closed properly. Both these conditions individually predispose the eye to get damaged, effect being more severe if both exist. The aim of management is to keep the eye clean, prevent its dryness and protect it from injuries due to dust and wind.

It is, therefore, necessary to build up a habit to look after the eyes. One has to develop a habit of blinking regularly with a voluntary conscious effort, i.e. 'think and blink'. The patient must remember to often close the eyes with effort from time to time. The eyes can be protected with spectacles or a shield while moving out in open and in the sun. If lagophthalmos is there, the eyes can be covered with an eyepad or head cloth while sleeping. The eyes should be washed with clean water twice daily and mopped gently with a clean cloth. Patient is told not to rub his/her eyes and report to the nearest health facility available if he/she notices any redness, irritation or pain in the eyes.

MANAGEMENT OF REACTIONS

The crucial elements in the proper management of reversal reaction are early recognition and prompt treatment. Neuritis associated with a reaction is an indication for starting corticosteroid therapy without delay. The dose of corticosteroid will depend on the severity of reaction, patient's body weight and response to treatment. It should be sufficient to relieve both nerve pain and tenderness. Administration of corticosteroid should be continued for several months. The actual duration of steroid therapy depends upon the individual circumstances.

MONITORING AND SELF-REPORTING

The patients can be taught to recognize reportable events like changes in eyes and vision, sensory motor functions, and nerve pain and to ask for help if required. But monitoring is still necessary in most cases because many patients are not aware of ongoing changes as in silent neuropathy. Plantar ulcers and their management are detailed in another chapter.

EVALUATION OF THE PATIENT AND ASSESSMENT OF DISABILITY

An assessment of disabilities and deformities in a patient is done at the time of his first visit and recorded before starting the treatment. This baseline information is helpful to assess the response to therapy and nerve functions.[27] A complete examination is carried out to find out the condition of skin, nerve trunks, sensory motor functions and joints. It is convenient to record this information in charts, containing outline drawings of hands and feet, so that these can be easily referred to in future, if required.

The skin of hands and feet is examined for texture, presence of mobility, sweating, fissures, ulcers and scars of previous injuries. The nerve trunks (ulnar, median, radial, common peroneal and posterior tibial) at the sites of their predilection, are palpated. The swelling and tenderness if found is noted down. An assessment of sensory-motor functions is done to find out the extent of manifest nerve damage. Evaluation of sensory functions in hands and feet is important. Methods to assess sensory and motor functions have been detailed elsewhere in the book.

Sensory system functions at subconscious level and therefore we take it for granted. It is only when there is sensory loss in palm and soles that we realize the importance of sensory inputs from these areas which perceive the environment around and keep the brain duly informed. These sensory inputs help the brain to develop a motor strategy to respond. If the stimulus is interpreted to be injurious, there is an immediate withdrawal. To appreciate finer details of an object, its texture, etc. intact sensory modalities are necessary. However, to appreciate noxious stimuli certain minimal sensory abilities are enough. This is called 'protective sensation' and is presumed to be essential so that the neurally impaired leprosy affected person can save himself from injuries and progressive damage to the tissues.

Average normal perception threshold for nylons at finger pulps is 0.217 g/mm^2 and levels of protective sensations are double the normal thresholds, i.e. 0.434 g/mm^2. For sole these values have been worked out to be 2.35 g/mm^2 and 5 g/mm^2, respectively.[28,29] Some other reports take responses to 10 g as cut off point to define protective sensations in sole.[30,31] The sole has a higher tactile threshold than hand due to thicker keratin layers in the plantar skin. Callosities, occupation, use of foot wear[32,33] and also the type of footwear seem to affect the plantar sensory thresholds and these factors should be kept in mind while interpreting the outcomes of testing. If sensations are lost, extra care is needed for this group of patients and they are to be educated and monitored for self-care practices.

The perception of touch decreases with age as a consequence of decrease in receptor density in the glabrous skin that occurs with age.[34] However, perception of pain remains same with age indicating that nociceptive free nerve endings do not decrease with age. Testing for pin prick pain has been widely used. In its basic form it is a nongraded test (yes or no replies). Modifications have been tried,[35] but have not been very popular. Since nonmyelinated fibers are first affected in the disease, testing for pinprick pain is essential. Since a potential risk of transmission of human immunodeficiency virus (HIV) and hepatitis is there, reuse of pins is discouraged.

Tip of ballpoint pens is used by majority of field workers to evaluate sensory loss and these have been reported to be comparable to monofilament nylons.[36-39] The ballpen test is universally available and simple to use. A light touch with a ballpoint pen can generate pressure of 4 g or more. Therefore, it may not be very useful to detect mild sensory deficits at least in the palm. However, the reliability of this method has been found to be satisfactory[37] and the method is capable of detecting major sensory changes while monitoring sensory functions.[39] Static two point discrimination, a test for innervation density, is reliable but slow to respond to changes as compared to monofilament nylons. Testing for temperature sensation, though potentially important to detect early cases is crude and not of much value in established cases of leprosy.

A simplified version of the voluntary muscle testing (VMT) is often used to detect gross paralysis which can be suitably modified to quickly assess the muscle strength. If any weakness is detected, the patients can be subjected to detailed assessment.[40] A rapid neurological evaluation must test sensibility, mobility and trophicity.[41-43] It is performed on each side (only six main nerve trunks are affected on each side in leprosy), in a sequence to save time.

Periodic assessment by voluntary muscle testing and response to graded monofilament nylons can be used to monitor progress of the patients preferably by the same observer as inter-observer variations do exist.[44-47] Of the various testing methods compared, for their efficacy to detect early nerve damage, nerve palpation and testing with 200 mg monofilament nylon were found better.[48] Palpation of nerves and testing with graded nylons gave comparable results as observed in another study also. In most situations, a combination of ballpoint pen testing and quick muscle testing appears to be a more practical option, detailed testing being reserved for cases with doubtful nerve function impairments.

ROLE OF PHYSIOTHERAPY

Physiotherapy is an integral part of management of leprosy and is needed to prevent the onset of disabilities and deformities and also to arrest the progression of those if already developed. It is required to relieve nerve pain and keep the integrity of muscle fibers intact till they are reinnervated, if palsy has set in. It also helps in the resolution of inflammation and edema of the extremities in leprosy reaction and keeps the joints mobile. Leprosy affected persons can be managed better if physiotherapeutic measures are added to the conventional MDT and other medical management. If surgical intervention is required for correction of deformities pre- and postoperative physiotherapy is mandatory.

TECHNIQUES OF PHYSIOTHERAPY AS APPLIED TO LEPROSY AFFECTED PERSONS

Commonly used physiotherapeutic methods in management of leprosy affected persons are hydro-oleo therapy, exercise, splinting, heat therapy and electrical stimulation.[49] These methods are simple and can be organized with very little inputs.

Soaking in Water and Oil Application

Due to autonomic nerve damage, the sweating is affected. The skin becomes dry and can crack resulting in fissures. Soaking in water and oil application is done to make the skin supple and soft. It can be practiced at least twice a day but is not advised if the part is acutely inflamed, has injuries or blisters and is infected.

The hands and feet are soaked in water at room temperature for 10–15 minutes in a suitable pot, like a plastic tub. After soaking, the skin is gently scrubbed with a thick cloth to rub off the dead keratin, taking special care around the fissures and ulcers to prevent damage to the delicate tissues lying in the depth of fissure. Any vegetable oil is then applied on wet skin in drops and lightly massaged so that it mixes well with the water on the skin and forms an emulsion film on the skin surface and helps to retain the moisture longer. To distract the insects and rats, camphor can be added to the oil to give it a smell.

While the oil is being applied and massaged, the finger joints are passively stretched 10–12 times each. If cracks or fissures are present in the digital creases, care is taken not to stretch them. The thumb web is also stretched by holding on to the head of first metacarpal and pulling it away from the index metacarpal. These maneuvers prevent the development of contractures. Oil massage is also preparatory to active exercises of the hands and feet.

Exercises

Active and resisted exercises are performed to increase the strength of the muscles and retain their tone. Active exercises are most useful in cases with early and incomplete motor paralysis. The exercise can induce hypertrophy of the remaining fibers increasing their power of contraction and may compensate for the damaged muscle fibers. These exercises also prevent disuse atrophy of the remaining muscles in a palsied limb and help overcome the mild joint stiffness and contracture. Since weak muscles get fatigued early, these should be exercised for relatively shorter periods.

Assisted active exercises are performed to prevent damage to the anatomical structures by adaptive postures, e.g. damage to extensor expansion of the fingers due to clawing and constant proximal interphalangeal (PIP) joint flexion. These exercises are called assisted because external support is used to stabilize the joints rendered unstable by muscle palsies, e.g. exercising PIP joints of fingers by supporting MCP joints in 90° flexion to prevent stretching and damage to extensor expansion.

Passive exercises, where joint movements are carried out with full outside support (instead of by the muscles which normally perform that movement), are aimed to put the joint through full range of movement so that contractures do not develop in opposite group of muscles and also in the joints. Mild to moderate established contractures can be overcome by forced passive movements. Such forced passive movements are gently performed in anesthetic extremities so that internal tissues are gradually stretched and do not get inflamed ending up with further scarring. Different exercises for the fingers and thumb are shown in Figures 38.2A to E.

The foot is massaged after properly cleaning the nails and interdigital spaces. The toe joints, subtalar joints and ankle are gently moved through full range of motion both actively and passively (Figs 38.3A and B). If facial muscles are weak eye closure exercises and blowing of the balloon is performed, 20–25 cycles two to three times a day, to strengthen these muscles. Different exercises that are commonly performed for the hand and foot and their benefits are listed in Table 38.6.

Splints and Splinting

Splints are external appliances which are worn over the affected part of the body to hold it in a desired position. These can be made from different materials.[50-52] Splinting is done to achieve different objectives individually or in combination, viz. to immobilize a part to relieve pain, to stabilize a joint, to retain the joint/part after release of contracture in a particular position, to prevent its movement in a particular direction and also to provide continuous gradual stretching.[52]

With innovative approaches, a variety of splints have been developed to serve a specific purpose. These are easy to carry, simple to apply and effective in preventing the progression of deformities in if these have developed.[51]

Claw Hand

The splints used to manage finger clawing can be static, that is to maintain the joint position or dynamic where some form of mechanism is incorporated to exercise the fingers.[53,54] The splints can be made of steel wire,[55] plaster of Paris, polyvinyl tubes[56] or thermoplastic materials. Prefabricated splints made of organic polymer, which have a screw mechanism incorporated in them, are now available. The screw can be manually tightened (half a

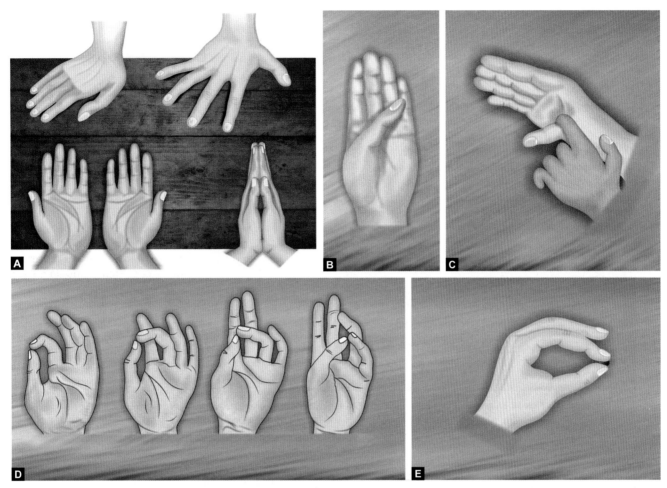

Figs 38.2A to E: Exercises for fingers and thumb. (A) Finger abduction and adduction exercises; (B) Thumb MCPJ joint flexion with IPJ extended; (C) Stretching of thumb web; (D) Apposition of thumb to pulp of individual fingers; (E) Pinching with index finger

turn in a day) to stretch the contracture especially of PIP joints. Since leprosy affected hands are anesthetic, using these splints is little risky. For this reason, these splints are not recommended to be used as a routine.

Common splints in use for hand deformities are: gutter splints, finger loop splints, opponens splints and adductor band (Figs 38.4 to 38.7). These splints can be easily fabricated at the local level.

Gutter splint is in the form of a half cut tube (made of thick, firm polyvinyl material) lined with felt and provided with Velcro fasteners at its either ends (Figs 38.5A and B). It is a static splint.

Loop splint consists of a loop of rexin or other suitable soft material having an eyelet at its end. Through this eyelet opening a rubber band is threaded and tied to itself. The other end of rubber band is tied to a wrist band at appropriate tension (Figs 38.6A and B). This is a dynamic splint and is used for exercising the fingers. It helps in strengthening the extensor systems of the fingers.

Opponens splint is similar to loop splint, the loop here is wider to accommodate for diagonal movement of the thumb (Figs 38.7A and B).

Adductor band consists of a straight band of appropriate dimensions at either end of which Velcro fasteners are stitched (Fig. 38.5C).

A simple spiral splint made out of 10 SWG galvanized steel wire sheathed with thick rubber sleeve is easy to fabricate and can be used by patient anytime (Fig. 38.4C). It stabilizes all four fingers.[55]

Serial splinting[50,54] involves repeated application of plaster of Paris casts to PIP joint(s) of the fingers at regular intervals to overcome the contractures gradually. The contracted finger is passively stretched and held in that position by a plaster of Paris cast, made by wrapping a wet plaster of Paris bandage (45 cm long and 5 cm wide) so as to form four to five layers around PIP joint, which is held in desired position till the cast is dry. Care is taken to apply the layers with moderate tightness so as not to impair the blood circulation and also not to press on knuckles otherwise skin in that area may necrose. The fingertip

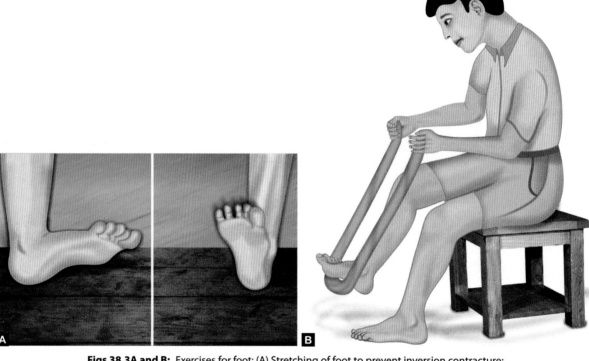

Figs 38.3A and B: Exercises for foot: (A) Stretching of foot to prevent inversion contracture; (B) Stretching of calf muscles and passive dorsiflexion of foot

Table 38.6: Benefits of different exercises of the hand and foot

Figure number	Exercises and its benefits
Fig. 38.2A	Finger abduction and adduction exercises strengthen the interossei and opens up the interdigital web space
Fig. 38.2B	Thumb MCP joint flexion with extended IP joint mobilizes MCP joint and prevents its contracture
Fig. 38.2C	Stretching of thumb web
Fig. 38.2D	Thumb approaches the pulp of individual fingers and in the process rotates through full range of movement
Fig. 38.2E	Helps in picking small objects and strengthens pulp to pulp pinch between index finger and thumb
Fig. 38.3A	Stretches the foot to prevent inversion contracture
Fig. 38.3B	Passive stretching of calf muscles and tendoachilles to prevent its contracture

is left exposed to monitor circulation (Fig. 38.8A). This cast is retained for a week. Then the cast is removed, wax therapy is given and the cast is reapplied with some more stretching. Minimum force is used while stretching so that circulation is not compromised and soft tissues are not injured. The process is repeated till the contracture is overcome. The release so obtained, is then maintained by gutter splints. For stretching the thumb web wedges of increasing angles, made of plaster of Paris, are applied at regular intervals as above (Fig. 38.8B).

Where to use and Which Splint?

When the palsy is just begun and little finger is not able to adduct, adductor band splint is used. For a hand with mobile finger clawing, loop splints are preferred. If the thumb is also paralyzed then opponens splint is used in addition. If the fingers have mild stiffness then loop splints are used during day time to exercise the fingers and gutter splints are used during night to maintain the stretched position of the fingers. For fingers with obvious contractures gutter splints are used. Similarly for the thumb interphalangeal (IP) joint, gutter splints are used.[51] If it can be managed, serial splinting gives better results in shorter period of time.

If thumb web has mild contracture, opponens splint will take care of it. However, if the thumb web had contracted, it can be stretched with plaster of Paris wedges of gradually increasing angles applied at periodic intervals.

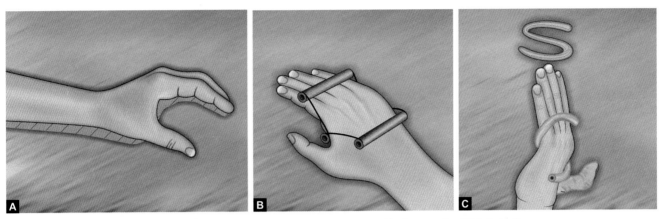

Figs 38.4A to C: Splints: (A) Wrist drop splint; (B) Knuckle duster splint; (C) Spiral splint

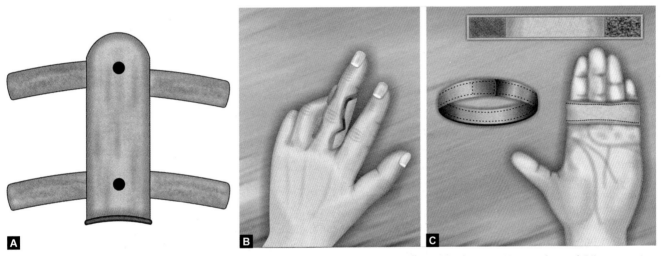

Figs 38.5A to C: Gutter splint and adductor band. (A) Standard gutter splint with Velcro fasteners; (B) Gutter splint with 'V' cut to accommodate PIPJ joint in cases having boutonniere deformity; (C) Adductor band

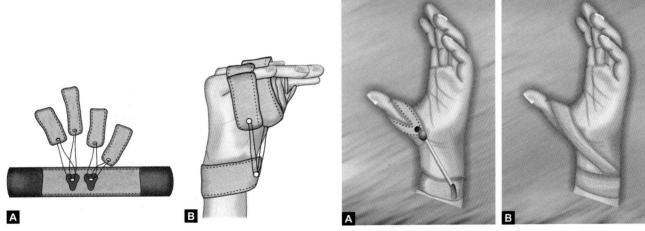

Figs 38.6A and B: Finger loop splint and its use. (A) Finger loop splint; (B) Splint in use

Figs 38.7A and B: Splints for the thumb. (A) Loop splint for opponens in use; (B) Static splinting of thumb in abduction using adhesive tape

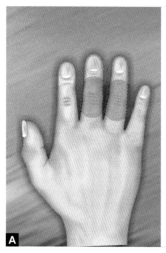 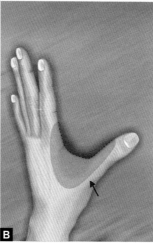

Figs 38.8A and B: Commonly used plaster of Paris splints;
(A) Cylindrical splint; (B) Thumb web splint

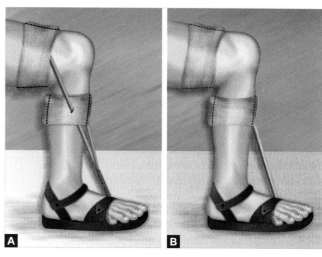

Figs 38.9A and B: Drop foot splints. (A) 'Y' strap with spring;
(B) Single elastic strap

Duration of Splinting

Even though it is difficult to predict the duration of splinting required for a particular case, majority of case have been observed to improve in 8–12 weeks time.[50,51,57] The splints are used till the improvement reaches a plateau and continued thereafter to keep the fingers mobile till the surgery is performed. If the patient is not willing to undergo surgery, he can continue using static splints during night.

Precautions to be observed while splinting the fingers and thumb: The adjustment of tension while applying splints to fingers is critical. In contracted fingers do not try to open up the fingers fully on the first day itself. The fingers should be stretched gradually. If redness or blisters occur on the dorsal aspect of the finger, discontinue the use of splints or loosen it. If patient complains of pain or swelling or bluish discoloration of nail or pulp occurs, the splint is immediately removed and its use discontinued till the condition is settled. Reapplication is done at a lower tension.

For loop splints the tension in the rubber bands is adjusted in such a way that metacarpophalangeal (MCP) joint is kept in 70–90° flexion. The rubber bands should not be over stretchable (beyond 10°) to prevent full MCP joint extension. The splints are not effective if the contracture has become fixed, i.e. it cannot be passively stretched by force. Such cases require a prior surgical release.

Foot Drop

Splinting for foot drop is aimed to prevent stretching of dorsiflexor muscles of the foot and prevent contracture of tendo-Achilles. A below knee slab of plaster of Paris, to keep the foot in neutral position, is adequate. It is important to wear the splint during night time because foot muscles can be unduly stretched by foot movements during sleep or while maneuvering the quilt or sheet to cover oneself. Alternatively a 'Y' strap with spring (Fig. 38.9A) or single elastic strap (Fig. 38.9B) can be used to provide lift to the forefoot while walking, prevent stretching of the dorsiflexors of the foot and prevent contracture of tendo-Achilles. This splint can be used while waiting recovery of muscles and also if the patient is not willing for surgery.[52,56]

Facial Palsy

The facial skin is appropriately splinted with hypoallergenic adhesive tape strips so that lower lid is not sagging due to gravity, and the angle of mouth is not deviated (Fig. 38.10). This is only a temporary measure and can be tried for few weeks, only if recovery is expected.

Splinting for Nerve Pain

The affected limb is placed in a splint made of suitable and easily available material so as to prevent the movement of nerve (joint across which the nerve trunk takes its course) and provide rest to the nerve. The joint is immobilized in such a position that the nerve is relaxed. For ulnar nerve (behind the elbow) the joint is kept at 110°, for median nerve the wrist is rested in neutral position, for common peroneal nerve knee is kept in 35–40° flexion and for posterior tibial nerve pain, the foot is kept in 15–20° plantar flexion (Figs 38.11A to D). For ulnar nerve at elbow the splint should extend up to mid arm, for median nerve up to mid forearm, up to lower third of thigh for common peroneal nerve and up to middle of the leg for posterior tibial nerve. The splint should be well-padded so that it does not press on the inflamed nerve. The splinting is continued till the pain subsides. When the pain has subsided, the joint position is gradually altered to gently stretch the nerve trunk so that it gains some freedom to move

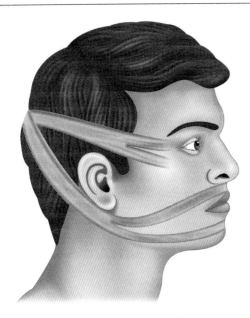

Fig. 38.10: Splinting for facial palsy

with joint movements. Total duration of splinting may vary from 3 weeks to 4 weeks, i.e. until tenderness subsides. If heat therapy is also given side by side, then splint is removed for the application of heat and then reapplied.

Heat Therapy

Superficial heating modalities like heating pads, hydrotherapy and paraffin baths which heat by conduction, are not able to heat past a depth of 2–3 cm because of the factors like patient tolerance, tissue resistance to heating and the body response to local heating. Of these, wax bath is most commonly used in leprosy because most of the tissues to be heated are within 2 cm from the body surface.

The physiologic effects of heat application are increased collagen extensibility, decreased joint stiffness, relief of pain and muscle spasm, increased blood flow and resolution of inflammatory infiltrates, edema and exudates. At 45°C, collagen is known to stretch irreversibly, proportional to the stress applied.[58] Several mechanisms have been postulated to explain the effectiveness of heat therapy including cutaneous

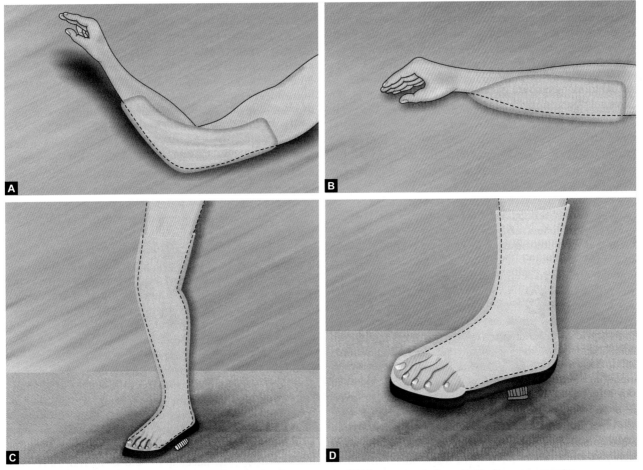

Figs 38.11A to D: Limb position for splinting for nerve pain. (A) Ulnar nerve at elbow; (B) Median nerve at wrist; (C) Common peroneal nerve at knee; (D) Posterior tibial nerve at ankle

counter-irritant action, vasodilatation with flushing of pain mediators, endorphin mediated response and altered cell membrane permeability. Elevated pain threshold has been documented with deep heating modalities.[59]

Wax bath is a method to give heat therapy where the part to be treated is covered with warm molten wax. It is useful in the treatment of nerve pain and stiff joints.[49] It is also used as an initiator before massage, exercises and splinting. It is also used before and after surgery for the hand deformities. Hot wax permits sustained heating of the part for a considerable period (up to 20 minutes or longer depending upon the ambient temperature).[60] In addition, it makes the skin supple, stimulates the sweat glands and improves blood circulation in the skin.

The heat of molten wax does not penetrate deep; therefore wax therapy has only marginal value in treating deep-seated pain. The main contraindication for wax therapy is presence of blisters and open sores. The temperature of the molten wax should be 42–45°C. The melting point of commercially available wax is about 65°C. It is lowered down by mixing wax with Vaseline and liquid paraffin in a ratio of 2:1:1. Portions of Vaseline and liquid paraffin are added to the molten wax and mixed till the desired melting point (42°C) is obtained.

The patients have to be careful not to touch the sides and the bottom of the bath. The part to be treated is dipped in the molten wax in such a way that a thick continuous coat of wax covers the part like a sleeve or glove. It requires about 6–8 dippings for getting a complete glove or else the molten wax can be poured over the part till it is fully covered. The outer layer of wax cools down to form insulation, preserving heat in deeper layers. After the coat is formed, the part is wrapped in a thick towel and is kept still for about 20 minutes. The coat is then peeled off and returned to the wax tub. The patient can practice oil massage and exercises after the wax therapy.

Electrical Stimulation

Electrical stimulating currents have low frequency and long wavelengths and easily penetrate human tissues. Electrical stimulation has been used for reduction of pain, stimulation of neuromuscular function and to stimulate the bone and soft tissue healing. Electrical stimulation of muscles has also been used to reduce edema and also to strengthen and re-educate the muscle.[61] Transcutaneous electrical nerve stimulation (TENS) has been widely used to treat acute and chronic painful conditions.[62] It has also been used in leprosy.[63] High frequency, low intensity TENS activates peripheral A beta fibers selectively, which blocks or modulates the pain carrying inputs at the level of the dorsal horn of spinal cord. Pain relief by TENS also occurs by release of endogenous opioids into the brainstem cerebrospinal fluid. It is also likely that afferent nociceptive inputs are blocked due to antidromic stimulation.

Physiologic tolerance to TENS may develop in due course of time.

Physiotherapy for special hand problems like reaction hand, recent motor palsies and finger contractures for hand has been discussed elsewhere in the book.

PREVENTION OF PROGRESSION OF DISABILITIES

The components of this activity include early detection of nerve damage and also the care for existing disabilities. Of these, severity of nerve damage decides the actual clinical outcome. More severe damage of shorter duration sometimes has better prognosis in contrast to a less severe damage of longer duration, viz. silent neuropathy which is chronic insidious type of nerve damage and has variable response to therapy.[9,64]

Problems faced by the patients having insensitive extremities (hands and feet) are: (1) problems of disuse or under use, (2) problems of misuse and overuse and (3) problems of protection.

Problems of disuse are seen in hands in patients having unilateral palsies especially where nondominant side is affected. Patients avoid using affected limb even if it is surgically restored until it is absolutely essential for them to use that.[65] This results in disuse atrophy of the muscles. In growing children disuse results in hypoplasia of the limb. The limb may also be neglected by the patient resulting in skin and joint contractures.

Problems of misuse and overuse are different in hands and feet. In hands, even if motor capability is there, the efficiency is reduced. The paralyzed hand adopts unnatural postures due to muscle imbalance and functionally convenient movement patterns for activities of daily living leading to contractures. The postures get some what fixed. In median nerve palsy pinch is badly affected. Even with simple anesthesia patients complain that they cannot hold the objects properly. They have a feeling that objects will fall down and therefore, tend to use much more force than what is actually required. This leads to gradual resorption of their fingertips. Fine manipulative activities cannot be performed. In cases with bilateral involvements it is a severe handicap. Blisters may develop on fingers and palm if they happen to hold hot objects like a cup of tea or while dipping the bread in hot gravy while taking food.

Patients keep standing on the same foot without changing postures for quite some time and walk briskly over long distances without resting their feet. Walking with large or wide steps, walking on hot pavements or in the presence of small pebble(s) in the shoes may also result in blisters on the sole, eventually leading to ulcer formation. Even if they have plantar ulcers they walk and injure the foot further in the process. The absence of pain is the root cause for all such misadventures. Surgically restored limbs are prone to injuries because patients are likely to carry a false impression that their limbs have become normal and do not require extra care anymore.

Problems of protected use are peculiar. Even if patients are aware of their deficiencies, psychological and social pressures come in their way. Also, there is an inherent desire in these patients to perform and behave like normal persons. As a result, they are likely to damage their hands and feet. The patients are shy to use appliances. At times it is because of social compulsions (to hide their disease and avoid social embarrassment) that they are not able to take protective measures.

Management

The patient needs to be properly examined and evaluated before a tailored scheme for his rehabilitation can be worked out.[66] A need based program has better chances to succeed. The evaluation includes, besides age and occupation, assessment of residual sensory motor functions and psychological state to find out his reaction and attitude toward his problems. The sensory evaluation begins by asking the patient to outline the area of sensory loss on his palm and sole. The presence or absence of protective sensations and use of hand by the patient for daily activities is assessed. Since no single test can completely assess the complexity of sensibility and dysfunctions, it is better to apply a battery of tests selected after initial examination.

Proper counseling is done in several sittings and options are suggested. It is for the patient to decide and choose the one that suits him the best under the circumstances. A constant feedback is obtained as it helps to check whether the patient understands his self-care routine and is carrying it out or not. During visits the patient can be asked to demonstrate his self-care skills. Special checks are to be made for 'think-blink' and footwear.

Health education is an important component of the management scheme and key to success. It should start from the day patient is brought under MDT umbrella and continue until he is ready to be released from control. Patient has to be told about the causation of injuries and ulcers. The role of sensory loss in this context has to be made clear. The patient should be explained the cause of anesthesia and also the methods to protect their hands and feet if affected. Simple and easy to follow instructions are important to ensure compliance. The patients must understand their physical limitations due to disease and accept that. Once this has been achieved, they can be empowered to adapt to the new situations.

Self-care is the responsibility of the individual who has NFI and he is expected to carry this out on daily basis. The healthcare workers are expected to educate and guide patients in self-care practices. The hydro-oleo therapy and passive exercises are prescribed to keep the skin supple and mobile. Looking for injuries, redness, blisters and impending ulcers in hands and feet on daily basis is essential. If found, prompt treatment, goes a long way in preventing mutilations.

The patients are taught protected use of hands and feet. They are advised to use visual feedback while using their hands for different tasks and use both hands with conscious effort. Use of tools and appliances with protective (molded) handles at home and at place of work can be suggested. Sensory re-education program can be tried in cases having some residual sensibility, especially in younger patients. With some training protective sensibility can be restored.

Constant use of proper fitting protective footwear is desirable. It is not a must to go in for conventional MCR footwear since it is not easily available in the market. As a matter of fact any footwear will reduce the walking foot pressure to the extent of 25%. The appropriate footwear should have a tough outer sole of 15–18 mm thick, soft inner sole of 18–22 mm thick and comparable firmness 15–20 shore. In addition to forefoot straps, a heal strap should also be there so that the footwear does not slip out of anesthetic foot. Ideally all the components of the footwear should have been stitched with thread or glued and have Velcro fasteners. Iron nails and buckles are to be avoided. Many commercial firms are making 'Raja Model' now and it is easily available. Earlier this 'Raja Model' (its MCR version was prescribed to leprosy affected persons) carried a stigma with it but now the design is very popular with the masses because of its comfort. Footwear is a cost-effective intervention in preventing plantar ulcers and its recurrences and along with self-care practices has done wonders for the patients. There might be some initial hesitation, but with time patients accept it realizing the benefits.

Treating and preventing disability should be an integral part of any control program and it is recommended that patients released from MDT programs should be followed up on a long-term basis with regard to appearance or worsening of disabilities. Only 10% cases are deformed, it means only one-tenth of the total cases need continued attention. In addition to early detection and provision of MDT, the process of POID has to be addressed at every level of care. A comprehensive concept of POID needs to be developed involving all areas of leprosy control, viz. early detection, MDT, nerve function assessments, identification of high-risk patients, prophylaxis, treatment, reconstructive surgery and rehabilitation.

Prevention of POID at the initiation and during MDT calls for proper recording of base line data and regular follow-up information about nerve function, detection of high-risk cases and management of reactions. Clinical diagnosis of leprosy is relatively simple, but the value of detailed records should not be undermined by presuming that 6 or 12 months of MDT is the answer for the disease and its related/associated problems. An initial record of disease when patient enters the MDT program is essential to keep track of events. The deformities and condition of the nerves should be carefully recorded so that we know how the patient is progressing. If the patient develops any reactive episodes and/or painful tender nerves, he needs management preferably under supervision. Regular testing should include accurate measurement of function in the eyes, hands and feet and recording of other disabling or stigmatizing signs in face. This is more important because activity of disease in nerve persists longer and may continue to exist even after skin is free from disease.

The physician must recognize the psychology of the person who has lost sensations in their limbs. Even intelligent patients continue to use their infected finger and continue to walk on wounds destroying their feet. Many patients who feel stigmatized by disease and by their deformity retain an immense desire to perform normally in the society. They want to walk faster, do other activities with their hands rejecting protective appliances that identify them as disabled. They love to do things with their own hands and even succeed at times at the expense of injury and infection. With a low self image, it is less likely for them to save their hands and feet. We have to spend some time to explain to them the physiology, pathology, mechanisms and psychology of their deformities and encourage them to believe that their limbs can be saved with some extra care.

DISABILITIES IN LEPROSY IN THE CONTEXT OF NEWER CONCEPTS

Leprosy-related disability is a challenge in endemic countries. The current concept of disabilities has undergone changes in recent years. The concept of health and wellness has expanded. Disability is more than a mere physical dysfunction and includes activity limitations, stigma, discrimination, and social participation restrictions. Disability is now conceptualized not as the presence of an illness or impairment but rather as the relationship between the disease/illness/impairment, the persons functioning within daily activities/social roles, and the social, cultural, and physical environments that enable or limit an individual's ability to participate fully in his or her community and daily lives. Several dimensions of disability are recognized in the International Classification of Functioning, Disability and Health (ICF): body structure and function (and impairment thereof), activity (and activity restrictions) and participation (and participation restrictions). The classification also recognizes the role of physical and social environmental factors in affecting disability outcomes. The ICF shifts the focus from the cause of disability to its effect, thereby emphasizing the role of the environment (physical, cultural, social and political) rather than focusing on disability as a 'medical' or 'biological' dysfunction.[67] The term includes mental and social disabilities as well.

Global disability measurement tools have been developed to measure these broad concepts.[68-70] A number of generic disability tools have been recommended and tried for disability assessment in lymphatic filariasis (LF).[71] These generic tools are suggested to be necessary and appropriate measures of disability impact for LF as they have been developed and validated internationally allowing for multicountry surveys. Leprosy related disabilities need assessment of the extent and its determinants among persons during and after release from multidrug treatment. It can be argued that a leprosy specific tool would allow greater sensitivity in the assessment of outcomes, particularly for patients in chronic stages of the disease where the physical impacts are irreversible and quality of life rather than cure becomes the aim of intervention.

Several scales have been developed applied and tested in leprosy. One such scale is Screening of Activity Limitation and Safety Awareness (SALSA), and it is a questionnaire that measures activity limitation in peripheral neuropathy (leprosy and diabetes),[72,73] has been validated and showed good correlations with another established scale to measure disability.[74] It is a cross-cultural tool, comprising 20 items of daily activities, related to the three domains of mobility, self-care and work. The questionnaire is administered by an interviewer. It is a subjective tool placing the interviewee at the center presenting how the client himself perceives his functional level. The SALSA group at Yahoo has been established to give information and facilitate communication between people who use or want to use the SALSA as a clinical tool or in research. SALSA scale is available in several Indian languages.

As a consequence of impairments, people affected by leprosy may experience limitations in activities of daily living.[75-77] To date, there is little insight into the impact of leprosy impairments on daily activities and social participation. To what extent, persons affected by leprosy also experience limitations in activities and perceive participation restrictions is not well-known, as these specific issues receive only limited attention during treatment.[78] Most studies have been performed in leprosy endemic countries and have focused only on impairments.[79-81] An International, Multicenter Study (in Brazil, China, India, Israel and Nigeria), in which an activity limitation questionnaire was used, showed a consistent increase in activity limitations with age and increased level of impairments.[69] Participation problems have been reported in leprosy endemic countries by a limited number of studies.[68,73,82,83] Major determinants of participation were severity of impairment and level of education, activity and stigma.[83] In leprosy, being a chronic disease, patients have time to adapt to the increasing impairments and limitations in activities. This adaptation may contribute to the mildness of the perceived restrictions in participation and autonomy. Probably for this reason 'Phantom limb' phenomenon is not common in leprosy affected people.[84] The severity of participation problems consistently increases with the severity of impairments.[78]

Future projections of the global leprosy burden show that 5 million new cases would arise between 2000 and 2020, and that in 2020 there would be an estimated 1 million people with WHO grade 2 disability.[85] There is very little data on the types of problems faced by people with leprosy-related disabilities (PLD) and the resulting needs they have for services. The current "enhanced global strategy to further reduce the disease burden due to leprosy" of WHO describes the necessary elements of prevention of disabilities and rehabilitation of persons affected by leprosy. Though much progress has been made in reducing the number of leprosy patients registered for MDT globally, relatively little is known about disability after release from treatment. Therefore, there is an urgent need for data on leprosy-related disability to assess the need for prevention of disabilities (POD) and rehabilitation services. Such data are also needed for program monitoring, evaluation and for advocacy.[86]

The development of a specific disability assessment tool, relevant to assess leprosy impact in the contexts and cultures of endemic areas, is vital for accurate reporting and measurement. A focus on morbidity management is increasingly required for leprosy related disabilities as we spend more years with elimination levels of disease. Reliable information about patient and community needs and the measurement of outcomes of the POD and POID activities is required to ensure best management for the prevention and alleviation of leprosy related disability.

The agencies working for leprosy continue to identify and prevent physical disability. However, there is limited motivation and financial support to develop substantial rehabilitation programs that support mental health and well-being, minimize barriers from stigma, provide adequate intervention for chronic disabilities to prevent their further progression and assist in re-engagement with daily activities which are important for patients both physically, mentally, and socially. The most commonly reported psychological issues, such as, feelings of shame, humiliation, low self-esteem, and fear are not measured by any tools. Likewise, the most commonly reported environmental issues are also not well-measured by the tools.

To improve daily life activities and social participation, leprosy affected persons may benefit from multidisciplinary rehabilitation treatment. Since impairments are important contributors to limitations in activities and participation restrictions, interventions such as footwear and devices to compensate for these impairments can be considered along with psychological counseling.

The most important determinant for future interventions appears to be impairment status at diagnosis. Deterioration in Nerve function impairment and disabilities can continue to occur after release from treatment. Eye, hand and foot (EHF) score has been suggested to be assessed at diagnosis, during MDT, reactional episodes and RFT.

This indicates a need for specific activities to prevent worsening of impairments also after RFT, especially surveillance of persons at high risk, training in foot and hand care, and provision of assistive devices. To improve social participation, interventions may be needed at different levels. At the personal and physical level, this would include measures such as improving education, income and activity, addressing physical impairments and rehabilitation; and at the societal level, reduction of stigma in the community and addressing other environmental barriers.

One such program, which involves the community and is cost-effective: integrated prevention of disability (IPOD) aims to improve the functional ability of the individual, reduce social and self-stigma and discrimination from the community.

In addition to physical impairment, the stigma of leprosy has a large impact on the lives of many people, affecting their physical, psychological, social and economic well-being. People with disability are often burdened with social stigma that promotes a cycle of poverty via unemployment, social discrimination and threats to mental health. Stigma has multiple causes; these should be addressed in partnership with communities and persons affected. Stigma reduction activities and socioeconomic rehabilitation are urgently needed in addition to strategies to reduce the development of further disabilities after release from treatment.

The biggest challenge lies ahead for the leprosy program managers to sustain interest and maintain services. They need to have a focused and coordinated approach to leprosy control at the primary health center level. Maintaining expertise for leprosy in health workers is another challenge since the disease is becoming relatively rarer. These issues need to be tackled appropriately.

REFERENCES

1. WHO Technical Report Series 1970, No 459:26-30.
2. WHO Technical Report Series 1988, No 768:35.
3. WHO. Leprosy disabilities: magnitude of the problem. Wkly Epidemiol Rec. 1995;70:269-75.
4. Gupte MD. Dapsone treatment and deformities: a retrospective study. Lepr India. 1979;51:218-35.
5. Tiwari VD, Mehta RP. Deformities in leprosy patients of Indian armed forces treated/reviewed at military hospital Agra (a retrospective study). Lepr India. 1981;53:369-78.
6. Kaur P, Singh G. Deformities in leprosy patients attending urban leprosy clinic at Varanasi. Indian J Lepr. 1985;57:178-82.
7. Srinivasan H, Noordeen SK. Epidemiology of disabilities in leprosy. Int J Lepr. 1966;34:170-4.
8. Wardekar RV. Sulphone treatment and deformities in leprosy. Lepr India. 1968;40:1-18.
9. Srinivasan H, Rao KS, Shanmugam N. Steroid therapy in recent: Quiet nerve paralysis. Lepr India. 1982;54:412-9.
10. Brand P. Temperature variation and leprosy deformity. Int J Lepr. 1959;27:1-7.

11. Brand P. Deformities in leprosy—orthopedic principles and practical methods of relief. In: Cochrane RG (Ed). Leprosy in Theory and Practice. London: John Wright & Sons Ltd; 1964: pp. 447-96.

12. Chacko CJ, Bhanu T, Victor V, et al. The significance of changes in nasal mucosa in indeterminate, tuberculoid and borderline leprosy. Lepr India. 1979;51:8-22.

13. Malaviya GN, Ramu G, Mukherjee A, et al. Synovial swellings over wrist in Leprosy. Indian J Lepr. 1985;57:350-3.

14. Ramu G, Balakrishnan S. Arthritis in lepromatous leprosy: clinical features and biochemical findings. Lepr India. 1968;40:62-9.

15. Pearson JM, Ross WF. Nerve involvement in leprosy: pathology, differential diagnosis, and principles of management. Lepr Rev. 1975;46:199-212.

16. Stefani MM, Martelli CM, Morais-Neto, et al. Assessment of anti-PGL-I as a prognostic marker in leprosy reaction. Int J Lepr. 1998;65:356-64.

17. Touw-Langendijk EM, Brandsma JW, Anderson JG. Treatment of ulnar and median nerve function loss in borderline leprosy. Lepr Rev. 1984;55:41-6.

18. van Brakel WH, Khawas IB. Nerve function impairment in leprosy: an epidemiological and clinical study—part 2: results of steroid treatment. Lepr Rev. 1996;67:104-18.

19. Sugumaran DS. Steroid therapy for paralytic deformities in leprosy. Int J Lepr. 1997;65:337-44.

20. Croft RP, Nicholls P, Anderson, et al. Effect of prophylactic corticosteroids on the incidence of reactions in newly diagnosed multibacillary leprosy patients. Int J Lepr. 1999;67:75-7.

21. Lockwood DN. Steroids in leprosy type I (reversal) reactions: mechanism of action and effectiveness. Lepr Rev. 2000;71:S111-4.

22. Anderson A. TRIPOD trial—prophylactic use of prednisolone, results at 4 and 6 months. Int J Lepr. 2001;69:S146-S14.

23. Ebenezer M, Andrews P, Solomon S. Comparative trial of steroids and surgical intervention in the management of ulnar neuritis. Int J Lepr. 1996;64:282-6.

24. Malaviya GN, Ramu G. Role of surgical decompression in ulnar neuritis of leprosy. Lepr India. 1982;4:287-302.

25. Srinivasan H. Surgical decompression of ulnar nerve. Indian J Lepr. 1984;56:520-31.

26. Kazen R. Role of surgery of nerves in leprosy in the restoration of sensibility in hands and feet of leprosy patients. Indian J Lepr. 1996;68:55-66.

27. Pearson JM. The evaluation of nerve damage in leprosy. Lepr Rev. 1982;53:119-30.

28. Malaviya GN, Husain S, Mishra B, et al. Protective sensibility—its monofilament nylon threshold equivalents in leprosy patients. Indian J Lepr. 1997;69:149-58.

29. Saltzman CL, Rashid R, Hayes A, et al. 4.50-gram monofilament sensation beneath both first metatarsal heads indicates protective foot sensation in diabetic patients. J Bone Joint Surg. 2004;86-A:717-23.

30. Birke JA, Simm DS. Plantar sensory thresholds in the ulcerative foot. Lepr Rev. 1986;57:261-7.

31. Hammond CJ, Klenerman P. Protective sensations in the foot in leprosy. Lepr Rev. 1988;59:347-54.

32. Stratford CJ, Owen BM. The effect of footwear on sensory testing in leprosy. Lepr Rev. 1994;65:58-65.

33. Malaviya GN, Husain S, Girdhar A, et al. Sensory functions in limbs of normal persons and leprosy patients with peripheral trunk damage. Indian J Lepr. 1994;66:157-64.

34. Conomy JP, Barnes KL. Quantitative assessment of cutaneous sensory function in subjects with neurologic diseases. J Neuro Sci. 1976;30:221-35.

35. Jain GL, Pasricha JS, Guha SK. Objective grading of the loss of pain and touch sensations in leprosy patients. Int J Lepr. 1986;54:525-29.

36. Brandsma JW. Basic nerve function assessment in leprosy patients. Lepr Rev. 1981;52:161-70.

37. Anderson AM, Croft RP. Reliability of Semmes-Weinstein monofilament and ball pen sensory testing and voluntary muscle testing in Bangladesh. Lepr Rev. 1999;70:305-13.

38. Birke JA, Brandsma JW, Schreuders T, et al. Sensory testing with monofilaments in Hansen's disease and normal control subjects. Int J Lepr. 2000;68:291-8.

39. van Brackel WH. Detecting peripheral nerve damage in the field our tools in 2000 and beyond. Indian J Lepr. 2000;72:47-64.

40. Brandsma JW. Monitoring motor nerve function in leprosy patients. Lepr Rev. 2000;71:258-67.

41. Fritschi EP. Field detection of early neuritis in leprosy. Lepr Rev. 1987;58:173-7.

42. Malaviya GN. Rapid neurological-evaluation of leprosy patients in field. Indian J Phys Med Rehab. 1991;4:4-9.

43. Palande DD, Bowden RE. Early detection of damage to nerves in leprosy. Lepr Rev. 1992;63:60-72.

44. van Brakel WH, Shute J, Dixon JA, et al. Evaluation of sensibility in leprosy: comparison of various clinical methods. Lepr Rev. 1994;65:106-21.

45. Lewis S. Reproducibility of sensory testing and voluntary motor testing in evaluating the treatment of acute neuritis in leprosy patients. Lepr Rev. 1983;54:23-30.

46. Lienhardt C, Currie H, Wheeler JG. Inter-observer variability in the assessment of nerve functions in leprosy patients in Ethiopia. Int J Lepr. 1995;63:62-76.

47. Brandsma JW, Van Brakel WH, Anderson AM, et al. Intertester reliability of manual strength testing in leprosy patients. Lepr Rev. 1998;69:257-66.

48. Prevention of disabilities. Lepr Rev. 2002;73 (Suppl 1):S35-S43.

49. Namasivayam PR. Physiotherapy in leprosy. Lepr India. 1963;35:65-73.

50. Selvapandian AJ, Menon MP, Palani N. Use of splints in the treatment of deformed hands in leprosy. Lepr India. 1964;36:20-43.

51. Shah A. Prevention and correction of claw hand by splintage—A new approach to deformity care. Bombay: Ciba-Geigy Leprosy Fund & Hindustan Ciba-Geigy Limited (1992).

52. Brandsma JW. Splinting in leprosy. Indian J Lepr. 2001;73:37-45.

53. Kulkarni VN, Mehta JM. Splinting of hand in leprosy. Lepr India. 1983;55:483-4.

54. Kulkarni VN, Mehta JM. Special features of physical therapy in the claw hand in leprosy. Lepr India. 1983;55:694-6.

55. Namasivayam PR. A spiral splint for claw fingers. Lepr India. 1976;48:258-60.

56. Theuvenet WJ, Ruchal SP, Soares DJ, et al. Advantages, indications and the manufacturing of melted PVC water pipe splints. Lepr Rev. 1994;65:385-95.

57. Koulamban SL. The role of static and dynamic splints, physiotherapy techniques and time in straightening contracted inter-phalangeal joints. Lepr India. 1969;323-8.

58. Lehmann JF, Masock AJ, Warren CG, et al. Effect of therapeutic temperatures on tendon extensibility. Arch Phys Med Rehabil. 1970;51:481-7.

59. Lehmann JF, Brunner GD, Stow RW. Pain threshold measurements after therapeutic application of ultrasound, microwaves and infrared. Arch Phys Med Rehabil. 1958;39:560-5.

60. Allis JB. Use of paraffin in leprosy. Lepr Rev. 1961;32:167-74.

61. Hamilton JM. The place of electrical stimulation in the physiotherapy of leprosy. Lepr India. 1977;49:197-206.

62. Long DM, Campbell JN, Gucer G. Transcutaneous electrical stimulation for relief of chronic pain. Adv Pain Res Ther. 1979;3:593-4.

63. Mehta JM, Nimbalkar ST, Thalayan K. A new approach in the relief of pain of leprous neuritis. Lepr India. 1979;51:459-64.

64. van Brakel WH, Khawas IB. Silent neuropathy in leprosy: an epidemiological description. Lepr Rev. 1994;65:350-60.

65. Malaviya GN. Unfavorable results after claw finger correction surgery as seen in leprosy. Indian J Lepr. 1997;69:43-52.

66. Malaviya GN. Rehabilitation of insensitive hands. Indian J Lepr. 2002;74:151-7.

67. WHO. (2011). World report on disability. [online] Available at http://www.who.int/disabilities/world_report/2011/en/. [Accessed June, 2014].

68. van Brakel WH, Anderson AM, Mutatkar RK, et al. The participation scale: measuring a key concept in public health. Disabil Rehabil. 2006;28:193-203.

69. Kelders R, van Brakel WH, Beise K, et al. Testing and validating a simplified scale to measure social participation of people with disabilities in Indonesia. Disabil Rehabil. 2012;34:638-46.

70. Melchior H, Velema J. A comparison of the screening activity limitation and safety awareness (SALSA) scale to objective hand function assessments. Disabil Rehabil. 2011;33:2044-52.

71. Lynne Z, Susan G, Marion G, et al. Disability measurement for lymphatic filariasis: a review of generic tools used within morbidity management programs. PLoS Neglect Trop Dis. 2012;6(9):e1768.

72. Ebenso J, Fuzikawa P, Melchior H, et al. The development of a short questionnaire for screening of activity limitation and safety awareness (SALSA) in clients affected by leprosy or diabetes. Disabil Rehabil. 2007;29:689-700.

73. Nicholls PG, Bakirtzief Z, Van Brakel WH, et al. Risk factors for participation restriction in leprosy and development of a screening tool to identify individuals at risk. Lepr Rev. 2005;76:305-15.

74. Wijk U, Brandsma WJ, Dahlstrom O, et al. The concurrent validity of the Amharic version of Screening of Activity Limitation and Safety Awareness (SALSA) in persons affected by leprosy. Leper Rev. 2013;84:13-22.

75. van Brakel WH, Anderson AM. Impairment and disability in leprosy: in search of the missing link. Indian J Lepr. 1997;69:361-76.

76. Tonelli N, Susilene M, Paschoal VD, et al. Limitations in activities of people affected by leprosy after completing multidrug therapy: application of the SALSA scale. Lepr Rev. 2012;83:172-83.

77. Ikehara E, Pedro HS, Paschoal VD. Characterization of the profession/occupation of individuals affected by leprosy and the relationship with limitations in professional activities. Indian J Lepr. 2012;84:1-8.

78. Slim FJ, van Schie CH, Keukenkamp R, et al. Effects of impairments on activities and participation in people affected by leprosy in The Netherlands. Rehabil Med. 2010;42:536-43.

79. Croft RP, Nicholls PG, Steyerberg EW, et al. A clinical prediction rule for nerve-function impairment in leprosy patients. Lancet. 2000;355:1603-6.

80. Shumin C, Diangchang L, Bing L, et al. Assessment of disability, social and economic situations of people affected by leprosy in Shandong province, People's Republic of China. Lepr Rev. 2003;74:215-21.

81. Richardus JH, Nicholls PG, Croft RP, et al. Incidence of acute nerve function impairment and reactions in leprosy: a prospective cohort analysis after 5 years of follow-up. Int J Epidemiol. 2004;33:337-43.

82. Cross H, Choudhary R. STEP: an intervention to address the issue of stigma related to leprosy in southern Nepal. Lepr Rev. 2005;76:316-24.

83. van Brakel WH, Sihombing B, Djarir H, et al. Disability in people affected by leprosy: the role of impairment, activity, social participation, stigma and discrimination. Glob Health Action. 2012;5:183-94.

84. Malaviya GN. Sensory perception in leprosy - neurophysiological correlates. Int J Lepr. 2003;71:119-24.

85. Richardus JH, Habbema JD. The impact of leprosy control on the transmission of M. leprae: is elimination being attained? Lepr Rev. 2007;78:330-7.

86. van Brakel WH, Officer A. Approaches and tools for measuring disability in low and middle-income countries. Lepr Rev. 2008;79:50-64.

Relapse in Leprosy

Devinder Mohan Thappa, Sowmya Kaimal, Divya Gupta

INTRODUCTION

Relapse of diseases, acute or chronic, caused by bacterial infections is quite common. Usually relapse indicates a failure to treat the infection thoroughly and this is compounded by irregular treatment, particularly in chronic diseases.

The treatment of leprosy, compared to other infectious diseases, is unique in terms of the fixed dose and duration of regimens and also in terms of the definition of "cure". Often, termination of treatment is based on the completion of recommended duration of treatment, rather than the disappearance of clinical signs and symptoms which led to initiation of treatment in the first place. Inadequate and incomplete treatment is the most important risk factor for reactivation and relapse, and it is quite often difficult to differentiate between the two.

Thus, the principal mode of assessing the efficacy of therapeutic regimens in leprosy is the "relapse rate". A very low relapse rate over an adequate period of observation indicates that the regimen used has been effective. The correct diagnosis of relapse and its differentiation from late reversal reaction (RR) is very important, particularly in the field conditions.

DEFINITION

The definition of "relapse" can be understood only in the context of the definition of "cure". In the era of dapsone monotherapy, a patient with multibacillary (MB) disease was declared "disease arrested" when skin lesions resolved and when three-monthly consecutive skin smears were negative for acid-fast bacilli (AFB), after which antileprosy treatment

was continued for another 5–10 years or even life time. A paucibacillary (PB) patient was declared "disease free" when all skin lesions resolved with no infiltration and no erythema; and nerves no longer painful or tender, after which antileprosy treatment was continued for 3–5 years.[1] With the advent of multidrug therapy (MDT), such rigid clinical criteria for cure have lost their importance. A leprosy patient is defined by the WHO, as the one who is found to have signs and symptoms of the disease and who has still not completed the prescribed duration of therapy. As of 1997, WHO recommends 1 year of MB-MDT for MB patients (12 pulses in 18 months) and 6 months of PB-MDT (6 pulses in 9 months) for PB patients. At any point of time during therapy, the patient should have ingested two-third of the pulses till that time. For operational purposes, once a patient receives adequate chemotherapy, he is considered "cured". Histopathological resolution of the lesions and clinical subsidence of the disease may take months to years after MDT is stopped.

Several definitions have been proposed for relapse in leprosy:

1. **Guide to Leprosy Control (WHO 1988)**
   A patient who successfully completes an adequate course of MDT, but who subsequently develops new signs and symptoms of the disease, either during the surveillance period (2 years for PB and 5 years for MB leprosy) or thereafter.

2. **Becx-Bleumink Lists Several Criteria for Relapse,[2]** which include:
   - New skin lesions
   - New activity in previously existing skin lesions

- Bacteriological index (BI) 2+ or more in two sets of skin smears
- New nerve function loss
- Histological evidence of relapse in skin or nerve biopsy
- Lepromatous activity in the eye(s).

3. **Relapse in Paucibacillary Patients**
   - Boerrigter et al.:[3] "Appearance of a new skin lesion or increase in size of pre-existing skin lesion, provided there is either strong clinical or definite histopathological evidence (or both) of leprosy in such a lesion".
   - Pandian et al.[4] proposed seven criteria for defining relapse in PB: (1) extension of the lesion, (2) infiltration, (3) erythema, (4) occurrence of fresh lesions, (5) pain and tenderness of nerve, (6) new paralysis of muscles, and (7) bacteriological positivity".
   - Linder et al.[5] defined relapse, as a case which has already received a course of specific antileprosy treatment and returns with signs of active disease which require a second course of treatment. Here a course of treatment is defined as 1 month less than the actual proposed minimum duration of MDT, e.g. 11 months for MB and 5 months of treatment for PB cases.

Regardless of the definition used for a case of relapse, it is important to remember that relapse in MB cases is relatively easy to recognize clinically, while in PB cases relapse may be difficult to distinguish clinically from late RR, occurring sometime after the therapy is completed.

Majority of the relapsed cases are in the age-group 30–44 years, followed by cases aged 45–59 years.[6] Relapses are frequent in males. During 2010, the sentinel surveillance network in 9 countries found a disparity in the sex of the 88 relapsed cases tested: 71 (81%) were male and only 17 (19%) were female.[6]

RELAPSE RATE

A reliable determination of the relapse rate is the single most important parameter determining the efficacy of MDT. The International Federation of Anti-Leprosy Associations (ILEP) suggests evaluating the effectivity of a control program by calculating the percentage of the number of patients treated for relapse versus the number of those treated for the first time in the same year. If this exceeds 5%, the control program should be reassessed.[5]

There are wide variations in the estimates of relapse rates in different regions. This is probably due to variations in the definition of relapse, proportions of previously dapsone-treated and untreated patients, range of skin smear positivity in MB cases, and differing durations of follow-up. The risk of relapse is very low, both for PB and MB patients after completion of MDT, and this is at least 10 times lower than with dapsone monotherapy.[1]

Also, often there is a lack of clear definition of relapse in the national guidelines and/or lack of awareness in the project staff about this definition, as a result of which the criteria for diagnosis are not applied in a uniform manner. This was borne out in a multicenter study on quality of routine data collection on relapses, where the overall rate of relapse per new patient treated varied from 0% to 29.4% in individual projects.[7]

The WHO has estimated a risk of relapse of 0.77% for MB, and 1.07% for PB patients, 9 years after stopping MDT. Various other studies using person-years (PY) of observation estimate relapse rates varying from 0.65% to 3.0% for PB, and 0.02% to 0.8% for MB leprosy.[1]

A prospective study on relapse rate from Phillipines included 300 smear-positive MB patients after being treated with MDT for 1 year. Each patient was followed up for a mean duration of 6.4 years. Only one case of relapse was detected 7 years after MDT, with an absolute relapse rate of 0.3% (0.52/1,000 patient-years at risk).[8]

A retrospective study of data from the Central Leprosy Teaching and Research Institute (CLTRI), Chengalpattu, Tamil Nadu, included 3,248 leprosy patients who completed WHO-MDT during the period 1987–2003.[9] The overall relapse rates for MB and PB leprosy were 0.84% and 1.9% respectively, while the rates for PY of follow-up were 0.86 and 1.92 per 1,000 respectively. Majority of the relapses occurred in the first 3 years after release from treatment (RFT). If an individual does not relapse within the first 5–6 years, his/her risk of relapsing is negligible.

In four consecutive follow-up surveys conducted in 1975–1977, 1978–1980, 1980–1982, and 1983–1985, among patients in South India, who had previously received dapsone monotherapy in 1973, relapse rates for leprosy were 106.1, 72.7 and 76.4 per 1,000 per year during the last three follow-up surveys, respectively. The age-specific relapse rates reduced from the first to the third follow-up survey.[10]

A cohort of 2,185 individuals was clinically evaluated for evidence of relapse, 2–7 years after RFT following WHO recommended MDT. There were 64 (2.9%) relapsed cases among them. Of the relapses, 75% and 95% of them occurred within 3 and 4 years after RFT respectively. Overall incidence of relapse per 1,000 PY was 6.7. Incidence of relapse per 1,000 PY was higher among men and in MB patients.[11]

In a recent retrospective analysis of relapse rate in China after 24 months of WHO MB-MDT for 2,374 MB patients, who were followed up for a mean duration of 8.27 years per patient, 5 patients with relapse were identified with an accumulated relapse rate of 0.21/1,000 person-years, which is quite low.[12]

Surprisingly, there were no confirmed relapses in 502 patients who completed fixed-duration MDT in the AMFES (ALERT MDT Field Evaluation Study) cohort, a descriptive study of leprosy in Ethiopia,[13] in a follow-up period of up to 8 years after completion of treatment. The study group included 57 cases with an initial average BI $\geq$ 4.0, 20 of whom have been followed for more than 5 years after ceasing MDT without any relapse. This again indicates that the relapse rates after MDT are low.

In a recent study from North India, the relapse rate in MB patients treated with 12 months of MB-MDT was found to be 1.7%, and 12 months of treatment was deemed sufficient.[14] Similarly, Deshpande et al. found that the relapse rate in those treated for 24 months was comparable to those treated for 12 months, and concluded that 12 months of MDT was both robust and adequate.[15]

Conversely, high relapse rate of 6.70 relapses/100 patient-years (RR = 9.80/100 patient-years if BI ≥ 2, RR = 5.60/100 patient-years if BI < 2; RR = 7.70/100 patient-years when treated for 24 months, RR = 5.70/100 patient-years when treated until smear negativity) was found in a Colombian retrospective cohort study on MB patients, who were followed up for 10 years from 1994–2004.[16]

MICROBIOLOGICAL ASPECTS

The conventional method of confirming activity or relapse in an infectious disease is demonstration and/or culture of the etiologic agent. These methods unfortunately have limited utility in leprosy because of the difficulty in demonstrating bacilli in PB cases and absence of a method of *in vitro* cultivation of *M. leprae*. Unlike PB leprosy, where the criteria for relapse depend heavily on clinical features, bacteriological parameters are useful mostly in MB leprosy.

Reappearance of positivity for AFB after the case has become negative has been considered a feature of relapse in both PB and MB cases. BI, persisting at the same level, an increase in BI of 2+, appearance of new active lesions with high BI, or BI becoming greater than what it originally was in the pre-existing lesion are some of the criteria for diagnosing relapse in MB leprosy. However, an increase in BI of even 1+ (checked repeatedly) should be considered as adequate supporting evidence for diagnosing relapse in patients who had earlier become negative, or were showing downward trend in BI after MDT.[17]

A number of *in vivo* and *in vitro* techniques are available for monitoring the progress of treatment in leprosy, which can also be used as additional objective criteria for confirming relapse.

In Vivo Techniques

Mouse Foot-pad Studies

This method measures the viability and includes cultivation of *M. leprae*.

In Vitro Techniques for Assessing the Viability

- Morphological index
- Fluorescein diacetate-ethidium bromide (FDA-EB) staining

- Laser microprobe mass analysis (LAMMA)
- Adenosine triphosphate (ATP) measurements
- Macrophage-based assays.

Molecular Techniques

- Deoxyribonucleic acid and ribonucleic acid targeting probes
- Polymerase chain reaction (PCR) for gene amplification[17]

A study conducted at the Schieffelin Leprosy Research and Training Center, Karigiri, India, tested biopsy samples of lepromatous patients who had completed 12 and 24 months of MB-MDT, for viable *M. leprae* by mouse foot-pad inoculation.[18] None of the skin or nerve biopsies from patients who completed 24 months of MDT showed any growth, while a small percentage (3.3%) of patients with a high BI were found to harbor viable bacteria in the skin after 12 doses of MDT. These patients need to be followed up for a longer period to ascertain whether or not they will relapse.

It may be possible to differentiate reinfection from relapse by molecular typing of *M. leprae*, based on amino acid sequencing, as well as to identify relapse at a very early stage using nucleic acid amplification techniques such as PCR.[19]

IMMUNOLOGICAL TESTS FOR RELAPSE

Although there are no widely available serologic tests for leprosy other than in a research setting, various immunological tests may be useful for monitoring patients on chemotherapy as well as for confirming suspected cases of relapse.

Phenolic Glycolipid 1 Antibodies

Lepromatous leprosy (LL) patients show a significant rise in titer of phenolic glycolipid 1 (PGL-1) immunoglobulin M (IgM) antibodies during the time of relapse. Tuberculoid leprosy (TT)/borderline tuberculoid (BT) cases who relapse to borderline lepromatous (BL)/lepromatous leprosy (LL) types may be detected by measuring anti-PGL-1 and anti-35 kD antibodies.[19]

The dipstick assay for detection of anti-PGL-1 antibodies has been used as a simple tool for classification of patients and for identification of those patients who have an increased risk of relapse.[20]

The Natural Disaccharide-Octyl-Bovine Serum Albumin Enzyme-Linked Immunosorbent Assay

This method [using the natural disaccharide (ND) of the phenolic glycolipid antigen of *M. leprae* linked to bovine serum albumin as antigen] is another useful test both for screening for early infection with *M. leprae* and for predicting a relapse, particularly in cured MB patients.[21]

Interleukins-based Assays

The Th1 and Th2 types of interleukin profile may be a useful method of identifying the type of relapsed leprosy. For example, when BL/LL patients relapse as TT/BT type, an upgradation of cell-mediated immunity (CMI) is expected, in the form of a Th1 type of immune response, which consists of a rise in levels of interferon gamma (IFN-γ), interleukin 2 (IL-2) and immunoglobulin G2 (IgG2) antibodies, in addition to a positive lepromin test. On the other hand, when TT/BT patients relapse to BL/LL types, a Th2 type of immune response is initiated, which should lead to a rise in IL-4, IL-5, IL-6, IL-10 and IgG1 production, and a concomitant fall in the levels of IL-2 and IFN-γ, and lepromin negativity.[19]

HISTOPATHOLOGY

Regular skin biopsies and skin smears, at least once in 6 months, from representative lesions should be studied during the period of treatment and the following 5 years after achieving negativity.

Histopathology of Relapsed Lesions in MB Leprosy[22]

Lepromatous leprosy lesions resolve under treatment, increasing number of macrophages become foamy, Schwann cells also show foamy change, there is reactive proliferation of the perineurium, and increasing fragmentation and granularity of the AFB in the granuloma. The granuloma gradually resolves, without any residual fibrosis or scar formation and there is fibrous replacement of the perineurium and hyalinization of the nerve parenchyma. Foam cell collections are known to persist for long periods in tissues, many years after the skin smears have become negative. A mild nonspecific chronic inflammation characterized by small focal collections of lymphocytes around skin adnexa can also persist in resolved LL lesions for several years.

In the early phase of relapse, small and large foci of newly arrived spindle-shaped macrophages with pink granular cytoplasm are identified along with a few small clumps of persisting foamy macrophages. Solid staining AFBs reappear in skin smears and biopsy specimens, in patients who may or may not have become completely smear-negative. Once the lesion is well-established, the foamy change becomes obscured by collections of spindle-shaped and immature macrophages. Skin adnexa are markedly atrophic and scanty, and dermal nerve bundles are few and show perineurial thickening and fibrosis. Macrophages, Schwann cells and endothelial cells are packed with solid staining AFBs.

Occasionally, there is infiltration by polymorphs, and it is also not uncommon to see LL patients relapsing with upgrading reactions, in the form of borderline lepromatous (BL) or rarely, borderline tuberculoid (BT) lesions.

Lesions of BL resolve much faster than polar LL cases and become bacteriologically negative much earlier.

Histopathologically, BL lesions leave behind a few focal collections of mononuclear cells around skin adnexae, and foam cells are not usually seen. Relapses in BL leprosy may manifest as LL, BL or rarely, as BT.

Histopathology of Relapsed Lesions in PB Leprosy[22]

Lesions in BT and TT leprosy are the result of a hypersensitive granulomatous response to the antigens of *M. leprae*, and are not directly due to the presence of *M. leprae*. With treatment, there is reduction in the size of the granuloma without any fibrous replacement of the skin adnexae. Dermal collagen is destroyed during the inflammatory process, leading to an atrophied and wrinkled appearance of healed skin lesions. Nerves undergo perineural and intraneural fibrosis. *M. leprae* get buried alive in these nerves and also in the arrector pili muscle cells, thereby serving as a possible focus for relapse.

The difficulty that arises in PB cases is the differentiation of relapse from type 1 reaction. Features that suggest a reaction include edema around the granuloma, dilated lymphatics and proliferating fibroblasts throughout the dermis. A true relapse can be detected histopathologically only after recording complete histological resolution of the lesion, which may take years. Relapse indicates that the bacilli have survived despite antileprosy therapy and have multiplied and released antigens to produce fresh granulomas. This manifests as appearance of solid staining organisms inside fibrosed nerve bundles (where there were none earlier), and the reappearance of a granuloma at the site of the original lesion. This granuloma usually begins as a small focus of lymphocytes and epithelioid cells, which often starts in the fibrosed nerve bundles or arrector pili muscle cells. Once the granuloma becomes well-established, it grows and involves large portions of the dermis, becoming indistinguishable from the original lesion. Therefore, in PB patients, regular 6-monthly biopsies showing disappearance of the granuloma will confirm "cure", and reappearance of the granuloma will identify "relapse". Rarely, PB cases will relapse as MB, and this is usually due to misdiagnosis of spectrum of the disease and the resultant inadequate treatment in the first place. In a follow-up of 100 released from treatment cases, 26 patients relapsed, of which, 10 PB cases relapsed as MB (38.5%).[23]

RELAPSE INTERVAL

Relapse interval is otherwise known as incubation period of relapse.[24] It is different with monotherapy and MDT.

Dapsone Monotherapy[24]

Majority (55.0–57.0%) of relapses occurred within:
- 3 years in nonlepromatous
- 5 years in borderline
- 6 years in lepromatous

Multidrug Therapy[24]

- *PB*: Same as with monotherapy
- *MB*: 9 years (median)

The implication of these figures is that PB patients should be under surveillance for at least 3 years and MB patients for 9 years, so that majority of the relapses can be detected.[24]

CLASSIFICATION OF RELAPSE

Kar et al. have classified relapse as follows:[25]
1. *Early relapse (0–3 years)*: Because of original misclassification resulting in inadequate/insufficient duration of chemotherapy or irregular treatment.
2. *Late relapse (3–10 years)*: Because of drug resistance, *M. leprae* persisters or reinfection.

PREDISPOSING FACTORS FOR RELAPSE[24]

Persisters

Persisting organisms or "persisters" consist of permanently or partially dormant organisms that have the capacity to survive in the host despite adequate chemotherapy. They have been identified in immunologically favorable sites such as dermal nerves, smooth muscle, lymph nodes, iris, bone marrow and liver. These organisms, which are responsible for relapse, are present in about 10% of MB patients, and their proportion may be higher in cases with higher BI.

Inadequate Therapy

This is usually the result of clinical miscategorization of MB leprosy with few skin lesions as PB cases, who receive 6 months of MDT instead of 12 months, initially respond to treatment, and eventually relapse.

Drug Resistance

This can be primary (infection with drug-resistant strains) or secondary (resistance develops as a consequence of irregular or monotherapy), and is an independent risk factor for relapse.[26] In one study, 6 out of 25 cases (24%) of relapse were due to drug resistance, and four out of these six patients (66.7%) showed high-degree resistance.[27] The WHO sentinel surveillance network found the prevalence of drug resistance in relapse patients to be 11.4% (10/88 cases).[6] Even in a nonendemic country like Malaysia, the prevalence of low level resistance was found to be 31%, and the level of intermediate and high level resistance was 22.1% by mouse foot-pad technique.[28] In a study from leprosy endemic Prata colony in Brazil, MB cases who had completed at least one MDT regimen and also their contacts, were investigated for drug resistance by direct sequencing of the *rpoB*, *folP1* and *gyrA* gene. Around 11% of pretreated individuals and 10% of

contacts were diagnosed with active disease. Clustering of *rpo*B and *fol*P1 mutation in this particular population was as high as 55%, indicating transmission of resistant strains among relapse cases and contacts. This indicates that disease control policies should focus on pockets of high endemicity of leprosy.[29]

Although surveillance network for drug resistance in leprosy are in place, the number of samples being tested for drug resistance remains low. Thus, we might be underestimating the role of drug resistance in relapsed cases.[30]

Irregular Therapy

Irregularity in ingesting self-administered clofazimine and dapsone either due to irregular supply of drugs or noncompliance on the part of the patient will effectively result in a scenario of rifampicin monotherapy. This will lead to rifampicin resistance, and subsequent relapse. Adherence with MDT is important to minimize the risk of relapse and avoid the emergence of drug resistance.[31] A retrospective analysis of 272 patients who were started on MDT revealed that upto 45.6% (124 patients) had defaulted on their MDT treatment. There was a significant relationship between the number of people who had grade I/II disabilities, gender (male more than females) and type of MDT (MB more than PB) and early defaulting. It is important that these groups be counseled regarding compliance to MDT at the beginning of treatment.[32]

Monotherapy

The relapse rate is high among patients who have received dapsone monotherapy, and did not later receive MDT. This is also due to the development and multiplication of resistant organisms.

High Initial BI

Patients who have a high BI initially, are at greater risk of relapse after fixed duration MDT compared to patients who are smear negative or have a low BI at registration. LL patients are four times more likely to relapse than those in the other spectrum.[16] These patients have a poor CMI, and hence, treatment cannot be stopped after 1 or 2 years, as persisters are likely to grow, resulting in relapse.[33]

Number of Skin Lesions and Nerves

The number and extent of lesions including nerve lesions, when multiple, i.e. more than five and covering three or more areas of the body correlate with higher relapse rate. Mycobacterial antibodies have been found in TT leprosy with a large number of lesions and in BT leprosy with more than

10 lesions. Since this is evidence of a fairly large number of organisms, these patients may not be truly PB, and treatment with two drugs for 6 months might be considered inadequate for these patients.

Lepromin Negativity

Borderline patients with a positive lepromin test have been observed to have a lower relapse rate than those with a negative response.

Antireaction Treatment

According to one study, patients who had taken antireaction treatment were five times more likely to relapse than those who had not. Persistence of bacilli was assumed to be the common factor that could explain both reactions and relapse.[16] In one study, nearly 50% of the relapsed patients had experienced previous recurrent erythema nodosum leprosum (ENL).[14]

Human Immunodeficiency Virus Infection

Although leprosy has now been reported to be presenting as an immune reconstitution disease among patients commencing highly active antiretroviral treatment, there is no evidence as yet to suggest an increased risk of relapse in patients with HIV coinfection.

Physiological Conditions

For example, pregnancy.

CLINICAL FEATURES

Age

In MB cases, relapse is more common in the older age groups.[6] PB leprosy with single skin lesions is more common in younger age groups, and relapse is less common in this group.[24,34]

Sex

Relapses are more common in males, possibly because of the higher prevalence of leprosy in males.[6] Relapses are seen in females in the setting of pregnancy and lactation.

Relapse in PB Leprosy

Skin Lesions

Previously subsided skin lesions show signs of renewed activity, such as infiltration, erythema, increase in extent, and appearance of satellite lesions. Often, there is an increase in the number of lesions as well.

Nerves

New nerves may become thickened and tender, accompanied by extension of area of sensory loss and insidious onset of motor deficit. Patients may complain of aches and pains along the peripheral nerves with or without evidence of nerve damage. Relapse may occur only in nerves without skin involvement (neural relapse), and there may be a change in the spectrum of disease on relapsing.

Relapse in MB Leprosy

Skin Lesions

Relapse may present as localized areas of infiltration over various parts of the body. Soft, pink, and shiny papules and subcutaneous nodules may be found at these sites, with or without a background of infiltration. Papules may enlarge to form plaques. They feel like peas in a pod, and increase in size with time. Skin smears from the overlying skin may be negative; hence, the scalpel should be plunged deep into the core of the nodule while taking smears. Relapse cases may present as histoid leprosy.

Nerves

Nodular swellings may occur along the course of cutaneous nerves and peripheral nerve trunks, in addition to fresh nerve thickening and/or tenderness, with insidious loss of function. Increase in area of sensory loss is noticed.

Ocular Lesions

Cases with pre-existing eye involvement may relapse with iris pearls or rarely, lepromata.

Mucosal Lesions

Papular or nodular lesions may be seen on the hard palate, inner lips and glans penis.

DIFFERENTIAL DIAGNOSIS

Differences Between ENL and Papules and Nodules of Relapse[24]

Papules and nodules that occur as part of relapse in the MB spectrum should be differentiated from the nodules of erythema nodosum leprosum (ENL). The most important point of difference is that ENL nodules are tender and evanescent, unlike lepromatous nodules. Additional differences are listed in Table 39.1.

Table 39.1: Differences between ENL and papules and nodules of relapse		
Feature	*ENL*	*Papules and nodules of relapse*
History of therapy	Episodes within 2 years of starting therapy in LL, LLs, and rarely BL	After completion of MB-MDT during surveillance in BB, BL, LLs, LL, and rarely BT
Onset	Sudden	Insidious
Constitutional symptoms	Present	Absent
Physical signs	Nodules are tender, warm, erythematous, blanchable on pressure, superficially located	Nontender, not warm, pink, do not blanch, involve full thickness of skin
Skin smears	Fragmented AFB, polymorphs	BI $\geq$ 2+, long solid staining AFB, globi±
Course	Change from red to bluish and dusky, evanescent subside within 48–72 hours	Pink changes to skin colored, consistency changes from soft to firm, in months

Table 39.2: Differences between reversal reaction and relapse		
Feature	*Reversal reaction*	*Relapse*
Time course	Usually within 6 months of release from treatment; in recurrent reactions up to 2 years	1 year or more after release from treatment
Type of disease	BT, BB, BL	All types
Skin lesions	Increased erythema, swelling, tenderness on pressure, succulent consistency; upward or downward change in the spectrum may occur; edema of hands/feet	Increase in extent and number of lesions, no tenderness, rubbery consistency; edema of hands and feet rare
Ulceration	Seen in severe reactions	Not seen
New lesions	Few, same morphology	Few to many
Nerves	Acute painful neuritis; nerves exquisitely tender; nerve abscess; sudden paralysis of muscles and increase in extent of sensory loss	New nerves involved; no spontaneous pain; tenderness on pressure; sensory and motor deficits slow and creeping
Skin smears	Continued decrease in BI. Granularity of bacilli increases in reactions	AFB positivity may occur in skin smear negative patients
Lepromin test	Progressively positive Mitsuda reaction	Mitsuda reaction corresponds to the type or spectrum of relapsed leprosy
Response to systemic steroids	Complete subsidence of lesions in 2–4 weeks; remain subsided with 2 adequate therapy	No response or partial response

Differences Between Reversal Reaction and Relapse

It is often a diagnostic dilemma to differentiate true relapse from a late RR in a PB case. Many studies on PB leprosy show falsely high relapse rates, possibly because of the inclusion of cases which are probably reactions and not really relapses.[24,34] Some of the features that will help in differentiating these two conditions are given in Table 39.2.

Relapse versus Resistance

Drug resistance is an emerging problem in leprosy worldwide, owing primarily to the chronicity of the disease and the long duration of treatment required.[24,34] Drug resistance may be primary, wherein lepra bacilli are resistant to the concerned drug from the onset itself, or secondary, wherein resistance develops as a result of mutant bacilli surviving in the setting of irregular therapy or monotherapy. Dapsone resistance is most common, owing to the earlier concept of dapsone monotherapy. Rifampicin resistance occurs in the setting of irregular therapy. Clofazimine resistance is very uncommon. Although mouse foot-pad studies are recommended for confirmation of drug resistance in leprosy, these facilities are not easily available, forcing clinicians to rely on clinical features alone. Drug resistance may itself be a reason for relapse, and it is important to differentiate the two, as outlined in Table 39.3.

Table 39.3: Differences between drug resistant leprosy and relapse

S. No.	Drug resistant leprosy	Relapse
1.	Due to primary or secondary drug resistance	Mainly due to persisters
2.	Initial amelioration followed by worsening	Recurrence after release from MDT
3.	Appearance of new lesions	Reappearance of lesions over old lesions
4.	Patient downgrades	Patient rarely downgrades

Abbreviation: MDT, multidrug.

Relapse versus Reactivation

Reactivation of lesions occurs due to incomplete treatment, i.e. premature termination of treatment or gross irregularity in treatment either due to noncompliance or irregular supply of drugs.[24,35] Reactivation occurs soon after subsidence of the disease while relapses occur after complete and sustained subsidence of the disease.

Relapse versus Reinfection

Recurrence of disease in a cured case may be due to reinfection.[24,35] Reinfection is an extremely difficult condition to prove, especially in an endemic area. It is a possibility when the time interval after RFT and occurrence of new lesions is beyond sufficient period of duration concordant with the incubation period of the disease, on relapse. When cured, leprosy patients continue to live in and around leprosy sanatoria or in hyperendemic areas, they may develop the disease again due to exogenous infection. Even after completing treatment, a lepromatous case does not become truly immunoincompetent, and hence, although the risk of reinfection is not high, there is a definite risk. When reinfection does occur, the incubation period is bizarre and fresh skin and nerve lesions do not correspond to the original lesions.

DIAGNOSIS

The diagnostic criteria for relapse are:[19,24]

1. Clinical Criteria

- Increase in size and extent of existing lesion(s)
- Appearance of new lesion(s)
- Erythema and infiltration in lesions that had completely subsided
- Nerve involvement (thickening or tenderness)

2. Bacteriological Criteria

Assuming a 0.5–1 log-unit/year fall in BI in a MB patient, the expected BI at the end of treatment can be calculated by subtracting the years after RFT from the initial BI (expected BI = initial BI - years after RFT). Thus, in patients with a positive BI, if BI increases by 2+ over previous smears at any two sites and continues to be so at two examinations, it is diagnosed as relapse, provided the patient has ingested 75% of the drugs. Positivity (in a smear negative patient) at any site in skin smears for AFB at two examinations during the period of surveillance is diagnostic of relapse.

Limitations of this criterion are:
1. Relapses presenting with a BI of < 2+ will not be diagnosed. This is relevant in early stages of re-multiplication and in patients with high immunity, which never present with a high BI.
2. The quality of the slit skin smears is "the weakest link in most leprosy control programs."[5]

3. Therapeutic Criteria

This is useful when RR is suspected. The patient may be treated with prednisolone (reaction dose being around 1 mg/kg/day), after which RR should subside completely in 2 months. If symptoms do not subside or only partially subside or lesions persist or increase under the cover of steroids, then relapse should be suspected.

In yet another limitation, Linder et al.[5] contend that treatment with steroids for reaction in an undiagnosed case of relapse can lead to multiplication of bacteria, and thus advocate combining it with antileprosy drugs. Therapeutic test with steroids is not performed in Linder's criteria for relapse.

4. Histopathological Criteria

This includes the reappearance of already regressed/regressing granuloma in PB cases; and increased macrophage infiltration with solid staining bacilli and increasing BI in MB cases.

5. Serological Criteria

In LL cases, the measurement of PGL-1 IgM antibodies is a good indicator of relapse.

The first three criteria are sufficient to make a diagnosis of relapse; criteria 4 and 5 are additional, and may be used wherever facilities are available.

Linder Scoring System for MB-Relapse in Leprosy[5]

This was shown to have higher sensitivity as compared to the WHO criteria. Basically it utilizes three criteria: (1) time factor, (2) risk factor, and (3) clinical presentation at relapse as given below:

I. Time factor:	
Time after release from treatment (RFT) (in months)	Score
≤ 12	0
13–24	1
25–60	2
> 60	3
II. Risk factor:	
If the initial BI is ≥ 3+	1
III. Clinical presentation at relapse:	
BI in a single lesion is ≥ 2+ higher than the expected BI*	1
Average BI is ≥ 2+ higher than the expected BI*	1
No signs of a reaction present[†]	1

Abbreviations: MB, multibacillary; BI, bacterial index.
*Expected BI = calculated BI with an assumed fall of 1 log-unit/year; if the initial BI was negative, a positive BI at relapse is sufficient to score.
[†]Clinical signs of inflammation of the nerve or the skin or erythema nodosum leprosum.

Relapses are diagnosed with a score of greater than or equal to 3; the maximal score equal to 7; the maximal score for the time factor equal to 3, the maximal score for the additional factors equal to 4, these scores are added to give the final score.

TREATMENT

Patients with a high initial BI of greater than or equal to 4.0 should preferably receive a longer treatment course and should be kept on a long-term follow-up.[5] Relapsed cases of leprosy should be identified and put back on chemotherapy as soon as possible to prevent further disability and transmission of infection.[36] Factors that should be considered in choosing an appropriate regimen are:
1. Type of leprosy (PB or MB)
2. Previous treatment history
3. Drug-resistance.

Type of Leprosy

Paucibacillary cases usually relapse as PB and MB cases as MB. However, PB cases occasionally relapse as MB, and such cases should receive MB-MDT.

Previous Therapy

- Patient previously treated with dapsone monotherapy—standard WHO-MDT is sufficient.
- Patient previously treated with clofazimine monotherapy—standard WHO-MDT is sufficient (clofazimine resistance is extremely rare).

Drug Resistance

Patients with known or suspected drug resistance pose a treatment problem only in the case of rifampicin resistance, which is rare (Table 39.4). MB patients who have received rifampicin as part of MDT are not at any significant risk of rifampicin resistance, unless they were infected with fully dapsone-resistant bacilli and either did not take their clofazimine or were not given another effective drug. Dapsone resistance occurs in the setting of prior dapsone monotherapy, and such cases respond well to standard WHO-MDT. Clofazimine resistance is extremely rare, if at all it occurs, these cases also respond to the other two drugs in the standard WHO-MDT.

Although drug resistance ideally is determined using the mouse foot-pad or other techniques, relatively few leprosy centers have such a facility available. Thus the decision on drug resistance most often is based on clinical information alone.

FAILURE TO RESPOND TO THERAPY

This group includes patients who do not show adequate bacillary clearance and subsidence of skin lesions in spite of receiving adequate treatment, or patients who actually show disease progression during therapy. The former group

Table 39.4: Recommended treatment regimens

Resistance	Scenario	Treatment
1. Relapse with *M. leprae* sensitive to all standard drugs	Relapse after a course of MB-MDT	Retreatment with WHO-MDT depending on the type of disease (PB or MB-MDT)
2. Relapse with dapsone-resistant *M. leprae*	Relapse after previous "cure" with dapsone monotherapy	Standard WHO-MDT
3. Relapse with rifampicin-resistant or rifampicin- and dapsone-resistant *M. leprae*	Primary or secondary dapsone-resistant MB cases who received standard WHO-MB-MDT but did not take their clofazimine (situation equivalent to rifampicin monotherapy)	Clofazimine 50 mg daily for 24 months plus two of the following drugs for 6 months: Ofloxacin 400 mg daily/minocycline 100 mg daily/ clarithromycin 500 mg daily, followed by: Ofloxacin 400 mg daily or minocycline 100 mg daily for the remaining 18 months

Table 39.5: Multidrug therapy regimens in the USA[39]

Type of leprosy	Dosage of drugs CLF may be added	Dapsone 100 mg after MDT for
Paucibacillary (I, TT, BT)	Dapsone 100 mg daily + Rifampin 600 mg daily for 6 months	3 years (I, TT) 5 years (BT)
Multibacillary (BB, BL, LL)	Dapsone 100 mg daily + Rifampin 600 mg daily for 3 years	10 years (BB) Lifelong (BL, LL)

contains potential relapse cases, but great care must be taken to rule out reaction and/or slow clearance of lesions and bacilli as a cause of poor response.

The WHO defines a "satisfactory result from MDT" in a patient who complies with treatment in which, after the start of therapy, bacilli begin to clear in MB cases and lesions generally though not necessarily rapidly improve in both PB and MB cases. Clearance of lesions is related more to the patient's immune response than to antileprosy treatment; all lesions and bacilli should eventually clear even though clearance may be incomplete at the time treatment is discontinued.[36] This was demonstrated in a study by Job et al.,[37] where 50% and 25% of patients treated with PB-MDT still showed histopathological activity after 6 months and 12 months respectively. In the same study, four patients had continued clinical and histopathological activity even at 23 months. This "delayed resolution" may lead to eventual treatment failures, and hence it may be desirable to follow-up high-risk patients for at least 2 years and if possible, 5 years.[37] The option of alternative antimicrobial regimen should be kept in mind for these high-risk patients, both from the outset, as well as upon relapse.[38]

Multidrug therapy regimens being used in the USA are more robust than the ones being recommended in developing countries by the WHO (Table 39.5). Although studies show that relapse rates are very low after WHO-MDT, the fact remains that relapses do occur. There is a possibility that more relapses in leprosy may develop if the WHO accepts uniform MDT. Unfortunately, it is not practical to introduce regimens like those in the USA on a large scale in a resource poor setting like India. However, clinicians may use their judgment and tailor treatment regimens for individual patients wherever practicable. In selected cases, longer regimens similar to those used in the US may be useful.

REFERENCES

1. The Leprosy Unit, WHO. Risk of relapse in leprosy. Indian J Lepr. 1995;67:13-26.
2. Becx-Bleumink M. Relapses among leprosy patients treated with multidrug therapy: Experience in the leprosy control programme of the All Africa Leprosy and Rehabilitation and Training Centre (ALERT) in Ethiopia; Practical difficulties with diagnosing relapses, operational procedures and criteria for diagnosing relapses. Int J Lepr. 1992;60:421-35.
3. Boerrigter G, Ponnighaus JM, Fine PE, et al. Four-year follow-up results of a WHO-recommended multiple-drug regimen in paucibacillary leprosy patients in Malawi. Int J Lepr. 1991;59:255-61.
4. Pandian TD, Sithambaram M, Bharathi R, et al. A study of relapse in non-lepromatous and intermediate groups of leprosy. Indian J Lepr. 1985;57:149-58.
5. Linder K, Zia M, Kern WV, et al. Relapses vs. reactions in multibacillary leprosy: proposal of new relapse criteria. Trop Med Int Health. 2008;13:295-309.
6. World Health Organisation. Surveillance of drug resistance in leprosy: 2010. Weekly Epidemiological Record. 2011;86:233-40.
7. Deepak S, Gazzoli G. A multi-centre study on quality of routine data collection on relapses. Lepr Rev. 2012;83:340-3.
8. Maghanoy A, Mallari I, Balagon M, et al. Relapse study in smear positive multibacillary (MB) leprosy after 1 year WHO-multi-drug therapy (MDT) in Cebu, Philippines. Lepr Rev. 2011;82:65-9.
9. Ali MK, Thorat DM, Subramanian M, et al. A study on trend of relapse in leprosy and factors influencing relapse. Indian J Lepr. 2005;77:105-15.
10. Arockiasamy J, Bhatnagar T, Mehendale SM, et al. Trends in incidence and relapse rates of leprosy during dapsone monotherapy era in south India. Paper presented at: 18th International Leprosy Congress; 2013 Sep 16-19; Brussels, Belgium.
11. Selvaraj V, Prabu R, Manickam P, et al. Incidence of relapse in a cohort of 2185 individuals released from treatment in south India. Paper presented at: 18th International Leprosy Congress; 2013 Sep 16-19; Brussels, Belgium.
12. Shen J, Liu M, Zhang J, et al. Relapse in MB leprosy patients treated with 24 months of MDT in south west China: a short report. Lepr Rev. 2006;77:219-24.
13. Gebre S, Saunderson P, Byass P. Relapses after fixed duration multiple drug therapy: the AMFES cohort. Lepr Rev. 2000;71:325-31.
14. Dogra S, Kumaran MS, Narang T, et al. Clinical characteristics and outcome in multibacillary (MB) leprosy patients treated with 12 months WHO MDT-MBR: a retrospective analysis of 730 patients from a leprosy clinic at a tertiary care hospital of Northern India. Lepr Rev. 2013;84:65-75.
15. Deshpande J, Chougule SG, Thakar UH, et al. Rate of relapse and reactions in MB leprosy patients after 24 and 12 months of MDT in Maharashtra. Indian J Lepr. 2004;76:229-30.
16. Guerrero-Guerrero MI, Muvdi-Arenas S, León-Franco CI. Relapses in multibacillary leprosy patients: a retrospective cohort of 11 years in Colombia. Lepr Rev. 2012;83:247-60.
17. Katoch VM. Microbiological aspects of relapse in leprosy. Indian J Lepr. 1995;67:85-98.
18. Ebenezer GJ, Daniel S, Norman G, et al. Are viable Mycobacterium leprae present in lepromatous patients after completion of 12 months' and 24 months' multi-drug therapy? Indian J Lepr. 2004;76:199-206.
19. Sengupta U. Immunological aspects of relapse in leprosy. Indian J Lepr. 1995;67:81-3.

20. Bührer-Sékula S, Cunha MG, Foss NT, et al. Dipstick assay to identify leprosy patients who have an increased risk of relapse. Trop Med Int Health. 2001;6:317-23.
21. Wu Q, Yin Y, Zhang L, et al. A study on a possibility of predicting early relapse in leprosy using a ND-O-BSA based ELISA. Int J Lepr Other Mycobact Dis. 2002;70:1-8.
22. Job CK. Histopathological features of relapsed leprosy. Indian J Lepr. 1995;67:69-80.
23. Vara N, Agrawal M, Marfatia Y. Leprosy beyond MDT: study of follow-up of 100 released from treatment cases. Indian J Lepr. 2010;82:189-94.
24. Ramu G. Clinical features and diagnosis of relapses in leprosy. Indian J Lepr. 1995;67:45-59.
25. Kar HK, Sharma P. New lesions after MDT in PB and MB leprosy: a report of 28 cases. Indian J Lepr. 2008;80:247-55.
26. Williams DL, Gillis TP. Drug-resistant leprosy: monitoring and current status. Lepr Rev. 2012;83:269-81.
27. Sekar B, Arunagiri K, Kumar BN, et al. Detection of mutations in folp1, rpoB and gyrA genes of *M. leprae* by PCR– direct sequencing—a rapid tool for screening drug resistance in leprosy. Lepr Rev. 2011;82:36-45.
28. Jamil A, Noor NM, Osman AS, et al. Primary dapsone resistant *Mycobacterium leprae* in a nonendemic country. Indian J Dermatol Venereol Leprol. 2013;79:527-9.
29. Rosa PS, Diório SM, Belone AF, et al. Evidence of active transmission of drug resistant *Mycobacterium leprae* strain in Brazil. Paper presented at: 18th International Leprosy Congress; 2013 Sep 16-19; Brussels, Belgium.
30. Saunderson P. Relapse and drug resistance in leprosy. Paper presented at: 18th International Leprosy Congress; 2013 Sep 16-19; Brussels, Belgium.
31. Weiand D, Thoulass J, Smith WC. Assessing and improving adherence with multidrug therapy. Lepr Rev. 2012;83:282-91.
32. Prakashkumar MD, Ebenezer M. Profile of defaulters and patterns of defaulting in a leprosy hospital in south India. Paper presented at: 18th International Leprosy Congress; 2013 Sep 16-19; Brussels, Belgium.
33. Munisamy M, Thappa DM. Fixed-duration therapy in leprosy: Limitations and opportunities. Indian J Dermatol. 2013;58:93-100.
34. Pfaltzgraff RE, Ramu G. Clinical leprosy. In: Hastings RC, Opromolla DV (Eds). Leprosy, 2nd edition. Edinburgh: Churchill Livingstone; 1994. pp. 237-87.
35. Desikan KV. Relapse, reactivation or reinfection. Indian J Lepr. 1995;67:3-11.
36. Jacobson RR. Treatment of relapsed leprosy. Indian J Lepr. 1995;67:99-102.
37. Job CK, Jayakumar J, Aschhoff M. Delayed resolution versus treatment failure in paucibacillary leprosy patients under six months fixed duration multidrug therapy. Indian J Lepr. 1997;69:131-42.
38. Gelber RH, Balagon VF, Cellona RV. The relapse rate in MB leprosy patients treated with 2-years of WHO-MDT is not low. Int J Lepr Other Mycobact Dis. 2004;72:493-500.
39. Jacobson RR. Treatment of leprosy. In: Hastings RC, Opromolla DV (Eds). Leprosy, 2nd edition. Edinburgh: Churchill Livingstone; 1994. pp. 317-49.

40
CHAPTER

Drug Resistance in Leprosy

Masanori Matsuoka

INTRODUCTION

Current leprosy control is solely based on early case detection and treatment by multidrug regimen recommended by WHO.[1] *Chaulmoogra* oil had been used for leprosy treatment since ancient time, but its efficacy was partial and relapse was common.[2] Modern chemotherapy for leprosy started by the introduction of promin (diamino azobenzene-4'-sulfonamide) in 1941.[3] A more effective sulfone, dapsone (4-4'-diamino diphenyl sulfone), replaced promin 6 years later.[4] Multidrug therapy (MDT) is highly effective for leprosy treatment and global leprosy prevalence has markedly reduced over two decades.[5] However, chemotherapy and drug resistance are two sides of the same coin. First, clinically suspected dapsone resistant cases were reported soon after introducing dapsone for leprosy treatment.[6] Dapsone resistance was experimentally proved by mouse footpad method in 1964.[7] Treatment by dapsone was life-long for some cases and such prolonged monotherapy led to emergence of daposne resistance. Bactericidal efficacy of rifampicin was recognized and introduced for leprosy treatment, but most cases were treated by rifampicin alone.[8,9] Monotherapy by dapsone or rifampicin alone lasted until multi-drug treatment was applied and many cases resistant to dapsone and rifampicin were reported from various regions of the globe.[9-11] Besides single drug resistance for dapsone or rifampicin, many multi-drug resistant cases have been reported subsequently.[12-15]

Spreading of drug resistant bacilli threatened leprosy control. Surveillance and awareness of level of drug resistance is essential to prevent spreading resistant strains and to keep MDT effective. Only mouse footpad method has been available for susceptibility assay since its development by Shepard.[16] The method is not practical to analyze susceptibility of many clinical samples and one has to wait over several months to know the results. Simple and reliable method to examine susceptibility to antibiotics for leprosy had been awaited for long time. Because of PCR development and increased knowledge of molecular background for drug resistance for dapsone, rifampicin and fluoroquinolones, molecular biological methods have been available for testing the anti-leprosy drug susceptibility since 2000s.[17-19] No drug resistant case caused by transduction, such as R-plasmid is known in *Mycobacterium leprae*. Longitudinal surveillance has been executed by WHO to monitor global trend of drug resistance using molecular biological methods.[20]

CHEMOTHERAPY

Current global leprosy control is mainly based on early case detection and MDT, which consist of dapsone, rifampicin, clofazimine, and ofloxacin to overcome the threat by drug resistance (Table 40.1).[21] Other second line antibiotics such as minocycline,[22,23] streptomycin,[24] clarithromycin,[25] fluoroquinolones,[26-28] ethionamide[29] are also effective in treating leprosy (See chapter on chemotherapy for details). Chemotherapy and drug resistance in leprosy have been reviewed by Matsuoka, and Williams.[30,31]

Antileprosy Drugs and Resistance

Dapsone

The first successful chemotherapy using promin (diamiono azobenzene-4'-sulfonamide) for leprosy was reported in 1943[3] at a leprosarium in Carville, LA, USA. Patients were

Table 40.1: WHO/MDT regimen for adults			
	Criteria	*Dose*	*Duration*
MB	≥ 6 skin lesions, or positive bacterial index	*Rifampicin*: 600 mg once a month *Dapsone*: 100 mg daily *Clofazimine*: 300 mg once a month and 50 mg daily	12 months
PB	≤ 5 skin lesions and negative bacterial index	*Rifampicin*: 600 mg once a month *Dapsone*: 100 mg daily	6 months

Abbreviations: MB, multi bacillary; PB, pauci bacillary. The report of 8th WHO expert committee on leprosy excluded single lesion pauci bacillary type (SLPB).[21]

intravenously administrated 5 mL of 30% promin solution for the treatment. A more effective sulfone, dapsone (4-4'-diamino diphenil sulfone, DDS), replaced promin and dapsone was used orally.[32] Since that time, dapsone is still a fundamental anti-leprosy compound even in the MDT era which started in the1980s.

Dapsone targets folic acid biosynthesis pathway and its effect is bacteriostatic. Dapsone is an analogue of p-aminobezoic acid (PABA) and acts as a competitive inhibitor of PABA. Dapsone binds to dihydropteroate synthase (DHPS), which is encoded by the *folP1* gene and inhibits folic acid synthesis.

A relationship between DHPS mutations and dapsone resistance has been demonstrated. Dapsone does not bind to DHPS by amino acid substitution in DHPS and bacilli acquire resistance to dapsone. Missense mutations at codon 53 (ACC) or 55 (CCC), coding threonine or proline, in *folP1* gene confer dapsone resistanc.[33,34] Figures 40.1A to C show a case of dapsone resistance caused by the mutation in codon 55. Table 40.2 shows mutations detected in drug resistance determining region (DRDR) in the *folP1*, *rpoB*, and *gyrA* genes of isolates of which resistance was confirmed by mouse footpad testing.[13,30,31,33-42]

Although the first dapsone resistant suspected cases were reported in 1953.[6] No methodology to confirm resistance was available until the mouse footpad assay was developed.[7,16,43] Using this assay method, three clinically suspected isolates of dapsone resistance were proved to be resistant to dapsone by the growth in the footpad of a mouse given a diet containing 0.1% dapsone[7]. The number of dapsone resistant cases increased after dapsone monotherapy during the 1960s and 1970s[10,11,44,45] including primary dapsone resistance. Primary dapsone resistance means a resistant strain from a patient without previous administration of any anti-leprosy drugs. Secondary drug resistance cases were detected in many areas.[40,42]

Rifampicin

High bactericidal effect of rifampicin 3-[[(4-methyl-1-piperazinyl)-imino]-methyl] was shown by mouse footpad model followed by confirmation in man.[46-49] Rifampicin is currently an integral part for leprosy treatment by MDT as

Table 40.2: Mutations detected in drug resistance determining region of drug resistant isolates	
folP1	*Reference*
53:Tre(ACC) → Ile(ATC)	13, 30, 31, 40, 41
53:Tre(ACC) → Val(GTC)	40, 42
53:Tre(ACC) → Ala(GCC)	40, 42
53:Tre(ACC) → Ser(TCC)	34
53:Tre(ACC) → Arg(AGG)	41
53:Tre(ACC) → Arg(AGA)	42
55: Pro(CCC) → Ser(TCC)	30, 35
55: Pro(CCC) → Leu(CTC)	13, 30, 33, 40, 41, 42
55: Pro(CCC) → Arg(CGC)	40, 41
55: Pro(CCC) → Ala(GCC)	34
rpoB*	*Reference*
407:Gln(CAG) Val(GTG)	38
410:Asp(GAT) → Tyr(TAT)	30, 36
420:His(CAC) → Try(TAC)	30
420:His(CAC) → Asp(GAC)	17
425:Ser(TCG) → Leu(TTG)	17, 30, 35, 37, 39
425:Ser(TCG) → Met(ATG)	17, 39
425:Ser(TCG) → Phe (TTC)	17, 39
409Met(ATG) → Insertion Lys, Phe(AGTTCA)	17, 39
gyrA	*Reference*
91:Ala(GCA) → Val(GTA)	13, 30, 35, 38

* Codons are numbered by *M. leprae* numbering system. Codon 516 in reference 36 corresponds to codon 410 in the table

shown in Table 40.1. A single dose of 1200 mg or a daily dose of 600 mg for three days presumably killed all bacilli as no bacillary growth was shown in mice inoculated with bacilli from these patients.[49]

Rifampicin targets the beta (β) subunit of RNA polymerase, which is encoded by the *rpoB* gene. Rifampicin binds to the β subunit and inhibits DNA dependent mRNA transcription. Correlation between rifamipicin resistance and missense mutations within highly conserved regions in the *rpoB* gene has been shown. Isolates shift to be rifamipicin resistance by harboring missense mutations at codon 407, 410, 420, 425 and 427 (Table 40.2). These missense mutations hinder rifampicin binding to the β subunit. Figures 40.1A to C show one case of mutation occurred in rifampicin resistant strain. Missense mutation Ser (TCC) to Lue (TCG) at codon 425 is most frequently observed for rifampicin resistant *M. leprae* and also *M. tuberculosis.* (Figs 40.1A to C)[30,37,39] One rifampicin resistant isolate harbored 6 bps insertion in the codon 409.[17,39]

Rifampicin had been administered as monotherapy or in combination with dapsone, and rifampicin resistance was reported in 1970s and early 1980s. The first rifampicin resistant case was reported in 1976, in an isolate from a relapsed patient on rifampicin monotherapy, who was previously treated with dapsone.[50] A susceptibility test for 45 relapsed cases treated previously by rifampicin alone or in combination with dapsone showed that 9 cases were rifampicin resistant and 7 isolates out of 9 rifampicin resistant cases were also resistant to dapsone.[51] Another study revealed that 19 out of 35 relapsed cases were resistant to both dapsone and rifampicin and 3 isolates were resistant to rifampicin alone.[9] Resistance to backbone antibiotics for leprosy treatment threatened leprosy control and this concern has led to the introduction of multi-drug therapy in the 1980s.

Ofloxacin

Ofloxacin (4-fluoroquinolone) is a moderate bactericidal antibiotic for *M. leprae*. The bactericidal activity for *M. leprae* was first demonstrated in 1986 by the mouse

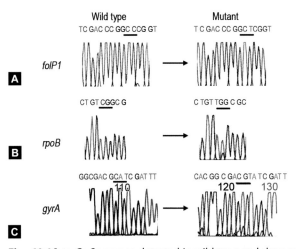

Figs 40.1A to C: Sequence detected in wild type and drug resistant mutants. Mutations in *folP1*, *rpoB*, and *gyrA* of *M. leprae* confer resistance to dapsone, rifampicin and quinolone, respectively. A; *folP1*: codon 55: CCC (Pro) → CTC (Leu), B; *rpoB*: codon 425: TCG (Ser) → TTG (Leu), C; *gyrA*: codon 91: GCA (Ala)→ GTA (Val)

footpad method and subsequently by a clinical trial.[26,52,53] Oflaxicin binds to the A subunit of DNA gyrase and inhibits DNA replication. Association between mutations within the highly conserved region of gyrA subunit coded by the *gyrA* gene and quinolone resistance was revealed in most resistant strains of mycobacteria.[54,55] The first ofloxacin resistant *M. leprae* was found in 1994 together with mutation detection in the *gyrA* gene by sequence analysis.[12] Two other cases of ofloxacin resistant *M. leprae* from Japanese relapsed cases were reported in 2000 and 2003.[14,35] Four possible ofloxacin resistant cases were found in Japan,[13] and one in Korea.[56] Recent studies indicate other fluoroquinolones are more effective for leprosy treatment.[57-59]

Three isolates confirmed to be resistant to ofloxacin harbored the mutation Ala-Val (GCA-GTA) at codon 91[12,14,35] in the *gyrA* gene (Figs 40.1A to C). One isolate for which the susceptibility could not be examined by the mouse footpad testing had the mutation Gly-Cys (GGA-TGC) at codon 89.[13] Two other amino acid changes, Ser at 91 and Asp at 94 (same codon numbers as *M. tuberculosis*), in *gyrA* of *M. tuberculosis* have been associated with quinolone resistance,[60] consequently it is predicted that mutations at codons 89, 92, and 95 in *gyrA* of *M. leprae* also confer quinolone resistance. No mouse footpad study results have been obtained for the isolate with mutation at codon 89 in gyrA up till now, but an *in vitro* molecular model study indicated mutation at this position causes quinolone resistance.[61] Although no case has been reported for mutation at codon 95, *in vitro* assay also strongly suggested that mutation at codons 95 confers quinolone resistance.[57] Another *in vitro* study indicated association between missense mutation at 464, 502, 504 in gyrB and quinolone resistance.[58] Prevalence of ofloxacin resistance is still low in some areas with high leprosy prevalence. No quinolone resistant isolate was detected among 78 isolates in Myanmar and 96 isolates in Cebu, Philippines.[42] Sentinel surveillance results also showed a very low prevalence of quinolone resistance in seven counties. Of 108 strains tested in 2009, two strains from India showed mutation in gyrA[62] no quinolone resistant case was found in 2010.[63]

Clofazimine

Clofazimine (B663, Lamprene) is [(3-p-chloroanilino)-10 (p-chlorophenyl)-2,10- dihydro-2- (isopropylimino) phenazine], bactericidal for *M. leprae*. The mechanism of action has not been fully elucidated. However, one of possible bactericidal mechanism is binding to GC rich domains.[64] Molecular background for drug resistance to clofazimine is still unclear due to the involvement of several different mechanisms. Clofazimine was first used for leprosy treatment in 1962.[65] Clofazimine is anti-inflammatory and is also used to control the type 2 reaction (erythema nodosum leprosum: ENL).

Although clofazimine has been used for leprosy treatment for over 4 decades, reported drug resistance is rare. Only one case in an article shows clear clofazimine resistance by mouse foot pad testing.[66] Other cases as clofazimine resistance are equivocal since bacillary growth is not clear or amount of clofazimine administrated is too little. Growth of some strains is inhibited in the footpad of mouse fed with 0.0001% of dapsone, but some strains grow in the footpad of mouse fed with 0.0001%, but not in foot pad of mouse treated with 0.01% and 0.001% diet, such case is regarded as dapsone resistance with low degree.[9,15] Some strains do not grow in footpad of mouse fed feed with 0.0001% of clofazimine but some other strains grow with very low concentration of clofazimine.[15,67,68] It seems concentration of 0.0001% is the critical concentration for mouse footpad susceptibility assay for both clofazimine and dapsone.

Dapsone resistant strain with low degree harbor no mutation but dapsone resistant strain with intermediate and high degree showed amino acid substitution in dapsone resistance determining region.[42] Of 6 low dapsone resistant cases, 5 strains showed no mutation in dapsone resistance determining region.[40] One exceptional case seemed due to technical error in mouse footpad assay. Feeding with 0.0001% is equal to dose of 1 mg daily for man. Taking these findings, it seems to be rational to exclude the assay for low concentration, 0.0001%, of clofazimine and dapsone by mouse footpad system.

Minocycline

Minocycline (7-dimethylamino-6-demethyl-6-deoxytetra-cycline) is the only tetracycline group active against *M. leprae*. Efficacy of minocycline against *M. leprae* was confirmed in 1987.[22,23] It is bactericidal and its activity is additive when combined with other anti-leprosy drugs.[69] Minocycline is used as second line anti leprosy drug according to the current MDT strategy by WHO.[21] Tetracyclines inhibit protein synthesis by binding to the 30S ribosomal subunit, blocking the binding of aminoacyl transfer RNA to the messenger RNA ribosomal complex.[70] To date, no minocycline resistant cases are known for *M. leprae*.

Nucleotide mutation in DRDR occurs spontaneously. The frequency of dapsone resistant mutants are estimated to be 1/10,[6] and the frequency for rifampicin and ofloxacin is estimated to be 1/10,[7] and 10^8 respectively.[31] The purposes of MDT are to enhance treatment efficacy and to kill the spontaneously induced drug resistant strains (which are resistant to one or two drugs) by the combination of more than two anti-leprosy compounds. Treatment with inappropriate regimens, drop outs and noncompliance are the main reasons for developing drug resistant leprosy cases by facilitating bacillary growth of mutants. For example, there were no authorized MDT regimens for leprosy treatment in Japan until 1997[71] and guidelines were provided by the Japanese

Leprosy Association in 2000.[72] Such inadequate conditions in defining treatment might be the cause of high prevalence of drug resistance among relapsed cases in Japan.[13]

Chemoprophylaxis has been conducted at many places to stop developing the disease.[73] A newly diagnosed untreated lepromatous case may harbor approximately 10^{10}-10^{11} bacilli.[73] Bacillary number in some people in latent phase of leprosy infection may be same in MB leprosy case. Most case of chemoprophylaxis use only rifampicin. Limited effect of chemoprophylaxis is supposed to be due to high bacillary load in some contacts, which are difficult to kill and clear by one shot of a drug.[73] Mutation conferred drug resistances occurs spontaneously with the frequency mentioned above. Monitoring drug resistance after chemoprophylaxis must be in place.[74]

METHOD FOR SUSCEPTIBILITY ASSAY

Mouse Footpad Method (MFP Method)

M. leprae is still not cultivable on axenic media *in vitro* and not only susceptibility testing but also microbiological studies had been hampered, until the development of the mouse footpad assay.[43] The first dapsone resistant case was confirmed with this method in 1964.[7] Some mutations are detected occasionally in DRDR which does not confirm whether these strains with such mutation are resistant to anti leprosy drugs, hence, footpad testing is still the gold standard for drug susceptibility in leprosy. A bacillary suspension is prepared from a biopsy sample containing bacilli. Mice are inoculated with 5,000–10,000 bacilli into the hind footpad and the bacillary number reaches 10^5 to 10^6 approximately, 25 to 30 weeks after inoculation. Mice inoculated with *M. leprae* are divided into groups of 10 to 20 mice each. One group is a control, and the remaining groups are administered drugs. Drugs are administered *per os*, either incorporated into the mouse diet (Table 40.3) or by gavage.[12,14,35,75,76] When bacillary growth is recognized in control mice at about 25–30 weeks, mice are sacrificed and bacillary growth is compared between the control group and each group of treated mice. An isolate is regarded as drug resistant when bacillary growth is present in the mouse footpads of treated mice. Results of bacillary growth for the isolate resistant to dapsone, rifampicin, and quinolones are shown in Figure 40.2. Although a diet with 0.0001% concentration are used for susceptibility assay for dapsone and clofazimine, strains grown in the footpad of mice treated with such diet does not seem resistant to these drugs as described in the discussion on clofazimine.

Mutation Detection by Sequencing

Although mouse foot pad method was breakthrough in the susceptibility test for *M. leprae*, the method is cumbersome and time-consuming, is not applicable to many strains, not

Table 40.3: Criteria for diagnosing drug resistance in the mouse	
Drug	*Concentration in the diet (%)*
Dapsone	0.0001; 0.001; 0.01*
Clofazimine	0.0001–0.001
Rifampicin	0.003–0.01
Ofloxacin	0.15
Sparfloxacin	0.02
Clarithromycin	0.03
Minocycline	0.08

*Low, intermediate or high level of resistance, respectively

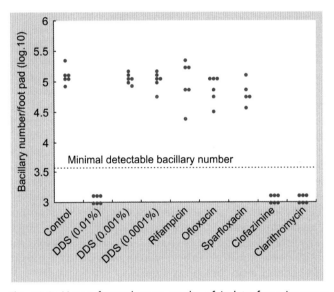

Fig. 40.2: Mouse footpad assay results of isolate from Japanese relapsed case. The strain is resistant to dapsone (of intermediate degree), rifampicin and quinolones[14]

suitable to obtain comprehensive data to monitor global level of resistance, and does not meet the needs of clinicians. The method requires viable bacilli and chilled samples are to be sent to the laboratory within a week, which is usually far from the field. Over the past two decades, mutations that lead to drug resistance to dapsone, rifampicin, and quinolones have been revealed as mentioned above. Missense mutations within a limited region in *folP1*, *rpoB*, and *gyrA* genes are in concordance with resistance to dapsone, rifampicin, and quinolones, as confirmed by mouse footpad testing. These regions are termed drug resistant determining regions (DRDR). Based on knowledge of molecular biology, DNA-based assays for detecting drug resistant *M. leprae* have been developed. Results of mouse footpad testing and sequence analysis are shown in Table 40.2.

Resistance to dapsone is classified into three grades according to bacillary growth in the mouse footpad assay with different concentrations of dapsone. Though Shepard *et al.* found that *M. leprae* obtained from untreated leprosy patients were consistently inhibited by 0.0001% dapsone in the diet,[77] Rees found that some isolates were not inhibited at this dapsone concentration.[78] Those isolates that grow in footpad of mouse treated with 0.0001% dapsone containing diet are classified into low degree resistance. No mutations were detected in *folP1* gene from 10 isolates with a low degree of dapsone resistance.[40,42] Dapsone resistance in the mouse at a concentration of 0.0001% is not associated with *folP1* gene mutations. However, such cases have no clinical significance, since administration of 0.0001g DDS per 100g mouse diet would be similar to humans receiving 1 mg DDS daily.[75] The usual dosage of DDS in MDT is 100 mg daily.[21] The mutation detection in DRDR indicated above predicts drug resistance to dapsone, rifampicin, and quinolones.

Clinical samples such as bacilli by slit skin method or biopsy are kept in 70% ethanol in room temperature. These samples are processed for DNA extraction. DRDRs are amplified by PCR and obtained PCR products are sequenced. Isolates with known missense mutation confirmed to confer drug resistance are regarded as drug resistant (Table 40.2).[20]

In mouse foot pad assay, some isolates do not multiply in control mouse footpads and their drug susceptibility cannot be determined by the MFP method. In contrast, DNA sequencing of PCR products is independent of the viability of *M. leprae*. Among 83 isolates, only 46 isolates could be tested for drug susceptibility by the mouse footpad method while 79 isolates could be sequenced and their susceptibility determined.[38] Results reveal usefulness of molecular biological method application for susceptibility testing. To prevent the spread of drug resistant isolates, comprehensive data on the magnitude of resistance is essential. The level of drug resistance in three South Asia countries, Indonesia, Philippines and Myanmar, was analyzed by PCR direct sequencing method.[42] Isolates which are primary or secondary resistant to dapsone and rifampicin were detected in Indonesia and Myanmar. Primary and secondary daspone resistance was detected in Cebu, Philippines, but no rifampicin resistant cases were found. No quinolone resistant case was detected in Philippines and Myanmar. Together with WHO's data[62,63] resistance to quinolone is still low in many areas with high prevalence of leprosy.

Mutation Detection by DNA Microarray

Direct sequencing of PCR products covering DRDR is a robust method to detect drug resistance, but implementation of sequencing is not easy in many developing countries where the prevalence of leprosy is still high. To overcome this disadvantage, some simple methods, which can be carried out without any special equipment such as sequencer, have been developed.

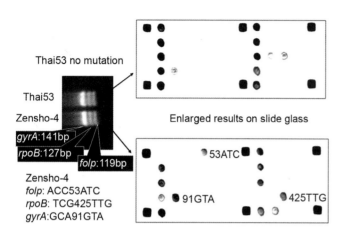

Thai53 no mutation

Thai53

Zensho-4

gyrA:141bp

rpoB:127bp

folp:119bp

Zensho-4
folp: ACC53ATC
rpoB: TCG425TTG
gyrA:GCA91GTA

Enlarged results on slide glass

53ATC

91GTA

425TTG

Fig. 40.3: Signal obtained with a susceptible strain Thai53[79] and Zensho-4[14] that has the following mutations: ATC (from ACC) in codon 53 in folP1, TTG (from TCG) in codon 425 in rpoB and GTA (from GCA) in codon 91 in gyrA. PCR products include drug resistance determining regions for three genes were amplified simultaneously in a tube

A method, LDS-DA, to detect mutations was exploited.[18] A series of oligonucleotide probes corresponding to each mutation detected in the folP1, rpoB, and gyrA genes for dapsone, rifampicin and ofloxacin resistance respectively, were selected and fixed on a glass slide as capture probes (Fig. 40.3). Biotin labeled PCR products were simultaneously amplified in a tube, denatured and hybridized with a probe corresponding to each mutation as shown in Table 40.2. Usefulness and validity of the methods was evaluated by applying them in Cebu and Myanmar. The high concordance obtained by this method in two countries with the results of nucleotide sequencing was shown. The method is feasible for testing drug susceptibility at a laboratory close to the field. These obtained data might be beneficial for both, the clinicians and patients by avoiding useless drug dosages.

Another method to detect mutation by reverse hybridization of PCR products, GenoType LepraeDR is available.[80] Probes to capture wild type and mutants are coated on the strip. PCR products for the folP1, rpoB, and gyrA genes are amplified followed by denaturation, hybridization with probes, conjugation with the enzyme alkaline phosphatase, and coloration. High concordance with in vivo assay results was confirmed. The kit is commercially available as DNA STRIP test (Hain Lifescience, Nehren, Germany).

A method without need for mutation specific probes was proposed.[81] The method is based on real-time PCR. Mutation is detected by Hetero-duplex formation and melt curve.

Buddemeyer Method

Buddemeyer method is based on detection of 14-CO_2 generation from 14-C- labeled palmitic acid in 7H12 medium with or without the metabolism by M. leprae.[82] The method requires large quantity, 10^7 of the bacilli, for one assay. The method is not applicable for susceptibility test of clinical material, but useful for screening efficacy of a compound for leprosy treatment.[83]

SENTINEL SURVEILLANCE BY WHO

Current MDT regimen consists of five drugs, dapsone, rifampicin, ofloxacin, clofazimine and minocycline. Resistance to dapsone, rifampicin and ofloxacin could be detected by molecular techniques. Although resistance to clofazimine and minocycline is not detected by sequence analysis of specific genes, frequency of drug resistance to clofazimine is negligible and no resistance to minocycline has been found. Therefore, most drug resistant cases to drugs used in MDT are detectable by mutation detection in DRDRs.

Emergence of drug resistance poses a threat to all the intervention programs. Understanding the magnitude of drug resistance is important to maintain current MDT strategy effective, and to prevent the spread of drug resistance. Although drug resistant cases or prevalence of resistance in some area have been reported occasionally, but no global comprehensive data are available. In this context, WHO started sentinel surveillance with PCR direct sequencing in 2008[20] The project aims to monitor longitudinally the level of drug resistance in both, patients who have not been treated previously and those who were previously treated and relapsed. Sentinel sites have been set in 16 countries with high leprosy incidence. Data obtained in 2009 and 2010 indicate that the level of drug resistance is still not faced with serious situation to threaten MDT regimes for leprosy control.[62,63] It is expected that comprehensive and longitudinal data for drug resistance worldwide will be obtained and lead to the pursuit of a better strategy for leprosy control.

RELAPSE AND PERSISTERS

Multi drug therapy (MDT) is effective for leprosy treatment and preventing drug resistance. However, recurrence of the disease occurs occasionally after release from MDT. Recurrence might be caused by two mechanisms. One is exacerbation of the disease by the indigenous bacillary growth which remained in the body after treatment completion. Such case is regarded as relapsed leprosy case. If bacilli from relapsed case are susceptible to drugs, the bacilli are termed as persister. Bone marrow or nerves are attributed to persistence of surviving susceptible bacilli.[84,85] Another mechanism of recurrence of the disease is due to the re-infection with exogenous bacilli. All studies on recurrence rate of the disease reported as of today did not take account on this point as no means were on hand to discriminate the bacilli between, from first time and the bacilli obtained after recurrence. Therefore, case studies for relapse rate include both persister and re-infection cases.

Differences in relapse rates depend on observation period. A total 22 patients relapsed from 927 patients, 5 years after release from MDT.[86] Observation for 16 years after MDT deduced cumulative risk of disease to be 6.6%.[87] Relapse rate observed in 424 patients for mean duration of 9.26 years, was 2.2 % or 0.2 per 100 person-years.[88] Although, high ratio of drug resistant case among relapsed cases are recognized,[9,13] one study showed many relapsed cases with drug susceptible strain.[89] Of the 15 strains form relapsed cases, mouse footpad assay showed that 14 were susceptible to rifampicin, clofazimine and dapsone. One case was of high degree dapsone resistance. A case of relapse with rifampicin and dapsone susceptible bacilli, together with a case with isolation of rifampicin susceptible and dapsone resistance bacilli was reported.[90] These cases were previously regarded as relapse with persister or with resistant strain, possibility of re-infection was neglected. Distinguishing relapse or re-infection is mandatory to evaluate the treatment efficacy. The methodology that meets such requirements has been awaited for long. Genotyping based on variable number tandem repeats (VNTRs) or single nucleotide polymorphisms (SNPs) enables to discriminate bacilli form each relapsed case.[91] Genotyping of 7 Brazilian relapsed cases showed different SNPs or VNTRs during first and second disease occurrence. The results suggest recurrence of disease with re-infection.[92] It was strongly suggested to collect and store slit skin smear and/or biopsy samples for later comparison of genotype with the bacilli from second episode.[93]

VIABILITY IN VARIOUS CONDITIONS

Determination of *M. leprae* viability is compulsory to evaluate efficacy of treatment or that of each anti-leprosy drug and recognition of bacillary growth capability in various conditions, such as in animal model, or out of body, which are the requirements for better experiments and leprosy control. Mouse footpad method devised by Shepard was a milestone for detecting viable *M. leprae*.[43] Bactericidal effect of rifampicin was revealed with mouse footpad method.[8] The method was applied to examine survival of the bacilli out of the body.[94] Bacilli survived for 9 days in a dried condition at 24–33°C, for 5 months after drying in the shade, 60 days in saline left at room temperature or in the Hanks' solution in a refrigerator, and 7 days with exposure to sunlight for 3 hours per day respectively. Additionally, the bacteria survived for 7 days in nasal discharge that had been discharged from a patient and dried.

A method of most probable-number calculation enables to measure proportion of viable bacilli in the bacterial suspension. The proportion of viable bacilli decreased with time after multiplication to 10^6 organisms per footpad. However, the method is labor intensive, time consuming and impractical.[95] Other methods were formulated to evaluate viability by fluorescent staining to analyze integrity of cell wall or radiorespirometry method to measure activity of the oxidation of palmitic acid.[82,96-98] These were applied to assess viability of the bacilli in macrophage, effectiveness of drugs, screening of anti-leprosy drugs, and to choose suitable bacterial specimens with high viability from nude mice for experiments.

Reverse transcription (RT) -PCR assays targeting messenger RNAs or 16s rRNA have been developed.[99-101] Assays are based on short half-life of prokaryotic mRNA, dead bacilli reduce the intensity of the PCR products. RT-PCR for mRNA of the 18-kDa protein tracked bacterial RNA changes in the biopsies, and RNA of *M. leprae* decreased in patients after MDT for 12 months.[101] Results mean declining of live bacteria by MDT. Some MB or PB patients showed RT-PCR, which detect 16s rRNA, after MDT for 6 months and results suggested desirability of a more prolonged treatment course.[102] Another study to assay amount of 16s rRNA also showed usefulness of the RT-PCR for monitoring viability and treatment efficacy.[103] Although early investigation to evaluate efficacy of rifampicin reported that a single dose administration is bactericidal in mouse footpad and even a single dose treatment of patients rendered the bacilli noninfectious for mice,[46, 47] the RT-PCR study revealed that rifapentine decreases the amount of mRNA of the bacilli in nude mice faster than rifampicin and rifampicin require up to 20 doses of 10 mg/kg to significantly decrease mRNA in nude mice model.[104] The study pointed out imperfect effect of chemoprophylaxis for contacts with high bacillary load as postulated in early report for the effect of chemoprophylaxis.[73]

Application of RT-PCR for environment materials suggested existence of live bacilli in soil.[105] Thus, RT-PCR might be more widely used to analyze dynamism of *M. leprae* and leprosy in near future.

REFERENCES

1. WHO study group Chemotherapy of leprosy for control programs. WHO, 1983 Technical Report Series. 675.
2. Jacobson RR. Treatment of leprosy. In Hastings R.H. (ed), Leprosy. Churchill Livingston, Edinburgh. 1994, pp.317-49.
3. Faget GH, Pogge RC, Johansen FA, Dinan JF, Prejean BM, Eccles CC. The promin treatment of leprosy: a progress report. Pub Health Rep. 1943;58:1792-41.
4. Lowe J. Treatment of leprosy with diamino-diphenylsulfone by mouth. Lancet. 1950;1,145-50.
5. Smith WCS. Epidemiology of leprosy. In Makino M. et al. (ed), Leprosy Science working towards dignity. Tokai University Press. Tokyo, 2011; pp 26-34. URL http://www.press.tokai.ac.jp.
6. Wolcotto RR, Ross SH. Exacerbation of leprosy during present day treatment. Int J Lepr Other Mycobact Dis. 1953;21:437-40.
7. Pettit JHS, Rees RJW. Sulphone resistance in leprosy. An experimental and clinical study. Lancet. 1964;26:673-74.
8. Levy L, Shepard CC, Fasal P. The bactericidal effect of rifampicin on *Mycobacterium leprae* in man: (a) single doses of 600mg, 900 and 1200mg; and (b) daily doses of 300mg. Int J Lepr Other Mycobact Dis. 1976;44:183-7.

9. Grosset JH, Guelpa-Lauras CC, Bobin P, Bruker G, Cartel JL, Constant-Desportes M, Flageul B, Frederic M, Guillaume JC, Millan J. Study of 39 documented relapses of multibacillary leprosy after treatment with rifampin. Int J Lepr Other Mycobact Dis. 1989;557:607-14.

10. Pearson JMH, Rees RJW, Waters MFR. Sulphone resistance in leprosy. A review of one hundred proven clinical cases. Lancet. 1975;12:69-72.

11. dela Cruz E, Cellona RV, Balagon MVF, Villaherrmosa LG, Fajardo TT Jr, Abalos RM, Tan EV, Walsh GP. Primary dapsone resistance in Cebu, The Philippines; Cause for concern. Int J Lepr Other Mycobact Dis. 1996;64:253-6.

12. Cambau E, Perani E, Guillemin I, Jamet P, Ji B. Multidrug –resistance to dapsone, rifampicin, and ofloxacin in *Mycobacterium leprae*. Lancet. 1997;349:103-4.

13. Maeda S, Matsuoka M, Nakata N, Kai M, Maeda Y, Hashimoto K, Kimura H, Kobayashi K, Kashiwabara Y. Multidrug resistant *Mycobacterium leprae* from patients with leprosy. Antimicrob Agents Chemother. 2001;45:3635-39.

14. Matsuoka M, Kashiwabara Y, Namisato Y. A *Mycobacterium leprae* isolate resistant to dapsone, rifampin, ofloxacin, and sparfloxacin. Int J Lepr Other Mycobact Dis. 2000;68:452-5.

15. Evenezer GJ, Norman G, Joseph GA, Daniel S, Job C K. Drug resistant-*Mycobacterium leprae* – Results of mouse foot pad studies from a laboratory in south India. Indian J lepr. 2002;74:301-21.

16. Shepard CC, Chang YT. Effect of several anti-leprosy drugs on multiplication of human leprosy bacilli in footpads of mice. Proc Soc Exp Biol Med. 1962;109:636-38.

17. Honoré N, Perrani E, Teleni A, Grosset J, Cole ST. A simple and rapid method for detection of rifampin resistance in *Mycobacterium leprae*. Int J Lepr Other Mycobact Dis. 1993;61:600-4.

18. Matsuoka M, Khin SA, Kyaw K, Tan EV, Balagon MV, Saunderson P, Gelber R, Makino M, Nakajima C, Suzuki Y. A novel method for simple detection of mutations conferring drug resistance in *Mycobacterium leprae*, based on a DNA microarray, and its applicability in developing countries. J Med Microbiol. 2008; 57: 1213-19.

19. Cambau E, Nevejans AC, Tejmar-Kolar L, Matsuoka M, Jarier V. Detection of antibiotic resistance in leprosy using GenoType®LepraeDR, a novel ready-to-use molecular test. PLoS Neg Trop Dis. 2012;6: e1739.

20. World Health Organization. Guideline for Global Surveillance of drug Resistance in Leprosy. EW-GLP 2009. Available from: http//www.searo.who.int/catalogue/2005-2011/pdf/leprosy/sea-glp-2009.2.pdf.

21. World Health Organization. WHO expert committee on leprosy, 8th report WHO technical report; no.968. Available from: http://www.searo.who.int/entity/global_leprosy_programme/publications/8th_expert_comm_2012.pdf.

22. Gelber RH. Activity of mynocycline in *Mycobacterium leprae* infected mice. J Infect Dis. 1987;186:236-9.

23. Gelber RH, Fukuda K, Byrd S, Murray LP, Siu P, Tsang M, Rea TH. A clinical trial of minocycline in lepromatous leprosy. Br Med J. 1992;9:91-2.

24. Gelber RH, Gibsone J. The killing potential of various aminoglycoside antibiotics for *M. leprae*. Int J Lepr Other Mycobact Dis. 1979;47:684-5.

25. Gelber RH, Siu P, Tsang M, Murry LP. Activities of various macrolide antibiotics against *Mycobacterium leprae* infection in mice. Antimicrob Agents Chemother. 1991;35:760-3.

26. Gelber RH, Iranmanesh A, Murry LP, Siu P, Sang M. Activities of various quinolone antibiotics against *Mycobacterium leprae* in infected mice. Antimicrob Agents Chemother. 1992;36:2544-7.

27. Chan GP, Garcia-Ignacio BY, Chavez VE, Livelo JB, Jimenez CL, Parrila MLR, Farazblau SG. Clinical trial of sparfloxacin for lepromatous leprosy. Antimicrob Agents Chemother. 994;38:61-5.

28. Gelber RH, Pardillo FE, Borgos J. Powerful bacterial activity observed in the first clinical trial of Moxifloxacian in leprosy. Abstracts 46th Interscience Conference on Antimicrobial Agents and Chemotherapy. 2006;43:371.

29. Shepard CC. Minimal effective dosage in mice of clofazimine (B663) and ethionamide against *Mycobacterium leprae* (34162). Proc Soc Exp Med. 1969;132:120-4.

30. Matsuoka M. Drug resistance in leprosy. Jpn J Infect Dis. 2010;63:1-7.

31. Williams DL, Gillis TP. Drug-resistant leprosy: Monitoring and current status. Lepr Rev. 2012;83:269-81.

32. Lowe J, Smith M. The chemotherapy of leprosy in Nigeria. Int J lepr and Other Mycobact Dis. 1949;17:181-95.

33. Kai M, Matsuoka M, Nakata N, Maeda S, Gidoh M, Meada Y, Hashimoto K, Kobayashi K, Kashiwabara Y. Diaminodiphenylsulfone resistance of *Mycobacterium leprae* due to mutations in the dihydropteroate synthase gene. FEMS Microbiol Lett. 1999;177:231-35.

34. Williams DL, Spring L, Harris E, Roche P, Gillis TP. Dihydropterote synthase of *Mycobacterium leprae* and dapsone resistance. Antimicrob Agents Chemother. 2000;44:429-32.

35. Matsuoka M, Kashiwabara Y, Zhang LF, Goto M, Kitajima S. A second case of multidrug-resistant *Mycobacterium leprae* isolated from a Japanese patient with relapsed lepromatous leprosy. Int J Lepr Other Mycobact Dis. 2003;71:240-3.

36. Zhang L, Namisato M, Matsuoka M. A mutation at codon 516 in the *rpoB* gene confers resistance to rifampin. Int J Lepr Other Mycobact Dis. 2004;72:468-72.

37. Williams DL, Waguespack C, Eisenach K, Crawford JT, Portales F, Salfinger M., Nolan CM, Abe C, Sticht-Groh V, Gillis TP. Characterization of rifampin resistance in pathogenic mycobacteria. Antimicrob Agents Chemother. 1994;38:2380-86.

38. Cambau E, Bonnafous P, Perani E, Sougakoff S, Ji B, Jarlier V. Molecular Detection of rifampin and ofloxacin resistance for patients who experience relapse of multibacillary leprosy. Clin Infec Dis. 2002;34:39-45.

39. Honore N, Cole ST. Molecular basis of rifampin resistance in *Mycobacterium leprae*. Int J Lepr Other Mycobact Dis. 1993;37:414-18.

40. Cambau E, Carthagena L, Cahuffour A, Ji B, Jarlier V. Dihdropteroate synthase mutations in the *folP1* gene predict dapsone resistance in relapsed cases of leprosy. Clin Infect Dis. 2006;42:238-1.

41. Williams DL, Pittman TL, Gillis TP, Matsuoka M, Kashiwabara Y. Simultaneous detection of *Mycobacterium leprae* and its susceptibility to dapsone using heteroduplex analysis. J Clin Microbiol. 2001;2001:2083-8.

42. Matsuoka M, Budiawan T, Khin SA, Kyaw K, Tan EV, dela Cruz EC, Gelber R, Saunderson P, Balagon MV, Pannikar V. The frequency of drug resistance mutations in *Mycobacterium*

leprae isolates in untreated and relapsed leprosy patients from Myanmar, Indonesia and the Philippines. Lepr Rev. 2007;78:343-52.

43. Shepard CC. The experimental disease that follows the injection of human leprosy bacilli into foot-pad of mice. J Exp Med. 1960;112:445-54.

44. Guinto RS, Cellona RV, Fajardo TT Jr, dela Cruz E. Primary dapsone-resistant leprosy in Cebu. Philippines. Int J Lepr Other Mycobact Dis. 1981;41:427-30.

45. Peason JMH, Hail GS. Primary dapsone-resistance in leprosy. Lepr Rev. 1977;48:129-32.

46. Rees RJW, Pearson JMH, Waters MFR. Experimental and clinical studies on rifampicin in treatment of leprosy. Br Med J. 1970;1:89- 92.

47. Shepard CC, Levy L, Fasal P. Rapid bactericidal effect of rifampin on *Mycobacterium leprae*. Am J Trop Med Hyg. 1972;21:446-49.

48. Shepard CC, Levy L, Fasal P. Further experience with the rapid bactericidal effect of rifampin on *Mycobacterium leprae*. Am J Trop Med Hyg. 1974;23:1120-24.

49. Levy L, Shepard CC, Fasal P. The bactericidal effect of rifampicin on *Mycobacterium leprae* in man: (a) single doses of 600mg, 900 and 1200mg; and (b) daily doses of 300mg. Int J Lepr Other Mycobact Dis. 1976;44:183-7.

50. Jacobson RR, Hastings RC. Rifampin-resistant leprosy. Lancet. 1976;2:1304-5.

51. Guelpa-Lauras CC, Grosset JH, Constant-Desportes M, Bruker G. Nine cases of rifampicin-resistant leprosy. Int J Lepr Other Mycobact Dis. 1984;52:101-2.

52. Saito H, Tomioka H, Nagashima K. In vitro and in vivo activities of ofloxacin against *Mycobacterium leprae* infection induced in mice. Int J Lepr Other Mycobact Dis. 1986;54:560-2.

53. Grosset JH, Ji B, Guelpa-Lauras CC, Perani EG, N'Deli L. Clinical trial of perfloxacin and ofloxacin in the treatment of lepromatous leprosy. Int J Lepr Other Mycobact Dis. 1990;58:281-5.

54. Takiff HE, Salazar L, Guerrero C, Phillip W, Huang WM, Kreiswirth B, Cole S, Jacobs WR Jr, Talentini A. Cloning and sequencing of *Mycobacterium tuberculosis gyrA* and *gyrB* genes and detection of quinolone resistance mutation. Antimicrob Agents Chemother. 1994;38:773-80.

55. Cambau E, Saugacoff W, Besson M, Truffot-Pernot C, Grosset J, Jarlier V. Selection of a *gyrA* mutant of *Mycobacterium tuberculosis* resistant to fluoroquinolones during treatment with ofloxacin. J Infect Dis. 1994;170:479-83.

56. You EY, Kang TJ, Kim SK, Lee SB, Chae GT. Mutations in genes related to drug resistance in *Mycobacterium leprae* isolates from leprosy patients in Korea. J Infect. 2005;50:6-11.

57. Yokoyama K, Kim H, Mukai T, Matsuoka M, Nakajima C, Suzuki Y. Amino acid substitution at position 95 in GyrA can add fluoroquinolone resistance to *Mycobacterium leprae*. Antimicrob Agents Chemother. 2012;56:697-702.

58. Yokoyama K, Kim H, Mukai T, Matsuoka M, Nakajima C, Suzuki Y. Impact of amino acid substitution in B subunit of DNA gyrase in *Mycobacterium leprae* on fluoroquinolone resistance. PLoS Neg Trop Dis. 2012;6:e1838.

59. Veziris N, Cahuffour A, Escolano S, Henquet S, Matsuoka M, Larlier V, Aubry A. Resistance of *M.leprae* to Quinolones: A question of relativity. PLoS Neg Trop Dis. 2013;67:e2559.

60. Cambau E, Jarlier V. Resistance to quinolones in Mycobacteria. Res Microbiol. 1996;147:52-9.

61. Matrat S, Cambau E, Jarlier V, Aubry A. Are all the DNA gyrase mutations found in *Mycobacterium leprae* clinical strains involved in resistance to fluoroquinolones? Antimicrob Agents Chemother. 2008;52:745-7.

62. World Health Organization. Surveillance of drug resistance in leprosy: 2009, Weekly Epidemiol Rec. 2010;85:281-4.

63. World Health Organization. Surveillance of drug resistance in leprosy: 2010, Weekly Epidemiol Rec. 2011;86:233-40.

64. Morrison NE, Marley G. Clofazimine binding studies with deoxyribonucleic acid. Int J Lepr Other Mycobact Dis. 1976;44:475-81.

65. Browne SG, Hogerzeil LM. "B663" in the treatment of leprosy. Preliminary report of pilot trial. Lepr Rev. 1962;33:6-10.

66. Shetty VP, Uplekar MV, Antia NH. Primary resistance to single and multipledrugs in leprosy—a mouse footpad study. Lepr Rev 1996;67:280-6.

67. Diepen TWV. Clofazimine –resistant leprosy, a case report. Int J Lepr Other Mycobact Dis. 1982;50:139-42.

68. Levy L. Clofazimine-resistant *M. leprae*. Int J Lepr Other Mycobact Dis. 1986;54:137-40.

69. Ji B, Perani EG, Grosset JH. Effectiveness of clarithromycin and miocycline alone and combination against experimental *Mycobacterium leprae* infection in mice. Antimicrob Agents Chemother. 1991;35:579-81.

70. Taylor DE, Chau A. Tetracycline resistance mediated by ribosomal protection: mini review. Antimicrob Agents Chemother. 1996;40:1-5.

71. Nakajima H, Nagao E, Ozaki M and Ishii N. Diagnosis of Hansen's disease, Guideline for the treatment. Ministry of Health, Tofu kyokai. 1997; (in Japanese)

72. Goto M, Ishida Y, Gidoh M, Nagao E, Namisato M, Ishii N and Ozaki M. Guideline for the treatment of Hansen's disease in Japan. Jpn J Lepr. 2000;69:157-77.

73. Moet F, Pahan D, Oskam L, Richardus JH. Effectiveness of single dose rifampicin in preventing leprosy in close contacts of patients with newly diagnose leprosy: cluster randomized controlled trial. Br Med J. 2008;336:761-4.

74. Oskam L, Mi B. Report of the workshop on the use of chemoprophylaxis in the control of leprosy held in Amsterdam, the Netherlands on 14 December 2006. Lepr Rev. 2007;78:173-85.

75. Ji B. Drug susceptibility testing of *Mycobacterium leprae*. Int J Lepr Other Mycobact Dis. 1987;55:830-5.

76. Rees RJW, Young DB. The microbiology of leprosy. *In* Hastings R.H. (ed), Leprosy. Churchill Livingston, Edinburgh, 1994; pp. 49-83.

77. Shepard CC, Rees RJ, Levy L, Pattin ASR, Ji B, dela Cruz EC. Susceptibility of Strains of *Mycobacterium leprae* Isolated prior to 1977 from patients with previously untreated lepromatous leprosy. Int J Lepr Other Mycobact Dis. 1986;54:11-5.

78. Rees RJ. Drug resistance of *Mycobacterium leprae* particularly to DDS. Int J Lep Other Mycobact Dis. 1967;35:625-36.

79. Matsuoka M. The history of *Mycobacterium leprae* Thai-53 strain. Lepr Rev. 2010;81:137.

80. Cambau E, Nevejans AC, Tejmar-Kolar L, Matsuoka M, Jarier V. Detection of antibiotic resistance in leprosy using GenoType®LepraeDR, a novel ready-to-use molecular test. PLoS Neg Trop Dis. 2012;6:e1739.

81. Li W, Matsuoka M, Kai M, Thapa P, Khadge S, Hagge DA, Brennan PJ, Vissa V. Real-time PCR and high resolution melt analysis for rapid detection of *Mycobacterium leprae*

drug resistance mutations and strain types. J Clin Microbiol. 2012;50:742-53.

82. Franzblau SG, Biswas AN, Jenner P, Colston MJ. Double-blind evaluation of BACTEC and Buddemeyer-type radiorespirometric assays for in vitro screening of antileprosy agents, Lepr Rev. 1992;63:125-33.

83. Franzblau SG, Biswas AN, Harris EB. Fusic acid is highly active extracellular and intracellular *Mycobacterium leprae*. Antimicrob Agents Chemother. 1992;36:92-4.

84. Job CK. Pathology of leprosy. In Hastings RH. (ed), Leprosy. Churchill Livingston, Edinburgh, 1994,pp.193-225.

85. Shetty VP, Suchitra K, Uplekar MW, Antia NH. Persistence of *Mycobacterium leprae* in the peripheral nerve as compared to the skin of multidrug-treated leprosy patients. Lepr Rev. 1992;63:329-36.

86. Barkel WV, Kist P, Noble S, O'toolle L. Relapses after multidrug therapy for leprosy: a preliminary report of 22 cases in West Nepal. Lepr Rev. 1989;60:45-50.

87. Balagon MF, Cellona RV, dela Cruz EC, Burgos JA, Abalos RM, Walsh GP, Saunderson PR, Walsh DS. Long-term relapse risk of multibacillary leprosy after completion of 2 years of multi drug therapy (WHO-MDT) in Cebu, Philippines. Am J Trop Med Hyg. 2009;81:895-9.

88. Shaw IN, Natrajan MM, Rao GS, Jesudasan K, Christian M, Kaavitha M. Long- term follow up of mulibacillary leprosy patients with high BI treated with WHO/MDT regimen for a fixed duration of two years. Int J Lep Other Mycobact Dis. 2000;68:405-9.

89. Cellona RV, Balagon MF, dela Cruz EC, Burgos JA, Abalos RM, Walsh GP, Topolski R, Gelber R, Walsh DS. Long-term efficacy of 2 year WHO multiple drug therapy (MDT) in multibacillary (MB) leprosy patients. Int J Lep Other Mycobact Dis. 2003;71:308-19.

90. Soares DJ, Neupane K, Britton WJ. Relapse with multibacillary leprosy caused by rifampicin sensitive organisms following paucibacillary multidrug therapy. Lepr Rev. 1995;66:210-3.

91. Matsuoka M. Recent advances in the molecular epidemiology of leprosy. Jpn J Lepr. 2009;78:67-73.

92. Rocha AS, Santos A AC, Pignataro P, Nery JA, Marianda AB, Soares DF, Fontes ANB, Milanda A, Ferria H, Boechat N, Gallo MEN, Sarno EN, Oliveira MLWD, Suffys PN. Genotyping of *Mycobacterium leprae* from Brazilian leprosy patients suggesting the occurrence of reinfection or bacterial population shift during disease relapse. J Med Microbiol. 2011;60:1441-6.

93. Oskam L, Dockrel HM, Brennan P, Gillis TP, Vissa V, Richardus JH, Members of the IDEAL consortium. Molecular method for distinguishing between relapse and reinfection in leprosy. Trop Med Int Health. 2008;13:1325-6.

94. Desikan KV, Sreevatsa. Extended studies on the viability of *Mycobacterium leprae* outside the human body. Lepr Rev. 1995;66:287-95.

95. Welch TM, Gelber RH, Murray LP, Ng H, O'nell M, Levy L. Viability of *Mycobacterium leprae* after multiplication in mice. Infec Immun 1980;30:325-8.

96. Bhagria A, Mahadevan PR. Rapid method for viability and drug sensitivity of *Mycobacterium leprae* calculated in macrophages and using fluorescent diacetate. Indian J Lepr.1987;59:9-19.

97. Lahiri R, Randhawa B, Krahenbuhl J. Application of a viability-staining method for *Mycobacterium leprae* derived from the athymic (nu/nu) mouse foot pad. J Med Microbiol. 2005;54:235-42.

98. Franzblau S. A rapid, microplate-based assay for evaluating the activity of drugs against *Mycobacterium leprae* employing the reduction of Alamar Blue. Lepr Rev. 2000; (71) Suppl: S74-76.

99. Patel BKR, Banerjee DK, Butcher P. Detection of *Mycobacterium leprae* viability by polymerase chain reaction amplification of 71-kDa heat-shock protein mRNA. J Infec Dis. 1993;168:799-800.

100. Kurabachew M, Wondimu A, Ryon J. Reverse Transcription-PCR detection of *Mycobacterium leprae* in clinical specimens. J Clin Micribiol. 1998;36:1352-6.

101. Chae GT, Kim MJ, Kang TJ, Lee SB, Shin HK, Kim JP, KO YH, Kim SH, Kim NH. DNA-PCR and RT-PCR for the 18-kDa gene of *Mycobacterium leprae* to assess the efficacy of multi-drug therapy for leprosy. J Med Microbiol. 2002;51:417-22.

102. Phetsksiri B, Rudeeneksin J, Supapku P, Wachapomg S, Mahotarn K, Brennan PJ. A simplified reverse transcriptase PCR for rapid detection of *Mycobacterium leprae* in skin specimens. FEMS Immunol Med Microbiol. 2006;48:319-28.

103. Martinez AN, Lahiri R, Pittman TL, Scollard D, Truman R, Moraes MO, Williams DL. Molecular determination of *Mycobacterium leprae* viability by use of real-time PCR. J Clin Microbiol. 2009;47;2124-30.

104. Davis GL, Ray NA, Lahiri R, Gillis TP, Krahenbuhl JL, Williams DL, Adams LB. Molecular assays for determining *Mycobacterium leprae* viability in tissue of experimentally infected mice. PLoS Neg Trop Dis. 2013;7:e2404.

105. Trunkar R, Lavania M, Singh M, Siva Sai KSR, Jadhav RS. Dynamics of *Mycobacterium leprae* transmission in environmental context: deciphering the role of environment as a potential reservoir. Inf Gen Evol. 2012;12:121-26.

Morbidity and Mortality in Leprosy

Ben Naafs, S Noto, PAM Schreuder

CHAPTER OUTLINE

- Morbidity
- Mortality

MORBIDITY

The exact morbidity of leprosy within a population is not known. It depends on genetic factors and the risk of infection. At present we have little influence on genetic factors, but may have some influence on the risk of infection.

Mycobacterium leprae is an obligate intracellular microorganism. A high proportion of mankind is genetically not able to sustain *M. leprae* in their cells. It is likely that in those people the bacillus cannot manipulate the host cell for its own benefit to create the appropriate environment for survival. Around 20% of the population is susceptible to infection, an estimate that is based on serology and epidemiological data.

Infection does not always lead to disease. Among the infected population, most people are able to develop an adequate immunity depending on genetic factors, the environment and the immunobiological history. Protective factors are: (1) vaccination—BCG vaccination offers some protection against leprosy—or, (2) contacts in the environment with antigenic determinants that enhance protection.[1] Negative factors include: (1) living in an area with a high risk of infection with a large inoculate, (2) being immunosuppressed,[2] (3) being in contact with antigenic determinants that promote infection.[1] The end result is that at most only a very small percentage of the infected individuals develop the disease.

Thus, the morbidity even in a highly infectious/endemic areas is low. However, when leprosy was first introduced into a number of Pacific islands in the early twentieth century, this lead to some instances of epidemics lasting several decades and up to 30% of the population became affected.[3,4]

Leprosy is nonrandom in its distribution.[3] In an area of high endemicity, leprosy patients are extensively clustered, but even within small communities not equally distributed.[5]

An indication of the magnitude of the present problem is that each year 400,000 individuals develop leprosy (an estimation) from which about 230,000 are reported (diagnosed) cases. In 2013, 95% of the 215,656 new cases were reported from 14 countries (Fig. 41.1).[6]

When an individual develops the disease, he or she manifests it in any one of the forms along a spectrum, as described by Ridley and Jopling.[7] As a complication, he or she may develop impairments in the eyes, nose, face, testes, hands and feet depending on the evolution of the disease. The nerve damage leading to these impairments with the permanent disability as consequence is the major problem in the course of leprosy infection. Were it not for this damage, leprosy would be a rather chronic but benign and innocuous skin disease.

Most of the nerve damage in leprosy occurs during the so called "reactions"; these are immunologically mediated episodes of inflammation, mostly acute, of nerves and skin, and particularly in the type 2 reaction [erythema nodosum leprosum (ENL)] of other organs too. Reactions belong to the natural history of the disease and may occur before, during and even after the treatment for leprosy has been stopped and the patient is declared "cured".[8]

The occurrence of reactions and disabilities depends on the form and the duration of the disease, the type of reaction and the quality of the leprosy treatment services, and may range from 10% to above 60%. Borderline [borderline tuberculoid (BT), borderline borderline (BB) and borderline lepromatous (BL)] leprosy patients have a high-risk of type 1 (reversal) reaction and its sequels; BL leprosy patients are at high-risk of developing either or both type 1 and type 2 reactions. Lepromatous (LL) leprosy patients may develop only type 2 reaction, but the risk is high. Most reactions are seen at diagnosis and during the first 6 months of treatment after which their number declines. There may be a temporary

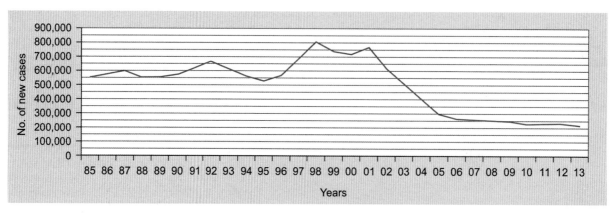

Fig. 41.1: Global new cases of leprosy (new case detection or NCD) 1985–2013

increased risk of reactions after treatment, the so-called late reactions.[9]

Good vision is critical, especially to a person who has lost sensory function in hands and feet, and developed visible deformities. In the course of the disease even, after the initial nerve damage, the disability may further increase due to loss of sensation, loss of muscle strength and damage to the eye and eyelids. Blindness is a catastrophic event and in leprosy several mechanisms like decreased corneal sensation, lagophthalmos leading to corneal damage due to exposure, subacute/acute iritis or iridocyclitis, cataract and glaucoma, etc. can lead to this event. The magnitude of ocular morbidity and blindness is to a large extent influenced by the clinical, demographic and social dimensions associated with the disease.

A longitudinal study of ocular leprosy (LOSOL) from India, Philippines and Ethiopia showed that 11% of patients already had leprosy related ocular complications at diagnosis[10] and a further 9% developed pathology during follow-up, and the process continued much longer after the completion of treatment.[11,12] These complications can persist and progress leading to blindness.[13]

The Global Leprosy Program has had a dramatic impact on the prevalence of registered cases of leprosy over the past 30 years through the wide spread introduction of multidrug therapy (MDT).[14] Together with the development of MDT for leprosy during the past few decades, there seems to be some decline in the ocular morbidity among the newly diagnosed and treated leprosy patients.

However, further advances in the field of leprosy are hindered by the lack of new tools to address the challenge of apparent persistence in transmission and incidence, and the long-term consequences of the disease.[14] In 2011, the ILEP board approved a new research strategy to develop new tools to prevent leprosy, improve patient care and reduce the consequences of leprosy.[14]

MORTALITY

Leprosy is not an immediate cause of death, but the prolonged effects of leprosy may lead to death. Those with the LL disease or sequels of the disease may have a four times higher risk of death than those in the general population. About 1–2 million people worldwide are irreversibly disabled because of the disease and are prone to septicemia, thromboembolism and consequently death.[15] We have to realize that today the treatment has curbed the number of deaths that could be directly caused by leprosy. However, the use of steroids have unveiled, in some patients fatal comorbidities like human immunodeficiency virus (HIV) infection, Chagas disease, hepatitis B infection, strongyloidiasis and latent tuberculosis.[16] Patients with a concurrent HIV infection are more prone to reactions and also the development of immune reconstitution inflammatory syndrome (IRIS).[17]

Many disabled patients live in destitute circumstances with little access to health services. Social impairment due to several conditions, including stigma, discrimination, poverty, disability and loss of independence, are still great obstacles to be overcome by people affected by leprosy.[18] The presence of prevalent restrictions in social participation of people affected by leprosy is associated with, among others, disabilities and low incomes, e.g. family income of less than three minimum salaries (US$ 160.50).[14] Visible impairments also affect the activities and attitudes of people affected by leprosy.[19]

In the past, the main cause of death of leprosy patients was tuberculosis. According to Mitsuda and Ogawa,[20] in Japan in the 1920s, more than half of the leprosy patients died from tuberculosis and more than 13% of renal problems (mainly due to amyloidosis). These renal problems were probably directly related to the disease, particularly to type 2 reactions. Septicemia was the cause in 9.3% and "cachexia" in 4%. They reported that their data were the same as those received from Lara, Culion, the Philippines, except for the data on septicemia, which was lower in the Philippines.[20] The data from the rest of the world would not have been much different. Other factors were also influencing the life of the patients and may have led to their death. These were isolation and separation from their families and communities, which unfortunately in some cases even assisted in their suicide[21] and sometimes went to the extent of actually killing of the patients by fire, drowning or bury them alive.[22-26] In China , suicide is the major cause of death after the patients have been diagnosed.[27,28]

Leprosy itself is not a killer. A few patients may develop renal problems and die. Very few patients with Lucio leprosy (Lepra bonita) develop Lucio phenomenon that leads to death. Lepra bonita is a form of leprosy reported in Central America and exceptionally in other regions. Moreover, the accompanying disabilities, particularly ulcers may lead to cachexia, septicemia and death. Chronic and recurrent ENL (type 2 reactions), and particularly its treatment with corticosteroids is another important cause of death.[29]

However, not only treatment of reactions may cause death, MDT may also be responsible; the dapsone syndrome, a severe allergic reaction to Dapsone (diamino difeny lsulfon, DDS) is highly prevalent in Eastern and Middle Asia, and often liver failure and electrolyte disturbances lead to death.[30] Rifampicin may cause liver problems or a so-called flu syndrome and clofazimine may cause enteric bleeding. However, the number of patients dying from these medications is very small.

The World Health Report (WHO, 2004) mentioned that in 2002 about 1,000 deaths from leprosy were reported from the Americas, 3,000 deaths from Southeast Asia, 1,000 deaths from Eastern Mediterranean and about 1,000 deaths by leprosy from the Western Pacific.[31] From data presented at the eighteenth World Leprosy Congress in Brussels, in 2013, it became clear how unreliable data on mortality are. Even if an ex-leprosy patient dies of old age, the cause of death may be recorded as leprosy and not, as for example, heart failure. Reliable mortality figures, because of leprosy, are not available.[31-33]

REFERENCES

1. Lyons NF, Naafs B. Influence of environmental mycobacteria on the prevalence of leprosy clinical type. Int J Lepr Other Mycobact Dis. 1987;55(4):637-45.
2. Massone C, Talhari C, Ribeiro-Rodrigues R, et al. Leprosy and HIV coinfection: a critical approach. Exp Rev Anti Infect Ther. 2011;9(6):701-10.
3. Fine PE. Leprosy: the epidemiology of a slow bacterium. Epidemiol Rev. 1982;4:161-88.
4. Bray G. The story of leprosy at Nauru. Proc R Soc Med. 1930;23(9):1370-4.
5. Bakker M, Hatta M, Kwenang A, et al. Epidemiology of leprosy among five isolated islands in the Flores Sea, Indonesia. Trop Med Int Health. 2002;7(9):780-7.
6. WHO WER 2000;75:225-232 (data 1985 - 1993) - WER 2002;77:1-8 (data 1994-2000) - WER 2007;82:225-232 (data 2001-2006) - WER 2013;88:365-80 (data 2007-2012).
7. Ridley DS, Jopling WH. Classification of leprosy according to immunity. A five-group system. Int J Lepr Other Mycobact Dis. 1966;34(3):255-73. Data are also available on line at: http://www.who.int/wer/archives/en/Accessed on August 2014.
8. Naafs B. Current views on reactions in leprosy. Indian J Lepr. 2000;72(1):97-122.
9. Kumar B, Dogra S, Kaur I. Epidemiological characteristics of leprosy reactions: 15 years experience from north India. Int J Lepr Mycobact Dis. 2004;72(2):125-33.
10. Courtright P, Daniel E, Sundar Rao PS, et al. Eye disease in multibacillary leprosy patients at the time of their leprosy diagnosis: findings from the Longitudinal Study of Ocular Leprosy(LOSOL) in India, the Philippines and Ethiopia. Lepr Rev. 2002;73(2):225-38.
11. Daniel E, Ffytche TJ, Sundar Rao PS, et al. Incidence of ocular morbidity among multibacillary leprosy patients during a 2 year course of multidrug therapy. Br J Ophthalmol. 2006;90(5):568-73.
12. Daniel E, Ffytche TJ, Kempen JH, et al. Incidence of ocular complications in patients with multibacillary leprosy after completion of a 2 year course of multidrug therapy. Br J Ophthalmol. 2006;90(8):949-54.
13. Parikh R, Thomas S, Muliyil J, et al. Ocular manifestation in treated multibacillary Hansen's disease. Ophthalmology. 2009;116(11):2051-7.
14. Smith WC, ILEP. A research strategy to develop new tools to prevent leprosy, improve patient care and reduce the consequences of leprosy. Five year leprosy research strategy approved by ILEP Board October 2011. Lepr Rev. 2012;83(1):6-15.
15. Pontes MA, Bührer-Sékula S, Penna ML, et al. Causes of death among patients of clinical trial for uniform multidrug therapy for leprosy patients in Brazil (U-MDT/CT-BR). Presented at: 18th International Leprosy Congress; 2013 Sept 16 – Sept 19; Brussels, Belgium. Abstract No. P-082.
16. Ooi W, Bilodeau M, Burns S, et al. Infectious comorbidities in Hansens disease (HD) patients in the US: implications for treatment. Presented at: 18th International Leprosy Congress; 2013 Sept 16 – Sept 19; Brussels, Belgium. Abstract No. O-082.
17. Lockwood D, Lambert SM, Nicholls P, et al. Leprosy HIV co-infection observational study in Ethiopa. Presented at: 18th International Leprosy Congress; 2013 Sept 16 – Sept 19; Brussels, Belgium. Abstract No. O-066.
18. Nardi SM, Paschoal VD, Zanetta DM. Social participation of people affected by leprosy after discontinuation of multidrug therapy. Lepr Rev. 2011;82(1):55-64.
19. Boku N, Lockwood DN, Balagon MV, et al. Impacts of the diagnosis of leprosy and visible impairments amongst people affected by leprosy in Cebu, the Philippines. Lepr Rev. 2010;81(2):111-20.
20. Mitsuda K, Ogawa MA. A study of 150 autopsies of cases of leprosy. Int J Lepr. 1937;5:53-60.
21. Skinsnes Law A. New perspectives on Kalaupapa's history as reflected in hundreds of letters petitions and newspaper articles translated from Hawaiian. Presented at: 18th International

Leprosy Congress; 2013 Sept 16 – Sept 19; Brussels, Belgium. Abstract No.O-171.

22. Richards P. The Medieval Leper and His Northern Heirs Chapter IX:83-88 Boydell & Brewer. 2000.

23. Campbell A. On the Custom of Burying and Burning Alive of Lepers in India. Transactions of the Ethnological Society of London; 1868.

24. Tanaka Y. Japanese Atrocities on Nauru during the Pacific War: The murder of Australians, the massacre of lepers and the ethnocide of Nauruans. 45-2-10, November 8 The Asia-Pacific Journal, 2010. http://www.japanfocus.org/-Yuki-TANAKA/3441#sthash.LVVlUFov.dpuf

25. Anonymous killing of lepers reported in China. Pittburgh Post-Gazette April 2, 1937.

26. The History of Leprosy in India. Presented at: Proceedings of the workshop on History of Leprosy in India; 2000 July 15 – July16; Mumbai, India.

27. Shen J, Liu M, Zhou M, et al. Causes of death among active leprosy patients in China. Int J Dermatol. 2011;50(1):57-60.

28. Weiss MG. Understanding stigma and self-esteem. Presented at: 18th International Leprosy Congress; 2013 Sept 16 – Sept 19; Brussels, Belgium. Abstract No. PL-005.

29. Walker SL, Lebas E, Doni SN, et al. There is a significant mortality associated with erythema nodosum leprosum (ENL) at ALERT hospital, Ethiopia–A five year retrospective study. Presented at: 18th International Leprosy Congress; 2013 Sept 16 – Sept 19; Brussels, Belgium. Abstract No. O-067.

30. Liu H, Zhang F. Establishment and application of risk prediction test for dapsone hypersensitivity syndrome-Preliminary report. Presented at: 18th International Leprosy Congress; 2013 Sept 16 – Sept 19; Brussels, Belgium. Abstract No. O-130.

31. World Health Organization. (2004). World Health Report 2004-Changing history. [online]. Available from: www.who.int/whr/2004/en/report04_en.pdf. [Accessed June, 2014].

32. Ramos RD, Ferreira S, Ignotti E. Death by leprosy as the underlying cause; Mato Grosso from 2000 to 2007. Presented at: 18th International Leprosy Congress; ; 2013 Sept 16 – Sept 19; Brussels, Belgium. Abstract No. P-213.

33. Rocha M, Soares RC, Levantezi M, et al. A descriptive study of Hanseniasis death in Brazil: the use of linkage to vital information. Presented at: 18th International Leprosy; 2013 Sept 16 – Sept 19; Brussels, Belgium. Abstract No. O-130.

42
CHAPTER

Recording-Reporting and Monitoring MDT Services

Pratap Rai Manglani

Health information is an integral part of any health program. It is a mechanism for the collection, processing, analysis and transmission of information required for organizing and operating health services and also for research and training. Information complementing routine leprosy information systems to address specific issues, such as epidemiological trends, completion rates, impact of interventions, changing patterns of leprosy and quality of services are useful to program managers for monitoring program activities. Wherever possible, trend analysis over the last five years should be used to assess the impact of leprosy control activities.

Monitoring the progress of an individual case and progress of the program at local, state or national level is based on records and monthly reports maintained regularly.

A WHO expert Committee identified the following requirements to be satisfied by the health information system:

- The system should be population based.
- The system should avoid the unnecessary agglomeration of data.
- The system should be problem-oriented.
- The system should employ functional and operational terms.
- The system should express information briefly and imaginatively.
- The system should make provisions for the feed-back of data.

In many countries including India, leprosy services are integrated into general health care. National Leprosy Eradication Programme (NLEP) information system in India was simplified in 2002 to suit to GHC system. 'Simplified Information System' (SIS) contained minimum data collection essential for monitoring the program. Case-card, treatment register, drug stock register, monthly progress report (MPR), quarterly and annual performance reports and indicators constitutes SIS. SIS was modified as Upgraded Simplified Information System (USIS) for NLEP India in 2013.

Review meetings at national and state/province level are very helpful in assessing the progress, difficulties in implementing the planned activities and fund utilization.

National Leprosy Control/Eradication Programmes need periodic independent evaluation of the structure, process and outcomes of the program so that an objective assessment can be made that would enable corrections and adjustments to be made in the strategies and activities.

TERMS USED

Monitoring can be defined as periodic collection and analysis of selected indicators. It is a process of measuring, recording, collecting and analysing data on actual implementation of the program and communicating it to program managers so that any deviations from the planned operations are detected, diagnosis for causes of deviation is carried out and suitable corrective actions are taken. Implementation of planned activities, quality of services and impact of services can be assessed and ensured through monitoring.

Data is the term used to describe basic facts and figures/statistics about activities of a project, which can be processed to produce information. Information is obtained by assembling items of data into a meaningful form.

Information is processed data. Processing is manipulation of facts, figures and statistics (data). The operation involved in the processing are: calculation, comparison, logic and decision taken.

Percentage is the number of units with a certain characteristic divided by the total no. of units in the sample and multiplied by 100.

Proportion is a numerical expression that compares one part of the study units to the whole. A proportion can be expressed as a fraction or in decimals.

Ratio is a numeral expression, which indicates the relationship in quantity, amount or size between two or more parts.

Rate is the quantity, amount or degree of something measured in a specified period of time.

Key Epidemiological Questions

What are the problems? Who is affected? How many are affected?

When did it take place? Where did it occur? Why did it happen?

How can we manage it? Which approaches are best?

Indicators

Indicators show to what extent targets are reached. Types of indicators are:

- Input (resources)
- Process (transforming)
- Output 1: coverage
- Output 2: quality
- Impact (health status)

Indicators (tools to measure progress and achievements under a program or project) used in NLEP India:

- Essential Indicators
  - Number and Annual New Case detection Rate (ANCDR) per 100,000 population
  - Number and rate of new cases with grade 2 disabilities per 10,00,000 population per year
  - Treatment Completion Rate (TCR) as proxy to cure rate
  - Prevalence Rate (PR)
- Additional Epidemiological Indicators
  - Number and proportion of Grade II disabilities among new cases
  - Number and proportion of females among new cases
  - Number and proportion of MB among new cases
  - Number and proportion of child (under 15 yrs) among new cases
  - Child rate per 100,000 population
  - Scheduled caste new case detection rate
  - Scheduled tribe new case detection rate
- Quality of Service Indicators
  - Patient month Blister calendar pack stock
  - Absolute number of patients made RFT
  - Number of relapse reported
  - Proportion of cases who developed new or additional disability after starting MDT

- Proportion of treatment defaulters
- Proportion of new cases correctly diagnosed

Each one of these indicators has been discussed in Box 42.1 indicating the following information:

i. Definition
ii. Numerator
iii. Denominator
iv. Source of data
v. Level of reporting
vi. Unit of analysis
vii. Frequency of data collection
viii. Frequency of analysis

It may be seen from the above table that source of all information will be the Primary Health Centres but District Hospitals/Medical Colleges/Other institutions will also provide requisite information.

Level of analysis varies from PHC to the State level depending upon the indicator. All data will be collected on monthly basis and compiled. However, frequency of analysis will vary from quarterly to yearly depending on various indicators.

- Definition of the indicators and formula to be used for their calculation are indicated below:
  - Annual New Case Detection Rate

Definition: It is the rate at which new cases (never treated before) are detected in a defined geographical area (Block, District) and in a given period of time.

$$\text{Calculation} = \frac{\text{Total number of leprosy cases newly detected} \times 100{,}000}{\text{Total population (midyear/census) of the area}}$$

- Number and rate of new cases with grade 2 disabilities per 10,00,000 population per year

Definition: It is the rate at which new disabilities are detected in the defined geographical population (area) in a given year

$$\text{Calculation} = \frac{\text{Total new cases detected with Gr II disabilities} \times 10{,}00{,}000}{\text{Total population (midyear/census) of the area}}$$

- Treatment Completion Rate

Definition: It is the rate of patients who complete their treatment on time as a proxy for cure rate. Cohort analysis of PB and MB cases are done separately.

$$\text{Calculation} =$$

$$\text{PB TCR} = \frac{\text{Number of new PB cases who completed MDT in 9 months} \times 100}{\text{Number of new PB cases who started MDT in a year}}$$

$$\text{MB TCR} = \frac{\text{Number of new MB cases who completed MDT in 18 months} \times 100}{\text{Number of new MB cases who started MDT in a year}}$$

S. No.	Indicator	Source	Reporting		Frequency of	
			Level	Unit of analysis	Data collection	Analysis
1.	No. and annual new case detection rate (ANCDR)	PHC	PHC Block PHC	Absolute number	Monthly	Yearly
			District State Country	Rate		
2.	Number and rate of grade II disability per million population	PHC	PHC compiled at District, State and Country	Rate	Monthly	Yearly
3.	Treatment completion rate (TCR)	PHC	District State Country	Rate	Yearly	Yearly
4.	Prevalence rate (PR)	PHC	PHC Block PHC	Absolute number	Monthly	Yearly
			District State Country	Rate		
5.	Number and proportion of grade II disability among new cases	PHC	PHC, Districts, State and Country	Absolute number and proportion	Monthly	Quarterly
6.	Number and proportion of female among new cases	PHC	PHC Districts State Country	Number and proportion	Monthly	Yearly
7.	Number and proportion of MB among new cases	PHC	PHC compiled at Districts, State and Country	Number and proportion	Monthly	Quarterly
8.	Number and proportion of child among new cases	PHC	PHC compiled at Districts, State and Country	Number and proportion	Monthly	Quarterly
9.	Child rate per 100,000 population	PHC	PHC compiled at District, State and Country	Rate	Monthly	Yearly
10.	Number and scheduled cast new cases detection rate	PHC	PHC compiled at Districts, State and Country	Number and rate	Monthly	Yearly
11.	Number and scheduled tribe new cases detection rate	PHC	PHC compiled at Districts, State and Country	Number and rate	Monthly	Yearly
12.	Patients month blister calendar pack stock	PHC	PHC compiled and analyzed at Districts, State and Country	Number of BCP/ patient	Monthly	Quarterly
13.	Absolute number of patients made RFT	PHC	PHC compiled at Districts, State and Country	Absolute number and proportion	Monthly	Yearly
14.	Number of relapses reported	PHC and District hospital	PHC, District, State, and Country	Absolute number	Monthly	Yearly
15.	Number and proportion of cases with new disability after starting MDT	PHC	PHC District and State	Rate	Monthly	Yearly
16.	Number and Proportion of defaulters from treatment	PHC	PHC, District, State and Country	Rate	Yearly	Quarterly
17.	Proportion of new cases correctly diagnosed	PHC	District State	Rate	Monthly	Quarterly

Box 42.1: A summary of the information from Sl. No. (iv) to (viii) is given below for ready reference

- Prevalence Rate

Definition: It is the total number of leprosy cases on record (under treatment) at a given point of time in an area.

$$\text{Calculation} = \frac{\text{Total number of leprosy cases on record} \times 10,000}{\text{Total population in the given time/mid year/census in an area}}$$

- Proportion of grade II disability among new cases

Definition: It is the proportion (%) of new leprosy patients with grade II disability among total new cases detected.

$$\text{Calculation} = \frac{\text{No. of grade II disabled cases detected in a year} \times 100}{\text{Total new case detected in a year}}$$

- Proportion of female among new cases

Definition: It is the proportion (%) of new female patients among total newly detected cases.

$$\text{Calculation} = \frac{\text{Number of new female patients} \times 100}{\text{Total no. of newly detected cases}}$$

- Proportion of multibacillary (MB) among new cases

Definition: It is the proportion (%) of new patients diagnosed as MB among newly detected cases

$$\text{Calculation} = \frac{\text{Number of new MB cases} \times 100}{\text{Total no. of newly detected cases}}$$

- Proportion of child among new cases

Definition: Proportion (%) of new leprosy patients up to 14 years of age among newly detected patients.

$$\text{Calculation} = \frac{\text{No. of child leprosy cases detected} \times 100}{\text{Total no. of newly detected leprosy cases}}$$

- Child rate per 100,000 population

Definition: The rate of new child leprosy cases (up to 14 years) detected among the population of the area in a year

$$\text{Calculation} = \frac{\text{No. of new child cases (up to 14 years) detected in a year} \times 100,000}{\text{Population of the area}}$$

- Scheduled caste (SC) new cases detection rate

Definition: Total number of new cases detected among the SC population in a given time in an area.

$$\text{Calculation} = \frac{\text{Total number of SC cases newly detected in a year} \times 10,000}{\text{Total SC population in an area}}$$

- Scheduled Tribe (ST) new cases detection rate

Definition: Total number of new ST cases detected among the ST population in given time in an area

$$\text{Calculation} = \frac{\text{Total number of ST cases newly detected} \times 10,000}{\text{Total ST population in an area}}$$

- Patients month Blister calendar pack (BCP) stock

Definition: Stock of BCPs in months, according to the number of patients expected to be treated in the next quarter.

$$\text{Calculation} = \frac{\text{Number of blister packs of each category [PB(A/C) MB(A/C)]}}{\text{No. of cases under treatment in each category [PB(A/C), MB(A/C)]}}$$

- Absolute number of patients made RFT

Definition: Number of patients released from treatment during the year. The number should include both the new and the other cases treated in a year.

- Number of relapses reported.

Definition: No. of relapse cases recorded in the PHC, District Hospitals, Medical Colleges and other institutions in the district during the given time.

- Proportion of cases with new disability after starting MDT

Definition: Proportion (%) of cases who developed new or additional disability after starting MDT.

$$\text{Calculation} = \frac{\text{No. of cases developed new or additional disability during treatment} \times 100}{\text{No. of cases put under MDT during the year}}$$

- Proportion of defaulters from treatment

Definition: Defaulter is an individual who fails to complete treatment within prescribed period. When PB patient misses 3 or more doses and MB patient misses 6 or more doses will be termed as defaulter. Proportion (%) of patients who defaulted from completion of treatment

$$\text{Calculation} = \frac{\text{No. of cases who missed 3 or more pulses in PB and 6 or more pulses in MB} \times 100}{\text{No. of PB or MB cases put under MDT during the year}}$$

- Proportion of new cases correctly diagnosed

Definition: Proportion (%) of cases diagnosed correctly out of cases validated in a given time

$$\text{Calculation} = \frac{\text{No. of correctly diagnosed cases} \times 100}{\text{No. of new cases validated}}$$

RECORDS

Six records are to be maintained under the Upgraded Simplified Information System under NLEP. These are:

ULF 01 — Patient Card (*Annex. I*)
ULF 02/A — Treatment Register for New cases (*Annex. II*)
ULF 02/B — Treatment Register for Other cases (*Annex. III*)
ULF 03 — MDT Drug Stock Register (*Annex. IV*)
ULF - 04 — DPMR Assessment Card (*Annex. V*)
ULF - 05 — DPMR Record (*Annex. VI*)

Patient Card

This card (ULF 01) has been designed to keep information on the case diagnosed as leprosy and to keep record of its treatment. The card will be initially prepared by the Medical Officer in the Health Centre where the patient has been diagnosed and will initiate treatment with 1st dose of MDT. The Medical Officer will then put his signature on the card and send the same to the concerned sub-centre from where the patient can take subsequent doses. The patient should also be informed from where he can collect the remaining doses of MDT.

Treatment Record

The treatment record should be kept in registers in all Primary Health Centers/Block PHC (CHC) wherever leprosy cases are diagnosed and treated. As discussed earlier, at first the patient card is prepared by the medical officer diagnosing the case of leprosy. The information will thereafter be filled up in the treatment register. Each center will have to maintain following two treatment registers:

1. *Treatment register for new cases (ULF 02/A):* All new cases detected in the indigenous population of the area are to be recorded in this register.
2. *Treatment register for other cases (ULF 02/B):* All cases who are immigrants and have registered themselves elsewhere. Other cases to be recorded here are cases needing treatment for categories of relapse, re-entered for completion of treatment, referred cases and cases with change in classification.

The Annual Serial Registration Number should match with the patient card, which will also be available from these registers. The Medical Officer I/C of PHC/CHC, etc. should give this responsibility to one of the General Health Care Staff working in the Health Centre. All information entered should be exactly similar to those recorded in the patient card.

Leprosy MDT Drug Stock Record

The MDT Drug Stock Record (ULF 03) is to be maintained in all PHC/ Block PHC where MDT is supplied from the District and stocked. This is to be maintained in a register. Separate pages should be used for each of the 4 types of MDT Blister packs supplied, viz. MB (Adult), MB (Child), PB (Adult) and PB (child).

DPMR Assessment Card

Disability Prevention and Medical Rehabilitation (DPMR) is an important component of the National Leprosy Eradication Programme. Each case of Leprosy need to be properly assessed for disability and nerve function. The results of DPMR assessment is to be maintained in the DPMR assessment card (ULF 04).

The format is at Annexure – V.

REPORTS

The data recorded in different centres need to be periodically collected and put in a predesigned format for submission to the next higher level for further use. These are called the reporting formats.

Under NLEP following reports are to be submitted at different periodicity:

Monthly Progress Report (MPR)

- *ULF 06* — NLEP monthly reporting form PHC/Block PHC report (*Annex. - VII*)
- *ULF 07* — NLEP monthly reporting form District/State report (*Annex. - VIII*)

Quarterly Progress Report (QPR)

- *ULF 08* — NLEP quarterly reporting form on training (*Annex. - IX*)
- *ULF 09* — NLEP quarterly reporting form on IEC (*Annex. –X*)
- *ULF 10* — Elimination status in 209 high endemic Districts (*Annex.–XI*)

Annual Reports

For the fiscal year from April to March every year.
- *NLEP-01* — Districts-wise information as on 31st March – (*Annex. XII*)
- *NLEP-02* — Block-wise information as on 31st March (*Annex. XIII*)
- *NLEP-03* — Urban Locality wise information as on 31st March (*Annex. XIV*)
- NLEP-04 — District-wise information on search Activities (*Annex. XV*)
- NLEP-05 — District-wise information on leprosy fortnight (*Annex. XVI*)

Monthly Reports

NLEP—Monthly reporting form–PHC: The ULF 06 form will be utilized by the Primary Health Centre, which is the basic reporting unit under NLEP. This form will be filled up from the data available in the treatment registers, the drug stock record and disability register maintained at the PHC. The same format also will be used by the hospitals providing primary care services.

NLEP—Monthly reporting form–Block PHC: At the Block PHC, the report received from the PHC/Hospitals/NGO Institution will be compiled including from their own PHC record and the total information will be entered in the ULF 06 – Block report.

NLEP—Monthly reporting form–District: The ULF 07 form will be utilized by the office of the District Leprosy cell. The basis of filling this form will be the reports received from all the Block PHCs in the district, plus any report received by the District directly from any urban municipality hospitals/ Private Hospital/Medical College, etc.

NLEP—Monthly Reporting Form–State

The ULF 07 form will be utilized at the state level, where compiled information received from all the districts will be entered.

Quarterly Reports

The quarterly reports are to be submitted by the districts to the State Leprosy cell and after compilation at the State Leprosy Cell to Central Leprosy Division. These report are on Training, IEC and elimination status of Districts. All these informations are essential to monitor achievement of target set by the program. Reports are to be submitted to the CLD by 20th of July, October, January and April for 1st, 2nd, 3rd and 4th quarter respectively.

NLEP—Quarterly reporting form on training: The ULF–08 form is to be used for this report by the Districts and the State Leprosy Cell.

NLEP—Quarterly reporting form on IEC: The ULF–09 form is to be used for this report.

NLEP—Quarterly report on elimination status of districts: The ULF –10 form is to be used for this report for submission by all the State/UT in each quarter.

Annual Reports

The annual reports are to be submitted by the State/UT leprosy Cell to the Central Leprosy Division. These reports provide information on New cases detected, Gr. II deformity cases and balance cases under treatment at the end of fiscal year, in all Districts, Blocks and Urban areas. Two other reports are on search activities and on leprosy fortnight activities, for each district covered. The reports are to be submitted to CLD by 30th April each year.

Districtwise information as on 31st March: The NLEP-01 form is to be used for this report.

Blockwise information as on 31st March: The NLEP-02 form is to be used for this report.

Urban localitywise information as on 31st March: The NLEP-03 form is to be used for this report.

Districtwise information on search activities: The NLEP-04 form is to be used for this report.

Districtwise information on anti-leprosy fortnight: The NLEP-05 form is to be used for this report.

Flow of Reports

- NLEP monthly report are originated in the recording units, namely Primary Health Centres. Similar reports are also originated in hospitals/NGO institutions. Sub-centers are providing MDT services on behalf of the PHCs, but basic records are maintained and regularly updated at the PHCs. Therefore, no monthly report is to be collected from the subcenter for this purpose.
- PHCs/Hospitals/NGO institutions will send their monthly report to the Block PHCs in ULF 06 by 4th of the next month.
- The report from PHC/Hospital/NGO Institution under the jurisdiction of the concerned Block PHC will be compiled and the Block PHC report, in the same ULF 06 format, will be sent to the District Leprosy Cell by 7th of the next month of the reporting month.
- The district office will compile all the Block PHC reports and add any report received directly from urban institutions and then prepare the District monthly report in ULF 07 format, The District report will then be sent to the State Leprosy cell by 12th of the month next to the reporting month.
- The State Leprosy cell will then compile the data from all the Districts and prepare the State monthly report in Form ULF 07. The State cell will send the monthly report to the Central Leprosy Division by 20th of the month next to the reporting month by E-mail and also send a signed copy by registered post.
- The leprosy division will compile the information submitted by the State Leprosy cell by the 25th of month of receipt of reports as indicated above. Example—Report for the month of September 2013 by 25th October 2013.
- Quarterly reports are to be sent to the Central Leprosy Division by the State/UTs by 20th of July, October, January and April for 1st, 2nd 3rd and 4th quarter respectively, each year.

- The annual reports are to be sent to the Central Leprosy Division by the State/UTs by 30th April each year.

Report analysis and feedback: On receipt of the monthly reports at the level of Block PHC, District, State and Centre the same will be examined by the concerned official immediately. Any shortcoming like incomplete information, wrong filling up of forms, mistake in calculation, etc. should be intimated in writing to the concerned office asking for the requisite correction/clarification immediately.

At Block PHC and district level such deficiencies should also be discussed in the monthly review meeting and proper guidance should be given to avoid mistakes in future.

Nonsubmission of report on time should be viewed seriously and immediate feedback should be sent to the defaulting unit by the District, state and central level to avoid lapse in information collection. Even zero reporting with NIL information must be sent regularly.

VALIDATION MECHANISM AT DIFFERENT LEVEL

The essence of a successful information system is meticulous collection and reporting of correct data. It is therefore important to regularly crosscheck and validate the data collected and reported. To achieve this, there should be inbuilt mechanism for validation within the system at all levels.

Validation of New Cases

Correct diagnosis of the newly detected cases is the essence of the correct record and reports, based on which the programme is assessed. The newly detected cases are therefore invariably needed to be validated within 2 months of diagnosis and starting treatment. The District Nucleus Teams are to carryout the validations routinely at field level. In low endemic situations all the cases should be validated. In high endemic areas at least 10% of the new cases are to be validated.

Result of validation should be recorded in the following format:

Date of Validation	Name of PHC/ Block PHC	No. of new cases validated	Results			
			Not a case	Wrongly typed as MB/PB	Reregi-stered	Correctly diag-nosed

The record in the treatment register need to be corrected on the spot in consultation with the medical officer of the Health Centre.

This should be a component of the monthly report of the District Nucleus Team to the State Leprosy Cell.

Validation of Records

At the subcenter: From the patient card, validate treatment completion. This has to be done by the Medical Officer or the Supervisor.

At the primary health center: Validate the diagnosis, classification and treatment completion on a sample of patients. Also check the drugs record. Validation should be done by Block PHC/ District Officers.

At the district level: Validate drug records, monthly report consolidation and monitor the progress of integration through the record of visit by District Nucleus Teams. Validation to be done by the state level officers, Regional office for Health and FW (ROH and FW), GOI officers and NLEP Consultants.

At the state level: Validate drug records, monthly report consolidation and monitor the progress of integration. Validation to be done by the ROH and FW/GOI in the state and Central Leprosy Division.

Validation of Reports

Primary health center: The monthly report will be prepared from treatment records, DPMR records and drug stock records by the person authorized by Medical Officer. The Health Supervisor in the PHC will validate the correctness of information before it is signed by the Medical Officer Incharge.

Block primary health center: The reports from the Primary Health Centres will be validated at the Block PHC level by Senior Health Supervisor. He will also validate the compiled report prepared at the Block PHC before it is signed by the Medical Officer Incharge.

District level: The reports received from the Block PHCs/ Hospitals /NGO Institutions will be validated by the Health Supervisor in the office of the District Leprosy Officer. He will compile the Block PHC reports and prepare the district monthly report. The District Leprosy Officer will ensure correctness of the report before putting his signature.

State level: The reports from District will be validated at State level by the State Leprosy Officer on receipt of the same. The district reports will then be compiled and the State monthly report will be prepared. The State Leprosy Officer will ensure correctness of the state report before putting his signature.

National level: Reports from the States will be examined for correctness of data, proper filling of the format and then same will be compiled and analysed at the Central Leprosy Division.

PERFORMANCE ASSESSMENT

Performance under the program will be required to be assessed quarterly and annually at each District and State/UT level, during the quarterly meetings. Two forms have been designed for this purpose as below:

- *ULF 11*—Quarterly Performance Assessment (*Annex. XVII*)
- *ULF 12*—Annual Performance Assessment (*Annex. XVIII*)

These forms are meant for internal performance assessment at District and State level. These are not reporting form and should be kept only at the respective District/State HQ.

For District level assessment Block-wise data need to be filled up in both the formats. For State level assessment District-wise information should be filled up. Indicators in the formats should be calculated as per guidelines given in the booklet.

Geographical Information System

Geographical information system (GIS) is a computerized, integrated system used for compiling, storing, manipulating and mapping spatial data.

Conceptually, a GIS can be envisioned as a stacked set of map layers, where each layer is aligned in relation to all other layers. Typically, each layer contains a unique geographic theme or data type. By sharing mutual geography, all layers in the GIS can be combined or overlaid in any user-specified combination.

A GIS provides a hybrid database that contains both spatial and attribute data. Spatial data describe the location of objects with respect to a known coordinate system, while attribute data describe the nature or characteristics of spatial phenomena. Data flows through a GIS via a series of system functions. Data can be manipulated in a GIS using a series of functional programs called "tools" that operate on mapped data. Users can also elect a series of output options for communicating the results of their analyses to the users.

GIS can be used for planning and monitoring the health services and health status of the community and find the cause of any discrepancy in the collected information. Some of the uses have been enumerated.

- Design the functions of health care services and administrative services.
- Monitor health status and service need.
- Set priorities for the allocation of health care resources.
- Evaluate health program and health care outcomes, e.g. changes in health status as a result of any intervention in the health care program.
- Identify environmental, socioeconomic and other risk factors, which influence health, under serviced, poor, inaccessible areas and other geographic and demographic factors.
- Generate "thematic maps" (ranged color maps on proportional symbol maps to denote the intensity of a mapped variable).
- Allow for overlaying of different pieces of information.
- Create buffer areas around selected features (e.g. a radius of 10 km around a Health Center to denote a catchment area).
- Calculate distances between two points.

GIS permits dynamic link between databases and maps so that data updates are automatically reflected on maps and also permit interactive queries of information contained within the map, table or graph.

Computerized Information System

Computerized information system for Leprosy Control Programme are designed to facilitate monitoring of program and individual patient also. Once the primary data related to each patient is fed into computer, processing of these data becomes easy, quick and correct and report generation is without delay and information can be used for decision making in time. Computerized data base and patient tracking system, if programed will monitor the individual patients and program as well.

Annexure I

NATIONAL LEPROSY ERADICATION PROGRAM (NLEP)

PATIENT CARD

Subcenter			PHC				
Block/CHC		Districts			State		
Registration number				SC	ST		Others
Name				Age	Female		Male
Address (with mobile no.)							
Duration of (signs/symptom in months)			.... Duration of disability if any				
Mode of detection			Voluntary/by ASHA/Referred by other/by contact survey/other mode				
Classification		PB	MB	New case	Other type (specify)		
Disability		Gr.-I	Gr.-II	EHF score			
Date of first dose							
AFTER ENTERING ABOVE INFORMATION IN THE PHC TREATMENT RECORD, THIS PATIENT CARD IS TO BE TRANSFERRED TO SUBCENTER FOR DELIVERY OF SUBSEQUENT DOSES				Signature of Medical Officer			

Date of subsequent doses

2	3	4	5	6 PB (Final)	7	8	9	10	11	12 MB (Final)

Date of discharge		Date		RFT/Otherwise deleted (specify)	
End status		EHF score		Follow-up required (after RFT)/for reaction, deformity, ulcer or eye care	
THIS CARD IS TO BE MAINTAINED AT SUBCENTER. AFTER EVERY DOSE. UPDATE THE PHC TREATMENT RECORD. AFTER ACHIEVING END STATUS, THE MPW SHOULD SIGN THIS CARD AND RETAIN AT SUBCENTER FOR FUTURE REFRENCE				Signature of subcenter MPW	

Guidelines to fill-up this card

Mode of detection	ASHA/Health worker/contact survey/search/voluntary reporting	
Contact survey in MB/child case	No. examined	Cases detected MB-PB

Record of Lepra Reaction/Neuritis

Type–I/II	**Neuritis–Yes/No**
Prednisolone doses issued with dates at PHC/District hospital	
Dates of MCR footwear if issued	
Date of referral for RCS	
Contact examination done on ...., new cases suspected/confirmed	

NB: This patient card is for use for the new cases as well as other cases. In urban situation, this card can be used by changing subcenter/PHC/CHC with appropriate health unit/area/region.

ULF 02/A

Annexure II

TREATMENT REGISTER FOR NEW CASES

PHC _____ Block PHC/CHC _____

Districts _____ State/UTs _____ Fiscal year _____

Reg. no.	Sub-center	Name	Address with mobile /Tel. number	Age	Sex M/F	ST/ SC	PB/ MB	Disability grade I/II	Date of first dose	Date of subsequent doses											Date of RFT
										2	3	4	5	6 (PB final)	7	8	9	10	11	12 (MB final)	

Annexure III

TREATMENT REGISTER FOR OTHER CASES

ULF 02/B

PHC _____ Block PHC/CHC _____

Districts _____ State/UTs _____ Fiscal year _____

Reg. no.	Sub-center	Name	Address and mobile number	Age	Sex M/F	ST/ SC	PB/ MB	Disability grade I/II	Date of first dose	Date of subsequent doses					6 (PB final)	7	8	9	10	11	12 (MB final)	Date of RFT	Category of case*
										2	3	4	5										

* Category of case: Relapse, re-entered for treatment completion, referred and changing in classification of MB/PB

ULF 03

Annexure IV
NLEP – LEPROSY MDT DRUG STOCK RECORD

Use separate page for each category of MDT [MB(A)*/MB(C)**/PB(A)*/PB(C)**] – Specify category : _____

(Same format to be used at PHC/District/State levels – Please specify level with name along with next highest level up to State)

PHC _____ State _____ Fiscal year _____

District _____ Block PHC/CHC _____

Transaction date	RECEIPT						EXPENDITURE						Balance in hand	Stock in patient month
	Quantity received	From where	Vide ref. no.	Batch no.	Expiry date		Quantity issued	Vide ref. no.	To whom	Batch no.	Expiry date			

* A = Adults
** C = Child

Annexure V

SENSORY ASSESSMENT

Date/Assessor	Palm		Sole		Comments
	Right	Left	Right	Left	

Key : (Put these mark/icon on the site where lesion is seen)

✓ Sensation present within 3 cm   S Contracture   Scar/Callus

✗ Anesthesia   Wound   Shortening Level

∧ Clawing   Crack

Annexure V (Continued)

Assessment of Disability and Nerve Function

Name _____ Village _____ Date of registration _____

S/o, W/o, D/o _____ Subcenter _____ Date of RFT _____

Age/Sex _____ Registration no _____ Referred by _____

Occupation _____ MB/PB _____ Date of assessment _____

Right									Left					
						← Date →								
						Vision (0, 2)								
						Light closure lid gap in mm.								
						Blink present/absent								
						Little finger out								
						Thumb-up								
						Wrist extension								
						Foot up								
						Disability grade–Hands								
						Disability grade–Feet								
						Disability grade–Eyes								
On date														
Max. (WHO) Disability grade														
EHF score														
Signature of Assessor														

Muscle power:
S = Strong
W = Weak
P = Paralysis

Score of vision: Counting fingers at 6 meters
0 = Normal
1 = Blurring vision
2 = Unable to count fingers

This form should be filled-in at the time of registration and repeated after 3 months (once in 2 weeks in case of neuritis/reaction).

ULF 05

Annexure VI

Disability Register

PHC/CHC _____ District _____ State/UTs _____

S. No.	Name of the patient	Age/Sex	Address village/Sub-center/PHC with phone number	New/UT/Old case	MB/PB	New cases (NC)/UT case/RFT	Disability grade I/II	Site of disability					
								Eye		Hand		Foot	
								Gr 0	Gr II	Gr I	Gr II	Gr I	Gr II
1	2	3	4	5	6	7	8	9	10	11	12	13	14

Ulcer simple/ Complicated	EHF score	Neuritis	Reaction Type-I/ Type-II	DPMR services provided				Refer with date				New disability developed after starting of prednisolone			Referral services provided/ follow-up taken up/ remarks
				Steroid/ dose/du- ration	Self-care practice	Ulcer treatment	Other if any	RCS	Complicated ulcer	Eye	Reaction not responding to steroid	Eye (Gr II)	Hand (Gr I/ Gr II)	Foot (Gr I/ Gr II)	
15	16	17	18	19	20	21	22	23	24	25	26	27	28	29	30

Annexure VII

NLEP Monthly Reporting Form PHC/Block PHC Report

PHC _____ Block _____
Districts _____ State _____
Reporting month _____ Year _____

					1.1 New cases	1.2 Other cases	
1.	No. of balance cases at the beginning of the month		PB				
			MB				
			Total				
2.	No. of new leprosy cases detected in the reporting month				During reporting month		
					PB	MB	Total
			Adult				
			Child				
	Among new cases – number from other states		Total				
3.	Among new leprosy cases detected during the reporting month, number of		Female				
			Disability	Grade-I			
				Grade-II			
			SC				
			ST				
4.	Number of new leprosy cases deleted during the month		RFT				
			Otherwise deleted				
			Total				
5.	Number of new leprosy cases under treatment at the end of the month (1.1 + 2 - 4)						
6.	Number of "other cases" recorded and put under treatment		(i) Relapse				
			(ii) Re-entered for treatment				
			(iii) Referred				
			(iv) Reclassified				
			From other State				
			Total				
7.	No. of "other cases" deleted from treatment		RFT				
			Otherwise deleted				
			Total				
8.	No. of "other cases" under treatment at the end of reporting month (1.2 + 6 -7)						
9.	Total number of cases under treatment at the end of month	New + Others (5+8)					

10. Leprosy drug stock at the end of the reporting month (if required use extra sheets)

Blister pack	Quantity	Expiry date	Total stock	No. of patient under treatment (new and others)	Patient months BCP
MB(A)					
MB(C)					
PB(A)					
PB(C)					

NB: Please calculate patient-monthly blister packs for MB(A), MB(C), PB(A) and PB(C) quarterly in the month of March, June, September and December and indicate the same in that respective monthly report.

Remarks, (if any)

Signature of Medical Officer

NLEP Monthly Reporting Form PHC/Block PHC

S. no.	Indicators	During reporting month		
		PB	MB	Total
1.	No. of new leprosy cases recorded			
2.	No. of reaction cases managed at PHC			
3.	No. of reaction cases referred to Dist. Hosp./other Instt.			
4.	No. of relapse cases suspected and referred by PHCs			
5.	No. of relapse cases confirmed at district hospital			
6.	No. of cases developed new disability after MDT			
7.	No. of patients provided with footwear			
8.	No. of patients provided with self-care kit			
9.	No. of patients referred for RCS			
10.	No. of new cases confirmed at PHC out of referred by ASHA			
11.	No. of case completed treatment through ASHA			
12.	No. of ASHA paid incentives			
13.	No. of contacts examined			
14.	No. of cases detected amongst contacts			
15.	No. of cases voluntarily reported, out of new cases recorded (S. no. 1)			

Signature of Medical Officer

Annexure VIII

NLEP Monthly Reporting Form District/State Report

(* Delete the level District/State whichever not applicable)

District		State/UT		Reporting Month/Year		
Population of the District/State			Total	SC		ST

				1.1 New cases		1.2 Other cases	
1.	No. of balance new cases at the beginning of the month						
		PB					
		MB					
		Total					

				During reporting month			Cumulative from 1st April		
2.	No. of new leprosy cases detected in the reporting month			PB	MB	Total	PB	MB	Total
		Adult							
		Child							
		Total							
	Among new cases – no. from other States	Total							
3.	Among new leprosy cases detected during the reporting month, number of	Female							
		Disability	Grade-I						
			Grade-II						
		SC							
		ST							
4.	Number of new leprosy cases deleted during the month	RFT							
		Otherwise deleted							
		Total							
5.	Number of new leprosy cases under treatment at the end of the month (1.1 + 2 – 4)								
6.	Number of "other cases" recorded and put under treatment	(i) Relapse							
		(ii) Re-entered for treatment							
		(iii) Referred							
		(iv) Reclassified							
		Total							
7.	No. of "other cases" deleted from treatment	RFT							
		Otherwise deleted							
		Total							
8.	No. of "other cases" under treatment at the end of reporting month (1.2 + 6 – 7)								
9.	Total number of cases under MDT at the end of month (5 + 8)								

10 Drug stock at the end of the reporting month (if required use extra sheets)

Blister pack	Compiled PHC/Distt. stock		District/State store stock		Total in the District/State		
	Quantity	Expiry date	Quantity	Expiry date	Quantity	No. of UT patient (new and other)	Patient month BCP
MB(A)							
MB(C)							
PB(A)							
PB(C)							

NB: Please calculate patient-t month blister packs for MB(A), MB(C), PB(A) and PB(C) quarterly in the month of March, June, September and December and indicate the same in that respective monthly report.

Remarks, (if any) –

Signature of DLO/SLO

NLEP Monthly Reporting Form District/State Report

S. no.	Indicators		During the month			Cumulative total from April till date		
			PB	MB	Total	PB	MB	Total
1.	No. of new leprosy cases recorded							
2.	No. of reaction cases managed at PHC							
3.	No. of reaction cases referred to Dist. Hosp./other Instt.							
4.	No. of relapse cases suspected and referred by PHCs							
5.	No. of relapse cases confirmed at district hospital							
6.	No. of cases developed new disability after MDT							
7.	No. of patients provided with footwear							
8.	No. of patients provided with self-care kit							
9.	No. of patients referred for RCS							
10.	No. of new cases confirmed at PHC out of referred by ASHA							
11.	No. of case completed treatment through ASHA							
12.	No. of ASHA paid incentives							
13.	No. of contacts examined							
14.	No. of cases detected amongst contacts							
15.	No. of cases voluntarily reported, out of new cases recorded (S. No. 1)							
16.	No. of institutes providing RCS	Govt.						
		NGO						
		Total						
17.	No. of persons – RCS done	Govt.						
		NGO						
		Total						

Signature of the DLO/SLO

Annexure IX

NLEP Quarterly Report on Training

Name of State/UT _____

Report for the quarterly ending – June/September/December/March (Year)

S. no.	Categories of persons trained	Type of training	Target for the year	Trained during the quarter	Cumulative progress during the year
1	2	3	4	5	6
1.					
2.					
3.					
4.					
5.					
6.					
7.					
8.					

Signature of the SLO

Annexure X

NLEP Quarterly Report on IEC

Name of State/UT _____

Report for the quarter ending – June/September/December/March (Year)

S. no.	Type of IEC activity	Target for the year (if any)	Completed during the quarter	Cumulative progress during the year
1	2	3	4	5
1.				
2.				
3.				
4.				
5.				
6.				
7.				
8.				
9.				
10.				
11.				

Signature of the SLO

Annexure XI

NLEP Quarterly Progress Report on Elimination Status of Districts

Name of State/UT _____

Report for the quarter ending – June/September/December/March (Year)

Total no. of Districts	No. of Districts achieved elimination	No. of Districts with prevalence rate (PR) – > 1/10,000 population
Name of Districts with PR > 1/10,000	**S. no.**	
	1.	
	2.	
	3.	
	4.	
	5.	
	6.	
	7.	
	8.	
	9.	
	10.	
	11.	
	12.	

Signature of the SLO

NLEP 01

Annexure XII

National Leprosy Eradication Programme
District-wise Information as on 31st March (Year)

Name of State/UT _____

S. no.	Name of District	Estimated population March (Year)	Total new cases (Year)	ANCDR/100,000	Total Grade–II disabled cases (Year)	Percentage of Gr II against new cases	Balance cases as on March (Year)	PR/10,000
1	2	3	4	5	6	7	8	9
1.								
2.								
3.								
4.								
5.								
6.								
7.								
8.								
9.								
10.								
11.								
12.								
13.								
14.								
15.								
	Total							

State Leprosy Officer

NLEP 02

Annexure XIII
National Leprosy Eradication Programme
Block-wise Information as on 31st March (Year)

Name of State _____

S. no.	Name of District	S. no.	Name of Block PHC	Estimated population of block, March (Year)	Total new cases (Year)	ANCDR/100,000	Balance cases as on March (Year)	PR/10,000
1	2	3	4	5	6	7	8	9
1.								
2.								
3.								
4.								
5.								
6.								
7.								
8.								
9.								
10.								
11.								
12.								
13.								
14.								
15.								
Total								

State Leprosy Officer

NLEP 03

Annexure XIV

National Leprosy Eradication Programme
Urban locality-wise Information as on 31st March (Year)

Name of State _____

S. no.	Name of District	S. no.	Name of urban locality	Estimated population of locality, March (Year)	Total new cases (Year)	ANCDR/100,000	Balance cases as on March (Year)	PR/10,000
1	2	3	4	5	6	7	8	9
1.								
2.								
3.								
4.								
5.								
6.								
7.								
8.								
9.								
10.								
11.								
12.								
13.								
14.								
15.								
Total								

State Leprosy Officer

Annexure XV

National Leprosy Eradication Programme
Report on Active Search (Year)

NLEP 04

Name of State/UT _____

Period for search activity _____

S. no.	Name of District	No. of block PHC covered	Population		Leprosy cases detected			No. of disability in cases detected			No. of child cases in cases detected		
			Enumerated	Examined	MB	PB	Total	Gr I	Gr II	Total	MB	PB	Total
1	**2**	**3**	**4**	**5**	**6**	**7**	**8**	**9**	**10**	**11**	**12**	**13**	**14**
1.													
2.													
3.													
4.													
5.													
6.													
7.													
8.													
9.													
10.													
11.													
12.													
13.													
14.													
15.													
	Total												

State Leprosy Officer

NLEP 05

Annexure XVI

National Leprosy Eradication Programme
Report on Anti-leprosy Fortnight (Year)

Name of State/UT _____

Period of active search _____

S. no.	Name of District	No. of block PHC covered	Population		Leprosy cases detected			No. of disability in cases detected			No. of children in cases detected		
			Enumerated	Examined	MB	PB	Total	Gr I	Gr II	Total	MB	PB	Total
1	**2**	**3**	**4**	**5**	**6**	**7**	**8**	**9**	**10**	**11**	**12**	**13**	**14**
1.													
2.													
3.													
4.													
5.													
6.													
7.													
8.													
9.													
10.													
11.													
12.													
13.													
14.													
15.													
Total													

State Leprosy Officer

ULF 11

Annexure XVII
Quarterly Performance Assessment

District _____

Quarter ending _____

State _____

Year _____

S. no.	Name of Block/District	Prevalence Rate/10,000	MB (%)	Child (%)	New Gr II disability (%)	ASHA involvement (%)	No. of new cases with disability			Patient month BCP status of MDT				Corrective action taken
							MB	PB	Total	MB (A)	MB (C)	PB (A)	PB (C)	
1.														
2.														
3.														
4.														
5.														

ULF 12

Annexure XVIII

Annual Performance Assessment

District _____ State/UT _____ Year _____

S. no.	Block/District	Prevalence	ANCDR/100,000	MB (%)	Child rate/100,000	New Gr II District/% mil	ST rate/100,000	SC rate/100,000	RFT/%		ASHA		Patient month BCP status of MDT			
									New case	Other case	No. involved	No. patient detected	MB (A)	MB (C)	PB (A)	PB (C)
1	2	3	4	5	6	7	8	9	10	11	12	13	14	15	16	17

Case validation	Training		IEC			Fund			Corrective action taken
No. Correct diagnosis	Target	Achieved	Target	Achieved %	Allocated	Expenditure	%	
18	19	20	21	22	23	24	25	26	27

SECTION 8

Rehabilitation and Social Issues

43
CHAPTER

Rehabilitation

D Kamaraj

INTRODUCTION

Most of the estimated 650 million people living with disabilities around the world lack access to appropriate medical care and rehabilitation services, especially those living in low and middle income countries. As a consequence, people with disabilities experience greater challenges in attaining and maintaining optimum independence and health. Lack of services creates a barrier to full inclusion and participation in all aspects of life.

Rehabilitation and habilitation are processes intended to enable people with disabilities to reach and maintain optimal physical, sensory, intellectual, psychological and/or social functions. Rehabilitation encompasses a wide range of activities including rehabilitative medical care, physical, psychological, speech and occupational therapy, and other support services. People with disabilities should have access to both general medical care and appropriate rehabilitation services.

Rehabilitation includes all measures aimed at reducing the impact of disability on an individual, enabling him or her to achieve independence, social integration, a better quality of life and self-actualization.

Rehabilitation usually includes the following types of services:

- Early detection, diagnosis and intervention;
- Medical care and treatment;
- Social, psychological and other types of counseling and assistance;
- Training in self-care activities, including mobility, communication and daily living skills, with special provisions as needed, e.g. for the hearing impaired, the visually impaired and the mentally retarded;
- Provision of technical and mobility aids, and other devices;
- Specialized education services;
- Vocational rehabilitation services (including vocational guidance), vocational training, placement in open or sheltered employment;
- Follow-up.

LEPROSY REHABILITATION

Historically, people with leprosy-related disability have been ostracized from their communities and have rarely been able to access integrated disability services, which includes all disability schemes provided by the government and nongovernmental organizations (NGOs) in general. They preferred the services offered by dedicated leprosy NGOs in the vertical approach. This institution-centric approach and the stigma surrounding leprosy meant that communities had little involvement in the rehabilitation process of people affected by leprosy.

However, in recent years there has been a change in attitude towards leprosy. The stigma associated with the disease has lessened. People affected by leprosy now often remain within their families and communities. As a result, involving the family and community members is now seen as a key strategy to empower people affected by leprosy, encouraging them to play an active role in their rehabilitation.

Changing Scenario of Leprosy Rehabilitation

Even though the strategies in leprosy rehabilitation have been modified to suit the present situation for some time now, it is still unclear as to who needs rehabilitation and which services are best suited for different groups of patients. In an analysis of studies on leprosy, Srinivasan reported that 21–45% of all persons affected by the disease deteriorated economically. A high proportion of this group had deformities, yet not all persons with deformities deteriorated economically. Conversely, some persons without deformities also deteriorated economically. The dilemma is to identify "who amongst leprosy affected persons need community level rehabilitation to address the economic and other psychosocial impact of the illness. Are they the persons with deformities or are they leprosy affected persons with some other parameters that are not yet identified"?

Likewise, it is yet not clear what kind of rehabilitation is the most acceptable to a leprosy affected person. For example, only a very small number of people with deformities are actually fit and willing for reconstruction surgeries. Similarly, a substantial number of economically deteriorated leprosy affected people show no interest in seeking available rehabilitation schemes. Objective evidence pertaining to acceptance and appropriateness of rehabilitation services in leprosy is scanty and is an area of concern. The transition of leprosy rehabilitation from medical to psychosocial and from institutional to community based processes requires certain changes in governance.

Traditionally, healthcare institutions used to have a "top-down" approach in service delivery and governance. In some cases the systems became so autocratic that "needs" of clients were ignored and they never became empowered to choose their goals. In contrast, "community based organizations" do not have highly differentiated structures or systems of communication that are imposed on clients. They use a "bottom-up" approach that allows client participation in strategy development. The major difference between institutions and community-based organizations is that institutions used to discourage people from accessing services if they did not agree with the institutional goals. In community-based organizations, any such differences are settled through a change in program plan to make it more client-centered. Until recently, leprosy rehabilitation was more institutional and top-down. However, of late, some programs have become "bottom-up" in approach, and as a result have started using "participatory needs analysis", "participatory decision making" and so on. These are approaches that are quite different from what these institutions were used to earlier (Fig. 43.1).

COMMUNITY BASED REHABILITATION

Community based rehabilitation (CBR) is recognized as the best practice in addressing the needs of people with

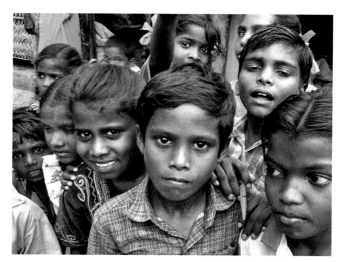

Fig. 43.1: Focus on leprosy awareness among children to stop transmission of stigma to generation next

disabilities, including those affected by leprosy. The definition recognized by the International Labor Organization (ILO), *United Nations Educational, Scientific and Cultural Organization* (UNESCO) and World Health Organization (WHO) describes CBR as follows: *"CBR is a strategy within general community development for the rehabilitation, equalization of opportunities, poverty reduction and social inclusion of all people with disabilities. CBR is implemented through the combined efforts of people with disabilities themselves, their families, organizations and communities, and the relevant governmental and nongovernmental health, education, vocational, social and other services".* The basic needs of all people, including people with disability and people affected by leprosy, are the same—food, health, education, shelter and so on. CBR facilitates access to basic needs, and at the same time promotes equal opportunities and equal rights. It is therefore, a multisectoral strategy with some key principles to enable people with disabilities to participate in the whole range of human activities.

One of the aims of CBR is to ensure that people with disabilities get the same rights and opportunities as all other community members. This includes rights such as equal access to healthcare, education, skills training, employment, family life, social mobility and political empowerment. A successful CBR aims at meeting the needs of people affected by leprosy and promoting their quality of life. Therefore, CBR is highly relevant to the rehabilitation of people affected by leprosy.

Moreover, just as leprosy control activities have been integrated into general health services, likewise rehabilitation services for people affected by leprosy can also be main streamed to general rehabilitation programs for greater sustainability and coverage. This would mean that in a leprosy-endemic area where only a leprosy-related program is available, it would take up other disabilities and vice versa.

Basic Principles of Community Based Rehabilitation

The principles outlined below are overlapping, complementary and interdependent.

Participation

Community based rehabilitation focuses on abilities, not disabilities. It depends on the participation and support of people with disability, family members and local communities. It also means the involvement of people with disabilities as active contributors to the CBR program, from policy-making to implementation and evaluation, for the simple reason that they know what their needs are.

Case study (participation): "Shiv Kranti Apang Bachat Gat" is the first self-help group (SHG) for the disabled persons in a village in Amravati district of Maharashtra (India). The group comprises of six members belonging to different age group and disability category. Among them are four males of age group 50–60 years, one adult female, and a girl 7 years old who is studying in a normal school. They have opened their bank account in Amravati District Central Cooperative Bank, Amravati.

The group members are actively working as unpaid volunteers in their village. They go in a group conducting survey of the disabled in Kurha village. Their main motive of doing this survey is to:

• Provide information about the government schemes to the individuals as per their age group and capabilities.
• To provide information about the importance and benefits of SHG and there of motivating them to form SHG on behalf of their own project(s).
• Their future plan is to start a ration shop in their village from the loan which they will be getting from the bank.

A SHG, which was formed for the socioeconomic rehabilitation of the group members, is now helping the other disabled in the community voluntarily, and is a positive role model for people with disabilities as active contributors for their own and for the society at large.

Empowerment

Local people—and specifically people with disabilities and their families—ultimately may make the program decisions and control the resources. This requires people with disability taking leadership roles within programs. It means ensuring that CBR workers, service providers and facilitators include people with disabilities, and that all are adequately trained and supported. Results are seen as restored dignity and self-confidence.

Case study (empowerment): The community participation in Prem Nagar leprosy colony in Janjgir-Champa district of Bilaspur, Chhattisgarh (India) has been very successful.

People in the community have helped in conducting the general survey and leprosy survey. Prevention of disability training of leprosy-affected volunteers of the colony was one of the highlights in the project, and then using them as supervisors and trainers in the self-care groups was very effective. Successful outcome of the 5 days training workshop had encouraged these 13 volunteers to share the knowledge and skill of self-care to others and increased their own confidence as well. Fifty one self-care groups have been organized in the colony. In the beginning, the project staff faced difficulty getting the people to practice self-care at home, but after organizing the self-care groups, there were amazing results. The members reprimanded each other if they had not cared for themselves properly and shared any trouble they were having in their families or community. The result has been significant. It has led to improvement in prevention of disability, increasing numbers of people using protective footwear, reduction in the recurrence of ulcers and reduction in hospital admittances (Fig. 43.2).

Raising Awareness

Community based rehabilitation addresses attitudes and behavior within the community, developing understanding and support for people with disabilities and ensuring sustainable benefits. It also promotes the need for and benefit of inclusion of disability in all developmental initiatives.

Self-advocacy

Community based rehabilitation consistently involves people with disabilities in all issues related to their well-being. Self-advocacy is a collective notion, not an individualistic one. It means self-determination. It means mobilizing, organizing,

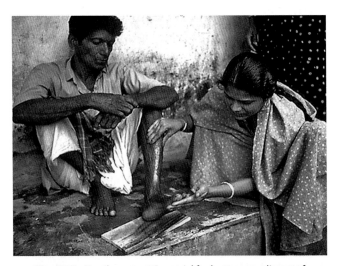

Fig. 43.2: Family support is crucial for better compliance of homecare program and, thereby, prevents further disability

representing, and creating space for interactions and demands.

Case study (awareness and advocacy): Bhusan Mahato is a 60-year-old man living at Simonpur village, a leprosy colony in Purulia district of West Bengal (India). Due to the disease leprosy and associated stigma, he lost his job. This put his family in a very difficult situation. They had to struggle even to get their daily bread. One day, following a community awareness meeting, Bhusan was very enthusiastic about all that he had heard that he decided to apply for a disability certificate and later approach the government for the benefits. But he was soon turned away and was not able to get a disability certificate. He approached the staff of the project team instead. The team advised him that first he has to apply to the medical board for the disability certificate. He was soon able to get a leprosy cured certificate and then after nearly 8 months was issued a disability certificate. With this, he was able to apply for the government benefits. Today, he receives a monthly pension with which he is able to support his family. There was screening camp of the Indian Red Cross Society in his area and he was gifted a tricycle, which today helps him to be mobile. Having received the right help at the right time, Bhusan has come a long way and is living a life of contentment.

Gender Sensitivity and Special Needs

Community based rehabilitation is responsive to individuals and groups within the community with special needs.

Case study (gender–women self-help group): The Laxmi Mahila Self-Help Group is based at Nangchui, Kota district of Bilaspur, Chhattisgarh (India). Initially, people were unaware of the concept of such a group. There were several visits by CBR workers and repeated sessions with the women to explain how SHGs function. After a certain level of rapport was established, the women were willing to give it a try. In March 2006, 11 members got together to form the group. There were two leprosy affected women, two with physical disability and seven others who were living below the poverty line. The group meets regularly in the meetings and each member contributes ₹ 20 and, therefore, a collection of ₹ 220 in a month is gathered from the group. The local government, that is the *panchayat*, gave them the responsibility of a mid-day meals project. Later, they went on to get involved in a fisheries project. Today, these stand as very successful income generating programs. The SHG made a profit of about ₹ 8,500 in mid-day meal program and from fisheries got a profit of ₹ 6,690. In the month of July, 2007, SHG women purchased 15 kg fish seed worth ₹ 3,000 and the members are carrying out inter lending and raising ₹ 21,000.

The Laxmi Mahila Self-Help Group has helped improve the standard of living of these 11 women and has also given them a sense of purpose, which has changed their outlook on

life. It also had a wider impact in the village. Seeing the good work of the SHG, the gramin bank is ready to give financial help according to the government scheme.

They have also started making plates out of palm leaves and are trying to get a good market for it. Having enjoyed many benefits, the women are enthusiastic to take up new challenges and move forward (Fig. 43.3).

Partnerships

Community based rehabilitation depends on effective partnerships with community-based organizations, government organizations and other organized groups.

Sustainability

Community based rehabilitation activities must be sustainable beyond the immediate life of the program itself. They must be able to continue beyond the initial interventions and be independent of the initiating agency. The benefits of the program must be long-lasting.

Case study (partnerships and sustainability): A good example for partnerships and sustainability is seen in the Mega *Mela* for the disabled persons organized at Ramachandrapuram, Andhra Pradesh (India), in 2005 (Table 43.1). The highlight is that most of the resources for the mela were drawn from the local community itself (Fig. 43.4).

Community Based Rehabilitation Guidelines and Matrix

The history of CBR dates back to 1978 following the declaration at the international conference on Primary

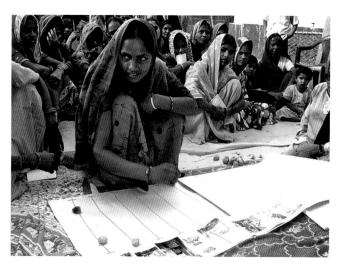

Fig. 43.3: Women are potential partners of family and community development

Table 43.1: Resources for the Mega *Mela* for the disabled persons organized at Ramachandrapuram, Andhra Pradesh (India), in 2005

1. Organizing Camp	Krushi Orthopedic Society, Vizag and the community project
2. Food	Sri Chetanya Rice Mills
3. Venue (Mandapam)	Lions club (at a subsidized rate)
4. Technical support	Krushi Orthopedic Society, AVFTD, Bhagwan Mahavir Seva Samiti (Rajasthan)
5. Mobility aids	Bhagwan Mahavir Seva Samiti (Rajasthan)
6. Miscellaneous	New Hope Loving Mission

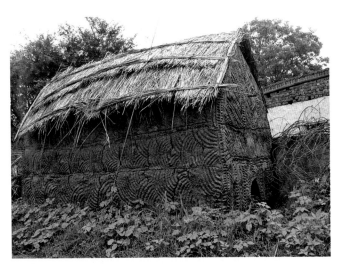

Fig. 43.4: Sustainable measures identify with the existing environment and respect the local culture

Health Care held at Alma Ata. CBR was initiated by the World Health Organization (WHO) as a strategy to improve access to rehabilitation services for people with disabilities in low and middle income countries using the available resources of the community. In 30 years, CBR has grown several folds and it has now evolved into a multisectoral strategy covering broader needs of people with disabilities classified into five components as per the CBR guidelines released by WHO, in 2010. They are health, education, livelihood, social and empowerment. It is clear that health alone is not sufficient for a person, but there are other crucial areas that can have an impact on the "health" which needs to be comprehensively addressed.

The guidelines promote CBR as a strategy or key to the implementation of the United Nations Convention of Rights of People with Disabilities (UNCRPD), and of disability inclusive national legislation, and which can support community-based inclusive development.

It is also acknowledged that all communities are different in terrain, culture, their political systems, socioeconomic conditions and many other factors. Therefore, there cannot be one model of CBR for the whole world. It may not be the same even within one country. There are many models of CBR programs; each is unique to its own situation. This is the uniqueness and at the same time the challenge of CBR programs. However, from experience, it has been realized that there need to be some basic norms for a valid CBR program. Evidence is needed that the particular CBR strategy being used is the most effective and efficient approach to enhance the quality of life for people with disabilities and their family members.

The matrix illustrates the topical areas which can make up a CBR strategy (Flow chart 43.1). It consists of five components, each divided into five elements. Each of these elements will have a dedicated chapter in the guidelines. The elements are sub divided into content headings. Each element has between 4–8 key content headings. The principles are in no way just theoretical or abstract but intended to be translated into tangible ways of working and should be observable in program activities. The CBR guidelines were released at the African CBR conference in Nigeria, in October 2010, and are available at: www.who.int/disabilities/cbr/guidelines/en/.

Examples of Implementing Part of the Matrix and Scaling-up

The matrix represents the topical areas, which an effective CBR program may contain, depending on local circumstances. The CBR practitioner may choose:

- The most practical entry point for the program, for example, an initiative on primary schooling or organizing parents of children with disabilities.
- The next logical steps to build up the program, for example, an initiative on antenatal and primary healthcare.
- And so on...until a coherent program of appropriate components and elements is formed, supported by a strong set of cross-sector alliances and partnerships.

Community Based Rehabilitation Challenges

- Community based rehabilitation (CBR) has become a community development process. The debate whether it should be initiated by outsiders or started by the community has been of interest. Votaries of the former view advocate starting delivery of services without waiting for the community to participate, because community ownership, where people take responsibility for planning, implementing, monitoring and risk sharing, is a slow process. The alternate view is that concerned groups themselves should initiate CBR because it is a developmental process. If CBR is externally initiated, communities can remain passive and do not develop capacity to manage their own affairs.

Flow chart 43.1: Community based rehabilitation strategy

Goal: Human rights ~ Socio-economic development ~ Poverty alleviation

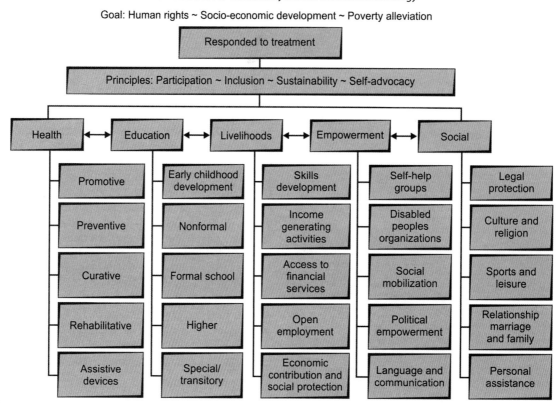

- "Community participation" is the central and essential tenet in the social model. However, communities are often quite heterogeneous, with wide differences in socioeconomic, educational, religious and ethnic status. This diversity can cause friction because some groups have different needs and priorities compared to others. Similarly, needs and priorities of people with disabilities are not always at the forefront when competing issues occur simultaneously.
- People in some developing countries also expect benefits from their governments as doles and, as a result, show a reluctance to take charge of their affairs. Decentralization and "bottom-up" strategies become difficult to implement in these circumstances.
- The emphasis in CBR today is on integrating disability into the developmental processes. Votaries of integration conclude that it is cost-effective, promotes better social integration and ensures access to people with disabilities as much as others in the community. Besides, community participation is greater when the majority rather than only a minority share its benefits. At the same time, unplanned integration of disability into development can ignore "real rehabilitation" needs of people with disabilities and segregate them further. During the last few years, integration of disability into community development programs has shown some tangible benefits and some

problems. Poor organizational capacity to integrate two functionally different streams of interventions and lack of familiarity with rehabilitation on the part of community development organizations have acted as major barriers for integration.
- Lack of mobility, education and other skills also prevent disabled people from being part of the broader development process.
- Integration of rehabilitation into development programs needs a high degree of coordination and collaboration between different sectors such as health, education, employment and others. Barriers in this process have to be removed before such collaboration can succeed and make the social model of CBR effective.
- CBR was promoted to gain wider coverage at affordable costs. In order to reduce costs, many interventions were shifted to families of disabled persons and community. Although CBR appears to be cheaper, in reality much of the costs are transferred to the consumers. If the costs to the consumers are also included in computing the expenditure, it may turn out to be much higher than what is generally assumed. Many families in developing countries do not have the means to support their disabled members. In an environment of increasing difficulty to access resources, these families are more likely to choose their "normal" members to support than their disabled relatives.

- About 30% of people with disabilities in CBR have severe and multiple disabilities. Sometimes severely disabled persons get neglected while CBR focuses on issues such as "community participation" and equal "rights". When they are neglected, programs tend to gloss over their shortcomings as a "limitation of CBR".
- Women with disabilities are another group whose needs are not adequately addressed. They face unique disadvantages simultaneously, such as difficulties in performing traditional gender roles, participating in community life and accessing rehabilitation services provided by male service providers.
- The problems of community volunteers illustrate how difficult it is to translate a theme like "community participation" into practice. Volunteers are difficult to find, their turnover is high, large resources are required to train them continuously, they lack motivation and do not perform if incentives or the small salaries are not paid regularly. However, there are programs that have successfully used volunteers, though they are exceptions.

Arrangements for the Delivery of Community Based Rehabilitation Services

Arrangements for the delivery of primary-level CBR services vary according to the local situation. Depending on which organizations exist, CBR services may be delivered through some or all of the following: Community-based organizations; organizations of people affected by leprosy or other disabilities; voluntary, nongovernmental organizations; government services.

Intervention

Interventions are activities agreed between CBR workers and clients that seek to address an agreed need or problem related to individuals or communities. They take many different forms, such as:
- Supplying information to clients or communities about resources and opportunities available in and around them;
- Counseling or social work to address psychological or social problems;
- Formation and development of SHGs or advocacy groups;
- Educational activities to enhance social harmony or to promote an inclusive society;
- Advocacy to promote equal opportunities and equal rights in the society;
- Negotiating access to local government services, schools, pensions or benefits;
- Promoting the participation of people with disabilities in community development activities;
- Small projects that provide income without the risk of aggravating disabilities;
- Developing home-based care programs—preferably self-care;

- Providing assistive devices to overcome physical disabilities;
- Encouraging people with disabilities to join mainstream SHGs;
- Skills training and income-generating activities.

As can be seen by the interventions listed above, income generation is just one of the many types of interventions. Clients and public healthcare (PHC) staff may identify other forms of intervention that are appropriate to the specific needs of the client. Some or all interventions may be arranged through referral to services provided by other organizations.

Choosing an intervention: The choice of intervention is central to the client's individual rehabilitation plan. The intervention should match the needs, skills, expectations and resources of the client, and other family and community members involved. The objective is to identify an appropriate activity to meet an agreed priority need, whether physical, psychological, social or economic. The result may be an intervention with the community, the family or the client. In choosing an intervention, it is important that clients recognize the risks and costs, as well as the opportunities and benefits.

Promoting Community Awareness and Participation

Experience has shown that impairment is only one limiting factor in the life of a person with disability. Attitudinal, institutional and other barriers have a strong influence on the level of disability experienced and limit the opportunities of people with disabilities. While the first step for many people with disabilities is a fundamental change in their mindset—from passive receiver to active contributor—removal of the barriers that deny them full participation in their communities is a key step in the rehabilitation process. Community-oriented interventions are needed that increase knowledge, change attitudes, mobilize resources, and encourage participation in rehabilitation activities (Fig. 43.5).

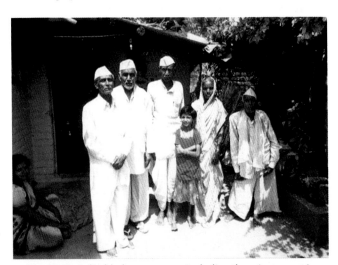

Fig. 43.5: A disabled or any group including them is an asset in community based rehabilitation

5 Evaluation
Monitor actions and evaluate the
results throughout the cycle and
decide what further action is
appropriate or how advocacy
could be done differently in the future.

1 Issue identification
Identity the problem that needs
to be addressed.

2 Research and analysis
Gather the necessary information and
ensure that the causes and effects of
the problem are understood.

4 Action
Take action, using the range of methods
and activities available. This will need to
be agreed and co-ordinated with all those
involved.

3 Planning
When advocacy has been
identified as an appropriate way
of addressing the problem, a strategy
needs to be formulated.

Fig. 43.6: Advocacy cycle

Source: Gordon G. Practical action in advocacy. Blackman R (Ed). Teddington: Tearfund; 2002. pp.1-84.

Advocacy

Activities commonly associated with advocacy include large-scale education programs or lobbying for changes in society to address injustice. Advocacy begins when individuals or groups contact the relevant authority and raise a specific issue, such as the need to enroll a disabled child in a local school, to access credit, to access housing benefit etc. (Fig. 43.6)

Networking with Community and Other Organizations

Being aware of the services available in the community for people with disabilities is important information for the rehabilitation process. Networking among potential partner organizations provides the opportunity to share information on local services, reduce duplication and open new ways to respond to rehabilitation needs. It ensures that rehabilitation programs and their clients gain access to the services they need. Organizations may represent the community or groups within the community. They may represent the interests of people with disabilities. They may provide resources or services, such as loans, vocational/skills training, marketing opportunities or other services or expertise (Fig. 43.7).

SAMPLE REFERRAL FORMAT

See Table 43.2

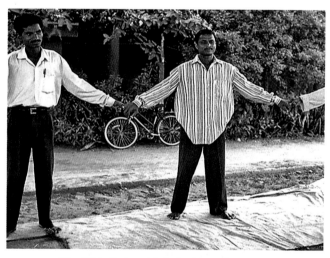

Fig. 43.7: Partnership helps to see the person
as a whole and look-out

REHABILITATION SERVICES FOR DISABLED PERSONS UNDER THE MINISTRY OF SOCIAL JUSTICE AND EMPOWERMENT

Physical, occupational, social rehabilitation and financial assistance for purchase of aids and appliances are provided under Ministry of Social Justice and Empowerment with the basic objective to bring the target groups (disadvantaged

Table 43.2: Referral format (Sample)

EDUCATION	Interventions	Select	Where to Refer?	Select
S/he could not pursue education (or) dropped-out due to leprosy/ disability related reasons? YES - NEXT COLUMN → NO - NEXT STAGE (LIVELIHOOD) ↓	ICDS (Balwadi)		*Anganwadi* worker	
			Women Self-help groups (select groups)	
	Primary education		Primary school (SSA)	
	Secondary education		Secondary school	
	Higher education		Higher secondary school/Inter-college	
	Counseling		Child-focus NGOs (incl.ILEP)	
			Philanthropists	
	Week-end/Evening tuition		Faith-based organizations (FBO)	
	Bridge courses		Self-help Groups (SHG)	
	Special school		District Disability Rehabilitation Centre (DDRC)	
	Distance education		Govt./Private universities	
LIVELIHOOD **Is she/he (with leprosy/disability) skilfully and/or gainfully employed?**	Job counseling		Vocational training centre - VTC (Govt.)	
	Nonformal vocational training like, Tailoring, Weaving, Carpentry, Bag/ Candle making		Vocational training centre (Private)	
			Vocational training centre (NGOs incl. ILEP)	
NO - NEXT COLUMN → YES - NEXT STAGE (AIDS and APPLIANCES) ↓	**Formal training** like Motor mechanic, Refrigeration, Radio and Television, Computers			
	Employment: Wage employment (Salaried)		Employment exchange (common/special)	
			Private sector	
	Self-employment and any other Socio economic Rehabilitation (SER) like Grants/Loans/ Subsidies		Banks	
			NGOs (incl. ILEP)	
			Philanthropists (Lions/Rotary club, etc.)	
			SHGs	
			FBOs	
AIDS and APPLIANCES **Does s/he (with leprosy/disability) have the necessary mobility aids and support devices?** NO - NEXT COLUMN → YES - NEXT STAGE (SOCIAL and EMPOWERMENT) ↓	MCR/Suitable footwear Splints Goggles Self-care kit Crutches Tricycle		DDRC	
			ILEP NGOs (leprosy)	
			Other NGOs	
			Philanthropists	
SOCIAL and EMPOWERMENT a. Does s/he enjoy being with family, friends, neighbors? b Is s/he aware of basic fundamental rights/disability rights. c. Can s/he get relevant information necessary for day-to-day life easily? d. Can s/he go to/use public places easily? e. Does s/he have a positive identity in the society? f. Can she contribute to the fullest potential in the society? g. Is s/he part of a people's group like SHG?	Counseling		DDRC	
	Awareness on basic fundamental rights of human-being + Rights of people with disabilities		Human Rights Institutions Like-minded NGOs Philanthropists	
	Advocacy		SHG	
	Capacity-building		FBOs	

and marginalized section of the society, viz., schedule caste, minorities, backward classes, persons with disability (PWD), aged persons, street children and victims of drug abuse, etc.) into the main stream of development by making them self-reliant. Provision of financial assistance for disabled persons is also available.

For information on the various disability schemes from the Central Government of India, a useful guide called *Information and Guidance Booklet for Persons with Disabilities,* January, 2004 was released and is available from Rehabilitation Council of India (RCI) Office, 23-A Shivaji Marg, New Delhi 110015, and also can be freely downloaded from: punarbhava.in/index.php?option=com_content&view =article&id=714&Itemid=483.

VOCATIONAL AND EMPLOYMENT SERVICES/ OPPORTUNITIES FOR PEOPLE WITH DISABILITIES UNDER THE MINISTRY OF LABOR

The Ministry of Labor of India has the responsibility for vocational training and economic rehabilitation of people with disabilities. Within the ministry, this responsibility is delegated to the Directorate General of Employment and Training. Both the National Council of Vocational Training (NCVT) and the Apprenticeship Training Scheme (ATS) reserve an unspecified number of places for people with disabilities. In addition, 2,000 industrial training institutes have set apart 3% of their vacancies for PWDs. The Ministry of Rural Areas and Employment runs the Training of Rural Youth for Self Employment (Trysem) scheme, which also guarantees to reserve 3% of places for PWDs. The ministry also runs 17 vocational rehabilitation centers that evaluate the physical, mental and vocational capacities of disabled persons, identify a suitable trade and aid people with disabilities in procuring admission to training, job or self-employment.

Moreover, the Directorate General of Employment and Training has identified 98 modules of modular employable skills (MES) under skill development initiative (SDI) suitable for PWD. This can be downloaded at: www.dget.nic.in/mes/ Downloads/disabilities.pdf.

The government launched the District Rehabilitation Centre (DRC) scheme in early 1995. Training for acquiring vocational training, job placement, etc., are some of the services provided in the scheme, which is operational in 11 different districts. Four regional rehabilitation training centers have been established to support the DRCs through training and manpower development as well as conducting training programs for communities, parents and PWDs.

The National Employment Service through 23 Special Employment Exchanges assists people with disabilities (specifically) in obtaining gainful employment and another 914 exchanges (employment exchanges) that cater to people with disabilities as well as people without such special needs.

Financial assistance is provided in the case of the special employment exchanges.

SERVICES FOR DISABLED PERSONS UNDER THE MINISTRY OF RURAL DEVELOPMENT

There is a growing thrust to integrate disability into mainstream development programs and schemes. The Government of India through its Ministry of Rural Development has introduced a 100-day employment guarantee scheme for rural India. The fourth edition of the operational guidelines of MG-NREGA 9.3.1 & 2 states; "The disabled or differently-abled persons defined under the PWD (Equal Opportunities, Protection of Rights and Full Participation) Act, 1995 (1 of 1996) as PWDs, the severity of which is 40% and above would be considered as special category of vulnerable persons for the purposes of MG-NREGA. The disabled persons as defined in the National Trust for Welfare of Persons with Autism, Cerebral Palsy, Mental Retardation and Multiple Disabilities Act, 1999 (44 of 1999) are also to be considered as disabled for the purpose of inclusion in MG-NREGA. Since this category of people is differently-abled, special conditions had to be created to facilitate their inclusion in MG-NREGA. It is estimated that around 5% of the population in rural areas will fall in the category of disabled and this group is one of the most deprived and vulnerable. More information about the identification of works, mobilization, adaptation of tools and equipments, etc., is available from the operational guidelines document downloadable from the link below: nrega. nic.in/netnrega/WriteReaddata/Circulars/Operational_ guidelines_4[th] Edition_eng_2013.pdf.

CONCLUSION

Rehabilitation of people affected by leprosy has become the focus area with the elimination of leprosy achieved in almost all the countries. Integration of leprosy control activities into general healthcare (GHC) has been effective with adequate training and support of the GHC staff. With the involvement of media and health promotion activities, the stigma related to leprosy is also gradually reducing. The general rehabilitation programs for people with other disabilities are gaining momentum with empowerment and economic sustainability. Now the time has come to integrate leprosy rehabilitation into mainstream rehabilitation programs. Sustained efforts are needed from all stakeholders (government, ILEP, NGO, corporate sectors, etc.) to bring this change.

BIBLIOGRAPHY

1. Do Prado GD, Prado RB, Marciano LH, et al. WHO disability grade does not influence physical activity in Brazlian leprosy patients. Lepr Rev. 2011;82(3):270-8.

2. Gautham MS, Dayananda M, Gopinath D, et al. Community based needs assessment of leprosy patients in Chamrajnagar District, Karnataka, India. Lepr Rev. 2011;82(3):286-95.

3. Jaeggi T, Manickam P, Weiss MG, et al. Stakeholders perspectives on perceived needs and priorities for leprosy control and care, Tamil Nadu, India. Indian J Lepr. 2012;84(3):177-84.

4. Khasnabis C, Motsch KH. Community Based Rehabilitation (CBR) Guidelines. Geneva: WHO Press; 2010. pp. 17-77.

5. Porichha D, Rao VN, Samal P, et al. Transfer of disability care of leprosy to the affected persons and the community members. Indian J Lepr. 2011; 83:81-6.

6. Thomas M, Thomas MJ. Challenges in Leprosy Rehabilitation. APDRJ. 2004;15(1):45-9.

7. United Nations enable. Objectives, Background and Concepts. World Programme of Action concerning Disabled Persons. [online]. Available from www.un.org/disabilities/default.asp?id=23#objectives. [Accessed June, 2014].

8. World Health Organization, ILEP. WHO/ILEP Technical guide on community-based rehabilitation and leprosy. Meeting the rehabilitation needs of people affected by leprosy and promoting quality of life. Geneva: WHO Press; 2007. pp. 1-57.

9. World Health Organization. (2014). Disabilities and rehabilitation. [online]. Available from www.who.int/disabilities/care/en/index.html. [Accessed June, 2014].

10. World Health Organization. Meeting Report on the development of guidelines for community based rehabilitation (CBR) programmes. Geneva: WHO Press (Switzerland); 2004 Nov. 1st and 2nd.

11. World Health Organization. Session 6: Rehabilitation. Workshop for health service managers in charge of leprosy control programmes. From global strategy to national action. participant guide. New Delhi: World Health Organization; 2007. pp. 128-33.

44
CHAPTER

Community-based Initiatives in Comprehensive Leprosy Work

PV Ranganadha Rao

INTRODUCTION

"Nothing about us without us",[1] as a principle vindicates the need of involving the community in general, and networks of persons affected in particular, to implement leprosy program and to strive toward a 'world free of leprosy and its suffering,' an aspired vision of all concerned with leprosy. This philosophy is echoed strongly in expressions of people affected. Mr Vagavathalli Narsappa, Chairman of National Forum Trust India (NFT India) of people affected by leprosy, argues emphatically that *"We know what we want and what can help us. We can play a key role towards the solution to the leprosy problem. If we are involved, we can make leprosy services comprehensive."*

Leprosy work, in fact, even before becoming a full-fledged public health program had an element of participation of people affected and the members of the community as a strong base for comprehensive health care. It is convincing to believe that "just pills alone" cannot restore holistic health as defined by the World Health Organization (WHO)[2] to a person affected by leprosy. Need of understanding the role and potential of the community as the primary stakeholder is elementary. Several community-based initiatives were reported; majority of them were from within the community, simple but crucial, filling the gaps in program implementation. Some initiatives were focused on addressing the needs of the people with disabilities due to leprosy, by groups, networks or fora (forums) of the people affected themselves, which gradually evolved into "community-based rehabilitation (CBR)". Some other community-based initiatives developed into community health program, and worked in unison with national leprosy program. These initiatives remained more or less local specific innovations complementing different components of leprosy work. It would perhaps be useful at this point in time to revisit some of those initiatives with a view to understand rationale, purpose, scope and principle and processes involved in making the leprosy work comprehensive.

Leprosy, though, usually starts as a skin patch, affects peripheral and cutaneous nerves; manifests with symptoms of nerve function deficit, such as loss of sensibility, reduced mobility of small joints and skin impairments like loss of hair, loss of sweating and altered skin color in the affected area. Leprosy also affects other organs, but involvement of hands and feet is marked by impairments like anesthesia and visible deformities, like clawing of fingers and toes. The type of deformities ranges from slight bending of fingers or toes (clawing) to severe forms of resorption of entire foot or hand. Eyes too get affected with structural and functional impairments ranging from loss of eyebrows to total loss of vision. Leprosy continues to challenge the medical professionals and social workers, because of its features like prolonged incubation period, varying presentations of the disease manifestation, episodes of exacerbations of disease symptoms, accompanied nerve involvement-impairment-damage, occurrence of deformities, and consequences due to deep rooted stigma and instances of discrimination in the community. Thirty years ago, till the advent of multidrug therapy (MDT), cure for leprosy was obscure and so were the perspectives about the disease in the community. MDT brought about a far-reaching change in the management of leprosy, making its inclusion in the list of curable diseases, decreasing the period of infectivity and reducing the chances of relapses. Making MDT available at all health centers is one of the critical factors responsible for all the achievements in leprosy program.

LEPROSY PROGRAM

Under the technical guidance of the WHO, national programmes implement leprosy control activities, and in India, the programme is referred to as National Leprosy Eradication Programme (NLEP). The 44th World Health Assembly (WHA), which met in Geneva in May 1991, adopted a resolution to eliminate leprosy as a public health problem by the year 2000.[3] Elimination of leprosy as a public health problem has been defined as prevalence rate of the disease to less than 1 case per 10,000 people. Most of the countries have already achieved this important milestone in leprosy control. MDT deserves a special mention in such a remarkable achievement, elimination of leprosy as a public health problem globally. Another testimony of success for MDT is reduction in the quantum of the disease burden. Since introduction of MDT, more than 16 million patients were cured of leprosy.[4] The reduction of disease burden is evident by the fact that in 1985 more than 122 countries were reporting large number of cases annually and as of today; only 16 countries have reported ≥ 1,000 cases.[5]

Achievements coexist with challenges and it is true with leprosy programme too. New cases continued to occur for long despite routine health interventions, after achieving the goal of elimination of leprosy as a public health problem. The number of new cases, barring a marginal decrease, continues to occur globally, ranging from 249,007 in 2008 to 215,656 in 2013 (Fig. 44.1). The stagnation of new case detection in spite of effective disease control activities raised concern among experts, programme managers and the people affected. The trends in new case detection globally in different regions are presented in the following illustration. Leprosy distribution is so patchy that 95% of leprosy is limited to 14 countries across the world and three countries, i.e. Brazil, India and Indonesia are home to 81% of the global disease burden. India, alone holds 60% of global leprosy.

Leprosy control is based on breaking the chain of transmission, a secondary prevention strategy from infected to the healthy members of the community by reducing the source of infection using MDT. Continued occurrence of new cases in a given community indicates the contrary, i.e. presence of source of infection. Early detection of patients—early enough before visible deformities appear—is another tenet of enhanced global strategy for further reducing the disease burden due to leprosy (2011–2015).[6] Numbers and rate of new cases with grade 2 disability or visible deformity (G2D) cases of recent history indicate delayed detection of cases (Fig. 44.2). Analysis of the trend of new G2D cases shows rather a marginal increase in number of new G2D cases in the year 2013 across the globe when compared to the figures from 2010.

Low awareness in the community and/or inadequate skills among the health staff to promptly diagnose leprosy is possible reasons for delay in diagnosis. Deformities *per se limit ability and function, but social implications affect participation of the persons affected, in the activities of daily living (ADL).*[7]

Community

Community by understanding is a group of people sharing same knowledge, resources and traditions and practices in ADL. *Community is defined as a group of people with diverse characteristics who are linked by social ties, share common perspectives, living together and practicing common ownership, sharing or having certain attitudes and interests in*

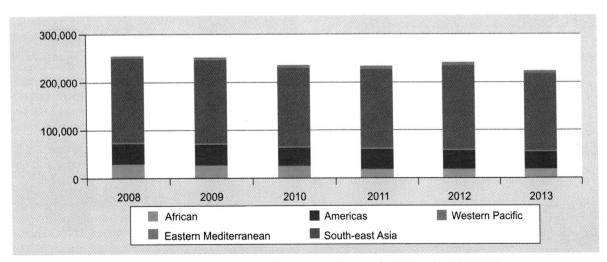

Fig. 44.1: Trends in the detection of new cases of leprosy, by WHO region, 2008–2013

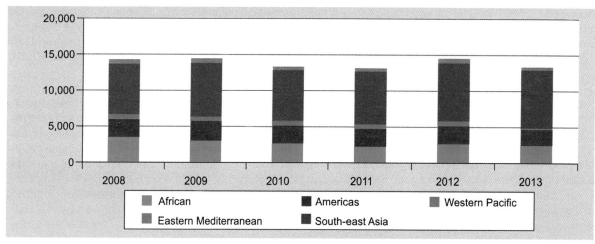

Fig. 44. 2: Trends in the detection of New G2D leprosy cases by WHO region. 2008–2013
Note: WHO regions: AFRO, African region; AMRO, American region; EMRO, Eastern Mediterranean region;
SEARO, Southeast Asian region; WPRO, Western Pacific region

common and engage in joint action in geographical locations or settings.

Dr PK Gopal, President of the International Association for Integration, Dignity and Economic Advancement (IDEA), says *"There are 700 leprosy colonies in the country (India) alone, where over two hundred thousand people live marginalised lives".*[8] Similar rehabilitation homes, colonies or institutions exist in many countries. The members dwelling in such isolation are significant too in terms of their experience, which can serve as a resource to evolve solutions to long-standing social, behavioral and attitudinal issues prevailing in the community and among the people affected. It is important to listen to the voices hitherto unheard particularly of the people affected.

RATIONALE AND PURPOSE OF COMMUNITY-BASED INITIATIVES FOR COMPREHENSIVE LEPROSY WORK

Community, by default, becomes the primary stakeholder as leprosy affects some members in the community; deformities and social stigma associated with the disease compounds the suffering of the people affected. Besides the people affected living in villages and urban locations, significant number of people live in self-settled leprosy colonies or rehabilitation homes and so constitute an important group among primary stakeholders. It is the need of mainstreaming the people affected, staying in the fringes of the society with in the community that warranted a movement of social mobilization.

Social mobilization has been brought to the fore of discussions in health management, because of the activism shown by users of health services. Movement by people living with human immunodeficiency virus (PLHIV) stands as a well-known example in patient activism. The potential

of a community in containing spread of infection in a disease control programme, and networks of people affected functioning as catalysts in improving reach and delivery of medical services has remarkably changed the philosophy, vocabulary and to a certain extent actions of policy makers in ministries of health. A phenomenal shift in believing that community is a partner to reckon and intending to delegate some of the health program functions is being witnessed in recent times, in many countries including India. Social movements, by second nature, bring people together, facilitate transmission of information and steer the society toward a social change. With particular reference to leprosy, the social movement is seen arising more out of frustration of the people affected due to deprived opportunities, instances of discrimination, and reduced participation due to deformities. Activism among the persons affected and the people in the community holds the key for social mobilization and enhances commitment of all stakeholders. The communities mobilized with such activism garner support from all stakeholders and complement national health programs to sustain the gains achieved in controlling leprosy and further reducing the disease burden.

COMMUNITY PARTICIPATION IN PRIMARY HEALTH CARE

Primary health care (PHC) aims to provide quality and comprehensive health care in a cost-effective and equitable manner, and is the foundation for strengthening health systems. PHC addresses inequity in health by advocating the following approaches:
- Universal coverage
- Intersectoral collaboration
- Community participation
- Appropriate technology.

Community participation is best achieved through educating and empowering the community in general and women in particular. Education, income generation and gender equality are some prerequisites for empowerment. Community education and empowerment not only lead to appropriate health behavior but also enable the community to demand good quality health care.[9]

People Affected by Leprosy and their Role in Leprosy Services

Persons affected by leprosy have a major role to play in leprosy services, especially in the areas of awareness, rehabilitation, advocacy and case finding. Organized efforts of the people affected are vital in promoting a positive public perception of and attitude toward the disease; to effect change in any legal measures that are discriminatory in nature; and in ensuring that leprosy control continues to occupy an important place in the health policy framework of the country.

Persons affected by leprosy also have a clear role and responsibility in enhancing community involvement and social action. The following areas can be strengthened by involving affected persons in the programme, either by including the activities as integral parts of leprosy control program or use the activities to complement the comprehensive leprosy care in the community and also in the program implementation. The potential key areas are:

- Feedback and regular information on implementation of leprosy activities
- Defining quality of services contextualizing to local circumstances
- Research and evaluations to give objective opinion on efficacy of leprosy control
- Contribute to reforming of leprosy services
- Ways to address issues related to stigma and discrimination.

Besides the above mentioned key recognized areas, people affected can be a crucial resource by virtue of experiencing the disease in reducing stigma and discrimination, counseling new patients for improving compliance to prescribed treatment and assisted interventions like physiotherapy and supporting residential care and self-care practices.

Community-based initiatives are well-positioned to complement the leprosy control, care and rehabilitation services. In some instances, they are in a better position to implement leprosy work holistically on their own. Evidence shows that it is possible and community-based initiatives need to be attempted with strong conviction. Community-based initiatives also leave a long lasting or sustainable change in the community with regard to health, subsequently resulting in improved quality of life. The Comprehensive Rural Health Project (CRHP), Jamkhed, Maharashtra state of India "Jamkhed Model", stands as an example for a comprehensive community-based health initiative.[10]

Comprehensive Leprosy Work

Articulation of a categorical definition of comprehensive leprosy work has been found challenging. But the conclusions from discussion about it include all interventions supporting the affected people from the stage of being a suspect with suggestive symptoms of leprosy to social reintegration of the ones with severe deformities living as residents of leprosy colonies on the fringes of the community.

A set of activities often surface during discussions as possible community-based initiatives which can complement leprosy program and make it a comprehensive care. These can be implemented through community-based initiatives with ease, whereas, it is quite challenging to include them in routine public health programs or medical treatment services. These initiatives are related to:

- Awareness raising
- Referral to health services
- Adherence to MDT
- Counseling to persons affected
- Home/community disability care
- Stigma reduction
- Advocacy for social entitlements
- Improving social accountability
- Networking and collectivization of people affected
- Fighting for human rights.

Diagnosis of leprosy and care of consequent deformities are based on available evidence on MDT and disability care protocols evolved from different experiences across the globe. In the absence of an objective test for diagnosis and cure, finding all leprosy cases and treating them with MDT remains the sole tool available for leprosy control program. Strategic issues identified in the guidelines for including persons affected by leprosy are discussed in terms of possible options and evidence available from field program experiences.

Purpose of Community-based Initiatives in Comprehensive Leprosy Work

The present trends of new case detection and marginal increase in new cases with G2D cases indicate stagnation of disease control process and needs strengthening of the health services in reaching undetected leprosy patients. Stagnation at a lower endemicity of a disease leads to lack of anticipated results, which gradually manifests in a health system as complacency. Once set, complacency subsequently leads to reduced interest in leprosy among health staff, program managers, policy makers and even in nongovernmental organizations (NGOs) working in small areas with dedicated focus on leprosy.

Innovative approaches increase demand for services by users, participation of all stakeholders, reach of the programme and activism among the people affected. These approaches work as a catalyst to trigger progress in implementation. The progress in implementation and recordable improvement of results gradually help to break the complacency and enhance the program performance.

OPPORTUNITIES FOR COMMUNITY-BASED INITIATIVES

Recognition of stagnation of disease control process is indicated by more or less static new case detection ranging from 240,000 per annum globally in 2005 to 215,656 in 2013. A marginal increase of number of new cases with grade 2 disabilities (13,289 new cases with visible deformities reported during 2013) has raised discussion for exploring possibilities of improving case detection particularly among the hard to reach populations/areas/districts/municipalities involving communities.

Patient activism initiated by IDEA, International and NFT India of the people affected also increased the demand for a good accountable quality of services to the affected. This made the national programs to look for appropriate suggestive approaches to get the community and the people affected involved in the national programs. Though not exhaustive, the following are a few policies and strategies, which encourage community-based initiatives to work in unison with leprosy program in order to further reduce social burden due to leprosy.

WHO Initiative to Strengthen Participation of Affected People in Leprosy Services

WHO organized a meeting at Manila, Philippines, in June 2010, inviting participation of individuals affected by leprosy, national program managers and various experts, to develop guidelines for increasing participation of leprosy affected persons in leprosy control activities.[11] Several areas and corresponding strategies were identified for empowerment of the people affected by leprosy in different aspects of life, including health, housing, social welfare, education and decision making as well as socioeconomic activities. The result of this enhanced participation and empowerment is assumed to be threefold, i.e. greater willingness of individuals affected by leprosy to seek diagnosis; completion of the prescribed treatment; and improved quality of life.

National Level Initiatives, India—National Rural Health Mission

Some national health programs have initiated community involved health programs. Government of India introduced National Rural Health Mission (NRHM) with a few key approaches enabling the community to take leadership on health and medical service related issues in the periphery at local level, i.e. village or revenue development blocks. Village Health and Sanitation Committees (VHSCs), known as *Gaon Kalyan Samitis* (GKSs) in some regions, at village level, *Panchayati Raj Institutions* (PRIs) at village/

block level, *Rogi Kalyan Samitis* (RKSs) at hospital levels were established as operational elements to enable the community to actively participate in health programs and manage certain interventions. Accredited Social Health Activist (ASHA) is a female volunteer working with the village community for enhancing access to PHC including all national health programs, to bridge the operational gap between community and health. The VHSC/GKS is entrusted with the responsibility of developing their respective village health plans and monitoring health interventions provided by public and private sector.

National Leprosy Eradication Programme

The NLEP in order to reach the unreached areas and enhance coverage through partnership from community-based organizations has announced NGO schemes. The schemes cover areas of leprosy services for early detection, treatment of reactions, disability care and rehabilitation of people affected by leprosy. Two particular schemes were designed to suit participation of the people affected.

Nongovernmental Organizations in Health Care

The NGOs working with communities in health and development introduced innovations within the community to bring about social change and thereby reduce poverty and disease. One such example is Comprehensive Rural Health Project (CRHP), Jamkhed, where the volunteers selected by the communities themselves, not only act as health workers, but also mobilize their communities to achieve better sanitation and hygiene, etc. Village health workers facilitate forming groups, for example, women's self-help groups (SHGs). These SHGs further work in their communities to identify illnesses, health care barriers and services needed and thereby participate in health care at village level. SHGs in some villages have improved remarkably health status of people by raising awareness about health, providing basic health care and linking up with service providers in public and private sector.[10]

A core committee was constituted by the Central Leprosy Division, NLEP, Ministry of Health and Family Welfare in December, 2012, comprising of key stakeholders to review the existing schemes in leprosy and propose need based schemes. The committee conducted a detailed review and proposed eight schemes based on the needs of NLEP and the strengths of the NGOs. The schemes have been outlined below:

Scheme 1A: Designated Referral Centers (DRC 1A)—outpatient facility

Scheme 1B: Designated Referral Centers (DRC 1B)—outpatient and inpatient

Scheme 1C: Designated Referral Centers (DRC 1C)—outpatient, inpatient and RCS

Scheme 2: Comprehensive care for underserved areas

Scheme 3:   Contact survey and home based self-care

Scheme 4:   Disability Care Center—leprosy colonies

Scheme 5:   Advocacy communication and social mobilization with activities to reduce stigma and discrimination in leprosy

Scheme 6:   Partnering with community for elimination of leprosy

National Forum India—an Opportunity to Take Up Community-based Initiatives

National Forum India (NFI)—a countrywide network of people affected was started informally in 2006, and subsequently registered as a trust in 2012.[12] NFI has a strong operational presence in 19 states, most of which are highly endemic. NFI thus stands as an opportunity and a partner to count on, for initiating community based comprehensive leprosy work. NFI in its operational plan expressed its future plans to create awareness about leprosy and eagerness to address challenges related to early case detection, disability care and stigma reduction.

SCOPE OF COMMUNITY-BASED INITIATIVES IN LEPROSY

A list of interventions related to medical treatment and health programs was identified through informal consultations with fora of people affected, and civil society organizations at district/state levels. For discussion purposes, the NLEP activities were grouped under six areas, i.e. case finding, case holding, disability care, reconstructive surgery, rehabilitation and empowerment of people affected and the communities. A schematic presentation of activities, which can be considered as potential areas for community based initiatives to complement national leprosy program is detailed in Table 44.1.

None of these activities singly treat or manage leprosy but are critical complements that can make leprosy work comprehensive in restoring health as defined by WHO to the person affected and mainstream them into the community. These potential interventions can be implemented singly or in combination of two or more of such activities as community based initiatives as part of national leprosy program. Some of the interventions can be carried out in partnership with people affected, NGOs and health department staff. Integration with other organizations is also a possibility.

EXPERIENCES OF COMMUNITY-BASED INITIATIVES IN COMPREHENSIVE LEPROSY WORK

Community-based initiatives, particularly the successful ones need to be documented, disseminated and discussed to understand the processes involved in developing the models. A few of such experiences are presented with a view to encourage replication and for further innovation of such initiatives.

Experience 1: The Comprehensive Rural Health Project, Jamkhed: "Jamkhed Model"

The CRHP, Jamkhed,[10] has been working among the rural poor and marginalized for over 40 years. Founded in 1970 by Dr Raj Arole and Dr Mabelle Arole to bring health care to the poorest of the poor, CRHP has become an organization that empowers people to eliminate injustices through integrated efforts in health and development. *The innovation of this approach lies in involving the communities themselves, especially those poor and marginalized, in deciding the needs and defining the parameters of community development.* CRHP works by mobilizing and building the capacity of communities to achieve access to comprehensive development and freedom from stigma, poverty and disease. Pioneering a comprehensive approach to primary community-based health care, CRHP has been a leader in public health and development in rural communities in India and around the world. CRHP achieved sustainable results in promoting health and development.

The indicators (Table 44.2) show the impact of the work.

"We divided the village into four sections, with one Mahila Vikas Mandal member responsible for the health of her section. She ensures that all children are immunized and all the pregnant women receive prenatal care. We also trained three women to be in charge of deliveries when I am not around. Every year we repeat the house-to-house survey." Sarubai, Village Health Worker, Jawalaka Village (Fig. 44.3).

The project initiated its work in 1979 covering 30 villages; the project had expanded to a region of over 250,000 people in the first 25 years. Within 5 years, the infant mortality rate fell to 52, the coverage of antenatal care increased to 80%, 74% of deliveries were considered to be 'safe', immunization coverage of children was 81%, and leprosy prevalence dropped to half. After 20 years, the infant mortality rate was 26 and prevalence of tuberculosis had fallen threefold (from 18 per 1,000 to 6). CRHP Jamkhed model stands as a testimony for comprehensive community based health care. Community based organizations may wish to emulate the model in their respective locations worldwide, but only if worked with strong conviction.

Experience 2: Pride and Prejudice: Women SHG in Comprehensive Leprosy Work[13]

"I will come and stay with my people when the community leaders and others come to me and ask." This was Lachu Bai's hurt lament when LEPRA India team met her, ostracized and alone, abandoned near the fringes of the woods away from

Table 44.1: Potential areas for community-based initiatives in comprehensive leprosy work

	Case finding	Case holding	Disability care	Reconstructive surgery	Rehabilitation	Empowerment
Leprosy program activities	Survey by health workers	Diagnosis	Treatment of reactions	Selection of patients	Selection of patients	Certification of disabilities
	Interface between program and community	Provision of MDT	Physiotherapy	Physiotherapy	Income generation schemes (IG)	Access to social entitlements
Potential areas for community-based initiatives in comprehensive leprosy work	Awareness raising	Interface between program and community	Foot care	Surgery, immediate hospitalization and care	Education, finance and employment support	Coordination with social justice
	Referral to health centers	Counseling	Interface between program and community	Social support – pension	Interface between program and community	Interface between program and community
	Education of patient contacts for examination	MDT adherence	Home-based care	Interface between program and community	Community-based rehabilitation	Networking
	Social mobilization	Referral on complications	Self-care groups	Enablement and employability training	Access to income generation schemes	Collectivization
		Defaulter tracing	Community care clinics	Motivation of other patients	Institutional support for rehabilitation	Decision making in leprosy program
						Social audit
						Fight for rights

Abbreviations: NLEP, National Leprosy Eradication Programme; MDT, multidrug therapy.

Table 44.2: Health outcomes in CRHP project villages over time: 1971–2011

Year	1971	1976	1986	1993	1996	2004	2011	India 2004
Infant mortality rate (IMR) n/1,000 live births	176	52	49	19	26	24	8	62
Crude birth rate (CBR) n/1,000	40	34	28	20	20	18.6	23.1	23.9
Antenatal care	0.5%	80%	82%	82%	96%	99%	99%	64%
Safe delivery	<0.5%	74%	83%	83%	98%	99%	99.4%	43%
Family planning	<1%	38%	60%	60%	60%	68%	*	41%
Immunization (DPT, polio) under 5	0.5%	81%	91%	91%	92%	99%	*	70%
Malnutrition in children under 5	40%	30%	30%	5%	5%	<5%	*	47%
Leprosy (cases per 1,000)	4	2	1	0.1	0.1	<0.1	*	0.24
Tuberculosis (cases per 1,000)	18	15	11	6	6	2	*	4.1

* Immunization is now being administered through government programs. Malnutrition, leprosy and tuberculosis are being monitored by CRHP, of which current data is being collected.

her village, Belsarampur in Adilabad district. Afflicted with leprosy, she was incapacitated and, as no treatment was provided, her condition worsened, visibly. Her husband, Lakku, solemnly gave into the decision of the village *panchayat*, to isolate and lodge her outside the village. LEPRA took Lachu Bai under its care and support and started treatment. Simultaneously, it started advocacy programs in the village about stigma and the implications of leprosy. A women SHG of the village, understanding the facts about leprosy, and the situation of Lachu Bai initiated consultation with village *panchayat* to motivate the community.

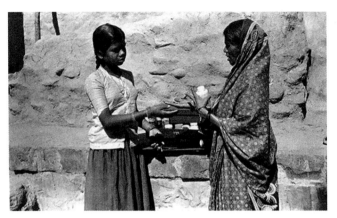

Fig. 44.3: CRHD, Jamkhed, community-based activity of reaching health services

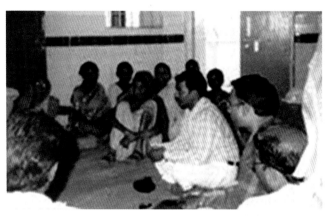

Fig. 44.4: Pride and Prejudice, Lachu Bai, being invited back to village by village elders as demanded by women SHG

Though a singular example, the instance raised awareness about the disease and its cure with MDT. The community responded by calling for a village meeting to reintegrate Lachu Bai into their village community. On 1st April 2005, a team including LEPRA workers went to bring her back into the village (Fig. 44.4). This was the final cure that every leprosy patient looks for—acceptance. Lachu Bai was not only accepted back in the community but was given a place as a village elder, to advice and guide the people with her wisdom that stemmed from pain, age and the life in the forest. She walked back home with a mixed sense of belonging and isolation.

Mainstreaming the affected persons into the community improves health, both physically and psychologically. Restoring an elderly woman to her family stands as an example of acceptance of persons affected by leprosy, and further reduces stigma in the community. Reduction of stigma and raising awareness about leprosy and MDT are integral components of comprehensive leprosy services.

Experience 3: Lokdoots and Sasakawa Memorial Health Foundation

Lokdoots: The concept of 'Lokdoots' was revised and introduced as 'community emissaries', who are the ones from people affected by leprosy groups or networks, work with the community to make the villages free of leprosy and its suffering. *Lokdoots* live in the community and support them in accessing services and fulfilling their needs. They help in reaching all persons with disabilities, disability assessment and counsel them for continuing self-care and physiocare practices and attend health posts whenever required.

A few districts were covered under a project named *Chetana*[14] collecting information about people living in the self-settled colonies and in the fringes of the society, identifying health and development needs of the people

affected. *Lokdoots* carry out a survey identifying needs of the people in various domains like education, health, livelihood training, economic assistance and support in general. Besides access to MDT, treatment for reactions, other activities related to health and development, the community benefitted with general support measures like having a library and facility to share challenges among themselves. *Lokdoots* initiative has covered 8 districts and 1,500 people affected by leprosy, ensured reach of medical services and linked up with development programs.

Experience 4: Bihar Health in Action Project; Implemented by LEPRA Society 2007–2010

Bihar Health in Action Project (BiHAP) was started in 2007 to strengthen community health fora (forums), community based organizations, community health resource centers (HRCs) and the health practitioners in addressing health issues at the community level in Bihar.

Strengthening of the communities in identifying and managing their health issues at the community level is one of the main agendas of LEPRA in Bihar. Village health forums (VHFs) of 10–12 members, including *Anganwadi Workers* (AWWs), auxiliary nurses and midwives and PRI members, have been formed in four districts of Bihar (Munger, Samastipur, Bhagalpur and Begusarai), particularly targeting difficult-to-reach areas. This has enhanced early case detection and timely referrals, and could be a sustainable approach toward community empowerment for villagers. VHF formed in 100 villages, serves as information point for diseases and active community participation. The village and sanitation committee got 520 cases registered for MDT and followed up till completion of treatment. All the healthy household contacts were examined by health staff. It was encouraging to note that in all the 100 villages, not a single instance of discrimination was noticed. The strategies of community involvement and formation of village health fora were found to be effective and self-functional, and are also actively participating in adjoining villages on issues of health.

Experience 5: Deformity Care by Community: The Bargarh Experience "Bargarh Integrated Community Health Project" LEPRA Society

"Leprosy Elimination Unit" was initiated in Bargarh in 2001, and the second phase of the project started in 2006 with an objective to support the district/block health administration in achieving the leprosy elimination covering a population of 650,000 with renewed emphasis on community involvement and participation. The project was later redesigned as "Bargarh Integrated Community Health Project (BICHP)".

The strategy emphasizing involvement of the community through 24 HRCs and 45 *Gaon Kalayan Samitis* provided disability care and services to 600 persons affected with ulcers. The project had enrolled 1,063 cases with G2D in the beginning of the year 2006, out of which 408 (38.4%) were with grade 1 deformity like sensory loss on hands and feet. Through Disability Care Clinics, Trialogue Reaching to the Communities–Advocacy, Education, Community Participation and Impact on Leprosy Programme-Dr N Murugesan, Health Administrator Vol : XVIII Number 2 : 73-77, pg. and prevention of deformity (POD) camps (an opportunity for patients, people and providers to interact and improve leprosy work, another example of community-based initiative) at *panchayat* and block levels, members of the HRCs were trained in disability care and on self-care.

As a part of this intervention, 300 like-minded people from different categories were identified as partners of the project and were facilitated to receive identity cards from the District Magistrate and Collector, Bargarh, as an acknowledgment of their good work and active involvement in providing voluntary leprosy services to needy clients.

An evaluation was conducted in 2009 to know the effectiveness of POD through self-care with community support, with a total of 115 affected persons and 25 service providers. The results indicate that 89.3% were convinced about cure, 98.2% are staying with family, 59.5% women are members in self-support groups and 25% expressed self-stigma.

Discussion

"It is (leprosy elimination) like two wheels of a motorcycle," Sasakawa said, "the front wheel is medical treatment and the back wheel is social solution. Both wheels should be equal in size and speed"[15]—Mr Yohei Sasakawa, the Goodwill Ambassador of WHO for Leprosy Elimination (Fig. 44.5). Community based initiatives to improve health of the people in general or addressing specific health issues like maternal and child health have been recorded in various examples. People affected, form part of the community, are integrated in it, and in certain situations are as a separate group of affected individuals or a network operating in the fringes of the community. An inclusive approach of integrating affected people, in fact, enriches the community in terms of information about leprosy and experience in dealing with it. Community based initiative by virtue of its base will be an opportunity to be utilized by health system in implementing leprosy programs. The strength in reaching the people affected and ensuring compliance to the medical services will be of much help. It would also be mutually beneficial for the groups or networks of people affected by leprosy and the community to develop community based initiatives in providing comprehensive care for leprosy work. Stagnation of disease control, enhanced political commitment to further reduce disease burden due to leprosy, rising activism of the community and people affected, increasing importance to public private partnerships particularly with civil societies are a few factors which argue for greater and meaningful involvement of communities and people affected.

Last mile of the race has been used as an analogy to the present leprosy situation. It is important to unite all the stakeholders in developing community based initiatives, in consultation with people affected and other stakeholders to work in tandem with national leprosy programs in order to reach the aspired goal of a world without leprosy. It would be prudent to recall Mahatma Gandhi's call on leprosy that "Leprosy work is not merely medical relief, it is transforming frustration of life into joy of dedication, personal ambition into selfless service". With these words, Mahatma Gandhi as an ideal leader who practiced more than what he preached, stands alive today in the minds of many professionals from both medical and social fields kindling interest in leprosy work (Fig. 44.6).

All concerned earnestly hope that such thoughts, words and expressions will lead the leprosy work through the last mile of leprosy control toward a world without leprosy and its sufferings.

ACKNOWLEDGMENTS

I gratefully acknowledge the opportunity given to me on behalf of Indian Association of Leprologists to present "LEPRA Society for the opportunity to develop the community based initiatives in leprosy work". I thank the staff of LEPRA Society for their contribution. I acknowledge the support extended to me by my family and professional colleagues, Dr D Porichha and Dr G Rajan Babu. The experiences quoted from organizations like CHAI, CRHP, LEPRA Society and National Forum India are duly acknowledged for their contribution to leprosy services.'

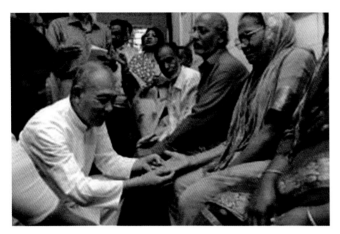

Fig. 44.5: Mr Yohei Sasakawa, interacting with persons affected showing the way forward

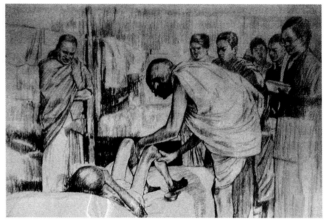

Fig. 44.6: Mahatma Gandhi Ji nursing a leprosy affected person in Sevagram—setting an example of acceptance

REFERENCES

1. The saying has its origins in Central European political traditions. It was the political motto that helped establish—and, loosely translated into Latin, provided the name for—Poland's 1505 constitutional legislation, Nihil Novi, which first transferred governing authority from the monarch to the parliament. It subsequently became a byword for democratic norms; [online] Available from http://en.wikipedia.org/wiki/Nothing_About_Us_Without_Us [Accessed June, 2014].
2. Preamble to the Constitution of the World Health Organization as adopted by the International Health Conference, New York, 19-22 June, 1946; signed on 22 July 1946 by the representatives of 61 States (Official Records of the World Health Organization, no. 2, p. 100) and entered into force on 7 April 1948.
3. The forty-fourth World Health Assembly (WHA), Leprosy Resolution WHA 44.9, May 1991.
4. Enhanced global strategy for further reducing the disease burden due to leprosy—questions and answers; SEA-GLP-2012.01.
5. Global leprosy situation 2012, an update; 88, No. 35, 365-380; WHO Weekly epidemiological record (WER) 30 August 2013, 88th year; [online] Available from http://www.who.int/wer [Accessed June, 2014].
6. Enhanced global strategy for further reducing disease burden due to leprosy: 2011-2015. Operational Guidelines (updated).
7. Activities of daily living evaluation. In: Krapp K (Ed). Encyclopedia of Nursing & Allied Health. Gale Group, Inc.; 2002. Enotes Nursing Encyclopedia. (2006). [online] Available from www.eNotes.com [Accessed June, 2014].
8. Leprosy continues to haunt India, social stigma remains. [online] Available from http://www.thehindu.com/news/national/leprosy-continues-to-haunt-india-social-stigma-remains/article4358263.ece [Accessed June, 2014].
9. Primary Health Care. The basis for health systems strengthening. WHO publication; August 2010. p. 14.
10. The Comprehensive Rural Health Project, Jamkhed (CRHP) "Jamkhed Model". (2013). [online] Available from http://jamkhed.org/ [Accessed June, 2014].
11. Report of the meeting to develop guidelines to strengthen participation of persons affected by leprosy in leprosy services, 9-10 June 2010, Manila Philippines, New Delhi, WHO Regional Office for South-East Asia, 2010 (SEA-GLP2010.3).
12. National Forum India, 14-15, Vol. 26, No. 9, September 2013, Health Action, Catholic Health Association of India (CHAI). [online] Available from www.hafa-india.org [Accessed June, 2014]. Acknowledged in the book.
13. Community and social reintegration: a rural example, Jayaramparasa, 22, Vol. 22, No. 2, February 2009; Health Action, Catholic Health Association of India (CHAI). [online] Available from www.chai-india.org [Accessed June, 2014].
14. Chetana project (lokdoots); Intervention to advocating Health and Socio-Economic issues of People Affected by Leprosy: 40-41, Vol. 26, No. 9, September 2013, Health Action, CHAI-India. [online] Available from www.hafa-india.org [Accessed June, 2014].
15. Help fight bias against leprosy victims: Sasakawa. [online] Available from http://ns.bdnews24.com/details.php?id=222389&cid=2 [Accessed June, 2014].

FURTHER READING

1. Abbatt F, McMahon R. Teaching Health-Care Workers: A Practical Guide, 2nd revised edition. Basingstoke: Macmillan educational Ltd.; 1993.
2. Chambers R. Rural Development: Putting the Last First. Harlow: Longman; 1983.
3. Community Mobilisation: Success and Prospects: Documentation of Experiences. Krishnatray P. Bhopal: Danlep; 2003.
4. Enhanced global strategy for further reducing the disease burden due to leprosy (plan period 2011-2015). WHO; SEA-GLP-2009.3.
5. First T. Don't Treat Me Like I Have Leprosy. London: International Federation of Anti-Leprosy Associations; 2003.
6. Guidelines for strengthening participation of persons affected by leprosy in leprosy services. New Delhi: WHO; SEA-GLP-2011.2.

7. I can do it myself! tips for people affected by leprosy who want to prevent disability: WHO; SEA/GLP/2007.2.

8. International Federation of Anti-Leprosy Associations (ILEP). Technical Guide: Facilitating the integration process. 2003.

9. International Federation of Anti-Leprosy Associations (ILEP). Technical Guide: Meeting the needs of people affected by leprosy through CBR. 2006.

10. Report of the International Leprosy Association Technical Forum. Paris, France, 22-28 February 2002. Int J Lepr Other Mycobact Dis. 2002;70(1 Suppl):S1-62.

11. Van Brakel WH. Measuring leprosy stigma—a preliminary review of the leprosy literature. Int J Lepr Other Mycobact Dis. 2003;71(3):190-7.

12. Werner D. Nothing About Us Without Us: Developing Innovative Technologies For, By and With Disabled Persons.

13. WHO/ILEP Technical guide on community based rehabilitation and leprosy. Meeting the rehabilitation needs of people affected by leprosy and promoting quality of life. 2007.

45

CHAPTER

Psychosocial Aspects in Leprosy

PK Gopal

INTRODUCTION

"The term *psychosocial* (Wikipedia)[1] refers to *psychological* development in and interaction with a *social environment.* The individual is not necessarily fully aware of this relationship with his or her environment. The term was first used by a psychologist Erik Erikson in his *Stages of Social Development.* Contrasted with *social psychology,* which attempts to explain social patterns of behavior in a *general* sense, the term "psychosocial" can be used to describe the unique internal processes that occur within the individual."

Psychosocial problems occur with the patients who suffer from a chronic illness like leprosy. Any chronic illness takes a long time to get cured and by that time the psychosocial problems set in the life of a patient. Unlike in many other diseases the social stigma in leprosy makes worse, the condition of the patients in their psychosocial behavior. Psychosocial support for leprosy patients through counseling, etc. was not the usual practice in the treatment facilities available in India.

STIGMA

"Stigma is a social process or related personal experience characterized by exclusion, rejection, blame or devaluation that results from experience or reasonable anticipation of an adverse social judgment about a person or a group. In health-related stigma, this judgment is based on an enduring feature of distortion of identity conferred by a health problem or health-related condition. It results into unjustifiable different treatment given to different people or groups by the society".[2] Social stigma in leprosy is widely prevalent not only in India but also in many other countries. The social acceptance of leprosy affected persons (LAPs) still remains a critical intervention for integration of these people in the society.

Leprosy affected children have difficulty in getting admission in schools. Employers do not like to employ leprosy affected persons. Leprosy affected persons have difficulties in accessing public services like transport, accommodation in hotels, etc. Marriage fixation with a member of a family where a LAP is also a part of the family is a big challenge because people think leprosy is a hereditary disease.

Still the undignified word "leper" is used to address the leprosy affected persons. In spite of best efforts by the government and voluntary agencies, social acceptance is still a problem being faced by leprosy affected persons. This is so because such acceptance depends on the mind-set of the community they live in or trying to integrate with.[3]

It may be difficult to ascertain the level of stigmatization by focusing only on the people with leprosy affliction. It is necessary also to know the level of stigma of many other diseases prevailing in the community in which the leprosy affected people are also living. When the person is diagnosed with leprosy, his normal psychological conditions are affected. The negative reaction of his family, friends and community aggravates his declining psychological condition. In many patients, suicidal thoughts came after the diagnosis of leprosy. Many patients have committed suicide in the hospitals and at homes as they had undergone extreme psychosocial burden. The social environment of the patient is responsible for damaging the psychological condition of the patient. The patient needs counseling as soon as the diagnosis of leprosy is made.

The psychosocial and economic problems of leprosy patients often continue even after they are cured from the disease. In many cases, the cure alone does not restore the normal psychosocial and economic conditions. Proper intervention by professionals at the right time is required to deal with such situations.

New Tools to Eliminate Stigma and Discriminations in Leprosy

On 21 December 2010, the General Assembly of the United Nations adopted Resolution A/RES/65/215 in which it took "note with appreciation" of the "Principles and Guidelines for the Elimination of Discrimination against Persons Affected by Leprosy and their Family Members" (Principles and Guidelines) that had been elaborated by the Human Rights Council. The General Assembly further encouraged "governments, relevant United Nations bodies, specialized agencies, funds and programs, other intergovernmental organizations and national human rights institutions to give due consideration to the principles and guidelines in the formulation and implementation of their policies and measures concerning persons affected by leprosy and their family members".

The Nippon Foundation, Japan, in 2011, initiated a project to disseminate and ensure effective implementation of the Principles and Guidelines throughout the world by organizing regional symposia in five regions, i.e. the Americas, Asia, Africa, Middle East and Europe. The governments and nongovernmental organizations (NGOs) should work to implement the "Principles and Guidelines" to eliminate stigma and discriminations which affect the leprosy affected persons and their families.

Social and Economic Rehabilitation

The overall objective of providing treatment to a patient is to enable him to stay with family while under treatment or return back to his family and community after cure if separated earlier for some reason or other and enjoy the same social and economic status which he was previously enjoying. Enabling a patient to achieve this status through socioeconomic rehabilitation measures cannot be neglected while implementing the Leprosy Eradication Programme.

At a time, when there is a great success in the treatment of the disease, it is also necessary to achieve socioeconomic integration in the society of the persons affected by leprosy, which would give a meaning for cure of the disease, in a real sense.

Since deformity is the main cause for social stigma in leprosy, it is most likely that majority of the cases having deformities are also subjected to psychosocial problems, and thus there are social and economic dislocations in their life in varying degrees. Therefore, measures should be introduced to identify the socially and economically displaced persons and rehabilitation facilities be provided to such persons to resolve also their psychosocial sufferings. To reduce the problem in the future, patients should be encouraged to come early for treatment so that the deformities can be avoided.

In no other disease the disease affected persons were made to leave their families and community to form themselves as a group to live separately. This happened with the segregated and isolated persons affected by leprosy. They started to live away from the community and these places have been called as leprosy colonies, leprosy homes, leprosy villages, etc., and they lived as outcasts, ostracized by the society.

Social and Economic Integration

The term "social" has a very broad meaning. The dictionary meaning for social is "living in company", "One who is not practicing solitary life", etc. The social process or socialization is a lifelong process. It begins with the family and is continued through school, contacts with relatives, friends, coworkers, etc. Every normal person desires to be useful to his family, social group and society in general. Each individual in the society has a role to play as father, mother, son, daughter, employer, and employee and so on. The society expects the individual to take up the responsibilities and perform them for self, and to help others, in fruitful coexistence of the family and community.

Leprosy interferes as a disease to disrupt the process of socialization in certain proportion of persons affected with the disease. For some, the disruption is for a short or long period and for some others it is lifelong disruption. To make them return to their original social and economic status or to bring them back to their own role in their society and establish themselves in order to lead a normal life is termed as social and economic reintegration.

Self-Settled Leprosy Colonies

Leprosy is a unique disease, which had rendered those affected, as a vulnerable target for discrimination around the world, regardless of country, religion or culture. It was the first disease which brought a division among people—segregating and isolating persons with leprosy.

The persons affected by leprosy had been segregated from their families and community compulsorily by law in some countries like USA, Japan and Korea to live a segregated life in isolation. They were denied normal living. They were unable to marry and prevented from having children. Their human rights were curbed. Those who violated the restrictions were severely punished, jailed, tortured, buried alive or even burnt.

In India, though there was no law to segregate them, the family and community abandoned the affected persons or forced them to leave their families. These persons had to resort to begging for their living. They joined together as a group and started to live in leprosy colonies away from the community. They married among themselves and had children.

With the support of the Nippon Foundation, Integration, Dignity and Economic Advancement (IDEA). India conducted a survey to know about the leprosy colonies in India. As per the survey there are about 778 such self-settled leprosy colonies, homes and sanatoria all over India where people are living a marginalized life (Table 45.1). The disease played

Table 45.1: State wise number of leprosy colonies in India

S. No.	Name of the State	Number of colonies
1	Andhra Pradesh	99
2	Bihar	57
3	Chhattisgarh	34
4	Delhi	28
5	Gujarat	17
6	Haryana	19
7	Himachal Pradesh	1
8	Jammu & Kashmir	1
9	Jharkhand	56
10	Karnataka	35
11	Kerala	4
12	Madhya Pradesh	31
13	Maharashtra	38
14	Orissa	59
15	Punjab	29
16	Rajasthan	14
17	Tamil Nadu	43
18	Uttar Pradesh	57
19	Uttarakhand	47
20	West Bengal	35
21	Asylums, Permanent Stay Homes, Sanatoria and Wards	74
	Total	**778**

a havoc, totally destroying the social fabric of the families of persons affected by leprosy.

REHABILITATION

What is Rehabilitation?

"Rehabilitation aims to provide reablement of physical function, readaptation in the existing physical condition to the life situations and reintegration with the family and community, resuming his/her normal social and economic living."

The World Health Organization (WHO) Expert Committee on leprosy defined rehabilitation as:

"The physical and mental restoration, as far as possible, of all treated patients to normal activity, so that they may be able to resume their place in the home, society and industry."

Rehabilitation in the field of leprosy requires greater efforts than the rehabilitation in the other types of disabled persons because the question of social acceptance does not arise in nonleprosy disabled persons. In the case of orthopedically handicapped, blind or deaf persons, their stay with the families are considered essential/obligatory but it is

prejudiced in the case of leprosy patients. This is due to the stigma attached to the disease. Therefore, one of the essential requirements in the socioeconomic rehabilitation is to create a suitable condition in the community for social acceptance of leprosy cured persons through effective health education measures.

Need for Separate Guidelines to Assess the Leprosy Disabilities

Though India has the largest number of leprosy affected persons in the world, there are no guidelines exclusively for leprosy to assess the disabilities in a person. At present, guidelines available for orthopedic disabilities are used to assess the leprosy disabilities. The loss of sensation and resulting deformities in foot and hands are not considered for gradation in the orthopedic disability assessment.

Institution Based Rehabilitation

In olden days, leprosy affected persons were segregated from the normal population and thereby leprosy villages and leprosy colonies sprang up. When institutions were started to take care of these patients, some of them were given permanent shelter in such institutions. The inmates of such asylums were engaged in different occupations like agriculture, animal husbandry, mat and cloth weaving, etc. mainly to meet the requirements of the institution. The approach was sympathy and charity based. In this system, the inmates developed a total dependency upon the institutions. They were not exposed to the society and its daily life situations. The inmates of such institutions preferred to stay in the institution even when cured rather than going back and face the society.

With the advancements in medical and surgical treatment procedures, such institution based rehabilitation has been outdated.

Community Based Rehabilitation

In community based rehabilitation, the leprosy cured person is helped to return to his own environment to live with his family and community. His family and community are involved in the rehabilitation process. He is encouraged and assisted to do a suitable, productive occupation to contribute to the economy of his family and thus live as a useful and self-supporting member of the community. Education, vocational training and employment are the main tasks which fall within the principles of community based rehabilitation.

In India, rehabilitation in the field of leprosy was provided in some places by few NGOs. Majority of the leprosy affected persons have not received the benefits of rehabilitation. The experiences gained by some of the organizations in the field of rehabilitation have shown clearly that leprosy cured persons could be successfully rehabilitated in the community and thereby their psychosocial and economic problems could be solved to a large extent.

Social and Economic Reintegration through Rehabilitation

Social and economic reintegration of persons affected by leprosy could be achieved through rehabilitation measures which would bring normalization in their life.

Rehabilitation means a return to a state of complete or near normalcy. This definition encompasses the need for social and psychological assimilation as a necessary complement to economic independence. Scientific knowledge about leprosy regarding its causation, cure and deformities has disproved the traditional beliefs, and this scientific information has to reach the public. Education of community is very important to bring normalization in the lives of persons affected by leprosy.

Normalization is a holistic goal. It cannot be achieved by addressing only the physical problems of persons affected by leprosy. It is necessary also to help them solve their disease related psychological, spiritual, social and economic problems.

The ultimate objectives of socioeconomic rehabilitation could be summarized as follows:

- Socially, the goal is to help persons affected by the disease to remain within their home communities, participating with the same rights and duties in the groups they would normally have participated, if they had never contacted the disease.
- The goal is to avoid all types of segregation which places persons affected by the disease in specialized leprosy institutions or bar them from general services provided by community institutions like schools, churches, housing, recreation facilities, hospitals, rehabilitation centers, homes for the elderly persons and disabled, etc.
- Economically, the goal is that persons affected by Hansen's disease continue to lead an economic life as similar to the one they would have led, had they never contracted the disease. This means that they have equal access to jobs and to vocational training opportunities for development of their skills. Access to economic assistance should be based not on the criteria of Hansen's disease but on more general factors such as age, disability level, financial need and availability of alternative sources of support.

Identifying the Target Groups for Socioeconomic Rehabilitation

In the field of leprosy, some data are available on physical disability, but the data on social and economic disability of leprosy affected persons are not generally available.

It is quite obvious that not all leprosy affected persons need rehabilitation. In a sample study conducted by the author in India in 1988, among 53,000 leprosy affected persons nationwide, it was found that 34% of them need some kind of social and/or economic rehabilitation assistance.[4] In the endemic countries, the number of leprosy affected persons treated so far is very high. It is necessary to select the leprosy affected persons who need rehabilitation. After selection it is also necessary to list them in priority based on their needs, capacity, available resources, etc.

The persons who would need rehabilitation also differ considerably in many ways. The person may be a male or female, young or old, educated or uneducated, rich or poor, etc. These wide variations among leprosy affected persons also emphasize the need of proper selection of needy persons for rehabilitation.

Socioeconomic rehabilitation is a major task involving different kinds of programs suitable for each category of persons. The problem of each individual is unique. Each person needs to be assessed and helped accordingly. It is necessary to broadly categorize the leprosy affected persons to find who would need, what type of assistance.

Based on the field experience in socioeconomic rehabilitation in India, a methodology was developed. This methodology is already in use in some projects in India. It is applied either in totality or with little modifications by most of the projects in many countries.

CATEGORIZATION OF LEPROSY AFFECTED PERSONS

All leprosy affected persons in the area need to be studied:

- Persons who do not have any deformity and do not have any social and/or economic problem and leading a normal life.
- Persons who have deformities but do not have any social and/or economic problem and leading a normal life.
- Persons who do not have any deformity but have social and/or economic problems just because they have/had leprosy.
- Persons with deformities whose social and economic life are under threat of dislocation.
- Persons who have deformities whose social and economic positions have been dislocated already and their normal life conditions are very much affected (dehabilitated).
- Persons who are aged and who have reached a state of destitution because of severe deformities; the end result of long sufferings, leading to dislocation of their socioeconomic life conditions.

As summarized in Table 45.2, the persons with first and second category of socioeconomic condition do not need any kind of rehabilitation.

The persons with sixth category are much disabled and not suitable for rehabilitation. Because of their old age and severe deformities, they need special care. This may be in the form of providing food, shelter and help/assistance in the daily activities, shopping, medical care, financial support, etc. Some of them have no money, no homes, no jobs and no family to take care of them. They may need institutional care.

Table 45.2: Categorization of leprosy affected persons in need of rehabilitation				
Category	**Deformity**	**Socioeconomic problems**	**Life condition measures needed**	**Rehabilitation**
1	Nil	Nil	Normal	Nil
2	Yes	Nil	Normal	Nil
3	Nil	Yes	Affected (due to stigma) Counseling	Psychological support
4	Yes	Threatened	Threatened rehabilitation	Investigation and suitable help
5	Yes	Dislocated	Seriously affected rehabilitation	Investigation and suitable help
6 (Severely incapacitated)	Yes	Totally dislocated	Seclusion and destitution	No rehabilitation, only food, shelter and general life support

The persons who fall in the third category need counseling and psychological support.

Persons in the fourth and fifth categories are very important. They need to be investigated and helped either to prevent dehabilitation or to provide socioeconomic rehabilitation.

The identification of eligible persons needing community based rehabilitation in an area is a major step in planning for rehabilitation. It is possible to identify the target groups for socioeconomic rehabilitation by this method.

EMPOWERMENT

The psychosocial problems of LAP should be relieved through engaging them in the process of achieving empowerment. Empowerment enables a person to make his own decisions about his life. Empowerment is not something which can be given to a person. On the other hand, a person must work to get himself empowered.

- Empowerment is strengthened by groups of individuals working together, realizing they have the potential to change their situation.
- The goal of empowerment is the inclusion of leprosy affected persons in family and community life and mainstream development programs.
- It beckons the group seeing the situation through different eyes and realizing the possibilities for change.
- The essence of empowerment is that leprosy affected persons and their families take responsibility for their development within the context of general community development. Ownership results from participation and involvement in decision making.

Responsibility and ownership are part of the empowering process. Empowerment is sustainable when based on understanding and skill. The understanding and skill can be applied again and again to solve further problems, and in turn this will generate a cycle of energy and creativity.

- Empowered people participate in family and community life; in learning, playing, working, in household activities, relationships and decision making, and in political and cultural activities.
- Change has to start with the people themselves. This means that the first step for many leprosy affected persons is a fundamental change in their mind-set from a passive receiver to an active contributor. The process starts from the time when they are given counseling to get relieved from their psychosocial problems.
- Once people with similar problems meet in socioeconomic empowerment workshops, they can realize that individual problems are common to the group and that there are common solutions for many. Being together helps to minimize isolation and to increase sharing and mutual support.

For any group to become empowered and to act effectively, they need to:

- Identify the common threads between the problems of the individuals.
- Recognize their strength in togetherness.
- Gather information to increase their understanding and knowledge.
- Fight against stigma and discrimination and to be free from psychosocial problems which would automatically improve the quality of life, to lead an integrated, dignified life.
- Receive support and opportunities from governments, NGOs and the community. The NGOs can play a major role in this process.

REFERENCES

1. Wikipedia, Free Encyclopedia (April 2008)—www.google.com, "psycho-social".
2. Upadhyay VS. "The Concept of Dehabilitation and Rehabilitation" paper presented at WHO seminar on Preventive Aspects of Rehabilitation Community Based approach, Gandhi Memorial Leprosy Foundation (GMLF), Wardha, 1990.
3. First T. "Don't Treat Me Like I Have Leprosy". London: ILEP; 1996.
4. Gopal PK. Methods to identify the leprosy patients needing rehabilitation. Indian J Lepr. 1997;69:438.

46
CHAPTER

Human Rights and Stigma in Leprosy

VV Dongre

IN THE FOOTSTEPS OF TIME...

Leprosy is an ancient disease, confined primarily to man. Man is a social animal, so, there are social dimensions to this disease.

- Prince Devashi (brother of Prince Shantanu) with leprosy could not become a crowned king in 5000 BC. (Mahabharata).[1]
- Supreme Court's verdict in September 2008 declared that a leprosy patient cannot contest an election. (Violation of Article 21 of human rights (HR) declaration).[2] The election rules in the state of Odisha are repealed and now leprosy patients can contest election in this state.
- Supreme Court's verdict in 1974 allowed divorce on the ground of leprosy.[3]
- International hostel denied admission to leprosy patients in New Delhi as recently as in November 2006. (News in Deccan Herald November 11, 2006).[4]
- A person who has no leprosy but is doomed because he lives in a leprosy colony in East Delhi with his parents, who have leprosy. He has been refused a driving license more than once and he stopped trying after being told, "Lepers should beg, not drive cars" (News in Hindustan Times dated, February 27, 2009).
  (*NB*: The motor vehicle Act 1989 does not debar a leprosy patient from getting a driving license.)
- Unfortunately, even persons who are concerned with Human Rights Commission at times make very wrong statements.

Chennai: Chairman of the Andhra Pradesh HR Commission has called for legislation to prosecute parents with diseases such as tuberculosis, HIV, leprosy and dyslexia, should they, knowing that they have the disease, have children.

The local doctors protested against this baseless statement, as tuberculosis and leprosy are not genetic diseases. (News in The Hindu dated, January 9, 2009).

In 1970, a member of the parliament (MP) tried to table a bill for the compulsory sterilization of leprosy patients. Dr RV Wardekar, Director, Gandhi-Memorial-Leprosy-Foundation (GMLF), Wardha, India fought tooth and nail against this damaging bill and saw to it that the bill was never tabled on the floor of the parliament.

In 1946, the father of nation Mahatma Gandhi, asked Dr Sushila Nayyar to contact an assembly member in Karachi (then in British India) to see that the bill for sterilization of leprosy patient does not materialize. The said bill was not passed.

The document is available in the archives of GMLF, Wardha.

SOCIAL ASPECTS

Societal attitudes, legal prescriptions and cultural perceptions are blended together to make social aspects.

(The news that appears in the print media creates a deep impression on the minds of the people. It is believed that the news are published after due confirmation of the facts. Needless to say that media should have accountability for whatever they publish.)

The Disease

The disease itself is mildly infectious and not hereditary, but, actually in the society it is believed to be infectious and hereditary and hence, the social stigma attached to it affects the children of the leprosy patients—both in the social sphere and in the cultural life.

Early detection and regular, adequate multidrug treatment (MDT) cures leprosy without deformities. 98% people have immunity against leprosy. Only 2% are susceptible to leprosy in the community. Only 8–10% of untreated leprosy patients are infectious, i.e. they can spread the disease in the society and the family mostly by droplet infection during coughing and sneezing or direct skin to skin contact under ideal conditions. They can be made noninfectious by MDT within a short period of time. One dose of rifampicin kills 99.99% germs of leprosy that are in the process of multiplication in the body of the patient under treatment.

Misconceptions in the Community

It is considered to be due to the sins committed in the previous incarnation and due to curse of God/Goddess. It is believed to be incurable. Assisted suicides were suggested to leprosy patients and many did happen. *Manusmriti*[5] condones suicide by an incurable leprosy patient with advanced disease. Relatives and friends were expected to be dutiful to help a leprosy patient to end his life by drowning or burying himself alive or burn himself to death.[6] The problem is not what the disease is, but what the people believe it to be![7] It is also a subject concerning the "human rights"!

Social Stigma and Its Effects

The disease itself has variegated forms and is on the decline due to multiple factors, such as MDT, prevention of deformity program, early case detection due to public education and the ultimate integration of leprosy services with general healthcare system, which helped to reduce the stigma. Unfortunately, some patients hide the disease because of the fear of dissociation by the family and the community—which delays the treatment and leads to deformities. Deformity is equated mostly with infectivity and hence the fear and associated social stigma.

MEDICAL IMPLICATIONS

Stigma impacts negatively on early diagnosis and treatment leading to increase in the transmission of the disease and prevalence of deformity.

ASPECTS OF DISCRIMINATION: HUMAN RIGHTS VIOLATIONS[8-10]

- *Community discrimination*: Violation of Articles 2 and 7 of HR declaration.
- *Religious*: Entry into temple forbidden, right of worship is denied (violation of Article 27 of HR declaration).

- *Social*: Visits to families of leprosy patients are avoided (violation of Article 27 of HR declaration).
- *Self-inflicted*: Visits to relatives and visits for social and cultural events are avoided by leprosy patients themselves (violation of Article 27 of HR declaration).
- *Educational*: School admission at times is denied to children of leprosy patients (violation of Article 26 of HR declaration).
- *Economic*: Jobs are not easily available to leprosy patients and their children (violation of Article 23 of HR declaration).
- *Health related*: Admissions in general hospitals to leprosy patients for treatment of other ailments are many a times denied (violation of Articles 2 and 7 of HR declaration).

All the above subjects involve HR issues.

Articles 38 and 41 of Indian Constitution provide the relevant ethos to the subject.

Consequences of Social Stigma

On the Intrafamilial Relation

The patient is not able to share meals with the family members. He is forced to live apart.

He is supposed to use separate articles, vessels and clothes of daily use. He is not allowed to touch family members. He cannot contribute to family decisions.

For him, marriage is not permissible and if already married, he is not permitted to have physical relationship with the spouse. The female patient is not allowed to bear a child or if already a mother, she is not allowed to fondle her child or breastfeed her child. Finally, the leprosy patient is "abandoned" by the family and divorce is asked for, on the basis of the disease.

Legitimacy for Social Ostracism

The dictums of religious books and traditional social codes or attitudes are more severe than any law. Societal attitudes are set in laws. The attitudes have roots in the religious books thus religion and law give the legitimacy for such a behavior.

The need for change was recognized and recommendations were proposed at the International Leprosy Congress in 1963 at Rio-de-Janeiro. Swaminathan committee of Government of India in 1982[11] and Gavai committee of Government of Maharashtra in 1982[12] also recommended to repeal outdated and outmoded Acts pertaining to leprosy patients, inflicting social injustice on them.

For social assimilation of leprosy patients, the retrograde legislation needs changes in the light of modern concepts of leprosy. All derogatory Acts adversely affecting the fundamental rights of a leprosy patient as a citizen should be repealed, where needed, without any delay. Connivance of the provisions in the Acts and laws amounts to their acceptance.[13]

The outdated, outmoded Indian Lepers Act of 1898 was repealed in October, 1984 in the state of Maharashtra and thereafter in the Union territories and other states of India. This Act considered leprosy patients as criminals for no crime of theirs. It did not protect the society at large from the infection or the disease nor did it help in any way for the control of the disease. On the contrary it perpetuated the social stigma. The patients used to hide the disease in the early stages for the fear of getting committed under the said Act.

Leprosy patients were not allowed to inherit ancestral property till 1956. The ancient literature like Koutiliya's *Arthashashtra* did support this tradition. The Hindu Succession Act of 1956 rectified this error and leprosy patients now are allowed to inherit ancestral property. However, on account of selfish motives, it is not so easy for a leprosy patient to get the due share of the ancestral property.

Laws on Matrimonial Alliance and Divorce

The present matrimonial Acts are negative and punitive in their approach toward leprosy patients which need to be revisited.

Manusmriti did not allow matrimonial alliance with leprosy patients as per the third chapter of the book. However, in the eighth chapter of the book Manu allows matrimonial alliance with a leprosy patient provided the disease is revealed to the spouse before marriage.

- Indian Divorce Act of 1869[14]
    - Clause 10 (iv) has for a period of not less than 2 years immediately preceding the presentation of the petition, been suffering from a virulent and incurable form of leprosy.
- Hindu Marriage Act of 1955[15]
    - Section 13 (iv), has been suffering from a virulent and incurable form of leprosy.
- Hindu Special Marriage Act of 1954[16]
    - Section 27 (g), has been suffering from leprosy, the disease not having been contracted from the petitioner.
- Muslim Marriage Act of 1939[17]
    - Section 2 (vi) that the husband has been insane for a period of 2 years or is suffering from leprosy or a virulent venereal disease.
- Indian Christian Marriage Act of 1872[18]
    - Section 10 (iv), virulent and incurable form of leprosy for a period of not less than 2 years.
- The objectionable terms used in the laws are "virulent and incurable forms of leprosy."

There is nothing like virulent form of leprosy and every form of leprosy is curable with MDT

Matrimonial Laws need Changes as:
- Leprosy is neither hereditary nor congenital
- All the types of leprosy are curable with MDT
- All the patients are not necessarily infectious

- Infectious patients can be made noninfectious by MDT within a short period of time.

PARSI MARRIAGE ACT OF 1936 (NO DIVORCE GRANTED ON THE GROUND OF LEPROSY)[19]

The grounds of divorce, dissolution and decree of nullity of marriage do not include leprosy.

[*NB*: Dr RV Wardekar, Director, GMLF, Wardha, who is the father of survey, education and treatment (SET) pattern of leprosy control, had a different view which was expressed in his letter dated, September 4, 1953 to Dr P Sen of School of Tropical Medicine, Kolkata, West Bengal. He has cited two case studies of two young, married female patients. In those days, bigamy was allowed. The husbands of both the female patients after abandoning their wives who had leprosy, got married again; but did not give divorce to their first spouses having leprosy. The unfortunate females, victims of leprosy, could not get married again as their previous husbands did not give them divorce. He expected that the law for divorce should be so flexible that the cases which are mentioned should get justice.]

(Copy of the original letter is available in the archives of GMLF, Wardha, Maharashtra state.)

Stigma in the Community

Most of the victims are 'abandoned' to their fate outside the court of law. The 'supreme committees' of different castes give verdict for divorce which is true till today (Article 16 violation of HR declaration).

Stigma in the Leprosy Hospitals

These hospitals were situated on the outskirts of the city/village. There were physical barriers which existed between the patients and the staff members. Leprosy phobia was the cause for the same. However, nowadays positive change is clearly visible in this respect.

Stigma in Leprosy Settlements/Leprosy Colonies

There used to be separate rows of huts for skin-slit smear positive and negative patients. The children used to get isolated in orphanages inside the settlements.

As these patients are outcasts from the society they lose their self-esteem.

Stigma: Admissions/Treatment in General Hospital

In the general hospitals, "no touch technique" is used most of the times by hospital staff members.

Circulars by Coroner of Mumbai,[20] Commissioner of Municipal Corporation of Greater Mumbai, Executive Health Officer—Municipal Corporation of Greater Mumbai[21-23] were sent to General Hospitals from time to time for admissions of needy leprosy patients for treatment for other ailments besides leprosy.

Leprosy was a notifiable disease according to Bombay Municipal Corporation Act,[24] under "Control of Communicable Diseases" which was incorrect as leprosy cannot be compared with diseases like cholera and typhoid.

Now, leprosy is not a notifiable disease in the areas of Municipal Corporation of Greater Mumbai. This is the latest repealing in the said Act of Municipal Corporation of Greater Mumbai.

Disposal of unclaimed dead bodies of leprosy patients is done in separate crematorium of Hindus and in separate areas of Christian and Muslim cemeteries in spite of a circular by Executive Health Officer—Municipal Corporation of Greater Mumbai 1983,[25] which orders all the crematoria to accept the dead bodies of leprosy patients for disposal.

Such a situation may be prevalent in other states of India, too.

EMPLOYMENT RULES

New recruits having leprosy find it difficult to get employment in the Government set-up. The State and the Central government rules[26,27] for leprosy patients to get re-employment after cure are not uniform.

Life Insurance and Leprosy Patients

Smear positive leprosy patients are not insured. Leprosy *per se* is not a cause of death and does not shorten the life of a patient (Violation of Article 22 of HR declaration).[28]

The petition committee has asked Life Insurance Corporation to do the needful.

Paradoxically, "Janashree Bima Yojna" includes leprosy patients with physical deformity/deformities.

Transports and Leprosy Patients

Maharashtra State Road Transport Corporation rules (1980) do not allow leprosy patients with recognizable deformity to travel with others. Usually the deformed patients are noninfectious (Violation of Article 13 of HR declaration).[29,30]

The petition committee has asked the authorities concerned to do the needful.

Similar laws may be prevalent in other states of India, too.

Paradoxically, concession is given to leprosy patients in the ticket fares when his or her disease is not in a recognizable form (Early infectious patients cannot be recognized so easily by anyone). However, nowadays, so many patients with leprosy come to hospital in public transport, many of them with obvious deformities and facies typical of leprosy, but nobody objects or throws them out. Though slowly, the stigma has reduced considerably not only among the family members; but also in the community following effective IEC program through NLEP. In villages also our experience of last 10 years shows that the active leprosy cases (on treatment); and those treated previously, live in the families, in the village itself, as a part of the society.

Indian Railways Act, 1989 (under section 56) empowers a railway servant on duty to ask a passenger with infectious disease to vacate the compartment before reaching the destination. Leprosy is included in the category of infectious diseases. This is again unscientific as leprosy is not a highly infectious disease. Railway authorities have explained to the Petition Committee that now leprosy is not included in the list of infectious diseases.

Leprosy patients do get concession in the ticket fares (e.g. 75% concession on rail travel), if they are holding a certificate from a medical officer as noninfectious patients.

Rehabilitation

It is difficult to get market for articles/merchandise made by leprosy patients due to leprosy phobia. Local Governmental organizations too do not purchase articles from rehabilitation centers of leprosy patients despite the Maharashtra Government Resolution, 1961, to that effect.[31]

The Persons with Disability Act of 1995[32-34] includes only cured leprosy patients with 40% deformities. Out of the 3% reserved jobs of physically handicapped persons, only 1% jobs are reserved for persons with physical deformities (besides vision impaired and hearing impaired) and leprosy patients.

Government of India has appointed a Committee for suitable amendments and the acceptance thereof is awaited.

Rehabilitation Council of India Act, 1992 needs to repeal in the clauses pertaining to definition of handicapped persons as the definition of handicapped persons does not include leprosy-affected.

Juvenile Justice and Care and Protection Act 2000, Section 48

This Act classifies leprosy as a disease that is communicable and inherently risky. This representation spreads wrong and adverse message about leprosy.

Prevention of Begging Act 1959 (Maharashtra)

After 2 years of tenure in the receiving homes, beggars who do not have leprosy are released from the receiving homes; whereas the beggars having leprosy are not released. This again is not justifiable. Similar laws may be prevalent in other states of India too.

WINDS OF CHANGE

Gloomy picture of leprosy is becoming rosy, but we have to offer roses without thorns to leprosy sufferers.

There are several welfare schemes under the state governments and the central government of India for the handicapped persons including those with leprosy. Unfortunately, they do not percolate to the needy patients. Nongovernmental organizations (NGOs) working for the welfare of handicaps should make an endeavor to extend such welfare schemes to the needy patients.

Fortunately, the walls are crumbling, clappers of leprosy patients are getting replaced by clapping with them by the people. Repeal of Acts pertaining to leprosy, in proper direction would change quality of life of leprosy patients. Early detection and regular, complete MDT have answered all questions raised in the legal context about incurability, infectivity and deformity.

At a recent meeting of the HR Commission in Geneva (January, 2009), representatives of the countries having leprosy problem, were allowed to project their views, experiences and suggestions before the commission and the ambassadors of the concerned countries were asked to take note of the same.

VOICE OF AWAKENING

During the International Leprosy Congress at Hyderabad, India in 2008, it was revealed that the discriminatory Acts, laws are currently in force only in Nepal and India. Nowhere in the world, are such laws existing at present. They were repealed or amended suitably in the light of modern concepts of leprosy. (Proceedings of the pre-congress workshop on "Stigma and Leprosy" held at the International Leprosy Congress, Hyderabad, January 2008).

The leprosy patients in Japan, who were incarcerated in leprosy homes, have been compensated financially as per the verdict of the Court of Law of Japan.

Human Rights Commission of the world had appointed a subcommission to look into the matter, who visited India and had discussions with the concerned authorities.

The International Leprosy Union, based at Pune, India did approach the HR Commission of India and submitted a memorandum on the said subject.

International Leprosy Union, Sasakawa Memorial Health Foundation and The Law Society of Pune have published their reports on the said subject during 2007.

Leprosy patients all over the world have formed an association of theirs. In India we have its chapter consisting of representation from nearly 700 self-settled leprosy colonies. A recent positive development-the association of Leprosy patients of India (IDEA-India) along with some NGOs have made an appeal to the speaker of Rajya Sabha (The Upper House of Parliament) in the form of a petition,[35-37] as a result, the petition committee of Rajya Sabha (headed by Shri Venkaiyya Naidu) visited some states for on the spot enquiry about the leprosy situation there. The report has been submitted by the petition committee to the speaker of Rajya Sabha for further action. The petition committee has referred certain queries to the respective departments for clarifications, e.g. Department of Revenue, Ministry of Finance and Ministry of Railways, etc.

Regionally also in India Society of Leprosy-Affected Persons—Andhra Pradesh (SLAP-AP) by Mr V Narsappa as Founder-President of SLAP was formed in 2006 with an aim to provide and promote quality of life as well as strive towards restoring hope and dignity to the leprosy-affected individuals and dependent families.

Strategies to Address the Social Aspects

- Integration of leprosy services with general healthcare system will increase early detection and good compliance of the treatment and help in reducing stigma.
- Successful community-based rehabilitation (CBR) of leprosy sufferers will help to reduce social stigma attached to the disease and help to solve rehabilitation and other related social issues.
- Empowerment of leprosy patients will increase their self-esteem.
- Behavior Change Communication (BCC) for legislators, medicos, administrators and people at large will hopefully help to change their attitude for good. Mass media and celebrities in the society have major role to play in this regard. Awareness and awakening about the disease will have to be undertaken by all the health functionaries. Advocacy role will have to be played by leprosy workers, general healthcare staff members and the school teachers as well as scientists working in the field of leprosy.
- Counseling for medical and social problems of leprosy sufferers will go a long way to improve the quality of their life.

If we want repeal of outdated Acts/Laws, few points need to be clarified by the scientists working in the field of leprosy without any credibility gap, to remove doubts, confusion, misconceptions about leprosy from the minds of the people at large including medical fraternity and the law makers.
- Is susceptibility genetically determined?
- How much period is required for an infectious leprosy patient to become noninfectious after starting MDT?
- What is meant by cure from leprosy?
- What is the magnitude of reinfection and relapse?
- Has the conjugal leprosy rate come down after the advent of MDT?
- Is there any test for detecting susceptibility?
- How much inoculum is needed to get infection?
- What is/are the mode(s) of transmission of the disease?
- What is the period of viability of the *M. leprae* outside the human body?

- What is the incubation period of leprosy?
- Can a cured leprosy patient donate blood? Or donate organs like kidney?

Provisions in laws may be affecting HR of leprosy patients but the exact number of legally handicapped leprosy patients is not available as hardly any leprosy patient knocks the doors of court of law for justice. Therefore, the unjustifiable provisions in the laws are like a sleeping dog, on awakening, it can bite an innocent person also. Hence, there is an express need for repeal of such outdated and outmoded provisions.

Social justice cannot be achieved by following the letters of law but only by proactive actions. Administrative and policy changes need to ensure the HR of the patients. There should not be step-motherly attitude toward leprosy problem by the authorities concerned. Ensure care after cure.

The Supreme Court has started inquiry regarding 19 Indian Acts and Laws inflicting social injustice on leprosy patients. The proceedings have directed the concerned ministries to have proper repeal/amendments of the said Acts.

United Nations General Assembly has adopted a resolution by the HR Council on 6th October 2010 and given principles and guidelines for the elimination of discrimination against persons affected by leprosy and their family members.

The Petition Committee of Rajya Sabha has published so far two reports concerning HR of Leprosy patients. The third report is awaited.

- Election rules are repealed in Odisha and Bihar, other states will follow suit
- Motor Vehicle Act 1990 does allow leprosy patients to drive cars
- Sasakawa India leprosy foundation is undertaking welfare activities in self settled leprosy colonies in India
- National forum of colony dwellers tackles the problems with the help of human right commission in each state
- Leprosy is included in general disability association of the world.

A synergistic joint action between the stake-holders namely, the patients, the providers, the people along with a positive "political will" will go a long way to remove the social stigma that is attached to leprosy for centuries. Then and then only leprosy will be considered as a disease like any other disease and violation of HR of the leprosy patient will come to an end.

REFERENCES

1. Maharshi Vyas. The Mahabharata.
2. The Hindu, Tamil Nadu, 24th Sept 2008 (Newspaper).
3. Karipurath P. Should leprosy be a ground for divorce? Lepr India. 1976;48(3):304-8.
4. Deccan Herald, 11/11/2006, (Newspaper).
5. Manusmriti, Dharmasindhu (Kashinath Shastri, pp. 636).
6. Ramu G. Indian Leprologists Look Back, Mumbai: Publication of RRE Society of Acworth Leprosy Hospital; 1990.
7. R K Mutatkar, GMLF Wardha, (Book - Society and Leprosy).
8. UNO, Universal Declaration of Human Rights, Dec. 10,1948 (A/HRC/8/L.18) International Covenant on Economic, Social and Cultural Rights1966 [GA res. 2200A (XX1)].
9. Convention on the rights of persons with disabilities, UN department of economic and social affairs, 2007.
10. The Elimination of discrimination against persons affected by leprosy and their family members, 18.06.2008.
11. Swaminathan Committee Report: Govt. of India, 1982.
12. Gavai Committee Report: Govt. of Maharashtra, 1982.
13. MS Mehendale (Health Education and Social Aspects in Leprosy work). Poona District Leprosy Committee, Pune.
14. Indian Divorce Act, 1869 Section-10 (iv).
15. Hindu Marriage Act, 1955, Section-13 (iv).
16. Hindu Special Marriage Act, 1954, Section-27 (g).
17. Muslim Marriage Act 1939, Section-2 (vi).
18. Indian Christian Marriage Act, 1872, Section-10 (iv).
19. Parsi Marriage Act, 1936.
20. Coroner of Bombay, 24/12/1960, No.2/1960 Circular.
21. Municipal Corporation of Greater Bombay — Municipal Commissioner, HO/41153/R-I of 15/3/84.
22. Director Health Services, Maharashtra, DHS/CELL/Lep/Medical Care/1990 (2/1/1990).
23. Surgeon General, Public Health, MISC-23185-G of 1969 (10-15/7/69).
24. Bombay Municipal Corporation Act, 1888, Clause 419.
25. Circular EHO MCGM, Public Health Dept. - Dead Body-No.HO/56708/R-I of 25/5/1984.
26. Employment Rules Govt. of Maharashtra, Urban Development Public Health & Housing Department, Resolution No. LEP/2571/77663-D, 14th Nov 1972.
27. Employment Rules Govt of India, No. A-17020/1/74-MG, 5/4/1974.
28. LIC Act 1956, 9 Nov 1987, Press Release.
29. Maharashtra State Road Transport Corporation, Traffic Circular No. 11 of 1980, 21/4/1980, No. ST/TD/CNS/208/5/79/2928.
30. Indian Railway Act, 1989 Section 56.
31. GR Govt. of Maharashtra — purchase of bandage cloth & bed-sheets, Industries & labour resolution no. STO-1059-21957-INDIII, Sachivalaya, Bombay 32, 11/4/1961 (Para 3).
32. Persons with Disability Act 1995, Govt. of India Section 2 (i) and (iii).
33. Prevention of Begging Act, 1959 (Maharashtra), The Rehabilitation Council of India Act, 1992 Section 2 (c).
34. The Juvenile Justice and Care & Protection of Children Act, 2000 Section 48.
35. Petition to Rajya Sabha by Ex-MPs, Mr. Ram Naik and others, Mumbai, which was admitted by the Hon. Chairman Rajya Sabha on 3rd April, 2008. The petition was reported to the council on 16th April, 2008, thereafter, it was referred to the committee on petitions for examination and report.
36. Report of Law & Leprosy 2006-07, by Indian Leprosy Union, Sasakawa Memorial Health Foundation and Indian Law Society, Submitted to Human Right Commission of India.
37. United Nations General Assembly resolution, 6th October 2010—principles and guidelines for the elimination of discrimination against persons affected by leprosy and their family members.

Migration and Leprosy

Mohammad Aleem Arif

CHAPTER OUTLINE

INTRODUCTION

As per the definition in Wikipedia,[1] "Human migration is movement by humans from one place to another, sometimes over long distances or in large groups". Migration could be within one's state/province/region, within the country or intercountry. Migration could be 'immigration' when people come into a place, region or country as residents, may be temporary also, other than one's native land or it could be 'emigration' when they migrate away from their homeland to settle in another. Reasons of migrating "away from the homeland" could be many: over population, illiteracy resulting in unemployment, lack of employment opportunities, discouraging working environment, lack of career advancements at homeland and these factors collectively are labeled as 'push factors' which are making people to leave their homeland while better employment opportunities, better salaries, better working arrangements, increased and varied employment/skill-development opportunities in other places are some of the 'pull factors' contributing to emigration (Fig. 47.1).[2]

These could be voluntary migration within one's own region, country or beyond. While in place of immigration, there are certain factors, which hold a person there, called 'stay factors', e.g. good living conditions, better career prospects, etc. Still there are factors, which attract the person to their point of origin called 'stick factors', e.g. parents, culture, etc.

There could be other reasons of migration (not in one's control) or involuntary migration (which includes the slave trade, trafficking in human beings, and ethnic cleansing). Small populations migrating to develop a territory considered void of settlement depending on historical setting, circumstances and perspective are referred to as settlers or colonists, while populations displaced by immigration

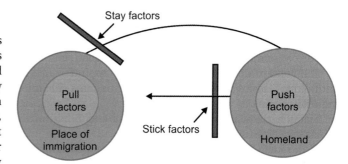

Fig. 47.1: Push and pull factors contributing in immigration and emigration

and colonization are called refugees. There are temporary migrations of travel, tourism, pilgrimages or the commute.

Familial reasons for movement are for marriage or separation, poor sanitation and environment, poor household structure, lack of privacy, caring for family members or employment for self or spouse.

People also migrate for better access to better treatment in their own country, but mostly from poor underdeveloped to rich developed countries. Present day medical/health tourism probably would fall in the same category.

Experiences of the immigrant group vary widely depending upon the city or region to which they migrate even within the same country. Transport option, employment opportunities and availability of healthcare and its quality, cultural, ethnic makeup of the area can all affect the experiences of an immigrant.

According to the "International Organization for Migration's" World Migration Report 2010, there were approximately 214 million international migrants in 2010.[3]

Migration and Leprosy

Movement of people affected by leprosy to seek solution to their problems is not a new phenomenon. The intended movement/migration after disease diagnosis is influenced by stigma, lifestyle, access to treatment, response to health policies and socioeconomic conditions. Though community people from same nationality may provide support system, but the preconceived ideas in the community may adversely affect the health seeking behavior. Migration of leprosy patients also led to creation of leprosy colonies in the past, particularly in urban areas.

In a study at a Delhi Urban Leprosy Center, it was found that 55.6% of patients were from Uttar Pradesh, 18.9% were from Bihar and only 10.17% were from Delhi itself.[4] In another study in Delhi slums it was found that 83.6% of the patients were from Bihar and Uttar Pradesh.[5] In an attempt to find out proportion of immigrant patients in NCT of Delhi, 2,536 leprosy cases were detected in the year 2012–2013, out of which 1,252 (49.37%) were from Delhi, 1,276 (50.31%) were from other states, while even eight cases (0.32%) were from other countries.[6] In a case control study in Maranhao, Brazil, it was noted that 23.5% cases migrated due to leprosy compared to 16.2% of the others migrated without the disease.[7] In another study by the same author in Tokantis state of Brazil, 20.9% individuals relocated after they were diagnosed with leprosy.[8] In a study in Dhaka, the capital city of Bangladesh 87% of the patients came from outside Dhaka while only 13% were living in Dhaka for more than 5 years.[9]

Shorter distance migration, however, allows migrants to maintain relationship with their home, community, etc. where relationships had been established.

EFFECTS OF MIGRATION ON LEPROSY CONTROL

Migrant population moves with the disease or carry leprosy bacilli, which may manifest as disease later. History of leprosy also tells us about its movement with migrant populations. Immigration of leprosy patients from neighboring high prevalent provinces/states/districts is increasing the case load of urban areas. This case load is increasing the infectious pool, additional work for the staff and delaying elimination of leprosy, a cause of concern for all of us. One of the factors in an urban setting is influx of population, from neighboring high prevalent states, which brings leprosy along with them.[10] Migration not only increases the case load but also increases burden on the health care system. The continuous flow of migrants into cities, from other states in search of jobs, family relations, etc. has certainly created major problems for the already crowded and subsidized health care system. This has to be tackled not only to help these patients but to check the spread of infection to the low endemic areas.[11]

Inflated Detection and Prevalence of Leprosy

Due to various reasons described above, continuous immigration and emigration is taking place in more developed/urban areas leading to distortion of data and incomplete picture of disease pattern, epidemiological situation/indicators. Some of the indicators which are affected due to migration are increased detection, low completion rate leading to high PR, which affects requirement of multidrug therapy (MDT) and other logistics under National Leprosy Eradication Programme (NLEP).

Low Completion Rate

National Leprosy Eradication Programme, which was launched by Government of India (GOI) in the year 1983 as a vertical program focused mainly on rural areas where drug distribution points (DDPs) were created and MDT services were provided by specially trained staff. During the period of vertical program implementation, few urban leprosy centers (ULC) were established mostly in hospital buildings to cater to leprosy patients. After integration of leprosy services into GHC system, these DDPs were dissolved and only ULCs situated in tertiary hospitals were expected to provide leprosy services to patients. In most of ULCs centers, there is no special staff to follow-up cases under treatment and thereafter. This leads to many defaulters and low completion rate in urban areas. Patients migrate to more developed and urban areas in search of job and livelihood opportunities and stay there till they have the job or engagement and leave the area whenever the job is over or they have to go back to their homeland for harvesting, without informing the dispensary/hospital staff or authorities. During the Leprosy Elimination Monitoring (LEM) exercise, cohort analysis was done by the monitors and it was found that overall defaulter rate was around 30%.[12] Without follow-up of defaulted or absentee patients and without updating registers, the PR reflected in the reports is not true prevalence but higher, and less than expected patients are getting cured. In a study at Bombay, Naik and More described annual dropout rate in 1989–1993 in the range of 35–55% and the dropout rate was higher, i.e. from 39% to 64% in non-Bombay resident patients.[13] Defaulter rate was also found to be higher in urban areas of Dhaka, Bangladesh.[9] In another study in urban area of Yangon, Myanmar the defaulter rate was 34.16%.[14] These findings reflect similarities in urban environment and similarities of problems of emigration. High defaulters and dropouts lead to less cure rates. Patients whose treatment is not completed may spread infection and may develop deformities if not followed up.

It can be seen from the Figure 47.2 that completion rates are low in a metropolitan city of Delhi, where immigration and emigration is high in comparison to urban areas of Uttar Pradesh, where migration is minimum.

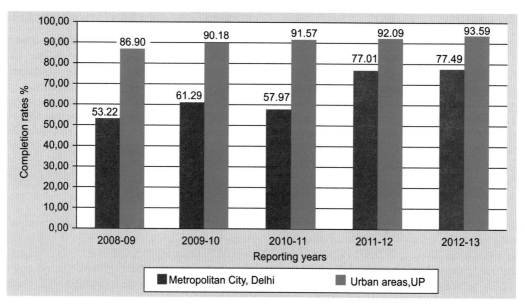

Fig. 47.2: Comparison of completion rates in cities with more migration and less migration
(*Source*: NLEP Delhi and Uttar Pradesh, 2013)

Re-registration

Re-registration should be understood clearly: It is registration of a case, as new, for the person who has already been treated elsewhere and declared cured. In most of the urban health centers, dispensaries and hospitals, patients are reporting voluntarily. Patients who have completed their treatment and declared cured in one center/area/city may migrate and get themselves registered again as new case in other area/centers/city or in different hospital or dispensary like in Delhi or Mumbai. Reason for this quest for more treatment is that the patch and disability do not go even after patient is considered cured. Sometimes, patients are not satisfied with the declaration of cure and services provided to them and migrate in search of better treatment. In a study in a cosmopolitan city of Chennai, Kumar et al. found that 11% of the patients were found to be dissatisfied with the services provided by the agency.[15] In the same study 35% patients had changed the agency for one or more times. Change of residences or migration was one of the major factors responsible for dropout or changing the agency. This was also found in a study in Delhi where 24% of women were not satisfied because of the persistence of patches.[16] This re-registration or double registration leads to appearance of names in both records and reports leading to inflated case detection and prevalence reported from the area.

In the hope of getting rid of the signs of leprosy, patients re-register themselves at another clinic sometimes even giving wrong information about their previous treatment. It is difficult for doctors and other leprosy staff to differentiate (in most cases) between the active signs in patients who have received treatment and those who did not receive treatment. Only very experienced leprosy workers or doctors can differentiate between treated and untreated cases, which is another subject of research to establish the possibility.

Re-registration was found to be 40.4% in Delhi and National Capital Region (NCR) of Delhi leading to inflation of detection rate.[12] Actual new case detection rate was found to be 2.4 compared to reported 4 per 10,000 population. The factors mentioned by the team were operational factors: wrong diagnosis or re-registration of cases. From the above discussion it can be concluded that re-registration is adding new cases, which truly are not the new cases. Re-registration is adding to increase in new case detection rate (NCDR), prevalence rate (PR) and delay in achieving elimination. With these inflated data assessing progress in the program is also difficult.

Duplication of Registration

Duplication means, a person is registered at one dispensary and is under treatment, he migrates to another location/city/state and gets registered as a new case there also. Leprosy services, in urban areas after involvement of general health care dispensaries and hospitals, are in the form of free consultations, investigation and provision of free MDT. Any patient can walk in and get registered for treatment. Also multiple agencies are involved in providing health services in an urban setting. Patients taking treatment in the area supported by one agency may also get themselves registered in the area supported by another agency, primarily because of migration and for their convenience and sometimes, when they are not satisfied by the treatment out comes, leading to duplication of registration and inflated new case detection and PR. This has an impact on over utilization of services and resource crunch on the part of the provider and opportunity costs to the consumer. During LEM[12] exercise the reported prevalence compared to the prevalence after applying standard definitions was found to be significantly higher in Delhi. Number of cases on record reduced by nearly 40% after applying standard definitions; actual prevalence found by the team was 2.6 per 10,000 population compared to reported prevalence of 4.3 for 10,000 population. During the same LEM exercise it was found that duplication of registration at different centers visited was found in the range of 17.1–29.4%. Some of the reasons for this duplication could be frequent immigration and emigration, relocation and displacement of slums. Patients sometimes register themselves in more than one center to avoid crowding and long waiting time. Duplication of registration or re-registration can also be seen from a study in Bombay, another mega city in India, where while finding the reasons for dropout, Naik and more found that 42% of cases were not true dropouts as they completed the treatment at other medical services center available in the city.[13]

During the same LEM, all the states the team visited reported a prevalence detection ratio of less than one but Delhi reported more than one. This means that prevalence is more than detection, i.e. still far more cases are registered, not cured, not deleted while detection is adding more cases to the records. With these inflated detection and PR, it is difficult for the program manager to evaluate and monitor the program and assess the logistics required to contain the disease.

MIGRATION, STIGMA AND HUMAN RIGHTS IN LEPROSY

There may be 'pull factors' or 'push factors', but immigration remains a serious concern for most of the developed places/nations where people from developing world try to settle legally, illegally, as asylum seekers, with a job or just like that. This leads to burden on the recipient governments as far as infrastructure, health care delivery and other services are concerned. As indicated by Soutar[17] in his paper that in many countries, leprosy is still a notifiable disease, the implication of which can have a direct impact on the rights of migrant workers and potential immigrants. Many countries have leprosy as a ground for refusal of visas and for inadmissibility of migrants. Countries having such discriminatory rulings include: Barbados, Hungary, Iraq, Namibia, the Philippines, Russia, Taiwan, Thailand, South Africa, the United Arab Emirates, United Kingdom and United States of America. In some countries migrant workers diagnosed with leprosy are routinely deported or at best offered one round of MDT before being sent home. It is unlikely that there is follow-up of those cases on their return to home countries and there is a

clear disincentive to workers to disclose or even present their body symptoms.

Immigrants because of language, culture, racism or ethnicity are itself not welcome in new areas and if they suffer from leprosy it is a further cause of stigma and discrimination. In an article by White[18] on immigration in United States, Dr Barbara Stryjewska, who works with the National Hansen's Disease Program in Baton Rouge, Louisiana, reported that a Marshallese man with leprosy who was living in Arkansas, USA, delayed seeking treatment in the US specifically because of a television news story broadcast and reactions of the participants labeling it as an impending uncontrollable epidemic of leprosy. He was afraid that he will be locked-up or quarantined, so he did not seek treatment until his symptoms worsened, thus putting himself at greater risk for nerve damage and serious disability. The problem of stigma and discrimination is further complicated by lack of knowledge and understanding of the disease, its curability and its transmissibility. With declaration of elimination of leprosy by WHO as a public health problem, interest of policy makers and the people and related knowledge has significantly gone down.

White, in her research work carried out on patient experiences with contemporary outpatient treatment in late 1990s in Rio de Janeiro, Brazil, observed that nearly every case of so called stigma or *preconceito* (usually the term equated with stigma or prejudice in Brazil) by people affected by the disease was not about others knowing they had leprosy, but about the difficulties they experienced as an indirect result of their illness within the socioeconomic and cultural context.[19]

CONCLUSION

International migration creates circumstances so that stigmatizing beliefs about leprosy (though not unique to migrants) are compounded by anti-immigrant sentiment, social and cultural differences in the host country and language barrier (especially with health workers) which can create difficulties in communication about diagnosis and treatment. Disease presence is used as a tool for racist or xenophobic attitudes. Negative stereotypes against a particular nationality, community, ethnic identity affected by a dreadful disease enhance such discriminatory attitudes. Disease in immigrants is used to bring back memories of policies of isolation. Politically motivated attempts have been frequently made to portray immigrants with leprosy as a threat to nation's safety. Racism, ethnocentrism and fears of the western world feature predominantly in leprosy confinement (leprosy colonies, leprosy homes, leprosaria) policies of the past.

The individuals with leprosy due to social customs and stigma might be separated from family and community and some of them in the past left the community entirely as migrants or otherwise. The International Federation of

Anti-Leprosy Associations (ILEP) review of leprosy research found that despite cultural differences across countries with a high incidence of leprosy, areas of life effected were similar.[20] Both self-imposed withdrawal and complete banishment from family and social networks has been noted in India[21] and Nepal.[22]

All these factors and association of leprosy with immigrants is a particularly effective means of generating anti-immigrant sentiment. This is a clear disincentive to patient to disclose or even present with early symptoms.

In nations where leprosy prevalence has historically been low, knowledge about the recognition of symptoms and treatment may also be low, which could result in misdiagnosis and delay in treatment. Some actions on the part of the physicians may even generate stigma.

Hansen's disease involves both medical and social aspects. From 2011 to 2015 WHO global strategy has rightly focused on not only reducing the burden of leprosy but also on ensuring equity, social justice, human rights, quality and sustainability of control activities.

The impact of IEC program in all endemic countries including India is gradually reducing the stigma related to leprosy, so also migration and other related factors including leprosy colonization.

REFERENCES

1. Wikipedia. (2007). Human migration. [online] Available from www.en.wikipedia.org/wiki/Human_migration. [Accessed June 2014].
2. Everett SL. (1966). A Theory of Migration. University of Pennsylvania. [online] Available from http://www.jstor.org/discover/10.2307/2060063. [Accessed June 2014].
3. International Organization for Migration. [online] Available from http://www.iom.int/cms/about-migration. [Accessed June 2014].
4. Sehgal VN, Ghorpade A, Saha K. Urban leprosy—an appraisal from northern India. Lepr Rev. 1984;55(2):159-66.
5. Pandhi RK, Khanna N, Sekhri R. Leprosy in resettlement colonies of Delhi. Indian J Lepr. 1995;67(4):467-71.
6. Directorate of Health Services. (2012-2013). Government of Delhi. [online] Available from http://www.delhi.gov.in/wps/wcm/connect. [Accessed June 2014].
7. Murto C, Chammartin F, Schwarz K, et al. Patterns of migration and risks associated with Leprosy among migrants in Maranhão, Brazil. PLoS Negl Trop Dis. 2013;7(9):e2422. doi: 10.1371/journal.pntd.0002422. eCollection 2013.
8. Murto C, Ariza L, Oliveira AR, et al. Motives and determinants for residence change after leprosy diagnosis, central Brazil. Lepr Rev. 2012;83(1):16-23.
9. Das KK. (2003). Leprosy read wrong News Age Metro. [online] www.bangla.net/newage/160603/met. [Accessed June 2014].
10. Vijayshankar P. Leprosy in urban setting. Lepr India. 1982;54(1):155-61.
11. Dambalkar K, Vashist RP, Ramesh V. Problems due to migration of leprosy patients into urban areas. Lepr Rev. 1995;66(4):326-8.
12. National Institute of Health and Family Welfare. Leprosy Elimination Monitoring (LEM) in Delhi. New Delhi: 2003.
13. Naik SS, More PR. The pattern of 'drop-out' of smear-positive cases at an urban leprosy centre. Indian J Lepr. 1996;68(2):161-6.
14. Myint T, Htoon MT, Win M, et al. Risk factors among defaulters in the urban leprosy control centre of Thaketa Township in the city of Yangon, Myanmar, 1986. Lepr Rev. 1992;63(4):345-9.
15. Kumar A, Sivaprasad N, Anbalagan M, et al. Utilization of Medical Agencies and Treatment Compliance by Urban (Madras) leprosy patients. Lepr India. 1983;55(2):322-32.
16. Kaur H, Ramesh V. Social problems of women leprosy patients—a study conducted at 2 urban leprosy centres in Delhi. Lepr Rev. 1994;65(4):361-75.
17. Soutar D. Immigration and human rights in leprosy. Lepr Rev. 2010;81(1):3-4.
18. White C. DejaVu: Leprosy and Immigration discourse in the twenty-first century United States. Lepr Rev. 2010;81(1):17-26.
19. White C. Leprosy and stigma in the context of international migration. Lepr Rev. 2011;82(2):147-54.
20. van Brakel W, Cross H, Declercq E, et al. Review of Leprosy Research Evidence (2002-2009) and Implications for current policy and practice. Lepr Rev. 2010;81(3):228-75.
21. Barrett R. Self Mortification and stigma of leprosy in northern India. Med Anthropol Q. 2005;19(2):216-30.
22. Heijnders ML. The dynamics of stigma in leprosy. Int J Lepr Other Mycobact Dis. 2004;72(4):437-47.

48
CHAPTER

Health Promotion, Education and Counseling

Manimozhi Natarajan

INTRODUCTION

This chapter deals with communication practices in the field of medicine. Health promotion, education and counseling are an essential component in the so called "treatment package" of the most successful health care interventions. Historically, this subject received little attention in medical colleges, where most of the medical and paramedical students were usually exposed to a superficial introduction to health education. This might be one of the main reasons behind the poor listening skills of most medics and paramedics. However, the ability to listen has more recently been acknowledged as an essential skill in the profession, especially for those programs dealing with patients affected by long-term conditions requiring relatively complex therapeutic interventions.

The chapter, although does not make any claim that Information, Education and Communication (IEC) programs could be sufficient in themselves to address such a complex problem as leprosy, it highlights the need to mainstream IEC into the existing service provision programs. This would ensure the achievement of essential targets, among which the following are regarded as priority targets: participation, voluntary reporting, treatment compliance, care of complications, quality leprosy services, management of disabilities and self-care.

PERSPECTIVES

With the paradigm shift from "leprosy elimination" (the elimination of leprosy as a public health problem) to the provision of quality, sustainable, integrated leprosy services utilizing all available resources in the national leprosy eradication programme (NLEP), there is currently a need for accelerating the pace to mainstream this new approach into the general health system (GHS).

Wider sharing of information about the disease status needs to be focused upon. IEC contents (messages) need to be redefined and used meaningfully based on the situation, result anticipation and intended action. Remedial actions against stigma and discrimination need to be initiated; political will for the NLEP should be strengthened and sustained. To ensure and provide denied dignity and "rights" to persons affected by leprosy, their voices need to be heard (Fig. 48.1). It was noticed that whenever there was a child case

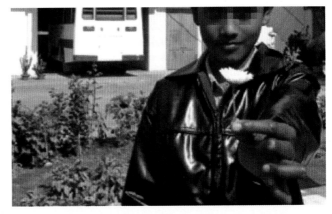

Fig. 48.1: Ensure and provide denied dignity and "rights" to persons affected by leprosy

of polio—the whole health system geared up. When a child presents with leprosy related disability/deformity, similar actions need to be undertaken—the idea is to "make noise" through effective communication channels to alert the health system and the community.

A passage from Harrison's Principles of Internal Medicine, by the editors of the first edition seems to articulate very well the responsibility of the physician in interacting with the patient. The passage reads as follows:

"No greater opportunity, responsibility, or obligation can fall to the lot of human being than to become a physician. In the care of the suffering (the physician) needs technical skill, scientific knowledge and HUMAN understanding. Tact, sympathy, and understanding are expected of the physician, for the patient is no mere collection of symptoms, signs, disordered functions, damaged organs and disturbed emotions. (The patient) is human, fearful, and hopeful, seeking, relief, help and reassurance."

Interpersonal communication, which can be established through doctor-patient interaction and communication, is presently acknowledged as an essential component of the care package. Formal training of medical and paramedical professionals needs to include communication skills development. The basis of medical interview is communication, and medical interview is itself the basis of medical practice. Effective communication can enhance patient compliance to treatment plans, contributes to augment the doctor's clinical competence and self-assurance, patient satisfaction and contribute to increase cost-efficiency and resource-effectiveness.

The doctor-patient relationship depends mostly on the understanding of the patient, as well as on mutual trust, which again are enhanced by communication skills.[1] Disclosing diagnosis to a person is a difficult task when the seriousness of stigma and discrimination are taken into serious consideration by the practitioner.

Declaration is a process of communication, "leprosy elimination" a scientific concept from global leprosy program and declaration of "leprosy eliminated", to the general public had led to constraints and complacency within the program. Program managers/decision makers had an understanding that leprosy as a disease was eliminated, but occasional press statement highlight that leprosy is back again. A better terminology than "elimination" could have averted the misunderstanding.

"Yaagaavaarayinum naakaaka kaavaakkal sokappar sol izhukkupattu"—Thirukkural (Meaning: whatever, whoever one could be in this world—failure to be vigilant and have control over their tongue, will lead to misery/trouble).

HEALTH PROMOTION

Health promotion focuses on addressing those determinants of health that can potentially be modified, such as individual health behaviors and lifestyle, income and social status, education, employment and working conditions, access to appropriate health services and the physical environment.

The Ottawa Charter for Health Promotion (1986) describes health promotion as the process of enabling people to increase control over and to improve, their health.[2]

Health promotion consists of a comprehensive social and political process. It aims to:
- Strengthen the skills and capabilities of individuals
- Change social, environmental and economic conditions to alleviate their impact on public and individual health. It is a process which enables people to increase control over determinants of health thereby improving the general health conditions of a population.

Expected outcomes of health promotion:
- People/patients with disabilities and their families are reached by the same health promotion messages, as are members of the general community
- Health promotion materials and programs are designed or adapted to meet the specific needs of people with disabilities and their families
- People with disabilities and their families have the knowledge, skills and support to assist them to achieve good levels of health
- Health-care personnel have improved awareness about the general and specific health needs of people with disabilities and respond to these through relevant health promotion actions

The community provides a supportive environment for people with disabilities to participate in activities, which promote their health

Community-based rehabilitation (CBR) program value good health and undertakes health-promoting activities in the workplace for their staff.

HEALTH EDUCATION

Evolution of Health Education

The concept of health education seems to have developed during the prehistoric era of mankind, while all the scientific approaches of health education are only few decades old and still in need of advancement. With the emergence of middle-class society in the 18th century, lifestyle became an issue as an important matter of concern toward food, shelter, cleanliness and other modalities, which focused around physical health.

By the 20th century, there was a boom in health recommendations with campaigns against serious infectious diseases, such as tuberculosis, venereal diseases, and cancer, and on topics like diet and addiction reflecting on biological and medical knowledge and its dissemination in various political systems in war and peace.[3]

Health education in leprosy encompasses all the activities, which are aimed to:

- Understand persons affected by leprosy in order to achieve early reporting and timely completion of treatment
- Ensure that people affected by leprosy learn taking care of their own disabilities and deformities along with the support of the health system
- Initiate and sustain the participation of the community at various levels through CBR.

Due to the complex sociocultural perceptions of the signs and symptoms of leprosy, "communication" is now regarded as one of the essential elements of any leprosy control program. Over the years, various approaches have been adopted in order to set up appropriate communication initiatives. Some of the approaches include: health education, IEC, behavior communication campaigns (BCC), and health education as a part of health promotion. All of them serve to achieve better health of the target population. Box 48.1 shows the health education terminology.

INFORMATION, EDUCATION AND COMMUNICATION

Information, education and communication (Fig. 48.2) is an inter-related triad of planned activities, which combine informational, educational, and communication processes. It aims to bring about objective behavioral, attitudinal, and participatory changes within a target population, based on a study of their needs and perceptions.

Information education and communication process should be clear, concise, and avoid the confusion that generally arises in dynamic situations related to health and disease. The objective is to foster change in health perceptions and behavior, taking into account the idiosyncratic challenges of the time and place.

An effective IEC program requires the support of an effective health system. In fact, it can only address communication-related problems, while the practical medical interventions remain indispensable for the treatment of leprosy as a disease.

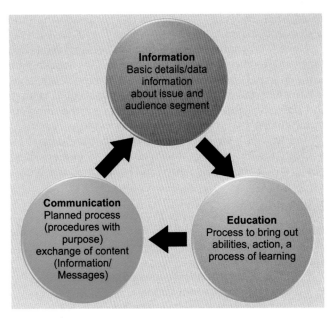

Fig. 48.2: IEC triad, information, education and communication a crucial cycle

Information

Facts provided/collected or learnt about something or someone—which includes a collection of useful briefs or detailed ideas, processes, data and theories that can be used for a certain period of time.[4] This needs focus and IEC gives ample scope to assess the actual situation for which interventions and remedial, educational activities followed by effective communication skills could be developed and implemented. An episode is given in Box 48.2.

Information (content/talking points) also refers to as what is conveyed or represented by a particular arrangement or sequence of things which includes the generation and dissemination of general and technical information, facts and issues, to create awareness among policy makers, administrators, academia and the general public, and of important developments in the country situation and policies of a country. It may involve public information activities

Box 48.2: An episode of session with patient

During one of the health education program in a clinic setting to a group of patients, the health worker very clearly and efficiently carried out his session, while doing so to check the attention of his audience, a question was posed to a particular person seeking its answer, for which the person was not responding and was only staring at the worker. The worker forced himself to repeat the question for which another person sitting next to the patient replied that he has speech and hearing disability which became an embarrassing situation for the worker:

Lesson learnt: Collect information before providing information.

to advocate necessary changes in policies, leadership and resource allocation.[5]

Leprosy programs collect information focusing on relevant target groups, their influence in the community, and program expectations. Once the data on target groups is available, information (talking points or messages) needs to be tailored for different target groups depending on the program expectations.

The Box 48.3 presents some points that are critical for a successful IEC strategy. Methodologies to address these points need to be individualized and made group specific.

Education

Education consists of systematic process of bringing out the ability to learn and apply knowledge.
These processes are:
- Selection of target groups (audience segmentation)
- Classifying them to various levels
- Formulating methods and approaches
- Designing of schedules and syllabi/curricula
- Teaching, training and learning activities by qualified competent staff.

Target Group: Audience Segment[6]

Target population (audience segmentation) need to be clearly demarcated dividing and organizing an audience into smaller groups of people having similar characters, communication-related needs, approaches/and identify several potential audiences for the communication strategy. Each audience consists of people who will directly benefit from the desired behavior changes. The task would be to determine the audiences on which to focus communication efforts in IEC strategies.

Audience Segments

- *Patients*, persons affected by leprosy, and all others in need of motivation for attention to specific issues; approach through interpersonal communication (IPC) counseling techniques, which offer a scope for better understanding and clarification.

Box 48.3: Situational analysis and planning for strategies

- Collection of data from and within community/client
- Review of literature
- Collection of information from other sources
- Survey and exploration to:
  - Determine needs
  - Influences on health
- Collection of data to explore opportunities for intervention.

- *Family and contacts*: For contact examination, dealing with children/differently abled, improved compliance, self-care practices through family-based care and for disability care activities.
- *Groups*: Gathering of two or more people with common interest for various activities, self-care groups, social welfare and women's organizations who can participate in supporting NLEP activities against discrimination, human rights violation and advocacy programs—these groups can be organized for discussions on various issues which are influencing the lives of affected persons and their families.
- *Community*: Community is a specific group of people, living in a defined geographical area and arranged in a social structure according to relationships that the community has developed over a period of time. Members of a community gain their personal and social identity through shared culture, beliefs, values and norms. All IEC work relies on good relationships with people in the community. Community members will also exhibit some awareness of their identity as a group; their common needs, and will have a commitment to meeting these needs. This segmented audience needs mass communication approaches to create awareness about various issues related to leprosy.
- *Institutions/Departments/Organizations*: An organization is a social unit of people, systematically structured and managed to meet to pursue collective goals on a continuing basis. These can be from public and/or private sector. These can be considered as a specific group for IEC activities to create network among interested partners willing to participate for the control of leprosy. The influence of this segment will support various issues related to leprosy control such as community mobilization/participation, creation of referral centers, community-based rehabilitation services, etc.
- *Underserved*, marginalized and those under special situations—geographically, sociopolitically, under-served areas, rescue operations during natural calamities, operations, such as relief, refugee camp, rehabilitation, resettlement, man-made mishaps, where special health services need to be strategically planned along with parallel IEC activities for immediate and urgent implementation.

Communication

The use of verbal and nonverbal means of communication is to express concepts, and to convey their meaning amongst participants while interacting. In its simplest form, communication involves exchange of information between people.

All three components of health promotion, i.e. health education, service improvement and advocacy involve communication in some form or the other. The main objectives of health promotion activities are to:

- Interact with communities (stakeholders) to promote health empowerment, developing their skills taking into account their beliefs
- Stimulate community participation
- Provide information about existing initiatives and opportunities
- Raise awareness and motivate the community for mobilization and participation
- Support communities to develop actions on health issues
- Improve competence of the health staff, manage, supervise and maintain sustained health activities
- Alert the decision makers to consider implementation and need-based modifications
- Network and develop public private partnerships.

Typically, a communication process is made up of a purpose (objective) and specific procedures (directions and activities that need to be undertaken).

Role Models and Nonverbal Information, Education and Communication Interventions.

An exemplary display by the medical doctor in the busy outpatient setting, welcoming a patient with a touch, a nonverbal display of positive behavior and attitude has shown effects among other patients and the person affected by leprosy. Sometimes actions speak louder than verbal means, which is an effect of IEC on undesirable situations due to lack of knowledge, ignorance with a wild play of "Forces".

Information, Education and Communication Implementation Approaches

The three basic IEC methods, such as mass (for a large groups-community), group (health providers, influencers, family members, and peer groups) and individuals (clients, patients), for interpersonal communications still hold well in planning IEC strategies.

Some target groups:

- *Health service sector:* Doctors, nurses, auxiliary staff, midwives, dressers, compounders, pharmacists
- *Public health sector:* Supervisors, health inspectors (male/female), *anganwadi* workers, accredited social health activists (ASHA) and others
- *Community level:* Panchayat Raj institutional members, leaders of all categories, traditional healers, spiritual leaders, women groups, youth groups, village administrators, nongovernmental organizations
- *Other sectors:* Those willing to participate could be mobilized.

Steps and Task Definition for Information, Education and Communication Activities

Step 1

Use broad categories to define the general field of activities the health workers are undertaking.

Categories should be comprehensive, in common usage to describe leprosy care.

- General community education activities about leprosy
- Case detection
- Diagnosis of leprosy
- Complete and regular treatment
- Release from treatment and post-treatment surveillance
- Prevention of deformities
- Reduction of stigma/discrimination (psychosocial), economic rehabilitation and integration of patient in community life (social and economic)
  (Involves combatting prejudice among employers, family counseling to prevent rejection of spouse, solutions to urban migration or other forms of displacement, and also mobilization of social and economic support for persons affected by leprosy in need).
- The preparation of other health workers for tasks in leprosy control.
  (This involves teaching leprosy to health workers including the IEC and psychosocial aspects. Campaigns to change the negative attitude and behavior of health workers toward patients and persons affected by leprosy).

Step 2

Within each category the expected IEC outcomes or indicators should be defined. (What can IEC activities achieve in each category? These indicators are used to assess the impact of IEC activities.)

Information, Education and Communication indicators are what we want to be the result of our IEC efforts and what they contribute toward the achievement of key goals in leprosy control, such as the number of cases who are detected early.

However, the IEC indicators may not be sufficient in themselves to explain the number of cases detected early, as other conditions intervene, such as, number of health workers capable of correctly diagnosing leprosy, frequency of case detection activities in specific target groups, etc.

Step 3

Once the indicators are defined, the question is what does a health worker need to do (as task performance) to achieve the indicator? What tasks are involved?

This step involves defining the tasks a health worker ought to carry out. Tasks are justified if there are reasonable grounds to accept that the task or tasks contribute to achieving the IEC indicator.

Step 4

The tasks defined in step 3 clarify the nature of the IEC tasks to be performed by the health worker. However, there is no indication of how to carry out the task. Step 4 answers this question and is called task analysis. Task analysis stipulates the subtasks or steps required to perform a particular task. The subtasks are listed in sequential chronological order and make explicit what the steps are, to successfully perform a particular task.

Subtasks are observable events (and therefore are used in more detailed checklists for assessing performance). Subtasks are also used to compose guidelines (written in detail and in sequential order).

Step 5

The tasks and subtasks define the IEC performance of the health worker.

Subtasks require that one has a certain knowledge, attitude and skill to carry out the subtasks correctly.

Step 6

Evaluation-assessment:
- Impact of health worker performance on the behavior, knowledge and attitude of patients, the public and other health workers. Use indicators as measures for assessment.
- Can be done with exit interviews, or through other special assessment projects. It is done informally in clinics, hospitals and the field through asking feed-back questions from target groups.
- How well the tasks or subtasks were performed by the health worker? Since tasks and subtasks are observable events, an observation checklist can be used in clinics or other situations where health workers perform.

The assessment of knowledge and attitudes as conditions for adequate task performance is usually done through written comprehension tests or by responses to items on a scale. This is done during the evaluation process of IEC activities.

Advocacy

Advocacy refers to persuading others to support an issue of concern to an individual, group or community. With relevance to IEC activities, advocacy consists of activities directed at the general public, but mostly at policy-makers, as they influence laws and policies concerning the allocation of resources, priorities for expenditure, direction of services and enforcement of laws. Advocacy is vital and necessary

part of IEC activities. It is essential for a program to have an impact. Its component of intervention will usually consist of a balanced mix of short-term and long-term activities.

Behavior Change Communication

The terms behavior change communication (BCC) and IEC are commonly used. What exactly do they mean and what is the difference between BCC and IEC (Table 48.1).

Providing people with information and telling them how they should behave ("teaching" them) are not enough to bring about behavior change. While providing information to help people to make a personal decision is a necessary part of behavior change, BCC recognizes that behavior is of having the appropriate information and making a personal choice (Box 48.4).

By carrying out BCC interventional activities, it is important to be clear about exactly whose behavior is to be influenced and which aspect of their behavior should be the focus for change. Communities are made up of different groups with different risk and vulnerability factors. Different target groups will require different approaches. Therefore, when making decisions about which target groups and which factors to address, it is necessary to consider:
- Which target groups are most vulnerable
- Which risk/vulnerability factors are most important
- Which factors may be related to the impact of conflict and displacement
- Which target groups and risk/vulnerability factors the community wants to address
- What could be motivators for behavior change
- What could be barriers to behavior change
- What type of messages will be meaningful to each target group.
- Which communication media would best reach the target group
- Which services/resources are accessible to the target group
- Which target groups and risk/vulnerability factors are feasible in terms of expertise, resources and time?

Table 48.1: Differences between IEC and BCC	
IEC	*BCC*
IEC is a process of working with individuals, communities and societies to: • Develop communication strategies to promote positive behaviors which are appropriate to their settings	BCC is a process of working with individuals, communities and societies to: • Develop communication strategies to promote positive behaviors which are appropriate to their settings. • Provide a supportive environment, which will enable people to initiate and sustain positive behaviors.

Box 48.4: Processes involved in behavioral changes

- Improved knowledge about leprosy and its consequences
- Improved awareness and changed behavior (self, family and community)
- Informed decisions to improve access to services (health, welfare and legal)
- Improved acceptance and reduced discrimination (social change)

Behavior change communication programs require careful analysis and pretesting of communication materials, which would be utilized[7] through integrated IEC approaches and methods (Table 48.2).

INTERPERSONAL COMMUNICATION

Counseling sessions, one to one.

Counseling[9]

Counseling is an advanced communication skill for a specific circumstance which is an interventional communication procedure aiming to stimulate the awareness and analysis of various available options. It is mostly used in health related activities to address psychosocial issues.

Qualities of a Good Counselor

A counselor should be compassionate, nonjudgmental, keeping note of the verbal and nonverbal communication.

Counselor should try and ensure that the clients have their rights to:

- *Information*: To learn about the benefits and availability of the services
- *Access*: To obtain services regardless of gender, creed, color, marital status or location
- *Choice*: To understand and be able to apply all pertinent information to be able to make an informed choice, ask questions freely, and be answered in an honest, clear and comprehensive manner
- *Safety*: A safe and effective service
- *Privacy*: To have a private environment during counseling or services
- *Confidentiality*: To be assured that any personal information will remain confidential
- *Dignity*: To be treated with courtesy, consideration and attentiveness
- *Comfort*: To feel comfortable when receiving services
- *Continuity*: To receive services and supplies for as long as needed
- *Opinion*: To express views on the services offered
- *Summary and confirmation*: End the session with clarity and confirmation that the information contents have been understood.

The Role of the Counselor

The counselor's role is to provide accurate and complete information to help the user make her/his own decision about which service (s) he will use. The role of the counselor is not to offer advice or decide on the service to be used. It

	Table 48.2: Integrated approaches/methods of IEC[8]	
1.	Collecting information	At the community level—collect information about the specific health problems. Use various data collection methods (ask who, when, where and how)
2.	Interpretational information	Discuss the problem with those concerned and outline focus area
		Select a priority problem and make an ordered list of other problems
3.	Action plan	Define what change is expected in the specific situation
		Analysis of influencing factors that might encourage or discourage the intended changes
		Discuss intended changes with all stake holders
4.	Implementation activities	Lead group discussions on main topic
		Develop audio-visual (and other) material, if needed
		Use innovative methods/techniques as appropriate
		Decide the "who, where , when and how" activates, which should be implemented
		Develop indicators to assess the impact of the intervention
5.	Supervision/Monitoring	Assess the impact of the activities carried out as a basis for ongoing planning of future steps and their evaluation

Source: TALC, UK.

becomes important during communications to consider environs, while focusing on realization more rather than just instructions informing to do and not to do to the patients.

Effective counseling requires understanding one's own values and not unduly influencing the user by imposing, promoting or displaying them, particularly in cases where the values of the provider and the user are different (Box 48.5).

Crucial Decisions

There are four crucial stages on which patients may take decisions, from the early onset of signs/symptoms of leprosy till the complete treatment and follow-up.

During this process, there could be desirable or undesirable decisions to be made, relating to issues such as:
- What to do when suspicious signs/symptoms are found by one self or others
- What to do if these signs/symptoms are diagnosed as leprosy and treatment is started
- How to follow regular treatment daily, and how to tolerate and manage complications, disabilities/deformities
- How to accept treatment termination while problems still persist. When to attend clinics for follow-up if needed, and accept several other personal/family decisions.

While decision-making is in progress during "interface" there are "positive" and "negative" forces at play, which might push an individual or community, back and forth from a desirable to an undesirable pathway.

Key Decisions Stages/Interface

What people do about leprosy may have desirable or undesirable effects on their health and the NLEP, depending on the kind of action they take. These actions are key decisions interfaced as stages to understand and to formulate IEC strategies. Leprosy control involves many different steps by health workers, patients, and by the people around. From the patient's point of view these steps represent decisions they take to solve their problems. From the program (health worker) point of view, the decision of a particular patient can be most appropriate or desirable or on the other hand can be most undesirable and lead to the severe disabilities and social problems of untreated leprosy.

Stages

- Suspect diagnosis
- Diagnosis and treatment
- Disability prevention
- Rehabilitation (postdischarge, after being released from treatment and follow-up). Discrimination and human rights violation.

Interface

Interface is the point where two people, organization systems meet and interact all through—leading to decision making.

Table 48.3 explains the itinerary of a patient passing through the key decisions stages of interface.

Forces

Positive forces like self-motivation and attitude, believes, and support from spouse/family/friends and committed health workers, etc. will lead the person to progress on a desirable pathway.

Negative forces like wrong beliefs, superstitions, wrong messages, denial, etc. could counter the push toward the desired pathway. Information about these forces could be collected from the patients during interviews and history taking. All efforts should be made to enhance positive forces and reduce or eliminate negative ones.

Good communication skills are essential for this purpose. It is essential to:
- Look at leprosy through the eyes of persons affected by leprosy and their community
- Identify and analyze the reactions of patients, family members, friends and others to leprosy
- Analyze the reasons why individuals/communities accept or reject participation in leprosy related activities.

Beliefs

Beliefs are the age old sanctions which help persons affected by leprosy to give meaning to events and make them more predictable and less threatening. Beliefs about health events are generally associated with beliefs about handling them. They can be useful, harmful or balanced. They are usually shared and passed on from generation to generation. Some Beliefs disappear over time, and some become stronger in terms of their sentimental and emotional undertones. When Beliefs have a component of spiritual faith, they become more sensitive and difficult to address (Box 48.6).

Box 48.5: Considerations of environs during communication
Space/zone while communicating:
Intimate zone = d"45 cm
Personal zone = 45 cm–1.2 m
Social zone = 1.2 m–3.5 m
Public zone = >3.5 m
During interpersonal communications (counseling sessions) it would be advisable to limit to personal zone/social zone if family members are included.
Communications as instructions v/s communication for realization
Focus communication skills on cause and effect

Table 48.3: Itinerary of a patient passing through the key decisions stages—of interface

Itinerary from early onset till the discharge from treatment and further; to rehabilitation and discrimination/human rights; there are desirable and undesirable decisions occurring in dynamicity all the time (4 stages and interface)

1. **Suspect diagnosis:** A patch/swelling/pain is detected by patient and/or a relative/friend or another person—"What to do" and make decision when faced with suspicious signs or symptoms.

Desirable pathway	Undesirable pathway	Program–outcome
• Patient goes to a health center with a health seeking behavior • Discusses problem with local health worker	Patient hides problem, ignores, seeks alternatives, migrates to other area	Early detection of leprosy (passive)

2. **Diagnosis and treatment including MDT:** What to do and make decision after the problem has been diagnosed as leprosy and treatment is initiated:

Desirable pathway	Undesirable pathway	Program-outcome
• Accepts diagnosis and starts treatment as prescribed • Reports to health facility whenever there are health related problems	• Denies/rejects, looks for alternative treatment, stops treatment, hides from health worker • Gets reactions and loses faith in treatment	Initial leprosy care

3. **Treatment and disability prevention and care:** Decides to be regular with treatment, takes precautions/ to prevent disability and deformity and takes proper care

Desirable pathway	Undesirable pathway	Program–outcome
Follows treatment for as long as indicated	Irregular at clinic, does not follow care for ulcers, does not report for follow-up	Treatment completion

4. **Rehabilitation–Discrimination and human rights violation:** Decides to take care of self and look for support, and if facing discrimination activities, demanding his/her deserved/denied rights

Desirable pathway	Undesirable pathway	Program–outcome
• Accept discharge and stops taking tablets • Pursues independent life	• Requests continuation of treatment • Seeks other centers for treatment • Looks for stay in leprosy colonies	Discharge from treatment

Abbreviation: MDT, multidrug therapy.

Attitudes, Norms and Values

Attitudes are approaches based on personal feelings and expressions toward persons, situations, events, disease, self, and the surrounding world. Attitudes influence decisions in positive or negative ways, thus leading to initiate an action of some sort, or none at all.

Values are a commonly accepted code of conduct, which are expressed to act or not in a certain way. For example, a person affected by leprosy is expected to behave in a certain way: like not to marry or share things with others.

These sanctions are powerful enough to influence the individual and the community to behave in a way that is not justifiable in terms of medical evidence, and even less in terms of human rights.

External Influence

Even when decision-making resides with just one individual, it is always influenced by external factors, such as threats, fear, personal experience, advice, suggestions, the local environment, financial considerations etc. More specifically, family members, friends, health workers, local elderly persons, and others often influence a person affected by leprosy. Their influence can sometimes be crucial in terms of decision-making. Time and money have also been identified as important factors for the acceptance or rejection of leprosy programs and services.

Factors influencing desirable course of actions: Positive forces which could be beliefs, attitudes, etc. need to be sustained and strengthened.

Box 48.6: Dealing with beliefs

- Collect and compile list of existing beliefs about leprosy, and assess their effects on decision-making.
- Make sure that the beliefs are respected and not ridiculed (since this could result in emotional situations and feelings of resentment). Stiff resistance to the proposed treatment could lead to inappropriate traditional medicine approaches.
- Provide simple facts to support medical world beliefs.
- Discuss about beliefs and their consequences, and allow time for change.
- Find out the guardians of belief system, contact them and explain the medical facts while respecting their thoughts and beliefs.

Denial

In situations of acute stress, individuals and communities sometimes react by pretending that the threatening situation is nonexistent (denial). This reaction is due to helplessness in the face of a threat that is felt as too overwhelming to be faced. The unconscious hope is that probably the resolution of the stressful condition will occur spontaneously. In many cases, denial leads to irrational choices, resulting in worsening of the situation.

Handling denial requires in the first place an understanding of the whole process of "denial". In the case of leprosy, for example, an individual could react in two ways: one by not accepting, withdrawing or denying the facts, and the other by coping with the situation by realizing, accepting, seeking support, adjusting and proceeding for management. It is essential to handle the situation using methods to promote the choice of a "coping process". The individual is assisted to find out reasonable solutions enabling him/her to make positive decisions.

Disclosing diagnosis to the patient: Disclosure is often an object of major debate. On one hand, it is a person's "right" to know about a problem. A competent health worker should be capable of breaking the news in a sensible and appropriate way.

The terminology at disclosure must be carefully selected. Phrases like "do not worry" should be avoided, as they automatically trigger a psychological reaction of uncertainty as to what will happen. Encouragement and emotional, empathetic support will suffice to control the problem much better than the suggestion not to worry. At this stage, some key strategies should be followed:

- Remember, and agree to the fact that "leprosy" is fearful for others (community, world) and that those around the patient may show unexpected reactions when informed of the disease (denial or coping mechanisms).
- Pause, by providing sometime as soon as diagnosis is disclosed. Keep observing the patient without making attempts to hurriedly explain the disease, its effects and management. All this talking shall be done at a later stage.
- Provide psychological reassurance and gain the person's confidence. Try to instil the feeling that the patient is in safe hands and provide a sense of security. Once the diagnosis is disclosed, a variety of emotional responses could be encountered, ranging from complete silence to desperate cry. This emotional relational episodes are to be expected, and are generally self-limiting. Provision of time is important at this stage. Patients may show: anger and hostile reactions. It should be kept in mind that patients are hostile and are expressing anger not toward the health personnel, but toward the situation. Health staff should not take this behavior personally. Provide time and allow the patient to get settled before resuming your work with him/her.

- Allow patients to express their thoughts freely at this stage. Encourage them to speak out, and show your appreciation for the fact that they are showing their feelings. This is the best way to gain information on their concerns and draw a plan on how to help.
- Provide support to normalize fear and denial by finding out the patient's main concerns. Provide examples on how the patient and family could overcome such pressures. Emphasize that it is normal to feel worried, and that such thoughts normally occur. Tell patients that they can come back to you again if they have more queries.
- Discuss the negative effects of denial and the positive effects of addressing the situation from the onset.

Motivation

Motivation could be regarded as a person's attitude and feelings toward a task ahead. Motivation will not necessarily be observable in a direct way. Often it can only be interpreted by observing the way in which patients behave and explain their own actions.

Motivation is a kind of energy, which is very vital and dynamic in nature. It is somehow a drive to fulfil basic needs. Such basic needs could be:

- Physiological—such as hunger, thirst, survival, safety and sex
- Social—such as self-esteem, body image, status of all kinds, self-image, relationships, religious/spiritual/nonreligious attachments, philosophy, etc.
- Hierarchical—need to occupy a specific place in the community
- Priority and precedence—where one needs to take precedence over another.

It becomes important for the health worker to identify needs that could generate positive energy leading to a motivational attitude.

CASE STUDY

Case study in brief: Figures from 48.3A to I, in sequence:

COMMUNICATION SKILLS

It is a fact that health professionals often lack training in communication skills. The importance of training and practice in communication skills cannot be underestimated. In leprosy programs it is extremely important to communicate with the patients and help them face their problems, the disease, its manifestations, as well as to identify complications at their onset. There are three important components in communication. These can be described as an interrelated triad; listening, observing and talking (LOT), when interacting at the interpersonal levels.

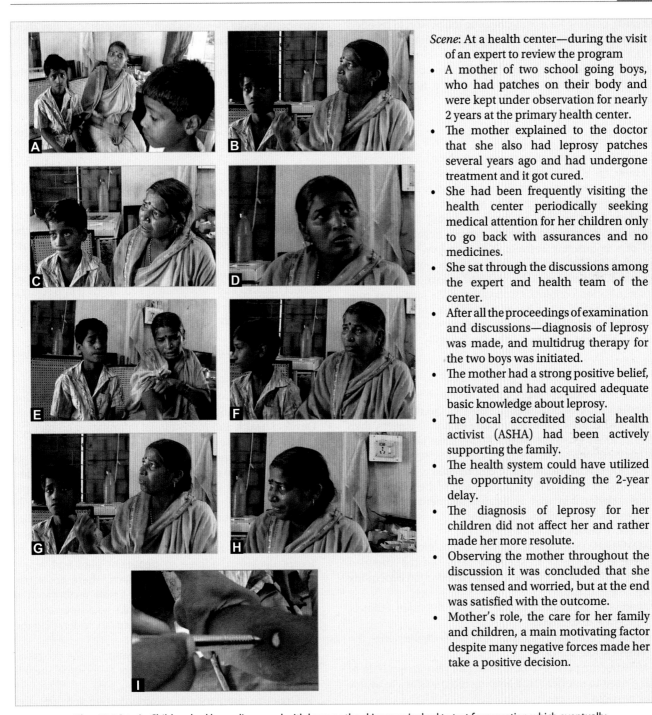

Figs 48.3A to I: Children had been diagnosed with leprosy, the skin was pinched to test for sensation which eventually became a scar. On examination both the boys had been confirmed with diagnosis of leprosy

Scene: At a health center—during the visit of an expert to review the program
- A mother of two school going boys, who had patches on their body and were kept under observation for nearly 2 years at the primary health center.
- The mother explained to the doctor that she also had leprosy patches several years ago and had undergone treatment and it got cured.
- She had been frequently visiting the health center periodically seeking medical attention for her children only to go back with assurances and no medicines.
- She sat through the discussions among the expert and health team of the center.
- After all the proceedings of examination and discussions—diagnosis of leprosy was made, and multidrug therapy for the two boys was initiated.
- The mother had a strong positive belief, motivated and had acquired adequate basic knowledge about leprosy.
- The local accredited social health activist (ASHA) had been actively supporting the family.
- The health system could have utilized the opportunity avoiding the 2-year delay.
- The diagnosis of leprosy for her children did not affect her and rather made her more resolute.
- Observing the mother throughout the discussion it was concluded that she was tensed and worried, but at the end was satisfied with the outcome.
- Mother's role, the care for her family and children, a main motivating factor despite many negative forces made her take a positive decision.

Listening

Developing the art of listening requires patience, interest, time and commitment. It is a process of paying attention to collect as much information as possible in order to provide appropriate services. In general, listening entails hearing all the messages conveyed, keeping silence while carefully keeping eye contact, asking questions (closed, open and a mixture of both) for clarification, acknowledging that attention is been paid (e.g. by summarizing what the patient just said), pausing for a while, helping the person to recollect and reorganize to speak, reflecting the feelings expressed by the person, initiating gestures like shaking one's head with sigh/words like hmmm! Ha ha! Is it so and so on. Time constraints/limitations at OPD could be a hindrance to a listening process.

Observing

During the communication process we share ideas, messages and thoughts with the other person. We also expect that they should pay attention to what is said while closely focusing on their vision—observing. There is a strong correlation between verbal and nonverbal interaction. Wrong interpretation and misunderstandings, could impact negatively at the end of a counseling session. It is therefore, important to observe a patient and try to grasp the person's nonverbal expressions. These should be analyzed as a whole with verbal communication contents. Observation skills play a key role. "What all is heard, and what all is seen may not be true, until thoroughly analyzed." Thorough analysis must be done by utilizing efficient listening and observing skills.

Talking

This activity usually takes most of the health worker's communication time. Although many of the messages sent out by the health workers are routine technical aspects, then a point comes when the patient finally must be informed of his/her condition.

Two aspects of talking can be emphasized:
1. The matter which is the actual content of the talk
2. The relationship that is established between the two parties (health staff and the patient)
   Effective talking will be promoted by:
- Making the participants feel free and comfortable, giving them enough time to spend to carry out the intended actions (e.g. taking consent, formal or informal depending upon the situation)
- Making an attempt to check whether the main point of concern is understood
- Keeping questions simple and not challenging the patient's statements
- Allowing the person to talk, asking for permission if there is a need to interfere, and keeping intermissions to as few as possible
- Instructions versus realization—the talk should depend upon the situation. It should not be the same all the time. It should not be a list of instructions, such as: "do this, do that, never do this".

Talking consists of a series of messages. Messages are the main core constituents of communication. Effective communication rests on four main cardinal components, content, appeal, relationship and emotions (CARE). These

components make messages more meaningful, as they show the communicator's concern and commitment.

Formulation of messages: While composing messages as talking points, the health worker should keep in mind the following:
- Whom the message is to be addressed to
- How it should be delivered and perceived
- The main idea to be conveyed to the patient must be clearly expressed.

PROGRAMME FOCUS IN RELATION TO LEPROSY

The main objective is to make the community aware of the disease, of its problems, and of the way in which the community can participate, so as to foster early case reporting.

Actions which could be initiated in a new community:
- Select the area and conveniently sub-divide it into sectors. This will:
  - Allow to carry out IEC activities on rotation basis/phases
  - Prevent an overload of suspect cases at the health centers
  - Guarantee the provision of better attention.
- Utilize all information gathered about the prevailing beliefs, notions and other related issues for the new area.
- Develop health and motivational information on medical facts and health service facilities.
- Pretest them under field conditions and modify as necessary prior to use (assess impact after implementation through indirect indicators, such as number of people with suspected skin lesions reporting voluntarily after IEC intervention, and analyze along with other program/epidemiological indicators). Communication is indispensable to help persons affected by leprosy to accept diagnosis, adhere to treatment plan and report immediately in case of complications. There are series of activities to be undertaken by all health facility staff to ensure the provision of patient friendly health services:
  - Create conditions (IEC) for patients to understand the importance of self-care
  - Support patients' active participation in the program. This will help them to adhere to positive health practices
  - Organize interpersonal communication activities and group discussions with peer groups, if necessary
  - Teach about self-care practices, prevention of disabilities (POD) and management of deformities. These represent a real challenge for IEC programs.

All IEC methods need to be adopted to achieve satisfactory results in self-care and prevention of disabilities. Health services also need to be strengthened in providing referral system in the management of disabilities/deformities.

KEY ISSUES IN COMMUNICATION FOR LEPROSY PROGRAMME (TABLE 48.4)

Understanding

The two main targets for the success of integrated programs are: Early case detection and completion of treatment without disabilities. In order to achieve these objectives, it is indispensable to ensure a robust communication program that can address the needs of the local community.

Leprosy program is no different from any other national program and requires three main components:
1. Competent staff (technical and operational)
2. Comprehensive health system to respond to the needs of the population
3. Participation of the affected persons, including the community.

To ensure active meaningful participation "communications" become crucially important, be it in the form of health education or BCC, with IEC becoming an important aspect of health promotion especially for diseases like leprosy.

Health workers must be aware that working with patients affected by leprosy could have negative implications for the lives of their patients if messages are not understood. The role of effective and positive communication should never be underestimated.

Perceiving

Health workers should be trained to develop instincts to ask, look and feel in terms of the community in which they work. POD activities require practice in asking one-self whether a patient is at risk of developing disability/deformity, whether early damage can be readily identified, whether the patient will be able to ask/seek immediate care in the existing rehabilitation services, if necessary.

Interfering with Patient's Habits

It is usually difficult for a person to adopt a new habit to prevent/manage disabilities. It might take some time to learn the practice and to realize that the new habit is valuable, until then, patients need support and motivation.

Family-based Support to Self-care Practices

It is important to plan and run group IEC/training programs for concerned family members. Their support can make a huge difference in the cure of leprosy and prevention of disabilities.

Self-care

Self-care practices are often a lifelong task for a person affected by leprosy. Individuals and families should be helped

	Table 48.4: Programme Guideline				
Step 1	State the IEC goals for the programme				
Step 2	Select target audience groups to be reached	Individuals (IPC) (A)	Groups (B)	Mass (C)	Other's (D)
Step 3	Define changes needed from each target groups to achieve the programme objectives				
Step 4	Determine which IEC activities (information, education, communication, institution building, advocacy, others) are needed to bring about expected changes				
Step 5	Outline key appropriate messages and message strategies				
Step 6	Identify the most appropriate combination of communication channels				
Step 7	Identify organizational and managerial strategies needed for implementation				
Step 8	*Budget*: Amount resources needed				
Step 9	Prepare Gantt Chart for time framed IEC activities				
Step 10	Monitoring/supervision evaluation procedures with indicators formulated.				
Step 11	Discuss the strategy in terms of critical factors and obstacles to be removed, revise it, and get it approved				

Source: SJ, C (1993). Developing information, education and communication (IEC) strategies for population programmes. New York: United Nations Population Fund (UNFPA).

to come to grips with the reality and be consistent in their self-care tasks.

Promoting Self-help

Patients and their families should be able to (1) listen to explanations about self-care techniques, (2) see the techniques being carried out and (3) practice them (role play exercises). Leprosy programs should propose self-care training in these three phases.

Not all problems are communication problems, but practice leads to perfection and effective communication can be learnt.

Information Education and Communication Strategy

National leprosy education programme implementation plan for the 12th plan period 2012–13 to 2016–17 (Box 48.7), had set 3 objectives which are:
1. Elimination of leprosy with prevalence of less than 1 case per 1,000 population in all the districts of the country
2. Strengthen disability prevention and medical rehabilitation (DPMR) of persons affected by leprosy
3. Reduction in the level of stigma associated with leprosy
   The IEC strategy during the 12th plan period will focus on communication for behavioral changes in the general public.

ACTIVITY PLANNING VERSUS STRATEGIC PLANNING

In general any program needs planning, and so do the health education program, focusing interventions not only towards results; but also against the causes of the problems. Activity planning forms the basis for strategic planning. It allows planners to break down the complex issues into smaller tasks while shifting from activity based to result oriented approaches with numerous uncertain causes. Therefore, strategic planning is particularly useful when the issues to be tackled are not clear and uncertain.

Leprosy is an unpredictable disease with intense psychosocial implications. As a result, activity planning is

Box 48.7: Crucial issues IEC-12th Planning Commission
• To develop communication material vis-a-vis the target
• To complement and support detection and treatment services being provided free of cost through the Government Health Services
• To remove the stigma associated with leprosy and prevent discrimination against leprosy affected persons
• To specially cover beneficiaries, health providers, influencers and the masses.

(*Source:* Central Leprosy Division)

particularly recommended for leprosy programs. According to this methodology, situational strengths, weaknesses, opportunities and challenges (threats) should be analyzed while preparing a plan of action. One should bear in mind that from the community/patient's perspective, leprosy could be quite different from what the medical staff regard as the actual health problem.

Some basic issues to be considered could be:
- "What do we need to know about persons affected by leprosy, and their attitudes and beliefs toward this disease?" These differ from person to person, and region to region, with some commonalities (like stigma and discrimination). It is essential therefore, that information is gathered and analyzed.
- "What could be done in relation to communication to promote acceptance of persons affected due to leprosy by the community?" How can we make them realize and follow advise/suggestions to take care of their disease, encourage early self-reporting when problems are suspected, motivate them for acceptance and adherence to treatment and self-care practices for prevention/management of disabilities and deformities. Effective communication at the patient as well as the community level will play an important role to tackle all the above issues. Therefore, the role of communication component in leprosy program should never be underestimated. Display of health education material at health centers could be organized with a proper plan. Information about various diseases and health problems/and related instructions are indiscriminately displayed in most of the health centers with no idea or plan. A well prepared and useful information materials often get muffled due to various other unsuitable displays.

It has been observed that there is poor medication adherence, an on-going issue in the management of outpatients,[10] and use of multiple methods assessing adherence to medication improves accuracy. Wider programs of counseling or direct support to patients and family members with increased community and social support had shown to improve adherence to treatment.[11]

All problems are not communication problems alone and IEC programs need support from service component. They go parallel, supporting each other to improve better participation, increased voluntary reporting, improved compliance to treatment, timely reporting to health center during occurrence of complications, improving quality leprosy services, bettering management of disabilities and self-care, understanding patients and service provider's perspectives, sharing of experiences; in all these, communication plays a vital role.

ACKNOWLEDGMENTS

I would like to thank Indian Association of Leprologists, Professor Dr.Bhushan Kumar, Professor Dr Hemanta Kumar

Kar, Dr CM Agrawal, ILEP colleagues, Arogya Agam, SLR & TC-Karigiri, AIFO and staff, Dr MV Jose, Dr Giovanni, Dr Sunil Deepak, Mr Sergio Zovini, Dr Daisy Kandathil, Dr Desikan, Dr S Arunthathi, Dr VK Pannikar, Dr P Vijayakumaran, Dr Rangandha Rao, Dr Rajan Babu, Dr Suman Barua, Mrs Chiara Carcianiga (editing), My parents, family, friends, finally to my beloved persons affected by leprosy for all their contributions and help. I express my sincere gratitude to my beloved teachers Dr V Ekambaram, Dr Mr and Mrs Paul Brand, Dr EP Fristchi, Dr M Christian, Dr Ramanujam, Dr Kumar Jesudasan and my almamater Kurnool Medical College.

REFERENCES

1. World Health Organization. Division of Mental Health. (1993). Doctor-patient interaction and communication. Geneva: World Health Organization. WHO/MNH/PSF/93.11. Available from www.who.int/iris/handle/10665/60263. [Accessed June, 2014].
2. World Health Organization (1986). Ottawa Charter for Health Promotion. Geneva. Available from http://www.who.int/healthpromotion/conferences/previous/ottawa/en/index3.html. [Accessed July 2014].
3. Arnold L. Gorske (2004). Health Education Program for Developing Countries. Available from http://www.hepfdc.info/files/EngHB2014Web.pdf. [Accessed June 2014].
4. Bosena Tebeje (2004). Lecture notes: Ethiopia Public Health Training Initiative. USAID, Jimma University. Available from www.share-pdf.com/2014/2/2/f8dbdb442f3e48ac86c6cb2814acee94. [Accessed June 2014].
5. Cohen SI (1993). Developing information, education and communication (IEC) strategies for population programmes/Tech paper no 1. Available from www.popline.org/node/342715. [Accessed June 2014].
6. NAHIP Toolkit_part12.indd
7. An approach to effective communication—Chapter 4. Undated: AIDSCAP Electronic library: AIDSCAP (n.d.). *HIV/AIDS Prevention and Control for Humanitarian workers - Course notes.*
8. TALC (Teaching Aids at Low Cost) publications. UK.
9. SI, C (1993). Developing Information Education and Communication (IEFC) strategies for population programmes. New York: United Nations Population Fund (UNFPA).
10. Weiand D, Smith WC, Muzaffarullah S. Qualitative assessment of medication adherence at an urban leprosy outpatient clinic in Hyderabad, India. Lepr Rev. 2011;82(1):70-3.
11. Weiand D, Thoulass J, Smith WC. Assessing and improving adherence with multidrug therapy. Lepr Rev. 2012;(83):282-91.

FURTHER READING

1. A Guide to Health Education in Leprosy: Neville PJ. TALMILEP teaching and learning Materials. ILEP,1993.
2. Education for health: A manual on health education in primary health care. WHO publication.
3. Graeff JA, Elder JP and Booth EM. Communication for Health and Behaviour Change: A Developing Country Perspective. San Francisco: Jossey-Bass Publications; 1993.p.205.
4. Health education in Leprosy work, A manual for Health workers: Van Parjis LG. Pub. Leprosy Mission International London, 1986.
5. Windahl S, Signitzer B, Olson JT. Using Communication theory. New Delhi: SAGE Publications; 2008.

49
CHAPTER

Role of NGOs in National Leprosy Eradication Programme

Thomas Abraham, Pankaj Sharma, Atul Shah, VV Pai, Mohammad Aleem Arif

INTRODUCTION

Involvement of nongovernmental organizations (NGOs) in the National Leprosy Eradication Programme (NLEP) is of vital importance; these had and still have an active role in health promotion in the community. Many patients even seek treatment through them. Though the Government of India (GOI) tackles the major burden of leprosy work, about 20–25% of the workload is handled by the NGOs. The significant role played by the NGOs in different leprosy-related activities is very well-acknowledged by the national program. The technical support rendered has facilitated the elimination of the disease and its integration with the General Health Services (GHS). The incidence of the disease presently is either stationery or declining very slowly. However, there still exist certain pockets with high prevalence. The major problems that still need attention are the detection of hidden cases at the earliest and put them on multidrug therapy (MDT), prevention and management of disabilities, rehabilitation, sustaining quality leprosy control activities including supervision and monitoring of programs at the district and sub-district level. The main role of NGOs is to support the NLEP to tackle these issues. Though the leprosy services are now provided through the general healthcare system, the GOI has established district leprosy cell in each district for proper operationalization of 12th five-year-plan under NLEP, by effective program planning, implementation of guidelines, recording and reporting, financial management and periodic program review.

MAJOR NGOs WORKING IN PARTNERSHIP WITH NLEP

International Federation of Antileprosy Associations (ILEP)

International Federation of Antileprosy Associations (ILEP) is an international federation of 13 autonomous nongovernmental antileprosy organizations with a powerful financial partnership, raising funds from public and institutional sources. Membership of ILEP enhances the capacity of these member associations to work toward the common goal of a "World without leprosy" (Table 49.1 and Fig. 49.1).

Their annual contribution to antileprosy work amounts to about €39 million globally. Members of ILEP work in partnership with the governments—international and local partners, supporting the development and sustenance of quality leprosy services.

International Federation of Antileprosy Associations globally supports leprosy field activities, including case finding, MDT, training, hospital care for complicated cases, research and socioeconomic rehabilitation. In India, ILEP contribution to leprosy services is around 600 million rupees annually.

International Federation of Antileprosy Associations Partners Working for Leprosy in India

- Aide aux Lépreux Emmaüs-Suisse ALES India (Swiss Emmaus Leprosy Relief Association)
- Associazione Amici di Raoul Follereau (AIFO India)
- American Leprosy Missions (ALM)
- Deutsche Lepta-und Tuberkulosehife Indien (GLRA India)
- Damien Foundation India Trust (DFIT)
- Fontilles India (Fontilles India)
- LEPRA India (Lepra India)
- The Leprosy Mission Trust India (TLMTI)
- Netherlands Leprosy Relief (NLR India Branch and Trust)

International Federation of Antileprosy Association member organizations active in India to support NLEP at national level by providing technical support to central leprosy division (CLD) by placing consultants in CLD, and support to states by placing state NLEP consultants. NLEP consultants provide technical support to the district staff at all levels through an experienced senior level medical

Table 49.1: Major International NGOs supporting leprosy programs: International Federation of Anti-leprosy Associations (ILEP)

S. No	Organization	Full name	Country
1.	AIFO	Associazione Italiana Amici di Raoul Follereau	Italy
2.	ALM	American Leprosy Missions	USA
3.	DAHW	Deutsche Lepra-und Tuberkulosehife	Germany
4.	DFB	Damien Foundation Belgium	Belgium
5.	FAIRMED	Fairmed	Switzerland
6.	Fontilles	Fontilles	Spain
7.	FRF	Fondation Raoul Follereau	France
8.	LEPRA	Lepra	United Kingdom
9.	NLR	Netherlands Leprosy Relief Association	The Netherlands
10.	SMHF	Sasakawa Memorial Health Foundation	Japan
11.	SLC	Le Secours aux Lépreux - Leprosy Relief Canada	Canada
12.	TLMI	The Leprosy Mission International	United Kingdom

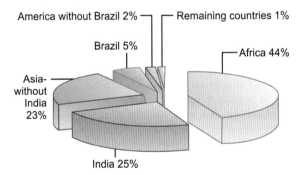

Fig. 49.1: Distribution of ILEP members' field support by region

ILEP a reasonably well-functioning mechanism of detecting, diagnosing and treating leprosy exists. In addition, ILEP has produced learning material in 12 different languages for various categories of government workers; trained the district nucleus (DN) teams and other staff in 590 districts in the country. One of the strong features of ILEP in India has been the healthy, reciprocally beneficial partnership with major players in leprosy field, which has resulted in remarkable progress in leprosy control and has become a model worthy of emulation.

Involvement of International Federation of Antileprosy Associations in the National Leprosy Eradication Programme (2013–2017)

International Federation of Antileprosy Associations agencies have signed another memorandum of understanding with GOI for a period of 2013-2017. The present support to NLEP is planned in line with the 12th five-year-plan of GOI and the new WHO enhanced global strategy and its operational guidelines, to sustain good quality leprosy services in the integrated scenario.

- The ILEP has significant role in providing National Disability Prevention and Medical Rehabilitation (DPMR) consultant to CLD who assist NLEP in planning, monitoring and evaluating DPMR activities in the country.
- Provides state level NLEP consultants for performing following functions:
  - Capacity building of district nucleus (DN) teams.
  - Advise and guide state in assessing training needs and defining strategy.
  - Assist in capacity building in states on managerial, analytical and supervisory skills.

officer with a vehicle for mobility. Besides this, they also support SLOs regional review meetings, provide technical support in developing and financial support in printing of learning material. Other support, provided by ILEP agencies, is: own projects and NGO-run projects. Own projects are generally hospitals which are operated directly by the concerned ILEP member organization and they provide a broad spectrum of services including management of leprosy and its complications, reconstructive surgery (RCS) and socioeconomic rehabilitation. The NGO-run projects are also hospitals, rehabilitation and field projects generally managed by a local NGO with total or partial support from ILEP member organization (Table 49.2).

The contribution of ILEP to leprosy control in India has been conspicuous, considerable and consequential. It has enabled the governments to establish and maintain integrated leprosy services in different states and districts of India. In all the districts of the country, thanks to the committed involvement of the government staff facilitated by

Table 49.2: Support by ILEP members's to leprosy work (in Euro) during 2013–2014

	Support to field projects	Support to research[1]	Indirect field support[2]	Total support
TLMI	97,21,634	1,42,004	0	98,63,638
DFB	77,09,246	1,38,434	0	78,47,680
DAHW	55,28,574	2,11,345	95,798	58,35,717
NLR	50,38,050	4,33,282	2,25,203	56,96,535
FRF	23,88,969	1,47,196	1,34,665	26,70,830
ALM	11,49,711	1,65,136	1,92,668	15,07,515
AIFO	12,46,623	1,500	0	12,48,123
FAIRMED	12,15,926	12,104	0	12,28,030
SMHF	7,16,993	35,955	3,45,612	10,98,560
SLC	6,97,157	37,731	31,073	7,65,961
LEPRA	6,55,126	21,982	0	6,77,108
SF	6,18,960	30,000	10,000	6,58,960
Total	**3,66,86,969**	**13,76,669**	**10,35,019**	**3,90,98,657**

[1] Including other scientific activities such as congresses and journals.
[2] Including support to training, consultancies and patients' associations.

- Advise and guide the state in establishing referral system.
- Analyze the data and advise the state leprosy society on implementation of the program.
- Participate in the surveillance system.
- Arrange for independent evaluation, etc.
- ILEP also provides technical inputs for the mid-term and independent evaluations of NLEP.
- Regional level review meetings for State leprosy officers (SLOs) are supported by ILEP to better monitor the program.
- Support operational research covering specific aspects of common concern related to provision of quality services/sustaining leprosy control activities/DPMR, etc.
- Assist in developing training curricula including DPMR for various categories of health staff. They also print and supply the learning material of DPMR for different categories of general healthcare staff.
- Involved in organizing SLO review meeting.
- The NLEP website was developed by ILEP in India for ready reference, which is now being updated by CLD.
- Supports CLD in organizing need-based, specific goal oriented workshops involving various stakeholders on specific issues of NLEP.
- ILEP-supported hospitals function as referral hospitals for treating complications of leprosy.
- The ILEP supports the NGO projects, which are functioning in accordance with GOI guidelines.
- ILEP assists in establishing reconstructive surgeries at Medical College hospitals by building the capacity of the surgeons in RCS through the visits of their core surgical teams.

- Continuing medical education (CME) for medical colleges:
  - Over the years, many goals have been achieved in NLEP including elimination of leprosy, integration of the vertical program with the GHS; and introduction of DPMR. To improve the students' knowledge on leprosy with the changing scenario, ILEP has decided to support holding seminars and CME programs on leprosy in Medical Colleges.
- Support to improve monitoring and supervision (including disease surveillance system):
  - The functional and structural integration has happened in all the states. In this scenario, it is necessary to improve monitoring and supervision of leprosy services. The ILEP plays a major role in facilitating this task by helping the DN through state consultants.
- Community-based rehabilitation (CBR):
  - ILEP agencies continue to participate in CBR activities to enable people affected by leprosy to gain a sustainable and improved quality of life. CBR is a multidisciplinary approach, implemented through the combined efforts of individuals with disabilities themselves, their families, disabled people's organizations, communities, governmental and nongovernmental, health education, vocational, social and other service organizations.

Involving the family and community members in the process of rehabilitation is a key strategy to empower people affected by leprosy, encouraging them to play an active role in their rehabilitation and to further reduce stigma. The central strategy of community-based rehabilitation is to facilitate community action; to ensure that people with disabilities have the same rights and opportunities as all other community members. This applies equally to people affected by leprosy. To improve rehabilitation coverage for people affected by leprosy, the CBR approach to facilitate integrative and participative rehabilitation with limited and locally available resources, to as many people as possible has been found as an effective tool. It is estimated that approximately 85% of rehabilitation needs of people with disabilities, can be met within the community.

International Leprosy Union, Pune

The International Leprosy Union (ILU), Pune, India was established in the year 1986 by voluntary organizations and leprosy workers from over 20 developing and developed countries, that recognized the need for linkage and networking among like-minded groups and individuals, actively pursuing the cause of eliminating leprosy and mainstreaming the leprosy affected in society. It has since worked as a catalytic agency with the unique objective not only to serve as the voice of NGOs active in developing countries but more importantly to give leprosy a human face.

The main objectives of ILU may be summarized as follows:
- To establish links between national and international voluntary organization working in the field of leprosy.
- To collect and disseminate information from various sources.
- To undertake advocacy program "To give leprosy a human face", the mission statement of ILU.
- To undertaking training programs for leprosy affected persons (LAPs) to empower them economically, to strengthen them and to build their self-confidence.
- To train, orientate and organize with general public, mix with public and LAPs on human rights of leprosy for redressal.

Ongoing activities:
- Field research on social aspects of leprosy.
- Advocacy and networking of NGOs working for leprosy.
- Human rights for leprosy affected persons.
- Publication of books, periodicals and educational materials.
- Community awareness program.
- Sponsorship of children under shadow of leprosy for higher studies.
- Organization of seminar/workshops at National and International level.

The ILU was granted official status by WHO in 1998 and Dr Gokhale SD, Chairman ILU, was appointed as a member of the Technical Advisory Expert Group of WHO in Geneva. Mr Ram Naik (former Petroleum and Railways Minister) took over as the president of ILU in1998. Mr Ram Belavadi continues with the post of Vice President and Mr Sharad Bhosale is the Executive Director of ILU. ILU has close collaboration and coordination with the GOI, WHO, Sasakawa Memorial Health Foundation, The Nippon Foundation, etc. and has been contributing to bring about remarkable changes in the social acceptance of leprosy affected in the community.

Gandhi Memorial Leprosy Foundation

The Gandhi Memorial Leprosy Foundation (GMLF) was established in the year 1951 with its national headquarter at Wardha to commemorate the thoughts and ideals of Mahatma Gandhi on leprosy and leprosy work in India.

The Sevagram, Wardha was the first unit to be established in 1951 which covered 27 villages in Wardha district. With special emphasis on health education, GMLF started its leprosy control units for the first time in the country in different regions. These units were located at Chilakalpalli (Andhra Pradesh) set-up in 1953; T' Narasipura (Mysuru district, Karnataka) in 1955 and Balarampur (West Bengal) in 1977. Ultimately, the units were handed over to the state governments.

Soon after its inception at Sevagram, the GMLF launched the pilot project to control leprosy in the country with the only drug 'Dapsone' available in those days. Thus, the survey, education and treatment SET pattern of leprosy work was evolved, which was adapted by GOI in 1955, by incorporating it in the five-year-plan, and that is how the National Leprosy Control Programme (NLCP) came into effect. Gradually, GMLF also developed the methodologies of Urban Leprosy Control Program, Community Awareness Program and establishment of referral hospitals for leprosy. The concept of socioeconomic rehabilitation for LAPs was also developed by GMLF and all these methodologies were incorporated by GOI in the national program.

Today, after integration, GMLF has suitably changed its strategy to collaborate its leprosy activities with the government policies and diversified its activities incorporating tuberculosis control, eye care, program for women development, imparting training in general health care, etc.

It is noteworthy that GMLF evolved the first leprosy training curricula for medical doctors, nurses and paramedical workers (PMW). The first training center was established by GMLF at Wardha in 1952 for the above cadres which created a team of trained leprosy workers throughout the country.

Hind Kushth Nivaran Sangh

The Hind Kushth Nivaran Sangh (HKNS), previously known as Indian Leprosy Association, is the premier voluntary organization working for the eradication of leprosy. In the British rule in 1925, the British Empire Leprosy Relief Association (BELRA) was established with a view to provide medical and social support to the leprosy sufferers. The branch of BELRA in India was called as Indian Council BELRA (ICBELRA), which soon after its formation was in position to function independently from its parent body on account of generous financial and other support gathered in India. After independence, it was renamed as Hind Kushth Nivaran Sangh and was registered in 1950 under Societies Registration Act, XXI of 1860. The honorable President of India is the President of the *Sangh*. The *Sangh* has a governing body of 41 members with its headquarters at Delhi. HKNS has at present its 18 branches in States and Union Territories headed by honorable Governors of respective states.

Objectives:

- Promote and coordinate voluntary work in leprosy in order to eradicate leprosy.
- Promote and support advocacy in leprosy.
- Promote and undertake information, education and communication (IEC) activities.
- Promote and support rehabilitation activities.
- Promote and support dissemination of scientific research through publication.

Delhi state branch of HKNS has been active in the field since its inception in 1961. Founded by Late Mr DC Aggrawal (a social activist and philanthropist), the main activities have been in distribution of MDT and providing rehabilitative services to leprosy patients (Fig. 49.2). The branch raises funds from sale of leprosy seals and from other voluntary donors (Fig. 49.3). There are arrangements of daily dressings of wounds and ulcers of patients, appointment of dressers in the leprosy colonies, supply of dressing materials; cotton, bandages, antiseptic solutions, creams, etc. There is also a regular supply of medicines for ulcers and others common ailments. Distribution of tricycles to patients with deformities, financial help to patients for social purposes like education of children, marriages of daughters, etc. are other notable activities of the branch.

Hind Kushth Nivaran Sangh publishes a research journal in India, "Indian Journal of Leprosy", which is widely circulated among the leprologists in India and abroad. Previously known as "Leprosy in India", it was started by Dr Ernest Muir in July 1929 and it retained this name till 1983. From January 1984 it was renamed as Indian Journal of Leprosy, by Dr Dharmendra, its Editor.

Missionaries of Charity, Gandhiji Prem Nivas, Titagarh

For those not loved, I give love. For those discarded, I give shelter and care.

— Mother Teresa

Gandhiji Prem Nivas Leprosy Center (mobile clinic) at Titagarh, 24-Parganas (West Bengal, India) was started by Mother Teresa in 1958. Later in 1960, the Titagarh municipality leased a piece of land to establish the permanent center for leprosy services, which included regular treatment and management of leprosy complications. The railway

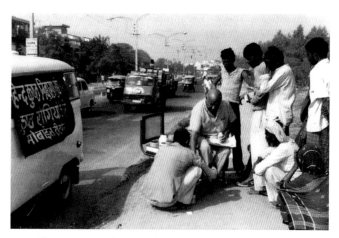

Fig. 49.2: Distribution of medicines by mobile treatment unit of HKNS (DSB)

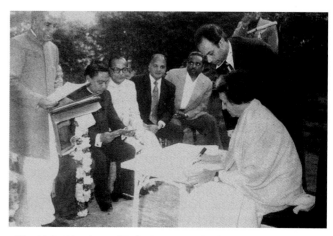

Fig. 49.3: Members of Delhi State Branch of HKNS with Smt Indira Gandhi on the occasion of leprosy seal campaigns
Courtesy: HKNS (DSB)

authorities donated a long stretch of land on the eastern side of railway track, between Titagarh and Kharda station where the Brothers have been offering distinguished services in the areas of counseling and rehabilitation.

Other facilities for leprosy affected:

- The outdoor clinic
- 200 bedded inpatient care center
- Surgical care (operation theater)
- Artificial limb center
- Footwear center
- Rehabilitation programs
  - Handloom center
  - Carpentry section
  - Tailoring unit.

Anandwan

Anandwan was the first of the three ashrams started by Baba Amte to treat and rehabilitate leprosy victims from the disadvantaged sections of society. After taking a leprosy orientation course at the Calcutta School of Tropical Medicine, Baba Amte began his fight against leprosy. He set-up about 11 leprosy clinics running weekly around Warora, in Chandrapur district (Maharashtra). Taking his work to the next level, he started the "Anandwan" (Forest of Joy) ashram in a remote jungle at Warora, in Chandrapur district of Maharashtra, about 100 km from Nagpur, to help rehabilitate patients. Anandwan was registered in 1951 and received a state land grant of 250 acres (1 km²) (Fig. 49.4).

The land was barren rocky, covered with scrubs and infested with scorpions and snakes. The nearest well was 2 km. away. Those days, leprosy was associated with intense social stigma and patients were disowned by society. It was then believed that the leprosy patients were sinners, paying for the sins they had committed. There was also a widespread fear that leprosy was contagious and could be spread by touch. Baba Amte strove to dispel these myths and once, even to the extent; that he allowed bacilli from a leprosy patient to be injected into him while participating as a volunteer in an experiment.

Later, Baba Amte also founded the *Somnath* and *Ashokvan* ashrams for treatment and rehabilitation of leprosy patients. The community development project at Anandwan in Maharashtra is recognized and respected around the world and has done much to dispel the prejudice against leprosy victims (Figs 49.4 to 49.6). The whole geosocial environmental milieu at Anandwan is of community living with farming, fruits, food and crops cultivation, cottage industries making household products, handicrafts, woven clothes, carpets, and decorative items.

Besides leprosy relief work, Baba Amte also made forays into other issues of social and public causes related to environment, human rights for which he was accorded several international awards which include Damien-Dutton Award, USA (1983), Magsaysay Award, Philippines (1985), UN Human Rights Award (1988), GD Birla International Award (1988). The National Awards include: Padma Shri (1971), Padma Vibhushan (1986), Welfare of Disabled Award (1988), and Jamnalal Bajaj Award (1979).

Pune District Leprosy Committee

No form of rehabilitation is complete without economic rehabilitation.

— Jal Mehta

Pune District Leprosy Committee (PDLC) was founded in 1957 by Late Dr Jal Mehta. He was an industrialist, the Vice-Chairman of Serum Institute of India (the premium institution in the production of vaccine in India) and a great philanthropist.

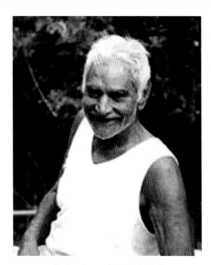

Baba Amte (1914–2008)

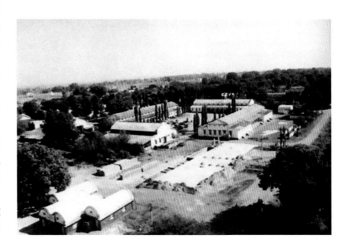

Fig. 49.4: The campus of Anandwan in present times
Courtesy: ©mss.niya.org

During his young age, Dr Jal Mehta was extremely influenced by the plight of the leprosy suffers in his area. He established Bandorawalla Leprosy Hospital which he named in fond memory of his father-in-law. The hospital is located on a big piece of land (over 100 acres) at Yeolewadi (Kondhwa) on the outskirts of Pune. There are 350 beds in the hospital, which is fully equipped with all the facilities for diagnosis and treatment of leprosy, reconstructive surgical care, physiotherapy and rehabilitation units. There are well-formed sections on artificial limbs, manufacturing special footwears and splints for leprosy patients. After the death of Dr Jal Mehta, due to paucity of funds, the hospital was handed over to state government in 2001.

Dr Jal Mehta's work in leprosy-medical, social relief, research and rehabilitation, during his tenure of more than 40 years of voluntary and honorary service, brought

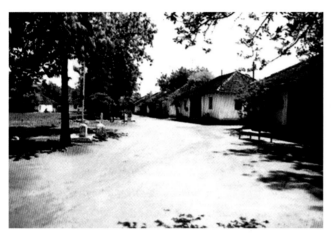

Fig. 49.5: Colony houses at Anandwan for leprosy affected residents
Courtesy: © mss.niya.org

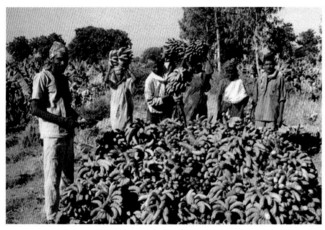

Fig. 49.6: Agriculture farmland crops at Anandwan
Courtesy: © mss.niya.org

the Dr Bandorawalla Leprosy Hospital and its associated rehabilitation and allied projects to national and international fame. By his rehabilitation work, he has raised these leprosy patients (from the weakest of the weaker section of society) to men and women; who can stand on their own feet, earn well, and this has increased their self-esteem equal to that of any other human being.

A big example of successful economic rehabilitation of leprosy patients has been presented by the rehabilitation units run by a cooperative body formed by leprosy cured patients, called as "Minoo Mehta Apangoddhar Sahakari Audyogik Utpadak Maryadit Sanstha (MMASAUS)" (Fig. 49.7). This Sanstha (organization) was set-up in 1983 by 55 leprosy cured patients (LCPs), and now has 110 members. Based at Yeolewadi in Kondhawa, the group is scaling greater heights with every passing day. The *Sanstha* was set-up under the

guidance of Dr Jal Mehta, who helped rehabilitate the LCPs after using innovative techniques of surgeries for correcting their deformities at the Bandorwala Leprosy Hospital.

In the rehabilitation units, 110 LCPs work in two shifts and earn between ₹ 4,500 and ₹ 5,500 per month. The machines have been designed in a manner for easy operation by persons with deformities. The organization has been manufacturing motor engine parts like chassis, cross box and clutch-plates for heavy vehicles and mounting bracket and assembly lever for light vehicles of Tata Motors in Pune. It is pleasing to note that the common popular vehicles of today (Indica, Sumo or Safari) are likely to have some vital engine components manufactured by a group of LCPs. The other clients of the organization include: Forbes Marshall, Lucas TVS, Poonawala Group, besides Tata Motors.

Bombay Leprosy Project: A Model NGO

Bombay Leprosy Project (BLP), an innovative concept in leprosy management was conceived on September 11, 1976 and has been in operation for over three and a half decades with the basic objectives of operational research in parts of Bombay and adjoining rural areas. Pioneering field oriented concepts in chemotherapy, disability care, rehabilitation, IEC and medical education have been the subjects of study and documentation. These innovations have become far more relevant in the current scenario of declining endemicity and integration of leprosy services in the background of dwindling funds from donor agencies.

Key Areas of Project Activities

Chemotherapy, Reactions and Nerve Damage: Bombay Leprosy Project was the first to introduce multiple drugs even before WHO MDT was implemented by NLEP in early 80s. In 1988, BLP reported that the initial intensive 21 days of rifampicin therapy recommended by Indian Association of Leprologists (IAL) had no added advantage over the WHO recommended monthly pulse therapy. Documentation of experiments with fixed duration treatment (FDT) for 24 and 12 months have helped to save cost and manpower. In 1986, BLP for the first time published data on bacteriological index (BI) decline in dropout patients. This finding helped reduction of treatment duration to 12 months.

Research trials with rifampicin and ofloxacin for 28 days (RO-28) showed that the rate of fall in BI is parallel to WHO MDT. BLP also published studies on single dose rifampicin–ofloxacin–minocycline (ROM) treatment for single lesions as well as 2–5 paucibacillary (PB) sessions.

The fact that relapses in multibacillary (MB) leprosy in FDT occurs mostly beyond 5 years was established through surveillance by volunteers in a cost-effective manner. More recently further observations on reactions and BI decline in clinical trials of moxifloxacin-based regimens have

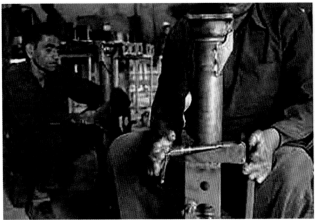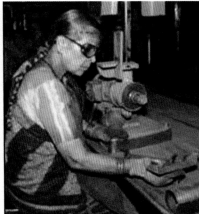

Fig. 49.7: Cured leprosy patients in role of mechanical workers at the MMASAUS rehabilitation units at Pune. The machine designs are such that even persons with deformities can operate.
Courtesy: Apoorva Gupte

been published for the first time. Results of the study of standardized regimens of steroid treatment in reactions in leprosy at referral center have also been published. Studies aimed to assess the magnitude of neuropathic pain in leprosy patients and the quantitative sensory testing (QST) profiles in India were published for the first time. Observations on the role of leukotriene inhibitors and newer immunosuppressant in leprosy reactions and thalidomide in type-2 reactions as maintenance therapy in leprosy have been published for the first time.

Disability Care

After years of field investigations in Andhra Pradesh inexpensive araldite grip aids (1982), prefabricated splints (1985), ulcer dressing kits, etc. were widely practiced (1985) by community volunteers.

A low-cost disability program was started in Mumbai slums (1994) and later in rural Maharashtra (1998) in which through massive campaigns; a high load of 1,250 disabled persons (Grade 2) (25–27 per 10,000 population) was unearthed in an adopted rural population of 476,970 covering 11 primary health centers in Thane district. Recently, at the request of DLO Thane, BLP has been offering prevention of disability (POD) training to Accredited Social Health Activists (ASHAs) under National Rural Health Mission (NRHM) scheme. A highly cost-effective model using village youth for door-step services has been established with a view to implement community-based rehabilitation (CBR) at a later stage. Consequent to consistent care and services in rural and urban areas, BLP has now attempted to assess the impact of these services in urban and rural areas.

Tertiary level care is also a part of this activity. BLP has broken ground in involving orthopedic and plastic surgeons of general hospitals and private nursing homes to perform reconstructive surgery.

Rehabilitation

In collaboration with general rehabilitation organizations working in Dharavi and other slums an integrated vocational rehabilitation training program was started in 1983 as a major step in abolishing stigma. The first attempt in CBR was made in Bharat Nagar slum in 1998. Community volunteers screened 74,000 slum dwellers and identified 173 disabled people, including those due to leprosy, and services were provided in collaboration with existing rehabilitation agencies (Fig. 49.8). The experiment was repeated in a part of Dharavi, the biggest slum in Asia. Out of 93,000 persons screened, 487 were found disabled. Appliances and mobility aids were provided with the help of All India Institute of Physical Medicine and Rehabilitation (AIPMR).

In year 2000, computer training was offered to leprosy disabled along with other physically challenged persons in the slum centers in an integrated manner. Many of these trained persons and other physically challenged persons are assisting BLP in work under its integrated rehabilitation program (Figs 49.9 and 49.10).

Information, Education and Communication Activities

In 1977, health education was used as a tool to identify leprosy patients, in Bharat Nagar. Nearly 54% of total cases and 82% of BI positive cases were spotted and identified by IEC technique. Later on BLP received an award for documenting this investigation. The immensely popular Ganapati festival was used to spread leprosy awareness in Dharavi, followed by a massive campaign in which 200 medical students of city colleges screened about 20,000 slum dwellers and detected 200 new leprosy cases.

The innovative campaign of BLP using local trains and Bombay Electric Supply and Transport (BEST) buses as a medium of public education for the first time, which was later followed by other NGOs.

Involving Medical Fraternity and Promoting Medical Education

Association with medical colleges and medical professionals by creative techniques has been a regular feature of BLP. A novel method of CME by displaying updates on leprosy scenario in 8 medical colleges through "Wall Journal" was instrumental in creating interest among the students and the faculty in the often sidelined subject of leprosy. A breakthrough achievement in this area was to get interns of

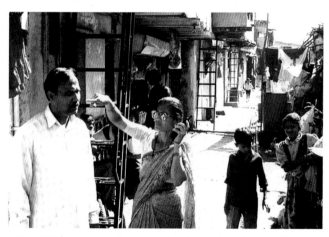

Fig. 49.8: A community volunteer using mobile phone in Dharavi

allopathic and nonallopathic (homeopathy, etc.) disciplines. Medical students as well as postgraduate (PG) students of dermatology departments were officially posted to BLP sites as a part of their academic curriculum (Fig. 49.11). They not only learn the subject, but also provide assistance in academic and research work. As it is expensive to employ full-time doctors, this strategy has proved to be highly cost-effective. Expert guidance has been provided to more than 25 PGs to write their dissertations.

The successful efforts of BLP have been:

- Organizing national conferences in medical college campuses (e.g. IAL Biennial Conference, two National Conferences of NGOs at the request of GOI and WHO/ NLEP meetings, etc.).
- Arranging guest lectures by visiting leprosy experts.
- Donating leprosy books, training materials and pamphlets to libraries.
- Organizing exhibitions of leprosy books and journals.
- Promoting PG students to present reviews and updates in seminars.
- Deputing interns and PGs to leprosy research institutions.
- Providing skin smear facility and POD services in private clinics.
- Offering special drugs like thalidomide to dermatologists and including them as partners in research.
- Organizing CME cum Workshops on practical aspects of leprosy, neurological assessment, smear taking and reporting for PG students of Dermatology in collaboration with Special Interest Group of Indian Association of Dermatologists, Venereologists and Leprologists (IADVL).

Other Highlights and Achievements

As a cost-effective method, BLP right from its inception has been engaging volunteers to assist trained PMWs in case

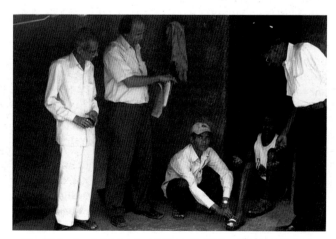

Fig. 49.9: A volunteer in rural area who is himself a cured leprosy patient, offers door-step rehabilitative services

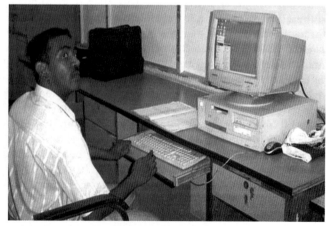

Fig. 49.10: A physically challenged person using the computer provides assistance in office work of BLP research activities

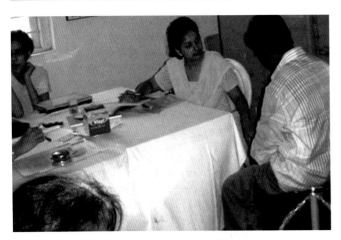

Fig. 49.11: Interns from medical colleges examine patients at BLP Referral Center

Novartis Comprehensive Leprosy Care Association

Novartis is at the forefront in the global fight against leprosy and its consequences, as a part of its corporate social responsibility. In addition to the role of Novartis collaborating with the WHO in supplying MDT free of cost worldwide, it established the comprehensive leprosy care project now called Novartis Comprehensive Leprosy Care Association (NCLCA) in India in 1989.

The objectives of the project were to enhance access to MDT, provide services for prevention, correction and care of disabilities; with rehabilitation, as a comprehensive package to the leprosy-affected. These activities are carried out in active collaboration with government healthcare personnel and other NGOs, to extend the coverage of DPMR services. It provides physical aid materials, technical support, RCS and rehabilitation articles for income generation activities, free of cost to patients besides training healthcare providers.

detection, supervised treatment and POD work, a procedure which long afterward received approval by the government and other funding agencies. First such volunteer was a Muslim girl in Bharat Nagar, who not only assisted surveys in 1976 but motivated her parents to run a BLP leprosy clinic in her own house in the slum.

Thorough surveys of slums, schools, factories, hospitals, leprosy colonies have led to the documentation of the quantum of infection and disability burden in the metropolis. Paramedical personnel and community volunteers were encouraged to be partners in academic work, write research papers and present them at conferences. More than 80 papers have been co-authored by 20 such staff members, out of the total of over 300 publications from BLP. Student volunteers were made to shed their stigma and were engaged to offer supervised MDT in nine leprosy colonies in 1982.

Bombay Leprosy Project has also exploited information technology methods in leprosy management. To cite one technique, mobile phones were used as early as 1998 by field workers to establish contact with the expertise available at the main centers, and so improve care at the periphery. In 2000, BLP hosted an academically oriented website which has not only motivated many students abroad to volunteer, but also has helped in fund raising.

Bombay Leprosy Project believes that NGOs functioning under severe resource constraints may continue to assist NLEP, provided they adopt creative strategies and effect savings. A cost analysis of BLP working system during 1976–1995 has shown that by following low cost techniques in field applications about 67% of the financial burden on donor agencies was relieved. BLP model of integration may be replicable in other metropolitan situations in India.

Key Modalities in Leprosy Care and Rehabilitation

- For health education about the importance of proper care of anesthetic hands and feet to prevent secondary deformities through injuries or burns, NCLCA has designed an educational pamphlet, which has been translated into many languages. It has also developed a booklet which deals with typical questions asked by patients, their families and the public.
- For physiotherapy NCLCA advocates a simple package of domiciliary physiotherapy in the form of "one exercise for each major deformity", which can easily be done at home by the patient. NCLCA uses the approach of "group therapy" where many cases are brought together and taught the measures of splint application and exercises they can do at home.
- Prefabricated standardized splints have proved to be highly effective in the prevention and correction of claw hand, a common deformity in leprosy (Fig. 49.12). The splints are made of durable and easily available material such as PVC, rexin and rubber bands. The public health program is leveraged to broaden the reach of prefabricated splints. Grip-aids with Modulan R epoxy resin have been innovated for patients with advanced deformities of the hands who have difficulty in holding and using articles of daily use. The instant Grip-aid kit developed by NCLCA is a tremendous boon in such instances (Fig. 49.13). The use of instant grip-aid in other disabilities like burns and amputation helps patients to adjust to their handicap remarkably. They increase the patient's quality of life and their self-esteem, because they enable them to perform many everyday tasks without the help of others.

- The most effective way of dealing with ulcers is by 'empowering patients' to take care of their own limbs. NCLCA conducts self-care empowerment camps to teach groups of patients the 'how's' and 'why's' of self-care. It has developed a special self-care kit (Fig. 49.14), containing sterile gauze pieces, scissors, sticking plaster, foot scraper, bandages, antiseptic cream and a simple moisturizing cream, which is distributed free at the self-care camps. Patients are also instructed to use the proper footwear. Follow-up clinics held after 2 months have clearly indicated good compliance with the self-care instructions, with nearly 60% reporting healing. The 'self-care kit' now forms a part of the POD guidelines endorsed by the GOI. Many other organizations have adopted its principles and are making their own kits with similar material.

- Novartis Comprehensive Leprosy Care Association has designed microcellulose rubber (MCR) footwear resembling commercially available patterns in order to overcome the reluctance of patients to use the typical leprosy footwear, which labels them as leprosy sufferers. This footwear is provided to patients free of cost.

- One of the key achievements of NCLCA is in the improved management of foot drop. NCLCA has prefabricated the Foot Drop Splints (FDS) and trained healthcare staff to provide it at the earliest sign of weakness in the leg to prevent complications. The FDS can be easily attached to the MCR footwear or patients own footwear with a buckle on the dorsal strap. Recently, prefabricated FDS made of thermoplastic material is given in cases where long-term use is indicated as it fits in the footwear making the walking comfortable.

- The "Camp and Workshop Approach for Reconstructive Surgery" by NCLCA has shown good results in Gujarat.

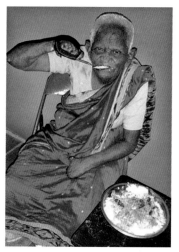

Fig. 49.13: Instant Grip-Aid

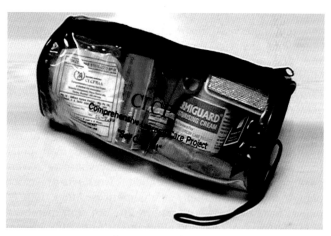

Fig. 49.14: Self- care Kit

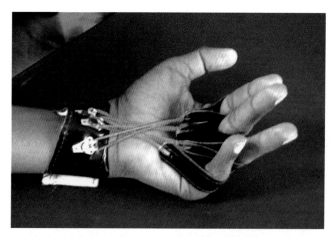

Fig. 49.12: Prefabricated finger-loop splint for correction of clawhand

This involves training of the local surgeons; deputing the field staff to inform, take the patients' consent and transport them to district or Medical College hospitals; involving the physiotherapists in postoperative care; and arranging for the admission of patients along with the stay of one relative (including food). The GOI has since named the approach—"The Gujarat Model". Since the inception of the project, thousands of cases have been benefited not only in Gujarat, but also in Goa and Sri Lanka.

- Appropriate "Economic Rehabilitation" aid, e.g. sewing machines, handcarts, kits for bicycle repair, carpentry, masonry work, agricultural tools, etc. is provided to patients, and in some cases their family members. The economic rehabilitation program has had a dramatic impact on the disabled individuals and has transformed the lives of hundreds of people (Fig. 49.15).

Achievements in Objectives and Components of the National Leprosy Eradication Programme

- The program was started by NCLCA at Borsad Taluka in Gujarat in 1989, as an activity of leprosy control primarily to improve access to disability care services. This was later adopted as the target for leprosy "elimination" when WHO announced its new approach with the definition of elimination (less than 1 case per 10,000 population). The target was achieved within 6 years.
- In Goa, from 1993 to 1999, NCLCA helped to bring down the prevalence rate from 10 to about 3 per 10,000 population thus paving the way for eventual elimination. Incidentally, Goa was one of the first states where Novartis Foundation provided blister calendar-packs (BCP) of MDT for nearly 3 years. Involvement of dermatologists of Goa Medical College was a pioneering step for eventual integration of leprosy services. RCS was pioneered at Goa Medical College by NCLCA.
- By supporting early new case detection through special survey drives, improving access to MDT and training the medical and health staff in "reaction management", the project has contributed to primary prevention of disabilities significantly. NCLCA has also helped to decrease the secondary deformities in the disabled cases. Close to

25,000 cases have directly benefited from the project over the years in India and nearly 2,000 cases have benefited in Sri Lanka. Over 100,000 patients have benefited indirectly through the services of the government staff trained by NCLCA.
- Novartis Comprehensive Leprosy Care Association supported by Novartis Foundation for sustainable development is committed to help bring about zero transmission of leprosy with MDT as well as with the prophylactic and therapeutic tools available.

Dr Atul Shah, Director, NCLCA (author of this part of the chapter) was honored with the Artificial Limbs Manufacturing Corporation of India (ALIMCO) award for designing the splints and the "instant Grip-aid kit" researched by Ms Neela Shah, Managing Director, NCLCA, which have now reached those in need as far as in Africa. The "self-care kit" has now become an integral part of ulcer care practice all over India. Training interested surgeons in RCS through the camp and workshop approach and transfer of technology has increased the acceptability of the leprosy-disabled into the general hospitals of the integrated set-up for surgical correction and medical rehabilitation.

Providing articles of income generation and economic rehabilitation has transformed the lives of more than a 1,000 patients who were the poorest of the poor, dejected

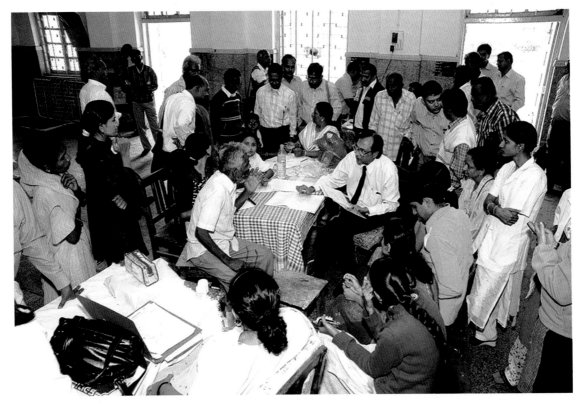

Fig. 49.15: Rehabilitation clinic in progress at CLCP

due to disease or its after effects and lacked moral support. Their ability to earn and support themselves, along with the use of the articles by their family members, has brought about increased income, better social acceptance and their integration and above all, heightened self-esteem.

Over the years, the key modalities practiced in the field area by NCLCA have been gradually accepted by the government and other nongovernment organizations. NCLCA has also undertaken assignments at Mexico, Myanmar, Tanzania and Sri Lanka embarking on its journey of restoring health and hope to leprosy patients. There have been many awards to the credit of NCLCA and its personnel, the most notable being the, Golden Peacock Award by the Institute of Directors of India for Innovative Products and Services; and the Reader's Digest Gold Award for Corporate Social Responsibility.

LOCAL VOLUNTARY ORGANIZATIONS

More than 250 local voluntary organizations are doing leprosy services in India, mainly on disability care and rehabilitation activities. We have been able to give description of the work carried by only a few of them.

CONCLUSION

Nongovernmental organizations have an important role in strengthening the NLEP through activities that include DN, DPMR and CBR. They also help in sustaining good quality leprosy services through the existing integrated health care system in line with the WHO Global Strategy Guidelines (2006–2010).

ACKNOWLEDGMENTS

Dr Arif MA, one of the authors of this chapter, would like to thank International Federation of Antileprosy Associations (ILEP) for their help with statistics and prompt revision of data.

Dr V Pai, another author of this chapter, is indebted to the Management of BLP for encouraging him to undertake all these activities and the staff for the assistance. GLTRA provided financial support for the basic routine control program and the infrastructure. This was helpful to raise funds from several other sources for various areas of research.

SUGGESTED READING

1. Anandwan through Dr. Y S Jadhav, Co-ordinator for Grip-Aid program and publications of Anandwan.
2. Hind Kushth Nivaran Sangh –Personal Communication from Dr. P R Manglani, Secretary HKNS.
3. International Federation of Antileprosy Association (ILEP) – working together for a world without Leprosy, ILEP Strategy, 2011-2015.
4. Memorandum of Understanding between Government of India and ILEP Members active in India. 2013.
5. Missionaries of Charity – information from various sources including personal visits by Atul Shah, Neela Shah and meeting with Mother Teresa.
6. Novartis Comprehensive Leprosy Care Association Annual Report, 2012-2013.
7. Novartis Foundation for Sustainable Development – Express News Letters – Dr. Ann Aertz, NFSD, 2013.
8. Pune District Leprosy Committee through personal evaluation of their socio-economic rehabilitation model by Atul Shah and disability care services camps at Bandorawala Hospital managed by PDMC.
9. Role of International Agencies in Leprosy Control – Studies on Leprosy by Bombay Leprosy Project, 1967-1986.

Future Prospects

CHAPTERS

50
CHAPTER

Leprosy: Future Challenges

Diana NJ Lockwood

CHAPTER OUTLINE

INTRODUCTION

Leprosy will continue to challenge many different health workers including clinicians, epidemiologists, scientists and health planners. The disease is still poorly understood in many aspects; we do not understand transmission well, diagnosis is often not easy and treatment of the immune-mediated reactions is difficult. Occurrence of peripheral neuropathy leaves patients at risk of development of disabilities even for decades. The stigma associated with leprosy is a global phenomenon and also needs to be challenged in different ways. This chapter will consider the evidence in these different areas and look at the ongoing research needs in leprosy.

Defining leprosy epidemiology is challenging because of the unusual clinical features of the disease. Leprosy has a variable incubation period ranging from 2 to 20 years. The presentation is also varied and there is often a delay in diagnosis especially in nonendemic countries. In London, we have demonstrated a significant delay in diagnosis[1] but even in India diagnostic delay has been shown in patients detected in integrated settings.[2] Diagnosis is also significantly affected by the awareness about leprosy and the level of service. When the chemoprophylaxis in leprosy (COLEP) trial was being setup in Bangladesh their population surveys revealed levels of leprosy up to seven times that recorded in the routine program.[3] Our current understanding of leprosy is that many persons in endemic areas have immunological exposure to *M. leprae* but only a few develop disease. However, it is difficult to verify this statement because there is no test for subclinical infection. A test of subclinical infection would be very helpful and could be used to test contacts of new leprosy patients to detect exposure. Since early leprosy is often self-healing including the tuberculoid type, such a test would need to be T-cell-based and measure cell mediated immunity

toward *M. leprae*. The T-cell tests currently available cannot differentiate between patients with tuberculoid disease and household contacts.[4]

It is important to look at leprosy epidemiology in India and try to understand disease patterns there. India has 60% of the global burden of disease and reports about 130,000 new cases annually.[5] This indicates that leprosy transmission is being sustained and it also means that leprosy will continue to be a significant problem in India for decades. However, there is evidence that leprosy is currently being under-reported in India.[6] In 2001, India was under pressure to reach the "elimination as a public health problem" target and so the measures outlined in the Kathmandu declaration in 2004 were adopted.[7] These included stopping active case finding, not registering single lesion cases, cease household screening, new cases only to be treated after validation by an external expert. These were all counterproductive to good public health measures. Leprosy case finding and management has also been integrated into primary health care. A national sample survey was conducted in 2010, but this has not yet been reported officially. The leprosy picture in India is complex with some states, e.g. Tamil Nadu, having low new case numbers whilst more new cases and those with deformities are concentrated in the Northern and Eastern states of Uttar Pradesh, Bihar, Odisha, Chhattisgarh and West Bengal. It is important that active case finding should be done here to improve case detection and to determine how many leprosy patients there are in India.

IMMUNOPROPHYLAXIS

The development of vaccines against leprosy has included Bacille de Calmette et Guérin (BCG) (a meta-analysis showed that childhood BCG vaccination gives about 50% protection against leprosy).[8] But a large scale protective study in South India found the protective effect to be very limited with no protective against smear positive disease.[9] In a comparative leprosy vaccine trial in South India, over 171,000 subjects were administered four vaccines: (1) BCG, (2) BCG + killed *M. leprae*. (3) Mw renamed as *Mycobacterium indicus pranii (MIP)* and (4) Indian Cancer Research Center (ICRC). After 5 years of follow-up ICRC vaccine was shown to provide the highest protection (65.5%) followed by BCG + killed *M. leprae*, BCG and MIP respectively.[10] This protection decreased considerably in a longer follow-up. The protection was, however, up to 60% in household contacts given MIP. Another larger field-based study using two doses of MIP also found a protective efficacy of 68% and 60% respectively after a 3 and 6 years of follow-up. This declined to about 40% in 8–10 years.[11] Chemoprophylaxis is also being explored as another tool for interrupting transmission of leprosy. The current evidence for efficacy is weak. In the COLEP trial in Bangladesh household and social contacts of leprosy patients were given a single 600 mg dose of rifampicin or placebo. Rifampicin did not protect against the development of leprosy in household members. It only protected significantly in social contacts of leprosy patients, protection was only against the development of paucibacillary (PB) disease and lasted only for 2 years.[12] These findings are consistent with rifampicin being effective only when the mycobacterial load is low at early disease stages. A trial of chemoprophylaxis was started in South India some years ago, but was abandoned due to operational difficulties. This highlights the need for other studies to be done on chemoprophylaxis to see if more effective regimens can be developed. These studies should also be replicated in other countries including India.

Our continued inability to grow *M. leprae* in the laboratory hampers our understanding of many aspects of the interaction between *M. leprae* and the human host as well as the environment. It also contributes to the difficulty in developing new antibiotics to treat leprosy. Since the genome has been sequenced our understanding of the transmission of leprosy has improved.[13] Leprosy probably originated in East Africa.[14] Recent work analyzing deoxyribonucleic acid (DNA) extracted from skeletons in Denmark and England have shown that the *M. leprae* genome present in medieval Europe has changed little since then and is similar to the strain currently found in the Middle East.[15] This has been very stable over centuries. This also suggests that even though *M. leprae* has lost many genes it has retained enough to survive and continue infecting people.

Why some people get leprosy is still unexplained. Poverty and overcrowding are risk factors, but weak ones. Many genetic studies have been done recently and linkage studies have identified associations with the genes coding for MHC II: *HLA–DR2, PARK2/PACRG, LTA*, chromosome 10p13.[16,17] Studies have also shown candidate gene associations with

genes for numerous immunological phenomena. A genome-wide scan on Chinese patients showed a gene-interaction network of five genes conferring susceptibility to leprosy.[18] However, none of these genes has shown a strong association with susceptibility to leprosy. No single factor has been shown to be universal and common to different population groups. So a polygenic susceptibility is more likely with each gene contributing a small amount to susceptibility. Although these studies have been very valuable in showing associations they need to be replicated in different geographical locations and with different populations with larger better powered studies with good clinical definitions. Looking for Genetic Associations for Developing Complications of Leprosy such as, Type 1 and erythema nodosum leprosum (ENL) reactions is important because these occur in defined disease groups and would be more likely to have genetic associations.

The interaction between *M. leprae* antigens, T-cells and macrophages is critical to the establishment of the immune response in leprosy. Various studies have been done looking at the polarized nature of the immune response; tuberculoid patients produce proinflammatory cytokines and lepromatous patients have increased levels of FOXp3 T regulatory cells that may inhibit the T-cell response in lepromatous leprosy (LL).[19]

DIAGNOSIS

The diagnosis of leprosy will remain clinically based and critically determined by the recognition of leprosy skin lesions. It is important that health staff be familiarized with the range of leprosy lesions and recognize the spectrum of lesions that can occur including the hypopigmented patches. Recognition of the nodules and plaques of LL is the key to diagnosing those patients. It is also important that the staff can palpate thickened nerves, as this has been shown to be a common feature in new leprosy patients in India. Study by Kumar et al. in Agra found that 40.3% of the patients with PB leprosy had thickened peripheral nerves.[20] It is also critical that health staff be able to asses nerve function in the hands and feet. When patients present with a neuropathy to general physicians the possibility of leprosy should always be considered. As leprosy becomes less prevalent, patients will present later and it is more likely that they will have nerve damage at diagnosis. Kumar et al. have shown that the risk of disability increases with increasing time to leprosy being diagnosed and also when more than three peripheral nerves are thickened.[21] Maintaining centers with the capacity for doing slit skin smears is also important so that bacterial load can be assessed easily and more so in patients referred from the field. It is also important to keep leprosy on the curriculum in Indian medical and nursing schools so that students are trained in recognizing and managing leprosy. Studies have shown that medical students have knowledge about the symptoms of leprosy, but are not well-informed about transmission and treatment.[22]

A small number of patients will continue to be diagnosed histologically because they have presented with unusual skin lesions. Skin biopsy has the advantage that a formalin-fixed biopsy can be sent anywhere for histological evaluation. It is also important to keep a critical number of histopathologists with expertise in leprosy so that there are experts who can review difficult or unusual histological features. The Karonga, Malawi study on early diagnosis comparing clinical and histological diagnosis showed that early leprosy is often difficult to diagnose and pathologists do not always agree, further highlighting the challenges of diagnosing early leprosy.[23] A study in India on the diagnosis of reactions showed that pathologists there also had similar discrepancies in the diagnosis of reactions.[24] It is therefore important to maintain collaboration between clinicians and histopathologists to facilitate diagnosis of difficult cases.

Serological tests for diagnosing leprosy have limitations because of the challenges posed to diagnose patients at different poles of the leprosy spectrum, having differing immune responses. Serological test based on detecting antibodies to the *M. leprae* antigen PGL-1 have been developed and are positive in patients with borderline leprosy (BL) and LL leprosy. However, they are negative in patients with tuberculoid leprosy. So having a negative test does not exclude the diagnosis of leprosy. Another limitation of using PGL-1 antibodies as a diagnostic test is that 18–39% of household contacts have detectable antibodies to PGL-1 without having disease.[25] In India, about 60% of the multibacillary (MB) patients have smear negative leprosy and majority of these patients would be negative on serological testing.[26] T-cell-based tests are being developed and these might be more promising in aiding diagnosis of patients with unusual skin lesions. However, the current T-cell-based tests were positive in both tuberculoid patients and household contacts and so cannot be used to identify patients. An ideal test would combine both a serological assay together with a T-cell-based test. This would detect both MB and PB patients. T-cell-based tests are being developed that use a new detection method for detecting interferon gamma production as a marker of a T-cell response using up-converting phosphor technology.[4] However, early testing suggests that these tests will not be useful for differentiating between a new PB patient and a household contact who has been exposed to *M. leprae* and developed protective immunity. It will be some years before such tests are available and in the meantime it is important to ensure that other simpler methods to support clinical diagnosis are maintained. If new tests are developed, it is important to consider how they can be used and what population screening might mean and how to interpret positive results. Previous experience with doing phenolic glycolipid-1 (PGL-1) antibody testing has shown that not all patients with positive serological test develop disease.

If household contact screening is done then it is important to have discussions with individuals and communities to establish what their preferences are when they are found positive in a screening test. Not everyone will be happy to take treatment for a possible early leprosy infection that might have self-healed.

It is fortunate that *M. leprae* remains very susceptible to anti-bacterial treatment with combination MDT and there is little evidence of drug resistance. The clinical effectiveness of MDT is good and the relapse rate remains about 1% or less.[27] Molecular testing for genes conferring drug resistance is now done regularly through a WHO collaboration. Fortunately, patients with bacteriological relapses can be retreated with standard MDT (rifampicin, clofazimine and dapsone). Very little work has been done on compliance. One study in Hyderabad showed that of patients attending clinic only 50% had evidence of dapsone metabolites in their urine which was used as a marker of compliance.[28] This and completion rates are areas that need more work. However, there are significant adverse effects associated with MDT and these have been little reported. When the early MDT studies were done no systematic monitoring of adverse effects was done. Recent studies show that up to 40% patients develop anemia whilst on MDT.[29] The skin pigmentation associated with clofazimine is a major problem for patients in India and Asia. Clofazimine pigmentation turns the skin brown and localization of pigment occurs in active leprosy lesions. This pigmentation is very disfiguring and when on the face causes patients to avoid contact with friends and isolate themselves at home. It also probably decreases compliance. Surprisingly no quality of life studies have been done on the patient perception of clofazimine pigmentation and this would be a useful study. There is a need to develop alternative nonclofazimine-containing regimens. A single monthly dose combination, rifampicin, ofloxacin and minocycline (ROM) has been tested in Philippines[30] and Brazil.[31] This regimen would have the advantage of avoiding clofazimine induced skin changes and the anemia associated with dapsone. It would also be easier to ensure that monthly doses of MDT were taken perhaps by using mobile phone technology to remind patients to take their MDT. A large MDT study done in India comparing clinical and bacteriological outcomes for patients with newly diagnosed leprosy and treated with either WHO MDT or with a ROM-based regimen would be a major contribution to developing simpler and easier regimens.[32]

Some data shows that there is already ofloxacin resistance in *M. leprae* in India probably caused by the high rate of antibiotic usage there. It would therefore, be prudent to test the new regimen with moxifloxacin replacing ofloxacin.

IMMUNOTHERAPY

From the times of Fernandez in 1939, through Shepard et al., Meyer et al., Samuel et al., and Convit et al. BCG and

BCG+ killed *M. leprae* have been reported to cause lepromin conversion and enhanced bacterial killing in experimental animals and humans. This has been subsequently confirmed in patients receiving MDT.[33] Similar results were obtained with Mw (MIP) when combined with MDT as compared to MDT given alone. Rapid killing and fall in bacteriological index (BI) was confirmed by mouse foot pad inoculation.[34] However, these studies need to be confirmed in carefully designed studies with close follow-up.

IMMUNOSUPPRESSION

Managing the immune-mediated inflammation associated with leprosy continues to be a major challenge and research is needed to define the best ways of managing these patients. It is important because the inflammation of nerves leads to disability and deformity and recurrent inflammation in skin lesions causes distress and stigmatization. Steroids are widely used to treat leprosy reactions and neuritis but there is little data from controlled clinical trials on their effectiveness. A recent Cochrane review was only able to include three trials and one of these did not use standardized methods for assessing outcomes.[35] One Indian study has shown that patients with reactions (skin inflammation and neuritis) had better outcomes with longer duration of treatment, 20 versus 12 weeks, with high- and low-dose regimens having similar outcomes, 60 mg versus 30 mg starting dose.[36] So the optimal regimen appears to be a 20 weeks regimen starting at 30 mg prednisolone. Other immune suppressants have been tested in leprosy reactions for improving outcomes. A randomized controlled trial was done in Nepal on patients with new reactions who received 1 gm of methyl prednisolone or placebo over 3 days at the start of treatment; methylprednisolone treatment did not show any benefit.[37] So this shows that short, high immune suppression is not beneficial in leprosy reactions. We have also studied longer immune suppression and have assessed the effects of adding azathioprine for 24, 36 or 48 weeks to a standard 20 weeks treatment with prednisolone. This study was done on patients in leprosy hospitals in North India, and skin and neurological outcomes were measured.[38] The improvements found were all associated with the prednisolone treatment and there was no evidence that adding azathioprine improved outcomes. Steroid treatment is effective in reducing skin inflammation and skin lesions improved by 80%, but neurological improvements were much smaller with sensory function remaining static in 65% patients and motor function in 50% of the patients. These data illustrate the modest effect that steroids have on nerve function. We also found a very high rate of recurrence with 37% patients requiring a further course of prednisolone. Skin inflammation was the most common type of recurrence. These studies illustrate the difficulty in switching off leprosy-driven inflammation. New work looking at gene expression in Vietnamese patients with T1R has shown that these patients have up-regulation of arachidonic acid pathway which is associated with the production of prostaglandins.[39] Further studies like this focusing on identifying the molecular mechanisms of T1R are essential if we are to understand these better and develop new interventions.

There is evidence that steroid treatment is associated with significant adverse effects, with 40% patients developing morphological features, such as moon face, 30% have infections and 20% have gastric irritation. Adverse effects due to steroids are probably underestimated in leprosy patients. Little work has been done on other adverse effects such as cataracts, osteoporosis, developing secondary infections or reactivation of latent infections.

ERYTHEMA NODOSUM LEPROSUM

Erythema nodosum leprosum is a regular complication of LL and borderline lepromatous (BL) leprosy and an Indian study has shown that up to 40% of patient with LL develop ENL.[40] Patients present with fever, painful skin lesions and systemic manifestations. The complications, such as orchitis, may cause infertility and the neuritis and bone pain are associated with significant morbidity. Patients need treatment with steroids, but frequently require prolonged courses extending over several years and develop steroid associated complications. A study from Addis Ababa in 2013 shows that patients with ENL have a mortality of 8%, compared with 1% for patients with T1R. Their deaths were due to complications associated with steroid treatment.[41] This highlights the severity of ENL and the life-saving role of other drugs. Thalidomide is available in India in many referral centers and a study from Chandigarh has shown that patients treated with thalidomide have significantly fewer episodes of ENL.[42] Women of child bearing age can be given thalidomide, but this should only happen when there is a strong policy effectively implemented to prevent pregnancy. This will include using dual contraception and having monthly pregnancy tests. It is also important that the patients taking thalidomide are warned not to share their drugs with anyone else. A new global network, the ENL International Study group (ENLIST) includes centers in India, The Philippines, Nepal, Ethiopia and Brazil.[43] This will facilitate the collection of new data on ENL. There is an urgent need to do studies on other immunosuppressants in patients with ENL so that second-line drugs can be defined. Drugs that should be tested include methotrexate, cyclosporine and azathioprine. Very little work has been done on the underlying immunopathology of ENL and studies using newer immunological investigations need to be done.

NEUROPATHIC PAIN

Neuropathic pain is being recognized as a complication of leprosy. A study found that 20% patients with treated leprosy who were attending a leprosy referral center in Mumbai had neuropathic pain which was defined as pain associated with a lesion of the sensory system.[44] Patients may have abnormal sensations in treated skin lesions such as burning or pricking pains. They may also have shooting pains in the arms and legs associated with previous peripheral nerve damage. These patients also had higher rate of depression than leprosy patients without pain. Detailed sensory testing of these patients shows impairment of thermal detection.[45] Neuropathic pain is probably also associated with previous nerve inflammation in dermal nerves and peripheral nerve trunks.[46] It is therefore another sequelae of leprosy reactions. It is important to ask patients if they have pain and this can be done using pain screening tools such as the Douleur Neuropathique 4 (DN4) questionnaire. The optimal management of neuropathic pain in leprosy patients needs to be defined. This will involve doing studies on nonanalgesic drugs such as amitriptyline.[47]

Prevention of disability is a core activity for leprosy programs. This activity requires the active input of many different professionals including doctors, physiotherapists, social workers, etc. It is critical that innovative ways of helping people to look after their neuropathic hands and feet are developed and assessed. This actually starts with early diagnosis, because if leprosy is diagnosed earlier then nerve damage is minimized. The other important medical aspect is through neurological examination so that sensory loss is looked for. This is often not done by nonleprosy specialists and it is important that the cultural issues around testing feet are overcome. Reactions need treating promptly to minimize new neurological damage. The important action is patient education so that patients protect their neuropathic hands and feet. Ulcers also need to be detected early. There is an absence of trials in this area and studies are needed to generate evidence on the best ways of preventing and treating ulcers.

Stigma continues to be strongly associated with leprosy and needs to be combated at many levels including the individual, community and at the national level.[48] Fortunately, there are new approaches which involve developing links with other people who experience stigma.[49] Community-based rehabilitation (CBR) is now recognized as a key part of leprosy work and new guidelines will help promote this work.

In a vast country like India, it was not economically viable to sustain a vertical leprosy control program especially with the dwindling number of leprosy cases. Integrating leprosy control program with general health services (GHS) was considered to have the potential of minimizing costs, expanding coverage and ensuring equity and sustainability, and to reduce stigma "reverse integration" could be a solution. There were also opportunities for partnership and integration at many levels including, surveillance, monitoring, drug distribution, treatment delivery, training, health information and promotion, program evaluation and research including greater synergy between leprosy, other tropical diseases, NGOs and the Government.

However, on the flipside, due to vast diversity in health and socioeconomic situation, a follow-up operational research to assess the integration related to referral services, training, diagnostic availability, MDT dispersal, etc. showed low training leading to missed cases, availability of MDT, etc. was nil to poor in some states.[50] If the missed case is of MB disease it may cause more problems in the future. However, in majority of the areas the proportion of bacteriologically positive cases did not change, which is a positive sign of effective coverage in the post integration era.[51]

With the decreasing prevalence, capacity and competence building and sustainability in leprosy is the essential responsibility of all the stake holders to fine tune the shift from a well-supported specialized program to the one integrated into GHS.

There are still significant challenges associated with leprosy. This review has noted many research areas that need to be addressed in relation to transmission, treatment of the infection, drug resistance, chemo/immunoprophylaxis, immunotherapy, treating reactions, enhanced patient education, CBR and strengthening post amalgamation services. Recommendation for more frequent use of slit-skin smear and histology are also made. All these areas need research done soon so that evidence is generated for national and local programs. These factors mean that leprosy needs to be kept on the agenda of medical schools, training programs and governments so that leprosy patients are diagnosed and treated early and accurately.

REFERENCES

1. Lockwood DN, Reid AJ. The diagnosis of leprosy is delayed in the United Kingdom. QJM. 2001;94(4):207-12.
2. Siddiqui MR, Velidi NR, Pati S, et al. Integration of leprosy elimination into primary health care in orissa, India. PLoS One. 2009;4(12):e8351.
3. Moet FJ, Oskam L, Faber R, et al. A study on transmission and a trial of chemoprophylaxis in contacts of leprosy patients: design, methodology and recruitment findings of COLEP. Lepr Rev. 2004;75(4):376-88.
4. Geluk A. Biomarkers for leprosy: would you prefer T (cells)? Lepr Rev. 2013;84(1):3-12.
5. Weekly Epidemiological Record (WER), WHO, 2013, Vol. 88, 35, PP365-380.
6. Lockwood DN, Shetty V, Penna GO. Hazards of setting targets to eliminate disease: lessons from the leprosy elimination campaign. BMJ. 2014;348:g1136. doi: 10.1136/bmj.g1136.
7. World-Health-Organisation. World Health Organisation Leprosy Elimination Project Staus Report, 2003-2004.
8. Setia MS, SteinmausC, Ho CS, et al. The role of BCG in prevention of leprosy: a meta-analysis. Lancet Infect Dis. 2006; 6(3):162-70.
9. Gupte MD. Vaccine trial against leprosy. Int J Lepr Other Mycobact Dis. 1998;66(4):587-9.
10. Gupte MD, Vallishayee RS, Ananatharamana DS, et al. Comparative leprosy vaccine trial in South India. Indian J Lepr. 1998;70(4):369-88.

11. Sharma P, Mukherjee R, Talwar GP, et al. Immunopophylactic effects of anti-leprosy vaccine in household contacts of leprosy patients: clinical field trials with a follow up of 8-10 years. Lepr Rev. 2005;76(2):127-43.

12. Moet FJ, Pahan D, Oskam L, et al. Effectiveness of single dose rifampicin in preventing leprosy in close contacts of patients with newly diagnosed leprosy: cluster randomised controlled trial. BMJ. 2008;336(7647):761-4.

13. Cole ST, Eiglmeier K, Parkhill J, et al. Massive gene decay in the leprosy bacillus. Nature. 2001;409(6823):1007-11.

14. Monot M, Honore N, Garnier T, et al. On the origin of leprosy. Science. 2005;308(5724):1040-2.

15. Schuenemann VJ, Singh P, Mendum TA, et al. Genome-wide comparison of medieval and modern Mycobacterium leprae. Science. 2013;341(6142):179-83.

16. Mira MT, Alcais A, Nguyen VT, et al. Susceptibility to leprosy is associated with PARK2 and PACRG. Nature. 2004;427(6975):636-40.

17. de Leseleuc L, Orlova M, Cobat A, et al. PARK2 mediates interleukin 6 and monocyte chemoattractant protein 1 production by human macrophages. PLoS Negl Trop Dis. 2013;7(1):e2015. doi: 10.1371/journal.pntd.0002015. Epub 2013 Jan 17.

18. Zhang FR, Huang W, Chen SM, et al. Genomewide association study of leprosy. N Engl J Med. 2009;361(27):2609-18.

19. Saini C, Ramesh V, Nath I. Increase in TGF-beta Secreting CD4(+) CD25(+) FOXP3(+) T Regulatory Cells in Anergic Lepromatous Leprosy Patients. PLoS Negl Trop Dis. 2014;8(1):e2639.

20. Kumar B, Dogra S, Kaur I. Epidemiological characteristics of leprosy reactions: 15 years experience from north India. Int J Lepr Other Mycobact Dis. 2004;72(2):125-33.

21. Kumar A, Girdhar A, Girdhar BK. Risk of developing disability in pre and post-multidrug therapy treatment among multibacillary leprosy: Agra MB Cohort study. BMJ Open. 2012;2(2):e000361.

22. Kanodia SK, Dixit AM, Shukla SR, et al. A study on knowledge, beliefs and attitude towards leprosy in students of Jaipur, Rajasthan. Indian J Lepr. 2012;84(4):277-85.

23. Fine PE, Job CK, McDougall AC, et al. Comparability among histopathologists in the diagnosis and classification of lesions suspected of leprosy in Malawi. Int J Lepr Other Mycobact Dis 1986;54(4):614-25.

24. Lockwood DN, Lucas SB, Desikan KV, et al. The histological diagnosis of leprosy type 1 reactions: identification of key variables and an analysis of the process of histological diagnosis. J Clin Pathol. 2008;61(5):595-600.

25. Barreto JG, Guimaraes Lde S, Leao MR, et al. Anti-PGL-I seroepidemiology in leprosy cases: household contacts and school children from a hyperendemic municipality of the Brazilian Amazon. Lepr Rev. 2011;82(4):358-70.

26. van Brakel WH, Nicholls PG, Das L, et al. The INFIR Cohort Study: investigating prediction, detection and pathogenesis of neuropathy and reactions in leprosy. Methods and baseline results of a cohort of multibacillary leprosy patients in north India. Lepr Rev. 2005;76(1):14-34.

27. Leprosy-global situation. Wkly Epidemiol Rec. 2000; 75(28):226-31.

28. Weiand D, Smith WC, Muzaffarullah S. Qualitative assessment of medication adherence at an urban leprosy outpatient clinic in Hyderabad, India. Lepr Rev. 2011;82(1):70-3.

29. Goulart IM, Arbex GL, Carneiro MH, et al. [Adverse effects of multidrug therapy in leprosy patients: a five-year survey at a Health Center of the Federal University of Uberlandia]. Rev Soc Bras Med Trop. 2002;35(5):453-60.

30. Villahermosa LG, Fajardo TT, Abalos RM, et al. Parallel assessment of 24 monthly doses of rifampin, ofloxacin, and minocycline versus two years of World Health Organization multi-drug therapy for multi-bacillary leprosy. Am J Trop Med Hyg. 2004;70(2):197-200.

31. Uras S, Diório SM, Carreira BG, etal. Estudio Terapeitico comparando a associaode rifampicina, ofloxacinaEminocyclinacom a assocacao rifampicina, clofazimiae dapsone em pacientes com hanseniase multibacilar. Hasenologia Internationalis. 2007; 32(1) 57-65.

32. Lockwood DN, Cunha Mda G. Developing new MDT regimens for MB patients; time to test ROM 12 month regimens globally. Lepr Rev. 2012;83(3):241-4.

33. Natrajan M, Katoch K, Bagga AK, et al. Histological changes with combined chemotherapy and immunotherapy in highly bacillated lepromatous leprosy. Acta Leprol. 1992;8(2):79-86.

34. Katoch K, Katoch VM, Natrajan M, et al. 10-12 years follow-up of highly bacillated BL/LL leprosy patients on combined chemotherapy and immunotherapy. Vaccine. 2004;22(27-28):3649-57.

35. Van Veen NH, Nicholls PG, Smith WC, et al. Corticosteroids for treating nerve damage in leprosy. Cochrane Database Syst Rev. 2007;(2):CD005491.

36. Rao PS, Sugamaran DS, Richard J, et al. Multi-centre, double blind, randomized trial of three steroid regimens in the treatment of type-1 reactions in leprosy. Lepr Rev. 2006;77(1):25-33.

37. Walker SL, Nicholls PG, Dhakal S, et al. A phase two randomised controlled double blind trial of high dose intravenous methylprednisolone and oral prednisolone versus intravenous normal saline and oral prednisolone in individuals with leprosy type 1 reactions and/or nerve function impairment. PLoS Negl Trop Dis. 2011;5(4):e1041. doi: 10.1371/journal. pntd.0001041.

38. Lockwwod D, Darlong J, Pitchimani G, et al. A randomised coontrolled trial of azathiopirine to treat leprosy nerve damage and reactions in India: main findings In Preparation. 2014.

39. Orlova M, Cobat A, Huong NT, et al. Gene set signature of reversal reaction type I in leprosy patients. PLoS Genet. 2013;9(7):e1003624.

40. Pocaterra L, Jain S, Reddy R, et al. Clinical course of erythema nodosum leprosum: an 11-year cohort study in Hyderabad, India. Am J Trop Med Hyg. 2006;74(5):868-79.

41. Walker S, Lebas, E, Doni SN, et al. The mortality associated with erythema nodosum leprosum in Ethiopia: a retrospective hospital-based study. PLoS Negl Trop Dis. 2014;8(3):e2690. doi: 10.1371/journal.pntd.0002690. eCollection 2014.

42. Kaur I, Dogra S, Narang T, et al. Comparative efficacy of thalidomide and prednisolone in the treatment of moderate to severe erythema nodosum leprosum: a randomized study. Australas J Dermatol. 2009;50(3):181-5.

43. Walker SL, Saunderson P, Kahawita IP, et al. International workshop on erythema nodosum leprosum (ENL)--consensus report; the formation of ENLIST, the ENL international study group. Lepr Rev. 2012;83(4):396-407.

44. Lasry-Levy E, Hietaharju A, Pai V, et al. Neuropathic pain and psychological morbidity in patients with treated leprosy: a

cross-sectional prevalence study in Mumbai. PLoS Negl Trop Dis. 2011;5(3):e981. doi: 10.1371/journal.pntd.0000981.

45. Haroun OM, Shetty VP, Shetty V, Pfau D, et al. Quantitative sensory testing (QST) profiles in leprosy patients in Mumbai-India 4th International Congress on Neuropathic Pain; Toronto, Canada 2013.

46. Haroun OM, Hietaharju A, Bizuneh E, et al. Investigation of neuropathic pain in treated leprosy patients in Ethiopia: A cross-sectional study. Pain. 2012;153(8):1620-4. doi: 10.1016/j.pain.2012.04.007. Epub 2012 Jun 22.

47. Moore RA, Derry S, Aldington D, et al. Amitriptyline for neuropathic pain and fibromyalgia in adults. Cochrane Database Syst Rev. 2012;12:CD008242. doi: 10.1002/14651858. CD008242.pub2.

48. Staples J. Interrogating leprosy 'stigma': why qualitative insights are vital. Lepr Rev. 2011;82(2):91-7.

49. van Brakel W, Cross H, Declercq E, et al. Review of leprosy research evidence (2002-2009) and implications for current policy and practice. Lepr Rev. 2010;81(3):228-75.

50. Pandey A, Rathod H. Integration of leprosy into GHS in India. A follow up study (2006-2007). Lepr Rev. 2010;81(4):306-17.

51. Daniel S, Arunthathi S. Rao PS. Impact of integration of the profile of newly diagnosed leprosy patients attending a referral hospital in South India. Indian J Lepr. 2009;81(2):69-74.

51
CHAPTER

Leprosy Scenario Beyond 2020

PS Sundar Rao

INTRODUCTION

In the earlier edition, the leprosy scenario beyond 2010 was predicted under three possible alternatives: the most pessimistic, the most optimistic and the most realistic. We are now 5 years beyond 2010 and the most realistic picture predicted seems true. In this revised chapter, an attempt will be made to look beyond 2020, when the 12th five-year plan of India would have been completed and also the WHO guidelines for enhanced leprosy control strategies for the period 2011–2015 would have been operationalized. The latest WHO report on global leprosy situation 2013 states: Leprosy control has improved significantly due to national and subnational campaigns in most endemic countries. Integration of primary leprosy services and effective collaborations and partnerships have led to considerable reduction in leprosy burden. Nevertheless, new cases continue to occur in almost all endemic countries and high burden pockets can exist against a low burden background.[1] Similar conclusions were drawn by the WHO expert committee at its eighth meeting.[2] And finally, the scientific presentations at the last international leprosy congress held in Belgium during September 2013,[3] generally confirm a rather disappointing and pessimistic picture of leprosy eradication under the prevailing conditions in most endemic countries. Thus, forecasting future scenario under such shifting data base will be fraught with many uncertainties and makes predictions rather difficult, especially when we look beyond 2020.

THE JOURNEY SO FAR

The National Leprosy Eradication Programme (NLEP) is a centrally sponsored health scheme of the Ministry of Health and Family Welfare, Government of India. The Programme is headed by the Deputy Director of Health Services (Leprosy) under the administrative control of the Directorate General Health Services, Government of India. While the NLEP strategies and plans are formulated centrally, the program is implemented by the States and Union Territories. The Programme is also supported as partners by the WHO, The International Federation of Anti-Leprosy Associations (ILEP) and few of the nongovernment organizations (NGOs). In 1955, the Government of India launched National Leprosy Control Programme (NLCP) based on Dapsone domiciliary treatment through vertical units implementing survey education and treatment activities as an integral part of its first five-year plan. Diaminodiphenylsulfone (DDS) or Dapsone was the antileprosy drug of choice, and the NLCP used this drug as its sheet anchor, recruiting one paramedical worker per 20,000 population, who carried out general household case-detection surveys once every 3–5 years. In addition, annual contact surveys, school surveys and special epidemiological surveys were also conducted. The voluntary case reporting was encouraged at innumerable field stations all over the country. One nonmedical supervisor (NMS) per 4–5 paramedical workers; and one leprosy medical officer were appointed at every 'taluk' level. Monitoring was done by estimation of prevalence rate (PR) of leprosy based on national population census done every 10 years till 1981. Mostly, it remained as an understatement due to recording of only cases with advanced leprosy, low self-reporting mainly due to stigma; and errors in coverage of population.

In 1981, the Government of India established a high power committee under chairmanship of Dr MS Swaminathan for dealing with the problem of leprosy, and when the multidrug therapy (MDT) came into use following the recommendation by the WHO Study Group, Geneva, in 1982, a new name was created as the National Leprosy Eradication Programme (NLEP) in 1983.

During early 70s, the specter of Dapsone resistance raised its head, when urgent research on efficacy and tolerability of multidrug therapy (MDT) started. Field trials on MDT began in late 70s and by 1984, most states in the country started initiating MDT. The dramatic effects of MDT were visible, and in the year 1991, the WHO issued a clarion call to eliminate leprosy as a public health problem by 2000. Except for 12 countries including India, globally this 'elimination' was reached by this date. Because of the heavy disease burden and extensive geographic areas involved, some in very difficult to access terrains, India could achieve elimination (leprosy prevalence of less than 1 per 10,000 population) only in December 2005, along with few more countries. The major feature of NLEP has been the active case detection campaigns to enable MDT to be administered to all patients as early as possible. MDT coverage of all districts was done in a phased manner and since there was shortage of infrastructure, only 201 districts could be covered till 1994. Contractual staff was provided to the remaining districts and all districts were covered by 1996. Case detection was recorded and reported by a large number of voluntary organizations till 2004. During the fifth five-year plan, case detection was also made through urban leprosy centers. Five modified leprosy elimination campaigns were visualized and implemented from 1997 to 2005. A special action plan for elimination of leprosy (SAPEL) was undertaken during 1997–2000. Leprosy elimination campaign (LEC) was also pushed through in urban localities during 1997–2000.

When the case load became manageable, the vertical component for leprosy control was removed and case detection is being conducted through general healthcare system since 2002–2003. Independent evaluations were also carried out during 2000, 2002 and 2005. Leprosy elimination monitoring (LEM) was conducted in 2002, 2003 and 2004. The sample survey-cum-assessment unit (SSAU) made a monthly visit report on LEM type study for state consumption.

Further, two Block Leprosy Awareness Campaigns (BLAC) were also undertaken in 2004 and 2005 with case detection component.

The impact of all these strong measures can be seen in the form of declining trends in the annual prevalence rates (PR) during the period from 1981 to 2011 as presented in Figure 51.1.

According to the WHO statistics, the new cases detected in India from 1992 to 2013 are depicted in Table 51.1 and Figure 51.2.[4,5]

From 517,000 in 1992 to less than 130,000 in 2013, is a dramatic achievement.

India registered 133,717 in 2009, 127,295 in 2011, 126,913 in 2013.[4,5]

THE CURRENT SCENARIO

From 2005 to 2013, the registered prevalence continued to show gradual decline nationally, although in some states of India, they were stagnant. On the other hand, the new case detection rate generally showed no decline and instead remained stagnant or reported some increase.

The trends in leprosy prevalence rates (PR) and the annual new case detection rates (ANCDR) in India from 1991 to 2013 are displayed in Figure 51.2.

The trend in PR shows remarkable decline during 2002–2006, but stabilized around 1.0 in the subsequent years. Similar dramatic reductions were seen for ANCDR from 2002 to 2006, which stabilized around 0.7 subsequently.

Relevant data on prevalence rate, new case detection rate, new cases according to type of leprosy, viz., PB or MB, percentage of new cases by MB, female, children, and grades of disability among the new cases from the Central Leprosy Division of the Directorate-General of Health Services, Government of India pertaining to the year 2012-13[4] are listed in Table 51.2.

There are great variations by states, and also in terms of multibacillary (MB) rate, child rate and female rate, as presented in the Table 51.2. Scientific papers published show that new case detection rate are more biased toward MB cases registering at integrated healthcare centers. Since active surveys have been discouraged, much of the statistics only reflect passive new case detections, majority of them reporting late after visible deformities occur.

Although elimination of leprosy at a national level was achieved by December 2005, one state (Chhattisgarh) and one union territory (Dadra and Nagar Haveli) have remained with PR between 2 and 4 per 10,000 population even in 2013, as given in the Table 51.3.

Further, three other States, viz. Bihar, Maharashtra and West Bengal, which have achieved elimination earlier have shown slight increase in PR (1.0–1.2) in the current year, perhaps due to special action programs during 2012, as presented in Table 51.4A.

As seen from the tables, wide variations are noted in the proportion of child cases, women and those with grade 2 deformities, reflecting perhaps more operational rather than epidemiological factors. The proportions of MB cases show even greater variability, and causes concern on the effectiveness of passive voluntary reporting at integrated health centers. Unless active surveys in vulnerable populations are undertaken, such as school children, tribals, urban slums and remote inaccessible areas, which constitute a significant part of our vast country, the picture from routine statistics as presented will be incomplete and probably misleading in terms of the new case detection rate, especially MB cases reporting late, especially after occurrence of visible deformities.

Further data on child rate and disability rate in each state and union territory during 2012-13 are presented in Table 51.4A. Four states and union territories which still have a high PR are listed in Table 51.4B.

In summary then, nationally, as of 2013, the PR was 0.73 per 10,000 population, ANCDR was 10.78 per 100,000 population,

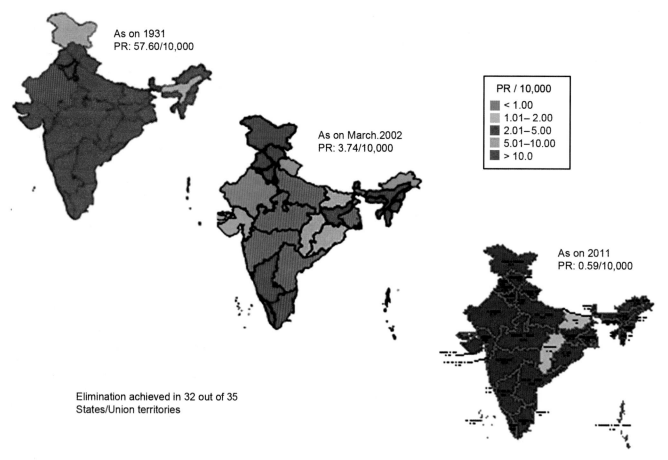

As on 1931
PR: 57.60/10,000

As on March.2002
PR: 3.74/10,000

PR / 10,000
■ < 1.00
■ 1.01– 2.00
■ 2.01–5.00
■ 5.01–10.00
■ > 10.0

As on 2011
PR: 0.59/10,000

Elimination achieved in 32 out of 35
States/Union territories

Fig. 51.1: Declining leprosy prevalence in India

an increase of 4% from previous year, MB leprosy was nearly 50% of new cases detected, 37% were female, 10% were children below 15 years, and visible deformity was present in 3.45%. The grade 2 deformity rate among new cases detected during 2012–13 works out to 3.72 per million population and grade 1 deformity an additional 4.14 per million population.

At the sub-state level, the annual new case detection rate (ANCDR) and prevalence rate (PR) among 649 districts as of March 2013 are listed in Tables 51.5 and 51.6 respectively, which reveal high endemic pockets all over the country.

Finally, the statistics of Government of India also show that the total number of leprosy cases released from treatment (RFT) during 2012–13 comes to 127,830 (92.5%) as against total deletion of 138,199 due to defaulting, loss of follow-up, deaths, etc. This brings the total number of persons affected by leprosy cured of the disease in the country with MDT from the beginning to date to an impressive total of 12.8 million.

While the accredited social health activists (ASHA) workers in the national rural health mission (NRHM) continue to be trained and involved in new case detection and case-holding

for completing MDT, the government also realized the need to carry out active surveys and intensified information, education and communication (IEC) activities in a small number of high endemic districts, which helped in detection of more than 20,000 new cases during 2012–13.

THE FUTURE

On 16 August, 2013, the Government of India and ILEP members active in India signed a new memorandum of understanding (MOU) providing a formal framework for collaboration between the Government of India and the nine ILEP members active in India, till the end of March 2017.[5]

International Federation of Anti-Leprosy Associations' members active in India have agreed to continue providing support to the NLEP. For the next five-year period, their support will be in line with the enhanced global strategy for further reducing the disease burden due to leprosy and the Government of India's 12th five-year plan with the aim of sustaining and improving quality leprosy services.[6] Support

Table 51.1: Annual new case detection in India 1992–2013	
Year	*New cases detected*
1992	517,000
1993	456,000
1994	414,894
1995	391,760
1996	415,302
1997	519,952
1998	634,901
1999	537,956
2000	474,286
2001	617,993
2002	473,658
2003	367,143
2004	260,063
2005	169,709
2006	139,252
2007	137,685
2008	134,184
2009	133,717
2010	126,800
2011	127,295
2012	134,752
2013	126,913

will be given at both the national and state level. At the national level for example, ILEP will supply a disability prevention and medical rehabilitation (DPMR) consultant to the central leprosy division, who will assist in planning, monitoring and evaluating the DPMR program. It will also continue to provide referral services and assist with developing guidelines on various elements of the NLEP, such as footwear provision.

At the state level, areas of support to be provided by ILEP include improving case detection, improving case management, increasing participation of persons affected by leprosy in society and reducing stigma.

From the background presented so far, it is clear that given adequate political support and necessary funding, the NLEP staff has reduced the leprosy burden, but sustaining the same level of focus and commitment will be a challenge, especially in low-resource settings where equity of access is an issue.[2,7-9] India practices the WHO recommended enhanced global strategy for further reducing the disease burden due to leprosy during its 11th five-year plan (2007–2011), which largely aims to reduce the grade 2 disability rate among newly detected leprosy cases by at least 35% by the end of 2015, compared with the baseline at the end of 2010. This approach underlines the importance of early detection and quality of care in an integrated health service setting.[10]

Given the historical background of leprosy in India and its strong association with sociocultural roots of stigma and health seeking habits, improvement of health services alone

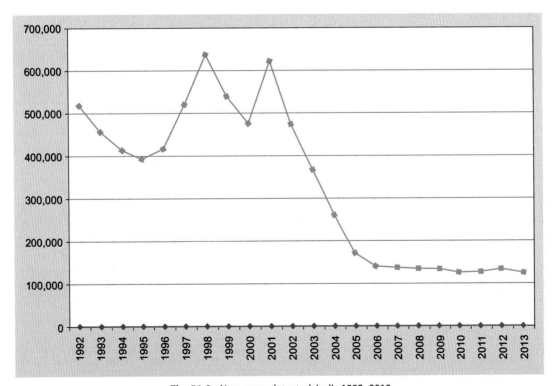

Fig. 51.2: New cases detected: India:1992–2013

Table 51.2: Prevalence and new case detection rate by State and Union Territories as of 2013

State/ UT	Census population as on March 2013	PR/ 10,000	ANCDR/ 100,000	Number of new cases detected			Percentage of new cases				
				PB	MB	Total	MB	Female	Child	Grade I	Grade II
Andhra Pradesh	86,469,955	0.61	9.59	4,223	4,072	8,295	49.09	41.15	11.34	3.38	4.97
Arunachal Pradesh	1,447,791	0.32	3.32	12	36	48	75	27.08	25	95.83	2.08
Assam	32,162,002	0.35	3.57	293	854	1,147	74.46	26.94	9.24	9.94	6.63
Bihar	108,549,626	1.2	20.27	13,692	8,309	22,001	37.77	38.78	15.88	1.62	2.32
Chhattisgarh	26,603,290	2.13	30.5	3938	4,177	8,115	51.47	37.33	6.72	5.19	5.72
Goa	1,480,846	0.25	3.71	19	36	55	65.45	43.64	1.82	0	0
Gujarat	62,540,126	0.96	14.42	4,997	4,022	9,019	44.59	48.71	9.39	4.37	2.84
Haryana	26,289,494	0.26	2.46	156	492	648	75.93	32	1.85	2.62	1.85
Himachal Pradesh	7,023,440	0.21	2.36	29	137	166	82.53	29.52	3.01	15.66	10.24
Jharkhand	34,324,980	0.66	10.75	1,882	1,809	3,691	49.01	36.74	7.5	3.09	1.41
Jammu and Kashmir	13,094,331	0.17	1.46	40	151	191	79.06	24.61	3.66	1.05	1.05
Karnataka	62,941,156	0.44	5.46	1,444	1,992	3,436	57.97	37.02	15.63	7.04	3.29
Kerala	33,708,968	0.24	2.47	327	505	832	60.7	100	12.86	7.93	8.77
Madhya Pradesh	74,581,916	0.72	8.58	2307	4093	6400	63.95	34.83	6.13	12.19	5.2
Maharashtra	115,746,634	1.09	16.17	8,411	10,304	18715	55.06	44.04	12.51	1.82	3.44
Manipur	2,816,190	0.08	0.85	5	19	24	79.17	37.5	12.5	8.33	8.33
Meghalaya	3,113,452	0.09	0.84	0	26	26	100	19.23	11.54	0	23.08
Mizoram	1,136,649	0.16	1.58	6	12	18	66.67	27.78	0	0	0
Nagaland	1,978,622	0.5	7.93	19	138	157	87.9	15.92	8.28	21.02	29.94
Odisha	43,062,077	0.98	19.1	4128	4,098	8,226	49.82	36.99	8.64	4.21	3.22
Punjab	28,429,228	0.21	2.46	172	528	700	75.43	8.86	4	2.86	1.43
Rajasthan	71,337,317	0.17	1.52	137	947	1,084	87.36	26.11	1.11	25.18	4.15
Sikkim	621,991	0.23	3.05	7	12	19	63.16	15.79	15.79	5.26	15.79
Tamil Nadu	74,260,793	0.39	4.78	1,740	1,810	3,550	50.99	28.42	10.76	4.31	4.85
Tripura	3,773,796	0.18	0.61	6	17	23	73.91	21.74	0	4.35	4.35
Uttar Pradesh	207,034,298	0.72	11.7	14,389	9,833	24,222	40.6	32.85	6.22	2.53	2.9
Uttarakhand	10,478,054	0.25	4.72	250	245	495	49.49	38.99	6.46	4.04	2.42
West Bengal	93,756,723	1.05	12.46	4,122	7,561	11,683	64.72	32.45	7.52	3.17	2.47
A & N Islands	384,899	0.36	3.64	8	6	14	42.9	35.71	7.14	14.29	0
Chandigarh	1,088,492	0.58	6.8	38	36	74	48.65	29.73	4.05	4.05	0
D & N haveli	374,476	3.61	98.27	283	85	368	23.1	58.42	26.09	6.25	0
Daman and Diu	264,656	0	0.38	0	1	1	0	0	0	0	0
Delhi	17,402,735	0.73	7.19	376	876	1,252	69.97	23.72	6.79	8.95	10.14
Lakshadweep	65,217	0	0	0	0	0	0	0	0	0	0
Puducherry	1,306,955	0.21	4.36	28	29	57	50.88	35.09	10.53	7.02	5.26

Abbreviations: ANCDR, annual new case detection rate; MB, multibacillary; PB, paucibacillary, PR, prevalence rate; UT, union territory; A & N, Andaman and Nicobar; D & N, Dadra and Nagar.

Table 51.3: Statement showing States/Union Territories not reaching elimination status as on March 2013

S. No.	State	Population as on March 2013	% of country's population	No. of cases on record	% of country's case load	PR/ 10,000	No. of new cases detected	% of country's new case	ANCDR/ 100,000
1.	D & N Haveli	374,476	0.03	135	0.15	3.61	368	0.27	98.27
2.	Chhattisgarh	26,603,290	2.13	5,656	6.17	2.13	8,115	6.02	30.50
	Total of 1 and 2	26,977,766	-	5,791	-	2.15	8,483	-	31.44
	Percentage	-	2.16	-	6.31	-	-	6.30	-

Abbreviations: ANCDR, annual new case detection rate; D & N, Dadra and Nagar Haveli; PR, prevalence rate.

Table 51.4A: States and Union Territories where elimination was achieved (PR < 1/10,000) as of March 2013 with some exceptions

S. No.	State	Population as on March 2013	% of country's population	No. of cases on record	% of country's case load	PR/ 10,000	No. of new cases detected	% of country's new cases	ANCDR/ 100,000
1.	Bihar	108,549,626	8.69	13,017	14.15	1.20	22,001	16.38	20.27
2.	Odisha	43,062,077	3.4	4,222	4.60	0.98	8,226	6.10	19.10
3.	Maharashtra	115,746,634	9.26	12,659	13.80	1.09	18,715	13.89	16.17
4.	Gujarat	62,540,126	5.00	5,981	6.52	0.96	9,019	6.69	14.42
5.	West Bengal	93,756,723	7.50	9,855	10.74	1.05	11,683	8.67	12.46
6.	Uttar Pradesh	207,034,298	16.57	14,865	16.20	0.72	24,222	17.98	11.70
7.	Jharkhand	34,324,980	2.75	2,276	2.48	0.66	3,691	2.74	10.75
8.	Andhra Pradesh	86,469,955	6.92	5,235	5.71	0.61	8,295	6.16	9.59
9.	Madhya Pradesh	74,581,916	5.97	5,369	5.85	0.72	6,400	4.75	8.58
10.	Delhi	17,402,735	1.39	1,262	1.38	0.73	1,252	0.93	7.19
11.	Nagaland	1,978,622	0.16	99	0.11	0.50	157	0.12	7.93
12.	Chandigarh	1,088,492	0.09	63	0.07	0.58	74	0.05	6.80
13.	Karnataka	62,941,156	5.04	2,789	3.04	0.44	3,436	2.55	5.46
14.	Tamil Nadu	74,260,793	5.94	2,930	3.19	0.39	3,550	2.63	4.78
15.	Uttarakhand	10,478,054	0.84	262	0.29	0.25	495	0.37	4.72
16.	Puducherry	1,306,955	0.10	27	0.03	0.21	57	0.04	4.36
17.	Goa	1,480,846	0.12	37	0.04	0.25	55	0.04	3.71
18.	A & N Island	384,899	0.03	14	0.02	0.36	14	0.01	3.64
19.	Assam	32,162,002	2.57	1,131	1.23	0.35	1,147	0.85	3.57
20.	Arunachal Pradesh	1,447,791	0.12	47	0.05	0.32	48	0.04	3.32
21.	Sikkim	621,991	0.05	14	0.02	0.23	19	0.01	3.05
22.	Kerala	33,708,968	2.70	810	0.88	0.24	832	0.62	2.47
23.	Punjab	28,429,228	2.27	605	0.66	0.21	700	0.52	2.46
24.	Haryana	26,289,494	2.10	692	0.75	0.26	648	0.48	2.46
25.	Himachal Pradesh	7,023,440	0.56	148	0.16	0.21	166	0.12	2.36
26.	Mizoram	1,136,649	0.09	18	0.02	0.16	18	0.01	1.58
27.	Rajasthan	71,337,317	5.71	1,185	1.29	0.17	1,084	0.80	1.52
28.	Jammu and Kashmir	13,094,331	1.05	219	0.24	0.17	191	0.14	1.46
29.	Manipur	2,816,190	0.23	23	0.03	0.08	24	0.02	0.85
30.	Meghalaya	3,113,452	0.25	29	0.03	0.09	26	0.02	0.84
31.	Tripura	3,773,796	0.30	69	0.08	0.18	23	0.02	0.61
32.	Daman and Diu	264,656	0.02	0	0.00	0.00	1	0.00	0.38
33.	Lakshadweep	65,217	0.01	0	0.00	0.00	0	0.00	0.00

Abbreviations: ANCDR, annual new case detection rate; PR, prevalence rate; A & N, Andaman and Nicobar.

					Table 51.4B: States and Union Territories with PR > 1/10,000 as of March 2014			
S. No.	State	Population as on March 2014	New cases detected	ANCDR/ 100,000 population	Prevalence end of March	PR/ 10,000 population	No. of cases with grade-II deformity	G2D rate per million population
1.	Dadra and Nagar Haveli	391,365	320	81.77	158	4.04	0	0.00
2.	Chhattisgarh	27,151,318	8,519	31.38	5,700	2.10	607	22.35
3.	Odisha	43,630,496	10,645	24.40	6,405	1.47	449	10.29
4.	Chandigarh	1,105,799	144	13.02	63	1.22	2	1.80

Abbreviations: ANCDR, annual new case detection rate; PR, prevalence rate.

			Table 51.5: Position of districts according to annual new case detection rate: 2012–13				
S. No.	State/Union Territories	Total no. of district(s)	ANCDR/100,000 in no. of districts (As on March 2013)				
			<10	10–20	>20–50	>50–100	>100
1.	Andhra Pradesh	23	14	9	0	0	0
2.	Arunachal Pradesh	16	16	0	0	0	0
3.	Assam	27	24	3	0	0	0
4.	Bihar	38	3	17	18	0	0
5.	Chhattisgarh	27	9	5	11	2	0
6.	Goa	2	2	0	0	0	0
7.	Gujarat	26	16	0	6	3	1
8.	Haryana	21	20	1	0	0	0
9.	Himachal Pradesh	12	12	0	0	0	0
10.	Jharkhand	24	9	15	0	0	0
11.	Jammu and Kashmir	22	22	0	0	0	0
12.	Karnataka	30	25	5	0	0	0
13.	Kerala	14	14	0	0	0	0
14.	Madhya Pradesh	50	36	10	4	0	0
15.	Maharashtra	34	12	10	9	3	0
16.	Manipur	9	9	0	0	0	0
17.	Meghalaya	7	7	0	0	0	0
18.	Mizoram	9	9	0	0	0	0
19.	Nagaland	11	10	1	0	0	0
20.	Odisha	31	8	10	11	2	0
21.	Punjab	20	20	0	0	0	0
22.	Rajasthan	33	33	0	0	0	0
23.	Sikkim	4	4	0	0	0	0
24.	Tamil Nadu	30	30	0	0	0	0
25.	Tripura	4	4	0	0	0	0
26.	Uttar Pradesh	72	35	28	9	0	0
27.	Uttarakhand	13	12	1	0	0	0
28.	West Bengal	19	10	3	5	1	0
29.	A & N Islands	3	3	0	0	0	0
30.	Chandigarh	1	1	0	0	0	0
31.	D & N Haveli	1	0	0	0	1	0
32.	Daman and Diu	2	2	0	0	0	0
33.	Delhi	9	7	1	0	1	0
34.	Lakshadweep	1	1	0	0	0	0
35.	Puducherry	4	4	0	0	0	0
	Total	649	443	119	73	13	1
	Percentage		68.26	18.34	11.25	2.00	0.15

Abbreviations: A & N, Andaman and Nicobar; D & N, Dadra and Nagar.

S. No.	State/UT	Total No. of districts	PR/10,000 in no. of districts (As on March 2013)					
			< 1	1–2	>2–5	>5–10	>10–20	>20
1.	Andhra Pradesh	23	22	1	0	0	0	0
2.	Arunachal Pradesh	16	16	0	0	0	0	0
3.	Assam	27	24	3	0	0	0	0
4.	Bihar	38	14	21	3	0	0	0
5.	Chhattisgarh	27	10	9	6	2	0	0
6.	Goa	2	2	0	0	0	0	0
7.	Gujarat	26	16	2	6	2	0	0
8.	Haryana	21	20	1	0	0	0	0
9.	Himachal Pradesh	12	12	0	0	0	0	0
10.	Jharkhand	24	21	3	0	0	0	0
11.	Jammu and Kashmir	22	22	0	0	0	0	0
12.	Karnataka	30	29	1	0	0	0	0
13.	Kerala	14	14	0	0	0	0	0
14.	Madhya Pradesh	50	42	7	1	0	0	0
15.	Maharashtra	34	19	10	4	1	0	0
16.	Manipur	9	9	0	0	0	0	0
17.	Meghalaya	7	7	0	0	0	0	0
18.	Mizoram	9	9	0	0	0	0	0
19.	Nagaland	11	10	0	1	0	0	0
20.	Odisha	31	18	9	4	0	0	0
21.	Punjab	20	20	0	0	0	0	0
22.	Rajasthan	33	33	0	0	0	0	0
23.	Sikkim	4	4	0	0	0	0	0
24.	Tamil Nadu	30	29	1	0	0	0	0
25.	Tripura	4	4	0	0	0	0	0
26.	Uttar Pradesh	72	60	11	1	0	0	0
27.	Uttarakhand	13	13	0	0	0	0	0
28	West Bengal	19	11	5	3	0	0	0
29	A & N Islands	3	3	0	0	0	0	0
30.	Chandigarh	1	1	0	0	0	0	0
31.	D & N Haveli	1	0	0	1	0	0	0
32.	Daman and Diu	2	2	0	0	0	0	0
33.	Delhi	9	7	1	0	1	0	0
34.	Lakshadweep	1	1	0	0	0	0	0
35.	Puducherry	4	4	0	0	0	0	0
	Total	649	528	85	30	6	0	0
	Percentage		81.36	13.10	4.62	0.92	0.00	0.00

Abbreviations: A & N, Andaman and Nicobar; D & N, Dadra and Nagar.

without active community involvement and intensified IEC activities will not be effective. Thus, India should also put into practice the UN resolution on the elimination of stigma and discrimination against persons affected by leprosy and their families. This strategy has to be worked out with increased empowerment of people affected by the disease, together with their greater involvement in the provision of services and in the community. Despite much high-sounding talks and resolutions, this strategy is yet to be worked out. Meanwhile, the specter of backlash by *M. leprae* in terms of relapses, recurrences and increased transmission will raise its ugly head, as seen in some parts of the country.[11]

A projection of new case detection rate up to 2020 is shown in Figure 51.3.

While leprosy is not likely to be eradicated by 2020, at least if there is a declining trend in the new case detection rate, there is hope of successful eradication.[12] All the efforts outlined above must be seriously followed even to keep the new case detection rate stable.[13] Failure can only result in an increase in the incidence of disease, which is disastrous for the country and wasteful of all the expenditures incurred on NLEP.

We now have about 5-6 years to correct existing deficiencies in our current health service policies, continue building up the capacities of our health workers, network effectively with the ILEP partners and other NGOs, strengthen the surveillance and monitoring mechanism to identify weak and vulnerable sections of the population, encourage more

special action programs and modified leprosy elimination campaigns, remove the ban and actively encourage vertical surveys among schools, urban slums, tribal areas and hard to reach communities, mobilize community support and active involvement of persons affected by leprosy in all these new case detection activities as well as eradication of misconceptions and stigma promoting wide use of MDT, cut the link between popular attitudes between leprosy and deformities, and generally initiate an almost military campaign against eradicating leprosy.

Is this possible? Realistic forecasting the leprosy scenario beyond 2020 depends on the answer to this question. In turn, we need to analyze the challenges and obstacles as well as opportunities and positive forces that can be used to our advantage to promote eradication of leprosy.

Medical and Clinical Aspects

Adequate information is available on the pathogen, methods of detection, some epidemiological factors, MDT as the best therapy so far, second line drugs, methods to prevent and manage deformities and reactions, methods for diagnosis of leprosy at a field level. Further knowledge on simpler methods of early diagnosis, molecular aspects of *M. leprae*, extra-human reservoirs, would be helpful. However, translation of existing knowledge has been poor and meagre, and if done seriously, would suffice to promote early detection and prompt effective antileprosy therapy and control of reactions.[7]

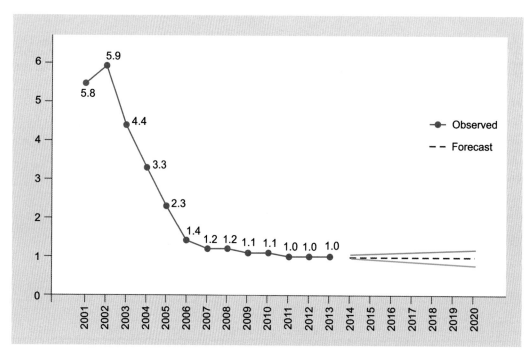

Fig. 51.3: Projected annual new case detection rate beyond 2013

Social and Psychological Aspects

More than adequate knowledge is available on the continuing high levels of leprosy stigma, both, perceived and enacted, and there is much documentation published and presented on the need to eradicate stigma and unjust discrimination. However, practical and effective methods to reduce stigma and educate society are still largely theoretical and insufficiently tested. Traditional IEC methods are still ineffectively used at great cost. Involving leprosy affected persons and community participatory approaches are still on paper only and rather meagre attempts are being made to test these strategies. Social science methods are poorly used in general to tackle this most crucial factor.[14]

Health and Leprosy Service Aspects

A very well, organized NLEP planned in 1983 by MS Swaminathan has been somewhat curtailed without adequate preparation for integration due to availability of MDT and pressure from WHO to eliminate leprosy as a public health problem by 2000. India with over 80% of the global leprosy burden managed to do so in 2005, but everyone knows that this was largely due to 'cleaning' of registers, and redefining prevalence in a narrow sense. Training of general health workers and building capacity to diagnose and classify leprosy was done, but not sustained.[3,8] It is also a well-known fact that the current classification of leprosy based on skin lesions alone results in at least 20% misclassification of MB cases as paucibacillary (PB), impacting not only on the duration of treatment, but premature release of MB cases from effective treatment. The almost exclusive reliance on passive reporting, which has been shown from reported statistics to be largely MB cases after appearance of visible deformities further complicates the vital issues of transmission of infection, as well as producing wrong statistics of prevalence and incidence of leprosy. Lack of sustained training and capacity building of general health workers, disruption and unavailability of blister packs for MDT, and poor monitoring have added to the inefficiency of the integrated leprosy services. The generous funding for MDT and certain other leprosy services, such as for reconstructive surgeries and medical rehabilitation, have been offset by the basic system failures, that has resulted in stagnant or slightly increasing new case detection rate. Thus, it is in the application of relevant knowledge that we have failed, especially in final push for eradication of leprosy.

The prediction for the future in the light of the above factors will depend on massive political will to overcome the grim situation and overhaul the health and development system at every level of administration from the state to village level, especially in the high endemic areas of our country. If not, the writing on the wall seems clear and dismal.

REFERENCES

1. WHO. Global Leprosy: Update on the 2012 Situation. WHO Weekly Epidemiological Record. 2013;88:365-78.
2. WHO Expert Committee on Leprosy-Eighth Report. WHO Technical Report Series No. 968, World Health Organization. Geneva; 2012.
3. Book of Abstracts 18th International Leprosy Congress-Hidden Challenges: Brussels, Belgium; September 2013.
4. Government of India: Directorate-General of Health Services, Central Leprosy Division: NLEP-Progress Report for the year 2012-2013. Nirman Bhawan, New Delhi.
5. Agrawal CM, Barkakaty BN. National Leprosy Eradication Program--Success and Future Planning. Health Action. HAFA National Monthly: 2013. pp. 4-5.
6. WHO: Enhanced Global Strategy for further reducing the disease burden due to leprosy, 2011-15 Operational Guidelines (updated) SEA.GLP.2009.4, WHO South East Asia Regional Office (SEARO), New Delhi.
7. Kuipers P, Rao PSS, Raju MS, et al. A conceptual protocol for translational research in the complex reality of leprosy. Lepr Rev. 2013;84(2):166-74.
8. Smith C, Editorial. The 18th International Leprosy Congress: Brussels 2013—a special event. Lepr Rev. 2013;84(2):115-8.
9. Novartis Foundation for Sustainable Development: How to curb the incidence of leprosy? Special Session by Aerts A, Cairns S, Noordeen SK, et al. 18th International Leprosy Congress. Brussels, Belgium; 2013.
10. Alberts CJ, Smith WCS, Meima A, et al. Potential effect of World Health Organization's 2011-2015 global leprosy strategy on the prevalence of grade 2 disability: a trend analysis in China, India and Brazil. Bull World Health Organ. 2011;89:487-95.
11. Kumar A, Girdhar A, Chakma JK, et al. Detection of previously undetected cases in Firozabad District (UP), India during 2006-2009: a short communication. Lepr Rev. 2013;84(2):124-7.
12. Sundar Rao PSS. Worldwide elimination of leprosy-A historical journey. Expert Rev Dermatol. 2012;7(6):513-20.
13. International Leprosy Summit-Overcoming the remaining challenges: The Bangkok Declaration towards a leprosy-free world. Bangkok,Thailand,24-26,July 2013. Global Leprosy Programme:http://www.searo.who.int/entity/glabal leprosy programme/Bangkok declaration/en/index.html.
14. Sasakawa Memorial Health Foundation. Leprosy in our Time-Everyone has a role to play in tackling stigma. The Nippon Foundation. 2013. pp. 6-11.

52
CHAPTER

Leprosy Scenario Beyond its Elimination

Marcos Virmond

INTRODUCTION

The present book through its various chapters, ascertains convincingly the status of leprosy being one of the oldest diseases known to mankind. Recently, archeological studies reveal absolute evidence of leprosy in an Egyptian skeleton of the 2nd century BC, although the earliest written records of the disease come from India which date back to 600 BC.[1,2] In this context, when the advances in medical sciences are considered, it is intriguing that this disease reaching the 21st century continues to affect large proportions of world population. The disease is caused by a slow, probably the slowest growing mycobacteria, and interestingly, despite the all-round improvements on medical technologies to fight leprosy, the progress toward the elimination also seems to be extremely slow. In fact, the time-line of the history of leprosy shows only a few major landmarks which are worth mentioning. Those are as follows:

- The identification of the causative agent by GA Hansen in 1874
- The introduction of sulfones[3] including dapsone for treatment, in the late 1940s[4]
- The Mitsuda skin reactivity for the prognosis of individuals exposed to *Mycobacterium leprae*[5]
- The *in vivo* growth of *M. leprae* in mice and later in armadillos[6,7]
- The introduction of the WHO recommended multidrug therapy (MDT) in the middle 1980s[8]
- The sequencing of the entire genome of the *M. leprae* in the end of the year 2000.[9]

However, the introduction of MDT in the treatment of leprosy has been considered as the most important development in the history of control of leprosy. Since then there has been a gradual, but significant change in the leprosy scenario both at the global and national level. The prevalence of active cases came down dramatically all over the world. Indeed, initial figures showed that within 2 decades there had been a marked decrease in the estimation of leprosy cases worldwide: from 10–12 million in the mid-1980s to 0.51 million in 2003.[10] Presently, the decrease is by far more impressive: the registered global prevalence for the beginning of 2013 stood at 215,656 cases. Another important achievement of MDT is the improvement in the organizational aspects of leprosy control programs, e.g. the improved quality of care and the relation of health team toward patients.

With the help of a robust therapeutic regime in hands and a strong political commitment envisaged by leprosy elimination strategy by the year 2000 as a public health problem, the leprosy scenario has changed progressively in various ways, among them, one deserves detailed discussion which is the concept of "cure of leprosy".

Recent studies indicate that leprosy stigma is still a global phenomenon, occurring in both nonendemic and endemic countries.[11] In the past, apart from disfigurement, the lack of an effective treatment has been pointed as important to the construction of heavy stigma against leprosy.[12,13] The incurability of leprosy was one of the negative features of the disease that MDT has definitely contributed to revert. On one hand, the WHOs concept of cure for leprosy, although objective, but is not strictly linked to a microbiological cure, because the concept is focused on a managerial achievement. On the other hand, the endless use of sulfone monotherapy was far from being a reasonable sign of a treatment in aiming for the cure of the disease. As a matter of fact, the concept of cure is still difficult to be fully understood among patients. Even today, the need for taking drugs for 6 or 12 months is conceived by some patients as a sign of an incurable disease.

Even notable that, the presence of any residual deformity is considered to be a clear sign that the disease is active in some patients.[14] Nevertheless, the MDT is a robust regimen for treatment and for the first time in the history of leprosy the disease has changed to a new concept, that leprosy is a curable disease.

THE ELIMINATION STRATEGY

The word 'elimination' in the context of leprosy has become a word of controversy, some believe in such concept and some do not. However, the successes with MDT lead WHO in 1991 to set the target of elimination of leprosy as a public health problem by the year 2000. Elimination was defined as achieving a prevalence level of less than 1 case per 10,000 population. Of course, elimination was not understood as eradication of leprosy, but to accept a residual number of cases. In an initial phase, it was related mainly with the reduction of the disease by treatment with MDT and a consequent decrease in the prevalence. In later phases, the disease reduction had to be attributed to the occurrence of fewer new cases owing to reduced disease transmission.[15]

As a matter of fact, after 12 years of the set target year of elimination, epidemiological figures for leprosy cases are striking. According to official reports coming from 105 countries and territories during 2013, the global registered prevalence of leprosy at the beginning of 2013 stood at 215,656 cases, while the number of new cases detected during 2011 was 226,626 (excluding the small number of cases in Europe).[16] Elimination of leprosy has been achieved in most of the past endemic countries and the problem is now restricted to a few countries in which the elimination in the district and subdistrict levels is still to be pursued, besides some pockets of high endemicity that still remain in some foci in Angola, Brazil, the Central African Republic, India, Madagascar, Nepal and the United Republic of Tanzania.

As a dynamic process the strategy of elimination moved on along the years and added some extra actions to enhance further to its basic principles. Among the actions undertaken one can mention the leprosy elimination campaigns, the leprosy elimination monitoring (LEM) and the special action projects for eliminating leprosy. Each one had its time and opportunity to assist managers and health personnel in progressing towards the goal of eliminating leprosy as a public health problem.

In 1999, the Global Alliance to Eliminate Leprosy (GAEL) was established to give a new breath into the elimination strategy whereby WHO joined the governments of major endemic countries and so also The Nippon Foundation, a major partner in the strategy, the Novartis Foundation for Sustainable Development, Danish International Development Agency (DANIDA) and International Federation of Antileprosy Associations (ILEP). As expected in such an embodied complex organizations, major conflicts emerged between some of the partners. In order to examine the extent to which the partnership has added the value to achieving the leprosy elimination goals, WHO invited an independent team of experts to evaluate the GAEL.[17] As the main outcome, the report recognized that the use of the word 'elimination' is problematic because it mean different things in different languages and the elimination really meant to most people the 'eradication'.

At the same token, the term also suggested that after the goal was met that there might not be important leprosy work to do. Another relevant point raised in the report was that collaborative leprosy efforts would focus more explicitly on the entire spectrum of leprosy activities from diagnosis to rehabilitation.

The GAEL experience was a critical turning point in the relations between WHO, NGOs, partners and governments, though the strategy of elimination has continued to be the official policy of WHO in regard to leprosy in the world. In the same way, ILEP continued to support worldwide leprosy programs in a broad range of areas, starting from detection, treatment, rehabilitation and up to research.

After that, important and ample meetings were organized by WHO convening all partners involved in the fight against leprosy. One of them was in 2009, which promoted the "2010–2015 Enhanced Global Strategy for further reducing the disease burden due to leprosy". In this document, it is possible to envisage some long-term result of the GAEL affair. It contains recommendations that greater emphasis is given to the need for an effective referral system, as the part of an integrated program. It is also emphasized that good communication between health team and patients is essential and that the control strategy continued to rely on early case finding and treatment with MDT. Most relevant, the document states that a greater emphasis on the assessment of disability at diagnosis should be given, so that those at particular risk can be recognized and managed appropriately. Another remarkable recommendation is the emphasis on the need for early recognition and timely management of leprosy reactions and neuritis. Prevention of disability and self-care practices has also been included and the wide array of care and social concern is depicted by the recognition that rehabilitation may include not only surgery but, in a broader scope, socioeconomic rehabilitation. A clear sign of a new route to the WHO strategy is the adoption of the number and rate of new cases with grade-2 disabilities per 100,000 population per year as one of the leading indicators for monitoring the epidemiologic trends of the disease.[18]

The WHO elimination strategy can thus be considered as the most remarkable and controversial event in leprosy control since the adoption of the compulsory isolation of cases. There are those that consider the elimination strategy as highly positive and those opposing as contrary to its implementation. Both groups have considerable evidences to support their positions.[19-28] However, the adoption of MDT seems to be a common ground of agreement between the groups. In fact, MDT is a key element of the leprosy treatment in any strategy due to its effectiveness and also because monotherapy with dapsone or any other antileprosy drug should be considered unethical practice.

Elimination of Leprosy by the Year 2000

In 2000, the WHO declared that leprosy had been eliminated as a global public health problem. The global prevalence fell from 5.35 million (12 per 10,000) in 1985 to 597,035 (1 per 10,000) at the end of 2000.[29] However, the two major endemic countries, Brazil and India, did not attain the proposed paradigm in the year 2000. The former, although with a marked reduction in prevalence[30] in the last decade, is still showing a prevalence rate of 1.51 per 10,000 as per January 2012. The latter has announced elimination in the national level by the end of 2005. Other smaller countries, such as Mozambique and the Democratic Republic of Congo, with a considerable burden of leprosy reached elimination at the national level in 2007. Those were joined by Timor-Leste by the end of 2010.[16] By the year 2012 all WHO regions had attained the elimination goal and there are just a few countries that did not manage to eliminate leprosy at the country level. Data reported to WHO on global prevalence rate as per March 2013 can be seen in Table 52.1.

Although central to the elimination concept, prevalence rate seems not to be the best indicator of the epidemiological course of leprosy. In fact, though prevalence has come down in all countries the same does not correlate with the detection rate of the disease. Moreover, there are evidences that slow decrease in detection rate may have started even before the adoption of the elimination strategy.[31] Although in a different time span, the curves for detection and prevalence rate for Brazil and India[32] (Figs 52.1 and 52.2) are similar to those projected for the world[33,34] (Table 52.2) which can be considered as a marked fall in the prevalence rate curve and

a steady linearity in the detection rate. This picture indicates strongly, that the elimination strategy has had little impact in the transmission of the disease, since the decrease of prevalence is attributed primarily to the discharged treated cases and defaulters and also to those within the fixed duration of treatment.[35]

Such stable detection rate and the lack of an effective vaccine to prevent the disease, indicates that leprosy will continue to be a public health problem of consequence in many countries in the decades to come. Consequently, an array of resources will be necessary to cope with a new challenge: leprosy in a new scenario beyond elimination.[36,37]

LEPROSY BEYOND ELIMINATION

One of the main reasons that support those who criticize the strategy of elimination is the fact that the terminology probably implied that after the goal has been met there would not be any important work associated with leprosy need to be undertaken as a follow-up. As a matter of fact, some problems regarding the control of the disease have been detected the reason for which may be attributed to a variety of causes. Among them, the new epidemiological feature of the disease with an outspread condition of low endemicity in many parts of the world has contributed to the assumption that leprosy is no more a concern of public health. This situation has led to new conditions and challenges that are the key factors in the new scenario of leprosy beyond elimination and should be with addressed carefully.

Decentralization and Integration

Decentralization and integration of leprosy service to the general health may be controversial, though mandatory to achieve broad control of a disease like leprosy. A possibility is that the decentralization of the vertical program and the integration to the general health system may lead to lack of

Table 52.1: Registered prevalence of leprosy and number of new cases detected in 103 countries or territories, by WHO Region, 2013

WHO Region[a]	Number of cases registered (prevalence/10,000 population), first quarter of 2014[b]	Number of new cases detected (new-case detection rate/100,000 population), 2013[c]
African	22,722 (0.38)	20,911 (3.50)
Americas	31,753 (0.36)	33,084 (3.78)
Eastern Mediterranean	2,604 (0.05)	1,680 (0.35)
South-East Asia	116,396 (0.63)	155,385 (8.38)
Western Pacific	7,143 (0.04)	4,596 (0.25)
Total	**180,618 (0.32)**	**215,656 (3.81)**

[a] No reports received from the European region.

[b] The prevalence rate is the number of cases on treatment/10,000 population at the beginning of 2014.

[c] The new case detection rate is the number of new cases/100,000 population during the year 2013.

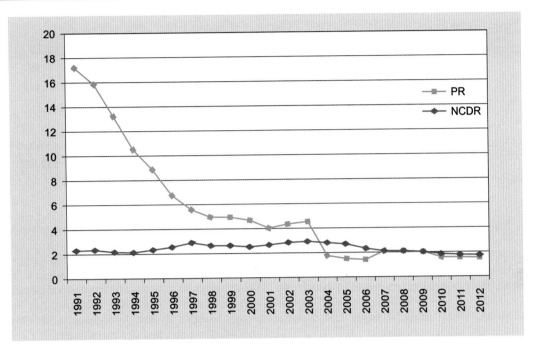

Fig. 52.1: Prevalence and detection rate in Brazil: 1991–2012
Source: SINAN - SVS - MoH - Brazil. Prevalence and detection rates per 10,000 in order to allow comparability.

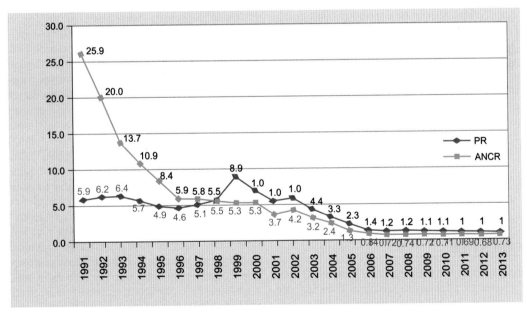

Fig. 52.2: Prevalence and detection rate in India: 1991–2013
Source: NELP, India. Prevalence and detection rates per 10,000 in order to allow comparability.

commitment by managers at the district and provincial levels. In fact, this has been pointed out as a problem of the post-elimination era in the integrated health system adopted in many countries, such as Brazil and India. The local managers have a workload of services dealing with the diagnosis of other diseases that are to be treated in their services, and the assumption that leprosy is no more a problem of concern makes them to divert their attention to other health needs but not leprosy. Of course, in those countries where leprosy is still controlled by vertical services the slackness in the

Table 52.2: Trends in the detection of new cases of leprosy, by WHO Region, 2006–2013

WHO Region[a]	2006	2007	2008	2009	2010	2011	2012	2013
African	34,480	34,468	29,814	28,935	25,345	20,213	20,599	20,911
Americas	47,612	42,135	41,891	40,474	37,740	36,832	36,178	33,084
Eastern Mediterranean	3,261	4,091	3,938	4,029	4,080	4,357	4,235	1,680
South-East Asia	17,418	171,576	167,505	166,115	156,254	160,132	166,445	155,385
Western Pacific	6,190	5,863	5,859	5,243	5,055	5,092	5,400	4,596
Total	**265,661**	**258,133**	**249,007**	**244,796**	**228,474**	**226,626**	**232,857**	**215,656**

[a] No reports received from the European region.

action toward leprosy control has not been felt. On the other hand decentralization and integration are essential to improve access of MDT services resulting in early diagnosis and adequate treatment, as well as contributing to decreased stigma.[38] In short, the essential components to concretely control or eliminate leprosy include the trained health personnel and drugs, which must be easily and friendly available near the house of a leprosy case.

Integration is more of a structural and managerial issue, despite certain logistical and technical issues which also need to be addressed simultaneously.[39] In this sense, to guarantee the quality of services it is needed to monitor and evaluate the integration process, which should be continuous and timely as provided at the national and provincial levels.[40] The main advantages of integration to general health services lay in its cost-effectiveness, in better perspective of local priority, in making services available directly to the person in need, and it helps to fight stigma and improve community involvement.[39] Consequent to this, leprosy will not be considered anymore a special disease, whose diagnosis and treatment are beyond the capacity of the general health services. Therefore, besides some very specific regional conditions that deserve tailored attention of a vertical approach, decentralization of services and integration into the general health system is the pragmatic approach to controlling the disease in the post-elimination era.

CLINICAL EXPERTISE

Leprosy is a clinical entity the diagnosis and management of which is mostly based on clinical examination. The adequate management of cases, including a correct classification, is based on clinical grounds integrated to the laboratory findings.

Due to the inherent characteristics of the disease, being treated by putting in isolation, leprosy historically has been a disease treated in clinics and hospitals devoted only to the disease. Therefore, doctors and nurses, working most of the time in these venues, were able to embody and maintain a sound knowledge on the diagnosis and treatment of this disease. With the adoption of the vertical program to control leprosy, this condition was further strengthened not only by increased participation of health personnel from the public health system but also the increasing group of scientists interested in investigation of the disease in its many aspects. Being primarily a disease of the peripheral nerves and with important skin manifestations, leprosy has been a disease largely handled by the dermatologists. In this basis, India and Brazil are the two countries in which a sound expertise in clinical leprosy was developed mostly because of the high endemicity and the extensive governmental approach to the problem that took place in these two countries in the mid-20th century, and on resulting in the construction of many leprosaria with their pertaining medical staff. Although European countries and the USA gave outstanding contribution to clinical and basic research in leprosy at that time, not to mention those devoted foreign leprologists working and living in topical countries, developments in clinical leprosy remained mostly in the hands of Brazilian and Indian scientists. In fact, in the last century, the clinical features of leprosy have been a major area of discussion among leprologists from these two countries, like Dharmendra, Luiz Marino Bechelli, Dinkar Palande, Eduardo Rabello, Srinivasan H, Ramanujam, Opromolla and Khanolkar VR.

With the introduction of MDT and its shorter regimens leading to an important reduction in prevalence, the medical interest in leprosy seems to be progressively fading away. A probable cause for this is the idea that leprosy is being eliminated, and even eradicated as a clinical entity, and, therefore, it is not a health problem of concern anymore. The decreased interest can be seen from another point of view—the lack of clinical expertise is noticed due to poor training and teaching, as well as the still prevailing stigma against the disease among professionals and teachers of medical schools.[41] However, one should remember that for a successful integration of leprosy services in the general health service, leprosy should be incorporated in the teaching of medical and nursing schools as well, as to sustain the leprosy expertise within the health services.

Unfortunately, leprosy has little space in the agenda of medical schools throughout the world,[42,43] and the expected result is misdiagnosis or delay in diagnosis, which are both detrimental to the patient care and the control of the disease at any time whether during elimination or post elimination periods. Some studies[44-46] have revealed the lack of skills among doctors and nurses regarding leprosy. It is remarkable to find that, one of the studies showed that, 32.5% of a group of leprosy cases were misdiagnosed in the first medical consultation[47] and surprisingly, 30.0–71.2% of the cases had to have more than five medical visits to have suspected leprosy for being definitely diagnosed.[48] Expertise among private practitioners seems also to be decreasing.[49] Therefore, one of the challenges for the post elimination era is to maintain a considerable degree of leprosy expertise. In those countries with a notable past prevalence and a relevant detection rate, leprosy should be part of the medical courses at graduation level as well as in the disciplines of dermatology, tropical medicine or infectious diseases at postgraduation level. Authorities in the Ministry of Health should be in charge of contacting medical societies/councils and medical schools to promote the inclusion of leprosy in the curricula of medical studies.

Another important need is to give full support to maintain international centers of excellence in leprosy studies around the globe to serve as a reservoir of the knowledge on leprosy and to provide teaching and training to doctors from countries where leprosy is no more a significant problem, although prevalent. In the past decades, there was a widespread fear that research and training institutions will have to reduce their activities or would even be closed with the attainment of the goal of elimination. This is not justifiable because, more than ever, these institutions have to play an important role now and in the years to come. With the integration of leprosy activities into the general health services, these institutions have to act as island of excellence and reservoirs of knowledge. In this regard, they should act as places to maintain alive the available knowledge on leprosy gathered so far and to function as reference centers for specially difficult cases to be treated in the periphery. Of course, those institutions that have a sound production of research must be strengthened in this direction following their own focus in research, but keeping an eye on the priority agendas of leprosy which was researched and proposed by WHO, ILEP, ILA and other international organizations.

It is reasonable to understand that at the levels of district, province or state units or hospital treating leprosy patients in an integrated base have no time available for personnel to cope with specific activities of special training and improvement of leprosy knowledge, because they are involved in treating and controlling other diseases besides leprosy. This is even more relevant with the reduction in the number of leprosy cases. In brief, leprosy will be regarded in general health services as a normal disease among others—not as a special condition in need of special arrangements to deal with. In some places or regions, leprosy could even become a rare condition. Therefore, these research and training institutions are unique

places to provide to workers of the general health services with continued training in order to adequately cope with a reduced but still present prevalence in the years beyond elimination.

These are the places where specialized and distinct expertise in clinical leprosy should be available to clarify doubts of peripheral units and, in some instances, to admit the patients for screening, to diagnose and for treatment of unusual or severe forms of leprosy.[50,51]

TRANSMISSION AND VACCINE

The remaining challenge of the post elimination era is the containment of transmission of leprosy. If MDT can cure people, it is rational to assume that early diagnosis and MDT will be the paramount for interrupting the chain of transmission. The data so far indicates that MDT did not have a striking effect in the reduction of leprosy transmission.[51-54] In fact, the global case detection rate has remained fairly static over the last decade in many countries. Causes for that are manifold, including BCG vaccination of population, epidemiologic definitions and operational factors related to control activities and geographical region.[54,55] Therefore, new strategies should be designed to interrupt transmission of *M. leprae.*[54,56]

A key point in this regard is the long duration of the disease incubation that, for leprosy, is uncertain and the infection is difficult to detect. Furthermore, transmission that took place before the case detection is therefore, likely to result in many more new cases in future. Research in this area is mandatory to develop practical diagnostic tools to detect levels of infection that can lead to transmission.[54] In the meantime, it is important to stress that basic control measures, such as early diagnosis and complete MDT treatment, are essential components to interrupt transmission. However, control of transmission is not solely dependent on the identification of subclinical infection by appropriate diagnostic tools and early treatment of cases, but also by improved housing conditions, sanitation and education. In addition, new studies reveal potential unusual means of transmission of leprosy and the disease can be discussed as being a zoonosis in some specific regions in the USA.[57,58]

Those who have studied leprosy control measures agree that having a vaccine with a high protective capacity and with few side effects, would greatly reduce the transmission of leprosy. So far, BCG vaccination used as prophylaxis is the most studied vaccine in leprosy and results are controversial since levels of protection ranges from 20% to 80%.[59] There were also attempts to use a therapeutic vaccine aiming to enhance leprosy chemotherapy which included *Mycobacterium w* (Mw), now renamed as MIP (*Mycobacterium indicus pranii*), and other vaccines in combination with BCG.[60,61] Besides improvements on some clinical features, results are not consistent to advocate at present, a general recommendation for any form of vaccine. Therefore, there is still room for further studies on the development of a vaccine with a potential for both prophylactic and therapeutic use.[62,63] Low endemicity in many countries makes it a difficult task in, designing of trials on a large scale to test efficacy of any kind of vaccine. In this context, focused groups in countries with large population should be the target of such studies.

Although difficult to attain, the availability of an effective vaccine would support the interruption of the chain of transmission of the disease, once the difficulty in detecting the subclinical infection by simple and reliable test for large scale application is overcome.

RESEARCH

There is a clear picture among leprosy workers that leprosy is not going to disappear anytime soon. Many challenges remain unsolved in different fields of the disease. Just to mention one, the causative agent is still not cultivable *in vitro*, though with limited success it has been achieved *in vivo*. Besides that, the precise mechanism of transmission of *M. leprae* is not clearly understood and extensive studies have not yet produced any practical and effective tool for early diagnosis. Furthermore, a highly effective vaccine has not yet been developed. Therefore, in case of leprosy, we face great limitations in the usual research approach adopted in case of most infectious diseases, such as:

- It is not easy to obtain great amounts of viable causative agent
- It is not possible to devise effective preventive measures due to the gaps in the understanding of the disease transmission
- Lastly, it is difficult to protect population due to nonavailability of an effective vaccine.

On the one hand, these arguments support the need for continued research on leprosy. On the other hand, the elimination strategy has been blamed for a drastic reduction of funds to research in leprosy as well as the shifting of research field by the scientists once engaged in the field of leprosy to the other diseases on the grounds that leprosy would not be any more a disease of concern. In fact, as the target of elimination approaches, governmental and NGOs personnel involved in disease control and research fear that, after attaining the goal of "elimination as a public health problem", leprosy services and of leprosy workers and researchers will be at high-risk for losing their positions.[64] However, one should remember that elimination is not eradication—it must be clear to everyone that leprosy will continue to exist even in areas where the elimination goal has been reached. In addition, the incidence trends for leprosy seem to be static in most countries, which reinforce the future need for patient care, health services and research.

In this context, the continuation of both basic and applied research is needed in the period beyond elimination. Priorities have been extensively discussed in an array of fora ever since, before the elimination date until today.[65-72] A common link between these reports include research for understanding the mechanism of transmission of the infection, for recognizing the mechanism for nerve damage and to test new and effective drug regimens to treat the infection, in particular more effective short duration remedies, such as uniform MDT. The relation of persistent bacilli and relapse is still an open field for study. Nerve damage, being the most feared and transcendent aspect of leprosy, has to be further investigated to better understand the mode of invasion and the immunological relations of *M. leprae* to nerve cells as a high priority. Here it is essential to include the mechanisms of reversal and erythema nodosum leprosum (ENL) reactions, definition of predictive biomarkers to reactions and development of new but less toxic and safe drugs for treatment of leprosy reactions as other research priorities. Thalidomide, still a gold standard for treatment of ENL, could be the focus of pharmacologic studies to better understand its damage to nerve tissues as well as to find a reshaped molecule to reduce its teratogenic adverse effect. Disabilities have a close relationship to all those above mentioned aspects as an undesirable outcome. A shorter duration of antileprosy treatments, i.e. short duration contact of patients with health services, may be a concern after MDT completion. Provision of prevention measures through counseling and regular post-MDT follow-up to detect new disabilities and to halt further worsening of cases with existing disabilities and availability of general rehabilitation services are a must.

Despite the improvement in field program management through the worldwide implementation of MDT services in the last decades, operational research is still the need. In fact, leprosy beyond elimination seems likely to continue to appear though in low numbers in many countries with unfavorable socioeconomic conditions. Scenarios that include poverty, malnutrition, unemployment, slums, illiteracy and political instability are a challenge to program managers and field personnel. Unfortunately, these conditions are still present in many countries where leprosy has been or was eliminated but the disease is still a major concern. Operational research has to offer tailor made solutions for these issues under local conditions. In this regard, cost-effective measure for prevention of disabilities, methods for improved adherence to, and completion of MDT treatment, strategies to maintain clinical expertise available at referral centers, studies on the abolition of social discrimination, stigma and human rights aspects of leprosy should be on the agenda of research to tackle the remaining challenges in the period beyond elimination.

CONCLUSION

M. leprae seems to be an earthly bacterium whose presence in the world is unavoidable. Despite the enormous accumulation of knowledge about its behavior in relation to the environment and man, the disease it causes seems to approach a stable condition. If one studies the burden of leprosy since the ancient times to the 21st century one cannot deny the tremendous improvements achieved in the treatment and control of the disease. In this sense, it is clear that leprosy in near future will be a disease of just a few cases, which, however, will deserve keen attention to its management. However, in the centuries to come, if the social conditions of the population improve due to the political improvement and with the access of this population to new technologies in the fields of agriculture, health and social sciences, leprosy will have only space in medical museums as a terrifying disease that had threatened human kind for many millennia. Leprosy will finally be a truly eliminated and eradicated disease from the surface of the earth and an average doctor would never have heard about the disease. Even though, I am quite convinced that in this late (far away) scenario, scientists will continue to be intrigued with many aspects of the biology of *M. leprae* that still remain unsolved.

ACKNOWLEDGMENT

I would like to express my deepest appreciation and thanks to Professor Pranab Kumar Das, Honorary Senior Research Fellow from the Birmingham University, UK, for his valuable suggestions to this text.

REFERENCES

1. Bryceson A, Pfaltzgraff RE. Leprosy, 3rd edition. Edinburgh: Churchill Livingstone; 1990.
2. Browne SG. The history of leprosy. In: Hastings RC (Ed). Leprosy. Edinburgh: Churchill Livingstone; 1989.
3. Faget GH, Johansen FA, Ross H. Public Health Reports, December 11, 1942: Sulfanilamide in the treatment of leprosy. Public Health Rep. 1975;90(6):486-9.
4. Lowe J. Treatment of leprosy with diaminodiphenyl sulphone by mouth. Lancet. 1950;1(6596):145-50.
5. Mitsuda K. On the value of a skin reaction to a suspension of leprous nodules. Hifuka Hinyôka Zasshi. (Jpn J Dermatol Urol), 1919;19:697-708. Reprinted in Int J Lepr Other Mycobact Dis. 1953;21:347-58.
6. Shepard CC. The experimental disease that follows the injection of human leprosy bacilli into foot-pads of mice. J Exp Med. 1960;112(3):445-54.
7. Kirchheimer WF, Storrs EE. Attempts to establish the armadillo (Dasypus novemcinctus Linn.) as a model for the study of leprosy. I. Report of lepromatoid leprosy in an experimentally infected armadillo. Int J Lepr Other Mycobact Dis. 1971;39(3):693-702.
8. World Health Organization. Chemotherapy of leprosy for control programmes. World Health Organ Tech Rep Ser. 1982;675:1-33.
9. Eiglmeier K, Parkhill J, Honoré N, et al. The decaying genome of Mycobacterium leprae. Lepr Rev. 2001;72(4):387-98.
10. World Health Organization. Global Strategy for Further Reducing the Leprosy Burden and Sustaining Leprosy Control Activities (Plan period: 2006-2010). Leprosy situation by WHO region at the beginning of 2004. WHO/CDS/CPE/CEE/2005.
11. Wong ML. Asia Pacific Disability Rehabilitation Journal. 2004;15:3-12.
12. Briden A, Maquire E. An assessment of knowledge and attitudes towards leprosy/Hansen's disease amongst healthcare workers in Guyana. Lepr Rev. 2003;74(2):154-62.
13. Luka EE. Understanding the stigma of leprosy. South Sudan Med. J 2010;3:45-8.
14. Santos AM, Gomes MK, Manoel BD, et al. Leprosy: the link between the disease and the concept of cure. 13th World Congress of Public Health. poster. 419, 2012. Available from https://wfpha.confex.com/wfpha/2012/webprogram/Paper10399.html. [Accessed June 2014].
15. Noordeen SK. Elimination of leprosy as a public health problem: progress and prospects. Bull World Health Organ. 1995;73(1):1-6.
16. World Health Orgnization. Leprosy today. Available at www.who.int/lep/en/. [Accessed June 2014].
17. Skolnik R, Agueh F, Justice J, et al. Independent evaluation of the Global Alliance for the Elimination of Leprosy. 2003.[online] Available at: www.gujhealth.gov.in. [Accessed June 2014].
18. World Health Organization. Enhanced Global Strategy for Further Reducing the Disease Burden Due to Leprosy Operational Guidelines (Updated) (2011-2015). India: 2009.
19. Nsagha DS, Bamgboye EA, Assob JC, et al. Elimination of leprosy as a public health problem by 2000 AD: an epidemiological perspective. Pan Afr Med J. 2011;9:4. Epub 2011.
20. da Cunha MD, Cavalieri FA, Hércules FM, et al. The impact of leprosy elimination strategy on an endemic municipality in Rio de Janeiro State, Brazil. Cad Saude Publica. 2007;23(5):1187-97.
21. Dogra S, Narang T, Kumar B. Leprosy—evolution of the path to eradication. Indian J Med Res. 2013;137(1):15-35.
22. Bechelli LM. Prospects of global elimination of leprosy as a public health problem by the year 2000. Int J Lepr Other Mycobact Dis. 1994;62(2):284-92.
23. Andrade V, Virmond M, Gilsuárez R, et al. New approach to accelerate the elimination of leprosy. Hansen Int. 1999;24:49-54.
24. Lockwood DN, Suneetha S. Leprosy: Too complex a disease for a simple elimination paradigm. Bull World Health Organ. 2005;83(3):230-5. Epub 2005 Mar 16.
25. East-Innis A. The quest for the global elimination of leprosy. West Indian Med J. 2005;54(1):1-2.
26. Fine PE, Warndorff DK. Leprosy by the year 2000—what is being eliminated? Lepr Rev. 1997;68(3):201-2.
27. Naafs B. Treatment of leprosy: science or politics? Trop Med Int Health. 2006;11(3):268-78.
28. Rani Z. Leprosy elimination strategy. J Pak Assoc Dermatol. 2007;17:1-3.
29. Sundar Rao PSS. Worldwide Elimination of Leprosy. Expert Rev Dermatol. 2012;7(6):513-20.
30. Penna ML, Penna GO. Trend of case detection and leprosy elimination in Brazil. Trop Med Int Health. 2007;12(5):647-50.
31. Fine P. Leprosy: what is being eliminated? Bull World Health Organ. 2007;85(1):2.

32. Sunda Rao PSS. Leprosy scenario beyond 2010. In: Kar HK and Kumar B. IAL Texbook of Leprosy. New Delhi: Jaypee Brothers Medical Publishers (P) Ltd.; 2010.

33. Feenstra P. "Elimination" of leprosy and the need to sustain leprosy services, expectations, predictions and reality. Int J Lepr Other Mycobact Dis. 2003;71(3):248-56.

34. Cunha SS, Rodrigues LC, Moreira S, et al. Upward trend in the rate of detection of new cases of leprosy in the State of Bahia, Brazil. Int J Lepr Other Mycobact Dis. 2001;69(4):308-17.

35. Global situation of leprosy control at the beginning of the 21st century. Lepr Rev. 2012;73:s15-16.

36. Duthie MS, Sauderson P, Reed SG. The potential for vaccination in leprosy elimination: new tools for targeted interventions. Mem Inst Oswaldo Cruz. 2012;107(Suppl 1):190-6.

37. Meima A, Richardus JH, Habbema JD. Trends in leprosy case detection worldwide since 1985. Lepr Rev. 2004;75(1):19-33.

38. Túlio Raposo M, Nemes MI. Assessment of integration of the leprosy program into primary health care in Aracaju, state of Sergipe, Brazil. Rev Soc Bras Med Trop. 2012;45(2):203-8.

39. Gupta AK. Integrated approach for leprosy elimination in India. Journal of Development and Social Transformation. 2004;1:31-6.

40. Siddiqui MR, Velidi NR, Pati S, et al. Integration of Leprosy elimination into primary health care in Orissa, India. PLoS One. 2009;4(12):e8351.

41. Ganapati R, Pai VV, Rao R. Dermatologist's role in elimination/post-elimination. Lepr Rev. 2007;78(1):30-3.

42. Crawford CL. Teaching leprosy to medical students. Br Med J. 1977;1(6061):643.

43. Karthikeyan K, Thappa DM. Modular teaching program on leprosy. Indian J Lepr. 2003;75(4):317-25.

44. Barreto JA, Conhecimentos de médicos sobre hanseníase e reflexos em sua epidemiologia. [online] Available from www.portal.cfm.org.br [Accessed June 2014].

45. Maia MAC, Oliveira AA, Oliveira R, et al. Conhecimento da equipe de enfermagem e trabalhadores braçais sobre hanseníase. Hansen Int. 2000;25:26-30.

46. Pires CAA, Viana ACB, Araújo FC. Avaliação de conhecimento em hansenologia de internos do curso de medicina do Estado do Pará. [online] Available from www.oxfordeventos.com.br. [Accessed June 2014].

47. Souza CS, Bacha JT. Delayed diagnosis of leprosy and the potential role of educational activities in Brazil. Lepr Rev. 2003;74(3):249-58.

48. Lastoria JC, Macharelli CA, Putinatti MS. Hanseníase: realidade no seu diagnóstico clínico. Hansen Int. 2003;28:53-8.

49. Kar HK. Leprosy free India: clinical perspectives and challenges ahead. Lepr Rev. 2007;78(1):38-9.

50. Virmond MC. Role of leprosy related research and training institutions in management and prevention of disabilities and rehabilitation. Hansen Int. 1999;24:38-42.

51. Vijayakumaran P, Jesudasan K, Mozhi NM, et al. Does MDT arrest transmission of leprosy to household contacts? Int J Lepr Other Mycobact Dis. 1998;66(2):125-30.

52. Meima A, Gupte MD, van Oortmarssen GJ, et al. SIMLEP: a simulation model for leprosy transmission and control. Int J Lepr Other Mycobact Dis. 1999;67(3):215-36.

53. Meima A, Smith WC, van Oortmarssen GJ, et al. The future incidence of leprosy: a scenario analysis. Bull World Health Organ. 2004;82(5):373-80.

54. Richardus JH, Habbema JD. The impact of leprosy control on the transmission of *M. leprae*: is elimination being attained? Lepr Rev. 2007;78(4):330-7.

55. Chiyaka ET, Muyendesi T, Nyamugure P, et al. Theoretical assessment of the transmission dynamics of leprosy. Applied Mathematics. 2013,4(2):387-401.

56. Araújo S, Lobatol J, Reis Ede M, et al. Unveiling healthy carriers and subclinical infections among household contacts of leprosy patients who play potential roles in the disease chain of transmission. Mem Inst Oswaldo Cruz. 2012;107(Suppl 1):55-9.

57. Lane, JE, Meyers WM, Walsh DS. Armadillos as a source of leprosy infection in the Southeast. South Med J. 2009;102(1):113-4.

58. Truman RW, Singh P, Sharma R, et al. Probable zoonotic leprosy in the southern United States. N Engl J Med. 2011; 364(17):1626-33.

59. Merle CS, Cunha SS, Rodrigues LC. BCG vaccination and leprosy protection: review of current evidence and status of BCG in leprosy control. Expert Rev Vaccines. 2010;9(2):209-22.

60. Katoch K, Katoch VM, Natrajan M, et al. 10-12 years follow-up of highly bacillated BL/LL leprosy patients on combined chemotherapy and immunotherapy. Vaccine. 2004;22(27-28):3649-57.

61. Kaur I, Dogra S, Kumar B, et al. Combined 12-month. WHO/MDT MB regimen and *Mycobacterium w*. vaccine in multibacillary leprosy: a follow-up of 136 patients. Int J Lepr Other Mycobact Dis. 2002;70(3):174-81.

62. Duthie MS, Gillis TP, Reed SG. Advances and hurdles on the way toward a leprosy vaccine. Hum Vaccin. 2011;7(11):1172-83.

63. Gillis T. Is there a role for a vaccine in leprosy control? Lepr Rev. 2007;78(4):338-42.

64. Faber WR, Klatser PR. Elimination of leprosy and its consequences for research. Adv Exp Med Biol. 2003;531:295-7.

65. Ginsberg AM. Leprosy research—setting priorities and facilitating collaborations: a personal perspective. Lepr Rev. 2000;71(Suppl):S183-7.

66. Fleury, RN. Priorities for leprosy research in Brazil (Editorial). Hansen Int. 2005;30:1-2.

67. World Health Organization. Global Strategy for Further Reducing the Leprosy Burden and Sustaining Leprosy Control Activities (Plan period: 2006-2010)WHO/CDS/CPE/CEE/2005.53.

68. ILEP. A research strategy to develop new tools to prevent leprosy, improve patient care and reduce the consequences of leprosy. [online] Available from www.leprosy-ila.org. [Accessed June 2014].

69. van Veen NHJ, McNamee P, Richardus JH, et al. Cost-Effectiveness of Interventions to Prevent Disability in Leprosy: A Systematic Review. PLoS One. 2009;4(2):e4548. doi: 10.1371/journal.pone.0004548. Epub 2009.

70. Martelli CM, Stefani MM, Penna GO, et al. Brazilian endemisms and epidemics, challenges and prospects for scientific investigation: leprosy. Rev Bras Epidemiol. [online], 2002;5(3):273-85.

71. World Health Organization. Major challenges and priority research needs; Report of the Scientific Working Group on Leprosy 2002;TDR/SWG/02.

72. Barua S. Leprosy: priority areas for research. In: Priority Areas for Research in Communicable Diseases. World Health Organization-SEARO. SEA-CD-197, 2009;77.

53
CHAPTER

Leprosy Recognition and Treatment in a Low Endemic Setting

David M Scollard

BACKGROUND

More and more patients with leprosy are being treated by physicians and medical officers with little or no experience with this disease. In the pre-dapsone era, leprosy was essentially incurable, and the common approach to prevention of the spread of infection was isolation in leprosaria. Physicians interested in this disease staffed these hospitals and, by experience, became "leprologists"; at some institutions, leprosy subspecialists developed in such areas as ophthalmology, otolaryngology and reconstructive surgery. These leprologists were familiar with many clinical manifestations of this disease and its complications.

With the discovery of the effectiveness of injectable sulfones in 1940s,[1] cure of *Mycobacterium leprae* infection became feasible, radically changing the prognosis for leprosy patients. By the early 1950s, oral dapsone had been proven effective,[2] and this inexpensive drug was distributed to leprosaria all over the world.

As a result of effective outpatient treatment, many leprosaria were closed over the following decades, and others were transformed into care facilities for those who were severely disabled, but were no longer infected with *M. leprae*. The implementation of chemotherapy and leprosy control was accomplished in many countries through "vertical" programs, with senior administrators in ministries of health and a staff of health workers dedicated to control of this disease. Often, these programs were descendants of the same ministries' administration of leprosaria. Beginning in the 1980s, the World Health Organization's leprosy elimination program promoted outpatient treatment and "horizontal" integration of leprosy care into the general health care system.[3]

The end of compulsory quarantine and the advent of routine outpatient management of this disease were great steps forward for patients and their families. But the closure of leprosaria has also meant the loss of centers for training physicians in the diagnosis and treatment of this disease, even though transmission of the infection continues. New cases are still diagnosed every year in almost every nation in the world, either due to transmission within the country or as a result of rapid travel and migration between countries. Over the decades, however, fewer and fewer physicians have had experience with this disease. Today, therefore, the problem with leprosy for physicians is not that it is incurable (as was believed in the past), but that to most doctors it is unimaginable that they will ever see a patient with this disease. As a result, too often it is not included in the differential diagnosis when patients present with chronic skin lesions, peripheral neuropathy, or with rheumatic and systemic symptoms of leprosy reaction.

WHAT IS LOW ENDEMIC?

Epidemiological criteria (see chapter No. 2 on Epidemiology of Leprosy), historical experience and geographic factors may all contribute to the working definition of a "low endemic" leprosy situation. The World Health Organization's Expert Committee in 1980 adopted a definition of the "elimination of leprosy as a public health problem" as a known prevalence of less than 1 case/10,000 population.[3] Since this has been the operating definition for national leprosy programs worldwide for more than three decades, a level below this may be considered an appropriate epidemiological definition of low endemicity.

Historical factors should probably also be considered. Countries such as India, which were highly endemic for centuries and which have only recently reached the goal of 1/10,000, represent situations in which a good case can be made for retaining some leprosy referral hospitals, since they may see a relatively large number of new patients as well as late complications of leprosy for some time to come.

The "low endemic" situation is becoming more common worldwide as treatment reduces the number of patients in many countries. Increasingly, diagnosis and treatment of leprosy will be organized on a "low endemic" model, continuing the de-emphasis of vertical types of programs with staff dedicated to this one disease, and emphasizing integration of leprosy care into the general medical program.

The old "vertical" approach—leprosy hospitals, leprologists, and dedicated nursing and administrative staff—is rapidly becoming obsolete. Experience with "horizontal" integration of leprosy services, however, has been fraught with problems and has often resulted in a reduction of access to care and quality of care. In many cases, the integration of leprosy work into the general health services has not been carefully planned and phased in. Major cultural concerns and stigma related to leprosy have been underestimated.

INTEGRATION OF LEPROSY SERVICES INTO GENERAL HEALTH CARE

Attempts to promote the treatment of this disease within any and all general medical facilities have also been problematic due to the over simplification of this disease and underestimation of the requirements needed to diagnose and treat it properly.[4] A realistic approach to leprosy in low-endemic settings must balance the facts that:
- Leprosy is a rare disease in these settings
- This is a complex disease for which some patients may require specialized expertise
- After cure of infection, neurological sequelae represent another set of chronic problems. Patients with neuropathy and disabilities will need periodic medical attention for the rest of their lives.

Although national medical systems in some countries assume and expect that patients will receive competent, appropriate care in all clinics, experience has indicated that health workers may find many excuses to delay or avoid treating leprosy patients. Patients and their families will greatly benefit if planning and policy-making accommodate the fact that some physicians are unwilling to manage patients with this disease over a long course of treatment, either because they are frightened or because they feel unprepared. Education is a powerful tool to combat both fear and ignorance, but not all physicians will take the time to learn about leprosy, given the myriad pressures and demands on physician time.

An alternative to either the "vertical" or "horizontal" approach to health care for neglected tropical diseases has recently been described by Dr. Jim Yong Kim, President of the World Bank, as a "diagonal" approach.[5] Such an approach adopts selected features of both vertical and horizontal programs.

GOALS AND REQUIREMENTS OF LEPROSY SERVICES IN LOW ENDEMIC SITUATIONS

Any contemporary plan for leprosy services must begin with the understanding that today the overall goal of leprosy treatment is to prevent or arrest the trajectory of disability due to nerve injury (Fig. 53.1). With currently available methods, the suggested paradigm for such a program is: *Early Diagnosis + Complete Treatment → Reduced Disabilities*. In settings in which leprosy is rare, the normal challenges of this disease are compounded by lack of awareness in the general population and among physicians as well. In such a setting, a national program must seek to accomplish the following objectives:
- Provide a high quality of outpatient care to all patients in all geographic areas:
  - Long-term medical treatment to cure the infection
  - Medical management of complications (reactions and neuritis)
  - Prevention of and rehabilitation for disabilities
- Maintain expertise in specialized areas such as:
  - Diagnosis and histopathology. The less experience a physician has with leprosy, the more valuable is biopsy confirmation and classification of the disease, as well as a biopsy at 1–2 years to assess resolution of the infection during treatment
  - Recognition and management of eye complications
  - Reconstructive surgery
- Maintain physician awareness throughout the country by continuous educational and training activities
- Maintain active research and collaboration with medical schools or other leprosy programs. This is essential in order to maintain intellectual vigor and to update standards of care resulting from new discoveries. Without such activities and collaboration, a program is likely to become isolated and ineffective, especially in a low endemic setting.

THE UNITED STATES EXPERIENCE AS A MODEL FOR MANAGEMENT OF LEPROSY IN A LOW ENDEMIC SITUATION: CARVILLE 2.0

The United States has always been a "low endemic" country for leprosy. This disease did not exist in the Western hemisphere until after European settlers arrived, but by the mid-1700s a few cases were described in what is now southern Louisiana.[6] A hospital for leprosy patients had

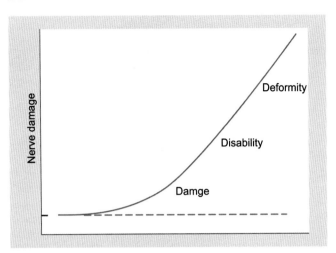

Fig. 53.1: Goal of leprosy services: to prevent or arrest the trajectory of disability in leprosy. The course of nerve function impairment in leprosy is shown schematically. The dotted line indicates the ideal result of no nerve impairment if leprosy is diagnosed early and treatment is completed. The solid line indicates the consequences if the disease is not diagnosed early or if treatment is delayed or incomplete, allowing nerve injury to progress to disability and deformity. "Disability" is used here to represent WHO Grade 1 disability (anesthesia), and "Deformity" to represent WHO Grade 2 disability (muscle weakness or paralysis with visible deformity)

been established at Carville, Louisiana, and in 1921 this became the national leprosarium, operated by the federal government. At its peak in the 1940s, 400–500 patients lived at Carville, where facilities had been built on the hospital grounds to offer long-term living accommodations, as well as churches, a theater and many other attributes of a small community. During the 1940s, doctors at Carville discovered the effectiveness of dapsone to treat infection with *M. leprae*, and by 1950 this treatment was standard at Carville. Subsequently, some patients were cured of the infection and were permitted to leave the hospital. At the same time, outpatient treatment of leprosy became more common and the number of new patients' admissions also declined. Since the 1970s, the number of new cases in the United States has ranged from 150–200 annually. The Laboratory Research Branch of the National Hansen's Disease Programs (NHDP) moved to the campus of Louisiana State University in 1992, and in 1999, the Clinical and Rehabilitation Branches moved into outpatient clinic facilities in Baton Rouge. Thus, after more than 100 years of inpatient care, the NHDP has become a fully outpatient program, with a network of clinics around the country.

Today there are two sources of patients in the United States. The majority of patients were born in or traveled to other countries in which leprosy is more highly prevalent (NHDP site). However, the single country from which the United States receives the largest number of patients is the United States itself (www.hrsa.gov/hansensdisease). Genotyping studies have provided convincing evidence that these autochthonous cases arise by transmission from wild-infected, nine-banded armadillos to humans.[7]

Although the overall number of cases of leprosy in the United States is relatively small, as a zoonosis it is highly unlikely that it can be eliminated. Thus, the United States will remain a low endemic country for the foreseeable future, and this may also be true for other countries in the Western Hemisphere. In other parts of the world, human-human transmission is likely to continue in some regions for a variety of reasons such as geographic isolation, regional conflict, and possibly in small populations with unique genetic susceptibility. In all of these situations, the need remains for the provision of good medical services for leprosy and sustaining medical expertise related to this disease.

In the United States, as in other large countries, a relatively small number of cases are distributed over a large geographic area (Fig. 53.2). Until the middle of the last century, patients from all over the United States were sent to the national leprosarium at Carville, Louisiana. After the discovery of the effectiveness of dapsone at Carville, treatment of leprosy in the United States became increasingly dependent on outpatient care. Admission of new patients to the hospital ceased, although patients with long-term disabilities continue to be cared for on an inpatient basis and an outpatient clinic remains at the headquarters of the National Hansen's Disease Programs in Baton Rouge, LA, not far from the historic site at Carville.

To effectively care for patients in other regions of the United States, a network of regional clinics has been established (Fig. 53.2). These operate under contracts from the NHDP, and are staffed by physicians who follow several patients and maintain expert skills in the diagnosis and management of leprosy. Most of these physicians are affiliated with medical schools and teaching hospitals; several of them are among the most outstanding physicians in their fields. These satellite clinics thus provide opportunities for teaching and training related to leprosy, attracting interest among students and medical residents. Importantly, for individual medical and scientific reasons these physicians have an interest in the treatment of this disease, and other physicians in nearby communities refer patients to them. Because of their individual interest and the referral of patients, their expertise in leprosy is maintained. These clinics also provide medication, regular sensory and muscle testing, and services for the prevention of disability, all supported by the NHDP at no cost to patients.

Increasingly, however, patients with leprosy in the United States are presenting to physicians far from these satellite clinics. These patients are cared for by individual physicians in their communities who indicate a willingness to do this,

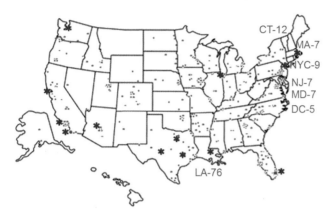

Fig. 53.2: Distribution of physicians caring for leprosy patients in the United States, 2000–2009. This map illustrates the wide geographic distribution of physicians treating leprosy patients in the United States over the decade from 2000–2009. Federally funded Hansen's disease clinics are located in cities indicated by blue stars. Individual physicians treating one or more patients are shown as red points. (Data are not shown for Hawaii, where several private physicians provide care coordinated by the State Department of Health)

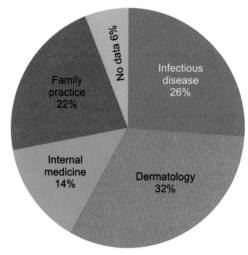

Fig. 53.3: Specialties of private physicians caring for leprosy patients in the United States. In 2010, a telephone survey was conducted contacting the last 100 private physicians who had been involved in treating Hansen's disease patients in the United States. The results indicate that physicians in four major specialties were involved in caring for patients (six physicians declined to provide information)

with support from the NHDP headquarters. A survey of 100 of these private physicians, usually treating only 1–2 patients, revealed that the majority of them are in dermatology, infectious disease, family medicine and internal medicine (Fig. 53.3). The unique medical, scientific and social aspects of leprosy are invariably intriguing to selected physicians who are inspired to work with patients who have this disease. This model builds on the interest of such physicians, rather than assuming that all physicians will have such an interest.

Through its federal funding, the NHDP headquarters offers specialized leprosy-related services at no cost to patients. This includes biopsy diagnosis and molecular diagnostic techniques, when indicated, and the provision of all anti-leprosy medication through their physician. Telephone and video consultations with NHDP clinicians are available as needed for patients who develop reactions, neuritis or other complications. Finally, for cases with complications beyond the capability of these physicians, short-term referrals to the NHDP can be arranged.

The NHDP recommends a more intensive multi-drug treatment (MDT) regimen than is recommended by the WHO and used in most countries (Table 53.1). Rifampicin and dapsone are recommended for tuberculoid (paucibacillary) patients, but both drugs are given daily; one full year of treatment is recommended. For lepromatous patients clofazimine is added to this regimen, also given daily, and the 3-drug combination is recommended for duration of 2 years. If any of these drugs cannot be used due to allergy, intolerance or interaction with other medications,

minocycline, clarithromycin or levofloxacin are substituted. A review of the United States' experience with these regimens, in patients followed for 15 years, found no relapse among 150 patients who had been treated with the recommended protocols, compared to one suspected relapse in 150 patients who had been treated with other protocols.[8]

The NHDP also conducts training programs of various types, including a comprehensive 2 days seminar, one-hour lectures at hospitals and medical schools, and instructional courses through the NHDP website. Web-based teleconferences have also been used to bring the expertise of the physicians in NHDP clinics to the benefit of physicians at other locations. Similar internet-based approaches are also being used in other countries.[9-11]

CONCLUSION

The combination of a central referral center, satellite clinics and teleconferencing has sometimes been referred to in the United States as "Carville 2.0". The central referral clinic can provide support and specialized expertise as needed. Physicians in satellite clinics see patients regularly and thus maintain their expertise. The result is a "diagonal" integrated approach. It does not imply that patients will be welcomed or treated appropriately at any clinic. The Hansen's disease clinic becomes known locally and regionally for this expertise and local physicians can refer patients to this clinic. This approach also addresses the issue of sustainability of expertise in leprosy diagnosis, treatment and rehabilitation.

Table 53.1: Multidrug treatment regimens: United States and World Health Organization

		United States[*]		WHO[**]	
	Medication	Dose	Duration	Dose	Duration
Tuberculoid (Paucibacillary)	Rifampicin	600 mg daily	12 months	600 mg monthly	6 months
	Dapsone	100 mg daily	12 months	100 mg daily	6 months
Lepromatous (Multibacillary)	Rifampicin	600 mg daily	24 months	600 mg monthly	12 months
	Dapsone	100 mg daily	24 months	100 mg daily	12 months
	Clofazimine	50 mg daily	24 months	50 mg daily + 300 mg monthly	12 months

[*]Additional information available at the NHDP website: http://www.hrsa.gov/hansensdisease/diagnosis/recommendedtreatment.html.
[**]Additional information available at the WHO website: http://www.searo.who.int/eg/Section10/Section20/Section2000.html.
Doses are reduced for children (see above websites).

Further experience will undoubtedly identify ways to use these capabilities more effectively, especially the use of videoconferencing and teleconferencing for both educational efforts and for consultations regarding individual patients. The greatest remaining challenge is to maintain the awareness of physicians that this disease does still exist and that good treatment is available. Even though most physicians in low-endemic settings will have limited experience with leprosy, with this integrated approach it is a reasonable goal that more and more physicians will be able to recognize leprosy, treat it with confidence and not be afraid of this disease.

ACKNOWLEDGMENTS

The author is grateful to Dr James Krahenbuhl, former Director of the NHDP, for his reading and helpful comments on the manuscript, and to Ms. Elizabeth Schexnyder, Curator of the National Hansen's Disease Programs Museum, for her assistance in historical research regarding Carville.

REFERENCES

1. Faget GH, Pogge RC, et al. Present status of promin treatment in leprosy. Int J Lepr. 1946;14:30-6.
2. Garrett AS. Mass treatment of leprosy with DADPS (dapsone). Lepr Rev. 1951;22(3-4):47-53.
3. World Health Organization. Chemotherapy of Leprosy for Control Programmes, in WHO Technical Report Series: Geneva; 1982.
4. Lockwood DN, Suneetha S. Leprosy: too complex a disease for a simple elimination paradigm. Bull World Health Organ. 2005;83(3):230-5. Epub 2005 Mar 16.
5. Kim JY, Chan M. Poverty, health and socities of the future. JAMA. 2013;310(9):901-2. doi: 10.1001/jama.2013.276910.
6. Badger LF. Leprosy in the United States. Public Health Rep. 1955;70(6):525-35.
7. Truman RW, Singh P, Sharma R, et al. Probable zoonotic leprosy in the southern United States. N Engl J Med. 2011;364(17):1626-33. doi: 10.1056/NEJMoa1010536.
8. Dacso MM, Jacobson RR, Scollard DM, et al. Evaluation of multi-drug therapy for Leprosy in the United States using daily rifampin. South Med J. 2011;104(10):689-94. doi: 10.1097/SMJ.0b013e31822d6014.
9. Trindade MA, Wen CL, Neto CF, et al. Accuracy of store-and-forward diagnosis in leprosy. J Telemed Telecare. 2008;14(4):208-10. doi: 10.1258/jtt.2008.071203.
10. Paixão MP, Miot HA, de Souza PE, et al. A university extension course in leprosy: telemedicine in the Amazon for primary healthcare. J Telemed Telecare. 2009;15(2):64-7. doi: 10.1258/jtt.2008.080704.
11. Ganapati R. Quality service to leprosy patients using mobile phones and pagers. Lepr Rev. 2009;80(2):232.

54
CHAPTER

Case Studies

Pankaj Sharma, Hemanta Kumar Kar, Ruchi Gupta

CHAPTER OUTLINE

- Childhood and Disease Detection
- Public Pressure for Isolation
- Shift away from the Native Land
- Choice of Profession
- The Social Mobilization of LAPS
- Family and the Children
- Embracing Christianity
- Social Implications of Disease
- No Family, Alone in the World
- The Children

- The Mission Factor
- The Religion
- Indirect Pressure for Extradition
- Treatment and Long Stays at Various Missionary Hospitals
- Move to Delhi (and no to Begging)
- Marriage and Children
- A Social Server by Heart and a Philanthropist
- The Changing Scenario
- Message

CASE STUDY NO. 1

Vitthal is a 60-year-old male, leprosy affected person (LAP) with deformities, living in a leprosy colony in Patel Nagar area in Delhi. He hails from village Madnoor (District Nizamabad, Andhra Pradesh) of South India. He got married at the age of 25 years age (around 1974), to Gango Bai, his maternal cousin. In his native area consanguineous marriages are common in the Hindu community as well. Few months after his marriage, he noticed a light colored patch over arm where he could not sense properly about touch. In 5-6 months times more similar patches developed in other body parts.

He was seen in the government hospital in Dichhpalli district in AP. That was the pre-MDT era of dapsone monotherapy, with high leprosy prevalence rates (around 18–25 per one thousand population) and dapsone was the usual drug regimen for leprosy. Also probably, isolation treatment in leprosarium was also prevalent, as seems from patient's statement that he stayed admitted in the hospital for 2 years. He remembers taking some red colored capsule once in a while, after which the urine color used to turn red for a day or two. In that period he also remembers several episodes of fever and painful nodular lesions developing (and clearing) over face and limbs.

While Vitthal was in hospital for leprosy treatment, his spouce Gango Bai never came to see him at hospital. Although she stayed at Vitthal's home, the marriage was somehow never consummated and no issues were produced out of the wedlock. By the time Vitthal came home after treatment, his wife had deserted the home. She did not reach even her parents home, instead found someone else as a life companion.

About 2–3 years later, Vitthal met Laxmi (a young woman around 17–18 years age) at Kukudpalli hospital in Andhra Pradesh. Laxmi was also a leprosy patient who used to come to the same hospital for treatment. She was also forsaken by her parents and left to herself (like Vitthal, mainly for the reason leprosy). During their acquaintance at hospital, both got friendly and started helping each other in managing their common illness. In view of the apathy seen by both, at their homes, they started living together, the bond they share even today (Fig. 54.1).

For the past around 25 years both are staying together (though their marriage could never be solemnized) as a family. They have two children, the elder is daughter, Venkatamma now around 28 years age, married to a farmer and staying in Andhra Pradesh with 3 children. The younger one is a son Raju, now around 24 years, working as shuttering

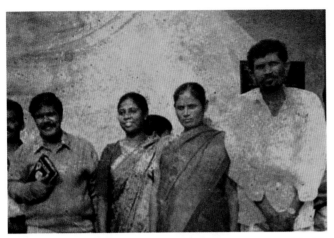

Fig. 54.1: Vitthal and his mate Laxmi (the two on extreme right) with Father of the Church and missionary workers

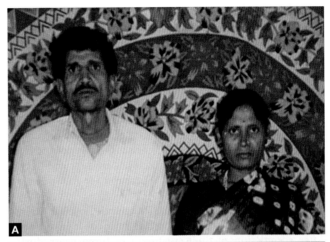

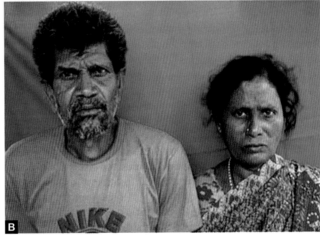

Figs 54.2A and B: Vitthal and Laxmi in the past and now (2009)

laborer in house construction business in Andhra Pradesh, he is married and has a son. All children of Vitthal and Laxmi, (Venkatamma and Raju) are healthy (and without any leprosy stigma attached to their parents), so are the grandchildren. They have settled with their families in the mainstream of society (Figs 54.2A and B).

Three years ago, the right leg of Vitthal had to be amputated below knee, for reasons of recurrent infections and subsequent gangrene, at a government hospital in east Delhi. He now wears an artificial limb, where he gets problem of stump ulcer off and on (Fig. 54.3).

Vitthal and Laxmi stay in a small colony house provided by a missionary welfare agency. They get a monthly pension (about ₹ 800 each) from the department of Social welfare, Delhi government. The medical team from Delhi state branch of Hind Kushth Nivaran Sangh (HKNS), an NGO active in the field of leprosy since 1963, visits the colony every 6 weeks and provides medication for common ailments. The arrangements are there for daily dressing of patients' ulcers, the regular supply of dressing bandages, cotton, antibiotic ointments is provided by HKNS (Delhi State Branch).

So leprosy the disease, which made Vithhal and Laxmi face apathy from home, also in a way brought them together. Their children and grand children remained free from leprosy and leprosy stigma, now well settled in the mainstream community.

CASE STUDY NO. 2

Mr P Mohan (simply called Mohan) is a 55-year-old male, treated leprosy patient living in a leprosy resettlement colony of Shalimar Bagh in Delhi. He lives with his wife Pavanamma around 50 years of age, his daughter and son-in-law, and 2 grand children also live next door.

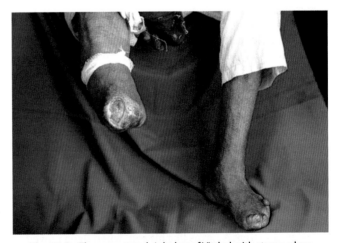

Fig. 54.3: The amputated right leg of Vitthal with stump ulcer, which troubles him off and on

We go back into past when Mohan was a young man of about 25 years (around 1979–80) living in Chingelput district of Tamil Nadu. The leprosy prevalence rates were very high in some states in those times, around 15–20 per one thousand population, Tamil Nadu being one of them. Like many other people in the area, Mohan also contracted leprosy for which he went to Chingelput leprosy hospital (Central Leprosy Training and Research Institute—CLTRI) for treatment. That was a time when it was not easy for a family to keep at home a member afflicted with leprosy (out of peer pressure from society, due to very deep stigma). Many leprosy affected patients (LAP) used to stay in leprosaria for treatment, so Mohan was also sent there.

During treatment period at Chingelput hospital Mohan met Pavanamma, who was also admitted in the leprosy home. After completion of their treatment of three years during 1980–83, both came under wedlock by simple exchange of garlands in the temple near the hospital residential complex. According to Mohan and Pavanamma, they used to come across many other patients (like them) tying the nuptial knot in the same temple, with the blessings of the hospital staff. They were blessed with two children during their stay in leprosarium, the elder one Jayanti (now 27 years age) and the younger Kumar, who died of fever at 10 years of age. However, he did not contract leprosy by then (Figs 54.4 and 54.5).

In the Mohan's native place there was no other leprosy case in his family. Pavanamma had a younger sister (Yelamma), also a leprosy patient, she received treatment from the same hospital. While on treatment at CLTRI she found a match in a hospital inmate (a leprosy patient) and married him, in the same temple at hospital area. Now she has two children (both healthy) and settled at Panipat district of Haryana.

It was not easy for Mohan and Pavanamma to go back to their native places, even after completion of their treatment, such was the stigma attached to leprosy at that time. Like many other leprosy patients, both moved to Delhi in 1989 and settled in a camp like slum colony on a piece of government land. After about 10 years of their shifting to Delhi, they found a suitable match for their daughter Jayanti and married her off to Amavas.

Amavas also had a similar trail of story behind him, he got leprosy patches when he was barely 11–12 years old. Both his parents had already died and he was staying at his maternal unlce's home in a village name Bawani (in Erode district of Tamil Nadu). He got his treatment from government hospital at Bawani, subsequently because of recurrent severe episodes of ENLs, he was referred to CLTRI, Chingelput, where he continued his treatment. After completion of his treatment, he came over to Delhi, along with another old leprosy affected person (called Baba) who used to stay at Chingelput hospital. Baba used to treat Amavas like his son, when Baba moved to Delhi, he took Amavas along (Fig. 54.6). After coming to Delhi they found a shelter in the same leprosy colony where Mohan and Pavanamma had put up.

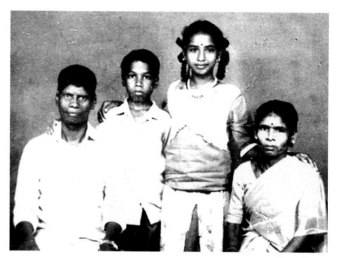

Fig. 54.4: Mohan and Pavanamma, with children Jayanti and Kumar (in 1992)

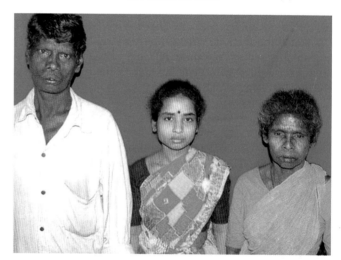

Fig. 54.5: P Mohan and Pavanamma, with their daughter Jayanti (in 2009)

Jayanti was healthy (free from leprosy) and after her marriage to Amavas, she gave birth to 2 children, Shivkamini (now 11 years and studies in class VII) and Raja now 10 years age and a student of class VI, both the children are healthy (Fig. 54.7). The colony of leprosy people at Shalimar Bagh has around 20 adults who had leprosy and some of them now live with their deformities. Around 10 of their children stay in Delhi and are day scholars in 'Nirmal Chhaya' a boarding school for children of leprosy patients, run by Department of Social Welfare, Delhi Government and located adjacent to Tihar Central prison campus.

Due to recurrent episodes of ENLs and neuritis at CLTRI, Chingelput, Amavas developed claw hands (Fig. 54.8). After he came to Delhi, he underwent reconstructive surgery done at leprosy mission hospital (Tahir Pur) in trans-Yamuna area of Delhi.

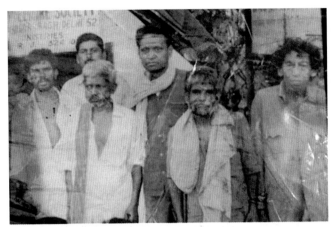

Fig. 54.6: The eternal bond of valued relationship. The man who brought Amavas to Delhi (the Baba), in front, (second from right, in blue shirt and pink scarf) and Amavas on extreme left. After Baba's death, his last rites were performed by Amavas

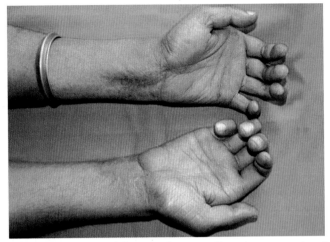

Fig. 54.8: Clawhand deformity of Amavas. Note the scar marks of reconstructive surgery over wrist areas, he underwent, which partially improved function of hands

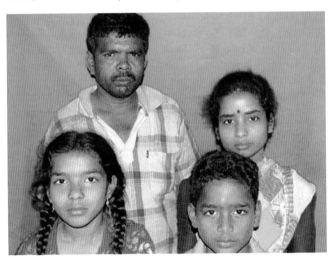

Fig. 54.7: Jayanti with husband Amavas, and children Shivakamini and Raja

It was observed that both Mohan and Pavanamma, had extensive body pigmentation after their treatment which is clearly evident in the photographs (Fig. 54.9).

It is a fact that Mohan, Pavanamma and Amavas, all suffered a lot in their lives because of leprosy, but the consolation is that their next generation is free from leprosy, and largely from the leprosy stigma. The elders hardly have anything to do other than the most usual occupation for them, i.e. begging. They start off from homes in the morning, go to their respective spots on the roads and come back by noon. Some of them again go to the begging spots in the evening also.

It may also be seen that Jayanti, who was healthy and free from leprosy, was not actually free from leprosy stigma. She married a leprosy patient with deformity (both claw hands), probably her parents did not have much option to choose a healthy match for her. But their children

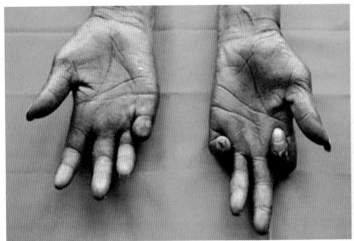

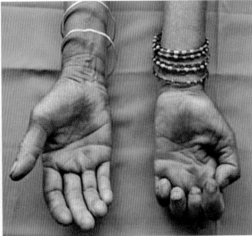

Fig. 54.9: Clawhand deformities of Mohan (left) and Pavanamma (right)

(the third generation) are going to school and would probably settle in their life with some respectable means of earning livelihood. It can be hoped they would not be carrying the burden of leprosy stigma, so it may also be hoped that, the society of the future would also be free of it. The leprosy stigma is also expected to wane out after the elimination of the disease is achieved (Fig. 54.10).

CASE STUDY NO.3

Narayan Choudhary is a 65-year-old leprosy affected person (LAP) presently living in a government set up leprosy colony of Delhi. At the first look, seeing his deformities we can make some idea/guess the problems and difficulties he must

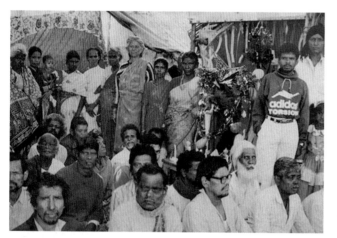

Fig. 54.10: An old picture of a community ceremonial gathering showing Mohan (sitting on left in red sweater), Pavanamma (standing back in pink sari) and Amavas (on right in brown Adidas T-shirt)

have been facing in his daily life, right from the morning till bedtime. What ... a long tale of physical and mental agonies he has faced in his life, one just can not imagine. The narration of his illness and apathy from the society surpasses all the tales of LAPs which have been heard by the authors themselves and for that matter (we believe) by all those doctors and health personnel who might have spent even 20–30 years of their career dealing with the leprosy patients.

CHILDHOOD AND DISEASE DETECTION

Narayan (a Hindu by religion) was born on 5th October 1944 in a family in Bidar district of Karnataka, which lies on the border area of three states—Maharashtra, Karnataka and Andhra Pradesh. His father was a landlord who had a large chunk of land under cultivation; he was also a fatherly figure for the whole village and the other surrounding villages. He used to support the people of the whole village with food from his grain store in the times of natural calamities like floods and famines. When Narayan was 9 years old (1953); a light colored patch was noticed by parents over his buttock region. At that time they did not have any idea about the nature of the disease, but with the passage of time it became clear that the disease he suffered from was none other than leprosy. Slowly, pressure started mounting from the villagers to isolate Narayan away from the home, and the village (Fig. 54.11).

PUBLIC PRESSURE FOR ISOLATION

Amid serious pressure from society to leave, Narayan continued to stay at home on account of show of family's financial stability and muscle power. He was also well aware of the fate of leprosy sufferers in his area at that time. They had to either leave the village voluntarily or face elimination.

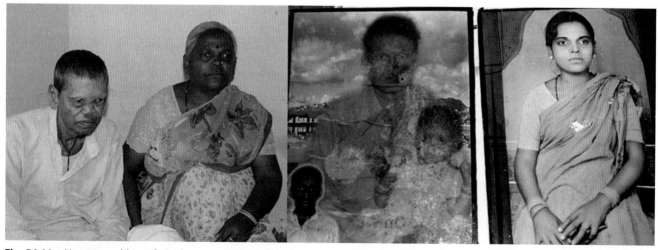

Fig. 54.11: Narayan and his wife Pushpa in 2009 (left). The old pictures of the two on the right (around 1975) when Narayan did not have deformities and Pushpa was pregnant with the eldest daughter (Ganga) and her patch on dorsum of left hand had resolved by then, after treatment with dapsone and Rifampicin

He narrated to the author, that at least 15–20 people with leprosy were burnt alive in the fields by villagers, during the time of his stay in the village. There was a collusion and secret understanding among the natives that no information about such killings used to reach the police authorities. While Narayan was at home, he kept on getting some form of treatment for his patch, which comprised some *desi* oral medicine and an oily injection (obviously he was referring to *Chaulmoogra* oil) which was injected at the periphery of the patch. After about 2 years of weekly injections the patch looked indistinct. In the meantime, his mother passed away when Narayan was just 12 years of age.

Survival by Rough and Tough Means

As the time passed by, the threat to his very existence on account of his disease was real, in spite of the treatment he took for his disease available at that time. In the process of putting stiff resistance to the society, slowly and steadily, he chose path outside the preview of the law. He got named in 14–15 cases of robbery, looting, arsoning but it was not easy for the police to book him. His modus operandi was like Robin Hood, he used to rob the riches and distribute the money to poor villagers. No one used to say anything against him to the police authorities, but ultimately the hands of the law reached him and he was imprisoned for 3 years in Bellary jail of Karnataka.

SHIFT AWAY FROM THE NATIVE LAND

By the time he came out of prison he was 23 years old, his father also expired during his imprisonment. He had virtually no family to go to, his land was also taken over by relatives. Then, on the advice of some leprosy sufferer whom he met at his native place, he moved to Delhi around 1968. He reached Delhi station, all alone in the city, had no money to feed. He stayed on the platform only, started doing the job of a coolie. He was happy to earn some quick money but this boon was also short lived. He was stopped by a policeman on duty there, on account of working as a coolie without a badge (unregistered worker); in the process he got into altercation with the policeman who was stopping him. The matter worsened as Narayan did not know Hindi and the policeman did not understand the language spoken by Narayan. Then a senior police officer (by chance a South Indian) came on the scene who understood both the languages. He pacified Narayan and made him understand that provision of carrying the badge by coolies is a must, it was meant to prevent theft of baggage by unauthorized persons on the platform. So it was not possible for Narayan any longer to stay on the railway station, he moved to a temple site in Chandni Chowk, situated opposite Red Fort.

CHOICE OF PROFESSION

Although he did not have any visible deformities due to leprosy at that time but he could identify the people with leprosy. He had developed a notion that only someone suffering from leprosy would listen to his plight in the city and would give him right advice. In front of the temple in Chandni Chowk, he met Bandhu Sen, a LAP who came from Moradabad and had settled on the pavement. His daily job (like so many other LAPs) was begging and he advised Narayan also to adopt this profession. The idea of begging did not find favor with Narayan and he preferred to work as a laborer. He joined as unskilled laborer with a contractor who was building Lajpat Rai market; the construction of which was inaugurated very recently, just across the road in front of the temple. He spent many years as a laborer in this construction work with the same construction contractor at different sites at Gandhi Nagar in trans Yamuna area and later at the new interstate bus terminus (ISBT) building near Kashmiri Gate. At ISBT work site, he came in contact with Marathi Baba, a LAP who worked as a priest and lived in Anandgram leprosy colony (Fig. 54.12). He used to move around different leprosy colonies all over Delhi for his social role as a mediator for marriage proposals among LAPs. In the same context he proposed the name of Pushpa to Narayan for marriage.

Marriage

Pushpa was a young girl of 16–17 years age (in 1973) living with her father at Anandgram, the first leprosy colony developed by missionary organization headed by Mother Teresa. Pushpa's father was a leprosy patient with severe deformities of hands and feet. She herself had a leprosy patch over dorsum of left

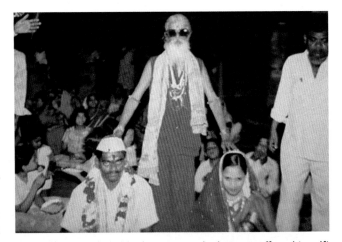

Fig. 54.12: Marathi Baba (the priest, and a leprosy sufferer himself) who made a match of Narayan and Pushpa, also solemnized the marriage of their son (performed again with Hindu rites)

hand for which she was taking treatment from the nearby municipal corporation of Delhi (MCD) dispensary at Tahir Pur. She remembers her doctor (Dr Chawla) in the dispensary who had a kind heart and was very popular among leprosy patients coming to the dispensary. The usual treatment at that time was a green colored tablet (from Ciba company, as mentioned by Pushpa), she had to go to the dispensary daily for consumption of the drug in the clinic itself, this treatment by taken by her for about 6 months. Years later, she also took Dapsone for about 4 months from Thangraj Leprosy Hospital, nearby, in the year 1982.

THE SOCIAL MOBILIZATION OF LAPS

In year 1974 Pushpa and Narayan came under wedlock and moved to a small place in Ghaziabad where Narayan opened a tea stall. In 6 months period they came to a place near Tahir Pur (close to the leprosy colony they reside now) and started a tea stall. Most of his customers were the LAPs and very few other persons (mainly those ignorant about leprosy) used to come to their teashop. While interacting with leprosy patients Narayan developed an idea to form a registered society of leprosy patients, so that they would get a piece of land to form a settlement colony with monetary help from Delhi government. He had a hard time persuading the LAPs to pay for the registration charges. He personally went to Wardha (Maharashtra), considered in those times the Mecca for LAPs, raised and maintained with the blessings of Mahatma Gandhi and Acharya Vinoba Bhave, to get the information regarding society registration. He even kept Pushpa's sarees and jewellery as security to raise money for registration fee. Ultimately the society was registered and the present day Kasturba Kushth colony came into existence at Tahir Pur, their home till date.

FAMILY AND THE CHILDREN

In the meantime, Pushpa gave birth to 5 children (four daughters and a son), the last two children being twins (Figs. 54.13 and 54.14). Narayan ran the teashop till 1994, wherein Pushpa also used to sit at for many hours to help him, besides looking after household work. Ultimately resorption of Narayan's hands and feet had progressed to a level of being nonfunctional. All his daughters completed their studies up to 10th class. The son (Parsram) could not study beyond 3rd class due to some infection persisting in the ears which made him deaf. He could not be helped for ear function much even by the reconstructive surgery. Later he learnt the job of motor mechanic. All the children were healthy, and in course of time all the daughters got married into the families who had no family member with leprosy. The son Parsram also got married to a girl without any disease in her family. Now son and daughter-in-law take care of Narayan, who has severe deformities. Narayan also owns an auto three wheeler which he lends on rent and has some earning daily.

EMBRACING CHRISTIANITY

Pushpa was from a Christian family but Narayan remained as Hindu till long. Once he had severe infection of arm (probably cellulites) he visited many doctors and even hospital, who all advised for amputation. He prayed before all Hindu Gods but his problem did not wane. Then Pushpa took him to her native place Baptala, in Vijaywara district of Andhra Pradesh to a missionary leprosy hospital (Fig. 54.15). He received treatment at that hospital for many months and his arm was saved from the suggested amputation. Moved by this severely emotional event of life, Narayan embraced Christianity

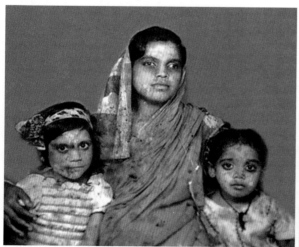
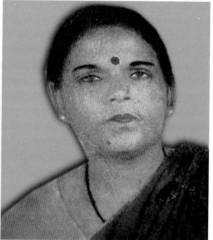

Fig. 54.13: Pushpa with two children (left) and in an old picture of time before marriage (right). She had a leprosy patch (paucibacillary) then and was taking dapsone, the only chemotherapy available at that time (around 1972)

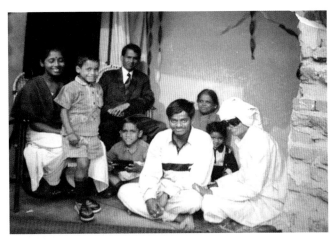

Fig. 54.14: Going without celebration? No way. Narayan celebrating 'Bara din' (X-mas) with son Parsram (sitting by him), and daughter Ganga (on chair)

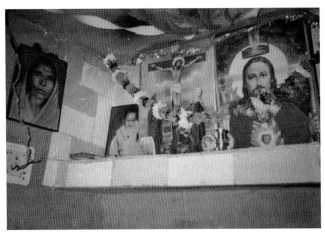

Fig. 54.16: Religion lies where heart finds solace and peace. The small 'Church' inside Narayan's house

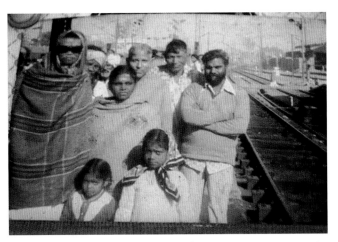

Fig. 54.15: Narayan with Pushpa and other family members in the wife's native place in Andhra Pradesh, when he was taken over there for treatment of his severe infection in arm

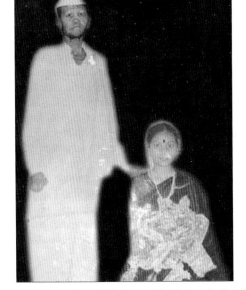

Fig. 54.17: Performed all the worldly duties of a father; with eldest daughter Ganga at her marriage

(Fig. 54.16). Of the five children of Narayan, eldest daughter Ganga is married into a Charistian family (Fig. 54.17), next 3 daughters are married in Hindu families and the son's wife is a Christian (Fig. 54.18).

Message

Narayan knew he had leprosy and the only job adopted by virtually all LAPs was begging, but he resisted this option. Rather he chose to work as a laborer, till his hands and feet remained functional. Later on when deformities and associated disabilities occurred, he changed over to lesser physically demanding work of running a teashop. He continued to take care of the tea shop till his hands and feet remained partly functional. He used his leadership quality to organize LAPs to form a society, traveled long distance all the way to Wardha for a public cause, married all his children into respectable families and remained independent throughout his life, never resorted to begging.

When society rejects someone, the new relations are made with those with similar destiny who provide some solace, irrespective of caste, religion and community. The present thrust on information, education and communication (IEC); and prevention and early detection of deformity and disability, their treatment and rehabilitation, in the newer strategy of NLEP would go a long way in preventing the similar situation, as happened with Narayan.

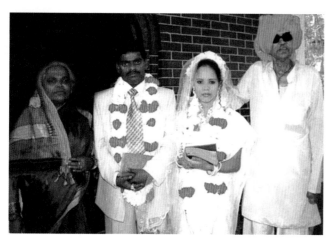

Fig. 54.18: Narayan and Pushpa at their son's wedding (according to Christian rites)

CASE STUDY NO.4

Note: The family discussed in this case study was extremely apprehensive of the social repercussions and adverse reaction from the society, especially fearfully concerned about their children who have now reached to socially reputable places in their careers. At their request, the names of characters have been changed, the names of places have been kept nonrevealing, and no photographs are presented.

Maharaj is a 60 years old (born 1949) LAP living with his wife in a colony of old leprosy patients in Delhi. He studied up to 10th standard in a leprosy mission school in Maharashtra. He was born in the family of a factory worker, long time after his parents' marriage, and so the jubilations. At the insistence of family members and friends, he was named Maharaj. After the early death of his mother Maharaj was brought up in the home of his maternal grandparents, since the age of 6–7 years, where, he joined in a local government school.

Disease Detection

At the age of around 9 years (when Maharaj was in his 3rd class) there came a health team from a government hospital for school health check-up of students. On examination Maharaj was found to have some patches over arms, which were totally asymptomatic. The disease of Maharaj was described as 'Maharog' by the health team leader and the school Principal was informed and advised to remove the child from the school immediately, lest it would be dangerous to others. In compliance with the usual practice in those days, the very next day Maharaj was sent back home where more problems were in store for him.

SOCIAL IMPLICATIONS OF DISEASE

The fact of disease was no more a secret among villagers. The grandfather of Maharaj was advised by village Pradhan, to

shift the habitat of the child to outskirts of the village for the best interest of the whole village, where there were some other people too with 'Maharog' already shifted out. In a difficult situation arising out of illness of Maharaj, the grandfather informed his father, who was living with his second wife, and working in a factory in Madhya Pradesh. On hearing about the news of Maharaj's illness, his father came and took him along. Maharaj started living with his stepmother. He used to be kept indoors completely for fear of his illness getting revealed in open. By this time Maharaj had developed sensory loss over hands and feet and other body areas, the patches were also increasing in number and size. He was allotted a separate small room in which he was made to sleep on floor. During sleep, he used to suffer rat bites, the fact coming to notice only on waking up in the morning by finding the blood stains over his clothes and on the piece of jute bed sheet on which he used to sleep.

But in course of time, Maharaj's illness was revealed to public. Soon the ladies in nearby households started advising the stepmother, to get rid of Maharaj anyhow, or else it could be dangerous to her own self. At home, Maharaj's father was also not oblivious to the fact, that his wife was adverse to keep Maharaj at home. From his side he always used to take personal care of Maharaj and make him sit for food, right with him. One day the child Maharaj noticed some hard grains in his rice, because of which he was not able to eat. He told about this to his father sitting by his side, who also tasted food in Maharaj's plate. It turned out to be powdered glass in the food, following which the father became very distressed and helpless, worrying about what to do with the child.

Leprosy Treatment

Under these gloomy circumstances in the course of discussion on "how to take care of the child" his father came across a fellow laborer working in the same factory, who knew about a leprosy mission hospital in Maharashtra. Immediately the 10-year-old Maharaj was taken by his father to that hospital. At the hospital some blood tests and skin smear examination were carried out which were all 'negative' (as described by the hospital staff). He was admitted to the hospital only for the management of ulcers. At that time *Chaulmoogra* oil was the only medication available for the treatment of leprosy. He used to get 15–16 injections every week, over different patches. Some time after the injections, the skin at the injection site turned black.

Schooling

He stayed in the hospital for 6–7 years, during which he remembered one important national event, i.e. the release of 'Naya Paisa' the new coin of one paisa by the Government of India in 1957, before that the English coins were in circulation. He had joined the school run by leprosy mission (located within the hospital campus) where he studied up to 10th class. This boarding school also admitted the children affected by leprosy from nearby villages and cities, whose parents were healthy but could not keep them at homes, out of social peer pressure. After treatment, once the children were declared cured, the children were either taken back home by the parents, or they used to spend years in the hospital complex, doing social service or working as laborers in the mission farm lands, where crops and vegetables were cultivated meant for consumption in the mission complex only. Some of them were engaged for other duties like washing and ironing clothes, as a dresser in the dispensary doing the dressings of patients, as the cook in the campus kitchen or for other such jobs in the campus. Unfortunately in the case of Maharaj, his father never visited him, once after he got admitted in the hospital.

NO FAMILY, ALONE IN THE WORLD

When Maharaj completed the study in 10th class at the age of about 17-18 years (around 1967), he came in contact with some other LAP visitors at hospital who told him that situations for LAPs were somehow better in Punjab. At that stage, he took a leap into outside world and reached in a city of Punjab where many colonies of LAPs were established with the financial contributions from many rich donors. Maharaj also landed up in one of them and he spent over 20 years in the same city, the main regular profession for LAPs was begging. After initial hiccup for roadside begging he also got engaged in this profession.

Marriage

Maharaj got married in 1979 at 30 year age with Harsha from West Bengal. The movement of LAPs used to be all over the country (but strictly within confines of the community) for social purposes like marriages, etc. The LAPs were well-informed about the eligible bachelors in the similar communities in other cities. In the process to find a match for himself, Maharaj reached West Bengal through some contact. Harsha was a young girl of 14-15 years getting treatment for leprosy from a local leprosy mission hospital. She was born in a very poor family, both her father and mother used to work as laborers. She had developed patches over the body at the age of 2-3 years but the matter remained unattended for long since the parents were not aware of the nature of illness. The only treatment administered to the child was 'Jhaar Phoonk' by the local 'Ojha' in the village. Years later when Harsha was around 14 years, she was suspected having leprosy by a leprosy patient; who happened to be a friend of her father. He took her to the same leprosy mission hospital where he himself was getting treatment, and the disease was confirmed and the treatment was started. The treatment for leprosy at that time (1979) was once a month Rifampicin capsule and

daily Dapsone. She started staying in the leprosy colony with her LAP uncle. Hardly a month passed and she was introduced to Maharaj who had gone there in search of a bride.

After marriage with Maharaj she moved to Punjab where the same treatment was continued at the local leprosy mission hospital which she took for 18 months. During the treatment in Punjab she had ulnar neuritis and developed clawing of both hands. Unfortunately this happened due to fear psychosis among patients, of using steroids for its presumed side effects; even though it was prescribed for neuritis by their doctor.

THE CHILDREN

Both Maharaj and Harsha stayed in Punjab for nearly 10 years. Begging was their main profession and both had their own begging points (spot locations) in the city. They were blessed with 2 children, elder one a boy and a girl. Concerned about the future of the children, and to keep them away from the leprosy stigma, they were sent to the missionary school in a hilly area of Uttar Pradesh. The school used to provide free education and boarding to the children of LAPs. After completion of schooling the children were fully supported for higher education in the outside (mainstream) institutions. So both children of Maharaj and Harsha completed their education up to graduation and postgraduate level, now both are settled in their respective professions.

THE MISSION FACTOR

During the study period of their children away from home, Maharaj and Harsha moved to Delhi in 1989 and settled in a leprosy colony. They got registered in the leprosy society and started getting the financial grant of ₹ 800 per month from the Department of Social Welfare (Government of Delhi). In Delhi, though Harsha went for begging for 2-3 years but Maharaj did not do so. With the financial help coming in from government, ultimately both stopped begging completely. In a long persevered thought about the role the leprosy mission played in their lives, and in the lives of their children, both Maharaj and Harsha (like far many other LAPs) feel extremely indebted and pay a thankful tribute to the mission.

In the extremely hard times for LAPs, 50–60 years ago, the mission arranged for leprosy hospitals, leprosy homes within the hospital campus or in nearby areas, schools for children of LAPs providing them free education and even hostel facilities. A fully organized chain was formed across the country. Besides, the children were well supported for higher education as well, into mainstream institutions. For example Harsha got care from mission institutions in West Bengal, Punjab, Delhi and their children got educational support from the mission in UP. So in a way it is evident how the mission was instrumental in providing care and support to those, forsaken even by their family and the society.

THE RELIGION

Both Maharaj and Harsha were Hindus and they are till date. The children, in a matter of upbringing in the mission institutions, are now baptized Christians. Both are settled in the mainstream of society and provide financial support to their parents. The parents still stay in their small quarter in the leprosy colony, away from their children lest the leprosy stigma affect their children's personal or professional lives.

Message

The earlier times portray a very gloomy picture of lives of LAPs. The job options were virtually nil (other than begging), partly on account of physical deformities due to leprosy, but more due to the attached stigma. Now the time seems to be changing, most of the new leprosy patients live with the families. The leprosy colonies in the cities now harbor old LAPs mostly burnt out cases with severe deformities. The children remain generally healthy and leading a happy prosperous life. Expectedly, in a matter of 20–30 years or less, as the older generations of LAPs will away wither from the scene, the leprosy stigma will also wane out slowly. By that time the new case detection is also expected to come down to meagre levels, and we can expect to see a leprosy free society, in real terms.

CASE STUDY NO. 5

This story describes the long run of life documentary seen by the lead character Kartik (Fig. 54.19). He is a 59-year-old (born 1950) hailing from a village in Sambalpur district of Odisha, from a farming family who owned some land in the village. The whitish patches were noted over his body at the age of 12 years, which remained undiagnosed until they were spotted by a small pox vaccination team during their visit to the village. The diagnosis of leprosy for Kartik soon came to the knowledge of villagers, and like we have seen in the previous case studies originating in other parts of the country, i.e. Maharashtra, Andhra Pradesh, Tamil Nadu and Karnataka, the same thing happened in this far eastern state of Odisha too, the pressure started building up for extradition of Kartik from the village.

INDIRECT PRESSURE FOR EXTRADITION

For the reason of robust position of Kartik's family in the village, it was not easy for the villagers to send him out of the village straightaway, instead they adopted a curvilinear course. It was known to some of the people that another leprosy affected person (LAP), was also living in village

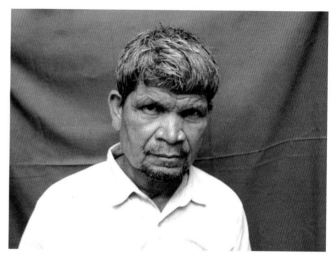

Fig. 54.19: Kartik as seen in 2009

clandestinely, with his illness under cover. In the heated environ arising out of Kartik's illness, the message also spread around about that LAP living in the village in hiding. Soon a '*Panchayat*' meeting was called, wherein it was decided to send that person out of village. Indirectly, it was a signal conveyed to the family that Kartik also could not stay in the village any longer.

Shifted to Madhya Pradesh (MP) in Search of Treatment

After leaving the village, Kartik reached a place called 'Chapa' in MP where he consulted in a private clinic. That clinic was known to be a 'specialized' clinic in the area, for leprosy treatment. No investigations were performed on Kartik and he was admitted for treatment. He received injection Penicillin, some particular soap for bath, in between he was also administered injection 'Calcium Sandoz' as recalled by Kartik. He stayed in that clinic for about 6 months and paid a sum of ₹ 22,000/- (rupees twenty two thousand was a big sum in those days around 1963, raised by the family from the sale of landed property in the village).

"Private Leprosy Hospitals" Minting Money, Well Organized Racket

Kartik used to go to a river for bath few kilometres away from the domiciliary clinic he was staying in. One day he came across some LAPs bathing at the riverside who were staying in a leprosy mission hospital, in the same city. They were well aware of the reality of the kind of leprosy clinics, Kartik was getting treatment from. There were many such residential clinics run by unscrupulous people guising as 'leprosy doctors' who (taking advantage of necessity of people to get their kin LAPs some habitat) used to charge exorbitant fee in lieu of the so called leprosy treatment. There were specially recruited agents of such hospitals whose job was to pull the new leprosy patients to the clinic, as soon as they entered the city. The agents used to place themselves at transit points like railway station, bus stands, and their main effort was to get the patients by any means to the clinic, they were working for, before the patient or his accompanying person get any hint or information about the mission hospital in the city, where treatment for leprosy was free.

The 'hospital' where Kartik got admitted comprised about 7-8 rooms accommodating 20-25 patients. At the meeting at riverside with people staying at mission hospital, they explained to Kartik that, if he really wanted to get treatment for his disease, he should either go to a mission hospital or to the government hospital at Jabalpur. Or else, these private hospitals are going to extract even the last penny from him and his family. He came back to the hospital and discussed the matter with a fellow patient and soon both of them decided to run away to Jabalpur government hospital, also called in the surrounding areas as the medical college.

They took a train for Jabalpur but at Katni railway station they were caught up by police. In those days there were instructions for police to arrest the leprosy patients from public places like bus stands, railway stations, etc. and get them admitted to the nearest government hospital for treatment. Initially, both of them got panicky where police would be taking them to, but they were relieved to know that police was taking them to the place, they themselves wanted to go to, i.e. Jabalpur Medical College.

Treatment at Jabalpur Medical College (1962–63)

Both of them were admitted to the hospital, first of all they were investigated. Slit-skin smear and biopsy were performed. By that time Kartik had developed ear lobes infiltration, and partial nasal deformity. A biweekly injection used to be given to patients. *Chaulmoogra* oil was given for massage and another ointment for application over hands and feet, which used to give a sensation of warmth. Kartik even now remembers the name of his doctor who was treating him at Jabalpur Medical College, Dr Devendra Gupta. Kartik stayed in the hospital for 4-5 months and then went back to his native village. There again, a '*Panchayat*' was called and he was allowed to stay in the village, but with some conditions. He was neither allowed to take bath in the village pond; nor was allowed to avail the services of the village barber for shaving and haircut, nor he could ask the village washerman to wash his clothes.

After staying in the village for some time, he was sent to his maternal uncle who used to live at a place called Ropia (near Sambalpur, Odisha) where he stayed for nearly one and a half year. At that place he started getting reactional episodes but there was no treatment for it in the village. He again went to Jabalpur and got admitted in the medical college and same treatment was resumed.

After some time he started working as a helper in a hotel nearby where he was happy to earn some money. One day, his treating doctor at the hospital Dr Devendra Gupta came to that hotel to have some snacks. He was happy to see Kartik working there and earning a livelihood for himself. Dr Gupta was a frequent guest at the hotel and the hotel owner was also friendly with him. Kartik can not recollect what transpired between Dr Gupta and the hotel owner, but the very next day Kartik lost his job.

He went to the residence of Dr Gupta in protest, under the impression that he was responsible for making him lose his job by revealing his illness. But Dr Gupta pacified him that it was not at all the matter, and the choice of keeping or not keeping a worker rests with the hotel owner. He also advised Kartik to go to the new missionary leprosy hospital at Sambalpur for further treatment, which would also be nearer to his native village, and convenient for him.

TREATMENT AND LONG STAYS AT VARIOUS MISSIONARY HOSPITALS

The usual treatment for leprosy at mission hospital at Sambalpur included *Chaulmoogra* oil orally (given with '*Batasha*'; a sweet preparation). *Chaulmoogra* oil was also given as intra-lesional injections. It may be noted, no dapsone was available. Tablet APC (a very popular combination of acetyl salicylic acid, phenacetin and caffeine, as a pain reliever tablet around 1960s to 1980s, especially in government hospital supplies) was the usual treatment for pain due to neuritis or reactions. Kartik stayed in that hospital for 3 years, subsequently he moved to the leprosy mission hospital at Naini, near Allahabad (UP). The treatment at Naini hospital comprised dapsone (called popularly by staff and patients as DDS) and it was available in three strengths, i.e. 25, 50 and 100 mg. Besides these, injection calcium gluconate was also given.

At hospital most of the admitted patients were engaged in community services in the hospital complex. Kartik worked as cook in the hospital kitchen at the salary of ₹ 3 per month. Subsequently he moved to mission hospital at Taran Taran in Punjab, with some fellow LAPs, where he stayed for 2 years and worked as laborer. He also traveled a lot with LAP friends to Bhav Nagar (Gujarat), Soroh (district Etah in UP), then to Shahjehan Pur (near Lucknow). In the last mentioned city he, for the first time, resorted to begging. He joined the group of LAPs engaged in begging, the gang was called among its members as the 'Company'. He started moving with the company from city to city, Nazibabad (UP), Moga (Punjab) and other cities, with the common job everywhere, begging. During his stay in Punjab, Kartik got the company of Vimla, a leprosy patient in the local colony, subsequently both started living together (Fig. 54.20).

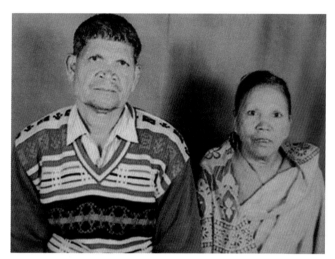

Fig. 54.20: Kartik with Vimla, whom he met in the leprosy colony in Punjab

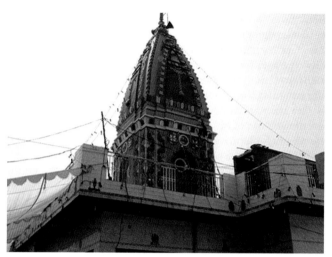

Fig. 54.22: The temple in the leprosy colony campus in Delhi, for which Kartik made considerable efforts in raising funds

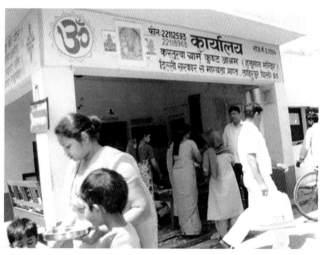

Fig. 54.21: The donors at the colony are the usual sites. Distribution of food grains, cooked food, clothes is regular

MOVE TO DELHI (AND NO TO BEGGING)

At the time of riots following assassination of PM Indira Gandhi (November 1984), he was in Punjab. After that he and Vimla moved to Delhi and landed up in the leprosy colony he is residing in even to this day. In Delhi they got registered in the society of leprosy affected people in the colony set up by Delhi Government (Fig. 54.21). Both started getting a monthly pension of ₹ 800 p.m., subsequently Kartik firmly made up his mind and stopped begging altogether, he never begged in Delhi.

Here in the colony, he got engaged in social work, mobilized donations from various donors and got a temple

constructed in the colony campus (Fig. 54.22). He helped many other leprosy affected persons in getting their pensions approved, helped in their papers and documentations, taking them to courts for affidavits, etc. He also helped in school admissions of many children of the colony.

In the meantime, Kartik and Vimla were blessed with a daughter. They sent her to local school where she grew up with good academic records. Now their daughter is a student of nursing at the Christian Nursing School at Jagadhari (Haryana). She never suffered from leprosy and is looking forward to settle in her life with a career as a nurse, free also from the leprosy stigma.

CASE STUDY NO. 6

Akbar Ali (born 1965) affectionately called Raju by all, basically hails from Dibrugarh district of Assam, where his father was a motor mechanic. He was the only child of his parents. After an early death of his father (Raju was barely 5 years of age then) his mother moved with him to Delhi in 1969 for making a livelihood. His mother started working as an 'Aaya' (governess) in a school and also stitching clothes at home. Raju was admitted in a mission school with hostel facility, where he continued his education till 8th class.

Disease Detection, Treatment as Hospital Inmate, in the Role of Patient and Server

When Raju was 10 years old few indistinct patches started appearing on his body but since there was no significant problem, they were ignored. About 5 years later, when Raju was in 8th class (15 years of age), he was sent to a charitable nursing home for check up and his illness was diagnosed as leprosy. Raju's illness was not disclosed to Raju or his mother, though it was revealed to the hostel in-charge. The hostel administration was not in favor of keeping Raju in the school hostel and he was referred to Mother Teresa Mission Hospital (Figs 54.23 and 54.24) in Nand Nagri (trans-Yamuna area), Delhi, for treatment. He got admitted for treatment in the hospital where besides his treatment, he also started learning the methods of dressing the leprosy patients. Soon he started working as a dressing helper in the hospital. He continued his further studies side by side from open school in which he continued till 10th class. During his tenure as a dresser in the hospital he was sent to Mission Leprosy Hospital and Training Centre at Chittaranjan (West Bengal) for a 6-month training course in physiotherapy. On his return he was positioned in the hospital in dual role as senior dresser and the physiotherapist. He worked in the hospital for 5 years, honorary—without taking any wages.

MARRIAGE AND CHILDREN

During his stay in job at the hospital he came in contact with 17 years old Rosy, who was not a leprosy patient but a worker as a cook in the hospital kitchen (Fig. 54.25). Hailing from a poor family from Tata Nagar (now in Jharkhand) she was left in the Hospital service by her parents. After some time both got married and Rosy (a Christian before) became Rosy Begum after marriage. After marriage, to meet the expenses of the family, both of them left the Mother Teresa hospital and settled in a leprosy colony at Tahir Pur, set up by Delhi Government. Raju started working as a building supervisor and was also engaged in social service, helping people in their various matters.

Raju and Rosy got blessed with 3 children, all of them were sent to school. The eldest daughter is now a nursing student in GTB Hospital School of Nursing, Delhi. The second child has been sent to Mission school at Dehradun and the youngest son is studying in 6th class (Fig. 54.26).

A SOCIAL SERVER BY HEART AND A PHILANTHROPIST

Rosy was also educated till 10th class and after settling in the colony both (Raju and Rosy) started giving tuitions at home to poor children of the colony free of charge for many years, and later at very nominal charges, the kind of social service which they do even to this day (Figs 54.23, 54.27 to 54.29). Raju works as a daily wages employee in Municipal Corporation of Delhi. He has a great passion of helping others and spends his free time in such activitie. Be it admission of child in school,

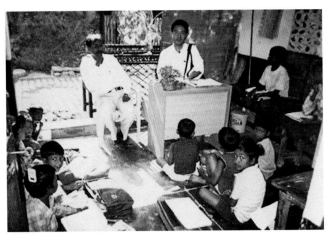

Fig. 54.23: A foreign visitor at the small school of Raju and Rosy

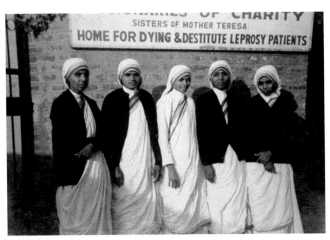

Fig. 54.24: Sisters of Mother Teresa leprosy hospital where Raju and Rosy worked and came under wedlock

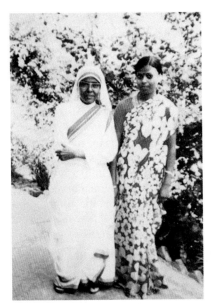

Fig. 54.25: Rosy (before marriage) with a Sister nun at Mother Teresa Hospital while she worked there as a cook

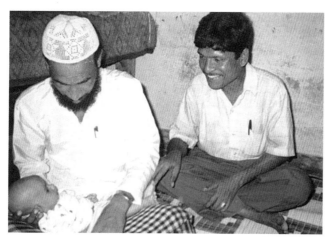

Fig. 54.26: Akbar Ali (Raju) at the naming ceremony of his son

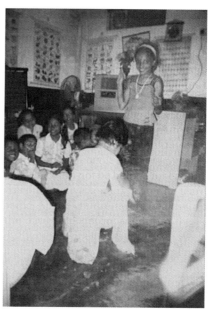

Fig. 54.28: Children performing at a function at the small school run by Raju and Rosy on charitable basis for the children of leprosy affected persons in the colony

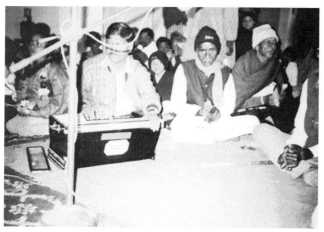

Fig. 54.27: Raju performing at a community function in the leprosy colony

or arranging for donors for some poor girl's marriage in the community, he is always ready and ahead.

The first author of this chapter also visits various leprosy colonies for social service at the weekends, as a Medical Officer of the mobile clinic team, run by Delhi State branch of Hind Kushth Nivaran Sangh. On follow-up the patients are looked after very well by Raju, from arranging for medication if a patient is not able to go to the market, taking the patients for investigations and reporting the author about any urgent development in the course of illness of any patient.

Leprosy Treatment Regime at Mother Teresa Hospital (Fig. 54.29)

Although in 1970–71 when Raju got the treatment for his disease, Dapsone, Rifampicin and Lamprene had become available, but the usual practice was administration of dapsone

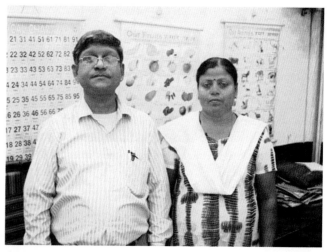

Fig. 54.29: Akbar Ali (Raju) with Rosy at the small class room in their house in the leprosy colony where children of leprosy affected persons from neighborhood are taught (tuition) at very nominal charges

monotherapy to all patients, and other two drugs only in cases when patches became red (in reaction). Other treatment for leprosy in practice was injection Calcium gluconate of which 10 mL used to be given I/V, the purpose being (as told to the patients) "to induce sweating" in the dry patches. For nerve pain, injection Neurobion, tablet B complex, and Tablet APC were the usual treatments. For deformities of hands and feet, hot wax bath and finger massage were the routine.

Mother Teresa Hospital, an Institutional Leprosy Care Home (Fig. 54.30)

As has been stated in previous case studies about the institutional nature of patient care at most of the mission hospitals providing treatment to leprosy patients, this hospital was also no exception. Most of the inmates were employed in the campus itself, in various occupations of farming, growing vegetables, ward boys, dressers (like Raju), security guards and so on.

Message

Raju lost his father at a very young age and had to move to Delhi with mother. He was the only child of his parents, both of whom were free from leprosy. His illness was limited, he got prompt treatment (whatever was available those days) and he never developed any deformity.

But the fact worth noting is that after spending so much time in the leprosy hospital, dealing with all sorts of leprosy patients, and subsequently after leaving the hospital and spending so many years living in the leprosy colony, he never developed any complex in his psyche of being a leprosy patient. Today most of the old leprosy patients with deformities are in the psyche of "takers" who begged all their lives. The reason could be that Akbar Ali did not have to face the discrimination on account of being in a big city like Delhi, when he developed the disease. Had he been in some remote rural areas (as like many other patients described in previous case studies), the things could have been different.

So it would not be inappropriate to say that leprosy debilitates the patient's body, but the stigma debilitates the mind and the patient's psyche as a whole, greatly shaking the patient's confidence and self-esteem. He is driven so much

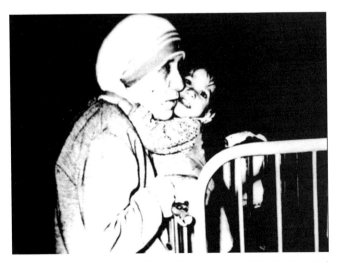

Fig. 54.30: Mother Teresa with a child during her visit to the hospital named after her, where both Raju and Rosy worked together

to the brink that he is left with no option except begging to earn a livelihood, the usual escape route to survival followed by most of the leprosy patients.

The persons with serving inclination and philanthropic thinking are difficult to come across in today's materialistic world. Both Raju and Rosy have set an example worth emulation not only for leprosy patients; but also the healthy members of the society.

CASE STUDY NO. 7

THE CHANGING SCENARIO

Mr Asad Mahmood was born in a middle class family of a small village in, Uttar Pradesh, India headed by his father Mr Mehfuz Ali who was a farmer by occupation and mother Mrs Rabia Khatoon who was house wife. He got good education in school till 12th when he got married to a beautiful girl of their community at the age of 18 and became father at the age of 20. Mr Asad got a clerical job in bank.

Disease Detection

At the age of 35 years Mr Asad started developing bending of little finger, after a few months he noticed that he was not able to feel anything on that finger. As it was his left hand he was not worried and the life went on by its usual pace.

After 6 years of relatively peaceful life, Mr Asad started noticing sensory loss and weakness in right hand too. He discussed this with his friend in bank who told him that this could be *kusht rog*. Due to stigma associated with disease he did not disclose his problem to any one in family but started maintaining distance from his wife and children. His son Fahim who was in class 12th noticed bending of finger of his father and told him that his friend's father also had similar illness for which he was undergoing treatment from health center and asked him to visit a doctor for check-up (Figs 54.31 and 54.32). But Asad did not listen to his son. Inspite of having good basic education stigma of being diagnosed as leprosy made him visit a *peer baba* who advised him to wear some *Taabiz* that could cure him. *Baba* told him, "*Beta Faalij Ka Asar Hai*" (Son it's a form of paralysis). *Baba* asked him to wait for few days for the results. The wait was very long and Asad gave up idea of waiting. He went to a local quack who gave him some powdered medications but that also did not work.

As the days of wait were prolonging, Mr Asad's hope of getting cured of the problem started dwindling. After about 6–7 months Asad started having pain and redness over face which was very horrible for him. His son who was seeing his father in a phase of agony decided to call a PHC Doctor, who was the father of his school friend. After a prolonged talk the doctor could convince Asad that it could be "*kusht rog* (leprosy)" which is completely curable and advised him

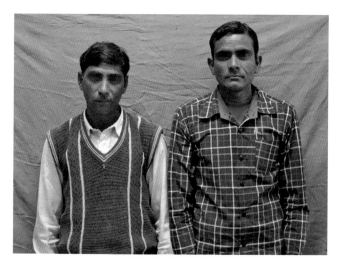

Fig. 54.31: Mr Asad (Left) with his son (Right)

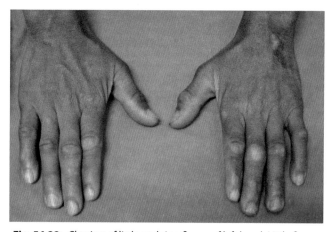

Fig. 54.32: Clawing of little and ring finger of left hand. Little finger of right hand is also showing clawing

to visit his PHC and Dr RML Hospital, Delhi for '*chamdi ki jaanch*' (slit skin smear and skin biopsy), for definite diagnosis, treatment and management of reaction.

The name of *kusht rog* was terrifying for Asad and he started maintaining a distance from his wife and children. Next week his son took him to Dr RML Hospital. Hours of waiting in Dermatology OPD might be too long, but seeing lots of people with multiple skin problems around him, gave him a feeling that he is not the only one cursed by God. Finally his wait was over and he was examined and counseled by the doctor about his illness. His son was also counseled. After relevant investigations he was started on MDT (multidrug therapy) and steroids for reaction on the same day. It was told to him that he could get MDT and steroid from the PHC doctor free of cost. However, he decided to come to Delhi for better follow-up (to see the progress) every month. His anxiety of transmitting his disease to his family members was also curtailed. All his family members were advised to visit nearest PHC doctor for complete check-up to exclude leprosy among family members. His son took all the family members to PHC for examination.

Asad came back to his village and started treatment from PHC where he got the treatment free of cost. The inflammation of face had a dramatic response in 3 weeks and that made Asad hopeful of getting completely cured.

He visited ULC of RML Hospital next month where the doctor was satisfied by his improvement of reaction and advised him to continue MDT and steroid from PHC. Necessary physiotherapy advice was given by the physiotherapist of the hospital for hand deformities. He completed his MDT and treatment for reaction including deformity without break. The happiness came back to family once again. At end of the year Asad was so happy that it was difficult to describe and became an brand ambassador for NLEP for his village and surrounding area.

MESSAGE

Stigma on leprosy not only exists among the poor and uneducated mass, but also among educated middle and higher class families. Constant endeavor must be stressed on IEC program. The help of cured patients must be taken for success of IEC program under NLEP.

Photo Gallery

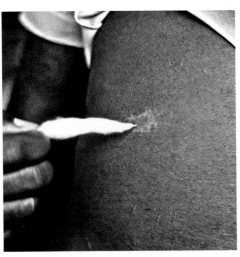

Fig. 1: Indeterminate leprosy evolving into tuberculoid leprosy

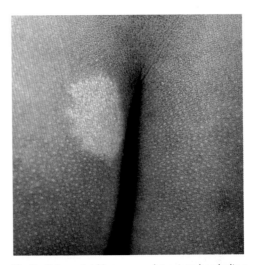

Fig. 3: Tuberculoid leprosy evolving into borderline tuberculoid leprosy

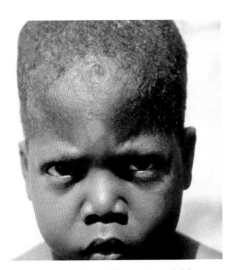

Fig. 2: Tuberculoid leprosy in a child

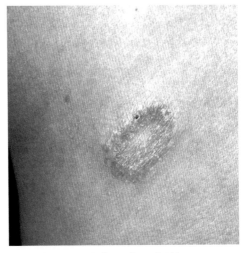

Fig. 4: Borderline tuberculoid leprosy

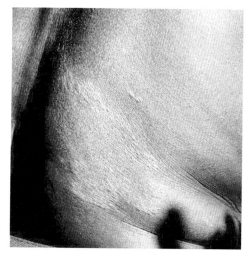

Fig. 5: Borderline tuberculoid leprosy

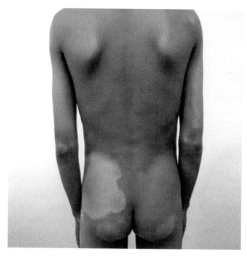

Fig. 8: Borderline tuberculoid leprosy (multiple lesions)

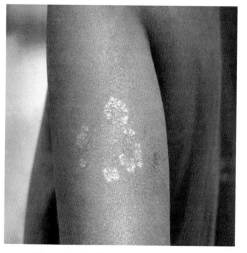

Fig. 6: Borderline tuberculoid leprosy

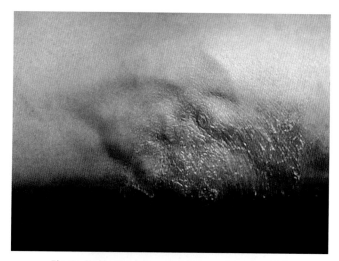

Fig. 9: Borderline tuberculoid in type I reaction (RR)

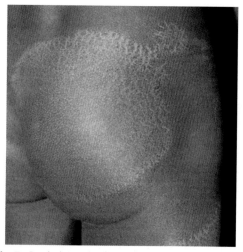

Fig. 7: Borderline tuberculoid leprosy (multiple lesions)

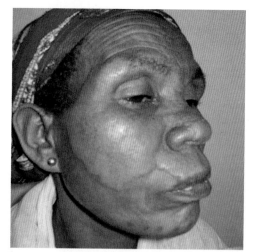

Fig. 10: Borderline tuberculoid in type I reaction (RR)

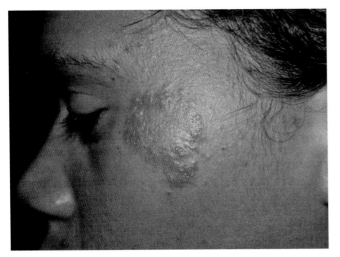

Fig. 11: Borderline tuberculoid in type I reaction (RR)

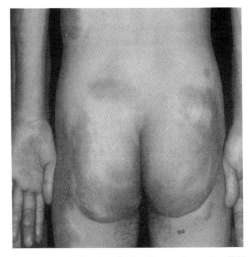

Fig. 14: Borderline borderline in type I reaction (RR)

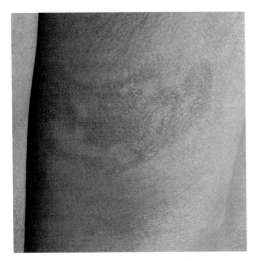

Fig. 12: Borderline borderline leprosy

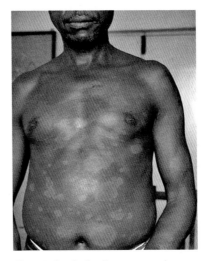

Fig. 15: Borderline lepromatous leprosy

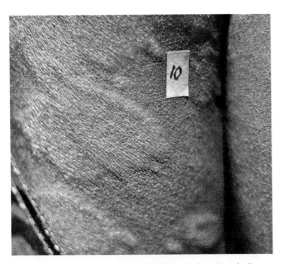

Fig. 13: Borderline tuberculoid/Borderline borderline in type 1 reaction (RR)

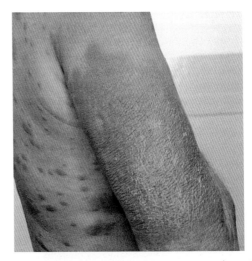

Fig. 16: Borderline lepromatous leprosy in reversal reaction

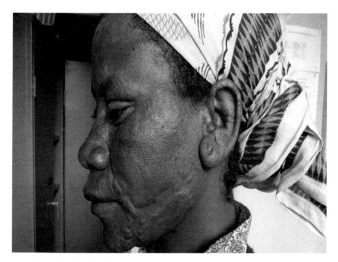

Fig. 17: Borderline lepromatous leprosy in reversal reaction

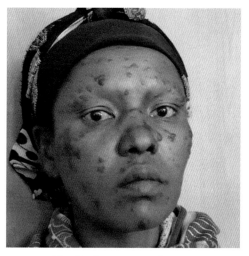

Fig. 20: Lepromatous leprosy

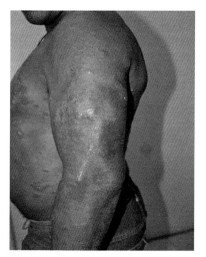

Fig. 18: Borderline lepromatous/lepromatous leprosy in type I and type II reaction

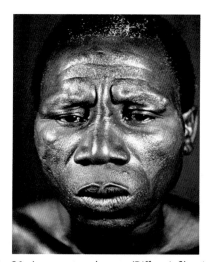

Fig. 21: Lepromatous leprosy (Diffuse infiltration)

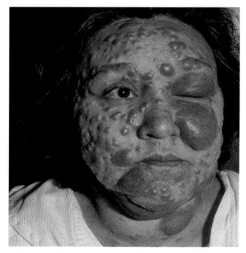

Fig. 19: Borderline lepromatous leprosy in reversal reaction

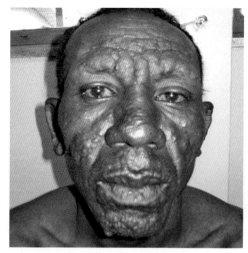

Fig. 22: Lepromatous leprosy (Nodular infiltrative lesions)

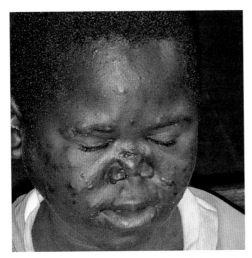

Fig. 23: Lepromatous leprosy with nasal destruction

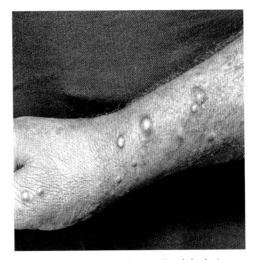

Fig. 26: Lepromatous leprosy (Nodular lesions resembling histoid lesions)

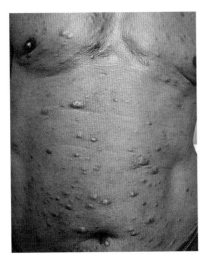

Fig. 24: Lepromatous leprosy (Nodular lesions)

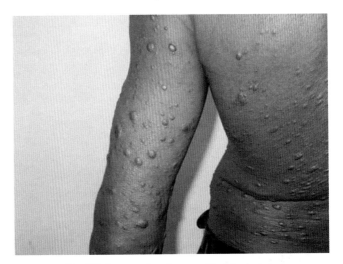

Fig. 27: Lepromatous leprosy (Nodular lesions resembling histoid lesions)

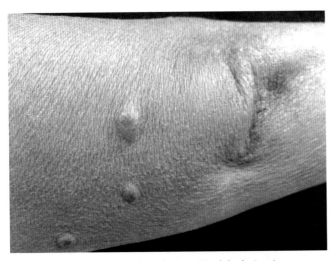

Fig. 25: Lepromatous leprosy (Nodular lesions)

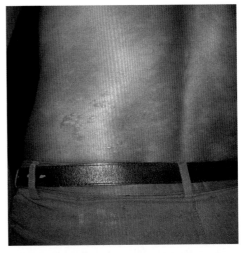

Fig. 28: Histoid leprosy in an HIV positive patient

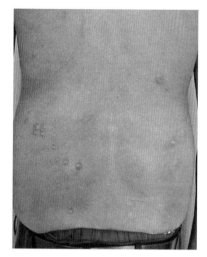

Fig. 29: Histoid leprosy

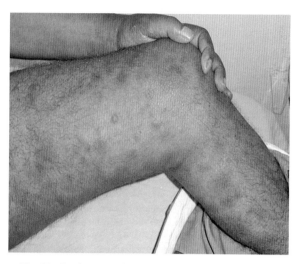

Fig. 32: Erythema nodosum leprosum (Nodular lesions)

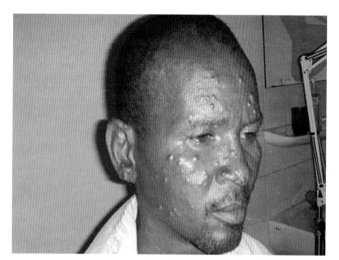

Fig. 30: Histoid leprosy in an HIV positive patient

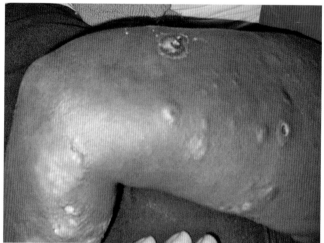

Fig. 33: Erythema nodosum leprosum (Necrotic lesions)

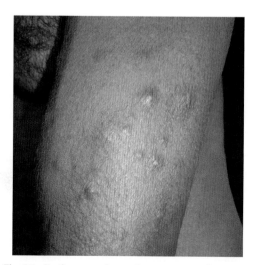

Fig. 31: Erythema nodosum leprosum–type II reaction (Nodular lesions)

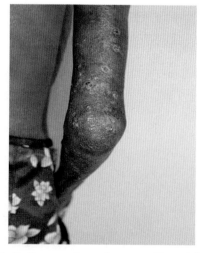

Fig. 34: Erythema nodosum leprosum (Necrotic lesions)

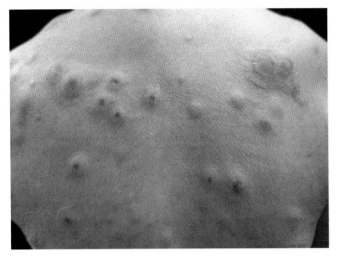

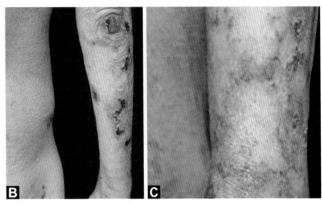

Figs 37B and C: Lucio phenomenon

Fig. 35: Erythema nodosum leprosum (EM like lesions)

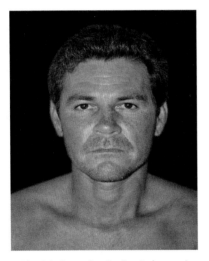

Fig. 36: Lepra bonita (Lucio leprosy)

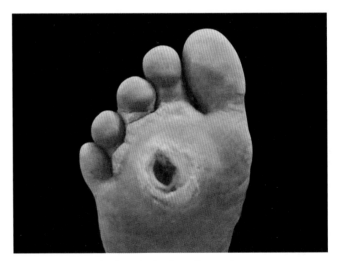

Fig. 38: Nonhealing plantar ulcer

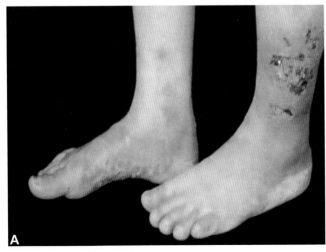

Fig. 37A: Lucio phenomenon

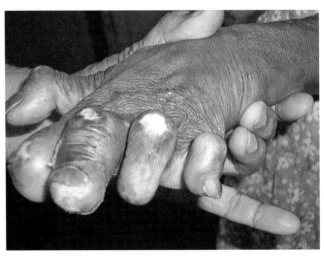

Fig. 39: Severe resorption of the fingers, proximal shifting of the nails with trophic changes

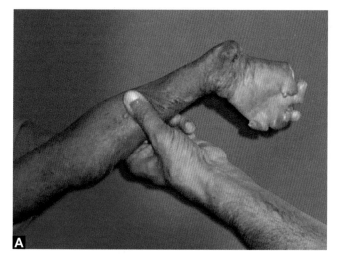 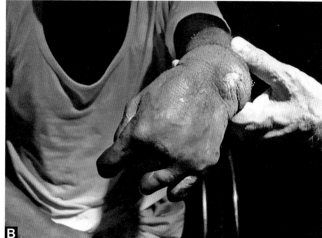

Figs 40A and B: Charcot neuropathic joint and severe resorption of the fingers with proximal displacement of nails

Photo Credits/Acknowledgments

- **Ben Naafs** - 1, 2, 3, 4, 5, 6, 7, 13, 14, 18, 19, 21, 28, 30, 34 and 35.

- **Saba Lambert** - 8, 9, 10, 15, 17, 20, 22, 23 and 32.

- **Luna Azulay** - 11, 12, 16, 24, 25, 26, 27, 29, 31, 33, 36A to C, 37A to C and 38.

- **Bhushan Kumar, Bella Devaleenal** - 39 and 40.

INDEX

Page numbers followed by *f* refer to figure, *fc* refer to flow chart, *t* refer to table and *b* refer to box, respectively